Absolute Pediatric Neurology

Yasser M. Awaad

Absolute Pediatric Neurology

Essential Questions and Answers

Springer

Yasser M. Awaad, M.D., M.Sc., FAAP, FAAN
Bloomfield Hills, MI
USA

ISBN 978-3-319-78800-5 ISBN 978-3-319-78801-2 (eBook)
https://doi.org/10.1007/978-3-319-78801-2

Library of Congress Control Number: 2018944124

Printed on acid-free paper

This Springer imprint is published by the registered company Springer Nature Switzerland AG.
The registered company address is: Gewerbestrasse 11, 6330 Cham, Switzerland

I am dedicating this work to my beloved family, especially my father, Mahmoud Awaad, mother, Galila Jad and children, Rania, Ammar and Emmad Awaad.

A very special dedication to my wife, Ola Abdellatif, who blessed me with unwavering support throughout my life journey.

Yasser M. Awaad

Contents

The original version of this book was revised: Copyright page text has been updated. An erratum to this book can be found at https://doi.org/10.1007/978-3-319-78801-2

Autism

Y. M. Awaad, *Absolute Pediatric Neurology*, https://doi.org/10.1007/978-3-319-78801-2_1

1

1. A 24 months old boy is referred for abnormal development and behavior. He has no use of speech to communicate his needs, has a limited repertoire of activities, and poor eye contact. He was diagnosed as autistic spectrum disorder by his primary care physician, but his parents are interested in finding out his specific diagnosis.
Which of the following tests can be used to best confirm his diagnosis and clarifying its type?
   - A. Blood lead level and serum IgG for gluten sensitivity
   - B. Chromosomal testing for 16p11.2 deletion/duplication
   - C. Checklist for autism in toddlers (CHAT) or modified checklist (m-CHAT)
   - D. Denver developmental screening test – revised (Denver II)
   - E. PDD assessment scale/ screening questionnaire

Correct Answer is: C
Environmental factors might contribute in many children with autistic spectrum disorders, such as lead exposure or celiac disease, but testing for those factors do not diagnose ASD. It is not the first test to do, 16p11.2 deletion/duplication is associated with autism, and is not a test to diagnose autism. The m-CHAT is a screening testing of both parental information and examiner observations, and it is for 16–30 month toddlers. The Denver II is a screening device, and is no longer recommended when screening for autism. The PDD Assessment scale/ screening questionnaire is not designed as a health care professional test. It is given to parents/ caretakers for reaching the diagnosing of their children.

Suggested Reading

- Article on PDD scale on ▶ Childbrain.com (▶ http://childbrain.com/pddq6.shtml). Diagnostic and statistical manual of mental disorders, 4th ed. Washington DC: American Psychiatric Association; 1994.
- Filipek PA, Accardo PJ, Ashwal G et al. International classification of diseases: diagnostic criteria for research, 10th ed. the World Health Organization. Practice parameter: screening and diagnosis of autism: report of the Quality Standards Subcommittee of the American Academy of Neurology and the Child Neurology Society. Neurology. 2000;55:468–479.

2. A 19 months old boy is referred for developmental delay evaluation. He was born at 37 weeks gestation as repeat cesarean section, birth weight of 3.0 kilograms. He rolled at 6 months, walked at 11 months, and said 3 words at 11 months. Currently he does not speaks any words, does not know body parts and will not follow one-step commands. Sleep habits are very poor, with frequent night awakenings. He has episodes of flapping movements of his hands and arms, last 20–30 min, but disappear if he was picked up, and reappear if he was put down. He will not point to objects and has variable eye contact.
Which of the following is the most likely diagnosis?
   - A. Hearing loss
   - B. Acquired auditory aphasia (Landau Kleffner syndrome)
   - C. Mental retardation
   - D. Autistic disorder
   - E. Childhood schizophrenia

Correct Answer is: D
Diagnosis of autistic spectrum disorders before the age of 2 years can be challenging, and other conditions should to be considered. Hearing loss is very important to rule out with formal hearing testing. This patient has a number of features that assist with making the diagnosis of autistic disorder, including restricted language and social skills and motor stereotypies.

Suggested Reading

- Zwaigenbaum L, Bryson S, Lord C, Rogers S, Carter A, Carver L, Chawarska K, Constantino J, Dawson G, Dobkins K, Fein D, Iverson J, Klin A, Landa R, Messinger D, Ozonoff S, Sigman M, Stone W, Tager-Flusberg H, Yirmiya N. Clinical assessment and management of toddlers with suspected autism spectrum disorder: insights from studies of high-risk infants. Pediatrics. 2009;123(5):1383–91.
- Wong V, Hui LH, Lee WC, Leung LS, Ho PK, Lau WL, Fung CW, Chung BA. Modified screening tool for autism (Checklist for Autism in Toddlers [CHAT-23]) for Chinese children. Pediatrics. 2004;114(2):e166–76.

3. An 8-year-old boy with "behavioral problems" and an intense preoccupation with trains that started at 3 years of age. There were no perinatal complications and normal early developmental milestones. He has no close friends, and difficulties in social settings at school. He has no problem in speech and language development, but he is unusually verbose, tangential or circumstantial, and at times exhibits inappropriate humor. He is extremely sensitive to stimulation, and has had difficulty falling asleep with intermittent awakenings during the night. He was inattentive during the evaluation, but his neurological examination was normal.
Which of the following is the most likely diagnosis?
   A. Autism
   B. Conduct disorder
   C. Asperger's syndrome
   D. Attention deficit hyperactivity disorder
   E. Depression

Correct Answer is: C
Asperger syndrome is an autistic spectrum disorder characterized by poor social interaction and the presence of restricted, stereotyped patterns of behavior and interests. Asperger syndrome patients often exhibit stereotyped behaviors and an intense preoccupation with a narrow activity or interest which is not required for diagnosis. In general, there is no delay in cognitive or language development, self-help or adaptive skills, or interest in the environment. Differential diagnosis includes autism, pervasive developmental disorder (not otherwise specified), attention deficit hyperactivity disorder, obsessive compulsive disorder, selective mutism, childhood disintegrative disorder.

Suggested Reading

- American Psychiatric Association. Diagnostic and statistical manual of mental disorders DSM-IV-TR. 4th ed. Washington DC: American Psychiatric Association; 2000.
- Khouzam HR, El-Gabalawi F, Pirwani N, Priest F. Asperger's disorder: a review of its diagnosis and treatment. Compr Psychiatry. 2004;45(3):184–91.
- McPartland J, Klin A. Asperger's syndrome. Adolesc Med Clin. 2006;17(3):771–88.

4. The choices are genetic or environmental risk factors for developing autism spectrum disorders and/or intellectual disabilities **EXCEPT**:
   A. More than 200 CGG trinucleotide repeats
   B. De novo mutations in the SCN2A (sodium channel, voltage-gated, type II, alpha), STXBP1 (syntaxin binding protein 1), SCN1A (sodium channel, voltage-gated, type I, alpha), or SYNE1 (synaptic nuclear envelope protein 1) genes
   C. TSC-1 (Tuberous Sclerosis Complex) gene mutations
   D. Deletions within the MECP2 gene
   E. Older parental age

1

Correct Answer is: E
Older paternal age at the time of birth has been considered as a risk factor for developing autism spectrum disorders (ASD), no sufficient evidence to validate this concern. Greater than 200 CGG trinucleotide repeats is diagnostic of Fragile X syndrome, it might have ASD manifestations and/or intellectual disability. TSC-1 mutations can cause Tuberous Sclerosis, which often has concomitant diagnoses of ASD and epilepsy. Deletions within the MECP2 gene are confirmatory of Rett Syndrome, which can manifest with ASD, intellectual disability, and epilepsy.

Suggested Reading

- Gardener H, Spiegelman D, Buka SL. Prenatal risk factors for autism: comprehensive meta-analysis. Pediatrics. 2011;128:344–55.
- Iossifov I, Ronemus M, Levy D, et al. De novo gene disruptions in children on the autistic spectrum. Neuron. 2012;74: 285–99.
- Sebat J, Lakshmi B, Malhotra D, et al. Strong association of de novo copy number mutations with autism. Science. 2007;316:445–9.

5. Which statement about autism spectrum disorders and epilepsy is true?
   A. The incidence of epilepsy autism spectrum disorders is similar for those with mild, moderate or severe manifestations
   B. The incidence and prevalence of epilepsy in autism spectrum disorders is independent of concomitant, co-morbid neurological disorders/diagnoses
   C. The biological and molecular mechanisms causing or leading to epilepsies or autism spectrum disorders are not similar and dependent
   D. EEG in autism spectrum disorders is not a useful test because of behavioral non-compliance
   E. The risk of epilepsy in children and adolescents with autism spectrum disorders ranges from 6–26%, and it is higher in patients with cerebral palsy or intellectual disabilities

Correct Answer is: E
The incidence of epilepsy in children and adolescents with autism spectrum disorders is higher in children with intellectual disabilities and cerebral palsy. Mortality rates increase in patients having autism associated with epilepsy. The growing evidence that epilepsies and ASD shares common biological etiologies and mechanisms, increase interest and research in devising interventions that can change the course of both diseases.

It is difficult to detect seizures in patients with autism spectrum disorders, and acquiring electroencephalograms can be challenging in individuals with behavioral challenges. With such individuals, utilization of behavioral interventions can be helpful, and technologies utilizing electrodes not requiring scalp abrasion, glues or pastes, allow for successful EEG acquisition, which can yield important information about clinical and subclinical epilepsies.

Suggested Reading

- Amiet C, Gourfinkel-AnI, Bouzamondo A, et al. Epilepsy in autism is associated with intellectual disability and gender: evidence from a meta-analysis. Biol Psychiatry. 2008;64:577–82.
- Bolton PF, Carcani-Rathwell I, Hutton J, et al. Epilepsy in autism: features and correlates. Br J Psychiatry. 2011;198:289–94.
- McVicar KA, Ballaban-Gil K, Rapin I. et al. Epileptiform EEG abnormalities in children with language regression. Neurology. 2005;65:129–31.
- Pickett J. et al. Mortality in individuals with autism, with and without epilepsy. J Child Neurol. 2011;26:932–9.

6. A 4 year old boy is here for a neurological evaluation. You noted that he does not have joint attention, makes minimal eye contact, has echolalia and repetitively spins instead of playing with the toys in the room. You consider the diagnosis of Autism Spectrum Disorder. In taking the history, the mother states that she had taken valproic acid and topiramate for severe migraines during the pregnancy. The valproic acid was added after the first trimester. She had also taken folic acid. She asked you if any of the medications could have contributed to the child's condition.

Your response would be:

A. Taking Valproic acid only increases the risk of spinal tube defects
B. Only thalidomide has been shown to increase the risk of Autism
C. Taking topiramate does not cause any birth defects
D. The risk of autism increased 3-fold for children born to mothers who took VPA during pregnancy
E. The risk of autism is similar to spina bifida; it only increases during first trimester exposure

Correct Answer is: D

Thalidomide and Valproic Acid have been shown to increase the risk of Autism in utero exposures. Valproic Acid exposure can increase the risk of neural tube defects is a well-known fact. The study by Christensen et al. and the commentary by Cynthia Harden revealed there "were an association of in utero VPA exposure and the risk of autism determined from a population-based study utilizing Danish national medical databases. Children born between 1996 and 2006 were followed for the documented occurrence of autism up to 14 years of age, with a mean follow-up of 9 years. Children born to mothers who took VPA during pregnancy, autism risk increased 3-fold and the risk of autism spectrum disorder (ASD) increased 5-fold over the general population risk. The absolute risk to VPA-exposed children was less than 5%, although the upper 95% confidence interval (CI) limit for ASD was 7.49%. There was no contribution of maternal epilepsy to the risk of VPA use. Hypospadias and spina bifida and occurs with first trimester exposure, but the autism risk was present in this study with VPA exposure starting at any trimester during pregnancy."

In Thalidomide exposure, there was a 50 fold higher rate of Autism in those with thalidomide embryopathy than in the general population.

The risk of oral clefts in infants exposed to topiramate during the first trimester of pregnancy has been increases according the data from the North American Antiepileptic Drug (AED) Pregnancy Registry. Infants exposed to topiramate as a single therapy experienced a 1.4% prevalence of oral clefts, compared with a prevalence of 0.38–0.55% in infants exposed to other antiepileptic drugs.

Suggested Reading

- Harden, C. In utero valproate exposure and autism: long suspected, finally proven. Epilepsy Curr. 2013;13(6):282–4.
- Christensen J, Grønborg TK, Sørensen MJ, Schendel D, Parner ET, Pedersen LH, Vestergaard M. Prenatal valproate exposure and risk of autism spectrum disorders and childhood autism. JAMA. 2013;309(16):1696–703.
- Strömland K, Nordin V, Miller M, Akerström B, Gillberg C. Autism in thalidomideembryopathy: a population study. Dev Med Child Neurol. 1994;36(4):351–6.
- Risk of oral birth defects in children born to mothers taking topiramate. FDA NEWS RELEASE, March 4, 2011.

1

7. An 11-year-old boy came for a neurologic evaluation because of "odd behavior". He and his family recently relocated from another state. He does not maintain good eye contact when you tried to engage him. His parents mentioned that he had no friends and is not very affectionate with family. He is methodical and rigid in his patterns, getting upset if there is a change in his routine. Also they mentioned that he is fixated on following the statistics of his favorite football team. He does very well in school. There is no history of language or cognitive impairment. **Which of the following is the most correct diagnosis?**
   - A. attention deficit hyperactivity disorder
   - B. autism spectrum disorder
   - C. Landau-Kleffner syndrome
   - D. Rett disorder
   - E. Tourette syndrome

Correct Answer: B
This patient has the main symptoms of autism spectrum disorder, including lack of social interaction, as well as restrictive and repetitive behaviors. The new DSM V eliminates the diagnosis of Asperger syndrome (which fits this patient best because of intact language function, which is characteristically impaired in DSM IV autism symptom complex) in favor of including these patients in the broader category of "autism spectrum disorder". This patient's presentation is not suggestive of ADHD. Rett syndrome is associated with regression of language abilities and hand stereotypies, typically seen in girls (X-linked dominant). Tourette syndrome is a tic disorder, commonly with comorbid ADHD and OCD.

Suggested Reading

- Pellegrino L, Liptak GS. Consultation with the specialist: asperger syndrome. Pediatr Rev. 2011;32(11):481–9.
- Sugden SG, Corbett BA. Autism-presentation, diagnosis and management. Continuum Lifelong Learning Neurol. 2006;12(5):47–59.

8. A 4-year-old boy presents with a speech delay. He was a full term, with no prenatal or perinatal complications. He began walking at 13 months of age, is able to feed himself with utensils. He says many different words during the day; however most of this speech is repetition of things he hears on the television or from his family. He has no interactive play and does not identify body parts. He has no chronic medical illnesses and takes no medication. No family history of developmental delays. There have been no difficulties with feeding or swallowing. He does not have eye contact and does not go to his parents for reassurance. He makes several grunting sounds; a brief echolalic speech is produced. When given blocks to stack, He arranges blocks in a straight line. The rest of his neurological exam is normal for age. Hearing testing was normal one month ago. **Which of the following diagnoses is most likely for the child's language delay?**
   - A. autism spectrum disorder
   - B. cerebral palsy
   - C. congenital perisylvian syndrome
   - D. Landau-Kleffner syndrome
   - E. Menkes disease

Correct Answer is: A
Delays in acquisition of language are common in the pediatric population. Although isolated expressive or mixed expressive and receptive language delays are two prominent developmental disabilities of childhood, often there are clues from the history or physical exam that suggest

another possible diagnosis. You cannot rely on hearing test to be performed to exclude congenital or acquired hearing loss, even if the newborn hearing screen was normal. If, in addition to the language delay, there is an impairment of social interaction (in this case suggested by poor eye contact, lack of sharing attention with caregiver (interactive play), an autism spectrum disorder is likely. Milder subtypes of the spectrum include pervasive developmental disorder (PDD) and Asperger syndrome. Patients with PDD may have normal nonverbal intelligence, and may have some segments of cognitive ability that are quite advanced. Patients with Asperger syndrome may have typically developed language skills, but are quite impaired in the social arena. There are multiple etiologies that may lead to an autistic phenotype, though in most cases a formal etiology is not discovered. When there is an associated severe intellectual disability present, testing to include chromosome microarray, fragile X evaluation and MRI of the brain may be considered. The incidence of autism clearly is increasing with time, likely due to genetic factors, though other environmental factors have additionally been proposed. Large meta-analytic studies have not shown vaccination to be a causative factor. Early identification of the child with autism is important, as the only clearly beneficial treatment is early institution of autism specific therapy such as applied behavioral analysis (ABA therapy). Even with early therapy, failure to develop language before the age of 5 is an extremely poor prognostic sign. Cerebral palsy is defined specifically by static delays in motor control due to an early insult or malformation of the brain. Though often associated with language and cognitive delay, this diagnosis strictly pertains to a motor disturbance (most commonly muscle spasticity). Congenital bilateral perisylvian syndrome is a rare, usually sporadic, disturbance in neuronal migration that results in a bilateral thickened cortex (pachygyria) in the sylvian and Rolandic regions. All affected children have not only a delay in language (presumably from the disorganized cortex in the Broca region) but also a prominent pseudobulbar palsy causing prominent dysphagia and feeding difficulties. Epileptic encephalopathies such as Landau-Kleffner syndrome (LKS) are quite rare, especially in comparison to the 1:150 incidence of primary autism disorders, though should be considered in a child who develops typical language and social skills prior to age 2, and then undergoes a period of regression between 2–4 years of age, often associated with development of clinical seizures. Occasionally the regression will ensue prior to the appearance of the ictal events. Electroencephalography in LKS demonstrates electrical status epilepticus of sleep (ESES). Treatment may be resistant to traditional anticonvulsants (such as valproic acid or levetiracetam) and may require high dose benzodiazepines nightly and/or corticosteroid treatment. Response of the electrical features of the syndrome usually leads to improvement in the encephalopathy, but early recognition and aggressive management are essential. Menke's syndrome is a disorder of copper metabolism and is apparent at birth with severe hypotonia and sparse, brittle hair and early onset of epilepsy. Seizures are also a commonly associated problem. Although it is important to expand the diagnostic evaluation of the child with autistic-like behavior associated with significant loss of previously acquired skills (regression), many of these patients will not have a specific etiology discovered and will be diagnosed simply with a regressive form of autism. Up to one-third of children with autism experience a regression in skills (typically restricted to language and social skills and sparing motor function) between the ages of 1 and 3 for reasons as of yet unknown.

1

Suggested Reading

Fenichel GM. Clinical pediatric neurology: a signs and symptoms approach. 6th ed. Philadelphia: Saunders Elsevier; 2005. p.119–21.

9. A 4-year-old boy was seen by his primary care physician. The family mentioned that he is "emotionless" as compared with his affectionate siblings. He never had eye contact. He does not like to be hugged or kissed and does not play with others. He prefers to sit alone in his room, playing with the racing cars, although he has several other toys. He often flaps his arms at his sides and sometimes when upset will repeatedly bang his forehead on the nearest piece of furniture or on a wall. He has few words in his vocabulary, but not as many as his siblings did at his age.
   What is your most likely diagnosis?
   A. Autism
   B. Avoidant personality disorder
   C. Depression
   D. Schizophrenia
   E. Schizoid personality disorder

Correct Answer: A

The most likely diagnosis is autism. Autistic spectrum disorder is characterized by the triad of impaired social skills, impaired communication skills, and restricted repertoire of activities and interests. Impaired communication skills include both verbal and nonverbal skills. Social skill abnormalities include lack of eye contact or atypical eye contact, failure to develop peer relationships, and lack of emotional reciprocity. Motor stereotypies, repetitive voluntary behaviors such as those described here, lack of flexibility, preoccupation with specific objects or part of an object, and ritualistic patterns of behavior occur. This spectrum is broad, ranging from high-functioning individuals as seen in Asperger disorder to nonverbal children with little interaction and sometimes no language skills. Cognitive delay is not a part of the diagnostic criterion but may be an associated feature, although supernormal IQs may occur in some. Some improvements occur in adolescence, although seizures, mood disorders, or other comorbidities may also emerge. A genetic basis has been considered based on the high concordance rates among monozygotic twins and increased incidence in families with another child with autism. Neuropathology seen in patients with autism include under-development of limbic structures and reduced cerebellar Purkinje cells. Other genetic and metabolic disorders have been associated with autism, including neurofibromatosis, Down syndrome, fetal alcohol syndrome, and peroxisomal disorders. A diagnostic workup might be indicated for these disorders. Personality disorder cannot be made at this time, although some of the personality disorders include rigid behavior.

This patient does not meet diagnostic criteria for depression and schizophrenia.

Suggested Reading

Comprehensive review in clinical neurology: a multiple choice question book for the wards and boards ©2011 Wolters Kluwer Health Lippincott Williams & Wilkins. All rights reserved.

10. A 20-month-old boy has been evaluated for evaluation severe expressive and receptive language delay. He cannot point and pulls his parents around the house to indicate his needs. He has eye contact occasionally. He lines up his toys and gets upset when they are taken out of order. He flaps his hands when he is excited. On physical exam, he has two hypo-pigmented macules on his back.
    What is your next step in his evaluation?
    A. Fragile X testing
    B. High resolution chromosomes
    C. EEG
    D. Modified Checklist for Autism in Toddlers
    E. Skull X-Rays

Correct Answer is: D

The child clinical presentation is classical for autism. Autism is a neurodevelopmental disorder characterized by impaired social communication, delayed expressive and receptive language and stereotypic behavior. The language disorder is a delay in the development of spoken language or difficulties sustaining speech. This is also a social disorder with marked difficulty in the use of nonverbal behaviors like gestures. There are restricted patterns of behavior like hand flapping, twisting or complex body movements. There may be absence of imaginative play. The cause for most cases of autism is unknown. Genetic disorders may be associated with autism spectrum disorders, Rett's syndrome, Fragile X and tuberous sclerosis complex. Early identification of Autism will allow specific interventions to improve the outcome. The Modified checklist for autism in toddlers is an easy tool to use for the pediatrician or primary provider. It is highly recommended that a multidisciplinary team that specializes in children with these disorders do the evaluation. The most common measures used include the Childhood Autism rating scales (trained observer), Gilliam Autism rating scale (parents report). The gold standard is the Autism Diagnostic Observation Schedule (ADDOS) or the Autism Diagnostic Interview-Revised (AID-R). The hypo-pigmented spots raise concern of tuberous sclerosis, so an MRI might be indicated.

Suggested Reading

- De los Reyes EC, Roach ES. In: Cecil's essential of medicine. Andreoli T. Benjamin I, Griggs R, Wing E, editors. Philadelphia: Saunder Elsevier; 2010 p. 1192–22.

11. The mother of a 5-year-old autistic boy is planning to have another child. She is asking you if there is a possibility that her next child will be affected with the same disorder. What testing would you do to help counsel the family?
    - A. Chromosomal microarray analysis
    - B. Mitochondrial point mutation testing
    - C. Head MRI
    - D. EEG
    - E. Serum amino acids

Correct Answer is: A

Genetic studies in families indicate a 5% recurrence rate. Although the cause of autism is not clear, most studies showed that the cause is most likely genetic. Comparative genomic hybridization (microarray or oligo array) offers high resolution genome wide screening of segmental genomic copy number variations. Microdeletions and duplications can be detected by this technique. De novo deletions and duplications offer insights to this well-recognized disorder. Due to its increasing widespread availability it has offered insight to the etiology of autism and autistic spectrum disorders. The most common abnormalities include maternally inherited duplication of Chromosome 15, de novo or inherited duplications of 16p 11.2.

Suggested Reading

- Shen Y, Dries KA, Holm IA et al. Clinical genetic testing for patients with autistic spectrum disorders. Pediatrics. 2010. 125:e727–35.

12. A 12-year-old boy with normal early developmental milestones comes to you for behavioral difficulties. He has long history of difficulties interacting with peers. He prefers adults and younger children. Lately, he became aggressive towards his classmates and even hit another child who was making fun of him. He has excellent grades in math but is failing in classes like English and reading. His favorite is Robotics. He has normal exam except monotonous, dysprosodic speech.

1

What is your diagnosis?

A. Asperger's syndrome
B. Sensory processing disorder
C. Pervasive developmental disorder
D. Mental retardation
E. Verbal apraxia

Correct Answer is: A

Asperger's syndrome is a neurodevelopmental disorder characterized by deficits in social interactions, pragmatic language and restricted interests. Usually children with the syndrome have normal acquisition of early developmental language skills with average cognitive skills. Diagnosis is usually around 6 years of age since the increasing social demands of school may lead to evaluation of the atypical behaviors. Language is characterized as "pedantic". Although verbal in specific topics of their interest, Asperger patients may have difficulty expressing their feelings or relating to others, especially with their peers.

Suggested Reading

- Levy SE, Hyma SL, Pinto-Martin J. Autism spectrum disorders. In: Accardo PJ, ed. Neurodevelopmental disabilities in infancy and childhood. Vol. 2, 3rd. Baltimore: Brooke's Publishing; 2008. p. 497.
- Place-Johnson C, Myers SM, Council on children with disabilities. identification and evaluation of children with autism spectrum disorders. Pediatrics. 2007. p. 1182–1215.

13. The family of a 6-year-old boy diagnosed with autism would like to know what the best treatment interventions are for their son. Physical exam is normal.

What is your advice to the family?

A. Behavioral intervention with Applied Behavioral Analysis
B. Hyperbaric oxygen treatments
C. Gluten and casein free diet
D. Chelation therapy
E. Vitamin and mineral supplements

Correct Answer is: A

Early diagnosis is recommended in children with autistic spectrum disorders. The management of autism is based on the principles of behavioral and educational intervention. Applied Behavioral Analysis is the process of applying interventions that are based on the principles of learning, derived from experimental psychology research, to systematically change behavior and to demonstrate that the interventions used are responsible for the observable improvement in behavior. ABA methods are used to increase and maintain desirable adaptive behaviors, reduce interfering maladaptive behaviors (or narrow the conditions under which they occur), teach new skills, and generalize behaviors to new environments or situations. Alternating program that is well accepted is structured teaching or the TEACCH program. The bases of the program, emphasize structure and organization. Other interventions include speech/language therapy and occupational therapy. However, these are not case controlled studies showed improvements on gluten and casein free diet. Media and certain parent groups have advocated the management of autism with multiple vitamins and supplements, however, there are no case controlled studies to determine efficacy.

Suggested Reading

- Myers S, Place-Johnson C, Council on children with disabilities. Management of children with autism spectrum disorders. Pediatrics. 2007. p. 1162–82.
- Filipek PA, Accardo PJ, Ashwal G et al. Practice parameter: screening and diagnosis of autism: report of the Quality Standards Subcommittee of the American Academy of Neurology and the Child Neurology Society. Neurology. 2000;55:468–79.

14. You evaluate A 9 years-old boy with a longstanding diagnosis of autism spectrum disorder-moderate/severe. His family describes occasional

"freeze episodes", characterized by a general cessation of movement in a fixed posture, during which time he is awake, alert but is not interactive or conversant. He has a history of seizures, happens approximately once a year while maintained on lamotrigine.

All the mentioned below differential diagnostic entities warrant consideration, which is most consistent with the boy's history:

A. GLUT-1 deficiency
B. Dravet's syndrome
C. Landau-Kleffner syndrome
D. Disorder of Cerebral Folate Metabolism
E. Fragile X syndrome

Correct Answer is: D

The history is consistent with recurrent episodes of catatonia-like episodes. Catatonia in individuals with autism spectrum disorders has been reported to be associated with Disorders of Cerebral Folate Metabolism, and in some cases can be improved with the administration of folinic acid. GLUT-1 deficiency can be associated with epilepsy and autism spectrum disorders, but usually intractable epilepsies relatively uncontrolled by antiepileptic drugs, but responsive to the ketogenic diet. Dravet's Syndrome is associated with genetic mutations of the SCN1A gene, and lamotrigine might worsen the seizures. Landau-Kleffner Syndrome is associated with language regression and autism spectrum disorders, with epileptiform activity seeing during sleep, and classically without observable seizure events. Fragile X syndrome is associated with intellectual disability, and can have associated with epilepsy or autism spectrum disorders. Other than Disorders of Cerebral Folate Metabolism, the other entities listed are not generally associated with catatonia.

Suggested Reading

- Ho A, Michelson D, Aaen G, Ashwal S. Cerebral folate deficiency presenting as adolescent catatonic schizophrenia: a case report. J Child Neurol. 2010;25:898–900.
- Hyland K, Shoffner J, Heales SJ. Cerebral folate deficiency. J Inherit Metab Dis. 2010;33:563–70.

15. A 5-month-old baby has refractory infantile spasms. A cardiac rhabdomyoma was diagnosed prenatally. Her skin has multiple hypomelanotic macules. Her Head MRI shows frontal cortical tubers. The EEG reveals multifocal temporal regions discharges.

What symptom in her history puts her at risk for developing autism?

A. Temporal lobe focus
B. Hypomelanotic macules
C. Cardiac rhabdomyoma
D. Age of developing infantile spasms
E. Frontal cortical tubers

Correct Answer is: A

Current evidence indicates that the likelihood of a child with tuberous sclerosis developing an autism spectrum disorder is greater if the child has a mutation in the TSC2 gene, although autism can and does develop in children with TSC1 mutations. The likelihood is also greater if the child has early-onset infantile spasms that are difficult to control, especially if there is an epileptiform focus in the temporal lobes. The emerging evidence is consistent with the notion that early onset electrophysiological disturbances within the temporal lobes has a deleterious effect on the development and establishment of key social cognitive representations concerned with processing social information, especially from faces.

Suggested Reading

- Bolton, PF. Neuroepileptic correlates of autistic symptomatology in tuberous sclerosis. Ment Retard Dev Disabil Res Rev. 2004;10(2):126–31.

1

16. A 6-year-old boy is referred by his school teacher because he is having difficulty with his peers. His mom reported that he does not interact with others. He only likes to talk about and play with the video game Minecraft. He does not understand peer teasing. He does not understand emotional cues. His mom states that he has a great vocabulary and is doing well academically. On examine, he has no eye contact, has limited facial expression and does not have joint attention. He cannot engage in a back and forth conversation but tells you about Minecraft. You consider whether he fulfills the criteria for an Autism Spectrum Disorder.

Which below choice is not included in the DSM V Criteria for Autism Spectrum Disorder?

A. Deficits in social-emotional reciprocity
B. Deficits in nonverbal communicative behaviors used for social interaction
C. Deficits in developing and maintaining relationships, appropriate to developmental level
D. Stereotyped repetitive movement, speech, or use of objects
E. Delays in language

Correct Answer is: E

The DSM V that was published in 2013 revealed changes in the criteria for ASD. The criteria no longer include language delays.

Diagnostic Criteria include:

1. **Persistent deficits in social communication and social interaction across multiple contexts, as manifested by the following, currently or by history (examples are illustrative, not exhaustive, see text):**
   1. **Deficits in social-emotional reciprocity, ranging, for example, from abnormal social approach and failure of normal back-and-forth conversation; to reduced sharing of interests, emotions, or affect; to failure to initiate or respond to social interactions.**
   2. **Deficits in nonverbal communicative behaviors used for social interaction, ranging, for example, from poorly integrated verbal and nonverbal communication; to abnormalities in eye contact and body language or deficits in understanding and use of gestures; to a total lack of facial expressions and nonverbal communication.**
   3. **Deficits in developing, maintaining, and understanding relationships, ranging, for example, from difficulties adjusting behavior to suit various social contexts; to difficulties in sharing imaginative play or in making friends; to absence of interest in peers.**

Specify current severity:

Severity is based on social communication impairments and restricted repetitive patterns of behavior.

2. **Restricted, repetitive patterns of behavior, interests, or activities, as manifested by at least two of the following, currently or by history (examples are illustrative, not exhaustive; see text):**
   1. **Stereotyped or repetitive motor movements, use of objects, or speech (e.g., simple motor stereotypies, lining up toys or flipping objects, echolalia, idiosyncratic phrases).**
   2. **Insistence on sameness, inflexible adherence to routines, or ritualized patterns or verbal nonverbal behavior (e.g., extreme distress at small changes, difficulties with transitions, rigid thinking patterns, greeting rituals, need to take same route or eat food every day).**

3. Highly restricted, fixated interests that are abnormal in intensity or focus (e.g., strong attachment to or preoccupation with unusual objects, excessively circumscribed or perseverative interest).
4. Hyper- or hypo reactivity to sensory input or unusual interests in sensory aspects of the environment (e.g., apparent indifference to pain/temperature, adverse response to specific sounds or textures, excessive smelling or touching of objects, visual fascination with lights or movement).

Specify current severity:

Severity is based on social communication impairments and restricted, repetitive patterns of behavior.

3. Symptoms must be present in the early developmental period (but may not become fully manifest until social demands exceed limited capacities, or may be masked by learned strategies in later life).
4. Symptoms cause clinically significant impairment in social, occupational, or other important areas of current functioning.
5. These disturbances are not better explained by intellectual disability (intellectual developmental disorder) or global developmental delay. Intellectual disability and autism spectrum disorder frequently co-occur; to make comorbid diagnoses of autism spectrum disorder and intellectual disability, social communication should be below that expected for general developmental level.

Note: Individuals with a well-established DSM-IV diagnosis of autistic disorder, Asperger's disorder, or pervasive developmental disorder not otherwise specified should be given the diagnosis of autism spectrum disorder. Individuals who have marked deficits in social communication, but whose symptoms do not otherwise meet criteria for autism spectrum disorder, should be evaluated for social (pragmatic) communication disorder.

Specify if:

- With or without accompanying intellectual impairment.
- With or without accompanying language impairment.
- Associated with a known medical or genetic condition or environmental factor.
- Associated with another neurodevelopmental, mental, or behavioral disorder.
- With Catatonia.

Suggested Reading

- Diagnostic and statistical manual of mental disorders: DSM-5

17. A 4-month-old baby girl has refractory infantile spasms. Prenatally she was found to have a cardiac rhabdomyoma. She has multiple hypomelanotic macules on her skin. Brain MRI reveals frontal cortical tubers. The EEG reveals multifocal discharges; predominantly in the frontal regions. **What factor puts her at risk for developing autism?**
    A. Having refractory infantile spasms
    B. Having hypomelanotic macules
    C. Having a cardiac rhabdomyoma
    D. Having frontal cortical tubers
    E. Having bifrontal discharges

Correct Answer is: A

Recent studies showed that the likelihood of a child with tuberous sclerosis developing an autism spectrum disorder is greater if the child has a mutation in the TSC2 gene, although autism can and does develop in children with TSC1 mutations. The likelihood will increase if the child has early-onset infantile spasms that are difficult to control, especially if there is an epileptiform focus in the temporal lobes. The emerging evidence is consistent with the notion that early onset electrophysiological

1

disturbances within the temporal lobes has a deleterious effect on the development and establishment of key social cognitive representations concerned with processing social information, perhaps especially from faces.

Suggested Reading

- Bolton, PF. Neuroepileptic correlates of autistic symptomatology in tuberous sclerosis. Ment Retard Dev Disabil Res Rev. 2004;10(2):126–31.

18. A 4-year-old boy with speech delay came to your office for an evaluation. He was born at full term, with no prenatal or perinatal complications. He walked at 14 months of age, is able to feed himself with utensils. He uses several words during the day; most of them is repetition of things he hears on the television or from his family. He has no interactive play and does not identify body parts. He has no history of chronic medical illnesses and takes no medication. He has no family history for any developmental delays. There have been no difficulties with feeding or swallowing. During his examination he does not make sustained eye contact and does not go to his parents for reassurance. He makes several grunting sounds; a brief echolalic speech is produced. When given blocks to stack, he puts them in a straight line. His neurological exam is normal for age. His hearing is normal and confirmed by an audiology examination one month ago.
What is most likely diagnose for the boy's language delay?
A. autism spectrum disorder
B. Landau-Kleffner syndrome
C. cerebral palsy
D. congenital perisylvian syndrome
E. Menke's disease

Correct Answer is: A
Language acquisition delays in the pediatric age group population is common. Although isolated expressive or mixed expressive and receptive language delays are two common developmental disabilities of childhood, usually there are clues from the history or physical exam that suggest another possible diagnosis. It is important for a hearing test to be performed to exclude congenital or acquired hearing loss, even if the newborn hearing screen was normal. If, in addition to the language delay, there is an impairment of social interaction (in this case suggested by poor eye contact, lack of sharing attention with caregiver (interactive play), an autism spectrum disorder is likely. Milder subtypes of the spectrum include pervasive developmental disorder (PDD) and Asperger syndrome. Patients with PDD may have normal nonverbal intelligence, and may have some segments of cognitive ability that are quite advanced. Patients with Asperger syndrome may have typically developed language skills, but are quite impaired in the social arena. There are multiple etiologies that may lead to an autistic phenotype, though in most cases a formal etiology is not discovered. When there is an associated severe intellectual disability present, testing to include chromosome microarray, fragile X evaluation and brain MRI may be considered. The incidence of autism is on the raise, likely due to genetic factors, though other environmental factors have additionally been proposed. Vaccination is not a causative factor based on a large meta-analytic studies. Early autism diagnosis is important, as the only clearly beneficial treatment is early institution of autism specific therapy such as applied behavioral analysis (ABA therapy). Even with early treatment, failure to develop language before the age of 5 is an extremely poor prognostic

sign. Epileptic encephalopathies such as Landau-Kleffner syndrome (LKS) are quite rare, especially in comparison to the 1:150 incidence of primary autism disorders, though should be considered in a child who develops typical language and social skills prior to age 2, and then undergoes a period of regression between 2–4 years of age, often associated with development of clinical seizures. Occasionally the regression will occur before the appearance of the ictal events. EEG in LKS demonstrates electrical status epilepticus of sleep (ESES). Treatment may be resistant to traditional anticonvulsants (such as valproic acid or levetiracetam) and may require high dose benzodiazepines nightly and/or corticosteroid treatment. Response of the electrical features of the syndrome usually leads to improvement in the encephalopathy, but early recognition and aggressive management are essential. Cerebral palsy is defined specifically by static delays in motor control due to an early insult or malformation of the brain. Though often associated with language and cognitive delay, this diagnosis strictly pertains to a motor disturbance (most commonly muscle spasticity). Congenital bilateral perisylvian syndrome is a rare, usually sporadic, disturbance in neuronal migration that results in a bilateral thickened cortex (pachygyria) in the sylvian and Rolandic regions. All affected children have not only a delay in language (presumably from the disorganized cortex in the Broca region) but also a prominent pseudobulbar palsy causing prominent dysphagia and feeding difficulties. Seizures are also a commonly associated problem. Menke's syndrome is a disorder of copper metabolism and is apparent at birth with severe hypotonia and sparse, brittle hair and early onset of epilepsy. Although it is important to expand the diagnostic evaluation of the child with autistic-like behavior associated with significant loss of previously acquired skills (regression), many of these patients will not have a specific etiology discovered and will be diagnosed simply with a regressive form of autism. Up to 1/3 of children with autism experience a regression in skills (typically restricted to language and social skills and sparing motor function) between the ages of 1 and 3 for reasons as of yet unknown.

Suggested Reading

- Fenichel GM. Clinical pediatric neurology: a signs and symptoms approach. 6th ed. Philadelphia: Saunders Elsevier; 2005. p. 119–21.

Behavior

Y. M. Awaad, *Absolute Pediatric Neurology*, https://doi.org/10.1007/978-3-319-78801-2_2

1. A 7-year-old and 9-year-old brothers, are being seen for their annual checkup by their PCP. The mother looks worn out and mentioned that her sons have always kept her busy. The younger brother has a lot of trouble with his school work. The mother said that he is smart, but he is not paying attention to anything, cannot concentrate for more than few minutes on his homework, is easily distractible, and never does what he is told, is constantly misplacing things, and even forgets to brush his teeth and shower sometimes if she does not remind him. The older brother also giving her trouble with his school work, he "just can't seem to sit still." At home, he is fidgety at the dinner table and while doing his homework. She was called several times to school because he leaves his seat and sometimes the classroom. He talks constantly, jumping from one topic to another, he does not wait his turn to answer, and is constantly butting into conversations.
What is your most likely diagnosis?
   A. This is a normal age appropriate behavior.
   B. Generalized anxiety disorder
   C. Oppositional defiant disorder
   D. Attention-deficit/hyperactivity disorder
   E. Conduct disorder

Correct Answer is: D
They have the classic symptomatology of attention-deficit/ hyperactivity disorder (ADHD). ADHD includes a predominantly inattentive type, as in the younger brother; a predominantly hyperactive type, as in the older brother a combined type. The diagnostic criteria for the inattentive type include six or more symptoms of inattention that have been present for the prior 6 months with at least some symptoms occurring before age 7 years that are leading to functional impairment and are not consistent with developmental level and include failure to pay attention to details in schoolwork or other activities, difficulty sustaining attention on a task or activity, not listening when spoken to and not following instructions, difficulty with organization, avoidance or dislike of tasks that require sustained mental activity, loss of objects necessary for tasks or activities, easy distractibility, and forgetfulness in daily activities. The diagnostic criteria for the hyperactive type include six or more symptoms of hyperactivity and impulsivity that have been present for the prior 6 months with at least some symptoms occurring before age 7 years that are leading to functional impairment and are not consistent with the developmental level and include frequent fidgeting or squirming, leaving a seat in situations when remaining seated is expected, running about or climbing excessively in inappropriate situations, or feelings of restlessness, difficulty engaging quietly in leisurely activities, talking excessively, blurting out of answers, difficulty awaiting a turn, and interruption of others. Although the etiology of ADHD is not clear, dysfunction in frontal-subcortical circuits has been implicated. Genetic studies have suggested involvement of genes involved in dopamine action or metabolism, though environmental factors play a role as well. Children of parents with ADHD and siblings of children with ADHD are more likely to be affected with ADHD than the general population.

Oppositional defiant disorder is a distinct entity from ADHD, but the two are often comorbid. Similarly, generalized anxiety disorder is also comorbid with ADHD, as are the disruptive behavior disorders. In childhood, academic failure and peer rejection are the major consequences of ADHD, whereas in adolescence, there is a threefold increase in substance use and abuse. Approximately 60% of patients with ADHD in childhood continue to be impaired in adult life; ADHD may also not be recognized

until adulthood. Adults with ADHD typically show instability with employment and relationships. The first line of treatment for ADHD are psychostimulants, including amphetamines and methylphenidates, of which there are various oral preparations. Common side effects include reduced appetite, weight loss, insomnia, and headaches. An electrocardiogram prior to initiation of stimulant medications is recommended to exclude underlying structural or conduction problems.

2. An 8-year-old white boy came to your office for evaluation of developmental delay. Pregnancy was unremarkable and he was a full-term at birth. He was at the regular nursery for 2 days because he had a feeding problem and jaundice. He was 7 lbs. 8 oz. (25–50%ile) and length was 22 in. (>95%ile) at birth. On your examination, he is tall and macro-cephalic (both > 97th percentile) with mildly dysmorphic facial features, including a high, broad forehead, down-slanting palpebral fissures, and a pointed chin. His hands and feet are enlarged. The rest of his neurologic examination is normal. No other similarly affected individuals in the family. **Which genetic test would you like to order?**
   - A. Chromosome microarray
   - B. FISH for chromosome 22q11 deletion
   - C. Karyotype
   - D. Methylation analysis of chromosome 15q
   - E. Nuclear receptor SET domain containing protein-1 (NSD1 testing)

Correct Answer is: D
Sotos syndrome (cerebral gigantism), is a genetic condition affecting 1: 10,000 to 1: 50,000 individuals. It is characterized by prenatal and postnatal overgrowth, macrocephaly, and characteristic facial features—specifically a high anterior hair line; frontotemporal hair sparsity, a long, thin face; frontal bossing; down slanting palpebral fissures; and a prominent mandible. Advanced bone age is common but is not a universal finding. Hypotonia and global developmental delay is a neurologic hallmarks, however mild intellectual disability is present in the affected adults exhibiting. Sotos syndrome can be caused by either intragenic truncating mutations or microdeletions that result in haplo insufficiency of the nuclear receptor binding SET domain protein 1 (NSD1), located on chromosome 5q35.3. More than 80% accounts for intragenic mutations in European-origin white patients, on the other hand microdeletions has a higher incidence in the Japanese population. The majority of cases are sporadic, though autosomal dominant pedigrees have been reported.

Suggested Reading

- Leventopoulos G, et al. A clinical study of Sotos syndrome patients with review of the literature. Pediatr Neurol. 2009;40:357–64.

3. A 7-year-old girl with a history of language difficulties. She was born full-term by normal spontaneous vaginal delivery following an uncomplicated pregnancy. Her milestones, walked at 10 months, said single words at 12 months, and combined words at 22 months. At age 5, her speech became progressively more telegraphic, and she started pointing or using sign language to indicate her needs. On your neurologic examination, she is able to follow simple commands. She has word-finding difficulties in spontaneous speech and on naming tasks and is unable to repeat short phrases. The rest of her neurologic examination is normal. Formal audiometric testing is normal.

Her family states that she occasionally stares off into space for 20 s to 1 min. No convulsive seizure was reported. She has no family history of epilepsy. **Most likely her EEG is going to show?**

A. Hypsarrhythmia with periods of electro decrement
B. Continuous, diffuse, polymorphic theta and delta slowing
C. Bilateral periodic epileptiform discharges (BiPEDs)
D. Electrical status epilepticus in slow wave sleep
E. Normal waking and sleep

Correct Answer is: D

In 1957, William L. Landau and Frank R. Kleffner reported a "syndrome of acquired aphasia with convulsive disorder in children" and postulated that persistent convulsive discharges were causing a functional ablation of brain areas concerned with language. Since then, many childhood epileptic encephalopathy syndromes it has become characterized by deterioration of one or more cognitive functions with or without motor, behavioral, and/or psychomotor decline in association with an EEG that shows strong activation of epileptic activity during sleep. At this point, electrical status epilepticus of slow wave sleep (ESES) and continuous spikes and waves during slow wave sleep (CSWS) are considered synonymous terms, and Landau-Kleffner syndrome (LKS) a distinct presentation of ESES/CSWS in which acquired aphasia is the core symptom.

LKS classically presents with language disturbance in normally developing children aged 3 and 8 years. Some have proposed that the language disturbance is in fact a verbal auditory agnosia (i.e. inability to comprehend spoken language in the absence of hearing difficulties). Over time, affected children experience a gradual deterioration in verbal comprehension and production, eventually leading to failure to respond to non-verbal sounds and mutism 20–30% of patients do not have any clinical seizure activity at all. There is no clear relationship between the severity of the seizures and the severity of the language deficits. EEG shows mainly bilateral posterior temporal spikes or spike-wave discharges that are activated by sleep. The clinical seizures are usually easy to control, with spontaneous resolution occurring in mid-adolescence. Treatment options include corticosteroids, levetiracetam, benzodiazepines, and valproic acid. Language function improves when the active phase of spike-wave discharges resolves; however, if the aphasia begins in early childhood and/or persists for more than 1–2 years, long-term language deficits are almost universal.

Suggested Reading

- Smith MC, Hoeppner TJ. Epileptic encephalopathy of late childhood. J Clin Neurophysiol. 2003;20(6):462–72.

4. A local school send a particularly difficult student for consultation. A 9 years old boy who has always been "hard-to-handle". His teachers have always assumed that his parents are excessively lenient with him, particularly because they lost his older brother when this boy was 6 years old. His classroom teacher reported that he refuses to do anything she asks and argues indiscriminately with other children in the class. He is very disruptive, throwing balled-up paper around the room while the children are supposed to be working on a science or math problem. She also mentioned that he seems quite bright, as he has an advanced vocabulary for age, including some words she would rather never hear in the classroom.

You are going to evaluate him for:
A. Attention deficit disorder
B. Oppositional-defiant disorder
C. Attention deficit disorder
D. Schizoaffective disorder
E. Autistic spectrum disorder
F. Obsessive-compulsive disorder

Correct Answer is: B
Children with disruptive, antisocial behavior should be evaluated for oppositional-defiant disorder. He might be showing difficulty paying attention or staying on task, but this is because of the intrusions of his need to "act out" and oppose requests or needs of others. The child in the case does not have the stero-typies or lack of social interaction of a child with an autism spectrum disorder. There is no description in this case of a thought disorder or perseverative compulsions.

Suggested Reading

- Althoff RR, Kuny-Slock AV, Verhulst FC, Hudziak JJ, van der Ende J. Classes of oppositional-defiant behavior: concurrent and predictive validity. J Child Psychol Psychiatry. 2014;55(10):1162–71.

5. A 4-year-old girl brought to your office for an evaluation for her developmental delay. She came with her maternal grandmother, who has custody of her because of parent neglect. Her physical exam showed, mild dysmorphic features with a head circumference at the 5th percentile and height/weight at 10th percentile. She has moderate to severe language delay. She has a thin upper lip with smooth philtrum.
Which of the following is the most likely diagnosis?
A. Down's syndrome
B. Autism
C. Fetal alcohol syndrome
D. Rett's syndrome
E. Trisomy 18

Correct Answer is: C
Clinical history of maternal exposure to alcohol and the physical appearance of the child can lead to the diagnosis of fetal alcohol syndrome. The diagnostic criteria recommended by the Research Society of Alcoholism Fetal Alcohol study group require: (1) Prenatal or postnatal growth retardation (2) CNS dysfunction, developmental delay or intellectual impairment; and (3) at least two of the following: microcephaly, microphthalmia and short palpebral fissures, or all 3 and hypoplastic philtrum with thin upper lip.

Suggested Reading

- Menke J. Toxic and nutritional disorders. In: Menke J, Sarnat H, Maria BL, editors. Child Neurology. 7th ed. Philadelphia: Lippincott Williams and Wilkins; 2006. p. 703–5.

6. A 6-year-old boy came to your office with his mother, who wants you to start him on methylphenidate for ADHD treatment. His medical history is remarkable for a speech delay, impaired social functioning with his school peers, restricted interests with a fascination for dinosaurs, and hand flapping behaviors when he is excited. In addition, his mother and teachers report that he has a very short attention span, poor impulse control, and hyperactive behavior. Another brother has been diagnosed with ADHD and has shown a dramatic benefit from methylphenidate treatment, with minimal adverse effects, but he does not have the same language and social difficulties as this boy.
Which of the following statements most accurately reflects the likelihood of positive and negative medication effects compared with his brother's response?

A. Equally effective with equal side effects
B. More effective but greater side effects
C. Less effective and greater side effects
D. Less effective but fewer side effects
E. More effective with fewer side effects

Correct Answer is: C
Autism spectrum disorder (ASD) is characterized by impairments in social functioning and communication, and restricted, repetitive behaviors and interests. On the other hand, ADHD is characterized by difficulties in maintaining attention and patterns of impulsive and/or hyperactive behavior. The DSM-IV-TR does not allow a comorbid diagnosis of ASD and ADHD, because ASD is the more severe disorder within the diagnostic hierarchy, so any inattention, hyperactivity, or impulsivity observed can be thought of as originating from the primary diagnosis of autism. This exclusion fails to account for the many individuals with ASD who also meet full criteria for ADHD; these individuals typically have more severe overall dysfunctions. Studies have shown that patients with both ASD and ADHD have a lower likelihood of favorable response with stimulant treatment (25–50%) when compared to patients with isolated ADHD; the incidence of adverse effects in this population is up to 60%, mainly agitation.

Suggested Reading

- Murray MJ. Attention-deficit/hyperactivity disorder in the context of autism spectrum disorders. Curr Psychiatry Rep. 2010;12:382–8.

7. 9-year-old female has a 6 month history of deteriorating school performance, disinhibited behavior, and agitation, and out of character compared to her premorbid, developmentally age-appropriate state. During your evaluation she describes episodes of non-command auditory hallucinations. There is no past medical history of head trauma or significant infectious illness. She is not taking any medications. Family history is non-contributory. She has a non-focal neurologic examination, but you noted occasional orofacial dyskinetic movements. There is a rise of 30 beats per minute of her heart rate when going from lying to standing.
Which of the following tests is most likely to be diagnostic?

A. Anti-DNase type B antibody and ASO titers
B. Magnetic resonance angiography of cerebral vessels
C. Pelvic ultrasound
D. Thyroid function testing (T4, T3 and TSH) with thyroid-peroxidase antibody (TPO) and anti-thyrotropin antibodies
E. Fasting lactate and pyruvate

Correct Answer is: C
Onset of childhood acute or subacute neuropsychiatric syndrome is indicative of Childhood Acute Neuropsychiatric Syndrome (CANS, also known as PANS or PANDAS). In females, the clinical findings of disinhibited behavior patterns, agitation and psychosis, associated with orofacial dyskinesias and autonomic dysfunction is indicative of anti-NMDA-receptor antibody encephalitis, a condition that can be associated with ovarian teratoma. This entity can also present with altered level of consciousness or seizures. For NMDA-receptor antibody encephalitis associated with ovarian teratoma, surgical resection of the tumor is usually curative. Streptococcal-associated CANS presents as Syndeham's Chorea (a major criterion of Rheumatic Fever, presenting with acute-onset of chorea and

obsessive-compulsive disorder) or possibly with "idiopathic" CANS. This latter category, initially reported as PANDAS, is described as presenting with acute onset of obsessive-compulsive symptoms as a primary criterion, although there may be an array of concomitant neuropsychiatric symptoms, and tics as a secondary criterion. Treatments can include antimicrobials directed at identifiable infectious agents, and immunomodulators. Hashimoto's thyroiditis more commonly presents in adolescence, and is commonly associated with more movement disorder phenomena (tremor, chorea, myoclonus, and ataxia). Identification of a non-infectious or para-infectious encephalitis/encephalopathy is important since treatment interventions can successful, albeit with variable success rates across cohorts.

Suggested Reading

- Kaur S, Juneja M, Mishra D, Jain S. Anti-N-methyl-D-aspartate receptor encephalitis: a case report and review of the literature. J Pediatr Neurosci. 2014;9:145–7.
- Singer HS, Gilbert DL, Wolf DS, et al. Moving from PANDAS to CANS. J Pediatr. 2012;160:725–31.

8. One of your patients on risperidone (Risperdal).
Periodically you should monitor him for:
A. Hemoglobin A-1-C
B. Lipid panel (fasting)
C. Prolactin level (AM)
D. Fasting blood glucose
E. All of the above

Correct Answer is: F
Neuroleptics side effects include the induction of tardive dyskinesias and other extrapyramidal dysfunction, hyperprolactinemia, hyperlipidemia, and type-II diabetes. All above choices are appropriate to monitor.

Suggested Reading

- Jerrell JM, Hwang T-L, Livingston TS. Neurological adverse events associate with antipsychotic treatment in children and adolescents. J Child Neurol. 2008;23:1392–9.

9. You evaluate an 8-year-old fourth grade boy for academic problems. He has a normal prenatal and perinatal course, and early neurodevelopmental milestones were achieved at an age appropriate time. Adequate grades were obtained through 3rd grade. In 4th grade, the mother and teachers have been complaining that he was inattentive and poorly organized. His teacher reported that he has difficulty with science and word problems, but good at reciting historical dates, and has trouble with math and reading comprehension. His family report that he can be awkward and has poor social skills, but is verbally expressive and verbose.
What is your next step in his care and management?
A. Head MRI
B. Trial of atomoxetine
C. Trial of mixed amphetamine salts
D. Psychiatric Consultation
E. Neuropsychological Evaluation

Correct Answer is: E
This is the clinical presentation of a non-verbal learning disorder (NVLD), which is characterized by discrepancies between verbal and non-verbal IQ, difficulties with conceptual learning and abstract thinking, poor social skills/development, visual-spatial deficits, and dyspraxia/incoordination. The strength areas, good rote memory skills, strong auditory learning skills, and eloquent expressive verbal abilities. Neuropsychological testing and evaluation will provide additional information concerning this patient's intellectual, cognitive and learning profile, and will have a higher yield than

psychiatric consultation in identifying a cognitive or learning disorder. Neuropsychological testing can empirically identify issues with cognitive processing, executive function, memory, and emotional contributors that might be causing or contributing to this patient's poor academic productivity.

In a struggling academic children, there is a tendency to diagnosis ADHD without a complete analysis of neuropsychological functioning to determine if there are other reasons for a child's poor academic function, and/or to confirm a clinical impression of ADHD. Over diagnosing ADHD in the United States has contributed to overprescribing of psychostimulant drugs. Although psychostimulants and nonstimulants such as atomoxetine can be useful for selected cases of individuals with ADHD, such a diagnosis should be established utilizing objective, empirical data rather than strictly "clinical impressions". Making or confirming a diagnosis of ADHD does not relay on the positive responses to psychostimulant medications. Since psychostimulant medications can enhance neurological functioning in all people, with or without ADHD, overuse can occur. Medication use in those with ADHD and associated academic productivity should be kept for selected cases. Atomoxetine is also useful for selected cases of ADHD, particularly in those with concomitant tics or anxiety.

Suggested Reading

- Graf WD, Miller G, Nagel SK. Addressing the problem of ADHD medications as neuroenhancements. Expert Rev Neurother. 2014;14:569–81.

10. The mother of an 8–year-old boy comes to your office for evaluation of possible seizures. Four months ago he was diagnosed by his pediatrician with attention deficit disorder and he was started on methyphenidate. The dose was slowly titrated with a good response in his inattentive symptoms. However, recently, the mother has noticed that he has seems more fidgety with repetitive eye blinking, shoulder shrugging, foot tapping and throat clearing. It is disruptive to his teachers. In the office, he makes these movements and noises almost continuously, but stops when he is being examined. **What is your next step in management?**
    A. Discontinue methylphenidate
    B. Brain MRI
    C. Obtain EEG
    D. Initiate fluoxetine
    E. Send antistreptolysin O titer

Correct Answer is: A
Stimulants, specifically, methylphenidate or amphetamine are the most commonly recommended medications for the treatment of attention deficit disorder. Behavioral therapy is also recommended. Approximately 15–30% of children experience tics which are often transient. However some of these movements may be persistent and bothersome to the patient and families. In addition, 50% of patients with Tourette's syndrome also have symptoms of attention deficit disorder.

Suggested Reading

- American Academy of Pediatrics. Subcommittee on attention deficit hyperactivity disorder. Committee on Quality Improvement.
- Treatment of the School-age children with Attention deficit hyperactivity disorder. Pediatrics. 2001;108(4):1033–44.

11. A10-year-old boy came to your office with his family for evaluation of frequent daydreaming. The family mentioned that he is disorganized

and tends to forget his homework. He has trouble at school. His primary care physician requested an electroencephalogram which was normal in the awake and asleep state. His physical exam is unremarkable.

What is the most appropriate next step in his evaluation?

A. Connor's questionnaire for parents and teachers
B. High resolution chromosomes
C. Head MRI with and without gadolinium
D. Serum lactate

Correct Answer is: A

Attention deficit disorder is an everyday problem seen by pediatricians, neurologist and psychiatrist. It may present at any period of a child's life. Also there is an increasing awareness of this condition in the young adult. The main symptoms are deficits in attention and vigilance as well as hyperactivity. The DSM-4 diagnosis requires the presence of six out of the nine symptoms of inattention and hyperactivity. There inattentive symptoms are inattention, poor organization, forgetfulness, failing to give attention to details. The hyperactive symptoms include talking excessively, blurting out answers, frequent interruption and intrusion. No laboratory or neurologic testing is indicated to diagnose ADHD unless there is an abnormal exam.

EEG was normal in this case. Absence seizure is a differential diagnosis for individuals who are noted to daydream.

Suggested Reading

- Pliska S, AACAP Work Group on Quality issues. Practice parameter for the assessment and treatment of children and adolescents with attention- deficit/hyperactivity disorder. In J Am Acad Child Adolesc Pyschiatry. 2007;46(7) 894–921.

12. A 4-year-old boy has language and social development delay, has a history of stereotypical self-stimulating behaviors like rocking his body and flapping his hands. No family history is available because he is adopted from Asia. He has microcephaly and blonde hair.

Which of the following metabolic conditions could be an explanation of his condition?

A. Glutaric Acidemia type 1
B. Maple syrup urine disorder
C. Phenylketonuria
D. Zellweger syndrome (cerebrohepatorenal syndrome)
E. Medium-chain acyl-coenzyme A dehydrogenase deficiency (MCAD)

Correct Answer is: C

Autism is highly associated with untreated phenylketonuria, and has the greatest body of literature and evidence to support this notion. Many of the others have early morbidity, or cause cognitive impairment without strong association with autism.

Suggested Reading

- Muhle R, Trentacoste S, Rapin I. The genetics of autism. Pediatrics. 2004;113(5):e472–86.
- Chen CH, Hsiao KJ. A Chinese classic phenylketonuria manifested as **autism**. Br J Psychiatry.1989;155:251–25.
- Lowe TL, Tanaka K, Seashore MR, Young JG, Cohen DJ. Detection of phenylketonuria in autistic and psychotic children. JAMA. 1980;243:126–8.
- Baieli S, Pavone L, Meli C, Fiumara A, Coleman M. **Autism** and phenylketonuria. J **Autism** Dev Disord. 2003;33:201–4.

13. A 15-year-old girl with primary generalized epilepsy well controlled on lamotrigine has a sudden onset of multiple paroxysmal episodes unlike her regular events. The mother

2

described a sudden startled look, followed by whole-body stiffening and arching in conjunction with "swimming" movements of the upper extremities and thrashing of the body. The events last 20 s to 3 min in duration and are followed by somnolence and she cannot remember the event. By history, there are no trigger factors, and lamotrigine serum level was normal. A prolonged video-EEG is obtained, showed occasional generalized polyphasic spike/wave discharges. One episode was captured during the recording and is associated with muscle artifact, with resumption of normal waking patterns after the event ends.

What is the most appropriate next step in management?

A. Switch to Valproic acid
B. Obtain psychiatry consultation
C. Decrease dose of lamotrigine
D. Start diphenhydramine
E. Head MRI

Correct Answer is: B
Clinical presentation strongly suggests psychogenic non-epileptic seizures, which is a form of conversion disorder. These include the following:Episodes are induced by stress, in certain settings, or by specific individuals.Seizures recur despite therapeutic antiepileptic drug levels. The ictus is of gradual onset and of unusually prolonged duration. There are thrashing/writhing movements, crying and/or screaming, pelvic thrusting, and rolling side-to-side.Movements are intermittent, arrhythmic, out-of-phase jerking, or with multiple periods of starting and stopping.

There is no loss of consciousness despite bilateral movements, and a lack of incontinence or cyanosis. This is not followed by post-ictal confusion or lethargyPresence of crying or shouting of obscenities.Eyes will be closed, and patients will tend to resist having their eyes forced open.The diagnosis of psychogenic seizures made primarily on video-EEG documentation of the non-epileptic nature of the clinical episodes of concern. While considered the definitive diagnostic test, video-EEG testing does not have perfect sensitivity and specificity. Some non-lesional focal epilepsies may be missed. 30–40% of patients having psychogenic non-epileptic seizures a have true epileptic seizures, making it extremely difficult to ascertain what are or aren't true epileptic events in the usual clinical settings, and even in the context of an emergency department visit. The presentation of the diagnosis of psychogenic non-epileptic seizures must be made with great care and sensitivity. The possibility of sexual abuse should always be considered.

Suggested Reading

- Bodde NM, Brooks JL, Baker GA, Boon PA, Hendriksen JG, Aldenkamp AP. Psychogenic non-epileptic seizures–diagnostic issues: a critical review. Clin Neurol Neurosurg. 2009;111(1):1–9.
- LaFrance WC Jr. Psychogenic nonepileptic seizures. Curr Opin Neurol. 2008;21(2):195–201.

14. A 10-year-old boy who is followed regularly for ADHD has developed frequent episodes of forced eye blinking and facial grimacing after being started on a stimulant medication. Although his parents report that it is very helpful for improving his attention and reducing hyperactivity, they are worried about

this eye blinking and the facial grimacing and asking if he can be on another medication. He is started on atomoxetine.

What do you have to monitor during treatment?

A. Complete blood count
B. Chest X ray
C. Suicidal ideation
D. Serum sodium
E. Electrocardiogram

Correct Answer is: C

The boy developed tics with a trial of stimulants. Hence, the family has requested another class of medications. Atomexetine, is a norepinephrine reuptake inhibitor. Its side effects include weight loss, anorexia and sleepiness. Acute liver failure has been reported as a rare complication. As with many neuroactive agents, there is a black-box warning about suicidal ideation, which should be monitored throughout therapy.

Suggested Reading

- Kinsbourne M, Wood F. Disorders of mental development. In: Menkes JH, Sarnat H, Maria B, editors. Child neurology. Philadelphia: Lippincott Williams and Wilkins. 7th ed. p. 1133–1140.

15. A 17-year-old girl is complaining of chronic headaches, problems falling asleep, upsetting dreams, and trouble at school, all of which have been worsening over the past several months. Her mother mentioned to you that her daughter has been losing interest in school activities and in socializing with her friends, and has been increasingly irritable, moody, and angry. By taking her history, you find out that her father was killed in a car accident six months ago and she broke up with her boyfriend after many verbal fights few months ago. She has been afraid to drive a car and has had nightmares about her father's death. Her headaches are "all over my head" and constant in nature. Their intensity does not vary over the course of the day or from day to day. Her neurological and general physical examination are normal.

What is your diagnosis?

A. Depression
B. Post-traumatic stress disorder
C. Bipolar disorder
D. Insomnia
E. Learning disability

Correct Answer is: B

Stressful events that lead to both emotional and physical consequences can be experienced by both children and adults. While reactions to stressful events are usually brief and associated with full recovery, exposure to catastrophic or repeated traumatic events can lead to unconscious mental dissociation, an emotional numbing to suppress the pain and trauma. It is important to realize that, since younger children have limited verbal skills and non-specific ways to react to stress, they may not always meet DSM criteria for post-traumatic stress disorder. Children generally exhibit more emotional lability after severe stress than do adults.

Suggested Reading

- Carrion VG, Weems CF, Ray R, Reiss AL. Toward an empirical definition of pediatric PTSD: the phenomenology of PTSD symptoms in youth. J Am Acad Child Adol Psych. 2002;41:166–73.

Genetic Disorders

Y. M. Awaad, *Absolute Pediatric Neurology*, https://doi.org/10.1007/978-3-319-78801-2_3

3

1. You are evaluating a 4-year-old boy with a diagnosis of cerebral palsy. His mother reports that he has been slow in walking and talking and has abnormal vision. His mother is 18-years-old with a history of substance abuse. There is no specific etiology for his CP. On examination, he has severe hypotonia, ataxia and dysmetria. He has nystagmus and frequently jerks his head to re-fixate. He does not talk but frequently sighs and then takes deep breaths. His brain MRI is shown and read as normal. He has no retinal response on electroretinogram.

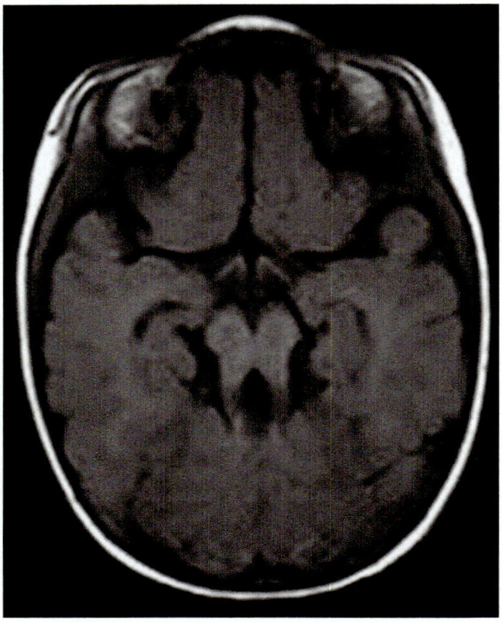

Fig. 3.1 Axial T2-weighted MRI. (Courtesy of Dr. Manikum Moodley and Dr. Gary Hsieh. Wikipedia)

What is the most accurate statement?

A. The problem is likely related to substance abuse, recurrence risk is low.
B. The child has a disorder that will lead to seizures and death with a 25% recurrence risk.
C. The child has a congenital disorder but exact determination of risk of recurrence requires specific genetic testing.
D. The child has a congenital disorder with the risk of recurrence being 25%.
E. The child has a congenital disorder that is sporadic and the risk of recurrence is minimal.

Correct Answer is: D
A child neurologist has to be fully aware of brain imaging as well as the features both clinically and radiologically of a genetically based disorder like Joubert Syndrom. The molar tooth sign is a diagnostic feature, that is frequently quite obvious, but not above being overlooked by the inexperienced radiologist or those not thinking about the clinical issues. Gene definition may be helpful particularly in confirming the diagnosis or recognizing the subtypes. The recent identification of retinal eletrophysiologic perturbation adds another feature to the complexity of Joubert.

Suggested Reading

- Khan AO, et al. Ophthalmic features of Joubert Syndrome. Ophthalmology. 2008;115:2286–9.
- Valente EM, et al.

2. You are seeing a 5-year-old girl with a history of mental retardation and lifelong seizures. Her seizures are recurrent generalized and focal seizures. She has poor seizure control in spite of using multiple anticonvulsant agents. On examination, she has a skull asymmetry with the right side being more prominent than the left. OFC is 54 cm. Her face is also large. Some hyperpigmentation is noted on the face and arm. She has hemiparesis on the left. EEG reveals prominent

persistent seizure discharge on the right and generalized slowing. Her MRI is shown.

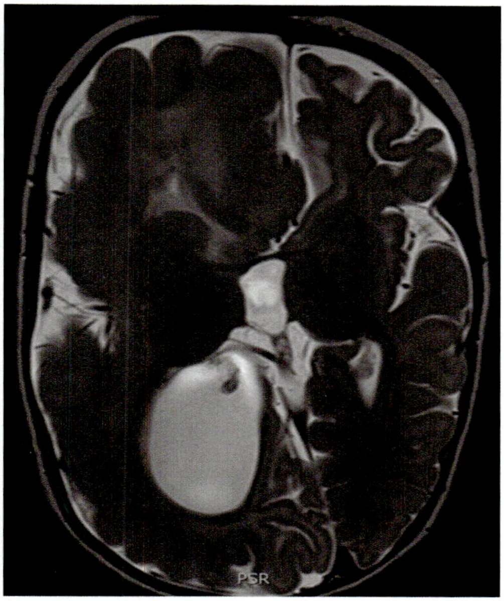

Fig. 3.2 With permission from ILAE.org. EpilepsyDiagnosis.org, Diagnostic Manual

What treatment option would you use to achieve optimal seizure control?

A. Corpus Callosotomy
B. Vagal nerve stimulator
C. Corticectomy
D. Hemispherectomy
E. Ketogenic diet

Correct Answer is: D

Patients with uncontrolled seizures secondary to hemimegencephaly should always be considered for surgery. The problem sometimes is recognizing the disorder. Many patients are obvious but more subtle or partial hemimegencephaly may be overlooked and the patient deprived of beneficial surgery. Any patient with uncontrolled seizures should be looked at critically in this regard. The ideal age for surgery has been a matter of debate. Early seems better than later. Focality on EEG and consonant MRI abnormality, in the uncontrolled epileptic should be sufficient impetus for serious surgical consideration.

Suggested Reading

- Di Rocco C, Battaglia D, Pietrini D, Piastra M, Massimi L. Hemimegalencephaly: clinical implications and surgical treatment. Childs Nervous System. 2006;22(8):852–66.
- Aicard J. Diseases of the Nervous System in Childhood, 3rd ed. Mac Keith press; 2009. p. 6.

3. A 14-year-old girl in foster care with no prior medical history came for an evaluation. The foster parents believe the child is autistic and perhaps mentally retarded. She drools excessively and does not swallow well. She does not socialize or smile. She has limited speech. She has significant behavior problem at home. On examination she does not blink to light. She cannot abduct either eye. She does not move her face.

What is your most likely diagnosis?

A. Poorly treated myasthenia gravis
B. Congenital myasthenic syndrome
C. Athapaskan brain stem dysgenesis
D. Moebius syndrome
E. Fazio-Londe Disease

Correct Answer is: D

The non-smiling ophthalmologic patient with no history can present an interesting set of problems. Moebius classical features are that of ophthamoparesis (especially abducens paresis) and facial diplegia. Lingual weakness and atrophy may also be a significant cranial nerve feature. Deafness is not a feature as it is in Athapaskan brain stem dysgenesis. Patients with Moebius syndrome may also have additional features which are important to know. They include scolio-

sis, muscle hypoplasia, mental retardation, hand and foot malformations. The psychological and social impact on the child who never smiles should not be overlooked.

Suggested Reading

- Verzijl HTFM, van der Zwaag B, Cruysberg JRM, Padberg GW. Moebius syndrome redefined: a syndrome of rhombencephalic maldevelopment Neurology. 2003;61: 327–33.

4. You are seeing a full-term baby girl who was born after uneventful labor and delivery. Her prenatal ultrasound performed at 34 weeks gestation showed posterior fossa cyst. Her examination is normal and she is feeding well. A brain MRI scan was ordered. **What is the most accurate diagnosis?**

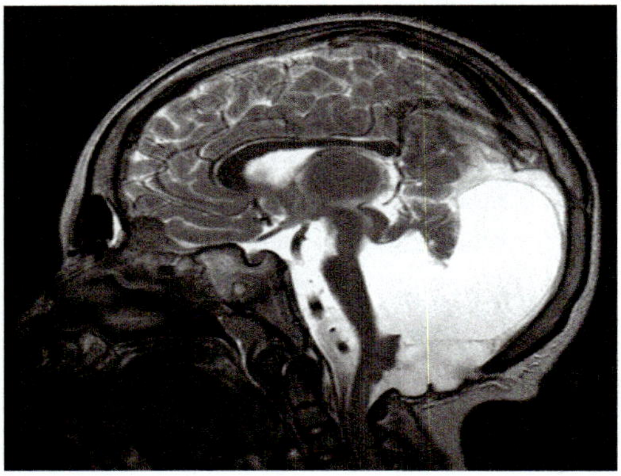

Fig. 3.3 Variant DWS with dysplasia of the pons and cerebellum in an 8-year old. T2 weighted sagittal MRI. Hellerhoff. Wikipedia

A. Cerebellar hypoplasia and arachnoid cyst
B. Enlarged cisterna magna
C. Dandy-Walker malformation
D. Type 1 Chairi malformation
E. Congenital cystic medulloblastoma

Correct Answer is: C

These radiological findings indicate Dandy-Walker malformation which is characterized by a dilated 4th ventricle with partial to complete agenesis of the cerebellar vermis. Hydrocephalus almost always develops in the first year but on rare occasions does not develop until adulthood. Other features include elevation of the tentorium and enlargement of the posterior fossa. Approximately 70% of cases are associated with other CNS malformations including agenesis of the corpus callosum. The etiology is thought to be due to improper closure of the ventral neural tube with failure of the foramina of Magendi to open. Despite the presence of normal foramina of Luschka CSF flow is disrupted. Treatment requires shunting of both the lateral and 4th ventricles. There is some suggestion that prognosis can be predicted by the degree of agenesis of the cerebellar vermis. The other causes for cysts in the posterior fossa, listed above, are not associated with dilation of the 4th ventricle.

Suggested Reading

- Klein O, Pierre-Kahn A, Boddaert N, Parisot D, Brunelle F. Dandy-Walker malformation: prenatal diagnosis and prognosis. Childs Nerv Syst. 2003;19: 484–89.

5. You are seeing a full-term infant was with a normal vaginal delivery. The mother had trauma at 34 weeks gestation, a prenatal ultrasound performed at that time and showed enlarged ventricles and a question of holoprosencephaly. The infant has a normal general and neurological exam, without dysmorphic features. A T2-weighted MRI scan is shown.
What is the most accurate diagnosis?

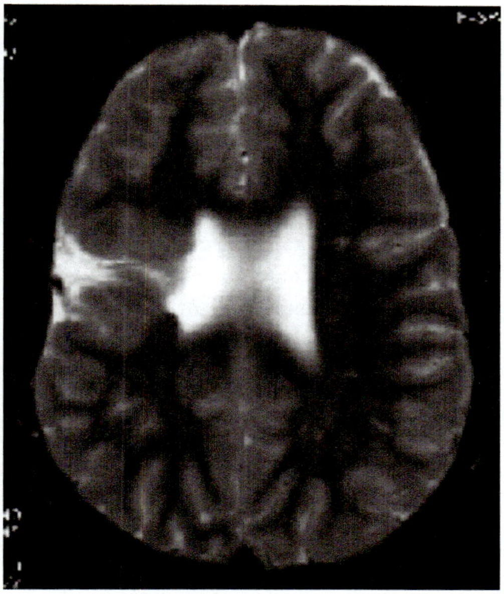

Fig. 3.4 With permission from ILAE.org. Epilepsy-Diagnosis.org, Diagnostic Manual

A. Lobar holoprosencephaly
B. Schizencephaly
C. Congenital hydrocephalus with arachnoid cyst
D. Lissencephaly
E. Agenesis of the corpus callosum with colpocephaly

Correct Answer is: B
The MRI shows right side schizencephaly. The condition is defined as cleft(s) involving the cortex and white mater from the ventricular ependyma to the pia. "Closed lip" schizencephaly refers to a cleft with the edges fused and "open lip" refers to clefts as in this case with CSF filling the space between the cortical surfaces. The condition is thought to arise in the second month and is characterized by migration defects in the area of the cortical ribbon lining the cleft. Other associated malformations including absence of the septum pellucidum, agenesis of the corpus callosum and septo-optic dysplasia. These other malformations are linked to a poorer prognosis. The etiology of this condition continues to be debated and is most often sporadic and linked to maternal trauma, intrauterine vascular accidents (such as the demise of a monozygotic twin), and intrauterine viral infection or is idiopathic. The incidence is estimated at 1 in 100,000. Since rare familial cases occur a genetic cause has been sought. Initial reports of mutations in the EMX2 homeodomain gene crucial to CNS development have not been found in further studies of groups of children with schizencephaly. The major manifestation is focal epilepsy and hemiparesis in unilateral cases. Bilateral cases can have a severe phenotype that includes mixed forms of epilepsy and spastic quadriparesis with severe developmental retardation.

Suggested Reading

- Denis D, Chateil JF, Brun M Brissaud O Lacombe D Fontan D Flurin V Pedespan J. Schizencephaly: clinical and imaging features in 30 infantile cases. Brain Dev 2000;22:475–83.
- Tietjen I, Bodell A, Apse K, Mendoza AM, Chang BS, Shaw GM, et al. Comprehensive EMX2 Genotyping of a Large Schizencephaly Case Series. Am J Med Genet 2007;143A:1313–16.

6. You are evaluating a 6-month-old boy for his seizures which started at his second day of life. He was born prematurely at 34 weeks gestation by normal vaginal delivery. Baby required oxygen after birth, but no artificial ventilation. His seizure was consisted of lip-smacking movements and arrest of behavior. Later the seizures were on the left side of his body. The mother has history of epilepsy treated with carbamazepine. He has developmental delay; he

3

cannot reach for objects nor roll over. On examination, he has inconsistent visual tracking, generalized hypotonia, and fewer spontaneous movements of his left limbs compared to the right. Brain MRI is shown.

What is the most likely cause of his seizures?

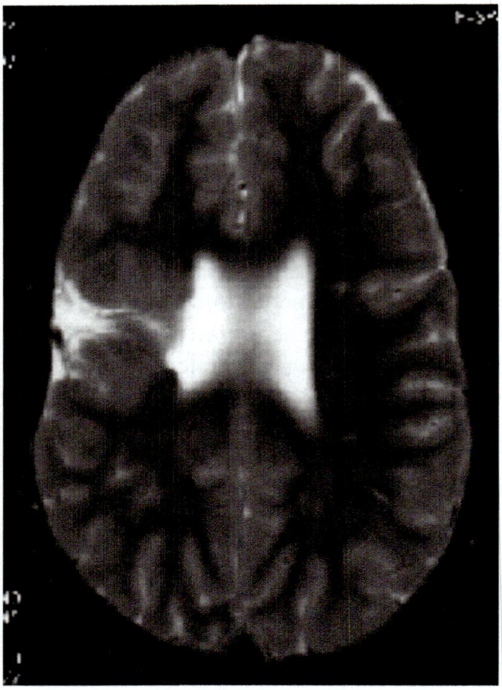

Fig. 3.5 With permission from ILAE.org. Epilepsy-Diagnosis.org, Diagnostic Manual

A. Hemimegalencephaly
B. Maternal carbamazepine use
C. Perinatal hypoxic ischemic brain injury
D. Prenatal stroke
E. Schizencephaly

Correct Answer is: E

MRI demonstrate Schizencephaly, which is a congenital brain malformation characterized by a cleft extending from the pial surface of the cerebral mantle to the ventricle. The cleft is lined by polymicrogyric cortex. The most common location involves the insula and adjoining pre/post central gyri. The clefts can be unilateral or bilateral, "closed-lip" (small defect) or "open-lip" (large defect). The etiology is heterogeneous and can be due to an early prenatal insult affecting the germinal zone prior to neuronal migration or can be genetic (mutation in the homeobox gene Emx2 has been identified in some cases). The presence of gyri and sulci (gray matter) radiating into the cleft aids in differentiating this condition from a late intrauterine or early postnatal MCA infarction. Patients with unilateral closed-lip type can be minimally affected or have hemiparesis and epilepsy. Those with open-lip type, especially if bilateral, have mental retardation, spasticity, epilepsy, and are severely compromised.

Suggested Reading

- Osborn AG, et al. Diagnostic imaging: brain. Salt Lake City, Utah: Amerisys Inc.; 2004. P I1 70–3.

7. You are seeing a 9-month-old baby boy for his developmental delay. He can roll over but cannot sit or scoot. His past medical history is remarkable for poor visual function and an ophthalmological assessment revealed hypoplastic optic nerves. On examination, he has severed generalized hypotonia, limited visual fixation and following, and nystagmus.

What other complications are you expecting in this boy in the future?

A. Deafness
B. Profound mental retardation
C. Growth impairment
D. Infantile spasms
E. Spastic quadriplegic cerebral palsy

Correct Answer is: C

This is a case of Septo optic dysplasia (Morsier syndrome). Optic nerve hypoplasia is part of the variable phenotype of Septo-optic dysplasia. This condition is defined loosely by any combination of the triad of optic nerve hypoplasia, midline neuro-radiological abnormalities (such as agenesis of the corpus callosum and absence of the septum pellucidum) and pituitary hypoplasia with consequent hypopituitarism. The reported incidence is 1/10,000 live births and affects males and females equally. Neurological deficit is common ranging from global developmental delay to focal deficits such as epilepsy or hemiparesis. Approximately 75–80% of patients exhibit optic nerve hypoplasia (bilateral in 88%) and is often the first presenting feature, with later onset of endocrine dysfunction. Hypothalamic-pituitary dysfunction may manifest as variable endocrine deficits ranging from isolated growth hormone deficiency (most common) to pan-hypopituitarism. Although neurological manifestations often occur, those listed above are not typically seen, while pituitary dysfunction is found in 62% of these patients.

Suggested Reading

- Kelberman D, Dattani MT. Septo-Optic Dysplasia- Novel Insights into the Aetiology. In: Horm Res 2008;69:257–65.

8. You are evaluating a 7-month-old boy for developmental delay and seizure-like spells. He was a product of uncomplicated full-term gestation. He is unable to roll over or sit, does not consistently visually regard or track objects, and does not reach for objects with his hands, but does put his hands in the mouth. On examination, head circumference is at 5th percentile. There are no dysmorphic features. Pupils are reactive to light but he does not track. Upon crying he has symmetrical facial movements. Neck and shoulder girdle muscle tone is decreased, but increased in the hands and ankles. DTRs are brisk, with bilateral ankle clonus. Axial T1 MRI is shown here.
What is the most likely mechanism to account for her condition?
   A. Congenital infection
   B. Inborn error of metabolism
   C. Migration brain anomaly
   D. Perinatal hemorrhage
   E. Prenatal ischemia

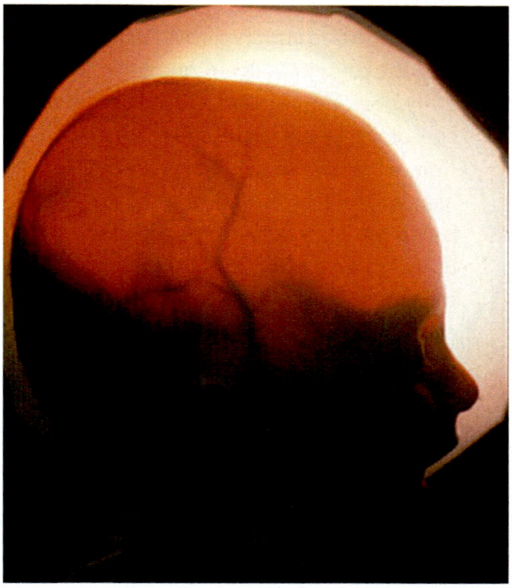

Fig. 3.6 Image of a baby with hydrancephaly, light passes through the skull indicating lack of forebrain. (*Courtesy of D. P. Agamanolis* ► http://neuropathology-web.org". Wikipedia)

Correct Answer is: E
This is a case of hydranencephaly, which is characterized by severe dysgenesis of the cerebral hemispheres, with relative preservation of the thalamus, cerebellum and brainstem. Advanced neurological imaging techniques have

showed that the affected regions are usually localized within the territories of the middle cerebral arteries. It has been suggested that hydranencephaly results from vasculopathy with carotid artery occlusion. This hypothesis was supported by the distribution of the marked hemispheric destruction observed in patients with hydranencephaly. Experiments entailing ligation of both the common carotid arteries and the jugular veins in monkeys during early gestation resulted in subsequent cerebral dysgenesis and focal destruction, with the regions supplied by the anterior and middle cerebral arteries being reduced to thin transparent membranes. The tissues supplied by the posterior cerebral arteries, which receive collateral blood flow from the vertebrobasilar system through the posterior communicating arteries, were usually mainly preserved. These findings support the proposed pathologic process in hydranencephaly.

Suggested Reading

- Tsai JD, Kuo HT, Chou IC. Hydranencephaly in Neonates. In: Pediatric Neonatal 2008;49(4):154–7.

9. You are seeing a 9-year-old girl with a 2 years history of seizure. Her seizures are described as unresponsiveness and lip smacking, sometimes also with jerking movements of the right arm. Her seizures have been partially controlled with carbamazepine, lamotrigine, and levetiracetam. She has a remarkable family history of generalized tonic-clonic seizure in her maternal uncle, started at her teens. She has unremarkable past medical history and she has normal development. She has normal examination. Her MRI is shown here.

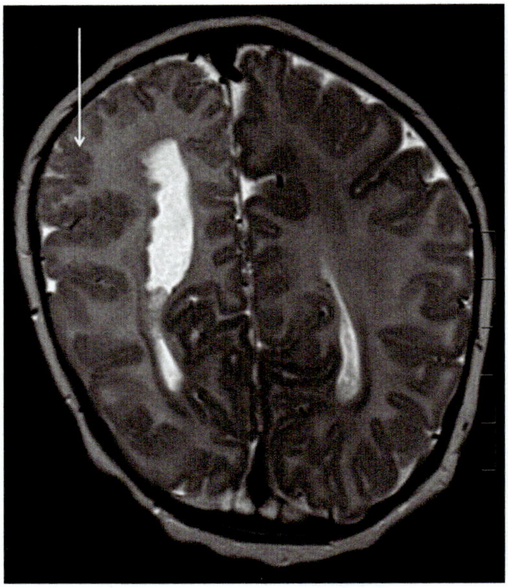

Fig. 3.7 With permission from ILAE.org. Epilepsy-Diagnosis.org, Diagnostic Manual

What is the most accurate description of the condition causing her seizures?

A. Band heterotopias
B. Idiopathic
C. Pachygyria
D. Polymicrogyria
E. Schizencephaly

Correct Answer is: D

MRI shows poly-microgyria, which is one of the most common malformations of cortical development. In this condition, the brain surface is irregular and the normal gyral pattern is replaced by an excessive number of small and partly fused gyri separated by shallow sulci. It is causally and histologically heterogeneous, resulting from a developmental disorder or injury that occurs toward the end of the period of neuronal migration and in the early phase of cortical organization. Causes include congenital infection (particularly CMV), localized or diffuse in utero ischemia,

or mutations. It can be focal or diffuse, unilateral (40%) or bilateral (60%). It can occur as an isolated lesion, in association with other brain malformations such as heterotopias or white matter lesions, or as part of several multiple congenital anomaly/mental retardation syndromes. The severity of clinical presentation and age at presentation depend mostly upon the extent of cortical involvement; bilateral involvement and involvement of more than half of a single hemisphere are poor prognostic indicators, portending moderate to severe developmental delay and significant motor dysfunction. The most common location is around the Sylvain fissure. Several distinct patterns of bilateral polymicrogyria have been described, including frontal, front parietal, perisylvian, lateral parietal, parasagittal parietooccipital (as in this case), and generalized Genetic mutation involving GPR56 has been identified in patients with bilateral front parietal form of polymicrogyria and is inherited in an autosomal recessive manner.

Suggested Reading

- Barkovich AJ. Current concepts of polymicrogyria. Neuroradiology. 2010;52:479–87.
- Jansen A, Andermann E. Genetics of the polymicrogyria syndromes. J Med Genet. 2005;42:369–78.
- Chang B, Walsh CA, Apse K, Bodell A. Polymicrogyria overview. GeneReviews [Internet], ► www.ncbi.nlm.nih.gov/books/NBK1329/.

10. You are evaluating a 5-month-old boy who developed of infantile spasms for the last 2 months. The spasm has been persistent despite treatment using Phenobarbital, levetiracetam, topiramate, and clonazepam. He has global developmental delay and has been unable to roll over or sit independently. He does not reach for objects and does not consistently visually track objects. On examination, he has poor head control, increased tone and reflexes in all limbs, and lack of visual regard.

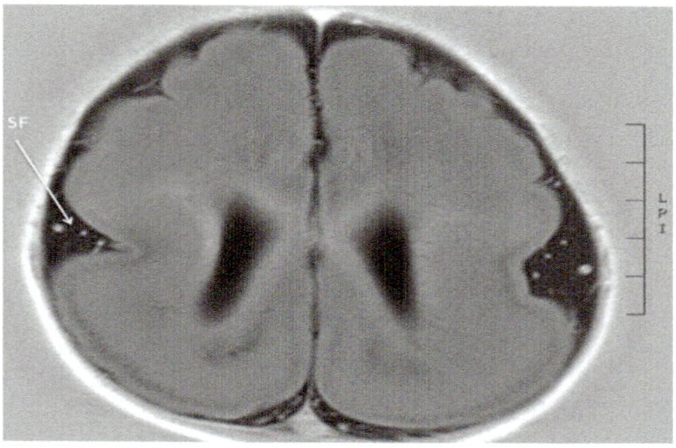

Fig. 3.8 With permission from ILAE.org. Epilepsy-Diagnosis.org, Diagnostic Manual

What is most likely genetic mutation responsible for her condition?

A. ARX
B. DCX
C. LIS1
D. MECP2
E. RELN

Correct Answer is: C
MRI shows characteristic of type 1 lissencephaly. Lissencephaly is a group of disorders characterized by an abnormally smooth surface of the cerebral cortex. Type 1 is also called "classic lissencephaly" while type 2 is known as "cobblestone complex". This severe brain malformation is associated with mutations in the LIS1 gene on chromosome 17p13.3. Mutations in this gene are associated with 2 clinical entities: Miller-Dieker syndrome and isolated lissencephaly sequence. The former is characterized by dysmorphic facial features including a prominent forehead, bi-temporal hollowing, and short nose with upturned nares,

protuberant upper lip, thin vermillion border, and small jaw. DCX, also known as doublecortin, is a gene located on the X chromosome and its mutation in male's causes' lissencephaly, but in female's leads to a much milder phenotype, including subcortical band heterotopias (double cortex syndrome). Both ARX and RELN are associated with "variant lissencephaly". ARX mutations are associated with agyria or pachygyria with posterior to anterior gradient of severity, thick cortex (not as thick as LIS1), and agenesis of the corpus callosum, abnormal white matter signals, and poorly defined basal ganglia. RELN is associated with generalized pacchygyria, severe cerebellar hypoplasia, and hippocampal abnormalities. MECP2 is associated with Rett syndrome.

Suggested Reading

- Mochida GH. Genetics and Biology of Microcephaly and Lissencephaly. Semin Pediatr Neurol. 2009;16:129–26.

11. You are seeing a 35-month-old South American girl for her delayed development. She had no prenatal care. Her birth weight was 3 kg. Delivery was complicated but the child had respiratory distress and jaundice in the neonatal period. Subsequently she had trouble swallowing and was followed carefully for nutritional deprivation. She is not regressing. She can cruise, but does not talk. Her examination shows a well-nourished child who is alert and sociable. She is hypotonic and is able to stand with support but has poor balance. She has prominent choreic and dystonic movements of the extremities. DTRs are intact and plantar responses are down going. Her MRI is shown.

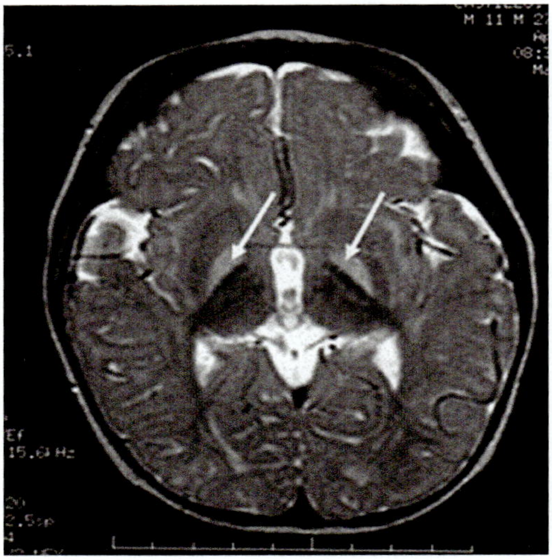

Fig. 3.9 MRI of the head. Hyperintense basal ganglia lesions on T2-weighted images. (de Gurrola GC, Araúz JJ, Durán E, Aguilar-Medina M, Ramos-Payán R, García-Magallanes N, Pacheco GV, Meraz EA. Kernicterus by glucose-6-phosphate dehydrogenase deficiency: a case report and review of the literature. *Journal of Medical Case Reports* 2008, 2:146 ► https://doi.org/10.1186/1752-1947-2-146. Gladys Cossio de Gurrola et al.)

What is the most likely explanation for her neurological condition?

A. Hypoxic-ischemic encephalopathy
B. Vitamin and nutritional deficiency
C. Leigh syndrome
D. Kernicterus
E. Methylmalonic aciduria

Correct Answer is: D
Nowadays, this condition has become relatively uncommon. Few cases still have been seen. This patient's neonatal experience was unique but her clinical presentation of kernicterus was not. The hypotonia, choreoathetosis, and lack of speech suggesting hearing impairment were all very characteristic and the diagnosis was confirmed by the MRI, which showed increased T2 signal in the globus pallidus. You have to be aware that a general radiologist reading the MRI may easily miss the diagnosis.

Suggested Reading

- Shapiro SM. Definition of the clinical spectrum of kernicterus and bilirubin-induced neurologic dysfunction (BIND). J Perinatol. 2005;25(1):54–9.

12. You are evaluating a 4-year-old because his mother and his Head Start teacher are concerned about his difficulty relating with others. He wanders around the room and hums during story time. He will flap his arms and spin when he is excited. He has a moderate speech delay and will be evaluated by speech therapy. He is a picky eater; he only eats chicken nuggets and French fries. On examination he has macrocephaly with an OFC of 57 cm.
Mutations in which of the following gene or chromosome regions are most likely responsible for the child's symptoms?
A. FMR1
B. PTEN
C. 22q11.2 deletion
D. ARX
E. 17p11.2 deletion

Correct Answer is: B
The boy has symptoms consistent with Macrocephaly/Autism Syndrome caused by mutations in the PTEN Gene. The *PTEN* (phosphatase and tensin homolog) gene was initially described as a tumor suppressor gene associated with a broad group of disorders referred to as *PTEN* hamartoma tumor syndrome which includes Cowden syndrome, Bannayan-Riley-Ruvalcaba syndrome, Proteus syndrome, and Lhermitte-Duclos disease. More recently, *PTEN* gene mutations have been associated with autism and macrocephaly. *PTEN* is recognized to play an important role in brain development, including neuronal survival and synaptic plasticity. The frequency of *PTEN* mutations as a cause of autism and macrocephaly range from 1% to 17%. Both *de novo* and familial *PTEN* mutations have been identified in this population. Children with ASD found to have a *PTEN* mutation generally have extreme macrocephaly ranging from + 3.7 SD to + 9.6 SD (average: +5.4 SD). In addition, mutation of *PTEN* is not specific for autism: Varga et al. [2009] found children with macrocephaly and intellectual disability but not autism who had a similar chance of having a *PTEN* mutation.

Suggested Reading

- Miles JH. Autism Spectrum Disorders. GeneReviews. 1993–2014.
- Macrocephaly/Autism Syndrome. OMIM # 605309.

13. Ocular manifestations are common in Lysosomal storage diseases.
The Lysosomal storage disease that is least likely to have a macular cherry red spot is:
A. Silicosis
B. GM 1 Gangliosidoses
C. Krabbe disease
D. Farber disease
E. Niemann-Pick disease

Correct Answer is: C
Krabbe disease is a lysosomal storage disease characterized by infantile-onset progressive neurologic deterioration and death before age 2 years (85–90% of individuals) or by onset between age 1 year and the fifth decade with slower disease progression (10–15%). Children with the infantile form appear to be normal for the first few months of life but show extreme irritability, spasticity, and developmental delay before age 6 months; psychomotor regression pro-

gresses to a decerebrate state with no voluntary movement. The onset and progression in the late-onset forms can be quite variable. Individuals can be clinically normal until weakness, vision loss, and intellectual regression become evident. The onset of symptoms and clinical course can be variable even among siblings.

In almost all individuals with Krabbe disease, galactocerebrosidase (GALC) enzyme activity is deficient (0–5% of normal activity) in leukocytes isolated from whole heparinized blood or in cultured skin fibroblasts.

Individuals with the infantile form of Krabbe disease can present with any or all of the following features. However, it is the least likely of all of the LSDs to have a cherry red spot:

- **Irritability**
- **Muscle hypertonicity**
- **Progressive neurologic deterioration**
- **Peripheral neuropathy**
- **Evidence of white matter disease on neuroimaging**
- **Elevation of cerebrospinal fluid (CSF) protein concentration**

Suggested Reading

- Wenger DA. Krabbe Disease. Gene Reviews. 2000.
- Hofman KJ. et al. Cherry red spot in association with galactosylceramide-β-galactosidase deficiency. J Inherit Metab Dis. 1987;10(3):273–4.

14. You are evaluating 3 days in the NICU for desaturation spells and neonatal seizures. His seizures are multifocal clonic spells. He was born full term, after uncomplicated pregnancy, labor or delivery. His brain MRI is shown below:

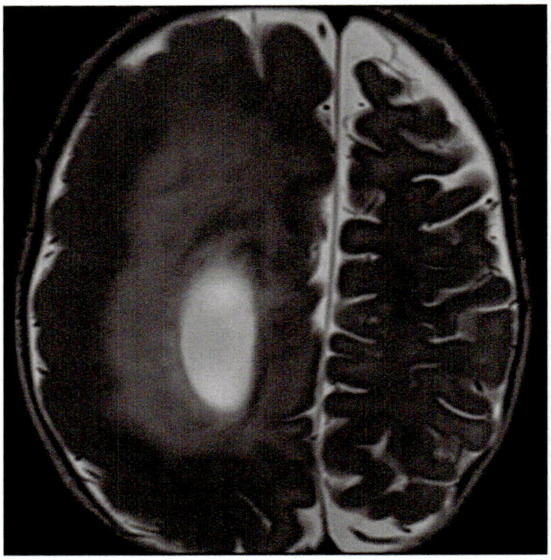

Fig. 3.10 With permission from ILAE.org. EpilepsyDiagnosis.org, Diagnostic Manual

What is the most likely diagnosis?

A. Right hemispheric infarction
B. Left chronic subdural hematoma
C. Hemimegaloencephaly
D. Lobar Holoprosencephaly
E. Neonatal adrenoleukodystrophy

Correct Answer is: C

There is an enlargement of the left hemisphere on the MRI consistent with hemimegaloencephaly. The left occipital lobe is so large that it crosses midline into the territory where the right occipital lobe occupies. This is called the "occipital pole sign" and is a seen in cases of hemimegaloencephaly. The cerebral cortex on the left is thickened and dysplastic.

Hemimegaloencephaly (HMC) is a congenital brain malformation that includes hamaromatous overgrowth of one hemisphere of the brain. Occasionally it can involve the cerebellum and brainstem. It presents as part of a

syndrome or in isolation. Usually it is associated with a neuro-cutaneous syndrome. These include Neurofibromatosis, Proteus syndrome, Klippel-Trénaunay-Weber syndrome and others. Other abnormalities of cortical development can be seen in associated with HMC including lissencephaly, pachygyria and polymicrogyria. Affected individuals typically present in infancy with intractable seizures, epileptic encephalopathy, and severe neurodevelopmental delay. Early hemispherectomy has been shown to an effective treatment for those with severe intractable epilepsy. The right hemisphere in this MRI is actually the normal hemisphere. There is no evidence of a chronic subdural hematoma. There is no evidence of abnormal fusion of the brain as seen with holoprosencephaly. Neonatal adrenoleukodystrophy is not felt to be associated with hemimegaloencephaly.

Suggested Reading

- Flores-Sarnat L. Hemimegaloencephaly: part 1. Genetic, clinical, and imaging aspects. J Child Neurol. 2002;17(5):373–84; discussion 384.

15. You are seeing a 2-year-old boy for hypotonia and abnormal eye movement. He has a history of having vomiting and diarrhea, and he has been choking on food and running into things. He has failure to thrive. On examination, he has hypotonic, abnormal eye movements, optic atrophy and difficulty with tracking, dystonia and an ataxic gait. His brain MRI shows symmetrical necrotic lesions in the basal ganglia, thalami and brainstem which appear hyper intense on the T2 weighted images.

    What is the most common genetic abnormality in this syndrome?

    A. Succinic semi aldehyde dehydrogenase deficiency
    B. Respiratory chain complex IV deficiency (COX)
    C. Coenzyme Q deficiency
    D. Carnitine deficiency
    E. POLG deficiency

Correct Answer is: B

This is a case of Leigh syndrome, which is a severe neurological disorder that typically arises in the first year of life. It is the most common clinical phenotype of mitochondrial disorders in childhood. The diagnostic criteria are (1) progressive neurological disease with motor and intellectual developmental delay; (2) signs and symptoms of brainstem and/or basal ganglia disease; (3) raised lactate levels in blood and/or cerebrospinal fluid (CSF); and (4) characteristic symmetric necrotic lesions in the basal ganglia and/or brainstem.

The most characteristic neuroradiological findings in Leigh syndrome are bilateral, symmetric focal hyperintensities in the basal ganglia, thalamus, substantia nigra, and brainstem nuclei at various levels on T2-weighted MRI.

There are at least 3 major causes of Leigh syndrome, each transmitted by a different mode of inheritance: X-linked recessive, mitochondrial, and autosomal recessive.

Disruption of complex IV, also called cytochrome *c* oxidase or COX, is the most common cause of Leigh syndrome. The most frequently mutated gene in COX-deficient Leigh syndrome is called *SURF1*. This gene, which is found in nuclear DNA, provides instructions for making a protein that helps assemble the COX protein

complex (complex IV). Mutations in the *SURF1* gene typically lead to an abnormally short SURF1 protein, resulting in the absence of functional SURF1 protein. The loss of this protein reduces the formation of normal COX complexes, which impairs mitochondrial energy production. The second most common cause is disruption of complex.

Suggested Reading

- Leigh Syndrome. Omim # 256000 Kartikasalwah et al. Leigh Syndrome: MRI findings in two children. Biomed Imaging Intervention J. 2010 Jan-Mar 2010.
- Morris et al. Deficiency of respiratory chain complex I is a common cause of Leigh Disease. Ann Neurol. 1996;40(1):25–30.

16. Angelman syndrome (AS) is a neurodevelopmental disorder characterized by severe mental retardation, absent speech, ataxia, sociable affect, and dysmorphic facial features. If genetic testing for the maternal deletion in the 15q11.2-q13 critical region was negative.
    What another genetic test should be considered?
    A. FMR
    B. UBE3A
    C. ARX
    D. LIS
    E. TSC

Correct Answer is: B
Angelman syndrome is a neurodevelopmental disorder characterized by mental retardation, movement or balance disorder, typical abnormal behaviors, and severe limitations in speech and language. Most cases are caused by absence of a maternal contribution to the imprinted region on chromosome 15q11-q13. Approximately 70% of AS cases result from de novo maternal deletions involving chromosome 15q11.2-q13; approximately 2% result from paternal uniparental disomy of 15q11.2-q13; and 2–3% result from imprinting defects. A subset of the remaining 25% is caused by mutations in the gene encoding the ubiquitin-protein ligase E3A gene (UBE3A).

Suggested Reading

- ▶ www.omim.org/entry105830

This question is part of a series of two questions

17. You were asked to see a 2-month-old girl after the infant was noted to be floppy and failure to thrive. The infant is brought to the ED for decreased oral intake over the last week. On examination, head is normo-cephalic but she has severe head lag and is floppy with muscle weakness. The infant has tachypnea. Her echocardiogram showed cardiomegaly. Creatinine kinase and Aspartate Aminotransferase were elevated.
    What is the next step in the evaluation?
    A. Lysosomal enzyme screen
    B. Serum lactate
    C. Serum Ammonia
    D. Muscle biopsy
    E. MRI of the brain

Correct Answer is: A
This is a case of Pompeo disease, Glycogen-storage disease type II (GSDII), an autosomal recessive disorder that results from the deficiency of acid alpha-glucosidase, (GAA). It is a rare (estimated at 1 in every 40,000 births), inherited and often fatal disorder.

Acid alpha-glucosidase is a lysosomal hydrolase that is required for the degradation of a 1–3% of cellular glycogen. Because the main pathway for glycogen degradation is not deficient in glycogen-storage disease type II disease, energy production is not impaired, and

hypoglycemia does not occur. However, the deficiency of this enzymatic activity results in the accumulation of structurally normal glycogen in lysosomes and cytoplasm in affected individuals.

In the infantile form, clinically significant storage occurs in the heart, resulting in progressive cardiomegaly with left ventricular (LV) thickening that eventually leads to outflow tract obstruction. Storage in skeletal muscle leads to hypotonia and weakness. The respiratory muscles are also affected, resulting in hypoventilation and progressive respiratory compromise. CNS involvement is primarily limited to the anterior horn cells of the spinal cord and brain stem nuclei, although intellectual performance remains normal.

Symptoms begin in the first months of life, with feeding problems, poor weight gain, muscle weakness, floppiness, and head lag.

Suggested Reading

- NINDS Pompe information page. Ibrahim J. et al. Genetics of Glycogen-Storage Disease Type II (Pompe Disease). Medscape. August 2014.

18. The parents of the patient above have questions regarding management and prognosis.
    Enzyme replacement therapy has been FDA approved in the all of the following Lysosomal Storage Disorders except:
    A. Gaucher types 1 and 3
    B. Mucopolysaccharidosis Types 1, 2 and 6
    C. Pompe Disease
    D. Metachromatic Leukodystrophy
    E. Fabry Disease

Correct Answer is: D
Enzyme replacement therapy (ERT) has been FDA approved for use in several Lysosomal Storage Disorders (LSDs) including Gaucher Types 1 and 3, Mucopolysaccharidosis Type 1 (Hurler, Hurler Schie Syndrome), Mucopolysaccharidosis Type 2 (Hunter Syndrome), Mucopolysaccharidosis Type 6 (Maroteaux-Lamy Syndrome), Fabry Disease and Pompe Disease. It involves replacement of the deficient enzyme by IV infusion of exogenous enzyme. It is recommended that it be used in LSDs without mental retardation because the exogenous enzyme does not cross the blood-brain barrier. ERT has proven to be effective in reducing many symptoms of LSDs.

Suggested Reading

- Bruni S., et al. Update on Treatment of Lysosomal Storage Diseases. Acta Myologica. 2007;XXVI: 87–92.

19. You were asked to see an infant who is having difficulty with sucking and has not passed meconium. On examination the infant is dysmorphic with a large fontanel, high forehead, high arched palate, right corneal opacity, palpable liver, hypotonic, floppy and does not react to visual or auditory stimuli.
    The signs that should raise suspicion of a peroxisomal disease include all of the following except:
    A. Faciocranial dysmorphic features
    B. Patellar calcifications
    C. Hirschsprung disease
    D. Renal cysts
    E. Neuronal Migration Defects

Correct Answer is: C
This is a clinical presentation of Zellweger syndrome, which is the most frequent and severe of the peroxisomal disorders in early infancy. It is a multisystem autosomal recessive disorder associated with a complete absence of peroxisomes in all tissues of the body and a generalized loss of peroxisomal

development. Signs of major diagnostic importance are the typical craniofacial dysmorphology, ocular abnormalities, renal cysts and patellar calcifications. In the typical patient, soon after birth it is noted that the child is hypotonic and has impaired hearing and diminished visual acuity. The craniofacial abnormalities include a high forehead, large fontanels and metopic suture, and high arched palate. Ocular abnormalities include cataracts and corneal opacities and retinal degeneration. Renal cysts occur in all patients. Patellar calcifications are present in half the patients. MRI may reveal abnormal neuronal migration.

Suggested Reading

- Lyon et al. Neurology of hereditary metabolic diseases of children. 2nd ed. 1996.

20. You are seeing a 10-year-old boy for Attention Deficit Hyperactivity Disorder evaluation. He has always been an excellent student but over the last year he has had difficulty paying attention in the classroom and has become hyperactive. He has a drop in his grades from A/B's to C's/D's. On examination, he is a thin adolescent without acute distress, but he has melanoderma on his skin examination. He has delayed processing, dysarthria, left hemiparesis and hemianopia on his neurological examination. Your admitted him urgently to the hospital and ordered a brain MRI, which shows increased signal intensity on T2-weighed and FLAIR sequences in the parieto-occipital region and the splenium of the corpus callosum.

    The most appropriate laboratory test would be:

    A. Creatinine Kinase
    B. Very long chain fatty acids
    C. Lactic acid
    D. Serum amino acids
    E. Urine organic acids

Correct Answer is: B
This is a case of an X-linked Adrenoleukodystrophy. X-ALD is a metabolic disorder characterized by impaired peroxisomal beta-oxidation of very long-chain fatty acids. Consequently, there is an accumulation of VLCFA in plasma and all tissues, including the white matter of the brain, the spinal cord and adrenal cortex. It is caused by mutations in the *ABCD1* gene located on the X-chromosome. Mutations in this gene cause the absence or dysfunction of ALDP, a peroxisomal transmembrane protein that transports VLCFacyl-CoA esters from the cytosol into the peroxisome. The onset of X-ALD is insidious, with deficits in cognitive abilities that involve visuospatial and visual-motor functions or attention and reasoning. In boys and adolescents, it initially results in a decline of school performance. These early clinical symptoms are often misdiagnosed as attention deficit hyperactivity disorder and can delay the diagnosis of X-ALD. As the disease progresses, clinical manifestations can include withdrawn or hyperactive behavior, apraxia, astereognosia, auditory impairment, decreased visual acuity, hemiparesis or spastic tetraparesis, cerebellar ataxia and seizures. There can also be adrenal insufficiency in which the patient presents with Addison's disease. The adrenal insufficiency can be subtle in which the only manifestation is bronzing of the skin. Usually death occurs 2–4 years after onset of symptoms. If X-ALD is suspected in a male with neurological symptoms or Addison's disease, elevated plasma VLCFAs confirms the diagnosis.

Suggested Reading

- Lyon et al. Neurology of Hereditary Metabolic diseases in children. 1996.
- Engelen et al. X-linked adrenoleukodystrophy (X-ALD): clinical presentation and guidelines for diagnosis, follow-up and management. Orphanet J. Rare Dis. 2012;7:51

21. You are seeing a newborn neonate in the nursery who has dysmorphic features, weak cry and suck. He has microcephaly, and he has a cataract and iris malformation. He has decreased movement and severe hypotonia on motor examination. His brain MRI shows cobblestone lissencephaly.
The most common defect in this congenital muscular dystrophy is:
    A. Merosin deficiency
    B. Collagen deficiency
    C. Abnormal dystrophin
    D. Abnormal glycosylation of alpha-Dystroglycan
    E. Defect in glycogen metabolism

Correct Answer is: D
This is a clinical presentation of Walker-Warburg Syndrome. It is the most severe of the dystroglycanopathies which are a group of disorders caused by abnormal glycosylation of alpha-dystroglycan. Alpha-Dystroglycanopathies include Fukuyama congenital muscular dystrophy, muscle-eye-brain disease, Walker-Warburg syndrome, and congenital muscular dystrophy type 1C. These disorders are associated with CNS pathology and structural eye abnormalities. Patients present with paralysis at birth, severe hypotonia, weak suck and cry and profound developmental delay. Brain abnormalities include microcephaly, hydrocephalus, cobblestone lissencephaly, severe hypoplastic cerebellum and brainstem, with a Dandy-Walker malformation in 15–20%. Ocular abnormalities include severe congenital myopia, glaucoma, and pallor of the optic discs, retinal hypoplasia, microphthalmia, cataracts, and iris malformations.

Suggested Reading

- Iannaccone ST, et al. Congenital muscular dystrophies and congenital myopathies. Continuum 2013;19(6):1509–34.

22. You are evaluating a 6 who was a floppy infant. Family states that he is not social, has repetitive behaviors, and is hyposensitive to pain. He has normal hearing and vision. On examination he has dysmorphic features; you note that he has a long narrow head, ptosis and prominent ears. He also has Autistic behavior, absent speech, and hypotonia. He has a normal head circumference.
Mutations in which of the following genes are most likely responsible for his condition?
    A. RAI1
    B. FOXG1
    C. PTEN
    D. SHANK3
    E. ARX

Correct Answer is: D
This patient has Phelan-Mc Dermid Syndrome- 22q13 deletion syndrome. Children with this disorder can have mild dysmorphic features.

Durand et al. (2007) reported evidence showing that abnormal gene dosage of SHANK3 is associated with severe cognitive deficits, including language and speech disorder and autism spectrum disorder. They reported 3 families with autism spectrum disorder and unambiguous alteration of 22q13 or SHANK3.

Mutations of RAI1 gene on chromosome 17 causes Smith-Magenis Syndrome (intellectual disability, behavioral problems and sleep disturbance).

Mutations of FOXG1 cause symptoms of an Autism Spectrum Disorder, developmental delay, and microcephaly.

Mutations of the PTEN cause symptoms of an Autism Spectrum Disorder, macrocephaly and hamartomas.

Mutations of the ARX gene cause X-linked mental retardation.

3

Suggested Reading

- Phelan-MC Dermid Syndrome. OMIM Entry # 606232. Genetics Home Reference.

23. You are evaluating a 7-year-old boy who has always been delayed but he is struggling in first grade although he is in special education. His past medical history is significant for failure to thrive, was "floppy" and had delays in motor development. Now he is overweight because he eats all the time and is always thirsty. He has been evaluated type 2 diabetes. On examination, he is obese, pleasant boy who is eager to interact with you. He has almond shaped eyes and small hands and feet. He has a large area of hypopigmentation on his face, and hypotonic. He cannot write his name but he is able to draw a picture of himself; the drawing is at a 3-year-old level.
What laboratory test is most likely would yield the diagnosis?
    A. Fragile X
    B. MRI of the brain
    C. DNA methylation of chromosome 15 q
    D. Neuropsychological testing
    E. FISH for chromosome 22q11 deletion

Correct Answer is: C
He has Prader Willi Syndrome (PWS). Prader-Willi (PWS) syndrome is characterized by severe hypotonia and feeding difficulties in early infancy, followed in later infancy or early childhood by excessive eating and gradual development of morbid obesity. Motor milestones and language development are delayed. All individuals have some degree of cognitive impairment. A distinctive behavioral phenotype (with temper tantrums, stubbornness, manipulative behavior, and obsessive-compulsive characteristics) is common. Short stature is common; characteristic facial features, strabismus, and scoliosis are often present, and non-insulin-dependent diabetes mellitus often occurs in obese individuals. Hypopigmentation can also be seen. The mainstay of diagnosis is DNA methylation testing to detect abnormal parent-specific imprinting within the Prader-Willi critical region (PWCR) on chromosome 15; this testing determines whether the region is maternally inherited only (i.e., the paternally contributed region is absent) and detects more than 99% of affected individuals.

Suggested Reading

- Driscoll DJ. Prader-Willi Syndrome. GeneReviews Internet. October 1998.

24. You are evaluating an 8-year-old boy for his developmental delay. His past medical history is remarkable of frequent ear infections and a heart murmur due to valvular disease. On examination, he has short stature, lordotic posture, slightly coarse facial features, and corneal clouding.
What laboratory test would most likely define this condition?
    A. Amino acid analysis
    B. 7-dehydrocholesterol level
    C. Lysosomal enzyme screen
    D. CSF neurotransmitter levels
    E. Uric acid level

Correct Answer is: C
The mucopolysaccharidoses (MPSs) are a group of rare inherited lysosomal storage disorders caused by the deficiency or absence of specific lysosomal enzymes. The absence of these enzymes leads to accumulation of complex carbohydrates in cells and tissues and in the cellular organelles, the lysosomes.

These complex carbohydrates are also known as mucopolysaccharides or glycosaminoglycans (GAGs) serve as the building blocks for connective tissues.

MPS III (Sanfilippo syndrome), is the most common of MPS disorders and results from the deficiency or absence of 4 different enzymes that are necessary to degrade the GAG heparan sulfate. Each enzyme deficiency defines a different form of Sanfilippo syndrome. Individuals with type A lack the enzyme heparan sulfate sulfatase. Individuals with type B lack the enzyme N -acetyl-alpha-D-glucosaminidase. Patients with type C lack acetyl-CoA alpha-glucosaminide acetyltransferase. Patients with type D lack the enzyme N- acetylglucosamine-6-sulfatase. The particular form of Sanfilippo syndrome cannot be determined based on clinical features, but rather must rely on enzymatic assays.

The neurological manifestations include mental regression beginning in the toddler years, coarse facial appearance, but may be mild, sleep disturbance and progressive myelopathy due to storage material in the spine. Seizures may occur. Initial clinical signs present as a change in behavior. Patients are hyperactive and display aggressive and destructive behaviors.

Suggested Reading

- Valstar MJ, Ruijter GJ, van Diggelen OP, Poorthuis BJ, Wijburg FA. Sanfilippo syndrome: a mini-review. J Inherit Metab Dis. 2008.

25. You are seeing a 7-year-old adopted boy because he has telangiectasias on his face and sclera and walks with a walker because he is ataxic. The adoptive family asking about the long-term implications of his genetic disease, you should tell them he is at higher risk than unaffected children of developing:
    - A. Tuberculosis
    - B. Inadequate responses to vaccinations
    - C. Sinus infection
    - D. Cancer
    - E. All of the above

Correct Answer is: E

This is a case of Ataxia-telangiectasia, which is a rare inherited disorder that affects the nervous system, immune system, and other body systems. This disorder is characterized by progressive ataxia beginning in early childhood. Telangiectasia, which occur in the eyes and on the surface of the skin, are also characteristic of this condition.

Mutations in the ATM gene, a gene the product of which is involved in DNA repair, cause ataxia-telangiectasia. Patients with ataxia-telangiectasia have immunoglobulin deficiencies and many develop chronic lung and sinus infections, including tuberculosis. They also have an increased risk of developing cancer, particularly leukemia and lymphoma. Affected individuals are very sensitive to the effects of radiation exposure. The life expectancy of people with ataxia-telangiectasia varies greatly, but affected individuals typically live into early adulthood.

Suggested Reading

- Perlman S, Becker-Catania S, Gatti RA. Ataxia-telangiectasia: diagnosis and treatment. Semin Pediatr Neurol. 2003;10(3):173–82.

26. You are evaluating a 16-year-old female for her progressive gait deterioration. She has a history of psychiatric symptoms including inattention, impulsivity, and anger outbursts for 1 year. Her past medical history is otherwise unremarkable and family history is noncontributory. On examination, she has a pale optic nerves, low amplitude deep tendon reflexes, increased tone and extensor planter responses. Her MRI is shown.

3

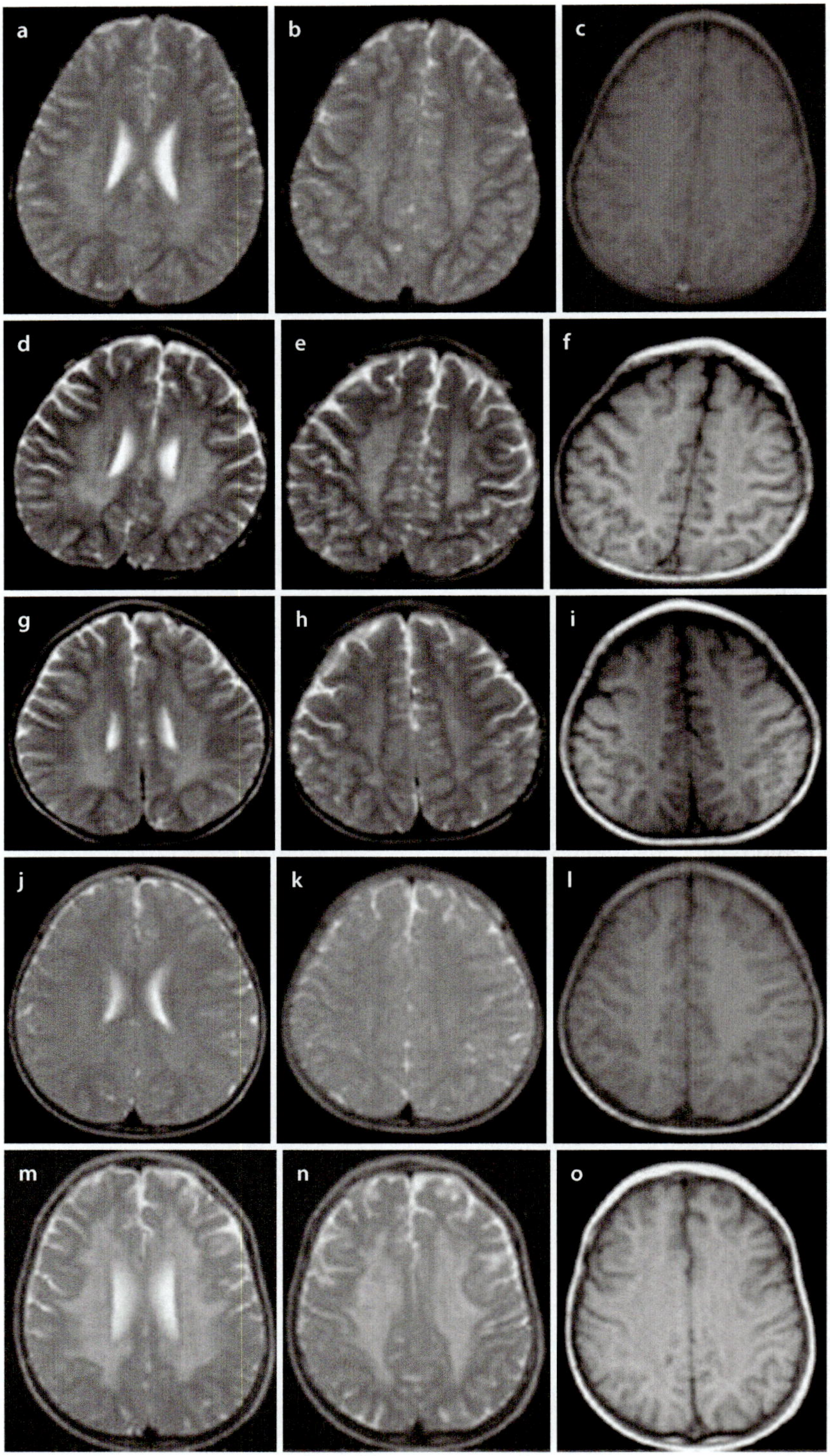

Fig. 3.11 Liaw, Hsiang-Ru, et al. "Late infantile metachromatic leukodystrophy: Clinical manifestations of five Taiwanese patients and Genetic features in Asia." Orphanet journal of rare diseases 10.1 (2015): 1. HR Liaw, HF Lee, CS Chi. This article is distributed under the terms of the Creative Commons Attribution 4.0 International License. **a–c** Patient #1; **d–f** Patient #2; **g–i** Patient #3; **j–l** Patient # 4; **m–o** Patient # 5

What is the most likely diagnosis?
A. Adrenoleukodystrophy
B. Krabbe's disease
C. Metachromatic leukodystrophy
D. Alexander's disease
E. Canavan's disease

Correct Answer is: C
This is a case of metachromatic leukodystrophy (MLD). MLD is due to Arylsulfatase A deficiency. There are three clinical subtypes: a late-infantile MLD, a juvenile MLD, and an adult onset form of MLD. The disease course may be from three to ten or more years in the late-infantile form and up to 20 years or more in the juvenile and adult forms. In the late infantile type, onset is between ages 1 and 2 years. Typical presenting manifestations include weakness, hypotonia, clumsiness, frequent falls, toe walking, and slurred speech. Later signs include inability to stand, difficulty with speech, deterioration of mental function, increased muscle tone, pain in the arms and legs, generalized or partial seizures, compromised vision and hearing, and peripheral neuropathy. In the final stages children have tonic spasms, decerebrate posturing, and general unawareness of their surroundings. Unexplained fevers and elevated CSF protein may be seen.

Suggested Reading

- Kaye EM. Update on genetic disorders affecting white matter. Pediatr Neurol. 2001;24(1):11–24.

27. The child shown in the picture below has history of global developmental delay and seizures. A similarly affected older sibling died at age 2 due to complications of sepsis. His CT scan is shown.

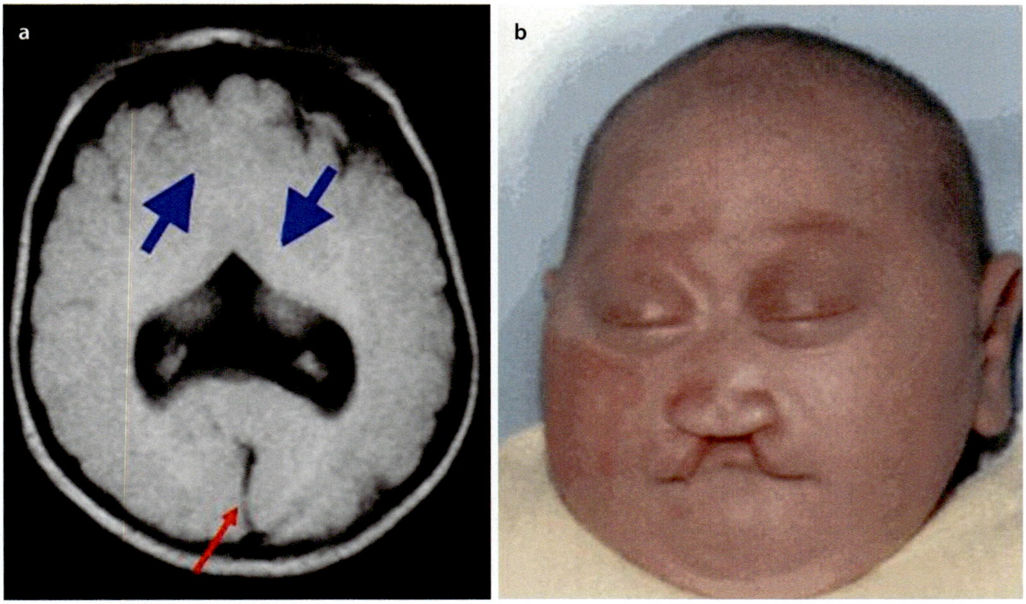

Fig. 3.12 **a** CT scan showing radiological findings of Holoprosencephaly. **b** A child is showing the facial anomalies associated with Holoprosencephaly. Courtesy of Max Muenke, M.D., NIH

What is the most likely diagnosis?
A. Aicardi syndrome
B. Fetal alcohol syndrome
C. Velocardiofacial syndrome
D. Lissencephaly
E. Holoprosencephaly

Correct Answer is: E
Holoprosencephaly (HPE) is the most common structural malformation of the developing forebrain in humans. It is characterized by failure of the forebrain to divide into the two separate hemispheres and ventricles. Holoprosencephaly encompasses a spectrum of brain malformations along a continuum based on the degree of non-separation of the hemispheres. This continuum includes alobar holoprosencephaly (a single ventricle and no separation of the cerebral hemispheres); semilobar holoprosencephaly (the left and right frontal and parietal lobes are fused and the interhemispheric fissure is only present posteriorly); lobar holoprosencephaly (most of the right and left cerebral hemispheres and lateral ventricles are separated but the most rostral aspect of the telencephalon, the frontal lobes, are not separated, especially ventrally), and syntelencephaly or middle interhemispheric variant (failure of separation of the posterior frontal and parietal lobes, with varying lack of cleavage of the basal ganglia and thalami, and absence of the body of the corpus callosum but presence of the genu and splenium of the corpus callosum).

Suggested Reading

- Muenke M, Gropman A. Holoprosencephaly, In: Genereviews. ▸ http://www.genereviews.org.

28. You saw a 4 weeks old girl for a big head. Her head CT is shown below. She is doing well clinically and so you decided to see her for follow up at 6 months of age, when she is noted to have "sun setting" eyes. A ventriculoperitoneal shunt is placed. Her head MRI after shunt placement is shown below:

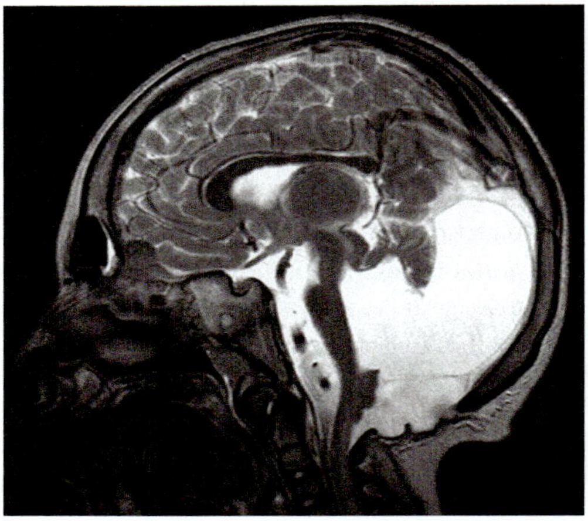

Fig. 3.13 Variant DWS with dysplasia of the pons and cerebellum in an 8-year old. T2 weighted sagittal MRI. Hellerhoff. Wikipedia

This child has a form of:
A. Arnold Chiari malformation
B. De Morsier malformation
C. Dandy-Walker malformation
D. Walker-Warburg malformation

Correct Answer is: C
This is a case of Dandy-Walker Syndrome, which is a congenital brain malformation involving the cerebellum and the fluid-filled spaces around it. The key features of this syndrome are an enlargement of the fourth ventricle, a partial or complete absence of cerebellar vermis, and cyst formation near the lowest part of the skull. An increase in the size of the fluid spaces surrounding the brain as well as an increase in pressure may also be present. The syndrome can appear dramatically or

develop unnoticed. Symptoms, which often occur in early infancy, include slow motor development and progressive enlargement of the skull. In older children, symptoms of increased intracranial pressure such as irritability and vomiting, and signs of cerebellar dysfunction such as unsteadiness, lack of muscle coordination, or jerky movements of the eyes may occur. Other symptoms include increased head circumference, bulging at the back of the skull, problems with the nerves that control the eyes, face and neck, and abnormal breathing patterns. Dandy-Walker Syndrome is frequently associated with disorders of other CNS areas, including absence of the corpus callosum, and malformations of the heart, face, limbs, fingers and toes.

Suggested Reading

- NINDS Dandy-Walker Syndrome Information Page. (Accessed 10-10-2014) ▶ http://www.ninds.nih.gov/disorders/dandywalker/dandywalker.htm.
- Correa GG, Amaral LF, Vedolin LM. Neuroimaging of Dandy-Walker malformation: new concepts. Top Magn Reson Imaging. 2011;22(6):303–12.
- Spennato P, Mirone G, Nastro A, Buonocore MC, Ruggiero C, Trischitta V, Aliberti F, Cinalli G. Hydrocephalus in Dandy-Walker malformation. Childs Nerv Syst. 2011;27(10):1665–81.

29. You are evaluating a 9-year-old healthy female in the ED with a history of vomiting and lethargy after a holiday party. She has unremarkable past medical history. Her developmental milestones were on target and she is an average student in the 3rd grade. Family history is remarkable for a maternal cousin who died in early infancy from an unspecified condition. When you examined her, she was obtunded. EEG shows slowing and triphasic waves.

What is the most appropriate next step in evaluation?

A. CSF exam
B. Ammonia
C. Plasma lactate
D. MRI of the brain with MRS
E. CT brain scan

Correct Answer is: B

Urea cycle disorders (UCDs) typically present in infancy, but the majority of individuals UCD present outside the neonatal period, frequently in childhood. Signs and symptoms are often vague, but recurrent; fulminant presentations associated with acute illness are also common. A disorder of urea cycle metabolism should be considered in children who have recurrent symptoms, especially neurologic abnormalities associated with periods of decompensation. Routine laboratory tests, including measurement of plasma ammonia concentrations, can indicate a potential UCD; however, specific metabolic testing and ultimately enzymatic or molecular confirmation are necessary to establish a diagnosis. Treatment with dietary protein restriction and medications may be challenging in children.

Suggested Reading

- Smith W, Kishnani PS, Lee B, Singh RH, Rhead WJ, Sniderman King L, Smith M, Summar M. Urea cycle disorders: clinical presentation outside the newborn period. Crit Care Clin. 2005;21(4 Suppl):S9–17.

30. You were asked to evaluate an 8-month-old boy for a history of periods of irritability, stiffness and regression of skills for 3 months. He has a normal birth and early development history. He also has periods of elevated temperature without evidence of infection. He has no dysmorphic

features on examination. There are episodes of opisthotonus in response to tactile stimulus. Muscle tone is increased and reflexes are absent. A spinal tap showed elevated protein but no other abnormalities.

What laboratory study would most likely be abnormal in this patient?

A. Phenylalanine hydroxylase
B. 7-dehydrocholesterol
C. Acid maltase
D. Galactocerebrosidase
E. Beta hexosamindase A

Correct Answer is: D

This is a clinical presentation of Krabbe disease. Krabbe disease is characterized by an infantile-onset progressive neurologic regressive disorder with death before age 2 years of age in the majority of individuals. Alternatively, onset may be between age 6 months and the fifth decade with slower disease progression. Children with the infantile form appear to be normal for the first few months of life but show extreme irritability, spasticity, and developmental delay before age 6 months; psychomotor regression progresses to a decerebrate state with no voluntary movement. In the late-onset forms, individuals can be clinically normal until weakness, vision loss, and intellectual regression become evident. The clinical course is variable even within the same family.

Stage I is characterized by irritability, stiffness, arrest of motor and mental development, and episodes of temperature elevation without infection, possibly caused by involvement of the hypothalamus. The child, apparently normal for the first few months after birth, becomes hypersensitive to auditory, tactile, or visual stimuli and begins to cry frequently without apparent cause.

In almost all individuals with Krabbe disease, galactocerebrosidase (GALC) enzyme activity is deficient in leukocytes isolated from whole heparinized blood or in cultured skin fibroblasts.

Suggested Reading

- Wenger DA, Suzuki K, Suzuki Y, Suzuki K. Galactosylceramide lipidosis. Globoid cell leukodystrophy (Krabbe disease). In: Scriver CR, Beaudet AL, Sly WS, Valle D, Childs B, Vogelstein B, editors The metabolic and molecular bases of inherited disease. 8th ed. New York: McGraw-Hill; 2001.

31. You are evaluating a 9-month-old girl for her seizure which is described as staring followed by a generalized convulsion lasting few minutes. Her past medical history is remarkable for hypotonia and developmental delay, is unable to roll over and does not reach for objects with her hands. On examination, her head circumference is above 95th percentile, while her weight and length are at 25th percentile. She has optic atrophy and nystagmus, central hypotonia and increased tone in the ankles, with clonus. Brain MRI shows increased signal in the white matter diffusely on T2-weighted images. Her MRS shows a strikingly elevated NAA peak.

What is your most likely diagnosis?

A. Krabbe leukodystrophy
B. Adrenoleukodystrophy
C. Mitochondrial encephalomyopathy
D. Canavan disease
E. Metachromatic leukodystrophy

Correct Answer is: D

The triad of hypotonia, macrocephaly, and head lag in an infant after the age of 3–5 months should raise the suspicion of Canavan disease. Diagnosis of Canavan disease in symptomatic individuals relies upon demonstration of very high concentration of N-acetyl aspartic acid (NAA) in the urine. NAA

concentration is also elevated in the blood and cerebrospinal fluid (CSF) of children with Canavan disease. In the brain, the elevated NAA can be visualized by 1H MRS as a single peak with a resonance of 2.01 ppm on the spectrum.

Suggested Reading

Janson CG, McPhee SW, Francis J, Shera D, Assadi M, Freese A, Hurh P, Haselgrove J, Wang DJ, Bilaniuk L, Leone P. Natural history of Canavan disease revealed by proton magnetic resonance spectroscopy (1H-MRS) and diffusion-weighted MRI. Neuropediatrics. 2006;37(4):209–21.

32. You are seeing a 15-old boy for microcephaly and developmental delay. He and his family migrated to the United States recently from Eastern Europe. His mother had 2 other children (from different fathers) who both have mild intellectual disability, microcephaly, and delay in linguistic development, congenital heart defects and severe growth retardation. The mother is a vegetarian since her childhood but currently does not practice any dietary restrictions. She barely graduated high school and has difficulty remembering appointments and paying bills.
What is the most likely explanation for this child's condition?
A. Chromosome disorder
B. Infantile autism
C. Leigh's disease
D. Maternal phenylketonuria
E. Urea cycle disorder

Correct Answer is: D
This is a case of phenylketonuria (PKU). PKU is an autosomal recessive disorder of amino acid metabolism affecting approximately 1/5000–10,000 infants in North America. It is most often due to deficiency of the enzyme phenylalanine hydroxylase which causes the accumulation of harmful metabolites, including phenylketones. If untreated, PKU leads to mental retardation, seizures, psychoses, eczema and a distinctive "mousy" odor. Pregnant women who have PKU and are not maintaining dietary restrictions are at risk of delivering infants with the effects of untreated maternal PKU and may also be at risk of developing neurologic symptoms themselves if they don't maintain lifelong dietary restrictions. The characteristic manifestations of maternal PKU syndrome include mental retardation, microcephaly, intrauterine growth retardation, and congenital heart defects. The risk for these defects is increased with maternal plasma phenylalanine levels > 20 mg/dL).

Suggested Reading

Bouchlariotou S, Tsikouras P, Maroulis G. Undiagnosed maternal phenylketonuria: own clinical experience and literature review. J Matern Fetal Neonatal Med. 2009;22(10):943–8.

33. You are evaluating a 7-month-old infant for his developmental regression with progressive opisthotonus, stridor, and swallowing difficulties. He was normal at birth. On examination, he has enlarged spleen, squint, head retro flexion, spasticity, and trismus.
Analysis of which of the following tissues would most likely define his condition?
A. Bone marrow
B. Blood leukocytes
C. Muscle
D. Skin
E. Liver

Correct Answer is: B
This is a clinical presentation of Gaucher disease. The diagnosis of Gaucher disease relies on demonstration of deficient glucosylceramidase enzyme

activity in peripheral blood leukocytes. Carrier testing by assay of enzyme activity is unreliable because of overlap in enzyme activity between carriers and non-carriers. Identification of two disease-causing alleles in GBA, the only gene known to be associated with Gaucher disease, provides additional confirmation of the diagnosis.

Suggested Reading

- Goker-Alpan O, Schiffmann R, Park JK, Stubblefield BK, Tayebi N, Sidransky E. Phenotypic continuum in neuronopathic Gaucher disease: an intermediate phenotype between type 2 and type 3. J Pediatr. 2003;143(2):273–6.

34. A pediatrician referred a 4-year-old boy because he felt the boy's liver 1 finger breadth below the right costal margin during a well-child check-up. Liver function studies were done and showed abnormal values: ALT, 70 U/L; AST, 100 IU/L. The mother reported that the child having trouble standing up when he has been sitting on the floor playing with toys.
If the lab has additional blood left over, you should ask the lab to test it for:
    A. Glucose-6-phosphate
    B. Bilirubin
    C. Alkaline phosphatase
    D. Creatine phosphokinase
    E. Prothrombin time

Correct Answer is: D
"Liver function tests" are tests for enzymes that are expressed at high levels in the liver, but are expressed in many other cell types, including muscle. As a consequence, elevated ALT and AST blood levels occur in neuromuscular disorders that involve lysis or high turnover rates of myocytes. Destruction of muscle in Duchenne muscular dystrophy is one such situation. It can be differentiated from the elevated ALT and AST of liver disease by the concomitant and disproportionate elevation of "muscle function tests", such as levels of CPK and/or aldolase.

Suggested Reading

- Korones DN, Brown MR, Palis J. "Liver function tests" are not always tests of liver function. Am J Hematol. 2001;66(1):46–8.
- Stein MT, Tipnis NA, Schultz P. Fatigue, decreased interest in play, motor delay, and elevated liver function tests in a 4-year-old boy. J Dev Behav Pediatr. 2002;23(1):37–41.

35. You are evaluating a 6-year-old male because his family complaining that he was completely normal until age 4, when he began bumping into things and not responding to visual cues. He was seen by a pediatric ophthalmologist who found that the child has retinitis pigmentosa. He is now legally blind. He started to have a change in his behavior 1 month ago. He will repeat asking the same questions several times and seemed not to be satisfied with the answer. The family reports that he is anxious. Last week, his teacher has questioned whether or not he understands what she is saying to him. He has official hearing testing which is normal. On examination, he perseverates on verbal and manual tasks, to be anxious, and to have occasional, single myoclonic jerks of one or the other of his arms or legs. His retinas have a tigroid appearance.
What gene testing would you like to order?
    A. Metachromatic Leukodystrophy
    B. Rett Syndrome
    C. Neuronal ceroid lipofuscinosis
    D. Morquio syndrome
    E. Zellweger syndrome

Correct Answer is: C
This is a presentation of Juvenile Batten disease, which is a neurodegenerative disorder that often has its onset in late toddlerhood or early childhood. It typically starts with pigmentary changes in the retina and progressive visual loss. This is followed by progressive dementia, myoclonus, and seizures. More than 60 different mutations in the CLN3 gene have been found associated with juvenile Batten disease. But the function of the CLN3 gene product is not completely understood. CLN3 protein is found in the membranes of many cell types; it appears to have some function related to lysosomal trafficking, pH, and size.

Suggested Reading

- Bennett MJ, Rakheja D. The neuronal ceroid-lipofuscinoses. Dev Disabil Res Rev. 2013;17(3):254–9.
- Cotman SL, Staropoli JF. The juvenile Batten disease protein, CLN3, and its role in regulating anterograde and retrograde post-Golgi trafficking. Clin Lipidol. 2012;7(1):79–91.
- Tuxworth RI, Chen H, Vivancos V, Carvajal N, Huang X, Tear G. The Batten disease gene CLN3 is required for the response to oxidative stress. Hum Mol Genet. 2011;20(10):2037–47.

36. You are seeing a 2-year-old developmentally delayed boy who has 3 different episodes type stared at 10 months of age. While he is propped up in a sitting position, his head just drops forward for a couple of seconds. Sometimes, without warning, he has a single, vigorous jerk of his whole body, extending his arms and legs, after which he is sleepy for up to an hour. Also, he has a generalized tonic-clonic seizure followed by sleepiness for hours. He has multiple spells per day. His past medical history is remarkable for infantile spasms between the ages of 2 and 6 months. His MRI scan is below.

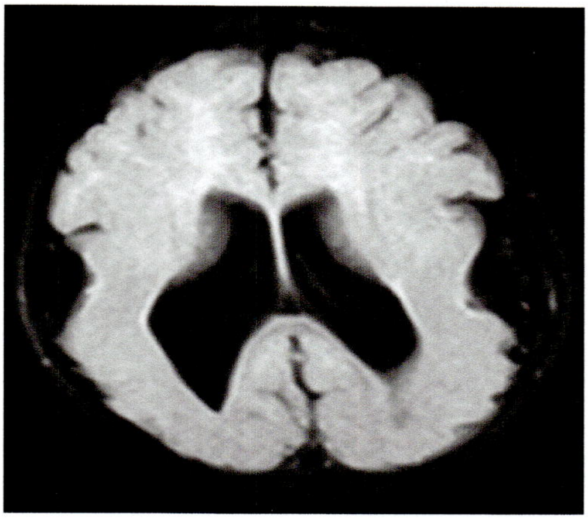

Fig. 3.14 MRI from Wikipedia, ▶ http://en.wikipedia.org/wiki/Lissencephaly, author: Ralpheig, accessed 10/5/2014

The child most likely has mutations in the gene that causes:

A. Fragile X
B. Miller-Dieker syndrome
C. Tuberous Sclerosis
D. Aicardi Syndrome
E. Joubert Syndrome

Correct Answer is: B
Mutations in the *PAFAH1B*1 (Miller-Dieker Syndrome), *DCX* (isolated lissencephaly), or TUBA1A gene can cause lissencephaly. PAFAH1B1 gene mutations are responsible for over half of isolated lissencephaly sequence cases; DCX gene mutations cause about 10% of cases; and TUBA1A gene mutations cause a small percentage of isolated lissencephaly sequence. These genes code for proteins that, through their interaction with microtubules, are involved in neuronal migration.

Suggested Reading

- Fry AE, Cushion TD, Pilz DT. The genetics of lissencephaly. Am J Med Genet C Semin Med Genet. 2014;166C(2):198–210.
- Reiner O, Sapir T. LIS1 functions in normal development and disease. Curr Opin Neurobiol.

37. You are seeing a baby boy in the NICU for episodes of clonic seizure activity involving left and right side independently lasting 30–60 s on several occasions. He is a product of full-term pregnancy, and born after an uneventful labor. He was depressed at birth with generalized hypotonia and hypoventilation. On exam, he has dysmorphic features consisting of micrognathia, broad nasal bridge, and high forehead, dolichocephalic skull with large anterior and posterior fontanelles. Liver edge was firm and 1 cm below the costal margin. He is hypotonic with poor gag and suck/swallow, absent reflexes and difficult to elicit Moro response. The EEG showed multifocal spikes on a mildly low voltage background without state change but no electrographic seizures. CT scan showed dilated posterior horns (colopocephaly).

What is the most likely diagnosis?

A. Prader-Willi syndrome
B. Zellweger's syndrome
C. Myotonic dystrophy
D. Spinal muscular atrophy
E. Congenital CMV infection

Correct Answer is: B

This is a clinical presentation of Zellweger's syndrome. It is an autosomal recessive disorder, is the severest form of the peroxisomal biogenesis disorders (PBD) and presents at birth with dysmorphic features, liver cirrhosis, severe hypotonia and neonatal encephalopathy with seizures. The diagnosis is suspected by the dysmorphic features and confirmed by analysis of very long chain fatty acids (elevated VLCFA C26:0, C26:1; abnormal ratios of C24/C22; C26/C22). Peroxisomes (which are missing in Zellweger's) process VLCFA which, if they accumulate abnormally, affect CNS and other cell membranes. CNS dysmyelination occurs and in the severe form leads to problems with radial glial guides and migration disorders (pachygyria, polymicrogyria, neuronal heterotopias, colopocephaly) resulting in severe encephalopathy and seizures. Mutations in twelve different PEX genes, those that encode peroxins, the proteins required for normal peroxisome assembly, have been identified in Zellweger's syndrome. Treatment is symptomatic and children fail to develop, with death usually in the first year. Other PBD are neonatal adrenoleukodystrophy, infantile Refsum disease (both considered part of the Zellweger's Syndrome Spectrum) and rhizomelic chondrodysplasia punctata. These disorders can be separated clinically and 80% of PBD are among the Zellweger's Syndrome Spectrum with an incidence of 1 in 50,000 births in the US.

Suggested Reading

- Steinberg SJ, Raymond GV, Braverman NE, Moser AM, and Moser HW. Peroxisome Biogenesis Disorders, Zellweger Syndrome Spectrum. Gene Reviews: ▶ http://www.ncbi.nlm.nih.gov/bookshelf/br.fcgi?book=gene&part=pbd.

38. You are examining a 5-month-old boy who was normal at birth has been startling easily for the past 2 weeks. Head circumference had been in the 50th percentile at birth, but is now in the 90th percentile. His retina photograph is shown.

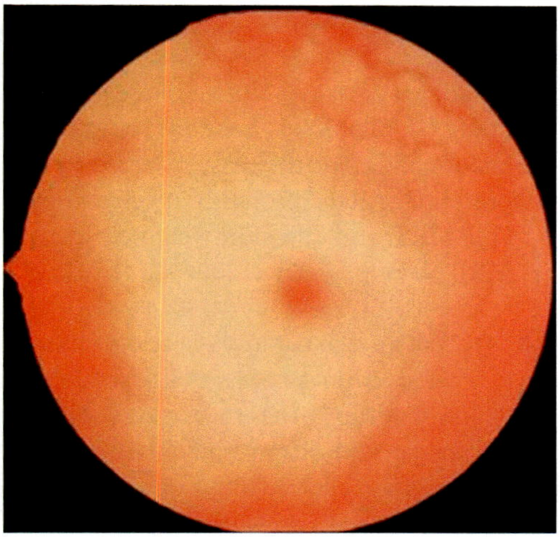

Fig. 3.15 Cherry-red spot as seen in the retina in Tay–Sachs disease. The fovea's center appears bright red because it is surrounded by a whiter than usual area. ▶ http://www.kellogg.umich.edu/theeyeshaveit/congenital/tay-sachs.html. Jonathan Trobe, M.D.

What would most likely be abnormal on laboratory testing?

A. Aryl sulfatase A activity
B. Beta galactosidase A activity
C. Beta-hexosaminidase A activity
D. Glucocerebrosidase A activity
E. Very long chain fatty acids

Correct Answer is: C

This photograph and the clinical presentation indicate Tay-Sachs disease, which is a fatal autosomal recessive lipid storage disorder in which the ganglioside GM2 build up in tissues and brain neurons. The condition is caused by insufficient activity of the enzyme beta-hexosaminidase A that catalyzes the biodegradation of acidic fatty materials known as gangliosides. Infants with Tay Sachs disease appear to develop normally in the first few months of life. As neurons become distended with storage material, the clinical course becomes one of relentless deterioration in which the child ultimately becomes blind, and deaf with seizures, encephalopathy and an increased startle to noise. A rarer form can be seen in young adults who present with a neuromuscular phenotype.

Suggested Reading

- Shapiro BE, Logigian EL, Kolodny EH, Pastores GM. Late-onset Tay-Sachs disease: the spectrum of peripheral neuropathy in 30 affected patients. Muscle Nerve. 2008;38(2):1012–5.

39. Children with Crouzon syndrome can develop cognitive impairment.
This is because of:
A. Cerebral dysgenesis
B. Hypoxia from airway dysgenesis
C. Abnormal calcium metabolism
D. Mitochondrial dysfunction
E. Multiple craniosynostoses

Correct Answer is: E

Management of the multiple simultaneous synostoses of the skull in Crouzon syndrome is an urgent matter, as they can restrict outward brain growth in all directions and limit CSF egress through occlusion of the foramina by impingement from inward-expanding parenchyma.

Suggested Reading

- Renier D, Lajeunie E, Arnaud E, Marchac D. Management of craniosynostoses. Childs Nerv Syst. 2000;16(10–11):645–58.
- Noetzel MJ, Marsh JL, Palkes H, Gado M. Hydrocephalus and mental retardation in craniosynostosis. J Pediatr. 1985;107(6):885–92.

40. You are evaluating a 4-year-old boy for motor delay. He was a product of 38 weeks gestation with uncomplicated pregnancy. He was normal for the first few months of life, but thereafter developed macrocephaly

3

and was delayed in his milestones. He has unremarkable family history. On examination, he is hypotonic and his head circumference is above the 95th percentile. His brain MRI scan is shown.

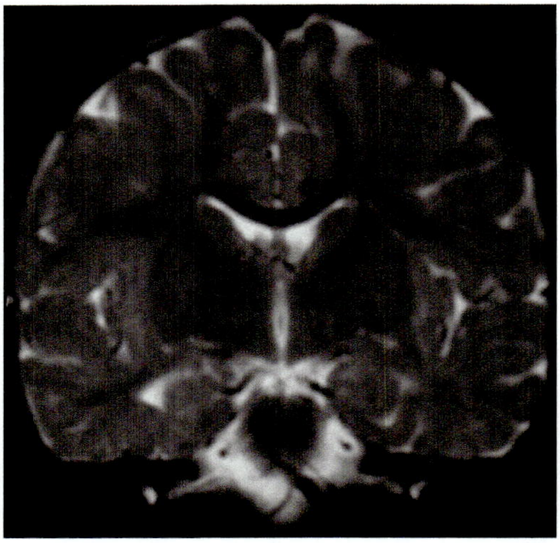

Fig. 3.16 Radiology picture of the day. (Dr. Laughlin Dawes. Canavan disease. Wikipedia)

What is the most likely diagnosis?

A. Adrenoleukodystrophy
B. Canavan disease
C. Krabbe disease
D. Metachromatic leukodystrophy
E. Vanishing white matter disease

Correct Answer is: B

The triad of hypotonia, macrocephaly, and head lag in an infant after the age of 3–5 months should raise the suspicion of Canavan disease. Diagnosis of Canavan disease in symptomatic individuals relies upon demonstration of very high concentration of N-acetyl aspartic acid (NAA) in the urine. NAA concentration is also elevated in the blood and cerebrospinal fluid (CSF) of children with Canavan disease. In the brain, the elevated NAA can be visualized by 1H MRS as a single peak with a resonance of 2.01 ppm on the spectrum.

Suggested Reading

- Janson CG, McPhee SW, Francis J, Shera D, Assadi M, Freese A, Hurh P, Haselgrove J, Wang DJ, Bilaniuk L, Leone P. Natural history of Canavan disease revealed by proton magnetic resonance spectroscopy (1H-MRS) and diffusion-weighted MRI. Neuropediatrics. 2006;37(4):209–21.

41. You are evaluating a 9-year-old autistic spectrum disorder (ASD) female with history of a recent seizure which began with staring and unresponsiveness and evolved into a generalized tonic-clonic convulsion. A picture of her face is shown.

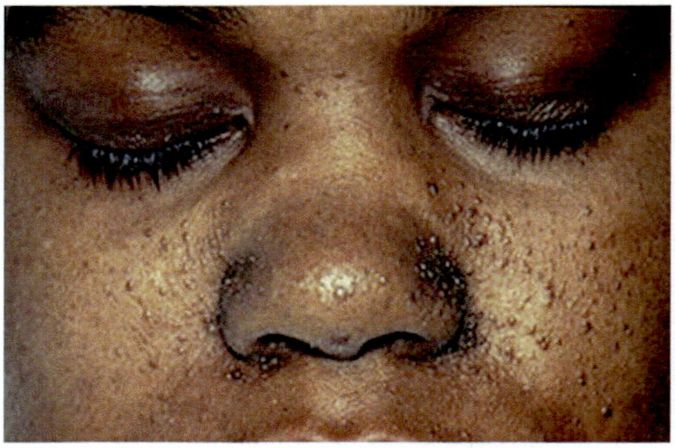

Fig. 3.17 A case of tuberous sclerosis showing facial angiofibromas in characteristic butterfly pattern. ► http://cnx.org/content/m14895/latest/. Herbert L. Fred, MD and Hendrik A. van Dijk

Which of the following is most likely to be present on further evaluation?

A. Conjunctival telangiectasias
B. Ash leaf spot
C. Family history consistent with recessive inheritance
D. Multiple café au lait spots
E. Pseudo arthrosis

Correct Answer is: B

This is a classic tuberous sclerosis (TSC) case. TS is a genetic disease with an incidence of about 1:40,000 that causes benign tumors to grow in the brain and other organs such as the kidneys, heart,

eyes, lungs, and skin. It commonly affects the central nervous system. In addition to the benign tumors that frequently occur in TSC, other common symptoms include seizures, mental retardation, behavior problems, and skin abnormalities. TSC may be present at birth, however, signs of the disorder can be subtle and full symptoms may take some time to develop. The most common skin lesion is the ash leaf spot.

Suggested Reading

- Gomez MR. Phenotypes of the tuberous sclerosis complex with a revision of diagnostic criteria. Ann N Y Acad Sci. 1991;615:1–7.

42. You electively admitted a 5-month-old boy to the hospital for evaluation of failure to thrive, developmental delay, and generalized seizures. His lab showed leukopenia. His evaluation includes urine organic acids and he is also found to have methylmalonic aciduria.

    He might have an abnormality involving utilization of:

    A. Vitamin D
    B. Vitamin E
    C. Vitamin C
    D. Vitamin B12
    E. Vitamin A

Correct Answer is: D

Vitamin B12-responsive methylmalonic academia (MA) is an inborn error of vitamin B12 (cobalamin) metabolism characterized by recurrent ketoacidotic comas or transient vomiting, dehydration, hypotonia and intellectual deficit, which responds to vitamin B12. There are three types: cblA, cblB and cblD-variant 2 (cblDv2).

To date, over 120 patients with cblA, 66 patients with cblB and 6 patients with cblDv2 have been reported. Prevalence of 1/48,000–1/61,000 have been reported for MA of all causes in North America, and 1/26,000 in China, but only a subset of this is vitamin B12-responsive MA.

Usually it starts in infancy or early childhood with manifestations including lethargy, failure to thrive, recurrent vomiting, dehydration, respiratory distress, muscle hypotonia, hepatomegaly and coma. They may also show signs of anemia (not megaloblastic), have potentially life-threatening ketoacidosis and/or hyperammonemia, and developmental delay and intellectual deficit, with metabolic stroke affecting the brain stem. MA frequently leads to end-stage renal failure by adolescence or adulthood. Patients with cblB are usually more severely affected than patients with cblA.

Suggested Reading

- Orphanet. ► http://www.orpha.net/consor/cgi-bin/Disease_Search.php?lng=EN&data_id=3260&MISSING%20CONTENT=Methylmalonic-acidemia--vitamin-B12-responsive&title=Methylmalonic-acidemia--vitamin-B12-responsive&search=Disease_Search_Simple. Accessed 10-10-2014.
- Manoli I, Venditti CP. Methylmalonic Acidemia. In: Pagon RA, Adam MP, Ardinger HH, Bird TD, Dolan CR, Fong CT, Smith RJH, Stephens K, editors. *GeneReviews®* [Internet]. Seattle (WA): University of Washington, Seattle; 1993–2014. 2005 Aug 16 [updated 2010 Sep 28].
- Parini R, Furlan F, Brambilla A, Codazzi D, Vedovati S, Corbetta C, Fedeli T, Merinero B, Pérez B, Ugarte M. Severe Neonatal Metabolic Decompensation in Methylmalonic Acidemia Caused by CblD Defect. J Inher Metab Dis Rep. 2013;11:133–7.

43. You are evaluating a 14-year-old male for severe generalized myoclonus, ataxia, and loss of color vision. Funds exam showed cherry red spots, and EEG demonstrated background

slowing, and photosensitive bilateral fast spike and wave activity.

What finding would establish the diagnosis?

A. An alpha-N-acetylgalactosami nidase deficiency
B. decrease in cultured skin fibroblast alpha-neuraminidase
C. A response to oral biotin
D. A hexoaminidase A deficiency
E. A muscle biopsy with ragged red fibers

Correct Answer is: B

An alpha-N-acetylgalactosaminidase deficiency is evident in Schindler disease, which is a rare autosomal recessive disorder with acute infant and chronic adult-onset forms. Infants demonstrate severe psychomotor deterioration with spaticity, cortical blindness, and myoclonic epilepsy with an exaggerated startle response. The adult form is characterized by mild cognitive deficits.

A presentation including severe generalized myoclonus, night blindness, and loss of color vision, ataxia, cherry-red spots, and generalized convulsions in an adolescent is characteristic of sialidosis type 1. As described above, the EEG shows progressive slowing and bilateral, photosensitive fast spike-wave discharges. A decrease in cultured skin fibroblast alpha-neuraminidase is diagnostic.

A response to oral biotin would be consistent with biotinidase deficiency. This disorder is characterized by hypotonia, generalized tonic-clonic and myoclonic seizures, rash, and alopecia, with onset in infancy. The EEG demonstrates multifocal spikes and slow waves.

A hexosaminidase A deficiency is evident in Tay-Sachs disease, with the onset of development delay, cherry-red spots, and "startle seizures" in infancy.

A muscle biopsy with ragged red fibers is indicative of myoclonic epilepsy with ragged red fibers (MERRF). The core features of this mitochondrial disorder include myoclonus, epilepsy, myopathy, intellectual disability, and cerebellar dysfunction. Patients may also have short stature, deafness, optic atrophy, cutaneous lipomas, and neuropathy. The onset is typically in childhood or early adulthood.

Suggested Reading

- Verma A, Moraes CT. Mitochondrial disorders. In: Bradley WG, Daroff RB, Fenichel GM, Jankovic J, editors. Neurology in Clinical Practice. 4th ed. Elsevier, Inc.; 2004. p. 781–808.
- Pastores GM, Kolodny EH. Inborn errors of metabolism of the nervous system. In: Bradley WG, Daroff RB, Fenichel GM, Jankovic J, editors. Neurology in Clinical Practice. 4th ed. Elsevier, Inc.; 2004. p. 1811–32.

44. You are seeing an18-year-old male with left-sided weakness and aphasia. CT head showed an acute ischemic infarct in the territory of the right middle cerebral artery. On exam, he is tall, thin, has long fingers, and high arched feet. His medical history is remarkable for lens dislocation, pigeon chest and osteoporosis.

What single blood test is likely to be of diagnostic use in this patient?

A. Peripheral blood smear
B. Thyroid-stimulating hormone
C. Homocysteine
D. Branched chain amino acids
E. Lactic acid

Correct Answer is: C

Genetics: AR; Cystathionine-13-synthase deficiency -- > elevation of blood and urine levels of homocysteine and methionine.

Symptoms and findings: Normal at birth; later developmental delay and intellectual disability. Seizures and psychiatric manifestations.

Collagen metabolism is affected -- > eye, bones, and the vascular system -- > Ectopia lentis and lens dislocation. Marfanoid habitus with tall and thin stature, pectus carinatum, pes cavus, genu valgum, and osteoporosis. Intimal thickening of the blood vessel walls and high incidence of thromboembolism, including strokes.

Diagnosis – elevation of plasma and urine homocysteine, methionine in the plasma and CSF.

Treatment – Majority of patient respond to pyridoxine, so give this first. Betaine, folate and vitamin 812 supplements. Low-protein diet, specifically low in methionine with cysteine supplementation.

45. You are seeing an 18-year-old female with a history of multiple abnormal movements, including a moderate frequency rest and postural tremor and a twisting and in-turning of her left foot. Her past medical history is remarkable for depression with suicide attempt and significant anxiety. A picture of her eye is shown below. She has elevated liver enzymes.

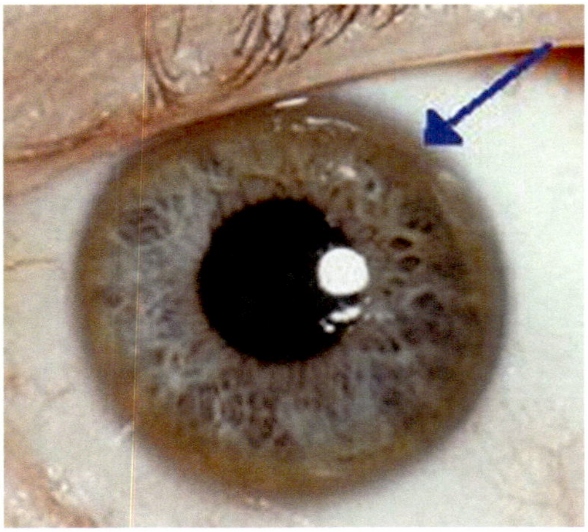

Fig. 3.18 A brown ring on the edge of the cornea (Kayser–Fleischer ring) is common in Wilson's disease, especially when neurological symptoms are present. ► https://commons.wikimedia.org/wiki/File:Kayser-Fleischer_ring.jpg. (Herbert L. Fred, MD, Hendrik A. van Dijk)

What is the most likely diagnosis in this patient?

A. Essential tremor
B. Tardive dystonia and tremor
C. Wilson's disease
D. Early-onset Parkinson's disease
E. A psychogenic disorder

Correct Answer is: C

This patient has Wilson's disease based on the history and MRI findings. It is an autosomal recessive disorder of copper metabolism resulting from mutations of the gene encoding the copper-transporting P-type ATPase (ATP7B) on chromosome 13. This enzyme normally binds to and transports copper across membranes. A defect in this enzyme leads to inability to excrete copper from the liver into bile, leading to copper accumulation. The presenting symptoms of the disorder can be neurologic, hepatic, or psychiatric, or a combination of these. Abnormal movements predominate the neurologic presentation, including Parkinsonism, dystonia, tremor, ataxia, as well as dysarthria. The tremor may have a variety of features, but classically, it is proximal and of high amplitude, giving the appearance of "wing beating" when the arms are abducted and the elbows flexed. A characteristic grin with drooling also occurs. Psychiatric symptoms include depression, anxiety, and less commonly psychosis. The liver disease may range from mild to fulminant hepatic failure. Laboratory findings in Wilson's disease include reduced serum levels of the copper-binding protein.

46. You are evaluating an 11-year old boy for his headaches. His headaches are exacerbated by lying down and associated with nausea and vomiting. On his MRI scan, a 1 centimeter enhancing mass is noted near the foramen of Monro. He has a His past medical

history is significant for cardiac rhabdomyoma, discovered at birth.

Which of the following is most likely true?

A. The patient has a mutation in the NF1 gene
B. The patient has a mutation in the TSC1 gene
C. The patient has a mutation in the PTCH1 gene
D. The patient has a mutation in the PTEN gene
E. The patient has a mutation in the NF2 gene

Correct answer is: B

This is a case of tuberous sclerosis complex. This disorder is caused by mutations in the TSC1 or TSC2 genes, coding for hamartin and tuberin, respectively.

Major features of this condition include facial angiofibromas, forehead plaques, ungula or periungual fibroma, 3 hypomelanotic macules, shagreen patch, retinal nodular hamartomas, cortical tubers, sub-ependymal nodules, sub-ependymal giant cell astrocytoma, cardiac rhabdomyoma and lymphangiomyomatosis/renal angiomyolipoma.

Minor features include hamartomatous rectal polyps, multiple pits in dental enamel that are randomly distributed, bone cysts, cerebral white matter radial migration lines, gingival fibromas, nonrenal hamartomas, retinal achromatic patch, confetti skin lesions, and renal cysts.

The diagnosis of definite tuberous sclerosis complex can be made in the presence of either 2 major features or 1 major feature and 2 minor features. The presence of 1 major feature and 1 minor feature is sufficient for a diagnosis of probable tuberous sclerosis complex. The presence of 1 major feature in isolation, or the presence of at least 2 minor features is suggestive of possible tuberous sclerosis complex.

The patient's enhancing brain mass, located near the foramen of Monro, is consistent with sub-ependymal giant cell astrocytoma (SEGA). This, and the patient's cardiac rhabdomyoma, allow for a diagnosis of definite tuberous sclerosis complex.

Mutations in the NF1 gene, encoding for the protein neurofibromin, cause neurofibromatosis type I. This is diagnosed in the presence of 2 of the following:(1) the presence of 6 cafe au lait macules (5 mm in diameter pre-pubertal, 15 mm in diameter post pubertal), (2) 2 neurofibroma or 1 plexiform neurofibroma, (3) freckling of the inguinal or axillary region, (4) an optic glioma, (5) 2:2 iris hamartomas, (6) osseous lesion (thinning of long bone cortex, sphenoid wing dysplasia) or (7) first degree relative with NF1.

Mutations in the PTCH1 gene encoding for Patched 1 are associated with nevoid basal cell carcinoma, or Gorlin syndrome. Major criteria for this condition include; 2 basal cell carcinomas (12: is sufficient for people under 20 years of age), odontogenic keratosis of the jaw, 3; palmar or plantar pits, bilamellar calcification of falx cerebri, rib abnormalities (bifid, fused, or markedly splayed), and a first degree relative with the condition. Minor criteria include (1) frontal bossing/hypertelorism/cleft lip or palate (2) springe deformity/pectus/syndactyly of digits, (3) bridging of sella turcica/hemivertebrae flame shaped radiolucensies (4) ovarian fibroma and (5) medulloblastoma. A diagnosis of Nevoid basal cell carcinoma can be made in the presence of either 2 major criteria or 1 major and 2 minor criteria.

Suggested Reading

- Jozwiak S, Migone N, Ruggieri M.The tuberous sclerosis complex. In: Ruggieri M, Pascual Castroviejo I, Di Rocco C, eds. Neurocutaneous Disorders Phakomatoses and Hamartoneoplastic Syndromes.

Morlenbach: Springer-Verlag/Wien; 2008:181–227.
- Tabori U, Laberge A-M, Ellezam B, Carret A-S. Cancer predisposition in children with brain tumors. In: Scheinemann K, Bouffet E, editors. Pediatric Neuro-Oncology. New York: Springer; 2015:127–38 .5. Lee J, Johnston DL. Chemotherapy. In: Scheinemann K, Bouffet E, editors. Pediatric Neuro-Oncology. New York: Springer; 2015:69–896.
- Glass TD, Cochrane D, Rassekh SR, Goddard K, Hukin J. Growingteratoma syndrome in intracranial non germinomatous germ cell tumors (iNGGCTs): a risk for secondary malignant transformation- a report of two cases. Child Nerv Syst. 2014;30(5):953–7.
- Bartels U, Singhal A. Central nervous system germ cell tumors. In: Scheinemann K, Bouffet E, eds. Pediatric Neuro-Oncology. New York: Springer; 2015: p. 149–62.
- Mach SC, Ramaswamy V, Wang X, Remke M, Sin-Chan P, Chan WSY, Bertrand KC, Merino D, Zayne K, Huang A, Taylor MD. Basic science of pediatric braintumors. In: Scheinemann K, Bouffet E, eds. Pediatric Neuro-Oncology. New York: Springer; 2015. p. 59–67.
- Jones DTW, Korshunov A, Pfister SM, Tayllor MD, Northcott PA. Medulloblastoma and CNS primitive neuroectodermal tumors. In: Cagle PT, Matthias KA, Zagzag D, editors. Molecular pathology of nervous system Tumors. New York: Springer; 2015. p. 121–42.
- Vanan Ml, Mehta V, Eisenstat, DD. Diffuse intrinsic pontine glioma. In: Scheinemann K, Bouffet E, editors. Pediatric Neuro-Oncology. New York: Springer; 2015. p. 117–26.
- Rutkowski S, Bode U, Deinlein F, Ottensmeier H, Warmuth-Metz M, Soeroenson N, Grade N, Emser A, Pietsch T, Wolff JE, Kortmann RD, Kuehl J. Treatment of early childhood medulloblastoma by post-operative chemotherapy alone. N Eng J Med. 2005;352(10):978.
- Geyer JR. Sposto R, Jennings M, Boyett JM, Axtell RA, Brieger D, Broxso E, Donahue B, Finlay JL, Goldwein JW, Heier LA, Johnson DM, Mazewski C, Miller DC, Packer R, Puccetti D, Radcliffe J, Tao ML, Shiminski-Maher T. Multiagent chemotherapy and deferred radiotherapy in infants with malignant braintumors: a report from the Children's Cancer. Group.J Clin Oncol. 2005;23(30):7621.
- Wells EM, Packer RJ. Pediatric Brain Tumors. Continuum: Lifelong Learning in Neurology 2015; 21(2):373–96. 14. Fleming AJ. Rare tumors of the central nervous system in children. In: Scheinemann K, Bouffet E, editors. Pediatric Neuro-Oncology. New York: Springer; 2015. p. 185–94.

47. A pediatrician refereed a 2-week-old child to you for evaluation. He has a distended abdomen and has had a few bowel movements in comparison to other children at his age. On examination, he has a distended abdomen with hypoactive bowel sounds. X-ray of the abdomen shows dilated loops of bowel with excessive fecal material. You suspect a diagnosis of Hirschsprung's disease.
Which of the following is not true regarding the enteric nervous system?
   A. The sub mucous plexus is predominantly involved in secretory functions of the gastrointestinal tract.
   B. Hirschsprung's disease is due to congenital absence of the sub mucous plexus.
   C. Hirschsprung's disease is often focal, though rare cases involve the entire colon.
   D. Hirschsprung's disease is due to congenital absence of the sub mucous plexus.
   E. Hirschsprung's disease is due to congenital absence of the myenteric plexus.

3

Correct answer is: E
The enteric nervous system consists of the myenteric (or Auerbach's) plexus that is located between the outer and inner smooth muscle layers of the gastrointestinal tract and the sub mucous (or Meissner's) plexus, which is located between the circular muscle layer and the mucosa. The myenteric plexus is predominantly involved in gut motility, whereas the sub mucous plexus is involved in secretory functions. Together, the myenteric and sub mucous plexus control the function of the gastrointestinal tract. Hirschsprung's disease is due to mal development of the myenteric plexus. Most commonly, focal congenital absence of the myenteric plexus in the internal anal sphincter or recto sigmoid junction occurs, though in rare cases, the myenteric plexus may be absent throughout the gastrointestinal system. Segments of the colon that lack myenteric plexus cannot relax leading to fecal retention and distention of proximal colonic segments. Some cases of Hirschsprung's disease are due to mutations in the RET proto-oncogene.

Suggested Reading

- Comprehensive Review in Clinical Neurology: A Multiple-Choice Question Book for the Wards and Boards

48. You are seeing a 10-year-old girl with a history of dystonia, dysarthria, and rigidity. Her MRI is shown. Genetic testing will most likely demonstrate a mutation in which of the following genes?

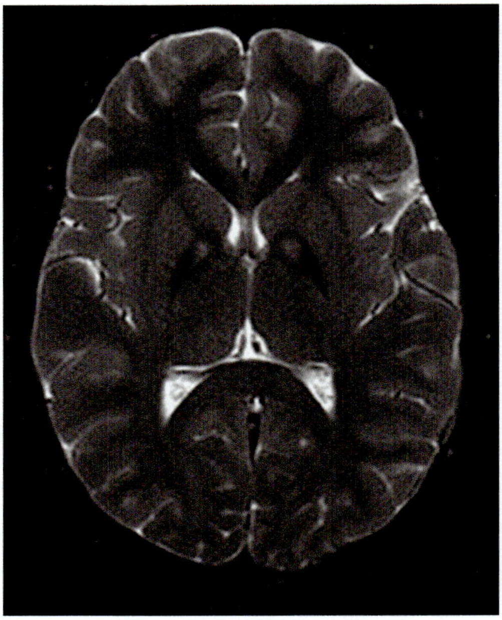

Fig. 3.19 MRI image shows iron deposits in the basal ganglia, the so-called eye-of-the-tiger sign (T2w GRASE sequence). (Enro2002. Wikipedia)

A. ATP1A3
B. GBA
C. MECP2
D. PANK2
E. PMP22

Correct Answer is: D
The clinical presentation and MRI showing the eye-of-the-tiger sign are diagnostic of pantothenate kinase-associated neurodegeneration (PKAN), a type of neurodegeneration with brain iron accumulation. The disorder results from mutations in the *PANK2* gene.

Deletions in *PMP22* are associated with hereditary neuropathy, with liability to pressure palsies, while duplications in this gene occur in Charcot-Marie-Tooth neuropathy type 1A.

***MECP2* mutations occur in Rett syndrome.**

Mutations in *GBA* are associated with Gaucher disease.

***ATP1A3* mutations cause rapid-onset dystonia-parkinsonism.**

Suggested Reading

- Gregory A, Hayflick SJ. Pantothenate kinase-associated neurodegeneration. Seattle (WA): University of Washington, Seattle; 1993–2013.

49. You are seeing a 2-day-old neonate with dysmorphic features including widely spaced eyes, low set ears, a short-upturned nose, and polydactyly. Echocardiogram shows a small ventricular septal defect and renal ultrasound shows a small left kidney and absent right kidney. MRI of the brain is shown.

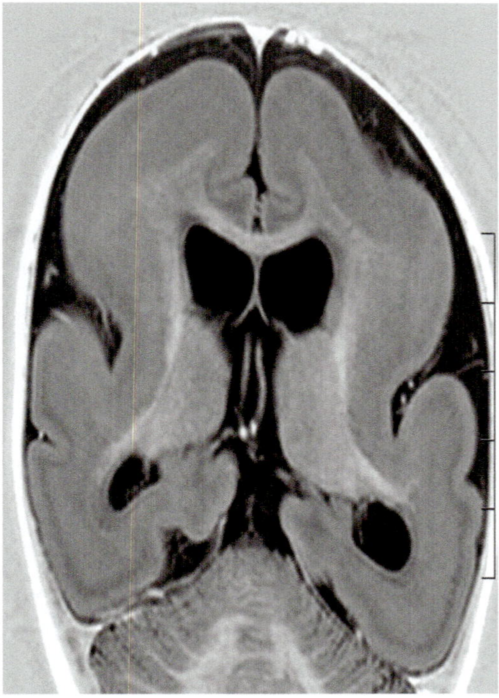

Fig. 3.20 With permission from ILAE.org. EpilepsyDiagnosis.org, Diagnostic Manual

What is the most likely diagnosis?

A. Double cortex syndrome
B. Hemimegalencephaly
C. Lissencephaly
D. Perisylvian syndrome
E. Polymicrogyria

Correct Answer is: C
The MRI shows lissencephaly with complete absence of cortical sulcation. The combination of lissencephaly and the above malformations and dysmorphic features is characteristic of Miller-Dieker Syndrome. Typical manifestations include a prominent forehead with bi-temporal hollowing, short nose with upturned nares, and thickened upper lip with thin vermilion upper border, widely spaced eyes, low set ears, and a small jaw. Other abnormalities include central hypotonia, heart malformations, omphalocele, inguinal hernia, duodenal atresia, pelvic and cystic kidneys, sacral tails, cryptorchidism, polydactyly, clinodactyly, camptodactyly, transverse palmar creases, and polyhydramnios during pregnancy. The underlying genetic abnormality is a deletion of the 17p13.3 locus, which involves LIS1 and YWHAE genes.

50. You are seeing an 18-year-old male a history of autism spectrum disorder and moderate mental retardation. He has epilepsy and takes topiramate and levetiracetam. His last seizure was 3 years ago. His brain T2 MRI scan is shown.
What skin findings would be expected in this man?

A. adenoma sebaceum
B. café-au-lait macules
C. linear nevus sebaceous in the scalp
D. lipoma over the lumbar spine
E. trigeminal distribution port-wine stain

3

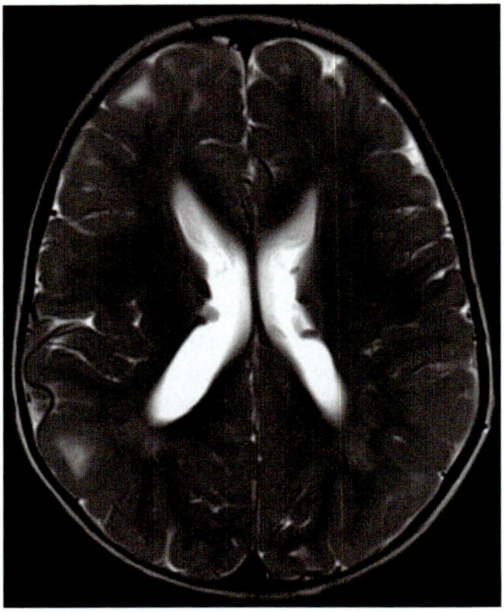

Fig. 3.21 With permission from ILAE.org. EpilepsyDiagnosis.org, Diagnostic Manual

Correct Answer is: A

A must part of the evaluation in patients such as this is detailed skin examination for evidence of a neruo-cutaneous syndrome. The MRI pictured shows evidence of hyper-intensities at the grey-white junction in multiple regions of the brain (tubers) and sub-ependymal nodules, two classic imaging features of tuberous sclerosis (TS). This disorder is inherited in an autosomal dominant fashion, though over 50% of cases represent spontaneous mutations and will not have affected family members. Two different genetic loci are responsible (with varying clinical phenotype depending on the gene involved) for encoding the proteins tuberin and hamartin. Seizures, in particular infantile spasms, are often the presenting feature of this disorder. Later in life multiple different seizure types present, often necessitating lifelong anticonvulsant therapy. Varying degrees of intellectual disability exist, often related to the number and size of the cortical tubers seen on MRI. These hyperintense regions represent regions of disorganized histogenesis of the brain. Subependymal nodules can enlarge rapidly and may evolve into an obstructive lesion near the foramen of Monro, called a subependymal giant cell astrocytoma (SEGA.) It is for this reason that serial MRI imaging is recommended for this patient population. Multiple organ systems are affected in tuberous sclerosis. Cardiac involvement is most common in early infancy, often with prenatal atrial myxomas identified on prenatal ultrasound. Though these lesions rarely cause obstructed atrial outflow the natural history for most of these lesions is to regress by the age of 12–24 months. Cutaneous findings are prevalent in TS. Early in life, hypo-pigmented macules (ash-leaf spots) are present, though may require use of a Wood lamp to identify in fair skinned individuals. With time, the patient may also develop some or all of the following: shagreen patch, adenoma sebaceum and periungual or gingival fibromas. Kidney, lung and ophthalmologic involvement is also common and should be looked for every few years to prevent complications. Diagnosis in the past had been made with clinical criteria; however, genetic testing is now available and especially used when the patient does not meet diagnostic criteria.

Six or more cafe-au-lait macules greater than 1.5 cm in size are one of the diagnostic criteria for neurofibromatosis. Linear nevus sebaceous syndrome presents with varying degrees of epilepsy and developmental delay and is associated with the nevus lesion, usually in the scalp or over the forehead. Often the seizure focus is ipsilateral to the skin lesion. Multiple different midline cutaneous lesions can be seen with underlying tethered cord syndrome to include tufts of hair,

port-wine stain or lipoma. Finally, a port-wine stain in the V1 or V2 distribution of the trigeminal nerve can be associated with Sturge-Weber syndrome. Realize that only 10% of the time is the port-wine stain associated with the full syndrome.

51. You are evaluating an 11-year-old boy for increasing frequent episodes of staring and unresponsiveness. On examination, he has difficulty with rapid movements of the right hand, brisk reflexes in the right arm and leg and a tendency to toe walk on the right. Examination of the skin and eyes is normal. MRI of the brain is shown.

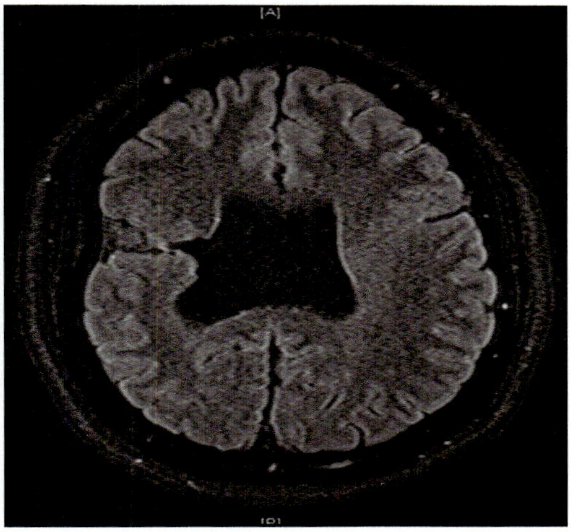

Fig. 3.22 American Academy of Neurology Institute, produced by permission

What is the most likely etiology of his epilepsy?

A. abnormal neuronal migration
B. calcium channel abnormality
C. perinatal stroke
D. sodium channel abnormality
E. tuberous sclerosis

Correct Answer is: A
The MRI pictured is consistent with an open lip schizencephaly. Schizencephaly is a type of abnormal neuronal migration characterized by a cleft that connects the cortical surface with the ventricular lumen. The cortical tissue is usually abnormal in its edges (either polymicrogyria, pachygyria or both); closed-lip schizencephaly occurs when the edges are juxtaposed, and open-lip schizencephaly when the edges are separated. Perinatal infarction of a branch of the middle cerebral artery could lead to the same clinical findings, though the imaging study would show encephalomalacia with an intact ventricular wall.

Patients with tuberous sclerosis can have various features of disordered neuronal migration, though not typically schizencephalic clefts, and notably absent in this case are the classic skin lesions (ash leaf macules) and hyperintensities on MRI at the cortical/subcortical junction (cortical tubers) that would suggest this as the correct diagnosis. Imaging studies in patients with calcium or sodium channel disorders would be expected to be normal.

Suggested Reading

- CONTINUUM: Lifelong Learning in Neurology: June 2013 - Volume 19 - Issue 3, Epilepsy – p 623–42 doi: 10.1212/01.CON.0000431379.29065.d3 Review Articles Neuroimaging in Investigation of Patients with Epilepsy Cendes, Fernando MD, PhD.

52. You are seeing a 15-year-old who complains of numbness, tingling, and pain in his arms and legs, problems with balance and coordination, and vision problems for the last year. He was also diagnosed by the school psychologist as learning disabled several years ago and placed in a special education class. He was previously healthy, takes no medications, and no previous hospitalizations. His vital signs are within normal limits.

3

On examination, he has proximal muscle weakness throughout the arms and legs, decreased peripheral vision, poor visual acuity, ataxia as well as sensory neuropathy in the extremities, and extraocular movements and eyelid movements are within normal limits.

What is your diagnosis?

A. Usher syndrome
B. NARP syndrome
C. Kearns-Sayre syndrome
D. Multiple sclerosis
E. Pompe's disease

Correct Answer is: B

Neuropathy, ataxia, and retinitis pigmentosa (NARP) is characterized by a constellation of symptoms including: proximal muscle weakness (neurogenic), sensory-motor neuropathy, ataxia, and retinitis pigmentosa (or other retinitis). It is an inherited disorder of mitochondrial DNA due to mutations in the MT-ATP6 gene. Prevalence is estimated to be around 1/100,000. In later stages, cerebellar atrophy can sometimes be seen on MRI.

Usher syndrome is characterized by hearing loss (secondary to inner ear abnormalities) and a gradual visual impairment (retinitis pigmentosa).

Kearns-Sayre syndrome (KSS) also known as oculocraniosomatic disease is a rare mitochondrial myopathy that presents usually before the age of 20. It is characterized by isolated involvement of the muscles controlling the eyelid: levator palpebrae and/or orbicularis oculi, as well as the extra-ocular muscles. This results in ptosis and ophthalmoplegia respectively. KSS also involves bilateral pigmentary retinopathy and cardiac conduction abnormalities. Other symptoms can include cerebellar ataxia, proximal muscle weakness, or deafness.

Suggested Reading

- Normal Lab Values (▶ https://s3.amazonaws.com/s3boardvitalsv3/exam_resources/normal_lab_values.pdf).

53. You ordered an autopsy on a 19-month-old boy who had a progressive neurologic disorder. He had macrocephaly, psychomotor retardation, spasticity and seizures. Figure shows a histopathologic specimen obtained at autopsy.

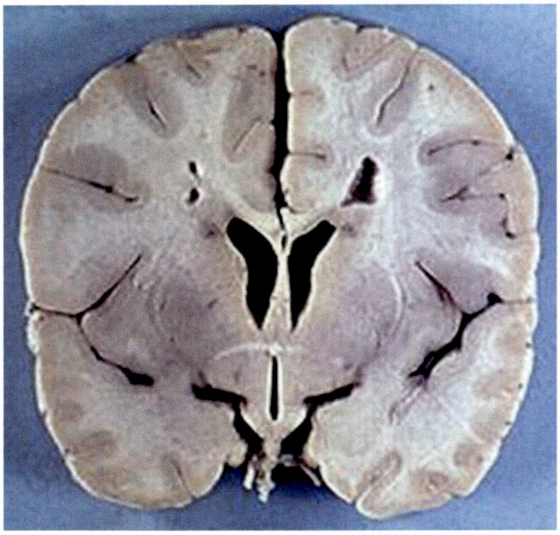

Fig. 3.23 Brain of a 4-year-old boy with Alexander disease showing macroencephaly and periventricular leukomalacia (note brownish discoloration around the cerebral ventricles). (Marvin 101)

What is the most likely diagnosis?

A. Canavan disease
B. Adrenoleukodystrophy
C. Alexander disease
D. Zellweger syndrome
E. Fabry disease

Correct Answer is: C

This is a case of Alexander disease, which is a progressive disorder of astrocytes caused by mutations in the gene for glial fibrillary acidic protein. It has

an autosomal dominant mode of inheritance, although this is controversial. There are infantile, juvenile, and adult forms.

Patients with the infantile form have megalencephaly, developmental delay, seizures, psychomotor retardation, spasticity, and quadriparesis. The juvenile form has onset in childhood, and these patients have more significant bulbar symptoms. The adult form manifests with bulbar signs, hyperreflexia, dysautonomia, ataxia, and sleep apnea. The brain MRI demonstrates diffuse white matter signal hyper-intensity, predominantly in the frontal lobes and anterior cerebral regions, with involvement of the U fibers. In the adult onset form, the "tadpole sign" on sagittal MRI results from dramatic thinning of the upper cervical spinal cord. The brains of these patients are large, and histopathologically, there are Rosenthal fibers. The specimen shown in the figure shows multiple Rosenthal fibers, which are elongated eosinophilic fibers seen on hematoxylin eosin, and they are diffusely distributed throughout the brain with clusters in the subpial, sub-ependymal, and perivascular areas. Rosenthal fiber deposition is associated with severe myelin loss and cavitation of the white matter.

They are not pathognomonic for Alexander disease and are seen in other conditions associated with gliosis. There is no specific treatment.

Suggested Reading

Comprehensive Review in Clinical Neurology: A Multiple-Choice Question Book for the Wards and Boards © 2011 Wolters Kluwer Health Lippincott Williams & Wilkins. All rights reserved.

54. Which of the following genetic changes is implicated in Williams's syndrome?
    A. Chromosome 22q11.21 deletion
    B. Maternal chromosome 1Sq11-q13 deletion
    C. Paternal chromosome 1Sq11–13 deletion
    D. Chromosome 7q11.23 deletion

Correct Answer is: C

The characteristic features of Williams's syndrome include, aortic stenosis, hypercalcemia, elfin facies, and mental retardation. It is caused by a chromosome 7q11.23 deletion. Individuals with this condition tend to be very social and musically talented. Cognitive dysfunction is not typically severe.

Velocardiofacial syndrome is caused by deletion of chromosome 22q11.21. It is characterized by hypocalcemia, conotruncal cardiac malformations, nasal speech, hypertelorism, and cognitive dysfunction. About a quarter of individuals with this condition develop psychiatric disease.

Maternal chromosome 1Sq-q13 deletion may lead to Angelman syndrome; known as "happy puppet" syndrome. This is characterized by microcephaly, mental retardation, speech difficulties, and seizures. Movements are often jerky in nature and patients may laugh inappropriately, hence the nickname "happy puppet" syndrome. Cerebral and cerebellar atrophy are preset; cerebellar atrophy is typically more severe.1.

Paternal chromosome 1Sq11–13 deletion leads to Prader Willi syndrome which is characterized by short stature, obesity, mental retardation, and the tendency to overeat. During infancy, patients may be hypotonic although this improves. Mental retardation may be severe.

Suggested Reading

- Menkes JH, Wilcox WR. Inherited metabolic diseases of the nervous system. In: Menkes JH, Sarnat HB, Maria BL. Child neurology. 7th ed. Philadelphia: Lippincott Williams and Wilkins. 2006 L. p. 29–142.

3

55. Which of the following genes is implicated in Friedreich ataxia?
    A. Ataxia telangiectasia muted ATM serine/ threonine kinase (ATM)
    B. Frataxin (FXN)
    C. Tocopherol (alpha) transfer protein (TTPA)
    D. Aprataxin (APTX)

Correct Answer is: B
Friedreich ataxia (FA) is caused by increased GAA repeats in the gene frataxin (FXN). FA is caused by repeats of over 66 although those with fewer than 300 repeats may not have symptoms until after age 25. It is characterized by ataxia, decreased deep tendon reflexes, positive Babinski, posterior column dysfunction, dysarthria, and nystagmus.

Mutations in ATM lead to ataxia telangiectasia. Patients present with ataxia, telangiectasias, immune deficiency, and increased risk of malignancy. Those patients are sensitive to ionizing radiation. Mutations in TIPA lead to ataxia with vitamin E deficiency. This is characterized by movement abnormalities, dysarthria, lower extremity areflexia, and peripheral neuropathy. Patients may also have retinitis pigmentosa. The alpha tocopherol transfer protein is necessary for processing of vitamin E in the diet. Mutations in the gene APTX are implicated in ataxia with oculomotor apraxia type 1. This gene is implicated in DNA repair and leads to increased cerebellar cell death. This is characterized by ataxia starting by age 5 with myoclonus, oculomotor apraxia, chorea, and neuropathy. Decreased albumin and increased cholesterol levels are characteristic. Mutations in the SETX gene lead to ataxia with oculomotor apraxia type 2. This is characterized by ataxia, in this case starting by age 15, oculomotor apraxia, myoclonus, chorea, and neuropathy. Elevated alpha fetoprotein and creatine phosphokinase are often present.

Suggested Reading

- National Library of Medicine (US). Genetics Home Reference [Internet]. Bethesda (MD): The Library; 2015 Dec 7. FXN; [reviewed 201O May; cited 2015 Dec 13]; Available from: ► http://ghr.nlm.nih.Gov/gene/FXN (► http://ghr.nlm.nih.gov/gene/FXN).
- National Library of Medicine (US). Genetics Home Reference [Internet]. Bethesda (MD): The Library; 2015 Dec 7. TIPA; [reviewed 2008 Apr; cited 2015 Dec 13]; Available from: ► http://ghr.nlm.nih.gov/genelTTPA (► http://ghr.nlm.nih.gov/genelTTPA).
- National Library of Medicine (US). Genetics Home Reference [Internet]. Bethesda (MD): The Library; 2015 Dec 7. Ataxia with vitamin E deficiency; [reviewed 2008 Apr; cited 2015 Dec 13]; Available from: ► http://ghr.nlm.nih.gov/condition/ataxia-with-vitamin-edeficiency (► http://ghr.nlm.nih.Gov/condition/ataxia-with-vitamin-e-deficiency).
- National Library of Medicine (US). Genetics Home Reference [Internet]. Bethesda (MD): The Library; 2015 Dec 7. Ataxia with oculomotor apraxia; [reviewed 2015 Apr; cited 2015 Dec 13]; Available from: ► http://ghr.nlm.nih.gov/condition/ataxia-with-oculomotor-apraxia (► http://ghr.nlm.nih.gov/condition/ataxia-with-oculomotor-apraxia).
- Bird TD, Jayadev. Genetic disease of the nervous system, In: Rosenberg RN editor. Atlas of clinical neurology. Philadelphia: Springer; 2009.

56. You are seeing a 15-year-old male with a progressive cerebellar ataxia, pigmentary retinopathy and a recent diagnosis of progressive external ophthalmoplegia.
What is the mode of inheritance in this case?
A. X-linked
B. Autosomal recessive
C. Autosomal dominate
D. Maternal

Correct Answer is: D
This is a case of Kearns-Sayre syndrome (KSS), which is a mitochondrial disorder. Inherited mitochondrial pattern follows maternal inheritance. Egg cells, not sperm cells, contribute mitochondria DNA to the developing embryo, only females pass mitochondrial conditions to their children. Mitochondrial disorders can appear in each generation of a family and affects both males and females, Fathers do not pass mitochondrial traits to their children.

1. **KSS is characterized by: Progressive external ophthalmoplegia.**
2. **Disease onset before age 20 and**
3. **At least one of the following; short stature, pigmentary retinopathy, cerebellar ataxia, heart block, and elevated cerebrospinal fluid protein (>100 mg/dl).**

Many cases of KSS are believed to be sporadic mitochondrial DNA deletions or duplications.

Inheritance by a gene on the X chromosome that causes the phenotype to be expressed in males who are hemizygous for the gene mutation and in females who are homozygous for the gene mutation (received copy of the gene on each of their two X chromosomes. Inheritance of a phenotype (or disease) requires the same copy of a gene in both copies a child receives each parent on an autosomal chromosome.

Inheritance of a phenotype (or disease) requires the only one (dominant) copy from either parent on an autosomal chromosome.

Suggested Reading

- Angelini, C. Kearns-Sayre syndrome. In: Genetic Neuromuscular Disorders. Springer International Publishing. 2014. p. 225–8.

57. You are evaluating a 2-year-old girl with progressive visual loss since infancy, associated with midface hypoplasia, enophthalmos and hypermetropia?
What is the likely diagnosis?
A. Leber congenital amaurosis
B. Bardet-Biedle syndrome
C. Wolfram syndrome
D. Pituitary adenoma

Correct Answer is: A
Leber congenital amaurosis (LCA) is a group of disorders of recessive retinal dystrophies and is the most common cause of congenital visual impairment. Characteristics of LCA are moderate-severe visual impairment at or near birth, along with nystagmus, and sluggish pupillary responses. Physical stigmata include mid-facial hypoplasia, enophthalmos, hypermetric and refractive errors. Retinal examination shows no abnormality in infancy and early childhood, but progressive retinal stippling and pallor of the disk gradually develop. Mental retardation may be associated.

Bardet-Biedle syndrome is characterized by pigmentary retinopathy, mental retardation, polydactyly, obesity and hypogenitalism.

Wolfram syndrome is characterized by optic atrophy, bilateral sensory hearing loss, diabetes insipidus and mellitus.

Pituitary adenomas account for 2% of childhood of all childhood intracranial

3

tumors. Optic atrophy occurs in up to 20% OF patients. Visual field deficits include unilateral temporal, bi-temporal hemianopia, or even homonymous.

Suggested Reading

- Weleber RG, Francis PJ, Trzupek KM, Beattie C. (2013). Leber congenital amaurosis. QID: 55258.

58. You are evaluating a 15- year-old male for a progressive sensorineural hearing loss over the last 2 years. Few months ago, he developed bilateral, asymmetrical moderate facial weakness and complained of trouble swallowing. He has tongue atrophy on neurological exam otherwise the rest of the cranial nerves are intact. He had a mild increase in muscle tone in his extremities.
   What is the most likely diagnosis?
   A. Facioscapulohumeral dystrophy
   B. Juvenile progressive bulbar palsy
   C. Pontobulbar Palsy with Deafness
   D. Juvenile myasthenia gravis

Correct Answer is: C
Ponto-bulbar Palsy with Deafness (Brown-Vialetto-Van Laere syndrome) is an autosomal recessive neuronopathy characterized by ponto-bulbar palsy affecting lower cranial nerves (primarily VII-XII).

Sensorineural deafness is often the leading sign, followed by facial weakness and dysphagia. Tongue atrophy occurs in most cases, but masseter and ocular motor palsies are uncommon. About 50% will have pyramidal tract dysfunction. Riboflavin supplementation has been reported benefit some patients. Patients mostly common die from respiratory insufficiency.

Facioscapulohumeral dystrophy begins in the second decade of life and includes facial weakness, but the shoulder girdle and humeral muscle weakness in more prominent.

Juvenile progressive bulbar palsy includes weakness of tongue, facial, pharyngeal and ocular muscles with a fluctuant course.

The most frequent clinical presentation of juvenile le myasthenia gravis is ptosis, which is often associated with other ocular symptoms namely unilateral or asymmetric ophthalmoplegia, strabismus, and lid twitch. Children with myasthenia gravis have lower frequency of acetylcholine receptor antibodies and a greater probability of achieving remission.

Suggested Reading

- Foley AR, et al. Treatable childhood neuronopathy caused by mutations in riboflavin transporter RFVT2. Brain. 2014;137(Pt 1):44–56.

59. What is the most likely diagnosis in a 4-year-old boy with congenital deafness, who now presents with a goiter?
   A. Pendred syndrome
   B. Infantile Refsum disease
   C. Hypomelanosis of Ito
   D. Vitiligo

Correct Answer is: A
Sensorineural hearing impairment is present at birth and is severe in about half of the cases of Pendred syndrome. A diffuse, non-nodular goiter most often develops during the first decade, often in infancy. No clinical signs of hypothyroidism are present. Growth and intelligence are usually normal.

Infantile Refsum disease is a disorder of peroxisome biogenesis and is characterized by early onset cognitive impairment, retinitis pigmentosa, sensorineural hearing deficit hepatomegaly, osteoporosis, failure to thrive and hypocholesterolemia.

Hypomelanosis of Ito (Ito syndrome) produces symmetric depigmented streaks or swirls on the skin. Some individuals can have wide set eyes or auricle anomalies, but hearing loss is not associated. Vitiligo is an autoimmune disorder characterized by depigmented patches of skin. Hearing loss is not associated with this condition.

Suggested Reading

- Smith RJ, Shearer AE, Hildebrand MS, Van Camp G. Deafness and hereditary hearing loss overview. 2014.

60. Polymicrogyria is associated with which one of the following conditions?
    - A. Chiari 1 malformation
    - B. Aicardi syndrome
    - C. Dandy walker malformation
    - D. Syringomyelia
    - E. Chiari II malformation

Correct Answer is: B
Polymicrogyria is some excessive, numerous small gyri. It may occur in combination with pachygyria. It is usually due to ischemic insult to the underlying parenchyma but can be due to defective migration. Other acquired intrauterine insults include infections such as toxoplasmosis and cytomegalovirus (and others, including rubella and herpes simplex). Associated with X-linked dominant Aicardi's syndrome and may occur in the context of specific inherited metabolic disorders, such as peroxisomal disorders (e.g., Zellweger's syndrome). Clinical presentation varies, depending on the associated condition. If involvement is focal, patients may be asymptomatic or present with seizures.

Aicardi syndrome is a disorder that occurs almost exclusively in females. It has three main features:

1. **Agenesis or dysgenesis of the corpus callosum.**
2. **Infantile spasms.**
3. **Choreoretinal lacunae.**

Additional brain abnormalities in Aicardi syndrome include – asymmetry between hemispheres, polymicrogyria, cysts, and microcephaly. Other ophthalmic abnormalities include – microphthalmia or coloboma, which can cause blindness. Facial features may include – small philtrum, a flat nose with an upturned tip, large ears, and sparse eyebrows. Other features include – small hands, scoliosis. They often have gastrointestinal problems such as constipation or diarrhea, gastroesophageal reflux, and difficulty feeding.

Suggested Reading

- Mowzoon, Nima, Kelly D. Flemming. Neurology board review: an illustrated study guide. Rochester, MN: Mayo Clinic Scientific, 2007. Print.

61. You are evaluating a 16-year-old with severe generalized myoclonus, ataxia, and loss of color vision. He has a cherry red spot on fundus exam. EEG demonstrated background slowing, and photosensitive bilateral fast spike and wave activity.
    What choice is correct to establish the diagnosis?
    - A. An alpha-N-acetylgalactosami nidase deficiency
    - B. A decrease in cultured skin fibroblast alpha-neuraminidase
    - C. A response to oral biotin
    - D. A hexosaminidase A deficiency
    - E. A muscle biopsy with ragged red fibers

Correct Answer is: B
Schindler disease is caused by a deficiency of alpha-N-acetylgalactosaminidase. It is a rare autosomal recessive disorder with acute infant and chronic adult-onset forms. Infants demonstrate

3

severe psychomotor deterioration with spasticity, cortical blindness, and myoclonic epilepsy with an exaggerated startle response. The adult form is characterized by mild cognitive deficits.

Sialidosis type 1 A manifestations include severe generalized myoclonus, night blindness, loss of color vision, ataxia, cherry-red spots, and generalized convulsions. In this case, the EEG shows progressive slowing and bilateral, photosensitive fast spike-wave discharges. A decrease in cultured skin fibroblast alpha-neuraminidase is diagnostic.

A response to oral biotin would be consistent with biotinidase deficiency. This disorder is characterized by hypotonia, generalized tonic-clonic and myoclonic seizures, rash, and alopecia, with onset in infancy. The EEG demonstrates multifocal spikes and slow waves.

A hexosaminidase A deficiency is present in Tay-Sachs disease, with the onset of development delay, cherry-red spots, and "startle seizures" in infancy.

A muscle biopsy with ragged red fibers is indicative of myoclonic epilepsy with ragged red fibers (MERRF). The core features of this mitochondrial disorder include myoclonus, epilepsy, myopathy, intellectual disability, and cerebellar dysfunction. Patients may also have short stature, deafness, optic atrophy, cutaneous lipomas, and neuropathy. The onset is typically in childhood or early adulthood.

Suggested Reading

- Verma A, Moraes CT. Mitochondrial disorders. In: Bradley WG, Daroff RB, Fenichel GM, Jankovic J, editors. Neurology in clinical practice. 4th ed. Elsevier, Inc.; 2004. p. 781–808.
- Pastores GM, Kolodny EH. Inborn errors of metabolism of the nervous system. In: Bradley WG, Daroff RB, Fenichel GM, Jankovic J, editors. Neurology in clinical practice. 4th ed. Elsevier, Inc.; 2004. p. 1811–32.

62. Which of the following conditions is associated with retinitis pigmentosa?
    - A. HARP syndrome
    - B. Glaucoma
    - C. Diabetic retinopathy
    - D. Multiple Sclerosis
    - E. Mc leod Syndrome

Correct Answer is: A
HARP stands for Hypoprebetalipoproteinemia, Acanthocytosis, Retinitis pigmentosa, and Pallidal degeneration. It is a rare disease of childhood similar to Hallervorden-Spatz disease in that there is a defect in the gene for pantothenate kinase (the first enzyme in the Coenzyme A synthesis pathway). Glaucoma and diabetic retinopathy are important causes of blindness but not retinitis pigmentosa.

Mcleod syndrome causes acanthosis, but not retinitis pigmentosa. The neuroacanthocytoses are a group of genetically diverse conditions that cause movement disorders, neurological problems and acanthosis (speculated red blood cells) including chorea acanthocytosis, Mc leod syndrome, Huntington's disease-like 2 (HDl2) and Hallervorden-Spatz (also called pantothenate kinase-associated neurodegeneration (PKAN)).

63. Which one of the following conditions is associated with Chiari type I malformation?
    - A. Myelomeningocele
    - B. Holoprosencephaly
    - C. Syringomyelia
    - D. Cerebellar atrophy
    - E. Corpus callosum agenesis

Correct Answer is: C
Chiari type I malformation: caudal displacement of cerebellar tonsils through the foramen magnum. Mean age at presentation: 41 years. Chiari type I malformation may be associated with:

Hydrocephalus, Intermittent increase in intracranial pressure, Syringomyelia, Klippel-Feil syndrome, basilar impression, and occipitalization of the atlas, Compression of brainstem structures and some rostral extension of the medulla. Patient may be asymptomatic. Presenting symptoms: headaches, especially brought on by neck extension or the Valsalva maneuver (most common presenting symptom), sometimes associated with tinnitus, nausea, and vomiting.

Various cerebellar symptoms, lower cranial nerve dysfunction, diplopia and downbeat nystagmus, dissociated sensory loss (loss of pinprick and temperature sensation and relative preservation of large fiber modalities), and possibly pyramidal tract involvement.

Surgical treatment: early surgery for symptomatic patients and observation for asymptomatic ones.

Suggested Reading

- Mowzoon N. Flemming KD. Neurology board review: an illustrated study guide. Rochester, MN: Mayo Clinic Scientific, 2007. Print.

64. You are seeing an 18-year-old male who has an acute ischemic stroke. His medical history is remarkable of cardiomyopathy of uncertain cause, severe hypertension, and end-stage renal disease. His first symptoms consisted of a burning sensation in his feet. His family history is remarkable of three brothers who died of end stage renal disease. His renal biopsy was obtained and showed birefringent lipid deposits in the glomeruli, and electron microscopy showed membrane bound lamellar deposits. **What is the most likely diagnosis?**
    A. Metachromatic leukodystrophy
    B. Fabry disease
    C. Niemann-Pick Type A
    D. Gaucher disease
    E. GM1 gangliosidosis

Correct Answer is: B
Fabry disease is an X-linked disorder caused by deficiency of the enzyme A-galactosidase, resulting in accumulation of ceramide trihexoside in epithelial, mesenchymal, and neural cells. The presenting manifestations start in childhood or adolescence, presenting with dysesthesias, lancinating pain, and episodes of burning sensation from small fiber neuropathy, which also may be associated with autonomic dysfunction. Dermatologic manifestations include the characteristic angiokeratomas, which are more prominent in the lower abdomen and legs, especially in the groins, hips, and periumbilical regions, and consist of cutaneous telangiectasias. Cardiac involvement manifests with valvular disease, arrhythmias, cardiomyopathy, and ischemic heart disease. There is also renal involvement from endothelial and glomerular damage, causing acute renal failure and eventually chronic renal disease leading to hypertension and uremia. Vascular compromise arises from endothelial and vascular smooth muscle involvement and is associated with ischemic stroke. Another frequent clinical finding is corneal opacity.

Pathologically, there is lysosomal storage of birefringent lipids, with membrane-bound lamellar deposits on electron microscopy.

Treatment includes enzyme replacement therapy.

Metachromatic leukodystrophy is caused by deficiency of arylsulfatase A.

Niemann-Pick Type A is caused by acid sphingomyelinase deficiency.

Gaucher disease is caused by deficiency of the enzyme glucocerebrosidase. GM1 gangliosidosis is caused by8-galactosidase deficiency.

3

65. You ordered a brain specimen obtained from an autopsy of a 10-month-old baby. The patient had irritability and hypersensitivity to stimuli at 3 months of age. He was also blind and had prominent regression by age 6 months. He also had developed stiffness of all four limbs and later of the trunk to the point that he was in an opisthotonic posture.

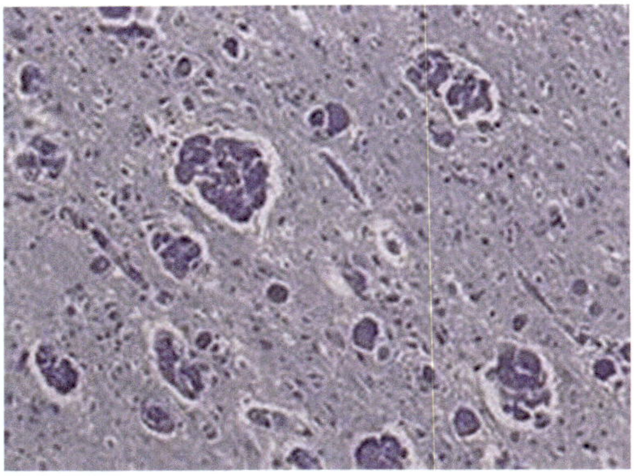

Fig. 3.24 Globoid cell leukodystrophy PAS – Mulinucleated macrophages ("globoid cells") and loss of myelinated fibers in a case of Krabbe's leukodystrophy. (Jensflorian. Wikipedia)

Which of the following is correct regarding this condition?

A. It is autosomal dominant
B. The deficient enzyme is 8-glucosylceramidase
C. There is demyelination with relative sparing of the U fibers
D. It is only seen in newborns, and all patients die by 1 year of age
E. The cause is deficiency of the enzyme A-galactosidase

Correct Answer is: C

This patient has Krabbe disease on the basis of the history and histopathologic findings. Krabbe disease or globoid cell leukodystrophy is a disorder with autosomal recessive inheritance, with the affected gene mapped to chromosome 14. This disorder is characterized by the accumulation of galactocerebroside in macrophages of the white matter in the CNS, leading to the formation of globoid cells and to progressive demyelination, but with sparing of the U fibers. The cause is a deficiency of the enzyme galactosylceramidase (also known as galactocerebroside galactosidase). It can involve the peripheral nervous system, leading to a demyelinating neuropathy, but affects predominantly the CNS.

There are three forms: –

1. **Infantile form: the most common variant and presents between 4 and 6 months of age with irritability, hypersensitivity to stimuli, increasing hypertonicity with eventual opisthotonos, unexplained low-grade fevers, and optic atrophy with blindness, psychomotor developmental arrest, and subsequent regression with loss of previously achieved milestones. These children also have a demyelinating polyneuropathy with arreflexia. They usually die by the age of 1 year.**
2. **Juvenile form: the onset is between 3 and 10 years of age, with vision loss, spasticity, ataxia, gait disturbance, and cognitive impairment.**
3. **Adult form: usually starts between the third and the fifth decade of life, with spastic paraparesis, weakness, vision loss, and evidence of neuropathy, but intellectual function tends to be normal.**

Pathologically, there is symmetric demyelination of the cerebral white matter, with relative sparing of the subcortical arcuate or U fibers. The pathologic specimen shown in the above figure is typical of Krabbe disease, demonstrating clusters of globoid cells, which are multinucleated macrophages with cytoplasmic accumulation of galactocerebroside.

Radiologically, there is symmetric periventricular white matter signal abnormality and cerebral atrophy.

NCS demonstrate slow conduction velocities and prolonged distal latencies.

CSF examination shows elevated protein levels.

66. You are evaluating a 15-year-old boy with growth retardation, generalized weakness, and ataxia. On examination, he has bilateral ptosis and restricted gaze in all directions. An electrocardiogram is obtained and shows complete heart block.
What is the most likely diagnosis?
    A. Kearns-Sayre syndrome
    B. Mitochondrial encephalopathy, lactic acidosis, and strokes
    C. Myoclonic epilepsy with ragged red fibers
    D. Leigh disease
    E. Myasthenia gravis

Correct Answer is: A
This is a presentation of Kearns-Sayre syndrome, which is a disorder caused by multiple mt DNA deletions. The diagnosis is made with the triad of progressive external ophthalmoplegia, onset before the age of 20 years, and at least one of the following: short stature, retinitis pigmentosa, cerebellar ataxia, heart block, and increased CSF protein (>100 mg/dl). Chronic progressive externalophthalmoplegia may be an isolated finding seen in some patients. Patients with Kearns-Sayre syndrome have a gradual progression of symptoms and most will have cognitive regression by third or fourth decade of life. Most cases are sporadic. An electrocardiogram is required to diagnose heart block, in which case, a pacemaker needed. Pathologically, patients may have muscles with ragged red fibers and white matter showing spongy myelinopathy without gliosis or macrophage reactions.

67. You are seeing a 10-month-old girl with hypotonia. Her medical history is remarkable to have low muscle tone at 6 months. She has attained few developmental milestones since that time and recently was noted to have an exaggerated started response to loud noises. On examination, she has an enlarged liver. She has been referred to an ophthalmologist for mild cornea clouding revealed a cherry-red spot.
What is the hereditary genetic pattern of this condition?
    A. Autosomal dominant
    B. Autosomal recessive
    C. X-linked
    D. Sporadic

Correct Answer is: B
Infantile GM1 gangliosidosis is an autosomal inherited disorder caused by a mutation in the GLB1 gene that produces beta-galactosidase.

This results in an accumulation of mucopolysaccharides in cells causing dysfunction and cell death. Onset is between 6 and 18 months. Hypotonia progresses to spasticity are accompanied with seizures, cognitive and visual impairment. Death usually occurs by 7 years of age. The absence of mucopolysaccharidiura and the presence of a cherry-red spot differentiate GM1 gangliosidosis from Hurler syndrome.

Tay-sachs disease (infantile GM2 gangliosidosis) may present with similar symptoms, but occurs almost exclusively in Ashkenazi Jews. Type II GM1 gangliosidosi s consists of intermediate forms of the condition. The third type of GM1 gangliosidosis is an adult form and is the mildest manifestation of the disease spectrum.

Suggested Reading

- Kannebley JS. Moryama LS, Bstos LOD, Guerreiro MM, Amato A, Min LL, Steiner CE. (2014, April). Clinical and radiologic features in 12 patients' with juvenile and adult GM1 Gangliosidosis. In: 13th International Child Neurology Congress (ICNC2014).

3

68. Which one of the following is associated with Chiari type II malformation?
   - A. Anencephaly
   - B. Encephalocele
   - C. Cerebellar atrophy with enlarged posterior fossa
   - D. Lissencephaly
   - E. Myelomeningocele

Correct Answer is: E

Chiari type II malformation: caudal displacement of cerebellar tonsils, cervico-medullary junction, pons, fourth ventricle, and medulla. Chiari type II malformation is associated with: Myelomeningocele; Hydrocephalus; Colpocephaly of the lateral ventricles; Elongated fourth ventricle; interdigitating gyri (associated with hypoplastic falx cerebri); Skull abnormalities: lacunar skull, hypoplastic; tentorium cerebelli, gaping foramen magnum. Other major findings: Medullary "spur" or "kink" as a result of caudally; displaced, elongated medulla. Tectal "beaking" of the midbrain due to pressure from herniated cerebellum. Hydrocephalus in 90% of patients.

Presentation: Variable age at onset usually neonatal to early childhood. Neonatal presentation with rapid neurologic deterioration, including weak or absent cry, respiratory failure, and strider, apneic spells, swallowing difficulties from involvement of the medulla. Hydrocephalus, weakness including facial weakness, lower cranial nerve abnormalities.

Treatment: surgical decompression and cerebrospinal fluid (CSF) shunt for hydrocephalus.

Suggested Reading

- Mowzoon N, Flemming, KD. Neurology board review: an illustrated study guide. Rochester, MN: Mayo Clinic Scientific, 2007. Print.

69. Which of the following is not true regarding periventricular nodular heterotopia?
   - A. Heterotopias are clusters of defective neurons in an area of otherwise normal cortex
   - B. It is a disorder of neuronal migration
   - C. It is more common in females
   - D. It is most commonly X-linked
   - E. Seizures are a common clinical manifestation

Correct Answer is: A

Heterotopia is a cluster of abnormally located neurons that are otherwise normal in morphology. Heterotopias result from abnormal neuronal migration. The most common form of heteropia is periventricular nodular heterotopia (also known as subependymal nodular heterotopia), located, as the name implies, near the lateral ventricles, but heterotopias can be found in various regions (such as subcortical nodular heterotopias, or transmantle heterotopias, which extend from the ventricles to the cortex).

In periventricular nodular heterotopia, neurons are thought to have never begun migration but rather remained in the sub-ventricular area (where cortical neurons originate). This disorder is most often bilateral, but it can also be unilateral. In more than half of cases, this disorder results from mutations in the FLNa gene on chromosome X. This FLNa gene encodes a protein involved in actin cytoskeleton reorganization, and abnormalities in this protein lead to disruption in cell migration by impeding

the generation of forces needed for cell movement. Periventricular nodular heterotopias may be seen in isolation or as part of a syndrome associated with multiple other anomalies. Epilepsy is a common clinical manifestation, with partial seizures being most common. Intelligence may be entirely normal; males are more likely to have developmental delay.

70. You were asked to see an infant who has moon-like facies, hypertelorism, microcephaly, low set ears, hypotonia, and a high-pitched cry.
What chromosomal analysis are you going to order?
   - A. 5p monosomy
   - B. Trisomy 13
   - C. Trisomy 18
   - D. Trisomy 21
   - E. Partial monosomy 13q

Correct Answer is: A
The clinical presentation indicates a 5p monosomy. The syndrome is known as "cri du chat," meaning "cry of the cat," reflecting the characteristic high-pitched cry. Associated manifestations include moon-like facies, low set ears, a small jaw, orbital hypertelorism, microcephaly, MR, hypotonia, low birth weight, and heart defects. Loss of the CTNND2 gene on chromosome 5 may be associated with particularly severe intellectual disability.

Trisomy 13, or Patau syndrome, consists of intellectual disability, microcephaly, holoprosencephaly, heart and spinal cord defects, seizures, and hypotonia. Other malformations include polydactyly, a single palmar crease, cleft lip and palate, low set ears, hernias, and cryptorchidism. Patients may have coloboma, microphthalmia, close-set eyes, or fusion into one eye. Many infants die shortly after birth, with only 5–10% living past 1 year.

Trisomy 18, or Edwards's syndrome, is characterized by intellectual disability, pointed ears, micrognathia, microcephaly, an occipital protuberance, a narrow pelvis, heart defects, and rocker bottom feet. Intrauterine growth retardation and low birth weights are common. Many infants die before or shortly after birth, with only 5–10% living past the first year.

Trisomy 21, or Down syndrome, has multiple systemic manifestations and a variable phenotype. Common findings include intellectual disability, hypotonia, characteristic facial features (e.g. upward slanted eyes, protruding tongue, flattened face, small nose with a depressed nasal bridge), and Brush field spots. Early onset Alzheimer's disease, heart defects, and an elevated risk for leukemia are also associated features.

Partial monosomy 13q occurs when a portion of the long arm (q) of chromosome 13 is deleted or monosomic. The phenotype is variable, depending on the size and location of the deletion. The syndrome may be characterized by low birth weight, craniofacial malformations, ocular abnormalities, defects of the hands and/or feet, urogenital malformations, and intellectual disability.

Suggested Reading

- Published 4/21/14. Accessed 4/28/14. ▶ http://ghr.nlm.nih.gov/condition/trisomy-13 (▶ http://ghr.nlm.nih.gov/condition/trisomy-13). Reviewed 11/13. Published 4/21/14. Accessed 4/28/14. ▶ http://ghr.nlm.nih.gov/condition/trisomy-18 (▶ http://ghr.nlm.nih.gov/condition/trisomy-18). Reviewed 3/ 12. Published 4/21/14. Accessed 4/28/14. Chen H. Down Syndrome. ▶ http://emedicine.medscape.com/article/943216-overview (▶ http://emedicine.medscape.com/article/943216-overview). Updated 4/10/14. Accessed 4/27/14.

71. A 5-month-old baby is referred to you because he has a small, midline tuft of hair over the lower lumbar region. His examination is otherwise entirely normal. You decided to see him for follow-up at 3 years of age, the child continues to have normal development and a normal neurologic examination.

Which of the following statements regarding this child is true?

A. On the basis of the finding of this tuft of hair, it can be concluded that he will eventually have significant cognitive delay, even if he has developed normally up until the age of 3 years

B. On the basis of the finding of this tuft of hair, it can be concluded that he will eventually have significant motor and cognitive delay even if he has developed normally up until the age of 3 years

C. This tuft of hair signifies a possible underlying defect in the posterior bony component of the vertebral column

D. This tuft of hair signifies the presence of a myelomeningocele

E. On the basis of the finding of this tuft of hair, it can be concluded that abnormalities in the spinal cord will definitely be seen on imaging

Correct Answer is: C

This is a clinical presentation of spina bifida occulta. This is a defect in the bony components along the posterior aspect of the vertebral column. It can often be asymptomatic, but an abnormal conus medullaris and filum terminale are possible. The presence of a tuft of hair, implying underlying spina bifida occulta, does not necessarily imply impending cognitive or motor delay. In fact, when early neurologic development is normal, it will typically continue to be so. However, associated neurologic dysfunction may present future neurologic impairment. When there is associated neurologic dysfunction in a child with a tuft of hair over the lumbar region but with no other evidence of neural tube defect, the disorder is named occult spinal dysraphism. In occult spinal dysraphism, a variety of developmental abnormalities may be seen involving the spinal cord or roots and posterior fossa, and associated findings may include dermoid or epidermoid cysts, intra-spinal or cutaneous lipomas, and tethered cord. Diastematomyelia, or splitting of the spinal cord, may also be seen. Rarely, a sinus tract connects the dura with the surface of the skin. In occult spinal dysraphism, neurologic manifestations vary widely and may range from minimal motor deficits and ankle hyporeflexia to bowel and bladder dysfunction, sensory loss, and paraparesis or paraplegia. Although patients may be initially asymptomatic, these neurological deficits can develop suddenly and be irreversible.

72. You are evaluating a 4-year-old girl. Her family reports that, she seemed to be a very happy baby early on life, she made eye contact and smiled and cooed all the time. She had met motor milestones similar to her siblings: holding her head up, crawling, and sitting unsupported. However, around the age of 18 months, she started to have difficulty sitting up and never developed any words. She later stopped smiling and laughing, and progressively lost use of her hands, constantly rubbing her hands against each other.

Which of the following statements is true regarding the most likely diagnosis in this patient?

A. It is more common in males but can also be seen in females
B. Macrocephaly is a common finding
C. It results from a mutation in the gene encoding the MeCP2 protein
D. It is autosomal dominant in inheritance
E. It results from mutations in mitochondrial DNA

Correct Answer is: E
This is a case of Rett syndrome, a syndrome of motor and cognitive regression with eventual severe disability. The presentation is one of early normal development with subsequent regression at approximately 6–18 months of age. Hand wringing and other motor stereotypies are a classic feature; patients with Rett syndrome often place their hands in their mouth or may hold their hands fisted, with their fingers flexed over their thumb. Arrest of head growth with eventual microcephaly, seizures, scoliosis, dysautonomia including respiratory dysfunction with apneas, and spasticity emerge as the disease progresses. It results from various types of mutations in the gene that encodes methyl CpG binding protein 2 (MeCP2), which is involved in binding to methylated DNA, modulating gene expression. It is most often seen in females, and it is thought to be most often fatal in boys, although cases of MeCP2 mutation in male infants and children with intellectual disability and other features have been identified. Another disorder of severe intellectual disability in females results from a mutation in the gene CDKLS.

73. You are seeing a 6-month-old boy with a 2-month history of irritability and hyper-startle responses that recently developed hypertonicity and was found to have a severe deficiency of galactosylceramide beta-galactosidase activity in his leukocytes?
What is your diagnosis?
A. GM1 gangliosidosis
B. Tay-Sacks disease
C. Globoid cell leukodystrophy
D. Sphingomyelin lipidosis

Correct Answer is: C
Globoid cell leukodystrophy, also referred to as Krabbe disease, is a rapidly progressive white matter demyelinating disorder that is transmitted by autosomal recessive inheritance of an enzyme defect in galactosylceramide beta-galactosidase. After 2–4 months after onset, the children typically regress and develop the position of opisthotonos.

GM1 gangliosidosis is caused by a defect in beta-glactosidase and presents with weakness and incoordination.

Tay-Sacks is caused by a deficiency in hexosaminase A and is associated with progressive cognitive function decline and severe spasticity by 1 year.

Sphingomyelin liposis is caused by a deficiency of sphingomyelinase that most commonly presents with feeding difficulty, failure to thrive and hepatosplenomegaly.

Suggested Reading

- Gieselmann V, Wenger DA, Krageloh-Mann I. Metachromatic Leukodystrophy and Globoid Cell Leukodystrophy. Lysosomal Storage Disorders: A Practical Guide, 2012. p. 70–9.

74. You are seeing a 5-month-old baby boy for psychomotor retardation. After birth, he was noticed to have prominent nystagmus, abnormal eye movements, and prominent incoordination. MRI demonstrates diffuse white matter changes sparing the U fibers, with a "tigroid" appearance.

3

Which statement is correct regarding this disorder?

A. It is inherited in an autosomal recessive fashion
B. The gene involved is PLP1
C. Central and peripheral myelin are affected
D. This patient has Alexander disease
E. The mutation is in the gene for glial fibrillary acidic protein (GFAP)

Correct Answer is: B

The presentation indicative of Pelizaeus-Merzbacher disease, which is a demyelinating disorder inherited in an X-linked recessive fashion. The gene involved is PLP1 on chromosome Xq22, and the mutation leads to abnormal synthesis of proteolipid protein 1. Mutations in this same gene also account for one form of hereditary spastic paraplegia. The onset of clinical manifestations is in the first few months of life, with intermittent nodding movements of the head, pendular nystagmus, and other abnormal eye movements. Ataxia, chorea, athetosis, dystonia, spasticity, and laryngeal strider also occur, and psychomotor development arrests with subsequent regression. Late manifestations include seizures and optic atrophy. Patients with later onset may have slower progression, and some patients survive into adulthood. The MRI demonstrates diffuse demyelination. Pathologically, there is a non-inflammatory demyelination sparing the U fibers and islands of white matter, giving it a "tigroid" appearance. Peripheral myelin is spared; and therefore, peripheral nerves are not involved. Genetic testing is available for diagnosis, and there is no specific treatment. This patient does not have Alexander disease, which is caused by a defect in the gene for glial fibrillary acidic protein (GFAP).

Suggested Reading

75. Which of the following statements is not true regarding Dandy-Walker malformation?

A. It includes cerebellar vermis hypoplasia
B. It includes fourth ventricle cystic dilatation
C. Lateral and third ventricular hydrocephalus is common
D. It may present in infancy with macrocephaly or may be asymptomatic into adulthood
E. It is associated with the "molar tooth sign" on imaging

Correct Answer is: E

The molar tooth sign is seen in various disorders associated with cerebellar hypoplasia, including Joubert syndrome, COACH syndrome (cerebellar vermis hypoplasia, oligophrenia, congenital ataxia, coloboma, and hepatic fibrocirrhosis), and Leber congenital amaurosis. However, this radiologic sign is not seen in Dandy-Walker malformation. Dandy-Walker malformation is characterized by cerebellar vermis hypoplasia, fourth ventricular cystic dilatation, and elevation of the torcula and the tentorium cerebelli. Posterior fossa enlargement and hydrocephalus are common. It is associated with various chromosomal anomalies. Neural tube defects, including encephalocele, and anomalies in other

organ systems, including the heart, may occur. Another association is with facial hemangiomas. Clinical presentation is variable and depends on the presence of hydrocephalus and associated anomalies. In severe forms, there is neonatal macrocephaly from hydrocephalus, brain stem dysfunction, and feeding and respiratory problems. Severe developmental delay and ataxia may be present. However, in other cases, no symptoms may be present and the malformation may be detected only incidentally on imaging in adulthood.

76. Globoid cells are characteristic of:
    - A. Metachromatic leukodystrophy
    - B. Krabbe disease
    - C. Zellweger syndrome
    - D. Adrenoleukodystrophy
    - E. Refsum disease

Correct Answer is: B

Krabbe disease, also known as globoid cell leukodystrophy, is a deficiency of galactosylceramide galactosidase.

This enzyme normally converts galactosylceramide to ceramide. Globoid cells are multinucleated macrophages that phagocytize the accumulated galactosylceramide in the CNS white matter. The disorder is inherited in an autosomal recessive manner, with mutations of chromosome 14. It results in fibrillary astrocytosis in regions of demyelination. In the infantile form, there is an exaggerated startle, low-grade fever, irritability, developmental regression, hyporeflexia, seizures, peripheral neuropathy, and spastic weakness resulting in opisthotonos. The juvenile form presents with cortical blindness, ataxia, developmental regression, and spasticity, in the absence of peripheral neuropathy. MRI is notable for diffuse demyelination.

Treatment is with bone marrow transplant prior to symptom onset.

Suggested Reading

- Fenichel GM. Clinical pediatric neurology. 5th ed. Philadelphia: Elsevier Saunders; 2005. p. 129, 140.

77. The triad of Kearns-Sayre Syndrome includes which visual abnormality?
    - A. Progressive external ophthalmoplegia
    - B. Bilateral optic neuropathy
    - C. Cortical blindness
    - D. Opsoclonus
    - E. Jerk nystagmus

Correct Answer is: A

Kearns-Sayre Syndrome (KSS) consists of the triad of: 1) Progressive external ophthalmoplegia (PEO), causing ptosis and impaired eye movements. 2) Onset prior to 20 years of age, and, 3) At least one of the following symptoms: short stature, pigmentary retinopathy, cerebellar ataxia, heart block, and/or elevated cerebrospinal protein levels. Patients may also have intellectual disability, muscle weakness, deafness, renal disease, and diabetes. Muscle biopsy reveals ragged red fibers. The disorder is caused by sporadic mutations of mitochondrial DNA.

Suggested Reading

- Verma A, Moraes CT. Mitochondrial disorders. In: Bradley WG, Daroff RB, Fenichel GM, Jankovic J, editors. Neurology in clinical practice. 4th ed. Elsevier, Inc.; 2004. p. 1833–46.
  ▶ http://ghr.nlm.nih.gov/condition/kearns-sayre-syndrome (▶ http://ghr.nlm.nih.Gov/condition/kearnssayre-syndrome). Reviewed 12/11. Published 5/26/14. Accessed 5/29/14.

78. Which of the following statements is not true regarding the abnormality depicted in the figure?

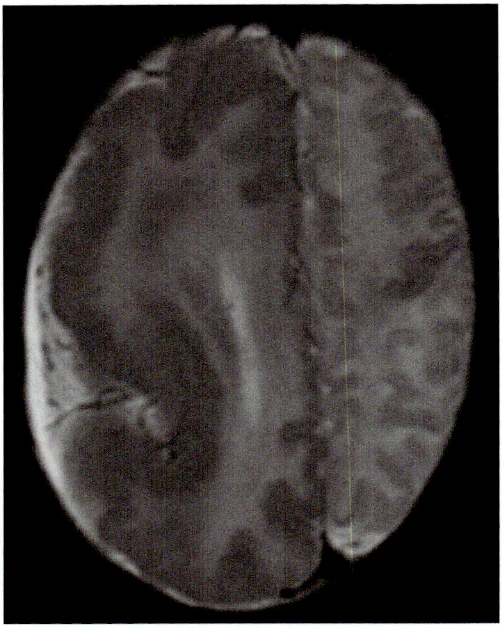

Fig. 3.25 With permission from ILAE.org. EpilepsyDiagnosis.org, Diagnostic Manual

A. Hemimegalencephaly frequently presents with seizures
B. Macrocephaly may be due to hydrocephalus or megalencephaly
C. Hemimegalencephaly rarely leads to motor manifestations
D. Megalencephaly is an oversized brain, with brain weight greater than 2 standard deviations above the mean
E. Megalencephaly may be a benign finding in some cases

Correct Answer is: C
This is the radiological manifestation of left hemispheric hemimegalencephaly, which frequently leads to contralateral hemiparesis. Microcephaly is defined as head circumference less than 2 standard deviations below the mean. A variety of causes of microcephaly exist. It can be a normal variant that is often hereditary, without clinical implications. When pathologic, causes include in utero infections, toxin exposure (such as alcohol, tobacco, and prescription drugs such as chemotherapeutic agents and anti-epileptics), hypoxic-ischemic injury, birth trauma, and metabolic disorders such as prolonged hypoglycemia. A wide variety of hereditary disorders including enzyme deficiencies can lead to microcephaly, as can chromosomal abnormalities. Clinical manifestations depend on the underlying cause and can range from none (asymptomatic microcephaly) to severe developmental delay and seizures. Macrocephaly is defined as a head circumference greater than 2 standard deviations above the mean. Macrocephaly may be a normal variant that is often hereditary, may result from increased CSF, as in hydrocephalus due to a variety of causes, from mass lesions such as tumors or subdural hematomas, or may result from megalencephaly, an oversized brain (brain weight greater than 2 standard deviations above the mean). Causes of megalencephaly include storage diseases such as mucopolysaccharidoses or Tay-Sachs disease, Canavan disease, Alexander disease, genetic disorders including Sotos syndrome, and others. In the latter disorders, eventual cell loss with subsequent atrophy typically occurs. Megalencephaly may also be a benign familial finding. Clinical manifestations depend on the underlying cause. Neurologic deficits may be absent in the benign familial form. Hemimegalencephaly, or enlargement of only one brain hemisphere, as in this case, invariably presents with seizures and hemiparesis. Hemimegalencephaly is associated with various genetic dis-

orders, including Beckwith-Wiedemann syndrome, which is characterized by gigantism, macroglossia, and midline abdominal wall defects.

79. You are evaluating a previously healthy 8-year-old boy for his abnormal gait, in the last few months he has been "walking funny". His mother reports that he has been clumsier, tripping frequently as well. The child started to have slurred speech a week ago. On exam, he has a wide-based slow gait and steppage gait. His motor strength in the distal lower extremities is 2/5 and proximal is 3/5. Lower extremity DTRs are absent. There is an extensor plantar response, and his feet are significant for high plantar arches. He has scoliosis on spine exam.
In what way this disorder is acquired?
A. X-linked
B. Autosomal dominant
C. Autosomal recessive
D. Post-infectious
E. Random (non-infectious and non-genetic)

Correct Answer is: C
This is a Friedreich's Atax ia (FA) case. It is an autosomal recessive disease caused by a mutation on chromosome 9 in the gene encoding the protein frataxin. Therefore, it occurs in males and females equally. An important thing to know is that it is the only disease caused by a GAA trinucleotide repeat. The more GAA repeats, the more profound the deficit in frataxin protein. Patients with Friedreich's Ataxia usually present between the ages of 5–15, though cases do occur even younger than this. Late-onset FA usually presents in the 2nd or 3rd decades. Presenting symptoms and signs include ataxia, motor weakness, scoliosis/kyphoscoliosis, dysarthria, high arches or pes cavus, diabetes in 20%, dysphagia, absent DTRs, muscle wasting, an extensor plantar response, nystagmus, cardiac involvement (cardiomegaly, cardiomyopathy). Treatment is symptomatic, and aims to support and maintain ambulation as long as possible. Most patients with FA are wheelchair-bound by age 15.

80. You are seeing a 9-month-old baby for his significant developmental delay with psychomotor retardation and failure to thrive. On examination, he also has a cherry-red spot on retinal examination and hepatosplenomegaly. Bone marrow specimen demonstrates foam cells. He carries a diagnosis is of Niemann-Pick disease.
What is correct regarding this diagnosis?
A. This patient has Niemann-Pick Type A
B. This patient has Niemann-Pick Type C
C. The activity of the enzyme acid sphingomyelinase is increased
D. The cause is a defect in intracellular cholesterol trafficking
E. Interstitial lung disease does not occur in any of the types of Niemann Pick disease

Correct Answer is: A
This patient has Niemann-Pick type A. Niemann-Pick types A and B are caused by acid sphingomyelinase deficiency, leading to accumulation of sphingomyelin. This disorder is autosomal recessive. Type A involves the CNS and other viscera and manifests in infancy with feeding difficulty, failure to thrive, psychomotor retardation with regression, hypotonia, and failure to thrive. Cherry-red spot is com-

monly seen, and these patients have massive hepatosplenomegaly. Most children die by age 3. Type B is purely visceral and does not affect the CNS, presenting with hepatosplenomegaly and interstitial lung disease. In both types, bone marrow biopsy will demonstrate vacuolated histiocytes with lipid accumulation and foam cells, in which the sphingomyelin adopts the form of concentric lamellar bodies. The foamy histiocytes can be seen also in the spleen, lymph nodes, hepatic sinusoids, and pulmonary alveoli. The diagnosis is based on detecting deficient activity of acid sphingomyelinase.

81. A 5-year-old boy with a history of progressive neurologic deterioration. Symptoms started around 1 year of age with hypotonia and inability to walk, with subsequent visual and hearing loss. He is now unable to walk and has generalized spasticity and cognitive regression. Brain MRI shows T2 hyper intense signal changes in the periventricular and subcortical white matter sparing the U fibers. Arylsulfatase A deficiency is detected on leukocyte analysis.

    What is the most likely diagnosis?

    A. Metachromatic leukodystrophy
    B. Niemann-Pick Type C
    C. Niemann-Pick Type A
    D. Krabbe disease
    E. Tay-Sachs disease

Correct Answer is: A

Metachromatic leukodystrophy is an autosomal recessive disorder caused by deficiency of the lysosomal enzyme arylsulfatase A with accumulation of sulfatide, resulting in demyelination of the central and peripheral nervous system. There are three forms: an infantile form with onset between 1 and 3 years of age, a juvenile form with onset in late childhood and early teens, and the adult form with onset in the 20s or 30s. The infantile form manifests with clumsiness, frequent falls, slurred speech, and is associated with weakness and hypotonia. With progression of the disease, these children are unable to stand, and their tone increases. They have loss of vision and hearing, peripheral neuropathy, and progressive deterioration of mental function to a vegetative state and death. The juvenile form has a slower progression. The adult form presents with behavioral changes, psychosis, and dementia. MRI demonstrates T2 hyper-intense signal changes in periventricular and subcortical white matter, sparing the U fibers. Cerebellar white matter is also involved. Pathologically, there are confluent symmetric lesions in the white matter and later atrophy. Central and peripheral demyelination is seen, with accumulation of metachromatic material in macrophages. Nerve conduction velocities are initially normal, but slowing is seen later in the course. The diagnosis is suspected on the basis of typical MRI findings and confirmed by demonstrating deficiency of arylsulfatase A in leukocytes and/or fibroblasts. Treatment is supportive. Niemann-Pick Type C is a disorder of intracellular cholesterol trafficking. Niemann-Pick Type A is caused by acid sphingomyelinase deficiency disease is caused by deficiency of galactosylceramidase. Tay-Sachs disease is caused by hexosaminidase A deficiency.

Suggested Reading

- Comprehensive Review in Clinical Neurology: A Multiple-Choice Question Book for the Wards and Boards ©2011 Wolters Kluwer Health Lippincott Williams & Wilkins. All rights reserved.

82. Which of the following is not true regarding abetalipoproteinemia or Bassen Kornzweig syndrome?
    A. It is autosomal dominant
    B. There is demyelination of the posterior columns of the spinal cord
    C. There is demyelination of peripheral nerves
    D. There is vitamin E deficiency
    E. It is associated with fat malabsorption

Correct Answer is: A
Abetalipoproteinemia, or Bassen-Kornzweig syndrome, is an autosomal recessive disorder caused by a molecular defect in the gene for the microsomal triglyceride transfer protein, which is localized to chromosome 4q22.24. This protein normally catalyzes the transport of triglyceride, cholesteryl ester, and phospholipid from phospholipid surfaces. The defect of this protein results in fat malabsorption and liposoluble vitamin deficiency, especially of vitamin E, which is the culprit of most of the clinical manifestations. This condition manifests since birth, with failure to thrive, vomiting, and loose stool. During infancy, there is progressive psychomotor retardation with cerebellar ataxia and gait disturbance. Proprioceptive sensation is lost in the hands and feet, with less compromise of pinprick and temperature sensation. Deep tendon reflexes are depressed. This is likely from demyelination of posterior columns and peripheral nerves. Visual disturbance is the result of retinitis pigmentosa, and nystagmus is common. Laboratory studies demonstrate acanthocytosis, absence of very low-density lipoproteins, absence of apolipoprotein B, low levels of vitamin E, and severe anemia. Treatment involves the restriction of triglycerides in the diet, and large doses of vitamin E with supplementation of vitamins A, D, and K.

83. Which of the following gene is implicated in congenital neuronal ceroid lipofuscinosis?
    A. Ceroid lipofuscinosis neuronal 2 (CLN2)
    B. Ceroid lipofuscinosis, neuronal 3 (CLN3)
    C. Ceroid lipofuscinosis, neuronal 6 (CLN6)
    D. Ceroid lipofuscinosis, neuronal 8 (CLN8)
    E. Ceroid lipofuscinosis, neuronal 10 (CLN10)

Correct Answer is: E
Ceroid lipofuscinosis, neuronal 10 (CLN10) codes for the lysosomal aspartic protease cathepsin D; CLN10 is also referred to as Cathepsin D (CTSD). This is diagnosed in the neonatal period and patients often pass away within the first week. Seizures, microcephaly, and a lack of reflexes may be present.

The infantile form of neuronal ceroid lipofuscinosis is caused by mutations in CN1; onset is usually within the first year of life. This is characterized by visual loss, seizures, cognitive decline, motor decline, and spasticity. Alterations in the same gene are implicated in a form of late infantile onset disease; additionally, alterations in this gene may lead to a form of adult onset disease.

Mutations affecting CLN6 (also referred to as CLN4) are implicated in both a late infantile or adult variation of this disease (also called Kufs disease). In addition to CLN6/CLN4, mutations in DnaJ heat shock protein family (Hsp40) member CS (DANJCS) lead to an adult onset form of the disease. The latter is inherited in an autosomal dominant manner.

Mutations in CLN8 lead to late infantile onset disease. This often starts with seizures, occurring prior to the age of 10,

with decline of motor and cognitive function and visual loss. Defects in this gene can also cause prominent myoclonic seizures with cognitive and motor decline; in the latter phenotype, visual loss may not be present.

3

Suggested Reading

- National Library of Medicine (US). Genetics Home Reference [Internet]. Bethesda (MD): The Library; 2015 Dec 7. CTSD; [reviewed 2013 Jul; cited 2015 Dec 13); Available from: ► http://ghr.nlm.nih.gov/condition/congenital-neuronal-ceroid-lipofuscinosis (► http://ghr.nlm.nih.gov/condition/congenital-neuronal-ceroid-lipofuscinosis).
- National Library of Medicine (US). Genetics Home Reference [Internet]. Bethesda (MD): The Library; 2015 Dec 7. PPT1; [reviewed 2013 Aug; cited 2015 Dec 13]; ► http://ghr.nlm.nih.gov/gene/PPT1 (► http://ghr.nlm.nih.gov/gene/PPT1).
- National Library of Medicine (US). Genetics Home Reference [Internet]. Bethesda (MD): The Library; 2015 Dec 7. TPP1; [reviewed 2013 Aug; cited 2015 Dec 13]; ► http://ghr.nlm.nih.gov/gene/TPP1 (► http://ghr.nlm.nih.gov/gene/TPP1).
- National Library of Medicine (US). Genetics Home Reference [Internet]. Bethesda (MD): The Library; 2015 Dec 7. CLN3; [reviewed 2013 Aug; cited 2015 Dec 13]; ► http://ghr.nlm.nih.gov/gene/CLN3 (► http://ghr.nlm.nih.gov/gene/CLN3).
- National Library of Medicine (US). Genetics Home Reference [Internet]. Bethesda (MD): The Library; 2015 Dec 7. CLN6; [reviewed 2013 Sept; cited 2015 Dec 13); ► http://ghr.nlm.nih.gov/gene/CLN6 (► http://ghr.nlm.nih.Gov/gene/CLN6).

? 84. Which of the following options is true regarding Leigh disease?

A. It is a static encephalopathy
B. It is due to mitochondrial abnormalities
C. It is inherited in an autosomal recessive fashion
D. Lactate levels are reduced during episodic exacerbations
E. Clinical manifestations most commonly begin during late childhood

✓ **Correct Answer is: B**

Leigh disease or acute necrotizing encephalomyelopathy is a manifestation of mitochondrial disorders that can be sporadic or familial, with only some cases with the typical maternal inheritance pattern. This condition affects neurons of the brain stem, thalamus, basal ganglia, and cerebellum. Most of the affected patients have onset of neurologic manifestations in the first year of life, but there are forms with late onset. Clinical features manifest with decompensation associated with intercurrent illnesses. In infancy, patients present with hypotonia, loss of head control, poor sucking, vomiting, irritability, seizures, and myoclonic jerks. If the onset is beyond the first year, patients present with gait disturbance, cerebellar ataxia, dysarthria, psychomotor retardation, spasticity, external ophthalmoplegia, and nystagmus, abnormal movements with chorea or dystonias, and peripheral neuropathy in some cases with autonomic failure. The disorder is progressive with episodic deterioration. Lactate level is increased in blood and CSF. Lactate and pyruvate levels in blood are elevated during exacerbations. MRI of the brain demonstrates bilateral symmetric hyperintense T2 signal abnormalities in the brain stem and/or basal ganglia, and in some cases in the spinal cord. Treatment is supportive and symptomatic.

Suggested Reading

- Comprehensive Review in Clinical Neurology: A Multiple-Choice Question Book for the Wards and Boards © 2011 Wolters Kluwer Health Lippincott Williams & Wilkins. All rights reserved.

85. You are seeing a 17-month-old boy with a history of progressive motor dysfunction with hypotonia, started at 5 months. He lost his vision at 12 months of age and he now has refractory seizures. Neuronal ceroid lipofuscinosis is suspected.
Which protein is most likely abnormal in this case?
   A. Palmityl protein thioesterase 1 (PPT)
   B. Tripeptidyl peptidase 1 (TPP1)
   C. Cathepsin D (CTSD)
   D. Cysteine string protein alpha

Correct Answer is: A
The patient most likely has the infantile form of neuronal ceroid lipofuscinosis based on the age of onset and manifestations described above. This is caused by a mutation in ceroid lipofuscinosis 1 (CLN1) which codes for the protein palmitoyl-protein thioesterase. The gene is also referred to as palmitoyl-protein thioesterase 1 (PPT1). Clinical features are usually present by 6 months of age and patients typically die within the first decade of life. Patients usually have seizures, microcephaly, hypotonia, and visual loss. Defects in the same gene can lead to later onset disease, with symptoms appearing between ages 2 and 4; seizures, developmental arrest, and visual loss may be present. CLN1 mutations may lead to another, late onset form of the disease starting during adulthood (usually after age 19) with decline in cognitive function, visual loss, ataxia, and Parkinsonism.

Defects in Tripeptidyl peptidase 1 (TTP1) caused by mutations in CLN2 (also referred to as Tripeptidyl peptidase I (TPP1)) lead to the late infantile neuronal ceroid lipofuscinosis. Patients between the ages of 2 and 4 present with generalized tonic clonic, absence, or myoclonic seizures. Deterioration of cognitive function, visual loss, and ataxia are also present and death may occur by age 15. Mutations in this gene do not typically lead to the earlier onset, infantile form of the disease.

Mutations in CLN10 lead to dysfunction of Cathepsin D resulting in a congenital form of the disease. Patients usually die in the neonatal period and present with microcephaly and respiratory troubles. Mutations in CLN 10 do not typically causes the infantile form of the disease. Mutations in DNAJCS, coding for cysteine string protein alpha (CSPa) lead to an autosomal dominant adult onset disease. This starts after age 30 and visual loss is usually not present.

Mutations in ceroid lipofuscinosis neuronal 4 (CLN4) were initially thought to underlie most adult onset disease. It was then discovered that the gene affected is the same as that causing a late infantile onset variant of ceroid lipofuscinosis, (CLN6). Mutations in DNAJCS do not typically cause infantile onset disease.

86. Mutations of the ALD (ABCD1) gene are most likely to cause:
   A. Frontal white matter abnormalities
   B. CNS and renal neoplasms
   C. A deficiency of very long chain fatty acids
   D. Cerebral inflammatory demyelination
   E. Infantile hypotonia

Correct Answer is: D
Mutations of the ALD (ABCD1) gene on the X chromosome causes adrenoleukodystrophy. The gene encodes a peroxisomal protein (ALDP) involved very long chain fatty acid (VLCFA) oxidative degradation. Mutations lead to an accumulation of VLCFAs, and adrenal failure with a deficiency of androgens and glucocorticoids. This results in perivascular lymphocytes, and demyelination, beginning in the parietal and occipital lobes and sparing arcuate fibers. MRI demon-

strates T2-weighted hyper-intensities of the posterior white matter. Several clinical phenotypes may result, including childhood onset, adolescent onset, adult onset, adrenomyeloneuropathy, Addison's disease only, and women with symptomatic X-ALD.

1. **Childhood onset adrenoleukodystrophy: The age of onset ranges from 2.5–10 years. Symptoms include extensive CNS demyelination, hyperactivity, dementia, ataxia, vision loss, hearing deficits, and seizures, with endocrine dysfunction. The course is rapidly progressive.**
2. **Adolescent onset adrenoleukodystrophy: Symptoms become evident between ages 10 and 21 years, and are rapidly progressive, with CNS demyelination, behavioral and cognitive changes, and endocrine dysfunction.**
3. **Adult onset adrenoleukodystrophy: This phenotype consists of a rapidly progressive dementia, psychiatric changes (e.g. psychosis, affective disorders), CNS demyelination, endocrine dysfunction, and possible myelopathy or neuropathy.**
4. **Adrenomyeloneuropathy: The age of onset is typically in early adulthood with a progressive spastic paraparesis, bowel and bladder incontinence, sexual dysfunction, mild dementia, and psychiatric changes (i.e. affective disorders),as well as sensorimotor, primarily axonal neuropathy. This phenotype may be either slowly or rapidly progressive.**
5. **An Addison's only phenotype consists of isolated adrenal dysfunction.**
6. **Heterozygous females typically develop symptoms by age 60. The disorder is slowly progressive, and may present with peripheral neuropathy, fecal incontinence, and pain in the legs. White matter lesions and endocrine dysfunction are rare.**

Treatment for adrenoleukodystrophy involves glucocorticoids and bone marrow transplant. Dietary fatty acid supplementation ("Lorenzo's oil"), has been used, but with limited data to suggest efficacy.

Suggested Reading

- Engelen M, et al. X-linked adrenoleukodystrophy (X-ALD): clinical presentation and guidelines for diagnosis, follow-up and management. Orphanet J Rare Dis. 2012;7:51. Rai PVS, et al. Childhood adrenoleukodystrophy – Classic and variant – Review of clinical manifestations and magnetic resonance imaging. J Pediatr Neurosci. 2013;8(3):192–7.

87. You are evaluating an 8-year-old female with a history of multiple complaints gradually worsening over the last few months. She has chronic pain and numbness in her hands and feet that feels like "burning achy pins and needles". Also, she has chronic abdominal pains and diarrhea and feels her vision "isn't so good sometimes". She has kidney dysfunction by laboratory investigation.
What is your diagnosis?
A. Raynaud phenomenon
B. Multiple sclerosis
C. Fabry disease
D. Rheumatic fever
E. Lupus

Correct Answer is: C
Fabry disease in children can present with acroparesthesias, GI symptoms/pain, corneal opacity, hypohydrosis, angiokeratomas (which are often mistaken for petechiae), and tinnitus or hearing loss. It is an X-linked recessive disorder which often manifests variably severe symptoms even in heterozygous females (X-linked recessive with incomplete penetrance in heterozygous

females), and is caused by accumulation of a glycoprotein called globotriaosylceramide caused by a deficiency of alpha galactosidase A (AGA). It occurs in 1/40,000–120,000 live births. Renal and cardiac involvement is fairly common and are common causes of death in these patients, and many end up on dialysis or with renal transplants.

88. You are seeing a 6-month-old boy for his intractable seizures. On examination, he has a short small chin, thin upper lip, and low-set ears. He has spastic quadriparesis and requires a feeding tube because of recurrent aspirations. His brain MRI shows essentially smooth frontal, parietal, and occipital lobes, with a thick cortex and without sulci or gyri.
What is your most likely diagnosis?
A. Miller-Dieker syndrome
B. Lissencephaly type II
C. Subcortical band heterotopias
D. Cobblestone lissencephaly
E. Polymicrogyria

Correct Answer is: A
The clinical and radiological presentation consistent with Miller-Dieker syndrome, a form of lissencephaly type I. In lissencephaly type I (classic lissencephaly), the cortex is thick but consists of only four layers or less (often two or three layers, as opposed to the normal six neocortical layers). Lissencephaly is a malformation of cortical development resulting from abnormal neuronal migration resulting in impaired formation of gyri. It is characterized by the presence of reduced cortical gyration and, in the most severe form, no gyri, or agyria, resulting in a smooth brain. Associated malformations may include agenesis of the corpus callosum or hypoplasia of the cerebellum, with sparing of the thalamus and basal ganglia.

Miller-Dieker syndrome (MOS), one form of lissencephaly type I, is characterized by lissencephaly associated with microcephaly, typical facies including micrognathia, low-set ears, thin upper lip, and other features. Clinical manifestations include global developmental delay, hypotonia and later spasticity, and intractable seizures. Life expectancy is often not beyond 1 year. MDS has been associated with microdeletions on chromosome 17 in the LIS1 gene. LIS1 gene encodes a protein involved in regulation of microtubules and dynein function, and mutations interfere with microtubule-directed migration of neurons from the ventricular zone. Mutations in LIS1 gene can also lead to isolated lissencephaly (so-called isolated lissencephaly sequence, without other features of MDS). X-linked lissencephaly is another form that results from mutations in the DCX gene on chromosome X when occurring in males. This gene encodes for the protein doublecortin, which is involved in microtubule organization and stabilization. In another form of Lissencephaly that results from mutations in the gene ARX, which encodes for a transcription factor involved in non-radial migration of cortical interneurons, the basal ganglia are abnormal in addition to the cortex and corpus callosum. In some forms of lissencephaly, there may be an anterior to posterior (or vice versa) gradient of gyral formation (e.g. with some gyral formation in the anterior or posterior aspects of the brain). Cobblestone lissencephaly, also known as lissencephaly type II, is seen in several disorders including Walker-Warburg syndrome, Fukuyama muscular dystrophy, and muscle-eye-brain disease of Santavuori. In polymicrogyria, there are excess, abnormal gyri. Subcortical band heterotopia, also known as "double cortex"

syndrome, refers to a band of subcortical heterotopia neurons, located midway between the ventricles and the cerebral cortex. The disorder is seen primarily in females and typically causes varying degrees of intellectual disability and almost all of them have epilepsy.

89. Which of the following statements is not true regarding disorders that involve the skin and CNS?
    A. Multiple intracranial arteriovenous malformations are a manifestation of hereditary hemorrhagic telangiectasia (Osler-Weber-Rendu syndrome)
    B. Patients with pseudoxanthoma elasticum are at increased risk of cerebral arterial occlusive disease
    C. Ehlers-Danlos syndrome is associated with increased risk of intracranial aneurysms and carotid dissection
    D. Xeroderma pigmentosa is associated with peripheral neuropathy, cognitive decline, ataxia, and hyperkinetic involuntary movements
    E. Fabry disease is a multiorgan disorder associated with neuropathy and cerebral artery ectasia and results from a defect in the enzyme sphingomyelinase

Correct Answer is: E
Fabry disease is an X-linked disorder that results from a mutation in the gene encoding the lysosomal enzyme A-galactosidase. Multiple organs are involved; renal involvement leads to renal failure and cardiac involvement to cardiomyopathy. Cutaneous manifestations in Fabry disease include purplish angiokeratomas often occurring in the groin. Neurologic manifestations involve both the peripheral nervous system (including small fiber neuropathy with attacks of cold-induced painful paresthesia in the extremities, acroparesthesias) and the CNS.CNS manifestations include stroke and other vascular events related to vascular ectasia, with often marked dolichoectatic enlargement of the basilar artery.

Hereditary hemorrhagic telangiectasia, or Osler-Weber-Rendu syndrome, is an autosomal dominant disorder in which telangiectasia occurs in the skin, mucous membranes, and several organs including the retina and gastrointestinal tract. Recurrent epistaxis is a common manifestation. CNS involvement results from single or multiple arteriovenous malformations (AVMs) or cerebral embolization from pulmonary AVMs. It results from a mutation in the HHT1 gene on chromosome 9 that encodes for endoglin, a protein that binds transforming growth factor-B (TGF-B},or from a mutation in the HHT2 gene on chromosome 12. Wyburn-Mason syndrome is another neurocutaneous disorder in which multiple AVMs occur on the face, in the retina, and intracranially. In pseudoxanthoma elasticum (Gronblad Strandberg syndrome), a connective tissue disorder that may be autosomal dominant or recessive, yellowish xanthomas occur in various skin regions, on mucous membranes, and in the retina. Neurological manifestations relate to vascular occlusions and intracranial carotid artery aneurysms.

Ehlers-Danlos syndrome exists in 10 subtypes, with types I, II, and III being the most common. These subtypes share the occurrence of hyperelastic skin, hyper extensible joints, and vascular lesions. This syndrome results from mutations in various genes encoding for different types of collagen. The main neurologic significance of this disorder is the increased risk of intracranial aneurysms, carotid-cavernous fistulas (that may be spontaneous or due to mild trauma), and arterial dissection.

Xeroderma pigmentosum (XP) is a neurocutaneous disorder marked by sensitivity to ultraviolet light that predisposes affected individuals to skin freckling and multiple cutaneous malignancies including melanoma, basal cell carcinoma, and squamous cell carcinoma as well as other cutaneous and systemic tumors. Neurologic abnormalities include progressive cognitive dysfunction, hearing loss, tremor, chorea, and ataxia as well as peripheral neuropathy.

XP is autosomal recessive and results from mutations on chromosome 9 that result in abnormal DNA repair. Cockayne syndrome is a related disorder. Another disorder of DNA repair associated with neurologic features is ataxia telangiectasia.

Suggested Reading

- Comprehensive Review in Clinical Neurology: A Multiple-Choice Question Book for the Wards and Boards

90. You are evaluating an 11-month-old baby for regression started at 6 months of age. Initially, she had gained some developmental milestones. On examination, she has coarse facial features, generalized spasticity, and motor impairment. A retinal picture is shown in the Figure. Enzymatic analysis showed a B-galactosidase deficiency in leukocytes.

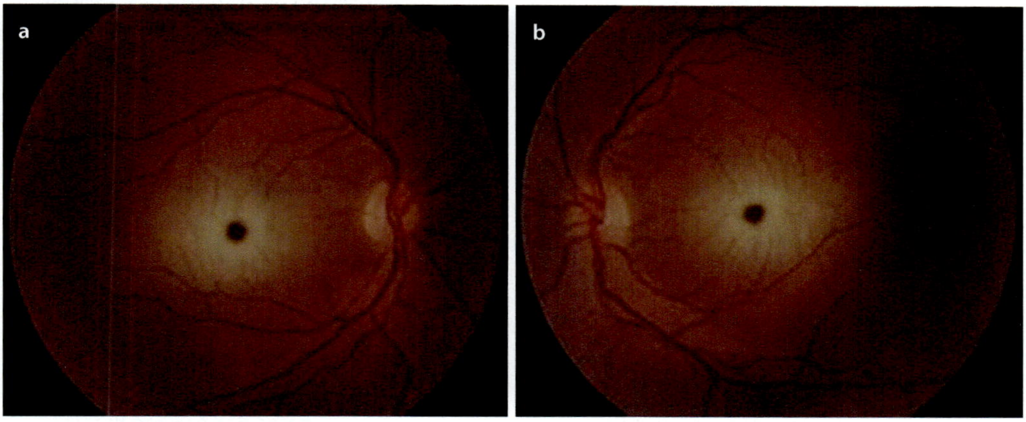

Fig. 3.26 **a** and **b** showing the accumulation of the gangliosides in the retina. JAMA Ophthalmology. Wikipedia

Which statement is correct?

A. This patient has GM2 gangliosidosis
B. Gangliosides accumulate in the brain and visceral organs
C. Sandhoff disease is caused by this enzymatic deficiency
D. Tay-Sachs disease is caused by this enzymatic deficiency
E. Mucopolysacchariduria is common

Correct Answer is: B

91. You are evaluating an 18-year-old male in hospital with a 12-h history of right-sided headache, nausea and light sensitivity, and had a generalized tonic-clonic seizure shortly before admission. His past medical history is remarkable for migraine. His family history is remarkable of a sister with history of diabetes mellitus, his mother and a maternal aunt had had strokes in their 40s. On examination, he was confused

with a GCS of 11. He had a left-sided homonymous hemianopia. Blood pressure was 175/95 mmHg but there were no other abnormalities. Work-up revealed: CBC/Electrolytes/ESR – Normal, Lactic acid – 14.2 mmol/L, Blood Glucose – Normal, MRI brain w/o contrast – Diffusion restriction on DWI in the right occipital lobe which appears hypo-intense on ADC.

What is your most likely diagnosis?

A. Familial hemiplegic migraine
B. Venous sinus thrombosis
C. cerebral autosomal dominant arteriopathy with subcortical infarcts and leukoencephalopathy
D. Mitochondrial encephalomyopathy with lactic acidosis and stroke-like episodes
E. Cerebral vasculitis

Correct Answer is: D

This is a clinical presentation of mitochondrial encephalomyopathy with lactic acidosis and stroke like episodes. Stroke like episodes are the hallmark feature of this disorder. Stroke like episodes may present with convulsions, visual abnormalities, numbness, hemiplegia, and aphasia. Episodes may be followed by transient hemiplegia or hemianopia, which lasts a few hours to several weeks. Patients may also experience episodes of seizures and visual abnormalities followed by hemiplegia.

Migraine or migraine-like headaches observed in these patients may also reflect the stroke like episodes. Pedigrees of patients with classic MELAS syndrome identify many members whose only manifestations are migraine headaches. Patients may have visual complaints due to ophthalmoplegia, and they may experience blindness because of optic atrophy and difficulties with night vision due to pigmentary retinopathy. Myopathy presents with hypotonia and weakness. Proximal muscles tend to be more involved than distal muscles. Additional features on neurologic examination may include ataxia, tremor, myoclonus, and dystonia, visual disturbances, and cortical blindness. Some patients may present with ophthalmoplegia and ptosis. On ophthalmologic examination, patients have presented with pigmentary retinopathy. Sensorineural deafness has been reported as part of the disorder in approximately 25% of patients with MELAS syndrome.

Cardiomyopathy with signs of congestive heart failure (CHF) may also be observed upon physical examination. Short stature may be the first manifestation of MELAS syndrome in many patients. Familial hemiplegic migraine may present in a similar manner but is not associated with seizures. Although subtle changes on MR imaging have been reported those shown here are far too extensive. Cerebral venous thrombosis may be clinically indistinguishable from this case, though the family history is not explained. MR findings are usually that of a hemorrhagic infarct not pertaining to a single arterial territory and CSF opening pressures were not elevated in this case. A diagnosis of CADASIL would be consistent with recurrent migraine and a dominant family history. Imaging in CADASIL shows deep white matter abnormalities, in contrast to the findings in this patient.

Suggested Reading

- Testai FD, Gorelick PB. Inherited metabolic disorders and stroke part 1: Fabry disease and mitochondrial myopathy, encephalopathy, lactic acidosis, and stroke like episodes. Arch Neurol. 2010;67(1):19–24.
- Scarpelli M, Zappini F, Filosto M, Russignan A, Tonin P, Tomelleri G. Mitochondrial sensorineural hearing loss: a retrospective study and a description of cochlear implantation in a MELAS patient. Genet Res Int. 2012;2012:287432.

- Singmaneesakulchai S, Limotai N, Jagota P, Bhidayasiri R. Expanding spectrum of abnormal movements in MELAS syndrome (mitochondrial encephalomyopathy, lactic acidosis, and stroke-like episodes). Mov Disord. Oct 2012;27(12):1495–7.
- Fayssoil A. Heart diseases in mitochondrial encephalomyopathy, lactic acidosis, and stroke syndrome. Congest Heart Fail. 2009;15(6):284–7.

92. Physical complications of spina bifida include which of the following?
    A. Allergy to latex
    B. Leg weakness and paralysis
    C. Club foot
    D. (B) and (C)
    E. (A) and (C)

Correct Answer is: E
68% of children with spina bifida have an allergy to latex, ranging from mild to life-threatening. The common use of latex in medical facilities makes this a particularly serious concern. Leg paralysis or weakness and orthopedic abnormalities such as club foot, hip dislocation or scoliosis, and urinary and bowel control problems are frequently present.

93. You are seeing an 8-year-old boy with a short stature due to growth hormone deficiency and is also being treated for hypothyroidism. He has a normal motor and cognitive development. He has reduced visual acuity. He has an absence of the septum pellucidum and hypoplasia of the optic nerves and chiasm on his MRI. The cortex and other areas appear normal. **What is your most likely diagnosis?**
    A. Holoprosencephaly
    B. Septo-optic dysplasia
    C. Lissencephaly
    D. Arrhinencephaly
    E. Cavum septum pellucidum

Correct Answer is: B
This is a clinical and radiological manifestations of septo-optic dysplasia. The malformations include hypoplasia or absence of the septum pellucidum, optic nerve and optic chiasm hypoplasia, dysgenesis of the corpus callosum and anterior commissure, and fornix detachment from the corpus callosum. Arrhinencephaly (agenesis of only the olfactory bulb and tract) and/or hypothalamic hamartomas may be associated features. Other less commonly associated abnormalities include cerebellar vermis defects and hydrocephalus. Septo-optic dysplasia can also be associated with lobar holoprosencephaly and other malformations of cortical development. Clinical manifestations include vision loss, ataxia when the cerebellum is involved, and symptoms of hydrocephalus when it is present, and endocrinology disturbances. Endocrinology disturbances can range from pan-hypopituitarism to isolated hormone deficiencies. Mutations in the transcription factors HESX1, a homeobox gene, and SOX may be implicated in this disorder. Cavum septum pellucidum, in which the septum pellucidum is not fused but rather exists in two separate pieces of tissue, is considered non-pathologic, with little clinical implications. The presence of normal cortex excludes holoprosencephaly, and lissencephaly. This patient has several features making septo-optic dysplasia the likely diagnosis rather than arrhinencephaly.

Suggested Reading

- Comprehensive Review in Clinical Neurology: A Multiple-Choice Question Book for the Wards and Boards © 2011 Wolters Kluwer Health Lippincott Williams & Wilkins. All rights reserved.

3

94. You are evaluating a 5-year-old boy with a history of behavioral problems with aggressiveness for 1 year. He has also had progressive cognitive deterioration and spasticity and visual loss. Plasma levels of very long-chain fatty acids are elevated, and MRI shows white matter T2 hyper-intensities, which are symmetric, involving posterior regions, and sparing the U fibers.

What is the most likely diagnosis?

A. Canavan disease
B. Adrenoleukodystrophy
C. Alexander disease
D. Zellweger syndrome
E. Fabry disease

Correct Answer is: B

Adrenoleukodystrophy is an X-linked disorder caused by a deficiency of the peroxisomal enzyme acyl coenzyme A synthetase, leading to the impaired ability to oxidize very long-chain fatty acids, with subsequent accumulation in tissues and plasma. There are four phenotypes: childhood cerebral type, adrenomyeloneuropathy, pure adrenal insufficiency, or asymptomatic. Female carriers may have mild symptoms of adrenomyeloneuropathy.

The cerebral type has an onset between 4 and 8 years of age, with behavioral changes progressing to cognitive impairment, spasticity, disturbances of gait and coordination, and vision and hearing loss. The prognosis is poor, and these patients die early. MRI demonstrates confluent T2 hyper-intensity in the white matter affecting more predominantly the parieto-occipital regions and the posterior corpus callosum. Pathologically, there is symmetric and confluent demyelination affecting initially the posterior regions and sparing the U fibers. There is involvement of other tissues, including the adrenal cortex and Leydig cells of the testis. Histopathological, cerebral lesions are characterized by the presence of perivascular cuffing, with predominance of T cells.

Adrenomyeloneuropathy is the most common phenotype and manifests with paraparesis that begins after age 20, and is slowly progressive into adulthood. There is also a sensory neuropathy in these patients. Some degree of cognitive impairment and adrenal insufficiency may be seen. Pathologically, there is long tract degeneration with axon and myelin loss. Peripheral nerve demyelination without inflammation also occurs. Patients with adrenoleukodystrophy have increased plasma levels of very long-chain fatty acids, and ACTH is increased secondary to adrenal insufficiency.

Treatment involves supportive care with steroid replacement therapy for adrenal insufficiency. "Lorenzo's oil", which consists of 4:1 glyceryl trioleate glyceryl trierucate, has been shown to reduce levels of very long-chain fatty acids in plasma. Dietary use of Lorenzo's oil may be beneficial in young asymptomatic patients but not in patients with neurologic deficits. Bone marrow transplantation may have a role in early stages of the disease.

95. You are evaluating a 3-year-old boy with a history of developmental delay and ataxia. On examination, he has extraocular muscle abnormalities, but visual acuity is unaffected and his irises appear normal. His brain MRI is shown in the figure.

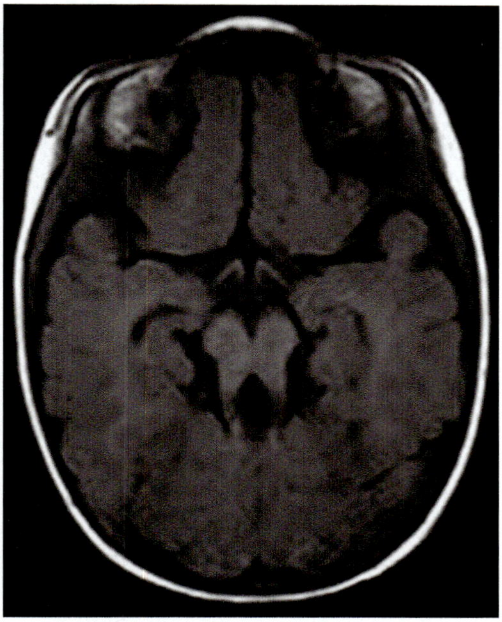

Fig. 3.27 Axial T2-weighted MRI. (Courtesy of Dr. Manikum Moodley and Dr. Gary Hsieh)

What is the most likely diagnosis?
A. Ataxia with oculomotor apraxia type I
B. Ataxia with oculomotor apraxia type II
C. Joubert syndrome
D. Leber congenital amaurosis
E. COACH syndrome

Correct Answer is: C
There is the molar tooth sign shown on the MRI, which results from cerebellar vermis hypoplasia with fourth ventricular enlargement, a large interpeduncular fossa, and abnormal superior cerebellar peduncles. It is seen in a variety of conditions associated with cerebellar hypoplasia, including Joubert syndrome. Joubert syndrome is an autosomal recessive disorder characterized clinically by developmental delay, ataxia, oculomotor abnormalities, and respiratory difficulties. The molar tooth sign is also seen in COACH syndrome (cerebellar vermis hypoplasia, oligophrenia, congenital ataxia, coloboma, and hepatic fibrosis), features of which are not present in this case. It is also seen in Leber congenital amaurosis, in which vision loss occurs due to rod and cone dystrophy. The molar tooth sign has not been associated with ataxia with oculomotor apraxia types I and II.

96. Which of the following statements is not true regarding polymicrogyria and schizencephaly?
A. Polymicrogyria is characterized by excessive abnormal gyri that are small and separated by shallow sulci
B. Schizencephaly is a deep cleft that extends from the pial surface to the ventricle and is lined with cortex
C. Polymicrogyria most often occurs in the perisylvian region
D. Porencephaly describes a type of schizencephaly
E. They are disorders of cortical organization

Correct Answer is: D
Porencephaly is distinguished from schizencephaly in that the cleft of schizencephaly is lined uniformly with gray matter. Porencephalic cysts are not due to malformations of cortical development but are rather CSF-filled cysts that most often result from in utero infarction or other insult. In malformations of cortical organization, neurons migrate relatively normally but formation of the cortical layers or cortical-cortical connections are

abnormal. These thus occur later in gestation. Malformations of cortical organization include polymicrogyria, in which there are excessive abnormal gyri that are small and separated by shallow sulci, and schizencephaly, a deep cleft that extends from the pial surface to the ventricle and is lined with cortex. These often co-occur in the same patient. Polymicrogyria can be unilateral or bilateral, generalized, perisylvian, predominantly frontal, or in a variety of other patterns. The perisylvian form is the most common. Polymicrogyria often occurs as part of various syndromes, either sporadically or in familial forms. Perisylvian polymicrogyria occurs particularly in the setting of peroxisomal disorders such as Zellweger syndrome. Several genetic mutations have been identified in association with polymicrogyria. Clinical manifestations depend on the location and the extent of the abnormality; epilepsy is common. Schizencephaly, or cleft brain, most often occurs in the perisylvian region but can occur anywhere. In closed-lip schizencephaly, the cerebral cortical walls on either side of the cleft are in contact. In open-lipped schizencephaly, the two walls are separated by CSF. Schizencephaly is most often an isolated finding or is associated with polymicrogyria but can rarely be seen in patients with septo optic dysplasia. Mutations in homeobox genes, which encode for transcription factors expressed during different times of embryologic development and modulate neuronal proliferation and migration, may be implicated in schizencephaly.

3

97. You are evaluating a 5-year-old boy for his progressive neurologic deterioration. It stared at 1 year of age with hypotonia and inability to walk, with subsequent visual and hearing loss. He is now unable to walk and has generalized spasticity and cognitive regression. There are T2 hyper-intense signal changes in the periventricular and subcortical white matter sparing the U fibers on brain MRI. Arylsulfatase A deficiency is detected on leukocyte analysis.

What is the most likely diagnosis?

A. Metachromatic leukodystrophy
B. Niemann-Pick Type C
C. Niemann-Pick Type A
D. Krabbe disease
E. Tay-Sachs disease

Correct Answer is: A

Metachromatic leukodystrophy is an autosomal recessive disorder caused by deficiency of the lysosomal enzyme arylsulfatase A with accumulation of sulfatide, resulting in demyelination of the central and peripheral nervous system. There are three forms: an infantile form with onset between 1 and 3 years of age, a juvenile form with onset in late childhood and early teens, and the adult form with onset in the 20s or 30s.

The infantile form manifests with clumsiness, frequent falls, slurred speech, and is associated with weakness and hypotonia. With progression of the disease, these children are unable to stand, and their tone increases. They have loss of vision and hearing, peripheral neuropathy, and progressive deterioration of mental function to a vegetative state and death.

The juvenile form has a slower progression.

The adult form presents with behavioral changes, psychosis, and dementia. MRI demonstrates T2 hyper-intense signal changes in periventricular and subcortical white matter, sparing the U fibers. Cerebellar white matter is also involved.

Pathologically, there are confluent symmetric lesions in the white matter and later atrophy. Central and peripheral

demyelination is seen, with accumulation of metachromatic material in macrophages.

Nerve conduction velocities are initially normal, but slowing is seen later in the course. The diagnosis is suspected on the basis of typical MRI findings and confirmed by demonstrating deficiency of arylsulfatase A in leukocytes and/or fibroblasts. Treatment is supportive.

Niemann-Pick Type C is a disorder of intracellular cholesterol trafficking. Niemann-Pick Type A is caused by acid sphingomyelinase deficiency disease is caused by deficiency of galactosylceramidase. Tay-Sachs disease is caused by hexosaminidase A deficiency.

98. You are seeing a 5-year-old girl with a history of intractable seizures. On examination, she has spastic quadriparesis and requires a feeding tube because of recurrent aspirations. Her brain MRI is shown.

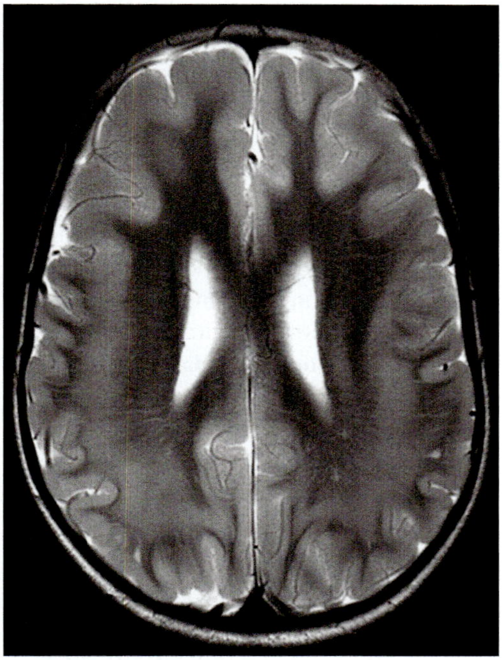

Fig. 3.28 With permission from ILAE.org. EpilepsyDiagnosis.org, Diagnostic Manual

What is your diagnosis?

A. Miller-Dieker syndrome
B. Lissencephaly type 11
C. Subcortical band heterotopia
D. Cobblestone lissencephaly
E. Polymicrogyria

Correct Answer is: C

The MRI shows subcortical band heterotopia. The neuronal migration disorder associated with muscular dystrophy is cobblestone lissencephaly. The lissencephaly syndromes result from neuronal migration abnormalities and include subcortical band heterotopia, or double cortex, in which there is relatively normal cortex with an underlying band of white matter, underneath which is a band of gray matter. This disorder results from a mutation in the DCX gene on chromosome X, which encodes for the protein doublecortin which is involved in microtubule organization and stabilization. The same mutation can lead to classic lissencephaly when occurring in males. This difference in manifestations in females as compared with males is thought to result from lyonization (random X inactivation) in females, such that in neurons in which the mutated gene is inactivated, normal migration occurs. Clinical features include intractable seizures, microcephaly, hypotonia, spastic quadriparesis, recurrent aspirations necessitating feeding tube, and shortened life expectance. Lissencephaly type I characterized by agyria or pachygyria rather than the presence of two bands of gray matter separated by a band of white matter. Cobblestone lissencephaly (rather than subcortical band heterotopia), or lissencephaly type II, is seen in several disorders, including Walker-Warburg syndrome, Fukuyama muscular dystrophy, and muscle-eye-brain disease of Santavuori. In polymicrogyria, there are excess, abnormal gyri.

3

99. You are evaluating a 15-year-old boy for growth retardation, generalized weakness, and ataxia. On examination, he has bilateral ptosis and restricted gaze in all directions. His EKG shows complete heart block. **What is the most likely diagnosis?**
    - A. Kearns-Sayre syndrome
    - B. Mitochondrial encephalopathy, lactic acidosis, and strokes
    - C. Myoclonic epilepsy with ragged red fibers
    - D. Leigh disease
    - E. Myasthenia gravis

Correct Answer is: A
This is a clinical presentation of Kearns-Sayre syndrome, which is a disorder caused by multiple mtDNA deletions. The diagnosis is made with the triad of progressive external ophthalmoplegia, onset before the age of 20 years, and at least one of the following: short stature, retinitis pigmentosa, cerebellar ataxia, heart block, and increased CSF protein (>100 mg/dl). Chronic progressive external ophthalmoplegia may be an isolated finding seen in some patients. Patients with Kearns-Sayre syndrome have a gradual progression of symptoms and most will have cognitive regression by third or fourth decade of life. Most cases are sporadic. An electrocardiogram is required to diagnose heart block, in which case, a pacemaker is needed. Pathologically, patients may have muscles with ragged red fibers and white matter showing spongy myelinopathy without gliosis or macrophage reactions.

100. You are seeing a 2-year-old child for his small head size noted by the child's pediatrician. The child's head size had been small at birth and the rate of growth had been below average over time. **Which of the following statements is correct regarding microcephaly?**
    - A. It always implies an underlying neurologic disorder and developmental delay is invariably present
    - B. Causes include infection, trauma, and hypoxic-ischemic insult
    - C. Microcephaly is defined as a head circumference less than 1 standard deviation below the mean
    - D. Seizures are infrequently seen in children with microcephaly
    - E. Maternal exposure to AEDs has not been associated with microcephaly

Correct Answer is: B
Microcephaly is defined as head circumference less than 2 standard deviations below the mean. A variety of causes of microcephaly exist. It can be a normal variant that is often hereditary, without clinical implications.

When pathologic, causes include in utero infections, toxin exposure (such as alcohol, tobacco, and prescription drugs such as chemotherapeutic agents and anti-epileptics), hypoxic-ischemic injury, birth trauma, and metabolic disorders such as prolonged hypoglycemia. A wide variety of hereditary disorders including enzyme deficiencies can lead to microcephaly, as can chromosomal abnormalities. Clinical manifestations depend on the underlying cause and can range from none (asymptomatic microcephaly) to severe developmental delay and seizures. Macrocephaly is defined as a head circumference greater than 2 standard deviations above the mean.

Macrocephaly may be a normal variant that is often hereditary, may result from increased CSF, as in hydrocephalus due to a variety of causes, from mass lesions such as tumors or subdural hematomas, or may result from megalencephaly, an oversized brain (brain weight

greater than 2 standard deviations above the mean). Causes of megalencephaly include storage diseases such as mucopolysaccharidoses or Tay-Sachs disease, Canavan disease, Alexander disease, genetic disorders including Sotos syndrome, and others. In the latter disorders, eventual cell loss with subsequent atrophy typically occurs. Megalocephaly may also be a benign familial finding.

Clinical manifestations depend on the underlying cause. Neurologic deficits may be absent in the benign familial form. Hemimegalencephaly, or enlargement of only one brain hemisphere, invariably presents with seizures and hemiparesis. Hemimegalencephaly is associated with various genetic disorders, including Beckwith-Wiedemann syndrome, which is characterized by gigantism, macrogloss ia, and midline abdominal wall defects.

101. You were asked to see a 6-month-old boy for intractable seizures. On examination, he has a short small chin, thin upper lip, and low-set ears. He has spastic quadriparesis and requires a feeding tube because of recurrent aspirations. His brain MRI shows essentially smooth frontal, parietal, and occipital lobes, with a thick cortex and without sulci or gyri. **Which of the following statements is not true regarding this disorder?**
   A. It results from abnormal neuronal migration
   B. The cortex in this disorder consists of six layers
   C. Associated malformations including corpus callosum agenesis may occur
   D. LIS1 mutation disrupts microtubule-directed neuronal migration
   E. Microcephaly and intractable seizures occur

Correct Answer is: B
Lissencephaly is a malformation of cortical development resulting from abnormal neuronal migration resulting in impaired formation of gyri. It is characterized by the presence of reduced cortical gyration and, in the most severe form, no gyri, or agyria, resulting in a smooth brain. In classic lissencephaly, or lissencephaly type I, the cortex is thick but consists of only four layers (or less often two or three layers, as opposed to the normal six neocortical layers). Associated malformations may include agenesis of the corpus callosum or hypoplasia of the cerebellum, with sparing of the thalamus and basal ganglia. Miller-Dieker syndrome (MDS), one form of lissencephaly type I, is characterized by lissencephaly associated with microcephaly, typical facies including micrognathia (small jaw), low-set ears, thin upper lip, and other features. Clinical manifestations include global developmental delay, hypotonia and later spasticity, and intractable seizures. Life expectancy is often not beyond 1 year. MDS has been associated with microdeletions on chromosome 17 in the LIS1 gene. LIS 1 gene encodes a protein involved in regulation of microtubules and dynein function, and mutations interfere with microtubule-directed migration of neurons from the ventricular zone. Mutations in LIS1 gene can also lead to isolated lissencephaly (so-called isolated lissencephaly sequence, without other features of MDS).X-linked lissencephaly is another form that results from mutations in the DCX gene on chromosome X when occurring in males. This gene encodes for the protein doublecortin, which is involved in microtubule organization and stabilization. In another form of lissencephaly that results from mutations in the gene ARX, which encodes

3

for a transcription factor involved in non-radial migration of cortical interneurons, the basal ganglia are abnormal in addition to the cortex and corpus callosum. In some forms of lissencephaly, there may be an anterior to posterior (or vice versa) gradient of gyral formation (e.g. with some gyral formation in the anterior or posterior aspects of the brain). Cobblestone lissencephaly, also known as lissencephaly type II, is seen in several disorders including Walker-Warburg syndrome, Fukuyama muscular dystrophy,and muscle-eye-brain disease of Santavuori. In polymicrogyria, there are excess, abnormal gyri. Subcortical band heterotopia.

102. You are seeing a 6-year-old boy for vision impairment because he bumps into things at home. His past medical history is remarkable of horizontal nystagmus at around 6 months of age and seizure disorder. He has not met developmental milestones with below average height. He has a low glucose levels. Ophthalmologic exam revealed small optic nerves and visual acuity of 20/200 both eyes.
What do you except to see on his brain MRI?
A. Occipital lobe stroke
B. Optic nerve tumor bilaterally
C. Absent septum pellucidum
D. Frontal lobe meningioma compressing optic nerves
E. Lissencephaly

Correct Answer is: C
This is a case of septo-optic dysplasia. Septo-optic dysplasia is described as absence or dysgenesis of the septum pellucidum with hypoplasia of the optic nerve (sometimes involving the optic chiasm) and pituitary infundibulum. It can be associated with either 1) Schizencephaly or 2) Constellation of diffuse white matter hypoplasia, ventriculomegaly, and abnormal hypothalamic-pituitary function. MRI of the brain will show - absent septum pellucidum; hypoplastic pituitary stalk; hypoplastic optic chiasm/optic nerves and globes. 60–90% of these patients present with blindness or symptoms of visual impairment. Signs related to visual loss include absent fixation, searching nystagmus, visual inattentiveness and strabismus. 75% of patients may have intellectual disability, epilepsy or cerebral palsy or attention deficit disorder or autism. Other developmental abnormalities include underdeveloped mid-facial structures, hypoglycemia, and hyperbilirubinemia, disturbance in temperature regulation, muscular hypotonia, microgenitalism, low Apgar scores and failure to thrive.

Suggested Reading

- Parker K, et al. J Pediatr Endocrin Metab 2002; 15:697–700. Lehnstein Campbell, C. Optometry 2003; 74:417–26.
- Phillips PH, Brodsky MC. Congenital optic ne abnormalities, In: Pediatric ophthalmology and strabismus, 2nd ed. Wright KW, Spiegel, PH, editors. New York: Springer, 2003. p. 918–22.
- Egan RA, Kerrison JB. Ophthalmol Clin N Am 2003;16:595–605.

103. You are evaluating a 6-month-old baby for seizures. He has multiple dysmorphic features and severe hypotonia, and brain MRI shows pachygyria. There is calcific stippling of the patella on skeletal radiographs. Very long-chain fatty acid levels are elevated in plasma.

Which of the following is not true regarding this condition?

A. This is a peroxisomal disorder
B. Liver cirrhosis occurs in these patients
C. Kidney cysts can be seen in these patients
D. White matter is not involved
E. Polymicrogyria may be seen in these patients

Correct Answer is: D

This is a clinical presentation of Zellweger syndrome, which is a peroxisomal disorder in which the white matter is involved. Peroxisomes are organelles involved in the biosynthesis of ether phospholipids and bile acids, oxidation of very long chain fatty acid, prostaglandins, and unsaturated long-chain fatty acids, and the catabolism of phytanate, pipecolate, and glycolate. The infantile syndromes of peroxisomal dysfunction include Zellweger syndrome, neonatal adrenoleukodystrophy, and infantile Refsum disease. Zellweger is the most severe form and is caused by mutations in the PEX genes, the majority with PEX1 resulting in abnormal peroxisomal biogenesis. Zellweger syndrome, or "cerebrohepatorenal syndrome", is characterized by dysmorphic features such as a high forehead, large fontanelles, flat supraorbital ridges, hypertelorism, epicanthal folds, broad nasal bridge, micrognathia, and flat occiput. These children have cataracts, retinal dystrophy, sensorineural hearing loss, severe hypotonia, decreased sucking and crying, hyporeflexia, deformities in flexion of the lower limbs with arthrogryposis, profound intellectual disability, and seizures. The brain demonstrates white matter changes and abnormalities in neuronal migration. There is liver dysfunction with cirrhosis and polycystic kidney disease. A very typical feature is chondrodysplasia punctata with bony stippling of the patella. Other congenital abnormalities have been reported, such as ventricular septal defects and other cardiac abnormalities.

Diagnostic workup demonstrates increased plasma very long-chain fatty acids, decreased red blood cell plasmalogens, and decreased or absent hepatic peroxisomes. Pathologically, the brain may be enlarged, and there is evidence of neuronal migration abnormality, white matter changes with lipid accumulation, and sometimes pachygyria and/or polymicrogyria. The treatment of Zellweger syndrome is symptomatic. Most of these patients die early. The other peroxisomal abnormalities are much milder. Neonatal adrenoleukodystrophy patients have liver cirrhosis, adrenocortical atrophy, and brain abnormalities such as polymicrogyria, subcortical heterotopia, and cerebellar dysplasia but no pachygyria. Infantile Refsum disease manifests with psychomotor retardation, sensorineural hearing loss, retinal degeneration, anosmia, and mild dysmorphic features and there may be cirrhosis and adrenal atrophy. In Refsum disease, phytanic acid levels are elevated and peroxisomes are reduced or absent. These patients may survive into adulthood.

104. You are seeing a 14-year-ofd boy with a history of migraines has short stature, ataxia, proximal weakness, mild cognitive impairment, deafness, and various types of seizures. He is admitted after a viral illness, becomes dehydrated, and is found to have lactic acidosis. He has been diagnosed with a progressive myoclonic epilepsy (PME); a muscle biopsy has been obtained and shown in the figure.

3

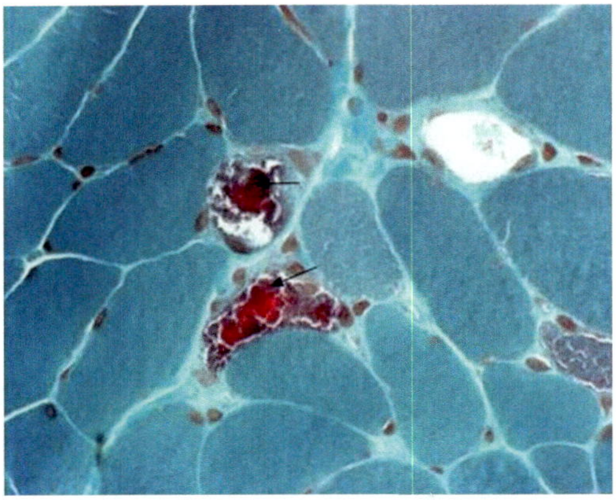

Fig. 3.29 Modified_Gomori_trichrome_stain_showing_several_ragged_red_fibers_.jpg. Abu-Amero KK, Al-Dhalaan H, Bohlega S, Hellani A, Taylor RW. derivative work: CopperKettle (talk)

Which of the following is a feature of this patient's condition?

A. Mutation affecting cystatin B
B. Cherry red spot on the fundoscopic examination
C. This is a mitochondrial disorder
D. EPM2 A mutation
E. Lafora bodies on skin biopsy

Correct Answer is: C

This is a case of myoclonic epilepsy with ragged red fibers (MERFF), which is a mitochondrial disorder. The patient has various characteristics suggestive of a mitochondrial disorder, including migraines, short stature, ataxia, cognitive impairment, deafness, epilepsy, and elevated lactate. He has generalized proximal weakness suggesting a myopathy. Mitochondrial disorders are a heterogeneous group of disorders that can affect both the peripheral and central nervous system. MERRF is a mitochondrial disorder that usually starts in the second or third decade of life, and is maternally inherited (like other disorders of mitochondrial DNA). CSF studies will show elevation of pyruvate and lactate, and the serum creatine kinase may be elevated. MRI of the brain usually demonstrates cerebral atrophy. Point mutations in mitochondrial DNA have been detected in this disorder.

Mutation affecting cystatin B is seen with EPM1 mutations in Unverricht Lundborg syndrome. Cherry red spot is seen in various conditions, including sialidosis, which is another progressive myoclonic epilepsy. EPM2A mutation is seen in Lafora body disease, in which Lafora bodies are also detected on skin biopsy.

Suggested Reading

- Delgado-Escueta AV, Ganesh S, Yamakawa K. Advances in the genetics of progressive myoclonus epilepsy. Am J Med Genet. 2001;106:129–38.
- Schmiedel J, Jackson S, Schafer J, et al. Mitochondrial cytopathies. J Neurol. 2003;250:267–77.

105. You were asked to see an 8-month-old boy who recently stopped visual tracking and nystagmus was noted. On examination, the pupillary response is sluggish and the reminder of his neurological exam is within normal limits.

What is your diagnosis?

A. Retinoblastoma
B. Craniopharyngioma
C. Kearns-Sayre syndrome
D. Leber Congenital amaurosis

Correct Answer is: D

This is a case of Leber congenital amaurosis, it is a retinal dystrophy and is the most common genetic cause of congenital visual impairment. Severe impairment begins in the first 3–4 months of life followed by nystagmus and sluggish pupillary responses. Visual acuity will rarely be better than 20/400 when they get older. Some children display midfacial hypoplasia and may have associated mental retardation.

Retinoblastoma features include unilateral progressive visual loss in a young child and strabismus. The most common initial sign is leucocoria, where the white

tumor reflects light and blocks view of the red colored retina.

Craniopharygioma is the most common non-glial tumor in children and most commonly occurs between the ages of 6–14. There is a 1–2-year history of progressive visual loss, delayed sexual maturation growth failure and bi-temporal hemianopia.

Kearns-Sayre syndrome is a mitochondrial disorder and consists of a triad of symptoms including: progressive external ophthalmoplegia, onset before age 20 and one of the following; short stature, pigmentary retinopathy, cerebellar ataxia, heart block, cerebellar ataxia, and elevated cerebrospinal protein.

Suggested Reading

- Weleber RG, Francis PJ, Trzupek KM, Beattie C. Leber congenital amaurosis. 2013.

106. You saw a baby who presented with irritability and hypersensitivity to stimuli at 4 months of age, but he died at 11-month of age and a brain specimen obtained from an autopsy is shown below. The baby was also blind and had prominent regression by age 6 months. He also had developed stiffness of all four limbs and later of the trunk to the point that he was in an opisthotonic posture.

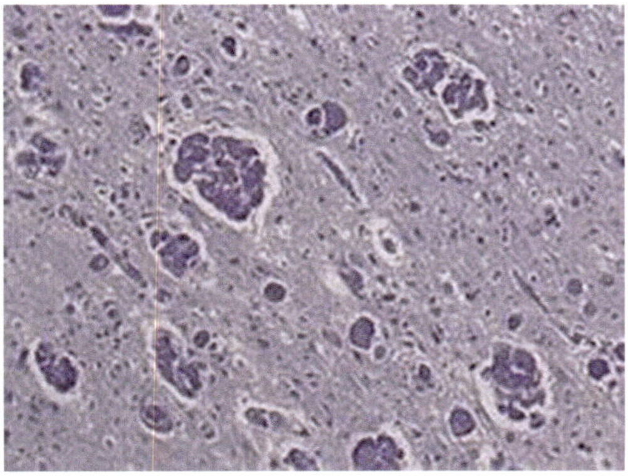

Fig. 3.30 Globoid cell leukodystrophy PAS – Mulinucleated macrophages ("globoid cells") and loss of myelinated fibers in a case of Krabbe's leukodystrophy. (Jensflorian. Wikipedia)

Which of the following is true regarding this condition?

A. It is autosomal dominant
B. The deficient enzyme is B-glucosylceramidas
C. There is demyelination with relative sparing of the U fibers
D. It is only seen in newborns, and all patients die by 1 year of age
E. The cause is deficiency of the enzyme A-galactosidase

Correct Answer is: C

This is a case of Krabbe disease on the basis of the history and histopathologic findings. Krabbe disease (globoid cell leukodystrophy) is a disorder with autosomal recessive inheritance, with the affected gene mapped to chromosome 14. This disorder is characterized by the accumulation of galactocerebroside in macrophages of the white matter in the CNS, leading to the formation of globoid cells and to progressive demyelination, but with sparing of the U fibers. The cause is a deficiency of the enzyme galactosylceramidase (also known as galactocerebrosidegalactosidase). It can involve the peripheral nervous system, leading to a demyelinating neuropathy, but affects predominantly the CNS.

There are three forms: - *Infantile form*: the most common variant and presents between 4 and 6 months of age with irritability, hypersensitivity to stimuli, increasing hypertonicity with eventual opisthotonos, unexplained low-grade fevers, optic atrophy with blindness, psychomotor developmental arrest, and subsequent regression with loss of previously achieved milestones. These children also have a demyelinating polyneuropathy with arreflexia. They usually die by the age of 1 year. -*Juvenile form*: the onset is between 3 and 10 years of age, with vision loss, spasticity, ataxia, gait disturbance, and cognitive impairment. - *Adult form*: usually starts between the third and the fifth decade of life, with spastic

paraparesis, weakness, vision loss, and evidence of neuropathy, but intellectual function tends to be normal.

Pathologically, there is symmetric demyelination of the cerebral white matter, with relative sparing of the subcortical arcuate or U fibers. The pathologic specimen shown in the Figure is typical of Krabbe disease, demonstrating clusters of globoid cells, which are multinucleated macrophages with cytoplasmic accumulation of galactocerebroside.

Radiologically, there is symmetric periventricular white matter signal abnormality and cerebral atrophy. NCS demonstrate slow conduction velocities and prolonged distal latencies. CSF examination shows elevated protein levels.

107. You are evaluating an 8-year-old girl with gait abnormalities and headache. On examination, she has nystagmus, and truncal and limb ataxia.

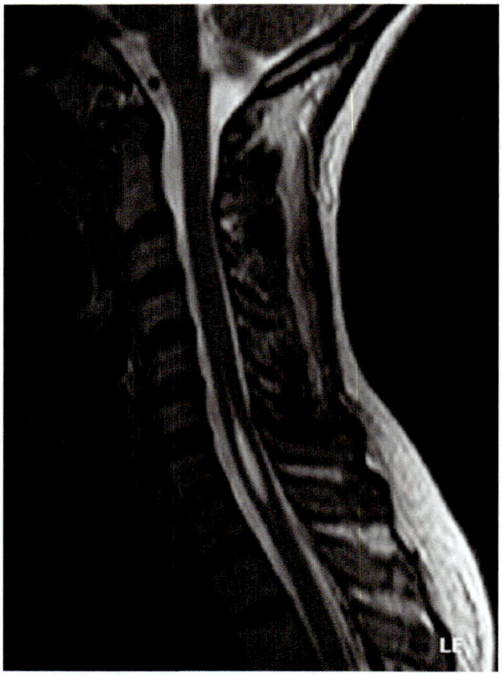

Fig. 3.31 Transferred from ▶ en.wikipedia to Commons. Cyborg Ninja at English Wikipedia

Which of the following statements regarding this patient's disorder is false?

A. Chiari 1 malformations may be asymptomatic and do not necessarily require surgical intervention
B. Myelomeningocele occurs in patients with Chiari II malformation
C. Hydrocephalus *is* a complication of Chiari malformation
D. Management of Chiari malformations may include sub-occipital decompression
E. Syringomyelia, which may occur in association with a Chiari I malformation, is an enlargement of the central canal of the spinal cord

Correct Answer is: E

While syringomyelia and hydromyelia are erroneously used interchangeably by some, the two are distinct by definition. Syringomyelia is a fluid-filled cavity within the spinal cord that is separate from the central canal; hydromyelia is the termed used to describe an enlargement in the central canal itself. Chiari 1 malformation is defined as displacement of the cerebellum and cerebellar tonsils downward through the foramen magnum. The MRI shows a Chiari I malformation with 1.3 cm downward displacement of the cerebellar tonsils. In minor downward displacement of less than 1 cm, the patient may be asymptomatic and care should be taken in attributing nonspecific neurologic symptoms to the Chiari malformation. In more severe downward displacement, as in this case, headache, cranial nerve abnormalities, and other brain stem symptoms, nystagmus, and ataxia may occur. Associated findings include syringomyelia. The pathophysiology of Chiari I malformation may relate to

posterior fossa overcrowding due to posterior fossa hypoplasia. In symptomatic cases, treatment includes posterior fossa decompression and duraplasty. Chiari II malformation, also known as Arnold-Chiari malformation, includes displacement of the cerebellar vermis and tonsils in association with a myelomeningocele. Brain stem dysfunction is often prominent, including prominent cranial nerve abnormalities, stridor, apnea, and feeding difficulties. Fourth ventricle compression leads to hydrocephalus.

Pathophysiological, Chiari II malformation is thought to be secondary to the presence of the caudal myelomeningocele, producing downward traction and hence herniation of the brain stem and cerebellum through the foramen magnum. Management of Chiari II malformation includes shunting for hydrocephalus and surgical intervention for myelomeningocele and may include posterior fossa decompression through suboccipital craniotomy.

Management of complications including seizures, feeding difficulties, and bowel and bladder dysfunction is also necessary. Chiari III malformation is cerebellar herniation into a cervical encephalocele. Chiari IV malformation is the term previously used to describe cerebellar hypoplasia but is no longer used.

108. A 12-year-old boy is found to have large orange-colored tonsils, hepatosplenomegaly, and sensory deficits in the upper limbs.
Which of the following is true regarding this condition?
   - A. It is caused by deficiency of low-density lipoproteins
   - B. It is autosomal dominant in inheritance
   - C. Peripheral nerves are not involved
   - D. It is caused by a mutation in the adenosine triphosphate cassette transporter protein
   - E. Total cholesterol level in the serum is very elevated

Correct Answer is: D
This is a presentation of Tangier disease, which is an autosomal recessive familial neuropathy, caused by mutation affecting the adenosine triphosphate cassette transporter protein, resulting in a deficiency of high density lipoprotein (HDL) and very low serum cholesterol and high triglyceride concentrations. Given the severely reduced HDL level, cholesteryl esters accumulate in various tissues, including tonsils, peripheral nerves, cornea, bone marrow, and other organs of the reticuloendothelial system. A typical clinical finding is the enlarged orange tonsils. Peripheral neuropathy is common and manifests with sensory loss to pain and temperature that may have a pattern in the upper extremities similar to that seen in syringomyelia and may affect the entire body. Motor involvement may manifest with weakness that affects the upper and lower extremities and particularly the hand muscles. A symmetric polyneuropathy is common; however, a mono-neuropathy presentation can also be seen. Deep tendon reflexes are depressed. Cranial nerves may also be involved. Premature atherosclerosis also occurs. The diagnosis is suspected on the basis of clinical features, and a lipid profile showing HDL deficiency, with low total cholesterol and high triglyceride levels. Foamy macrophages are present in the bone marrow and other tissues. There is no specific treatment.

109. You are evaluating a 16-year-old male with growth and psychomotor retardation, sensorineural hearing loss, frequent headaches, seizures, and multiple stroke-like episodes. CT scan and MRI from different time points are shown in the figure. Lactate level is found to be elevated.

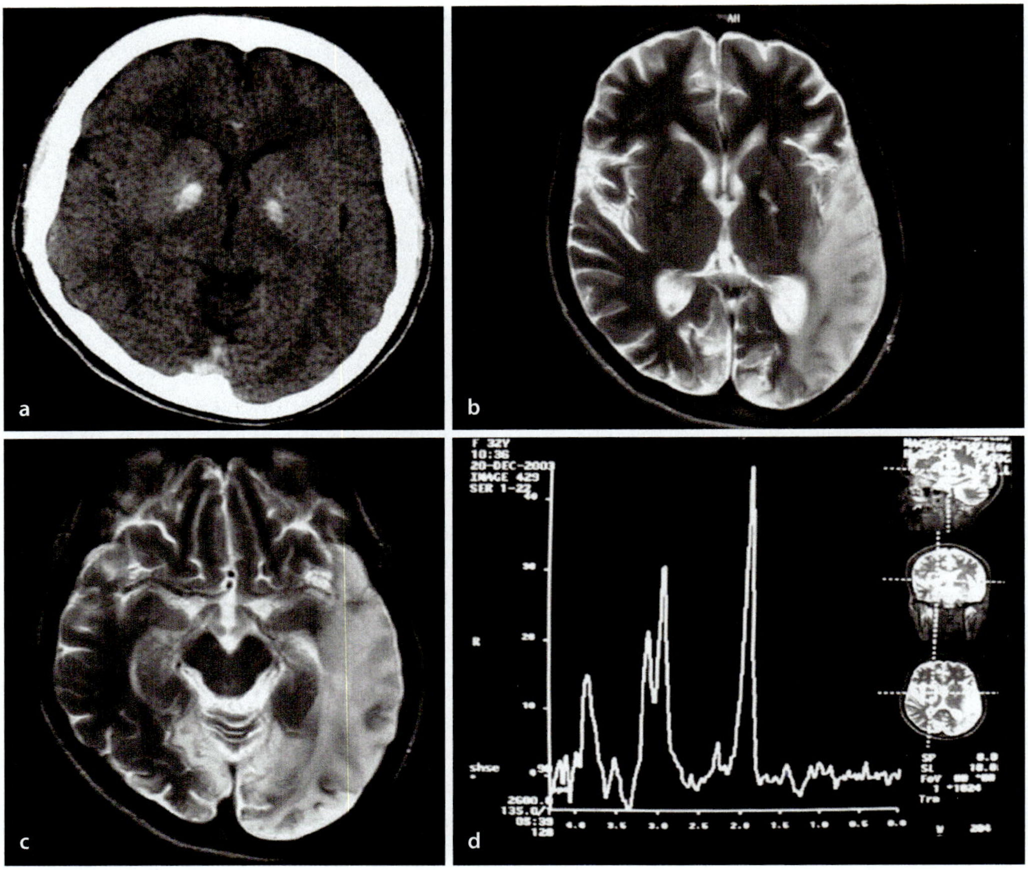

Fig. 3.32 **a** A computed tomography brain scan showing bilateral basal ganglia calcification; the cerebellum shows prominent folia indicating mild cerebellar atrophy. **b** Axial T2 brain magnetic resonance image scan showing left temporo-parieto occipital ischemic lesion. **c** Axial T2 brain magnetic resonance image scan showing the extension of the parietal temporal region to the occipital lobe, and also showing a right occipital lesion. **d** Magnetic resonance spectroscopy showing inversion of J-coupling phenomenon at 1.3 ppm, indicating lactate peak. (Abu-Amero et al. *Journal of Medical Case Reports* 2009 3:77 ► https://doi.org/10.1186/1752-1947-3-77). A patient with typical clinical features of mitochondrial encephalopathy, lactic acidosis and stroke-like episodes (MELAS) but without an obvious genetic cause: a case report. Abu-Amero KK, Al-Dhalaan H, Bohlega S, Hellani A, Taylor RW. Wikipedia

What is the most likely diagnosis?

A. Kearns-Sayre syndrome
B. Mitochondrial encephalopathy, lactic acidosis, and strokes
C. Myoclonic epilepsy with ragged red fibers
D. Leigh disease
E. Neuronal ceroid lipofuscinosis

Correct Answer is: B
Mitochondrial encephalopathy, lactic acidosis and strokes (MELAS) is a mitochondrial disorder with typical maternal inheritance; however, sporadic cases may occur. The most common mutation is in the mtDNA MTTL1 gene encoding for an mtDNA tRNA. The onset is often between 2 and 10 years of age, although symptoms may begin at any age, including adulthood. Patients are normal at birth, later manifesting with seizures, migraine headaches, vomiting with anorexia, exercise intolerance, and weakness. Failure to thrive, growth

retardation, and progressive deafness are common in these children. Stroke-like episodes occur, presenting with transient hemiparesis, cortical blindness, and altered consciousness, with cumulative residual effects leading to gradually progressive neurologic impairment, leading to mental deterioration and encephalopathy. The MRI shown in the figure demonstrates multifocal infarcts that do not correlate with definite vascular territories. Initially, the infarcts occur in the posterior cerebral regions, with eventual involvement of other cerebral and cerebellar cortices, basal ganglia, and the thalamus. The infarcts are extremely epileptogenic. Lactate level is elevated in the blood and CSF. Muscle biopsy may demonstrate ragged red fibers. There is no specific treatment. These patients may have some benefit from coenzyme Q10 and L-carnitine.

L-arginine may attenuate the severity of strokes and reduce the frequency of these events.

110. Which of the following options is true regarding Leigh disease?
   A. It is a static encephalopathy
   B. It is due to mitochondrial abnormalities
   C. It is inherited in an autosomal recessive fashion
   D. Lactate levels are reduced during episodic exacerbations
   E. Clinical manifestations most commonly begin during late childhood

Correct Answer is: B
Leigh disease or acute necrotizing encephalomyelopathy is a manifestation of mitochondrial disorders that can be sporadic or familial, with only some cases with the typical maternal inheritance pattern. This condition affects neurons of the brain stem, thalamus, basal ganglia, and cerebellum. Most of the affected patients have onset of neurologic manifestations in the first year of life, but there are forms with late onset. Clinical features manifest with decompensation associated with inter-current illnesses. In infancy, patients present with hypotonia, loss of head control, poor sucking, vomiting, irritability, seizures, and myoclonic jerks. If the onset is beyond the first year, patients present with gait disturbance, cerebellar ataxia, dysarthria, psychomotor retardation, and spasticity, external ophthalmoplegia, nystagmus, abnormal movements with chorea or dystonia, and peripheral neuropathy in some cases with autonomic failure. The disorder is progressive with episodic deterioration. Lactate level is increased in blood and CSF. Lactate and pyruvate levels in blood are elevated during exacerbations. MRI of the brain demonstrates bilateral symmetric hyper- intense T2 signal abnormalities in the brain stem and/or basal ganglia, and in some cases in the spinal cord. Treatment is supportive and symptomatic.

111. You are seeing a 5-month-old baby for evaluation of seizures. He has a prominent startle response and developmental delay. He had reached some developmental milestones but has started regressing now. It is also noticed that he is macrocephalic and spastic. A cherry-red spot is seen on ophthalmologic examination, and he also has prominent hepatosplenomegaly. There is suspicion for a GM2 gangliosidosis.
   Which of the following is true regarding this patient's condition?
   A. Hexosaminidase A is the only enzyme affected
   B. Both hexosaminidases A and B are affected

C. T-Galactosidase deficiency is the most common cause
D. Sphingomyelinase deficiency is the cause
E. This patient has Tay-Sachs disease

Correct Answer is: B
This patient has GM2 gangliosidosis, more specifically Sandhoff disease caused by deficiency of hexosaminidase A and B. Galactosidase deficiency causes GM1 but not GM2 gangliosidosis. Sphingomyelinase deficiency causes Niemann-Pick types A and B. GM2 gangliosidosis is caused by deficiency of hexosaminidase A in Tay-Sachs disease or hexosaminidase A and B in Sandhoff disease. Both are autosomal recessive. Tay-Sachs disease or infantile GM2 gangliosidosis is more common in Ashkenazi Jews but may also occur in other populations with less frequency, and the CNS is the only affected organ. Onset is between 3 and 6 months of age, with increased startle response and subsequent motor regression, spasticity, blindness with optic atrophy, and seizures. There is a delay in reaching developmental milestones, with subsequent regression. A cherry-red spot in the macula is commonly seen, and these patients have macrocephaly. Progression to severe intellectual disability occurs, and most children die by the age of 5 years. The diagnosis is suspected in patient with psychomotor retardation and a cherry-red spot and is confirmed with the detection of hexosaminidase A deficiency with normal activity of hexosaminidase B. Treatment is supportive. Sandhoff disease occurs from combined deficiency of hexosaminidase A and B. The clinical features are similar to those seen in Tay-Sachs disease; however, as mentioned, in Tay Sachs disease, the brain is the only organ involved, whereas in Sandhoff disease, the GM2 gangliosides accumulate in the brain and viscera, causing hepatosplenomegaly that is not seen in Tay-Sachs disease. The diagnosis is based on these clinical features and confirmed with analysis of the enzymatic activity of the enzymes involved.

112. You are seeing an 18-year-old female in the ED for severe abdominal pain, along with nausea, vomiting, fever, and tachycardia. She has been evaluated multiple times over the past year for similar symptoms and has undergone evaluation for appendicitis and other gynecologic causes, including exploratory laparoscopy in the past. There are no cutaneous manifestations. She has increased aminolevulinic acid and porphobilinogen (PBG) concentrations in the urine, with no increase in urinary or fecal coproporphyri n III.
Which of the following is true regarding this disorder?
A. The enzyme affected is PBG deaminase
B. The enzyme affected is coproporphyrinogen oxidase
C. The enzyme affected is protoporphyrinogen oxidase
D. Seizures can occur and should be treated with phenobarbital
E. A symmetric distal demyelinating polyneuropathy occurs predominantly in the lower limbs

Correct Answer is: A
This is a case of porphyria, likely acute intermittent porphyria (AIP) given the lack of cutaneous manifestations and the absence of increased coproporphyrin III in the urine and stool, therefore making variegate porphyria (VP) and hepatic coproporphyria (HCP) less likely. The enzyme involved in

AIP is porphobilinogen deaminase. Porphyrias are a group of metabolic disorders caused by deficiency of a specific enzyme involved in the heme biosynthetic pathway. Most of the porphyrias are inherited in an autosomal dominant fashion, except 5-aminolevulinic acid dehydratase deficient porphyria, which is autosomal recessive. AIP has primarily neurologic manifestations, HCP and VP have a combination of neurologic and cutaneous manifestations with photosensitivity, and porphyria cutanea tarda has cutaneous, with no neurologic, manifestations. The acute porphyrias manifest with attacks of neurovisceral symptoms, with markedly elevated levels of plasma and urinary concentrations of the porphyrin precursors aminolevulinic acid (ALA) and porphobilinogen (PBG). Levels are usually elevated during attacks and may be normal in between. The attacks may be triggered by drugs such as barbiturates, sulfonamides, AEDs, and hormones among other medications. Attacks may also be triggered by a low-carbohydrate diet, infections, or other intercurrent illnesses. AIP is the most common of the acute porphyrias with neurovisceral symptoms and is caused by deficiency of PBG deaminase, with the gene localized on chromosome 11. Onset occurs after puberty, with acute attacks of abdominal pain, sometimes associated with nausea, vomiting, diarrhea, fever, tachycardia, and leukocytosis. Commonly these patients experience limb pain and muscle weakness resulting from a peripheral neuropathy that is predominantly motor and axonal, affecting more proximal than distal segments and more the upper than the lower extremities. Deep tendon reflexes are depressed. The radial nerve has been described as being classically involved, and in severe cases, there may be bulbar, and respiratory involvement. Seizures can occur from neurologic involvement or may result from the hyponatremia that is seen in these patients.

Neuropsychiatric symptoms such as anxiety, insomnia, depression, disorientation, hallucinations, and paranoia may occur. The diagnosis is based on clinical suspicion and elevated urinary excretion of ALA and PBG during the attacks. Genetic testing and enzyme analysis are also helpful.

Management is focused on preventing attacks by avoiding precipitating factors. During attacks, these patients may need hospitalization for hydration and pain control. Carbohydrates decrease the synthesis of porphyrins, and an infusion may be required. Hematin infusions may be helpful. For seizures, clonazepam and gabapentin may be helpful.

Unfortunately, many AEDs precipitate attacks, especially barbiturates, which should be avoided. HCP is caused by coproporphyrinogen oxidase deficiency, and VP is caused by protoporphyrinogen oxidase deficiency. In both, the neurovisceral manifestations are similar to AIP, but in HCP and VP, there are cutaneous manifestations with photosensitivity, abnormal skin fragility, and bullous skin lesions on sun-exposed areas. HCP and VP cause increased urinary and fecal levels of coproporphyrin III.

❓ 113. An Ashkenazi Jewish family of 6-month-old boy brought the baby for evaluation of seizures. He has prominent startle response and developmental delay. He had reached some early developmental milestones but then began to regress. It is also noticed that he is macrocephalic and spastic, but there is no visceromegaly. A cherry-red spot is seen on ophthalmologic examination. There is suspicion for a GM2 gangliosidosis.

3

What is correct regarding this patient's condition?

A. This patient has Sandhoff disease
B. Hexosaminidase A is the only cause
C. It is autosomal dominant
D. It occurs only in Ashkenazi Jews
E. B-Galactosidase deficiency is the most common cause

Correct Answer is: B

The baby has a GM2 gangliosidosis, more specifically Tay-Sachs disease caused by hexosaminidase A deficiency. Galactosidase deficiency causes GM1 but not GM2 gangliosidosis. Sphingomyelinase deficiency causes Niemann-Pick types A and B. GM2 gangliosidosis is caused by deficiency of hexosaminidase A in Tay-Sachs disease or hexosaminidase A and B in Sandhoff disease. Both are autosomal recessive. Tay-Sachs disease or infantile GM2 gangliosidosis is more common in Ashkenazi Jews but may also occur in other populations with less frequency, and the CNS is the only affected organ. Onset is between 3 and 6 months of age, with increased startle response and subsequent motor regression, spasticity, blindness with optic atrophy, and seizures. There is a delay in reaching developmental milestones, with subsequent regression. A cherry-red spot in the macula is commonly seen, and these patients have macrocephaly. Progression to severe intellectual disability occurs, and most children die by the age of 5 years. The diagnosis is suspected in patients with psychomotor retardation and a cherry-red spot and is confirmed with the detection of hexosaminidase A deficiency with normal activity of hexosaminidase Treatment is supportive. Sandhoff disease occurs from combined deficiency of hexosaminidase A and B. The clinical features are similar to those seen in Tay-Sachs disease; however, as mentioned, in Tay-Sachs disease, the brain is the only organ involved, whereas in Sandhoff disease, the GM2 gangliosides accumulate in the brain and viscera, causing hepatosplenomegaly that is not seen in Tay-Sachs disease. The diagnosis is based on these clinical features and confirmed with analysis of the enzymatic activity of the enzymes involved.

114. Which of the following statements is correct regarding disorders of corpus callosum development?

A. They result from abnormalities in the third trimester of pregnancy
B. Most commonly, complete agenesis of the corpus callosum occurs
C. They result from abnormalities in the commissural plate
D. Corpus callosum agenesis is most often seen in isolation
E. Severe developmental delay is invariably present

Correct Answer is: A

During the fifth week of gestation, within the lamina terminalis, the commissural plate develops and serves as a bridge over which axonal processes decussate. The corpus callosum is fully developed by week 17th of gestation. Abnormalities in the commissural plate lead to agenesis or dysgenesis of the corpus callosum. Agenesis of the corpus callosum may be complete or more commonly partial and may occur in isolation or more commonly is associated with dysplasias of other prosencephalon derivatives and aplasia of the cerebellar vermis. It may also be seen in a variety of syndromes, including Aicardi syndrome, or may be associated with metabolic disorders such as nonketotic hyperglycinemia. Clinical manifestations may be absent, or there may be subtle cognitive or perceptual

abnormalities; developmental delay and seizures may also occur. Hypertelorism is seen in many. Coronal MRI shows vertically oriented lateral ventricles ("steer horn sign," or "racing car sign" on axial images).

115. Which of the following malformations is not paired with the appropriate underlying mechanism?
    A. Focal cortical dysplasia-disorder of cell proliferation
    B. Lissencephaly-disorders of neuronal migration
    C. Polymicrogyria-disorder of cortical organization
    D. Periventricular nodular heterotopias-disorder of cell proliferation
    E. Schizencephaly-disorder of cortical organization

Correct Answer is: D
Periventricular nodular heterotopia is a disorder of neuronal migration. Malformations of cortical development are divided into three categories based on the underlying cause: disorders of cell proliferation, migration, or cortical organization.

Disorders of neuronal proliferation include some forms of megalencephaly and focal cortical dysplasia.

Disorders of neuronal migration include lessencephaly, periventricular nodular heterotopias, and others.

Disorders of cortical organization include polymicrogyria and schizencephaly.

Focal cortical dysplasia may be seen in isolation or in the setting of tuberous sclerosis. One type of focal cortical dysplasia is characterized pathologically by the presence of balloon cells, which result from proliferation of abnormal cells within the germinal matrix. This is a common pathology in focal epilepsy, with the seizures often being intractable to medical therapy.

116. You are evaluating a 6-year-old boy for seizures. He has had gradual vision loss and progressive psychomotor retardation. Neuronal ceroid lipofuscinosis (NCL) is within the differential diagnosis.
    Which of the following is true regarding NCL?
    A. NCL occurs only in childhood
    B. It is autosomal dominant
    C. Myoclonic seizure is the least common type of seizure seen in these patients
    D. The infantile form is more common in Finnish people
    E. Electron microscopy is useless as there are no characteristic findings

Correct Answer is: D
Neuronal ceroid lipofuscinosis is a group of autosomal recessive disorders characterized by progressive psychomotor retardation, seizures, and blindness, which can present in infantile, late infantile, juvenile, and adult forms. Mutations in eight genes causing the disorder (CLN1 through CLN8) have been described. The most commonly involved genes are CLN1 and CLN2. CLN1 encodes for palmitoyl protein thioesterase 1 (PPT1), and CLN2 encodes for tripeptidyl peptidase 1 (TPP1). The storage products are saposins A and D in the infantile forms and subunit C of ATP synthase in the other forms. The infantile form is most common in Finland and is associated with CLN1 gene mutations. These patients are normal at birth, with onset of symptoms between 6 and 24 months, including microcephaly, hypotonia, myoclonus, seizures, ataxia, progressive psychomotor retardation, and blindness. Neurons accumulate membrane-bound osmophilic deposits (seen on electron microscopy) and neuronal loss with cortical atrophy will ensue. The late-infantile form presents between 2 and

4 years of age and is associated with CLN2 mutations, and these patients develop seizures, myoclonus, ataxia, involuntary movements, blindness, and psychomotor retardation. Neurons accumulate curvilinear bodies, which are seen on electron microscopy. The juvenile form begins between 4 and 10 years of age and is associated with CLN3 mutation, and these patients develop visual loss, seizures, myoclonus, psychomotor retardation, and focal neurologic deficits. The storage product consists of fingerprint bodies, which are seen on electron microscopy. The adult form is evident at approximately 30 years of age and is characterized by myoclonus, ataxia, behavioral abnormalities, and dementia. The storage material consists of a combination of fingerprint bodies, granular osmiophilic deposits, and rectilinear profiles. The diagnosis is based on the clinical presentation and supported with electron microscopic examination of lymphocytes or cells from other tissues. Enzyme activity studies for PPT1 and TPP1 are also available, as is genetic testing for all of the identified CLN genes. The treatment is symptomatic.

117. You are seeing a 6-year-old boy with short stature secondary to growth hormone deficiency and is also being treated for hypothyroidism. His motor and cognitive development has been normal. He has reduced visual acuity. He has absence of the septum pellucidum and hypoplasia of the optic nerves and chiasm on MRI. The cortex and other areas appear normal.
What is your likely diagnosis in this patient?
   A. Holoprosencephaly
   B. Septo-optic dysplasia
   C. Lissencephal
   D. Arrhinencephaly
   E. Cavum septum pellucidum

Correct Answer is: B
This patient's history and imaging findings are consistent with septo-optic dysplasia, a group of malformations that include hypoplasia or absence of the septum pellucidum, optic nerve and optic chiasm hypoplasia, dysgenesis of the corpus callosum and anterior commissure, and fornix detachment from the corpus callosum. Arrhinencephaly (agenesis of only the olfactory bulb and tract) and/or hypothalamic hamartomas may be associated features. Other less commonly associated abnormalities include cerebellar vermis defects and hydrocephalus. Septo-optic dysplasia can also be associated with lobar holoprosencephaly and other malformations of cortical development. Clinical manifestations include vision loss, ataxia when the cerebellum is involved, and symptoms of hydrocephalus when it is present, and endocrinologic disturbances. Endocrinologic disturbances can range from panhypopituitarism (with deficiencies in both anterior and posterior pituitary hormones) to isolated hormone deficiencies. Mutations in the transcription factors HESX1, a homeobox gene, and SOX may be implicated in this disorder. Cavum septum pellucidum, in which the septum pellucidum is not fused but rather exists in two separate pieces of tissue, is considered non-pathologic, with little clinical implications. The presence of normal cortex excludes holoprosencephaly, and lissencephaly. This patient has several features making septa-optic dysplasia the likely diagnosis rather than arrhinencephaly.

118. You are evaluating a 5-year-old girl for her involuntary writhing movements in her arms with small, random, superimposed twitches. Her past medical history is remarkable for asthma and frequent pneumonia

and sinusitis. On examination, she has hypometric saccades, forced blinking to initiate saccades, truncal ataxia, and choreoathetosis. Skin examination shows telangiectasias on the bulbar conjunctivae, on the tops of the ears, along the malar prominences of the face, and within the flexor creases of the elbows and knees.

What test is most likely to be diagnostic?

A. Alpha-fetoprotein (AFP) and carcinoembryonal antigen (CEA)
B. Chest radiograph
C. EMG/NCS
D. MRI of the brain and lumbar puncture
E. Urine for catecholamines

Correct Answer is: A

This patient has Ataxia telangiectasia (AT). This child has the classic triad of ataxia, telangiectasia, and frequent sinopulmonary infections, which suggests a diagnosis of ataxia telangiectasia (AT). AT is an autosomal recessive disorder affecting the ATM gene on chromosome 11, which is a gene involved in cell-cycle progression and DNA repair. Ataxia begins proximally and spreads distally, and choreoathetosis is frequent. Telangiectasias appear between age 2 and 10 years, and mild intellectual disability occurs. There is an increased tendency to develop malignancies, especially lymphomas and leukemias. The immune system is also impaired, accounting for recurrent infections. AFP is often elevated, CEA may be elevated, and IgG (especially subclasses 2 and 4), IgA, and IgE are depressed. Together these tests have up to 90% sensitivity.

Specific testing for the ATM gene is also available. Brain MRI may show cerebellar atrophy. Management of AT includes aggressive treatment of infections and avoiding radiation, including chest radiography and sunbathing. Heterozygotes are also at risk for malignancy, especially breast cancer.

Suggested Reading

- Perlman S, Becker-Catania S, Gatti RA. Ataxia-telangiectasia: diagnosis and treatment. Semin Pediatr Neurol 2003;10:173–82.

119. You are evaluating an infant with epileptic encephalopathy. He has microcephaly and prominent developmental delay. On CSF analysis, the glucose level is 30 mg/dl, whereas the serum glucose level is 112 mg/dl. Other CSF tests are normal.

What is correct regarding this condition?

A. Brain MRI usually suggests the diagnosis
B. It is caused by deficiency in the glucose transporter type 1
C. Phenobarbital is the treatment of choice
D. Ketogenic diet has been shown to be ineffective for seizure control
E. It is inherited in an X-linked fashion

Correct Answer is: B

This patient has a glucose transporter type 1 (GLUT-1) deficiency. The brain utilizes glucose as its primary source of energy. In fasting conditions, glycogen is exhausted within minutes, and since amino acids and fat cannot be used for the production of energy in the brain, ketones become the alternative fuel. Glucose crosses the blood brain barrier facilitated by GLUT-1, which is a membrane-bound protein encoded by the SLC2A 1 gene on chromosome 1p35–31.3. GLUT-1 deficiency syndrome is inherited in an autosomal dominant fashion and causes a defect in glucose transport across the blood-brain barrier

and into brain cells, manifesting as an epileptic encephalopathy with infantile-onset seizures, developmental delay, microcephaly, and complex movement disorders. CSF glucose level is low with a normal serum glucose level, and other CSF studies are normal, excluding other causes of hypoglycorrhachia (such as CNS infection). EEG may show 2.5–4 Hz spikes and waves and the inter-ictal EEG findings may improve with glucose. Neuroimaging does not show specific abnormalities. Later-onset forms with episodic movement disorders and ataxia, paroxysmal exertional dyskinesia, or early-onset atypical absence epilepsy have been described. A ketogenic diet should be started as soon as the diagnosis is suspected, since this treatment option improves seizure control and the abnormal movements; however, it is less effective for the psychomotor impairment.

Congenital

Y. M. Awaad, *Absolute Pediatric Neurology*, https://doi.org/10.1007/978-3-319-78801-2_4

4

1. You are evaluating a one-month-old baby for severe hypotonia since birth. His pregnancy and delivery were normal. On examination, he has a flat occiput, frontal bossing, large fontanelles, epicanthal folds, shallow supraorbital ridges and hepatomegaly.
What test is most likely to be diagnostic?
A. Chromosome analysis
B. CT scan of the brain
C. Plasma carnitine levels
D. Plasma very long chain fatty acid levels
E. Skeletal X-rays

Correct Answer is: D
Peroxisomes are cytoplasmic organelles in all mammalian cells except RBC; single membrane. They contain no nucleic acid; the proteins are encoded by nuclear genes and translated on free cytoplasmic ribosomes. They have many cellular anabolic and catabolic functions including degradation of very long chain fatty acids (C22, C24, and C26), early steps of plasmalogen biosynthesis, degradation of phytanic acid, selected steps in cholesterol biosynthesis, degradation of pipecolic acid, synthesis of bile acid intermediates, and glyoxylate metabolism. Peroxisomal disorders result from failure to form or maintain the peroxisomes or a defect in one of the enzymes normally found in the peroxisome.

Zellweger syndrome is due to total absence of liver peroxisomes. Patients present with dysmorphic facies, hypotonia, seizures, mental retardation, neuronal heterotopias, cataracts and/or glaucoma, and renal cysts; about 50% have epiphyseal calcifications. Death usually occurs by 6–12 months. The diagnosis depends on showing lack of all peroxisomal function. No peroxisomes would be seen on EM. Elevated VLCFA or low plasmalogens are good screening tests.

Suggested Reading

- Steinberg S, Raymond GV. Peroxisome biogenesis disorders, Zellweger syndrome spectrum. Gene Revi. At ► http://www.genereviews.org.

2. You are seeing a 2-year-old girl for her progressive neurological disorder. She was a full-term baby with normal and an uncomplicated pregnancy. She was reportedly normal at birth. She achieved her normal milestones in the first year of life, with walking and babbling by 14 months. But at 16 months of age, she began falling and became clumsy with her hands. At 18 months she stopped babbling and walking; subsequently she developed loss of visual function, myoclonic seizures, and progressive microcephaly.
What is the most likely diagnosis?
A. Methylmalonic academia
B. Mitochondrial disorder
C. Neuronal ceroid lipofuscinosis
D. Ornithine transcarbamylase deficiency
E. SCN1A gene mutation

Correct Answer is: C
The neuronal ceroid lipofuscinoses (NCLs) are the most common group of genetic storage disorders that lead to progressive diseases of children and young adults. They are characterized by neurological regression, epilepsy, and visual loss due to retinal degeneration. Pathologically, they are storage disorders with accumulation of an auto-fluorescent material, ceroid lipofuscin, in combination with the degeneration of neuronal cells. There are at least 10 genetically distinct NCLs, designated CLN1 to CLN10 and genetic testing is available for many of them. Several NCLs exhibit a widely variable clinical picture, depending on the severity of the individual mutation. NCL may

be suspected by the clinical history and supplemented by the finding of leukocyte inclusions on skin biopsy or buffy coat analysis.

Suggested Reading

- Kohlschütter A, Schulz A. Towards understanding the neuronal ceroid lipofuscinoses. Brain Dev. 2009;31(7): 499–502.

3. You are evaluating a 4-year-old boy for his motor delay. He was born at full term after normal and an uneventful pregnancy. He was normal at birth and in the first few months of life, but thereafter developed macrocephaly and was delayed in his milestones. He has no family history of such case. On your examination, he is hypotonic and his head circumference is above the 95th percentile. A brain MRI scan is obtained and is shown.

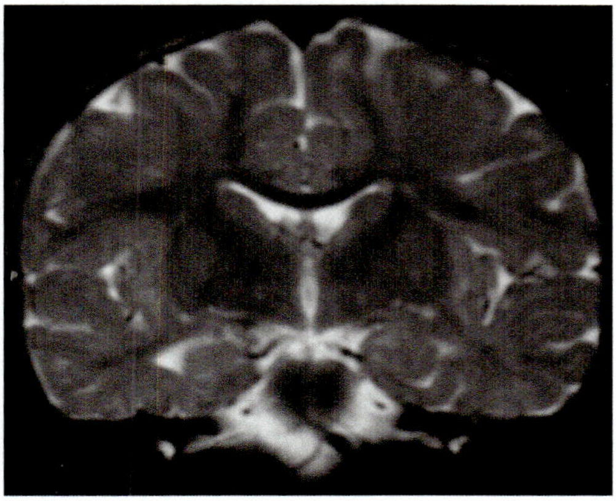

Fig. 4.1 Radiology picture of the day. Dr. Laughlin Dawes. Canavan disease. Wikipedia

What is the most likely diagnosis?

A. Adrenoleukodystrophy
B. Canavan disease
C. Krabbe disease
D. Metachromatic leukodystrophy
E. Vanishing white matter disease

Correct Answer is: B

This clinical presentation should raise the suspicion of Canavan disease because of the triad of hypotonia, macrocephaly, and head lag in an infant after the age of three to 5 months. Very high concentration of N-acetyl aspartic acid (NAA) in the urine is diagnostic of symptomatic Canavan disease patients. NAA concentration is also elevated in the blood and cerebrospinal fluid (CSF) of children with Canavan disease. The elevated NAA can be seen by 1H MRS as a single peak with a resonance of 2.01 ppm on the spectrum.

Suggested Reading

- Janson CG, McPhee SW, Francis J, Shera D, Assadi M, Freese A, Hurh P, Haselgrove J, Wang DJ, Bilaniuk L, Leone P. Natural history of Canavan disease revealed by proton magnetic resonance spectroscopy (1H-MRS) and diffusion-weighted MRI. Neuropediatrics. 2006;37:209–21.

4. You are seeing a 15-yr. old boy with history of intermittent falling for 2 years. His examination at that time revealed ataxia, dysarthric speech and multifocal myoclonus, and he was diagnosed with myoclonic seizures. One year ago, he developed intractable seizures including myoclonic and generalized tonic clonic seizures. He also complained of transient episodes of visual loss. He also developed progressive multifocal myoclonus at times brought on by auditory stimulation. Now, he lost his ability to walk and became non-ambulatory, has a tracheostomy to help with handling of secretions, is nonverbal and does not follow commands. Brain neuroimaging showed severe diffuse brain atrophy. His optical fundus examination was normal. A skin biopsy slid is shown.

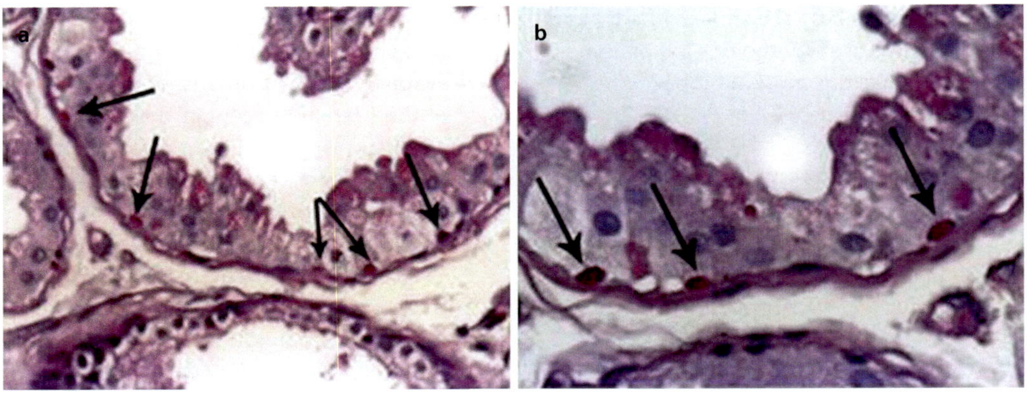

Fig. 4.2 Lafora bodies on skin biopsy. **a** Histopathologic examination of the skin biopsy taken from the axillary region reveals round-to-oval intracytoplasmic, periodic acid–Schiff-positive, diastase-resistant inclusions within the myoepithelial and acinar cells of sweat glands, corresponding to Lafora bodies (*arrows*). Periodic acid–Schiff stain, 200×. **b** Lafora bodies in a magnified view (*arrows*). Periodic acid–Schiff stain, 400×. Print ISSN: 0028-3878 Online ISSN: 1526-632X

What is the most likely diagnosis?

A. Neuronal ceroid lipofuscinosis
B. Lafora body disease
C. Dravet syndrome
D. Tay Sach's disease
E. Juvenile Myoclonic Epilepsy

Correct Answer is: B

At age 13 he developed progressive myoclonic seizures, progressive stimulus induced myoclonus and loss of milestones eventually leading to a vegetative state. This is consistent with a neurodegenerative disorder, specifically one associated with progressive myoclonic epilepsy. There are a group of disorders that fall into this description. These include neuronal ceroid lipofuscinosis, Unverricht Lundborg, Disease (ULD), Lafora Body Disease, myoclonic epilepsy with ragged red fibers (MERRF), and sialidosis. Lafora body disease patients have normal development until 13 to 17 years of age when they develop ataxia, dysarthria and eventually progressive myoclonus. They develop myoclonic epilepsy, occipital seizures with episodic loss of vision, and progressive myoclonus. They experience eventual loss of all acquired milestones, with progressive dementia and typically leading to a vegetative state. Initial Neuroimaging shows global atrophy in later stage which is normal initially. Electroencephalograms show paroxysmal spike wave bursts and poly spike and wave with an occipital predominance. Diagnosis can be made by skin biopsy with characteristic PAS positive eccrine duct deposits as shown in the picture below. The putative genes have been named EPM2A and EPM2B (epilepsy with progressive myoclonus).

Juvenile neuronal ceroid lipofuscinosis could present in a similar fashion, but typically presents at a younger age, around 5–8 yrs. of age; the retinal exam would show a pigmentary retinopathy, with progressive loss of vision occurring early on.

Dravet syndrome is a disorder, which typically presents in infants and children with a history of multiple febrile seizures, febrile hemiclonic status epilepticus and myoclonic seizures. There is slowing of development starting around the age of 2 years, and typically has a slower progression.

Juvenile myoclonic epilepsy is associated with early morning myoclonic jerks, typically nocturnal generalized tonic clonic seizures and poly-spike and wave on EEG. It is not typically associated with neurodegeneration.

Juvenile Tay-Sach's disease usually presents around 2–10 years of age. Symptoms include loss of cognitive milestones, difficulty with gait and at times seizures. It is related to a deficiency of hexosaminidase A. Progression is slower than Lafora Body disease and the skin biopsy would not show the results seen for this patient.

Suggested Reading

- Zhao X, Scherer SW, Ackerley CA, Berge A. Minassian Early-onset Lafora body disease. Brain. 135(9):2684–98.
- Anna C Jansen, MD, PhD and Eva Andermann, MD, PhD, FCCMG. Progressive Myoclonus Epilepsy, Lafora Type. Gene Reviews. Initial Posting: December 28, 2007; Last Update: November 3, 2011.
- Zupanc ML, Legros B. Progressive myoclonic epilepsy. Cerebellum. 2004;3(3):156–71.

5. What anticonvulsant is likely to cause life-threatening side effects in the patient with mitochondrial disorders?
   - A. Oxcarbazepine
   - B. Levitiracetam
   - C. Clonazepam
   - D. Valproic acid
   - E. Ethosuccimide

Correct Answer is: D

Valproic acid that, in their metabolism, generate reactive oxygen species can cause irreversible, and life-threatening liver disease in patients with mitochondrial disorders and other disorders of redox regulation.

Suggested Reading

- Nanau RM, Neuman MG. Adverse drug reactions induced by valproic acid. Clin Biochem. 2013;46:1323–38.
- Pronicka E, Weglewska-Jurkiewicz A, Pronicki M, Sykut-Cegielska J, Kowalski P, Pajdowska M, Jankowska I, Kotulska K, Kalicinski P, Jakobkiewicz-Banecka J, Wegrzyn G. Drug-resistant epilepsia and fulminant valproate liver toxicity. Alpers-Huttenlocher syndrome in two children confirmed post mortem by identification of p. W748S mutation in POLG gene. Med Sci Monit. 2011;17:CR203–209.

6. You are seeing a 5-month-old adopted Chinese boy because the family noticed episodes of inconsolable screaming, arching of his back and neck, and apparent lack of awareness of his surroundings right after they bring him home. On your exam, he has no deep tendon reflexes but has paradoxically increased tone both axially and appendicularly.
   What abnormalities would you expect to see on his brain MRI?
   - A. Skull
   - B. Grey matter
   - C. White matter
   - D. Venous sinuses
   - E. Basal ganglia

Correct Answer is: C

This a classic description of Krabbe disease (leukodystrophy). Because he was not born in the U.S., it explains the absence of the newborn testing that might have made this family aware of the diagnosis before the adoption.

Suggested Reading

- Kohlschütter A. Lysosomal leukodystrophies: Krabbe disease and metachromatic leukodystrophy. Handb Clin Neurol. 2013;113:1611–18.

7. You are seeing a 4-year-old girl South American for her progressive refusal to walk and absent deep tendon reflexes. When you examined her, you noticed that she keeps her hips and knees flexed, even when you support her from both axillae to hold her up in vertical suspension.

4

When you try to put the soles of her feet onto the examining table, she screams as if she is in pain. Rubbing the bottoms of her feet with your hands elicits the same response. When you lay her flat on the table and passively extend her legs, you notice they are bowed. Her family states that her diet consists of juice and chicken nuggets.

You think you know what is wrong and test your hypothesis by ordering:

A. An MRI of the brain
B. A serum lactates
C. Serum calcium, phosphate, alkaline phosphatase, and vitamin D
D. A somatosensory evoked potential study.

Correct Answer is: C

Longstanding vitamin D deficiency in toddlers causes a painful neuropathy, bowing of the legs, a low serum calcium, a low serum phosphate, and a high serum alkaline phosphatase. The neuropathy may be evident on an EMG/NCV study, but this study will not allow determination of the etiology of the neuropathy. The other studies would be expected to be unhelpful in this child.

Suggested Reading

- Elder CJ, Bishop NJ. Rickets. Lancet. 2014;383:1665–76.

8. You are evaluating a 4-month-old baby for muscle stiffness with hyperextension of his neck and back. He has had failure to thrive with swallowing difficulties. He might have a possible seizure. He is extremely irritable. Examination is notable for an irritable, cachexic infant with strabismus, bulbar dysfunction and hypertonia. There is hepatosplenomegaly. A previous child in the family had a similar presentation and died at age 3 years.

Activity of which of the following enzymes is most likely to be abnormal?

A. Arylsulfatase
B. Glucocerebrosidase
C. Hexosaminidase
D. Sialidase

Correct Answer is: B

Gaucher disease is the most common lysosomal storage disease. It is inherited as an autosomal recessive disorder due to deficiency of lysosomal glucocerebrosidase (gene locus 1q21). Type I is a non-neuronopathic (visceral) Gaucher disease and neuronopathic glucocerebrosidase deficiency was referred to as type II (acute neuronopathic) or type III (subacute neuronopathic). Meanwhile, it has been recognized that all forms represent a broad spectrum of manifestations rather than clearly distinguishable disorders. Neuronopathic type is found in less than 1:100,000 live births. So far, more than 200 mutations have been described, but lack a genotype-phenotype correlation. Patients with acute neuronopathic Gaucher disease exhibit severe neurological symptoms during the first year of life including stridor, strabismus due to palsy of the ocular muscles, and dysphagia. Some patients show affection of the pyramidal tract with spasm, retroflexion of the head or opisthotonus. Acute neuronopathic Gaucher disease is usually fatal within the first 2 years of life.

Suggested Reading

- Staretz-Chacham O, Lang TC, LaMarca ME, Krasnewich D, Sidransky E. Lysosomal storage disorders in the newborn. Pediatrics. 2009;123(4):1191–207.
- Hoffmann B, Mayatepek E. Neurological manifestations in lysosomal storage disorders – from pathology to first therapeutic possibilities. Neuropediatrics. 2005;36(5):285–9.

9. The girl shown in the picture has history of hypotonia and global non-regressive developmental delay with autistic features. She has poor school performance. She has cataracts on examination.

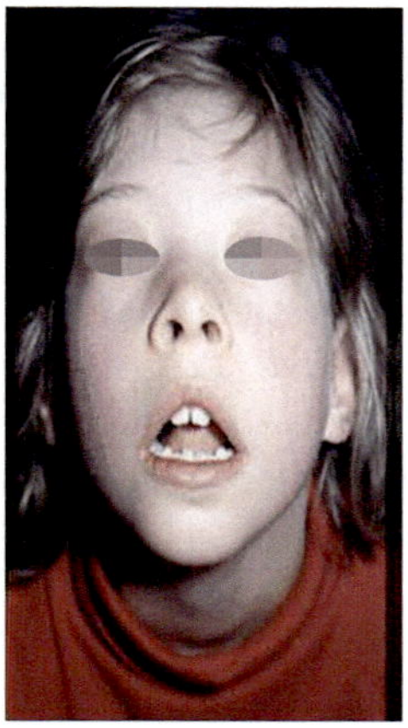

Fig. 4.3 Smith-Lemli-Opitz_syndrome. ▶ http://learn.genetics.utah.edu/content/disorders/whataregd/slos/index.html ▶ http://emedicine.medscape.com/article/949125-overview ▶ http://en.wikipedia.org/wiki/Smith-Lemli-Opitz_syndrome

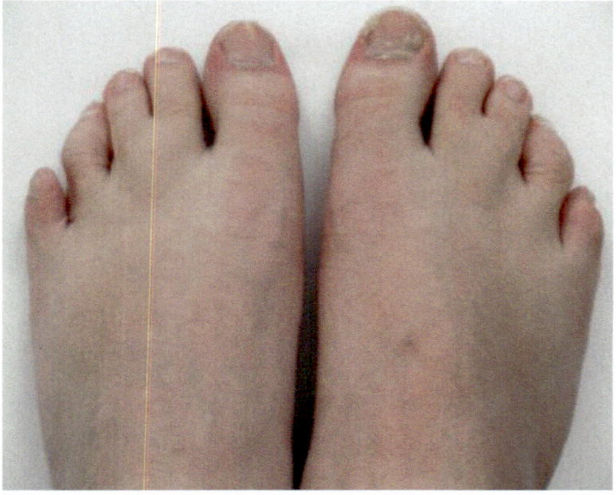

Fig. 4.4 My feet with limited partial syndactyly (and some other ugly defects). (AzaToth. Own work. Wikipedia)

What is the best diagnostic test to consider in this patient?

A. Mitochondrial point mutation and deletion panel
B. Microarray analysis
C. Very long chain fatty acids
D. 7 dehydrocholesterol
E. Buffy coat

Correct Answer is: D

This child has Smith-Lemli-Opitz syndrome (SLOS). It is a complex malformation syndrome with prenatal and postnatal growth retardation, microcephaly, moderate to severe mental retardation, and multiple major and minor malformations. The facial features can be subtle or severe. The malformations include distinctive facial features, cleft palate, cardiac defects, underdeveloped external genitalia in males, and 2–3 syndactyly of the toes. Many children present due to developmental delay and autism. The diagnosis is often missed. The defect lies in the final step of cholesterol metabolism. Testing for 7 dehydrocholesterol is diagnostic as many milder patients have normal plasma cholesterol levels. Testing of plasma cholesterol is not diagnostic.

Suggested Reading

- Pickler L, Elias E. Genetic evaluation of the child with an autism spectrum disorder. Pediatr Ann. 2009;38(1):26–9.

10. A pediatrician referred a 6-month-old male because he has periods of irritability, stiffness and regression of skills since he was 4 months of age. He has normal birth and early development history. He also has periods of elevated temperature without evidence of infection. Examination shows no dysmorphic features. There are episodes of opisthotonus in response to tactile stimulus. Muscle tone is increased and reflexes are absent. His CSF testing showed elevated protein but no other abnormalities.

Which of the following laboratory studies would most likely be abnormal in this patient?

A. Phenylalanine hydroxylase
B. 7-dehydrocholesterol
C. Acid maltase
D. Galactocerebrosidase
E. Beta hexosamindase A

Correct Answer is: D
this is a presentation of a Krabbe disease, which is characterized by an infantile-onset progressive neurologic regressive disorder with death before 2 years of age in the majority of individuals. Alternatively, onset may be between age 6 months and the fifth decade with slower disease progression. Children with the infantile form appear to be normal for the first few months of life but show extreme irritability, spasticity, and developmental delay before age 6 months; psychomotor regression progresses to a decerebrate state with no voluntary movement. In the late-onset forms, individuals can be clinically normal until weakness, vision loss, and intellectual regression become evident. The clinical course is variable even within the same family.Stage I is characterized by irritability, stiffness, arrest of motor and mental development, and episodes of temperature elevation without infection, possibly caused by involvement of the hypothalamus. The child, apparently normal for the first few months after birth, becomes hypersensitive to auditory, tactile, or visual stimuli and begins to cry frequently without apparent cause.In almost all individuals with Krabbe disease, galactocerebrosidase (GALC) enzyme activity is deficient in leukocytes isolated from whole heparinized blood or in cultured skin fibroblasts.

Suggested Reading

- Wenger DA, Suzuki K, Suzuki Y, Suzuki K. Galactosylceramide lipidosis. Globoid cell leukodystrophy (Krabbe disease). In: Scriver CR, Beaudet AL, Sly WS, Valle D, Childs B, Vogelstein B, editors. The metabolic and molecular bases of inherited disease, 8th ed. New York: McGraw-Hill; 2001.

11. You were asked to see a full-term baby boy in the NICU who was born after non-complicated labor but appeared depressed at birth with generalized hypotonia and hypoventilation. He started to have spells of clonic seizure activity involving left and right side independently lasting 30–60 seconds on several occasions. On your examination, he has micrognathia, broad nasal bridge, and high forehead, dolichocephalic skull with large anterior and posterior fontanelles. A firm liver edge was noted 1 cm below the costal margin. On neurological exam, he has sever generalized hypotonia with poor gag and suck/swallow, absent reflexes and difficult to elicit Moro response. His EEG showed multifocal spikes on a mildly low voltage background without state change but no electrographic seizures. CT scan showed dilated posterior horns (colopocephaly).
What is the most likely diagnosis?
A. Zellweger syndrome
B. Prader-Willi syndrome
C. Myotonic dystrophy
D. Spinal muscular atrophy
E. Congenital CMV infection

Correct Answer is: A
the child has Zellweger's syndrome. It is an autosomal recessive disorder, is the severest form of the peroxisomal biogenesis disorders (PBD) and presents at birth with dysmorphic features, liver cirrhosis, severe hypotonia and neonatal encephalopathy with seizures. The diagnosis is based on the dysmorphic features and confirmed by analysis of very long chain fatty acids (elevated VLCFA C26:0, C26:1; abnormal ratios of C24/C22; C26/C22). Peroxisomes (which

are missing in Zellweger's) process VLCFA which, if they accumulate abnormally, affect CNS and other cell membranes. CNS dysmyelination occurs and in the severe form leads to problems with radial glial guides and migration disorders (pachygyria, polymicrogyria, neuronal heterotopias, colopocephaly) resulting in severe encephalopathy and seizures. Mutations in twelve different PEX genes, those that encode peroxins, the proteins required for normal peroxisome assembly, have been identified in Zellweger's syndrome. Treatment is symptomatic and children fail to develop, with death usually in the first year. Other PBD are neonatal adrenoleukodystrophy, infantile Refsum disease (both considered part of the Zellweger's Syndrome Spectrum) and rhizomelic chondrodysplasia punctata. These disorders can be separated clinically and 80% of PBD are among the Zellweger's Syndrome Spectrum with an incidence of 1 in 50,000 births in the US.

Suggested Reading

Steinberg SJ, Raymond GV, Braverman NE, Moser AM, and Moser HW. Peroxisome biogenesis disorders, Zellweger syndrome spectrum. Gene Rev. ► http://www.ncbi.nlm.nih.gov/bookshelf/br.fcgi?book=gene&part=pbd.

12. You are evaluating a 5-month-old baby who was normal at birth, but has devolved regression with progressive opisthotonus, stridor, and swallowing difficulties. On examination, he has enlarged spleen, squint, head retroflexion, spasticity, and trismus.
What tissue analysis would most likely define his condition?
A. Bone marrow
B. Blood leukocytes
C. Muscle
D. Skin
E. Liver

Correct Answer is: B
Gaucher disease diagnosis is based on the demonstration of deficient glucosylceramidase enzyme activity in peripheral blood leukocytes. Carrier testing by assay of enzyme activity is unreliable because of overlap in enzyme activity between carriers and non-carriers. Identification of two disease-causing alleles in GBA, the only gene known to be associated with Gaucher disease, provides additional confirmation of the diagnosis.

Suggested Reading

Goker-Alpan O, Schiffmann R, Park JK, Stubblefield BK, Tayebi N, Sidransky E. Phenotypic continuum in neuronopathic Gaucher disease: an intermediate phenotype between type 2 and type 3. J Pediatr. 2003;143(2):273–6.

13. You are evaluating an 8-year-old boy for his developmental delay. His medical history is remarkable for frequent ear infections and a heart murmur due to valvular disease. On examination, he has short stature, lordotic posture, slightly coarse facial features, and corneal clouding.
What laboratory test would most likely define his condition?
A. Amino acid analysis
B. 7-dehydrocholesterol level
C. Lysosomal enzyme screen
D. CSF neurotransmitter levels
E. Uric acid level

Correct Answer is: C
the child has Sanfilippo syndrome. It is one of the mucopolysaccharidoses (MPSs) disorders. It is inherited lysosomal storage disorders caused by the deficiency or absence of specific lysosomal enzymes. The absence of these enzymes leads to accumulation of complex carbohydrates in cells and tissues and in

the cellular organelles, the lysosomes. These complex carbohydrates are also known as mucopolysaccharides or glycosaminoglycans (GAGs) serve as the building blocks for connective tissues.

MPS III, or Sanfilippo syndrome, is the most common of MPS disorders and results from the deficiency or absence of 4 different enzymes that are necessary to degrade the GAG heparan sulfate. Each enzyme deficiency defines a different form of Sanfilippo syndrome. Individuals with type A lack the enzyme heparan sulfate sulfatase. Individuals with type B lack the enzyme N -acetyl-alpha-D-glucosaminidase. Patients with type C lack acetyl-CoA:alpha-glucosaminide acetyltransferase. Patients with type D lack the enzyme N- acetylglucosamine-6-sulfatase. The particular form of Sanfilippo syndrome cannot be determined based on clinical features, but rather must rely on enzymatic assays. The neurological manifestations include mental regression beginning in the toddler years, coarse facial appearance, but may be mild, sleep disturbance and progressive myelopathy due to storage material in the spine. Seizures may occur. Initial clinical signs present as a change in behavior. Patients are hyperactive and display aggressive and destructive behaviors.

Suggested Reading

- Valstar MJ, Ruijter GJ, van Diggelen OP, Poorthuis BJ, Wijburg FA. Sanfilippo syndrome: a mini-review. J Inherit Metab Dis. 20.

14. A normal healthy 9-year-old female is brought to the ED with vomiting and lethargy after a birthday party. She has unremarkable past medical history. Her early developmental milestones were on target and she is an average student in the 3nd grade. Family history is remarkable for a maternal cousin who died in early infancy from an unspecified condition. On examination she is obtunded. Her EEG shows slowing and tri-phasic waves.

    What is your next step in evaluation?

    A. Ammonia
    B. CSF exam
    C. Plasma lactate
    D. MRI of the brain with MRS
    E. CT brain scan

Correct Answer is: A

this is a clinical presentation of ornithine transcarbamylase deficiency. Although classically associated with presentation in infancy, the majority of individuals with urea cycle disorders (UCDs) present outside the neonatal period, frequently in childhood. Signs and symptoms are unclear but recurrent; fulminant presentations associated with acute illness are also common. A disorder of urea cycle metabolism should be considered in children who have recurrent symptoms, especially neurologic abnormalities associated with periods of decompensation. Routine laboratory tests, including measurement of plasma ammonia concentrations, can indicate a potential UCD; however, specific metabolic testing and ultimately enzymatic or molecular confirmation are necessary to establish a diagnosis. Treatment with dietary protein restriction and medications may be challenging in children.

Suggested Reading

- Smith W, Kishnani PS, Lee B, Singh RH, Rhead WJ, Sniderman King L, Smith M, Summar M. Urea cycle disorders: clinical presentation outside the newborn period. Crit Care Clin. 2005;21(4 Suppl):S9–17.

15. You are evaluating an 8-year-old boy with a history of a progressive gait disturbance and abnormal involuntary movements for 1 year. He has unremarkable past medical history. On examination, he has remarkable dystonia and equinovarous deformity in his feet, rigidity in his legs, and chorea. His brain MRI is shown.

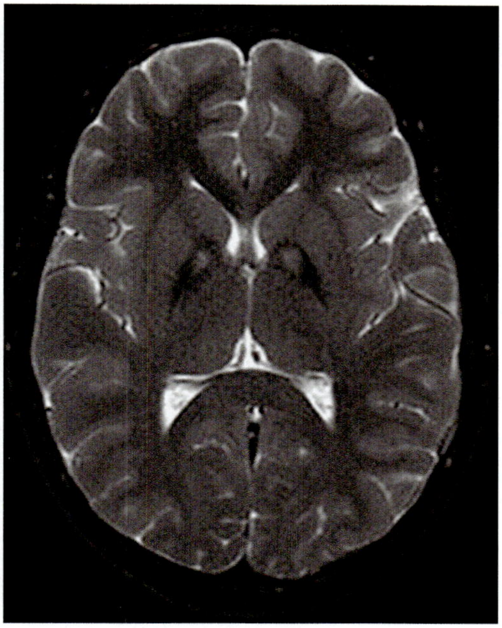

Fig. 4.5 MRI image shows iron deposits in the basal ganglia, the so-called eye-of-the-tiger sign (T2w GRASE sequence). (Enro2002. Wikipedia)

Which of the following metals can case this metabolic disorder?

A. Copper
B. Iron
C. Mercury
D. Lead
E. Zinc

Correct Answer is: B

This is a presentation of Pantothenate kinase-associated neurodegeneration (PKAN). It is a form of neurodegeneration with brain iron accumulation (NBIA formerly called Hallervorden-Spatz syndrome) characterized by progressive dystonia and basal ganglia iron deposition with onset that usually occurs before age 10 years. The most clinical manifestations include dysarthria, rigidity, and pigmentary retinopathy. About 25% of affected individuals have an 'atypical' presentation with later onset (after age 10 years), prominent speech defects, psychiatric disturbances, and more gradual progression of disease. Approximately 50% of the patients have identifiable mutations in the PANK2 gene. All individuals with NBIA who are found to have the 'eye-of-the-tiger' sign on T2-weighted magnetic resonance imaging have been found to have at least one mutation in PANK2.

Suggested Reading

- Gregory A, Polster BJ, Hayflick SJ. Clinical and genetic delineation of neurodegeneration with brain iron accumulation. J Med Genet. 2009;46(2):73.

16. You are seeing a 7-month-old girl with a history of a seizure described as staring followed by a generalized convulsion lasting 5 min. Her past medical history is remarkable of hypotonia and developmental delay, is not able to roll over and does not reach for objects with her hands. On examination, her head circumference is above 95th percentile, while her weight and length are at 25th percentile. She has optic atrophy and nystagmus, central hypotonia and increased tone in the ankles, with clonus. Her brain MRI shows increased signal in the white matter diffusely on T2-weighted images. Her MRS shows a strikingly elevated NAA peak.
What is the most likely diagnosis?

A. Krabbe leukodystrophy
B. Adrenoleukodystrophy
C. Mitochondrial encephalomyopathy
D. Canavan disease
E. Metachromatic leukodystrophy

Correct Answer is: D

Canavan disease diagnosis can be made based on the triad of hypotonia, macrocephaly, and head lag in an infant after the age of 3–5 months. Diagnosis of Canavan disease in symptomatic individuals relies upon demonstration of very high concentration of N-acetyl aspartic acid (NAA) in the urine. NAA concentration is also elevated in the blood and

cerebrospinal fluid (CSF) of children with Canavan disease. In the brain, the elevated NAA can be visualized by 1H MRS as a single peak with a resonance of 2.01 ppm on the spectrum.

Suggested Reading

- Janson CG, McPhee SW, Francis J, Shera D, Assadi M, Freese A, Hurh P, Haselgrove J, Wang DJ, Bilaniuk L, Leone P. Natural history of Canavan disease revealed by proton magnetic resonance spectroscopy (1H-MRS) and diffusion-weighted MRI. Neuropediatrics. 2006;37(4): 209–21.

17. A 14-year-old female with 1-year history of psychiatric symptoms including inattention, impulsivity, and anger outbursts came to your office for evaluation of progressive deterioration in her gait. She has unremarkable past medical history and noncontributory family history. Her examination demonstrates pale optic nerves, low amplitude deep tendon reflexes, increased tone, and extensor plantar responses. Her brain MRI is shown.
    What is your likely diagnosis?
    A. Adrenoleukodystrophy
    B. Krabbe's disease
    C. Metachromatic leukodystrophy
    D. Alexander's disease
    E. Canavan's disease

Correct Answer is: C

This is a case of Metachromatic leukodystrophy (MLD). It is due to Arylsulfatase A deficiency. There are three clinical subtypes: a late-infantile MLD, a juvenile MLD, and an adult onset form of MLD. The disease course may be from three to ten or more years in the late-infantile form and up to 20 years or more in the juvenile and adult forms. In the late infantile type, onset is between 1–2 years of age. Typical presenting findings include weakness, hypotonia, clumsiness, frequent falls, toe walking, and slurred speech. Later signs include inability to stand, difficulty with speech, deterioration of mental function, increased muscle tone, pain in the arms and legs, generalized or partial seizures, compromised vision and hearing, and peripheral neuropathy. In the final stages children have tonic spasms, decerebrate posturing, and general unawareness of their surroundings. Unexplained fevers and elevated CSF protein may be seen.

Suggested Reading

- Kaye EM. Update on genetic disorders affecting white matter. Reference: Pediatr Neurol. 2001;24(1):11–24.

18. Which of the following is correct regarding sialidosis?
    A. Sialidosis type I has infantile onset
    B. Sialidosis type II has adult onset
    C. A cherry-red spot is rarely seen in this condition
    D. Coarse facial features are almost never seen in sialidosis type II
    E. These patients have myoclonic epilepsy

Correct Answer is: E

Sialidosis is one of glycoproteinoses group, and myoclonic epilepsy is common in these patients. Glycoproteinoses are a group of lysosomal storage disorders of autosomal recessive inheritance, in which the enzymatic defect leads to accumulation of oligosaccharides, glycopeptides, and glycolipids. Accumulation in the brain and viscera leads to vacuolization of multiple cell types. There are multiple phenotypes depending on the enzyme affected. In general, these patients have coarse facial features, skeletal abnormalities, and psychomotor retardation. Sialidosis is caused by deficiency of lysosomal A-neuraminidase (sialidase), leading to increased urinary

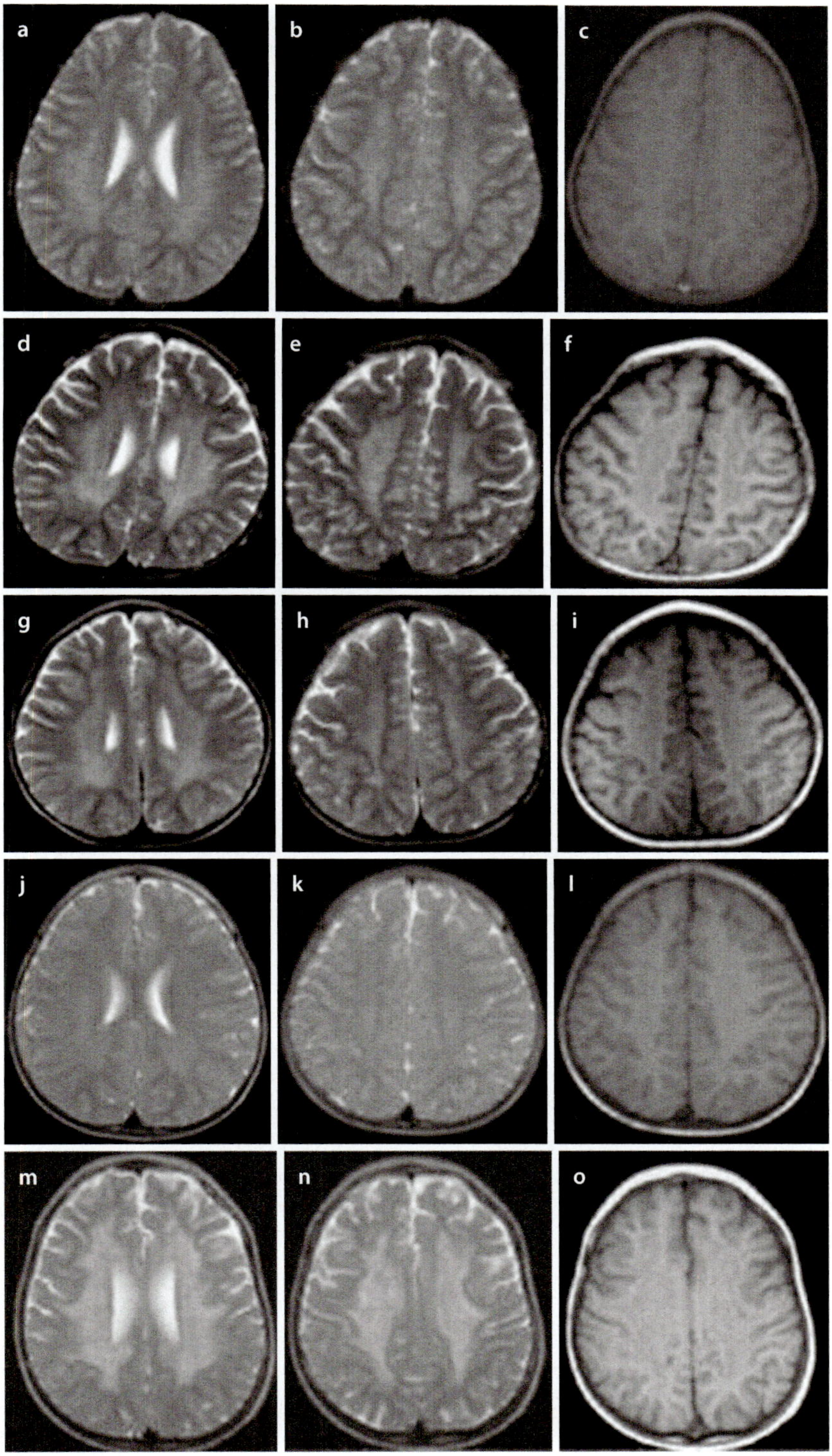

Fig. 4.6 Liaw, Hsiang-Ru, et al. "Late infantile metachromatic leukodystrophy: Clinical manifestations of five Taiwanese patients and Genetic features in Asia." Orphanet journal of rare diseases 10.1 (2015): 1. HR Liaw, HF Lee, CS Chi. This article is distributed under the terms of the Creative Commons Attribution 4.0 International License. (**a**–**c**) Patient #1, (**d**–**f**) Patient #2, (**g**–**i**) Patient #3, (**j**–**l**) Patient # 4, (**m**–**o**) Patient # 5

excretion of sialic acid-containing oligosaccharides.

Type I sialidosis (cherry red spot myoclonus syndrome) has its onset in adolescence to adulthood and manifests with myoclonic epilepsy, visual deterioration, and cherry-red spots without dysmorphism.

Type II is the childhood form, and these patients have not only myoclonic epilepsy and cherry-red spots in the retina but also severe neurologic abnormalities, coarse facial features, severe dysostosis, and psychomotor retardation.

The neonatal form is characterized by hydrops fetalis, nephrotic syndrome, and early death.

Other glycoproteinoses include A-mannosidosis caused by A-mannosidosidase deficiency, B-mannosidosis caused by B-mannosidosidase deficiency, fucosidosis caused by fucosidase deficiency, aspartylglucosaminuri a caused by aspartylglucosaminidase deficiency, and Schindler disease caused by A-N acetylgalactosaminidase deficiency.

Abnormal urinary excretion of oligosaccharides and glycopeptides, as well as vacuolated lymphocytes with membrane-bound vacuoles, can be seen. Definitive diagnosis is made with analysis of enzyme activity.

Suggested Reading

- Comprehensive review in clinical neurology: a multiple-choice question book for the wards and boards © 2011 Wolters Kluwer Health Lippincott Williams & Wilkins. All rights reserved.

19. Which of the following statements is not true regarding the abnormality shown in the Figure? Coronal T2-weighted MRI
    - A. Hemimegalencephaly frequently presents with seizures
    - B. Macrocephaly may be due to hydrocephalus or megalencephalyc.
    - C. Hemimegalencephaly rarely leads to motor manifestations
    - D. Megalencephaly is an oversized brain, with brain weight greater than 2 standard deviations above the mean
    - E. Megalencephaly may be a benign finding in some cases

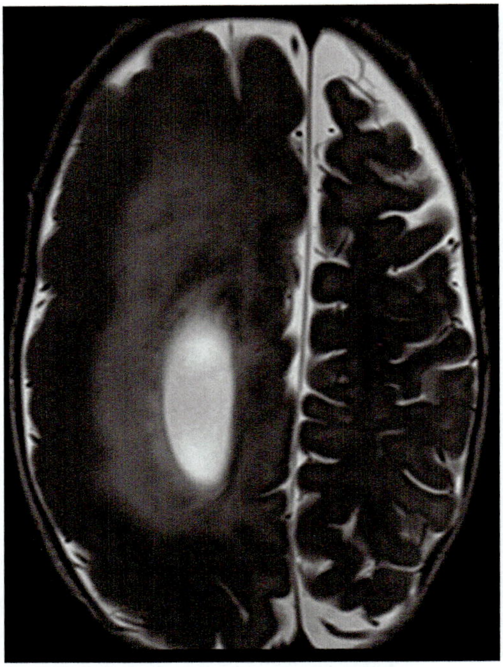

Fig. 4.7 Hemimegalencephaly From ► ILAE.org, ► EpilepsyDiagnosis.org, Diagnostic Manual

Correct Answer is: C

This is a radiological presentation of left hemispheric hemimegalencephaly, which frequently leads to contralateral hemiparesis. Microcephaly is defined as head circumference less than 2 standard deviations below the mean. A variety of causes of microcephaly exist. The hereditary form could be a normal variant, and has no clinical implications. In utero infections, toxin exposure (such as alcohol, tobacco, and prescription drugs such as

chemotherapeutic agents and antiepileptic), hypoxic-ischemic injury, birth trauma, and metabolic disorders such as prolonged hypoglycemia are the pathological causes for the microcephaly. A wide variety of hereditary disorders including enzyme deficiencies can lead to microcephaly, as can chromosomal abnormalities. Clinical manifestations depend on the underlying cause and can range from none (asymptomatic microcephaly) to severe developmental delay and seizures.

Macrocephaly is defined as a head circumference greater than 2 standard deviations above the mean. Macrocephaly may be a normal variant that is often hereditary, may result from increased CSF, as in hydrocephalus due to a variety of causes, from mass lesions such as tumors or subdural hematomas, or may result from megalencephaly, an oversized brain (brain weight greater than 2 standard deviations above the mean).

Causes of megalencephaly include storage diseases such as mucopolysaccharidoses or Tay-Sachs disease, Canavan disease, Alexander disease, genetic disorders including Sotos syndrome, and others. In the latter disorders, eventual cell loss with subsequent atrophy typically occurs. Megalencephaly may also be a benign familial finding. Clinical manifestations depend on the underlying cause. Neurologic deficits may be absent in the benign familial form.

Hemimegalencephaly, or enlargement of only one brain hemisphere, invariably presents with seizures and hemiparesis. Hemimegalencephaly is associated with various genetic disorders, including Beckwith-Wiedemann syndrome, which is characterized by gigantism, macroglossia, and midline abdominal wall defects.

Suggested Reading

- Comprehensive review in clinical neurology: a multiple-choice question book for the wards and boards ©2011 Wolters Kluwer Health Lippincott Williams & Wilkins. All rights reserved.

20. You are seeing a 6-month-old baby boy for his seizures. The family recently emigrated from Colombia, and he did not undergo newborn screening at birth. He has significant developmental delay, hypotonia, has failure to thrive, and is microcephalic. His urine has a musty odor.
    Which of the following is not true regarding this condition?
    A. Phenylalanine transaminase deficiency is the cause of this condition
    B. Tetrahydrobi opterin is a cofactor in the conversion of phenylalanine to tyrosine
    C. Dietary restriction of phenylalanine is the treatment for this condition
    D. Cognitive impairment and seizures are common
    E. The musty odor in the urine and sweat is caused by phenylacetic acid

Correct Answer is: A

This is a clinical presentation of phenylketonuria (PKU). It is a disorder of phenylalanine metabolism, caused by a deficiency of phenylalanine hydroxylase. This enzyme converts phenylalanine to tyrosine, and its deficiency leads to accumulation of phenylalanine, which is then metabolized by phenylalanine transaminase to phenylpyruvic acid, which is subsequently oxidized to phenylacetic acid, responsible for the musty odor of the sweat and urine of these patients. It is autosomal recessive disorder. Children with PKU are normal at birth, with a rise in the phenylalanine levels after initiation of feeding. These children will have developmental delay, cognitive impairment, microcephaly, seizures, hypotonia, and severe behavioral disturbances. A musty odor, as described, is characteristic. These children are fair, with blond hair, blue eyes, and pale skin given the lack of tyrosine and

melanin pigment production. Newborn screening detects hyperphenylalaninemia, and the diagnosis is made on the basis of elevation of phenylalanine levels in blood. Tetrahydrobiopterin is a cofactor for phenylalanine hydroxylase, and its deficiency may also produce hyperphenylalaninemia (and PKU). A reduction of phenylalanine levels in blood and urine after a trial of tetrahydrobiopterin is used to make the diagnosis of this condition. The treatment of PKU is dietary restriction of phenylalanine, and these patients should be placed on a low-protein diet and phenylalanine-free feeding formula as soon as possible after birth, which will prevent neurologic complication. Untreated patients have severe intellectual disability. Despite treatment, some patients still have varying degrees of mild to moderate cognitive delays. Tetrahydrobiopterin is used as a treatment adjunct in select patients.

21. You are evaluating a 6-year-old boy who reached his normal motor and cognitive development by 1 year of age, but at 16 months the child began to have frequent falls and looked "unsteady" when walking. He was seen by another neurologist at 2 years of age and he documented, ataxia, distal leg weakness and absent tendon reflexes. His brain MRI showed subcortical demyelination with a posterior predominance and sparing of the subcortical U-fibers. Since then he experienced significant cognitive decline, optic atrophy and progressive spasticity.
What is the most likely diagnosis?
    A. Krabbe disease
    B. Metachromatic leukodystrophy
    C. Adrenomyeloneuropathy
    D. Limb-Girdle myasthenia

Correct Answer is: B

This is a presentation of the late infantile form of metachromatic leukodystrophy, which is an inherited disorder of myelin metabolism and is caused by a deficiency of the enzyme arylsulfatase A. Segmental demyelination occurs in peripheral nerves and cell death in central oligodendroglia cells. Sparing of the subcortical U-fibers on MRI is found in other leukodystrophies (x-linked adrenoleukodystrophy andgloboid cell leukodystrophy) as well in the inborn errors of metabolism disorders, such as phenylketonuria, maple syrup urine disease, Lowe's disease and hypohomocysteinemia.

Krabbe disease, or globoid cell leukodystrophy, is caused by a deficiency of galactosylceramide beta-galactosidase and symptoms begin between 2–6 years with mental regression, cortical blindness and spasticity.

Adrenomyeloneuropathy is the most common phenotype of adrenoleukodystrophy and is caused by an inability to oxidize very-long chain fatty acids. Paraplegia begins after the age of 20 and slowly progresses throughout life.

Limb-Girdle myasthenia is an immune-mediated myasthenia gravis, with an age of onset after 10 years, and presents with progressive proximal weakness of the limbs.

Suggested Reading

- Von Figura K., Gieselmann V, Jaecken J. Metachromatic leukodystrophy: Lysosomal disorders. In: the metabolic and molecular bases of inherited disease 2011. p. 3695–724.

22. You are seeing a 5- years old with severe peripheral motor and sensory neuropathy, has tightly curled hair (unlike either parent) and cognitive impairment with a sural nerve biopsy remarkable for enlarged axons filled with disrupted neurofilaments.
What is the most likely diagnosis?
    A. Infantile neuroaxonal dystrophy
    B. Late infantile neuronal ceroid lipofuscinosis
    C. Giant axonal neuropathy
    D. Sub-acute necrotizing encephalomyelopathy

Correct Answer is: C

In giant cell neuropathy, the underlying pathology is disruption of intermediate filament organization that predominantly affects the neurofilaments. Usually the first symptoms to be seen before 5 years of age. Both central and peripheral axons are disrupted and manifest impaired function. Boys and girls are equally affected. Symmetrical distal atrophy is universal with impairment of vibratory sensation and proprioception with diminished tendon reflexes.

The neuropathology of infantile neuroaxonal dystrophy is characterized by the presence of large axonal eosinophilic spheroids, forming as a result of axonal swelling, in the cerebral and anterior horn cell grey matter.

Symptoms of late infantile neuronal ceroid lipofuscinosis begin between 2 and 4 years of age and include progressive cognitive impairment and abnormal movements. Visual impairment begins by 4 years of age and progresses to blindness.

Subacute necrotizing encephalomyelopathy (Leigh disease), present between 3 and12 months of age with neurological decompensation associated with lactic acidosis.

Suggested Reading

- Kuhlenbaumer G, et al. Giant axonal neuropathy. Gene Rev. October 9, 2014. ► http://www.ncbi.nlm.nih.gov/books/NBK1136/ (► http://www.ncbi.nlm.nih.gov/books/NBK11361).

23. You were asked to see a 2-year-old girl for developmental delay evaluation. Her parents reported that at 12 month of age the child was no longer able to stand with assistance. She has muscle wasting and weakness at her 18 months regular exam. Serum CK levels and an MRI of the brain were normal. She has a normal motor and sensory nerve conduction velocities 1 week ago. EMG showed neuropathic motor units. On your examination she had severe weakness, muscle atrophy and exaggerated tendon reflexes. Cranial nerves were intact, except for atrophy and fasciculation of the tongue.
Which of the following tests could confirm the diagnosis?
    A. Deficiency in hexosaminidase-A activity in cultured leukocytes
    B. Reduced erythrocyte galactose-1-phosphate uridyltransferase (GALT)
    C. Elevated dermatan sulfate and heparin sulfate
    D. Muscle biopsy evidence of fiber necrosis and regeneration

Correct Answer is: A

This is a presentation of GM2 gangliosidosis (Tay-Sachs disease), which may present with a variety of phenotypes. The initial features can be similar to spinal muscular atrophy. Wasting, weakness and cramps of proximal leg muscles are initial symptoms followed by distal leg weakness along with proximal and distal arm weakness. As the disease progresses there are both upper and lower motor neuron symptoms. Some children develop cerebral symptoms.

Galactosemia is a transference deficiency that presents with early signs of cataracts. Physical symptoms are provoked by the first feeding after birth including vomiting, diarrhea and jaundice. Even with diet modifications, developmental delays and truncal ataxia develops.

Elevated dermatan sulfate and heparin sulfate are present in mucopolysaccharidoses, including Hunter Syndrome. Cognitive regression occurs as a result of progressive neuronal storage of gangliosidosis after 2 years of age.

In this age group, fiber necrosis with signs of regeneration is most consistent with children born with congenital muscular dystrophy. They display hypotonia, poor suck and respiratory distress at birth.

Suggested Reading

- Scriver CR. Physician's guide to the laboratory diagnosis of metabolic diseases. In: Blau N, Duran M, Blaskovics ME, Gibson KM, editors. Springer Science & Business Media; 2012.

4

24. Mutations of the ALD (ABCD1) gene are most likely to cause:
    - A. Frontal white matter abnormalities
    - B. CNS and renal neoplasms
    - C. A deficiency of very long chain fatty acids
    - D. Cerebral inflammatory demyelination
    - E. Infantile hypotonia

Correct Answer is: D

Mutations of the ALO (ABCD1) gene on the X chromosome causes adrenoleukodystrophy. The gene encodes a peroxisomal protein (ALDP) involved very long chain fatty acid (VLCFA) oxidative degradation. Mutations lead to an accumulation of VLCFAs, and adrenal failure with a deficiency of androgens and glucocorticoids. This results in perivascular lymphocytes, and demyelination, beginning in the parietal and occipital lobes and sparing arcuate fibers. MRI demonstrates T2-weighted hyper-intensities of the posterior white matter. Several clinical phenotypes may result, including childhood onset, adolescent onset, adult onset, adrenomyeloneuropathy, Addison's disease only, and women with symptomatic X-ALD.

- **Childhood onset adrenoleukodystrophy: The age of onset ranges from 2.5–10 years. Symptoms include extensive CNS demyelination, hyperactivity, dementia, ataxia, vision loss, hearing deficits, and seizures, with endocrine dysfunction. The course is rapidly progressive.**
- **Adolescent onset adrenoleukodystrophy: Manifestations start between ages 10–21 years, and are rapidly progressive, with CNS demyelination, behavioral and cognitive changes, and endocrine dysfunction.**
- **Adult onset adrenoleukodystrophy: This phenotype consists of a rapidly progressive dementia, psychiatric changes (e.g. psychosis, affective disorders), CNS demyelination, endocrine dysfunction, and possible myelopathy or neuropathy.**
- **Adrenomyeloneuropathy: The age of onset is typically in early adulthood with a progressive spastic paraparesis, bowel and bladder incontinence, sexual dysfunction, mild dementia, and psychiatric changes (i.e. affective disorders), as well as sensorimotor, primarily axonal neuropathy. This phenotype may be either slowly or rapidly progressive.**
- **An Addison's only phenotype consists of isolated adrenal dysfunction.**
- **Heterozygous females typically develop symptoms by age 60. The disorder is slowly progressive, and may present with peripheral neuropathy, fecal incontinence, and pain in the legs. White matter lesions and endocrine dysfunction are rare.**

Treatment for adrenoleukodystrophy involves glucocorticoids and bone marrow transplant. Dietary fatty acid supplementation ("Lorenzo's oil"), has been used, but with limited data to suggest efficacy.

Suggested Reading

- Engelen M, et al. X-linked adrenoleukodystrophy (X-ALD): clinical presentation and guidelines for diagnosis, follow-up and management. Orphanet j Rare Dis. 2012;7:51.
- Rai PVS, et al. Childhood adrenoleukodystrophy – classic and variant – review of clinical manifestations and magnetic resonance imaging. J Pediatr Neurosci. 2013;8(3):192–7.

25. On which chromosome is the responsible gene located in a 7-year-old boy with a previous diagnosis of developmental delay and cerebral palsy that now presents with serious biting of his fingers, lips and cheeks?

A. 3
B. 21
C. X
D. Unknown etiology

Correct Answer is: C

The hallmark sign of Lesch-Nyhan disease is self-mutilation. This is a disorder of hypoxanthine guanine phosphoribsyltransferase deficiency mapped to the gene locus Xq26. Uric acid in the blood and urine is elevated.

Patients usually appear normal at birth, then develop hypertonia and delayed motor milestone attainment. Progressive spasticity frequently leads to an initial diagnosis of cerebral palsy. Occasionally aggressive behavior towards caretakers is also present.

Syndromes associated with chromosome 3 include van Hippel-Landau, 3-methylcrotonyl-CoA carboxylase deficiency and Charcot-Marie-Tooth disease.

The most common childhood disorder associated with chromosome 21 is Down's syndrome.

Cerebral palsy can be a manifestation of many disorders and often a specific etiology is not known.

Suggested Reading

- Torres RJ, Puig JG, Jinnah HA. Update on the phenotypic spectrum of Lesch-Nyhan disease and its attenuated variants. Curr Rheumatol Rep. 2012;14(2):189–94.

26. You are seeing a 3-year-old boy for his follow-up visit. He has a history of developmental delay and intellectual disability since early in life and has developed torticollis and spasticity in his limbs. He also has a history of seizures and aggressive behavior. He began biting himself to the point of bleeding and constantly self-inflicts injuries. He has had kidney stones and hyperuricemia.

Which of the following is not correct regarding this condition?

A. The genetic defect is in the gene HPRT1
B. It is autosomal recessive
C. Hypoxanthine guanine phosphoribosyltransferase is the deficient enzyme
D. It is caused by an enzymatic defect in the purine salvage pathway
E. Patients may have choreoathetotic movements

Correct Answer is: B

This is a case of Lesch-Nyhan syndrome (LNS), which is inherited in an X-linked fashion and is caused by deficiency of the enzyme hypoxanthine guanine phosphoribosyltransferase (HGPRT), which participates in the salvage pathway of purines. HGPRT is encoded by the gene HPRT1 on chromosome Xq26, and deficiency of this enzyme leads to the accumulation of purines with their subsequent conversion to uric acid.

There is a wide presentation of the disease, ranging from the classic LNS form to milder forms without neurologic manifestations. The classic LNS form may manifest in the newborn period with severe hypotonia. These children will have delayed motor development, progressive limb and neck rigidity with dystonia, choreoathetotic movements, facial grimacing, seizures, spasticity, and intellectual disability. These patients have aggressive and severe self- mutilation behavior.

Milder forms include those with less severe neurologic disease, and those in which there are no neurologic manifestations, presenting with hyperuricemia, gout, and nephrolithiasis. The clinical picture, including neurologic manifestations, self-mutilation behavior, and hyperuricemia suggests the diagnosis.

HGPRT activity can be assessed in fibroblasts, and genetic testing can also be used.

Treatment includes purine restricted diet, hydration to prevent kidney stones, allopurinol to decrease the production of uric acid, and supportive care to prevent self-inflicted injuries and control abnormal movements. Levodopa and tetrabenazine have been tried for the neuropsychiatric manifestations.

27. You are evaluating a 6 -year-old boy in your office. On examination, he has coarse facial features, short stature with dysmorphic appearance, prominent psychomotor retardation, hepatosplenomegaly, and several nodular lesions that are ivory colored on his upper back. The activity of iduronate sulfatase in leukocytes is almost absent.

    Which of the following is correct regarding this condition?

    A. It is inherited in an X-linked fashion
    B. Corneal clouding is a prominent feature in this syndrome
    C. He has Hurler syndrome
    D. Heparan sulfate, but not dermatan sulfate, will be elevated in the urine
    E. This patient has mucopolysaccharidoses type

Correct Answer is: A

These are the manifestations of Hunter syndrome. It is inherited as an X-linked disorder. Patients with Morquio syndrome have no intellectual disability. Mucopolysaccharidoses (MPS) are due to impaired lysosomal degradation of glucosaminoglycans, which are long unbranched molecules of repeating disaccharides. Many enzymatic defects lead to the accumulation of glucosaminoglycans in lysosomes and the extracellular matrix. All MPS are autosomal recessive except for Hunter disease, which is X-linked. In general, MPS are a group of progressive multi-systemic disorders that affect the cornea, cartilage, bone, connective tissue, reticuloendothelial system, and nervous system. Hurler syndrome is MPS type I and is caused by a-L-iduronidase deficiency. The gene is localized to chromosome 4, and there is accumulation of both dermatan and heparan sulfate. Children are normal at birth, but within the first 2 years of life, they will develop coarsening of facial features, with progressive skeletal dysplasia with dysostosis multiplex and growth impairment (dwarfism). Those children have restricted range of motion of the joints, hearing loss, corneal clouding, macroglossia, hernias, visceromegaly, valvular heart disease, and prominent intellectual disability. Mild MPS type I is also known as Scheie syndrome, and the intermediate form is known as Hurler-Scheie syndrome. Most recently, MPS type I has been classified as severe MPS type I and attenuated MPS type I. The diagnosis of MPS type I is based on elevated urinary excretion of dermatan and heparan sulfate and confirmed with enzyme analysis in leukocytes and fibroblasts. Pathologically, there are cells with vacuolated appearance, expansion of perivascular spaces in the CNS, and neuronal lipidosis. Electron microscopy demonstrates reticulogranular material in epithelial and mesenchymal cells, and lamellar material in neurons, some of which adopt a layered appearance and are called zebra bodies. Enzyme replacement therapy can be used to treat non-central nervous system manifestations of the disease. Stem cell transplantation can be potentially helpful.

Hunter syndrome or MPS type II is due to a defect in iduronate sulfatase, with accumulation of dermatan sulfate

and heparan sulfate. These patients have the Hurler phenotype but lack the corneal clouding and have characteristic nodular ivory-colored lesions on the back, shoulders, and upper arms. These children have short stature, macrocephaly, macroglossia, hoarse voice, hearing loss, visceromegaly, dysostosis multiplex, joint contractures, entrapment neuropathies such as carpal tunnel syndrome, and intellectual disability. The diagnosis is based on mucopolysacchariduria and confirmed with analysis of the enzyme activity. Treatment is symptomatic.

28. You are seeing a 4 years old boy for his developmental delay, hypotonia, and dysmorphic features. On examination, he has inverted nipples and prominent fat pads in the buttocks area. A diagnosis of a congenital disorder of glycosylation is suspected.
Which of the following is not true regarding this condition?
   - A. It affects multiple organ systems
   - B. Analysis of transferrin glycoforms can help make the diagnosis
   - C. Patients can present with stroke-like episodes
   - D. Some patients may have hypogonadism
   - E. It is inherited in an X-linked fashion

Correct Answer is: E

Congenital disorders of glycosylation (CDG), previously known as carbohydrate-deficient glycoprotein syndrome, are a group of genetic disorders inherited as an autosomal recessive disorder. It is a multiple- systems disorder, especially the CNS. The defect is abnormal synthesis, transport, modification, and/or processing of the carbohydrate moieties or glycans of glycoproteins, therefore affecting protein components in many tissues. Type I CDGs are caused by abnormal synthesis of these glycans. Clinical features are widely variable, with multiple subtypes, including combinations of failure to thrive, developmental delay, dysmorphic features, hypotonia, ataxia, and weakness, and retinitis pigmentosa, short stature with skeletal abnormalities, polyneuropathy, and stroke- like episodes, liver dysfunction, hypogonadism, and multisystem involvement.

Lipodystrophy with prominent fat pads in the buttocks and suprapubic area and inverted nipples are distinctive features. Type II CDGs are caused by abnormal processing and modification of glycans and lead to profound intellectual disability but no cerebellar ataxia or peripheral neuropathy.

CDGs are characterized by the presence of a carbohydrate-deficient transferrin in the serum and CSF, and the analysis of the glycoforms of this protein is a diagnostic test. Genetic confirmation is available. Treatment is supportive.

Suggested Reading

Comprehensive review in clinical neurology: a multiple-choice question book for the wards and boards © 2011 Wolters Kluwer Health Lippincott Williams & Wilkins. All rights reserved.

29. You are seeing a 5-year-old trisomy 21 girl for her annual checkup.
Which of the following statements is not true regarding this disorder?
   - A. Intellectual disability of varying degrees of severity may be present
   - B. Patients with trisomy 21 are at increased risk of leukemia
   - C. MRI of the brain would show hypertrophy of the frontal lobes, with macrocephaly
   - D. There is increased risk of atlanto-axial dislocation
   - E. Early dementia with Alzheimer type pathology is seen

Correct Answer is: C

MRI findings in Down syndrome, or trisomy 21 are, the frontal lobes are small and under developed, and the superior temporal gyri are small and thin.

Developmental delay is defined by performance on standardized tests of function, that is, 2 standard deviations below the mean. Intellectual disability is a diagnosis made on the basis of testing intelligence quotient (IQ) and is characterized as mild, moderate, or severe on the basis of the IQ, the degree of impairment, and the level of assistance in daily activities and other activities that are required. Mild intellectual disability is defined by an IQ of 55 to 70, whereas severe intellectual disability is defined by an IQ of 25 to myriad of causes for developmental delay exist, including but not limited to genetic disorders, toxin exposure, and metabolic disorders. Down syndrome, or trisomy 21, results from trisomy of the 21st chromosome or, less commonly, chromosomal translocations. Diagnosis is made in the majority through karyotyping. Increased maternal age is a risk factor. The frontal lobes are small and under-developed, and the superior temporal I gyri are small and thin. Clinical manifestations include presence of medial epicanthal folds, slanting palpebral fissures, micrognathia (small mouth) leading to an apparently large tongue, the so-called simian crease (in which there is a single palmar crease), Brush field spots (white spots of depigmentation in the iris), clinodactyly (incurving of the fingers), short stature, and other features. In addition to varying degrees of intellectual disability, seizures, hematologic malignancies, and congenital heart defects occur. Early dementia with Alzheimer type pathology is seen, as the B-amyloid gene is on chromosome 21. These patients are at risk of cervical spinal cord compression due to atlantoaxial instability.

4

Trisomy 13 or Patau syndrome is characterized by microcephaly, microphthalmia, iris coloboma, low-set ears, cleft lip and palate, polydactyly (excess number of fingers), prominence of the heels, and cardiac abnormalities. Life expectancy is typically not beyond early childhood.

Trisomy 18 is characterized by microcephaly, ptosis, overlapping of the third finger over the second finger, rocker-bottom feet, umbilical hernia, congenital heart disease, and other findings. Life expectancy is typically not beyond early infancy.

In Klinefelter syndrome, two X chromosomes are present in a male: XXY. Clinical features include intellectual disability, a wide arm span, high-pitched voice, gynecomastia, and small testes.

30. You are evaluating a 6-year-old boy who has coarse facial features, short stature with dysmorphic appearance, prominent psychomotor retardation, hepatosplenomegaly, and several nodular lesions that are ivory colored on his upper back. The activity of iduronate sulfatase in leukocytes is almost absent.

    Which of the following is correct regarding this condition?

    A. It is inherited in an X-linked fashion
    B. Corneal clouding is a prominent feature in this syndrome
    C. He has Hurler syndrome
    D. Heparan sulfate, but not dermatan sulfate, will be elevated in the urine
    E. This patient has mucopolysaccharidoses type I

Correct Answer is: A

This is a case of Hunter syndrome (MPS type II) is caused by a defect in iduronate sulfatase, with accumulation of dermatan sulfate and heparan sulfate. These patients have the Hurler phenotype but lack the

corneal clouding and have characteristic nodular ivory-colored lesions on the back, shoulders, and upper arms. These children have short stature, macrocephaly, macroglossia, hoarse voice, hearing loss, visceromegaly, dysostosis multiplex, joint contractures, entrapment neuropathies such as carpal tunnel syndrome, and intellectual disability. The diagnosis is based on mucopolysacchariduria and confirmed with analysis of the enzyme activity. Treatment is symptomatic.

Other MPS include types III, IV, VI, VII, and IX as follows: - MPS type III or Sanfilippo syndrome has several subtypes (A, B, C, and D) and is associated with accumulation of heparan sulfate only. The main manifestation is intellectual disability. - MPS type IV or Morquio syndrome has two subtypes (A and B), and they manifest with corneal clouding, dysostosis multiplex, and heart disease, with normal intelligence. - MPS type VI is also known as Maroteaux-Lamy syndrome and manifests with normal intelligence, dysostosis multiplex, corneal clouding, heart disease, and other features similar to Hurler syndrome. - MPS type VII is also known as Sly syndrome, and these patients have hydrops fetalis, intellectual disability, dysostosis multiplex, corneal clouding, and other features of Hurler syndrome.

Suggested Reading

- Comprehensive review in clinical neurology: a multiple-choice question book for the wards and boards ©2011 Wolters Kluwer Health Lippincott Williams & Wilkins. All rights reserved.

31. You are evaluating a 4-year-old female for her developmental delay. By family report, she seemed to be a very happy baby early on, she made eye contact and smiled and cooed all the time. She had met motor milestones similar to her siblings: holding her head up, crawling, and sitting unsupported. By on year of age, she started to have difficulty sitting up and never developed any words. She later stopped smiling and laughing, and progressively lost use of her hands, constantly rubbing her hands against each other.
Which of the following statements is correct?
A. It is more common in males but can also be seen in females
B. Macrocephaly is a common finding
C. It results from a mutation in the gene encoding the MeCP2 protein
D. It is autosomal dominant in inheritance
E. It results from mutations in mitochondrial DNA

Correct Answer is: C
This is a presentation of Rett syndrome, a syndrome of motor and cognitive regression with eventual severe disability. The presentation is one of initially normal development with subsequent regression at approximately 6 to 18 months of age. Hand wringing and other motor stereotypies are a classic feature; patients with Rett syndrome often place their hands in their mouth or may hold their hands fisted, with their fingers flexed over their thumb. Arrest of head growth with eventual microcephaly, seizures, scoliosis, dysautonomia including respiratory dysfunction with apneas, and spasticity emerge as the disease progresses. It results from various types of mutations in the gene that encodes methyl CpG binding protein 2 (MeCP2), which is involved in binding to methylated DNA, modulating gene expression. It is most often seen in females, and it is thought to be most often fatal in boys, although cases of MeCP2 mutation in male infants and children with intellectual disability and other features have been identified. Another disorder of severe intellectual disability in females results from a mutation in the gene CDKLS.

4

32. Which of the following is not true regarding abetalipoproteinemia or Bassen Kornzweig syndrome?
    - A. It is autosomal dominant
    - B. There is demyelination of the posterior columns of the spinal cord
    - C. There is demyelination of peripheral nerves
    - D. There is vitamin E deficiency
    - E. It is associated with fat malabsorption

Correct Answer is: A

Abetalipoproteinemi a, or Bassen-Kornzweig syndrome, is an autosomal recessive disorder caused by a molecular defect in the gene for the microsomal triglyceride transfer protein, which is localized to chromosome 4q22 0.24. This protein normally catalyzes the transport of triglyceride, cholesteryl ester, and phospholipid from phospholipid surfaces. The defect of this protein results in fat malabsorption and liposoluble vitamin deficiency, especially of vitamin E, which is the culprit of most of the clinical manifestations. This condition manifests since birth, with failure to thrive, vomiting, and loose stool. During infancy, there is progressive psychomotor retardation with cerebellar ataxia and gait disturbance. Proprioceptive sensation is lost in the hands and feet, with less compromise of pinprick and temperature sensation. Deep tendon reflexes are depressed. This is likely from demyelination of posterior columns and peripheral nerves. Visual disturbance is the result of retinitis pigmentosa, and nystagmus is common. Laboratory studies demonstrate acanthocytosis, absence of very low-density lipoproteins, absence of apolipoprotein B, low levels of vitamin E, and severe anemia. Treatment involves the restriction of triglycerides in the diet, and large doses of vitamin E with supplementation of vitamins A, D, and K.

33. You are evaluating a 9-month-old baby for his hypotonia, growth retardation and poor psychomotor development. He also has a history of episodes of incoordination, especially with high-carbohydrate meals and during systemic infections. On laboratory evaluation, he is found to have elevated levels of lactate and pyruvate, with a low lactate: pyruvate ratio. Deficiency of the enzyme pyruvate dehydrogenase (PDH) is detected.
    Which of the following is not true regarding this condition?
    - A. PDH is responsible for oxidative decarboxylation of pyruvate to carbon dioxide and acetyl coenzyme A
    - B. Only inherited in an autosomal recessive fashion
    - C. Can present with severe neonatal acidosis
    - D. High-carbohydrate diet can precipitate episodes of ataxia
    - E. Ketogenic diet has been used to treat patients with this condition

Correct Answer is: B

Pyruvate dehydrogenase (PDH) deficiency is caused by defects of the PDH complex, which is responsible for the oxidative decarboxylation of pyruvate to carbon dioxide and acetyl coenzyme A. This enzymatic complex has three main components called E1 (A and B subunits), E2, and E3. E1 deficiency is the most common and is inherited in an X-linked fashion, whereas the other defects are autosomal recessive. Since the brain derives energy primarily from glucose oxidation, neurologic dysfunction is one of the main clinical features. The clinical presentation is variable, ranging from severe neonatal lactic acidosis with death in the neonatal period, to less severe forms that are manifested in infancy, in which patients have lactic and

pyruvic acidosis, and episodic or progressive ataxia, nystagmus, dysarthria, lethargy, weakness with arreflexia, hypotonia, and psychomotor retardation, which can be profound. These patients have periodic exacerbations, which can be spontaneous or triggered by infections, stress, or high-carbohydrate meals. Some patients may have a presentation of Leigh disease. The diagnosis is suspected in children with clinical manifestations as described and with elevations of lactate and pyruvate levels, with a low lactate: pyruvate ratio. Enzyme analysis can be performed in leukocytes, cultured fibroblasts, muscle, or liver biopsy specimens. Pathologically, there may be cystic lesions in the white matter and basal ganglia, and certain cases of the neonatal form may have agenesis of the corpus callosum. Management of PDH deficiency includes ketogenic diet (high fat with low carbohydrates) and thiamine supplementation. Carnitine, coenzyme Q10, and biotin supplementation may be given, but their efficacy is not well established. Acetazolamide may be used for the treatment of episodes of ataxia.

34. You are seeing an 8-year-old boy who is referred to you because his funny walk for the last few months. His mother reports that he has been clumsier, tripping frequently as well. While you are examining him, you notice that his speech seems slightly slurred, and his mother states this just started a week ago. On examination, he has a wide-based slow gait and steppage gait. Motor strength in the distal lower extremities is 2/5 and proximal is 3/5. Lower extremity DTRs are absent. There is an extensor plantar response, and his feet are significant for high plantar arches. Also, he has scoliosis.
What is the mode of inheritance in this disease?

A. Autosomal dominant
B. Autosomal recessive
C. Post-infectious
D. Random (non-infectious and non-genetic)

Correct Answer is: B
This a case of Friedreich's Ataxia (FA). It is an autosomal recessive disease caused by a mutation on chromosome 9 in the gene encoding the protein frataxin. Therefore, it occurs in males and females equally. It is the only disease caused by a GAA trinucleotide repeat. The more GAA repeats, the more profound the deficit in frataxin protein. Those patients usually present between the ages of 5 to 15, though cases do occur even younger than this. Late-onset FA usually presents in the 2nd or 3rd decades. Presenting symptoms and signs include ataxia, motor weakness, scoliosis/kyphoscoliosis, dysarthria, high arches or pes cavus, diabetes in20%, dysphagia, absent DTRs, muscle wasting, an extensor plantar response, nystagmus, cardiac involvement (cardiomegaly, cardiomyopathy). Most patients with FA are wheelchair-bound by age 15.

Treatment is symptomatic, and aims to support and maintain ambulation as long as possible.

35. You are seeing a 7-month-old boy with history of seizures and developmental delay for follow-up visit. He has had increased head circumference, progressive psychomotor retardation, spasticity and qudriparesis for the last 2 months. His brain MRI showed white matter hyperintesity mainly in the frontal lobes and anterior cerebral regions, involving the cortical U fibers.
What is the most likely etiology for his presentation?

A. Hexosamindiase A deficiency
B. Galactocerbrocidase beta-galactosidase deficiency
C. Gene mutation for glial fibrillary acidic protein (GFAP)
D. Aspartocylase deficiency
E. Mitochondrial DNA deletion

Correct Answer is: C
This is a patient of Alexander disease. Etiology is gene mutation for glial fibrillary acidic protein (GFAP). It is a progressive disorder of astrocytes. There are three forms: Infantile form – features include megalencephaly, developmental delay, seizures, psychomotor retardation, spasticity, and quadriparesis.

Juvenile form - in childhood, more significant bulbar symptoms.

Adult form – features include bulbar signs, hyperreflexia, dysautonomia, ataxia, sleep apnea.

MRI shows diffuse white matter signal hyperintensity, mainly in the frontal lobes and anterior cerebral regions, involvement of U fibers. In the adult-onset form, the "tadpole sign" on sagittal MRI results from dramatic thinning of the upper cervical spinal cord.

Histopathology, there is Rosenthal fibers - elongated eosinophilic fibers seen on H&E, and they are diffusely distributed throughout the brain with clusters in the sub-pial, sub-ependymal, and perivascular areas. Severe myelin loss and cavitation of the white matter is seen.

Suggested Reading

- Mowzoon N, Flemming KD. Neurology board review: an illustrated study guide. Rochester: Mayo Clinic Scientific; 2007. Print.

36. You are seeing a 6 years old boy for his abnormal gait which started at 4 years of age, and followed by toe walking. He has a history of frequent falls with a subtle loss of hand grasp strength. On examination, he has enlarged calf muscles.

What the inheritance of this condition?

A. Sporatic/unknown
B. Most common in Ashkenazi Jews
C. Autosomal dominant
D. Autosomal recessive
E. X-linked

Correct Answer is: E
Duchenne Muscular Dystrophy (DMD) and Becker Muscular Dystrophy have variable phenotypic expression of the gene defect on Xp21. In DMD the gene product dystrophin is present at 0–5% of the normal level and in BMD between 5–20%. The incidence of DMD is 1 per 3500 male births and typically presents earlier than BMD. Mutation analysis is now routine for diagnosis, carrier detection and fetal diagnosis. At the time of diagnosis, the serum concentration is usually 10 times normal in boys with DMD.

Dystrophin analysis on muscle biopsy can aid in differentiating the two forms of the condition. Several of the inherited metabolic disorders are more common in the gene pool of Ashkenazi Jews.

Suggested Reading

- Yiu EM, Kornberg AJ. Duchenne muscular dystrophy. J Pediatr Child Health. 2015.

37. Which of the following statements is not true regarding the syndromes of cobblestone lissencephaly?

A. Muscle-eye-brain disease of Santavuori is most often seen in Finland
B. Fukuyama muscular dystrophy is most often seen in Japan
C. Muscular dystrophy is seen in all these syndromes
D. Eye abnormalities seen include retinal hypoplasia and glaucoma
E. They are autosomal dominant in inheritance

Correct Answer is: E

The cobblestone lissencephalies are mainly autosomal recessive in inheritance although X-linked forms have also been identified. Cobblestone lissencephaly, or lissencephaly type II, is a neuronal migration disorder in which the cortical gray matter has reduced number of gyri and sulci that appear like cobblestones. There is reduced and abnormal white matter, and the cerebellum and brain stem are hypoplastic. Microscopically, the cortex has no recognizable layers. Hydrocephalus frequently occurs because of the presence of fibroglial bands and abnormal vascular channels disrupting the subarachnoid space. It has three autosomal recessive syndromes: Walker-Warburg syndrome, Fukuyama muscular dystrophy, and muscle-eye-brain disease of Santavuori. These three syndromes share similar clinical features, including microcephaly, global developmental delay, epilepsy, hypotonia, and evidence of muscular dystrophy. Walker-Warburg is the most severe form. Several gene mutations have been identified in patients with Walker-Walburg and muscle-eye-brain disease of Santavuori. Eye abnormalities in the latter two conditions include retinal hypoplasia, optic nerve atrophy, glaucoma, and cataracts. Muscle eye-brain disease of Santavuori is seen most commonly in Finland but also occurs in other European populations. Fukuyama muscular dystrophy, which results from a mutation in the gene fukutin, is most common in Japan and is rare in other populations. It has the least amount of cortical abnormalities, but the muscular dystrophy is severe with progressive weakness and joint contractures. An elevated level of serum creatine kinase is seen.

38. You are seeing a 9-month-old baby in the ED for a new-onset seizure. She has been healthy, with no fever or other signs of illness. On examination, she has a reddish patch over her right eyelid and forehead. Her head circumference is 45 cm, her anterior fontanelle is soft and small, and no other dysmorphic or cutaneous features are noted. You ordered a MRI, which shows a left posterior leptomeningeal angioma with prominent, tortuous veins coursing toward the vein of Galen.
What is the inheritance pattern of this disorder?
A. Autosomal dominant
B. Autosomal recessive
C. Maternal mitochondrial
D. Sporadic
E. X-linked

Correct Answer is: D

This is a case of Sturge Weber syndrome (SWS). It is a "congenital, non-familial disorder of unknown incidence and cause." In Takeoka's article the incidence is estimated at 1 per 50,000. The neuroimaging findings can be unilateral or bilateral, even with unilateral skin findings, though if unilateral, it is generally on the same side as the port wine stain. Glaucoma can be present at birth or develop later.

Suggested Reading

- ► http://www.sturge-weber.org/about-sws/conditions/12-sturge-weber-syndrome.html.
- Sturge-Weber Syndrome. On ► http://emedicine.medscape.com/article/1177523-overview, author M Takeoka. Updated Jan 5, 2010.

39. You are seeing a 6-year-old boy for his motor development delay. His history is remarkable of unsteady gait ever since he started to walk independently at 3 years of age. Also, he has frequent involuntary movements in his arms and hands. On examination he has choreoathetoid movements in the upper extremities. He prefers to turn his head rather than his eyes during horizontal tracking. He has decrease sensation to all modalities and absent deep tendon reflexes. Gait and

coordination examination revealed both limb and truncal ataxia. Eye exam showed that he has prominent blood vessels in the conjunctiva.

What is correct regarding this patient's most likely diagnosis?

A. The clinical picture is consistent with a pure cerebellar ataxia.

B. It is associated with the Fragile X chromosome.
C. This condition is secondary to a GAA repeat expansion.
D. Patients with this condition typically have hypogammaglobulinemia.
E. Serial CT scans of the head should be performed to monitor the progression of cerebellar atrophy.

Correct Answer is: D

This a presentation of ataxia–telangiectasia, an autosomal recessive disorder that presents in early childhood with ataxia. The telangiectasias are venous plexuses that are commonly present in the bulbar conjunctiva, ear lobes and other areas. It is important to know that these hallmark cutaneous signs may not be present until several years after the neurologic features of the disorder. In addition to the truncal and limb ataxia, affected patients may have frequent choreoathetoid movements, oculomotor apraxia (evidenced by a defect of initiation of spontaneous saccades forcing a patient to compensate by head-thrusting in the desired direction) and signs of a diffuse neuropathy. Mutation in the ATM gene on chromosome 11 is the cause of the disorder, and in addition to the neurologic phenotype, results in impaired DNA repair leading to an increased risk of hematologic and other malignancies. Hence exposure to radiation even for routine procedures is strongly discouraged. MRI may show signs of progressive cerebellar atrophy. Patients usually have hypogammaglobinemia and are prone to infections. In fact, malignancies and recurrent infections are the most common cause of death in these individuals eventually. Freidreich's ataxia is another autosomal recessive ataxia syndrome in children, results from a GAA expansion in the frataxin protein coding region. Patients with this genetic condition typically have a later onset of ataxia (between ages 10–15) and do not have the above mentioned cutaneous changes or the extrapyramidal or ocular features (though signs of dorsal column and peripheral nerve dysfunction are also present.) Fragile X typically leads to severe intellectual disability in children. Adults with milder phenotypes may present with ataxia as part of the Fragile X- Tremor- Ataxia syndrome.

Suggested Reading

- Ropper A, Samuels M, Klien J. Adams and Victor's Principles of Neurology. 10th ed. New York: Mcgraw Hill; 2014. p. 946.
- Pandolfo M, Manto M. Cerebellar and afferent ataxias. Continuum Lifelong Learning Neurol. 2013;19(5):1312.

Demyelinating Disorders

Y. M. Awaad, *Absolute Pediatric Neurology*, https://doi.org/10.1007/978-3-319-78801-2_5

5

1. Which of the following is inconsistent with a diagnosis of Guillain-Barre syndrome
   A. Sensory involvement
   B. Persistent asymmetry of weakness
   C. Cranial nerve palsies
   D. Dysautonomia
   E. Increased cerebrospinal fluid protein levels for >1 week

Correct Answer is: B

Acute inflammatory demyelinating polyradiculoneuropathy (AIDP), or "Guillain-Barre syndrome," is an autoimmune, areflexic, ascending weakness with mild sensory changes that progresses over a few weeks' time. It is classically a demyelinating process, although axonal damage may occur in cases of severe demyelination.

Predominantly axonal variants also exist (e.g. Miller-Fisher syndrome, acute motor axonal neuropathy). It is often associated with a preceding respiratory infection, gastrointestinal infection, surgery, or vaccination.

Characteristic manifestations include:

- **Progressive upper and lower extremity weakness, which may also involve facial, oropharyngeal, and respiratory muscles**
- **Areflexia or hyporeflexia**
- **Progression over days to weeks. By definition, progression ends 4 weeks after onset**
- **Symmetry of weakness**
- **Mild sensory changes**
- **Inter-scapular or low back pain**
- **Cranial nerve palsies (45–75% of cases), most often bilateral and involving the facial nerves**
- **Dysautonomia (e.g. orthostasis, anhidrosis, urinary retention, arrhythmias), occurring in approximately two-thirds of patients**
- **Lack of fever**
- **Elevated cerebrospinal fluid protein levels persisting beyond the first week of symptoms, in the absence of pleocytosis ("albuminocytological dissociation")**
- **Nerve conduction slowing or block on nerve conduction studies**
- **Recovery over week**

Findings that are inconsistent with a diagnosis of Guillain-Barre syndrome include:

- **Persistently asymmetric weakness**
- **A clear sensory level**
- **Severe bowel or bladder dysfunction at the onset of symptoms**
- **A marked cerebrospinal fluid pleocytosis should also raise suspicion for an alternative diagnosis.**

2. A 15-year-old female came to the ED with a 2 days history of right eye blurry vision that has rapidly progressed to an inability to read print with that eye. This morning, she had complained of a frontal headache, pain with eye movement, and flashing lights in her central visual field, which she attributed to migraine. She had an upper respiratory tract infection 2 weeks ago with full recovery. On examination, her visual acuity is 20/20 OS and finger counting at 3 feet OD. She has a right afferent pupillary defect and elevation of the right optic nerve head. Head MRI is shown. CSF analysis is unremarkable.
   Admission to the hospital with high-dose methylprednisolone treatment is recommended for which of the following reasons?
   A. Preventing blindness
   B. Preventing involvement of the unaffected eye
   C. Speeding recovery of the affected eye
   D. Preventing the subsequent development of multiple sclerosis
   E. Treating status migrainosus

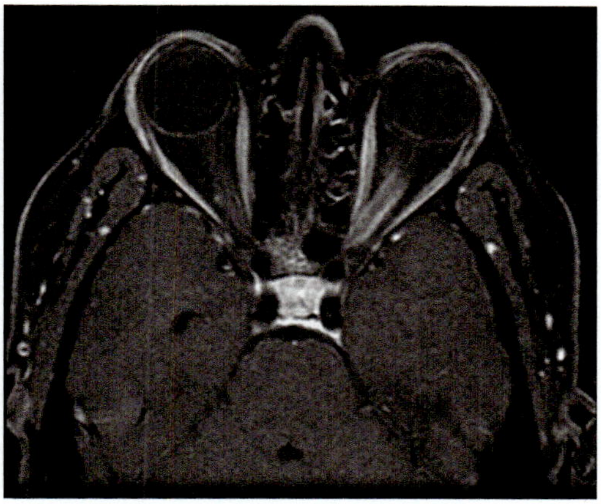

Fig. 5.1 Optic Neuritis (Transferred from en.wikipedia to Commons. Topperdoc at English Wikipedia)

Correct Answer is: C

Optic neuritis is an acute inflammatory condition of the optic nerve. It occurs as a separate entity or as a manifestation of many other demyelinating diseases (multiple sclerosis, neuromyelitis optica, and acute disseminated encephalomyelitis) and collagen vascular disorders (lupus). There are no controlled trials regarding the treatment of optic neuritis in children; however, the Optic Neuritis Treatment Trial (ONTT) demonstrated that treatment with high-dose intravenous methylprednisolone shortened the time to initial recovery but did not change the long-term visual course in adults. Most physicians treat pediatric optic neuritis with intravenous methylprednisolone at a dose that is comparable to that used in the ONTT.

Suggested Reading

- Brady KM, Amarpreet SB, Lee AG, Coats DK, Paysse EA, Steinkuller PG. Optic neuritis in children: clinical features and visual outcome. J AAPOS. 1999.

3. An 8-year-old boy is brought by his family to the ED because he has been sleepy and confused since waking up this morning. He vomited several times and has complained of headache and neck pain. He has unsteady gait and needed help to walk. Past medical history is unremarkable, but he had an upper respiratory illness with sore throat and cough 1 week ago. He has no known allergies and taken no medications. On examination he is afebrile with normal vital signs. He is lethargic and does not follow commands. He has mild neck stiffness and complains of headache. Cranial nerves are intact. Tendon reflexes are brisk in the right limbs and the right plantar response is extensor. He is unable to walk. EEG shows diffuse slowing and MRI is shown. CSF exam shows protein 62 mg/dL, glucose 60 mg/dL, 35 lymphocytes/hpf, and 0 RBC/hpf.

What is the most likely diagnosis?

A. Acute disseminated encephalomyelitis
B. Herpes simplex virus encephalitis
C. Measles encephalitis
D. Multiple sclerosis
E. Mitochondrial encephalomyopathy

Correct Answer is: A

Acute disseminated encephalomyelitis (ADEM) is an immune-mediated demyelinating disease which most commonly affects children (mean age 7 years). It most commonly presents in winter and spring. Majority of patients have history of a recent infection with a mean latency of 2 weeks. Encephalopathy is a must symptom; typical symptoms include headache, vomiting, confusion, drowsiness, and meningismus, symptoms which are uncommon in multiple sclerosis. Other neurologic signs relate to the specific areas of white matter involvement and can include pyramidal, cerebellar, and brain stem signs. Distinguishing ADEM from multiple

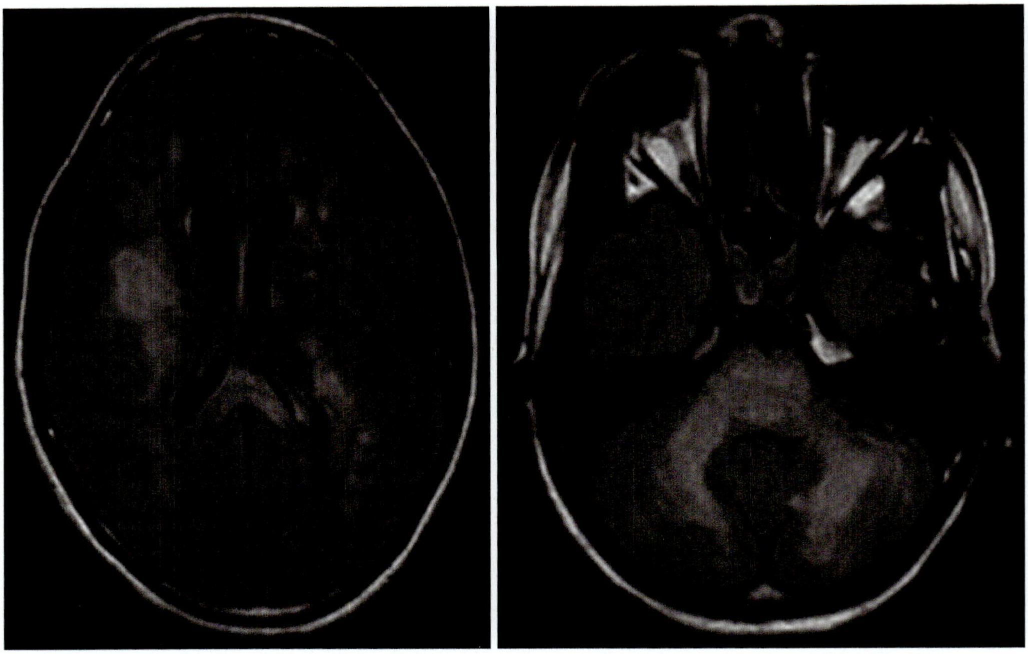

Figs. 5.2 and 5.3 MRI showing white matter changes in ADEM disease. American Academy of Neurology Institute, produced by permission

sclerosis (MS) can be difficult. In MS, CSF usually shows intrathecal synthesis of oligo clonal bands. The MRI shows multifocal white matter lesions in both ADEM and MS, but there are differences. Lesions in ADEM tend to have less distinct margins, do not involve the periventricular white matter, but do involve deep gray matter. Lesions in MS typically have distinct margins (plaques) and are most commonly seen in the periaqueductal, corpus callosum, and periventricular white matter. Repeat MRI scans 6 months after presentation most often show complete or partial resolution of the lesions and no new lesions in ADEM. Treatment of ADEM usually involves 10–30 mg/kg/day intravenous methylprednisolone for 3 days followed by a 2–6 week tapering course of oral prednisolone.

Suggested Reading

- Dole RC, Branson JA. Acute disseminated encephalomyelitis or multiple sclerosis: can the initial presentation helps in establishing a correct diagnosis? Arch Dis Child. 2005;90:636–9.
- Menge T, Kieseier BC, et al. Acute disseminated encephalomyelitis: an acute hit against the brain. Curr Opin Neurol. 2007;20(3):247–54.

4. A 4-year-old female started having trouble walking for 2 days. Today, she is not able to bear weight, has trouble raising her arms above her head, and cannot crawl. She is not complaining of any pain at rest but when you performed the Kernig and Brudzinski maneuvers on her, there is discomfort in the thighs. She is areflexic but her cranial nerves are intact. She has a normal MRI.
What are you going to do to confirm the diagnosis?
A. CSF protein
B. Repetitive nerve stimulation study
C. MRI of the spine with contrast
D. Nerve conduction velocity study
E. Response to IVIG infusion

Correct Answer is: D
The nerve conduction studies are the best studies to confirm acute demyelinating polyneuropathy. Typically, conduction velocity is slowed but there may be prominent delays in F waves and conduction blocks as well. CSF protein may not be elevated early in the clinical course and thus is not reliable for diagnostic confirmation. On occasion MRI may identify inflamed nerve roots but this is not a reliable way to make the diagnosis. Repetitive stimulation would be normal in these patients as there is no defect in neuromuscular transmission. Response to treatment is not a reliable approach to diagnosis, particularly a nonspecific therapy such as immunoglobulin.

Suggested Reading

- Soliven B. Acute demyelinating polyradiculoneuropathy In: Gilman S, Goldstein GW, Waxman SG, editors. Med link. 12th ed. San Diego: Arbor Publishing; 2007
- Bromberg MB. Comparison of electrodiagnostic criteria for primary demyelination in chronic polyneuropathy. Muscle Nerve. 1991;14(10):968–76.

5. A 16-year-old female complains of acute onset of numbness in her right arm, which disappeared few days later. Her medical history is unremarkable and she takes no medications. A brain MRI is obtained. A FLAIR Sequence sample is shown.
Which of the following test results listed below is needed to diagnose MS?
   A. Demonstration of abnormal SSEPs
   B. Demonstration of abnormal VEPs
   C. Monoclonal antibodies in the CSF
   D. Five or more lesions on T-2 weighted MRI
   E. T-2 weighted MRI showing lesions in the spine

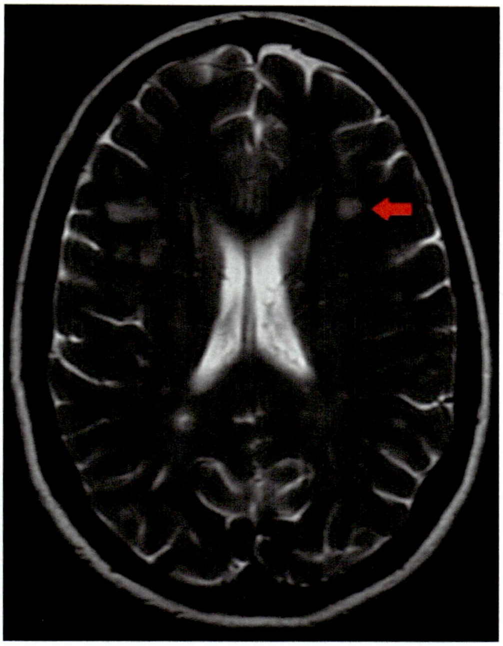

Fig. 5.4 MRI showing white matter changes in Multiple sclerosis. (James Heilman, MD. Wikipedia)

Correct Answer is: D
Typically, the diagnosis of MS requires the identification of more than one episode of neurological dysfunction with more than one locale within the central nervous system. The increasing use of MRI and the variability of the clinical presentation in the pediatric age group have led to a change in the diagnostic criteria for MS in this population.

The criteria for MS on MRI in pediatrics requires 2 of the following three features;

1. **Five or more lesions on T-2 weighted MRI scans.**
2. **Two or more periventricular lesions.**
3. **At least one lesion in the brainstem.**

The importance of making a firm diagnosis of MS, even in the pediatric age group is enhanced by the fact that there are now therapies available which have the potential to modify the long-term outcome of these patients.

5

Suggested Reading

- Callen DJ, et al. Role of MRI in the differentiation of ADEM from MS in children. Neurology. 2009;72:968–73.

6. You are seeing a 9-year-old female in the ED for her gait disturbance and drowsiness. 2 days ago, she woke up with walking difficulty, veering to the right side. By the end of the day, she became drowsier and has to stay in bed. She has an absence seizure disorder which began last year and is being treated with Lamotrigine. 1 week ago, she had cough and congestion and she was treated with amoxicillin, otherwise she is a health girl. She has normal vital signs. She is drowsy, but you can awaken her with vigorous stimulation. She is not speaking or following commands. Her pupils are 6 mm and sluggish. She has normal fundus exam. Muscle tone is normal and tendon reflexes are brisk, with bilateral extensor plantar responses. A brain MRI is obtained and is shown here.

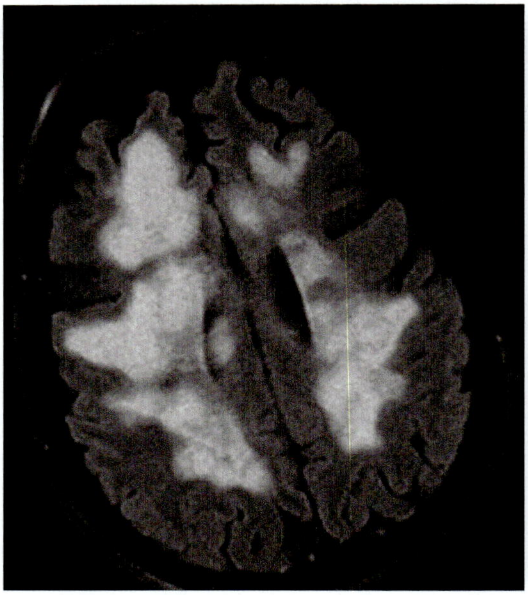

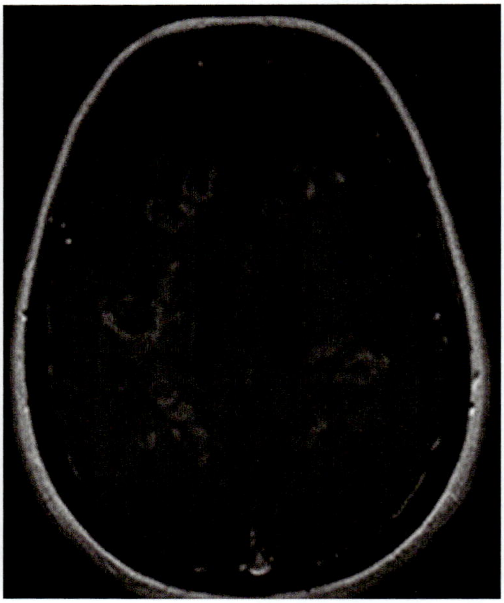

Figs. 5.5 and 5.6 MRI showing white matter changes in ADEM. American Academy of Neurology Institute, produced by permission

What is your explanation for her condition?

A. Acute demyelinating encephalomyelopathy
B. Herpes simplex encephalitis
C. Clinically isolated syndrome
D. Multiple sclerosis
E. Tuberculous meningitis

Correct Answer is: A

Acute demyelinating encephalomyelopathy (ADEM) is defined as a first episode of inflammatory demyelination with multiple CNS sites neurological deficits most often accompanied by encephalopathy (defined as altered behavior or consciousness). MRI features of diffuse, bilateral lesions are supportive, but not diagnostic, of ADEM. ADEM occurs more commonly in children less than 10 years of age. ADEM may be preceded by infectious symptoms, although a specific pathogen is rarely found. Meningism, fever, and seizures are more commonly seen in ADEM than in

"clinically isolated syndrome". Complete recovery is expected in approximately 70%. This patient's drowsiness and lack of prior neurological events distinguish ADEM from either clinically isolated syndrome or multiple sclerosis. Herpes simplex encephalitis typically affects the temporal lobe rather than the brainstem. The MRI findings and her clinical course are much more characteristic of ADEM than tuberculous meningitis.

Suggested Reading

- Dale RC, Brilot F, Banwell B. Pediatric central nervous system inflammatory demyelination: acute disseminated encephalomyelitis, clinically isolated syndromes, neuromyelitis optica, and multiple sclerosis. Curr Opin Neurol. 2009;22:233–40.

7. A 4-year-old boy has been evaluated for his first left onset partial seizure with secondarily generalization. EEG showed right sided spike and sharp wave and also slowing on the same side. Because his high peripheral white blood cell count at 18.5, you ordered a lumbar puncture which showed 18 WBC/uL and a protein of 45 mg/dl. His MRI is shown here. **What is your next step in his management?**
   A. Administer Fosphenytoin 20 mg/kg
   B. Administer high-dose intravenous corticosteroid medication.
   C. Administer intravenous acyclovir.
   D. Begin plasmapheresis.
   E. Send CSF for HSV PCR.

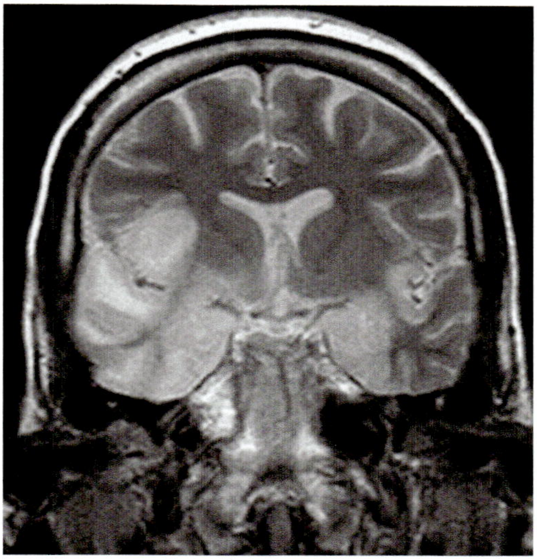

Fig. 5.7 Herpes encephalitis. Coronal T2-weighted MR image shows high signal in the temporal lobes including hippocampal formations and parahippogampal gyrae, insulae, and right inferior frontal gyrus. A brain biopsy was performed and the histology was consistent with encephalitis. PCR was repeated on the biopsy specimen and was positive for HSV. (▶ http://www.radpod.org/2007/03/24/herpes-simplex-encephalitis/. dr Laughlin Dawes)

Correct Answer is: E
The clinical presentation is most likely ADEM but it is very important to rule out herpes encephalitis. One should also consider visual fields and visual acuity testing and inquire about the status of the spinal cord function. Antiepileptics are not indicated after his first seizure, particularly if it is secondary to a known process. One might also consider an MS panel on the CSF, because in children under 10 years of age multiple sclerosis more often has large white matter lesions and more often has seizures associated with the onset.

Suggested Reading

- Aicardi J. Diseases of the nervous system in childhood. 2nd ed. Cambridge University Press; 1998. p. 444.

8. You are evaluating a 5-year-old boy for his irritability and unsteadiness in walking and using his arms for the last 2 days. He was crying from pain in his legs and back and now he is unable to walk without assistance. He had gastroenteritis 1 week which has been resolved with no treatment. He takes no medications. His family history is

unremarkable. On your examination, he has normal ocular movements and pupillary reactions. He has mild facial weakness, and mild weakness in both shoulders, but a good handgrip. He has action coarse tremor when reaching for objects. He cannot support his own weight and is unable to sit unsupported. He is areflexic and plantar responses are flexor. Sensation is intact.

5

What is your diagnosis?

A. Acute cerebellar ataxia
B. Acute transverse myelitis
C. Botulism
D. Guillain Barre Syndrome
E. Polymyositis

Correct Answer is: D
The association of facial and limb weakness with areflexia of acute onset and rapid progression are most compatible with acute inflammatory demyelinating polyradicuopathy, although a significant subset of these patients have an axonal form rather than demyelinating. Guillain Barre Syndrome is an eponym for acute or chronic, axonal or demyelinating inflammatory neuropathy. Presentation can be different in young children than in adults. 1/3 of pediatric cases occur in less than 3 years of age children. In the pediatric group, pain is a common presenting complaint, involving the back or limbs. Ataxia and disturbances of equilibrium are more common in children than adults. Electrophysiological studies performed in the first week of the illness most often demonstrate prolonged or absent F-responses (88%), prolonged distal latency (75%), conduction block (58%), and reduction in conduction velocity (50%).

Suggested Reading

- Delanoe C, Sebire G, et al. Acute inflammatory demyelinating polyradiculopathy in children: clinical and electrodiagnostic studies. Ann Neurol. 1998;44:350–6.

9. A 13-year-old female has been evaluated because of her vertigo, nausea, vomiting, and visual disturbances which started 2 weeks ago after a basketball game. She reported that she felt unsteady just before starting the game, but she did not pay too much attention to it. She was struck by the ball in the face and felt stunned. Two hours later, she noticed a spinning sensation associated with nausea and vomited several times. The following day, her vertigo continued and she was unable to walk. Two days later she began to experience double vision. An MRI was performed and results are not available. Her symptoms started to resolve gradually over the following 2 weeks. You examined her today and she has normal exam. **What is the most likely diagnosis?**

A. Acute demyelinating encephalomyelopathy
B. Multiple sclerosis
C. Clinically isolated syndrome
D. Neuromyelitis optica
E. Traumatic brain injury

Correct Answer is: C
The girl has a first episode of neurological dysfunction, the onset of which predated the basketball injury. Multiple sclerosis diagnosis would require a second demyelinating event. ADEM diagnosis requires encephalopathy (altered behavior or consciousness) as a clinical feature. Neuromyelitis optica is characterized by sequential or concomitant optic neuritis and transverse myelitis, patient does not have either. Clinically isolated syndrome (CIS) is the most accurate diagnosis for this patient. CISs are more common than ADEM in children, particularly in those > 10 years of age. CIS is a clinically heterogeneous entity and has a higher incidence of subsequent MS diagnosis than ADEM. CIS can be mono-focal affecting

a localized part of the CNS (optic neuritis, transverse myelitis, brainstem syndrome, hemispheric syndrome) or multifocal but must not include encephalopathy.

Suggested Reading

- Dale RC, Brilot F, Banwell B. Pediatric central nervous system inflammatory demyelination: acute disseminated encephalomyelitis, clinically isolated syndromes, neuromyelitis optica, and multiple sclerosis. Curr Opin Neurol. 2009;22:233–40.

10. **The following scenario is part of a 7-question series, Discussion & References included at the end of series.**

    The following 7 questions pertain to the patient history below:

    A 10-year-old boy is complaining of 5 days history of frontal headache which affected him playing his last volleyball game. He also complains of blurred vision. His visual acuity is count fingers on the left and 20/60 on the right, with color desaturation on the left.

    Given this patient's history, which of the features below is most likely to be seen?

    A. Optic nerve (ON) pallor
    B. Macular Star
    C. Bilateral papillitis
    D. Cells in the vitreous
    E. Increased cup to disc ratio

Correct Answer is: C

This is a clinical presentation of acute optic neuritis. Bilateral papillitis will be the most expected findings on his exam. Optic nerve pallor is indicative of a chronic process, and therefore is less likely to be seen in acute ON. While a macular star might be seen in extreme cases of inflammatory optic neuritis, it is not the most likely finding. A macular star may be seen in some cases of severe optic nerve edema, but this finding indicates neuro-retinitis. It may be seen in association with infectious etiologies as well as non-infectious etiologies, including multiple sclerosis, sarcoidosis and other inflammatory disorders. Inflammatory cells in the vitreous may suggest uveitis: this finding is not suggestive of optic neuritis. An increased cup-to-disc ratio is seen in glaucoma, and is indicative of increased intraocular pressure.

11. **The following scenario is question 2 of the 7-question series, Discussion & References included at the end of this series.**

    Imaging is performed:

    Image 1: axial T2-FLAIR image of the brain.

    Image 2: T2-weighted image of orbits.

    Image 3: T1-weighted image of the orbits with contrast.

    Image 4: T2-weighted sagittal image of the spine.

    What findings are you seeing on the MRI?

    A. T2 hyper intensities of the ON with gadolinium enhancement; T2 lesion in the spinal cord, brain normal
    B. T2 hyper intensities of the ON bilaterally, Brain, and Spinal Cord, with leptomeningeal enhancement
    C. Brain, spine and ON within normal limits
    D. Bilateral ON hyper intensities with gadolinium enhancement, brain and spine within normal limits.
    E. Longitudinally extensive spinal cord lesion, ON within normal limits, brain within normal limits

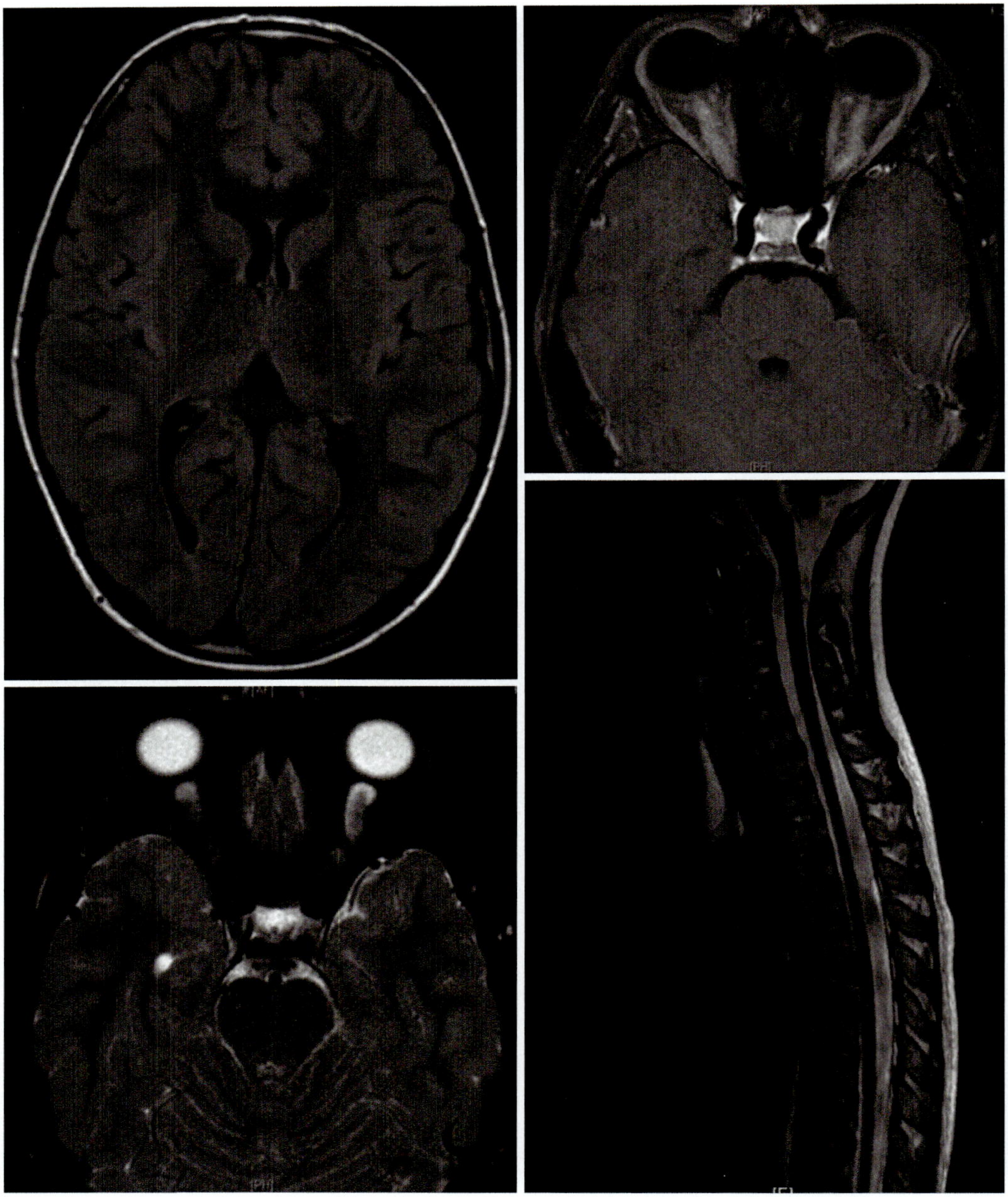

Figs. 5.8, 5.9, 5.10 and 5.11 Bilateral ON hyper intensities with gadolinium enhancement in ► Fig. 5.9, all other figures are normal. By permission from Radiopaedia

Correct Answer is: D
Imaging shows bilateral optic nerve T2 weighted hyper intensities with gadolinium enhancement on T1 weighted imaging bilaterally. The other imaging is normal.

12. **The following scenario is question 3 of the 7-question series, Discussion & References included at the end of this series.**
What might be seen on visual field testing?

A. Normal visual fields
B. Bilaterally increased blind spot
C. Bilaterally decrease blind spot
D. Bilateral quadrantanopia
E. Homonymous homonopsia

Correct Answer is: B
The most common visual field abnormality seen in bilateral optic neuritis is an enlarged central scotoma, or on field testing, bilaterally increased blind spot.

13. The following scenario is question 4 of the 7-question series, Discussion & References included at the end of this series.
Testing is performed.
Which key serological test may be important in this case?
A. ANA
B. CRP
C. ESR
D. NMO-IgG
E. NMDAR ab

Correct Answer is: D
NMO-IgG. Neuromyelitis optica is characterized by severe optic neuropathy and longitudinally extensive transverse myelitis. It is positive in approximately 3/4 of children with a clinical diagnosis of relapsing neuromyelitis optica.

Suggested Reading

- Banwell et al. Neurology. 2008 Jan 29;70(5):344–52. Epub 2007 Dec 19.

14. The following scenario is question 5 of the 7-question series, Discussion & References included at the end of this series.
The parents ask what percentage of children who have the disease being evaluated for in the question above have a positive serum test. What would your answer to this family be?
A. 1/3
B. ½
C. ¾
D. 1/8

Correct Answer is: C
In a small series of children with clinically established recurrent NMO, about ¾ (78%) are positive for the antibody.

Suggested Reading

- Banwell et al. Neurology. 2008 Jan 29; 70(5):344–52. Epub 2007 Dec 19.

15. The following scenario is question 6 of the 7-question series, Discussion & References included at the end of this series.
What would you expect the visual evoked potential to show in this child?
A. Bilaterally decreased amplitude
B. p100, no response on the left, markedly delayed on the right
C. W-wave bilaterally
D. Delay of n75 bilaterally

Correct Answer is: B
The child has bilateral optic neuritis with severe involvement of the left and moderate involvement on the right. Prolongation of the p100 is the classical finding on PRVEP in optic neuritis.

16. The following scenario is question 7 of the 7-question series, Discussion & References included at the end of this series.
What would your first line treatment of choice for this acute presentation be?
A. IVIG 1 g/kg per day for 2 days
B. Solumedrol 30 mg/kg/day for 3 days
C. Cyclophosphamide 750 mg/m2
D. Plasmapheresis, 5 cycles

Correct Answer is: B
The first line therapy of choice is pulse IV steroids, other treatments might be used in severe optic neuritis. The optic neuritis treatment trial suggests that the use of pulse IV Solumedrol for 3 days speeds recovery of ON in comparison to placebo and oral prednisone at a dose of 1 mg/kg/d. Beck et al. N Engl J Med. 1992 Feb 27;326(9):581–8.

Pulse steroid dosing in the pediatric population is 20–40 mg/kg/d for 3 days. While recovery may be hastened, there is no evidence for long term benefit of steroids over placebo for return to normal VA (Gal RL, Vedula SS, Beck R, Corticosteroids for treating optic neuritis, Cochrane Database Syst Rev. 2012 Apr 18;4:CD001430. doi: ► https://doi.org/10.1002/14651858.CD001430.pub3.).

5

Suggested Reading

- Beck et al. N Engl J Med. 1992 Feb 27;326(9):581–8.
- Gal RL, Vedula SS, Beck R, Corticosteroids for treating optic neuritis. Cochrane Database Syst Rev. 2012;(4):CD001430. ► https://doi.org/10.1002/14651858.CD001430.pub3.

17. The following scenario is part of a 7-question series.

The following 7 questions pertain to the patient history below:

You are seeing a 14-year-old boy with an 8-week history of behavioral changes and hallucinations. He was previously healthy and a good student at school. He has no history of psychiatric problems, and no family history of psychiatric problems. His parents got separated recently. What is in the history might point to an autoimmune etiology?

A. Presence of mood disturbance
B. Acute or sub-acute onset
C. Diagnosis of borderline personality
D. Insight into symptoms

Correct Answer is: B
Small percentage of children have underlying neurologic disease for their acute psychosis. Several series of patients with first onset schizophrenia, depression, and borderline personality have not revealed an increased likelihood of pathologic antibodies to the NMDA-receptor (NR1 IgG) in these patients.

Suggested Reading

- Kayser et al. JAMA Neurol. 2013 September 1;70(9): Of the answers provided, an acute or sub-acute onset might point to an autoimmune etiology, but is not adequate in itself to suggest this (Suleiman et al. Epilepsia 54(6)1036–45, 201).

18. The following scenario is part 2 of a 7-question series, Discussion & References included at the end of series.

The family reports occasional transient facial twitching not accompanied by loss of consciousness. You order an EEG. Which EEG feature may point specifically to an autoimmune encephalitis?

A. Frontal predominance of sharp waves
B. Focal slowing
C. Extreme delta brush
D. Intermittent rhythmic delta
E. Triphasic waves

Correct Answer is: C
Extreme delta brush has been reported specifically in NMDAR patients and is usually not present in other encephalopathies.

Suggested Reading

- Schmitt et al. Neurology. 2012 Sep 11;79(11):1094–100. ► https://doi.org/10.1212/WNL.0b013e3182698cd8. Epub 2012 Aug 29.

19. **The following scenario is part 3 of a 7-question series, Discussion & References included at the end of series.**
    You see a suggestive pattern on EEG.
    What test might be helpful?
    A. Rheumatoid factor
    B. Anti-TTG
    C. NMO IgG
    D. NMDAR antibodies
    E. Anti-gliadin antibodies
    F. Oligo clonal bands

Correct Answer is: D
NMDAR antibodies may be helpful in this case, although the testing should not be limited to this. The story suggests the presence of an autoimmune encephalitis, and the behavioral changes suggest the possibility of a limbic encephalitis. This story, combined with extreme delta brush on EEG, suggests the need for testing for NMDAR antibodies. The other antibody/rheumatologic tests listed (RF, anti-TTG, Anti gliadin ab, NMO-IgG) have not been associated with autoimmune encephalitis).

20. **The following scenario is part 4 of a 7-question series, Discussion & References included at the end of series.**
    The child's testing is positive.
    What would you use as a first line therapy?
    A. Cyclophosphamide
    B. IVIG 1 g/kg x 2 days
    C. Interferon beta 1a
    D. Solumedrol 30 mg/kg/d x 3 days
    E. Glatiramer Acetate

Correct Answer is: D
While no clear prospective evidence for therapy for NMDAR encephalitis is available, retrospective analyses suggest that first line therapy with pulse steroids is effective in half of patients.

Suggested Reading

- Dalmau et al. Lancet Neurol. 2011 Jan;10(1):63–74. ► https://doi.org/10.1016/S1474-4422(10)70253-2; Titulaer MJ et al. Lancet Neurol. 2013 Feb; 12(2):157–65. ► https://doi.org/10.1016/S1474-4422(12)70310-1. Epub 2013 Jan 3.

21. **The following scenario is part 5 of a 7-question series, Discussion & References included at the end of series.**
    Which ancillary testing should you ordered?
    A. Pulmonary function tests
    B. Abdominal ultrasound
    C. Ultrasound of the pelvis
    D. Chest CT
    E. Thyroid scan

Correct Answer is: C
NMDAR encephalitis was first described in relation to ovarian teratoma (Dalmau 2004); while the likelihood of teratoma is lower in the pediatric population (6% of one large series), resection is curative.

Suggested Reading

- Tuzun et al. Acta Neuropathol. 2009;118(6):737–43. ► https://doi.org/10.1007/s00401-009-0582-4; Dalmau et al. Lancet Neurol. 2011;10(1):63–74. ► https://doi.org/10.1016/S1474-4422(10)70253-2.

22. **The following scenario is part 6 of a 7-question series, Discussion & References included at the end of series.**
    Based on presently available knowledge.
    What will you tell the family about risk of recurrence?
    A. 20%
    B. 10%
    C. 30%
    D. 40%
    E. 50%

Correct Answer is: B
Risk of recurrence is 10% in large series.

Suggested Reading

- Dalmau et al. Lancet Neurol. 2011;10(1):63–74. ▶ https://doi.org/10.1016/S1474-4422(10)70253-2; Titulaer MJ et al. Lancet Neurol. 2013;12(2):157–65. ▶ https://doi.org/10.1016/S1474-4422(12)70310-1. Epub 2013 Jan 3.

23. **The following scenario is part 7 of a 7-question series, Discussion & References included at the end of series.**

    The family asks you whether recovery is expected.
    What would you tell the family?
    A. 70% of children suffer from irreversible cognitive impairment
    B. 50% chance of seizures long term
    C. Ongoing behavioral problems in greater than half of children
    D. Full recovery seen in 75% of patients
    E. Recurrent disease is seen in 50% of children

Correct Answer is: D
Full recovery is seen in 75% of children.

Suggested Reading

- Dalmau et al. Lancet Neurol. 2011;10(1):63–74. ▶ https://doi.org/10.1016/S1474-4422(10)70253-2.

24. A 12-year-old boy is complaining of double vision for 1 day. When you examine him you find internuclear opthalmolplegia. An MRI is performed.

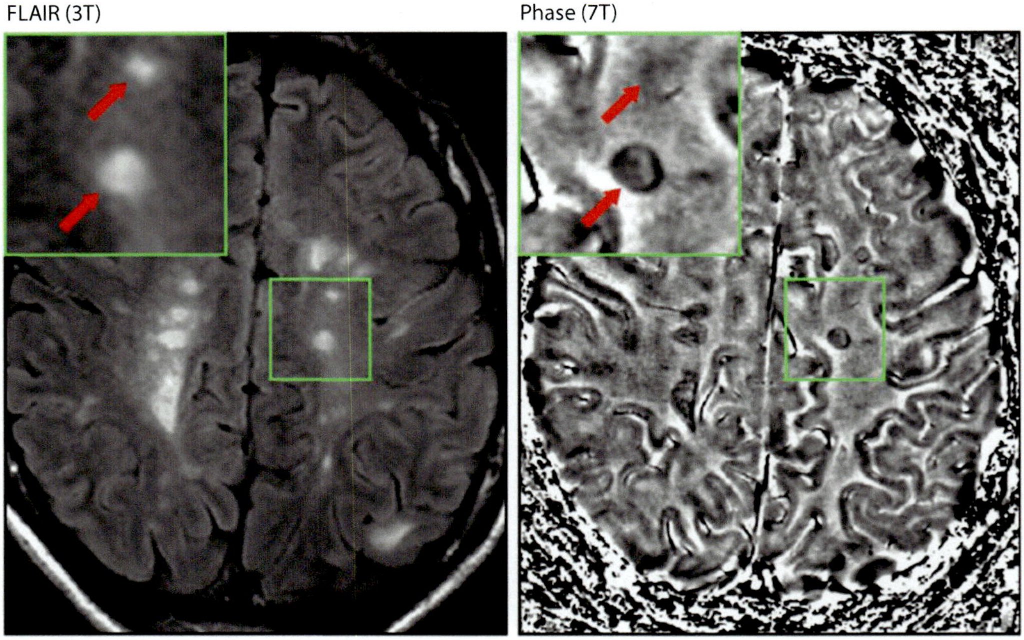

Figs. 5.12 and 5.13 MS. FLAIR (3 T) and GRE phase (7 T) images of a patient with active relapsing-remitting MS.FLAIR images show numerous white matter MS lesions of which 2 are magnified (inset, red arrows). Phase imaging at 7 T phase/GRE reveals a hypointense ring corresponding with one lesion on FLAIR. The other lesion is not visible on 7 T GRE (inset, arrows). (Mehta V, Pei W, Yang G, Li S, Swamy E, et al. (2013) Iron Is a Sensitive Biomarker for Inflammation in Multiple Sclerosis Lesions. PLoS ONE 8(3): e57573. ▶ https://doi.org/10.1371/journal.pone.0057573. ▶ http://www.plosone.org/article/info:doi/10.1371/journal.pone.0057573#pone-0057573-g005. Veela Mehta, Wei Pei, Grant Yang, Suyang Li, Eashwar Swamy, Aaron Boster, Petra Schmalbrock, David Pitt)

Given the T2 FLAIR Axial and Sagittal MRI brain images below, what will allow you to make the diagnosis of MS?

A. 3 more lesions in the brain
B. A lesion in the spinal cord and a gadolinium enhancing lesion
C. One gadolinium enhancing lesion and one hypo intense lesion on T1 weighted imaging
D. White blood cells in the CSF and black hole
E. Increased opening pressure on LP and black hole

Correct Answer is: C

Current diagnostic criteria for MS, the revised McDonald Criteria (reference Polman et al. Ann Neurol. 2011 Feb; 69(2):292–302. ► https://doi.org/10.1002/ana.22366), are acceptable for use in pediatric cases of multiple sclerosis over 12 years of age (Krupp et al. Multiple Sclerosis Journal 2013 ► https://doi.org/10.1177/1352458513484547).

These criteria allow for the MRI diagnosis of multiple sclerosis at first clinical event, as long as there is evidence for dissemination in space and time on the MRI scan in children older than 12 years of age. The 2010 revision of the McDonald Criteria specifies that one new enhancing or non-enhancing lesion be seen in order to make a diagnosis of MS.

In this case, the boy has had one clinical attack and would need MRI evidence for dissemination in time. This would be fulfilled with another lesion which was enhancing on T1 weighted imaging or evidence for an old lesion, as represented by a hypo intense lesion on T1 weighted imaging ("black hole").

The following are specific pediatric diagnostic criteria for MS. Note the importance of having more clinical episodes in the young child with a first presentation of acute disseminated encephalomyelitis.

1. **MS Diagnosis, from Krupp et al. MS Journal 2013. Two or more nonencephalopathic (e.g. not ADEM-like), clinical CNS events with presumed inflammatory cause, separated by more than 30 days and involving more than one area of the CNS.**
2. **One nonencephalopathic episode typical of MS which is associated with MRI findings consistent with 2010 Revised McDonald criteria for DIS and in which a follow up MRI shows at least one new enhancing or non-enhancing lesion consistent with dissemination in time (DIT) MS criteria**
3. **One ADEM attack followed by a nonencephalopathic clinical event, three or more months after symptom onset that is associated with new MRI lesions that fulfill 2010 Revised McDonald DIS criteria**
4. **A first, single, acute event that does not meet ADEM criteria and whose MRI findings are consistent with the 2010 Revised McDonald criteria for DIS and DIT (applies only to children 12 years or older)**

Suggested Reading

- MS Diagnosis, from Krupp et al. MS J. 2013.

25. A 12-year-old boy woke up this morning noticing that he could not see out of his left eye. He complains of blurry vision in the left eye and rubbing the eye or squinting did not make it better. He had no pain in the eye. He has no medical history of previous trauma, fever, respiratory symptoms, or headache. The mother made an appointment with an optometrist for him to be seen today. While he is waiting to be seen, the mother had to take him to the ED because the boy complained of mid-back pain and rapidly developed difficulty urinating,

stiffness of his legs, and tingly sensation when he ran his hand over his abdomen below his belly button. ED attending admitted him for evaluation and treatment.

The attending most likely checked him for:

A. Anti-NMDA receptor antibodies
B. Anti-microsomal antibodies
C. Anti-thyroid antibodies
D. Anti-aquaporin 4 antibodies
E. Anti-neuronal antibodies

5

Correct Answer is: D

Neuromyelitis optica (NMO) is an uncommon disease syndrome of the central nervous system (CNS) that affects the optic nerves and spinal cord. Individuals with NMO develop optic neuritis and transverse myelitis. NMO leads to loss of myelin.

Historically, NMO was diagnosed in patients who experienced a rapid onset of blindness in one or both eyes, followed within days or weeks by varying degrees of paralysis in the arms and legs. In most cases, however, the interval between optic neuritis and transverse myelitis is significantly longer, sometimes as long as several years. After the initial attack, NMO follows an unpredictable course. Most individuals with the syndrome experience clusters of attacks months or years apart, followed by partial recovery during periods of remission. This relapsing form of NMO primarily affects women. The female to male ratio is greater than 4:1. Another form of NMO, in which an individual only has a single, severe attack extending over a month or two, is most likely a distinct disease that affects men and women with equal frequency. The onset of NMO varies from childhood to adulthood, with two peaks, one in childhood and the other in adults in their 40s.

In the past, NMO was considered to be a severe variant of multiple sclerosis (MS) because both can cause attacks of optic neuritis and myelitis. Recent discoveries, however, suggest it is a separate disease. NMO is different from MS in the severity of its attacks and its tendency to solely strike the optic nerves and spinal cord at the beginning of the disease. Symptoms outside of the optic nerves and spinal cord are rare, although certain symptoms, including uncontrollable vomiting and hiccups, are now recognized as relatively specific symptoms of NMO that are due to brainstem involvement.

The recent discovery of the anti-aquaporin 4 antibody in many individuals with NMO gives doctors a reliable biomarker to distinguish NMO from MS. The antibody, known as NMO-IgG, seems to be present in about 70 percent of those with NMO and is not found in people with MS or other similar conditions.

Suggested Reading

- Wingerchuk DM, Weinshenker BG. Neuromyelitis optica (Devic's syndrome). Handb Clin Neurol. 2014;122:581

26. A family of previously healthy 6-year-old boy brought him to the ED because he cannot walk. For the last few days he has developed progressive weakness of both legs, ataxia, left facial weakness, blurred vision, lethargy, and an epileptic seizure. He has no medical history of any sickness. He was seen by his pediatrician 10 days ago and had his routine vaccinations. On examination, he is somnolent, and cannot sit up in bed. He has brisk reflexes in all 4 extremities with an up-going Babinski response bilaterally. MRI scan of the brain is shown.

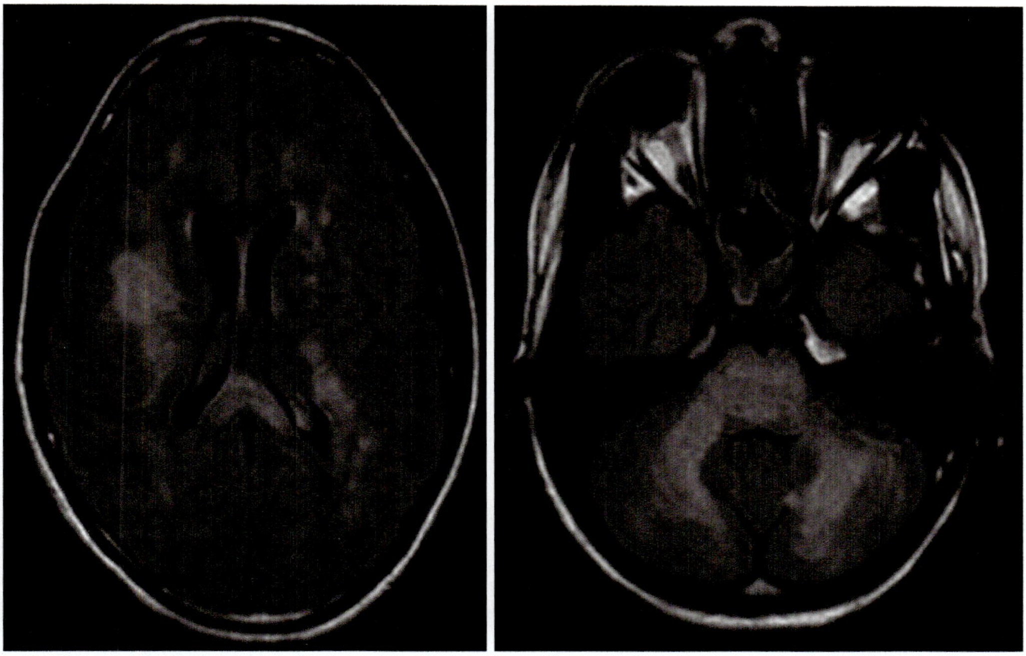

Figs. 5.14 and 5.15 MRI showing white matter changes indicating ADEM disease. American Academy of Neurology Institute, produced by permission

What would be the most reasonable treatment for him at that time?

A. Albendazole
B. Beta-interferon
C. Methylprednisolone
D. Pyridostigmine
E. Temozolomide

Correct Answer is: C

The presentation is consistent with acute disseminated encephalomyelitis (ADEM), supported by the clinical and radiographic findings. ADEM is an immune-mediated, demyelinating disease of the CNS that presents typically in children, often following a defined viral illness or vaccination. Although there are no randomized, controlled treatment trials for ADEM, standard clinical practice involves some type of immunosuppresant therapy, such as high dose steroids or intravenous immunoglobulin, or attempts at removal of the responsible antibody (not typically known) via plasmapheresis. Most cases are monophasic, although 11% can be multiphasic over time. Beta-interferon has been used anecdotally for recurrent ADEM but not for acute monophasic ADEM. Pyridostigmine, which acts at the neuromuscular junction, is used in the treatment of myasthenia gravis, and have no use in ADEM. Albendazole is a benzimidazole used to treat cysticercosis and other parasitic infections, not ADEM. Temozolomide is an alkylating chemotherapy drug used to treat glioblastomas and other tumors, not ADEM.

Suggested Reading

- Tenembaum S, Chitnis T, Ness J, Hahn JS. Acute disseminated encephalomyelitis. Neurology. 2007;68(16 suppl 2):S23–36.
- Chitnis T. Pediatric demyelinating diseases. Continuum (Minneap Minn). 2013;19(4):1023–45.

27. You are seeing a 9-year-old girl in the PICU for mental status changes and worsening headache for the last 2 days. Her mother reports that she has been increasingly lethargic and confused with a diffuse continuous headache which improves only slightly with acetaminophen. Her mother also report that she is weak, unable to sit or stand on her own. She has a flu-like illness 2 weeks ago. Her immunization is not up-to-date. She came to the US with her family from South America 2 years ago. Her maternal aunt has multiple sclerosis. On examination, she is febrile with temperature of 38.5 °C; pulse 90/min; respirations 20/min; blood pressure 110/65. She is asleep but when you stimulate her vigorously she will open her eyes. She will not speak nor follow commands. Cranial nerves are intact with no papilledema. Movements are symmetric but diffusely weak. DTR are 3+ and symmetric with flexor plantar responses. Brain MRI is shown. CSF shows 8 lymphocytes/mm 3, protein 65 mg/dL, glucose 70 mg/dL.

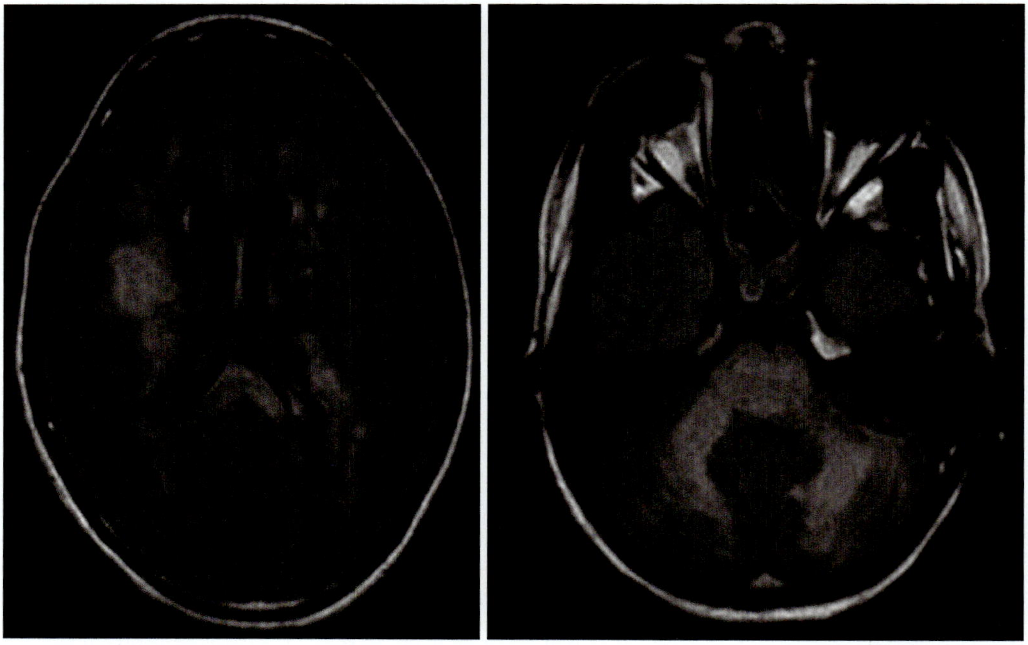

Figs. 5.16 and 5.17 MRI showing white matter changes indicating ADEM disease. American Academy of Neurology Institute, produced by permission

What is the most likely diagnosis?

A. acute disseminated encephalomyelitis
B. herpes encephalitis
C. multiple sclerosis
D. neurocysticercosis
E. subacute sclerosing panencephalitis

Correct Answer is: A

This girl has an acute encephalopathy following a predated illness. The clinical presentation in association of CSF and MRI findings is most indicative of acute disseminated encephalomyelitis (ADEM). Herpes encephalitis has a predilection for the temporal lobes, which

does not show up on MRI. Because this is her first episode of neurologic symptomatology makes multiple sclerosis (MS) an inappropriate diagnosis. Distinguishing between patients with ADEM and those with a first demyelinating episode which eventually becomes MS can be very difficult. Studies of children after a first episode of demyelination have identified disease onset in adolescence, intrathecal oligoclonal bands and optic neuritis as associated with a higher MS risk; whereas prepubertal onset, presence of multifocal features with encephalopathy and transverse myelitis have been associated with a lower risk of subsequent MS. Although she is from South America where parasitic diseases like neurocysticercosis are common, most such patients present with seizures and the MRI finding is not supportive. Despite not being immunized against measles the likelihood of subacute sclerosing panencephalitis is much lower than ADEM.

Acute disseminated encephalomyelitis (ADEM) is an immune-mediated inflammatory disorder of the CNS, commonly preceded by an infection and mainly affecting the brain and spinal cord white matter. In the absence of specific biologic markers the diagnosis of ADEM is based on the clinical and radiologic features. Although ADEM usually has a monophasic course recurrent or multiphasic forms have been reported, raising diagnostic difficulties in distinguishing these cases from multiple sclerosis (MS). ADEM can occur at any age but it is more common in pediatric patients than in adults. A seasonal distribution in the winter and spring months has been found in studies conducted in the US. ADEM is classically described as a monophasic disorder which typically begins within 2 days to 4 weeks after a predated illness. Approximately 70% to 77% of patients report a clinically evident predated infection or vaccination during the prior few weeks. The typical symptoms and signs of ADEM include a rapid onset encephalopathy associated with a combination of multifocal neurologic deficits. A prodromal phase with fever, malaise, headache, nausea and vomiting may be observed shortly before the development of meningeal signs and drowsiness. The clinical course is rapidly progressive and usually develops over hours to maximum deficits within days (mean: 4.5 days). There is a wide variation in the severity of the illness. Occasionally ADEM can present as a subtle disease with nonspecific irritability, headache and somnolence, or may show a rapid progression of symptoms and signs to coma and decerebrate rigidity. Respiratory failure secondary to brainstem involvement or severely impaired consciousness occurs in 11% to 16% of cases.

Neuroimaging is extremely important in establishing the diagnosis of ADEM. MRI abnormalities are most frequently identified on T2-weighted and fluid-attenuated inversion recovery (FLAIR) sequences as patchy, poorly marginated areas of increased signal intensity. Lesions in ADEM are typically large, multiple and asymmetric. They typically involve the subcortical and central white matter and cortical gray-white junction of both cerebral hemispheres, cerebellum, brainstem and spinal cord. The gray matter of the thalami and basal ganglia are frequently involved, typically in a symmetric pattern. The periventricular white matter is also frequently involved, being described in 30% to 60% of cases. Lesions confined to the corpus callosum are less common.

There is no standard therapy for ADEM. Most treatment approaches have employed some form of nonspecific immunosuppressant therapy similar to that used for MS and other autoimmune diseases, including steroids, IV immunoglobulin (IVIG) or plasmapheresis. Most of the data describing treatment for ADEM are derived from case reports and small series. To date there have been no randomized, controlled trials for the treatment of ADEM in either children or adults.

5

Suggested Reading

- Tenembaum S, Chitnis T, Ness J, et al. Acute disseminated encephalomyelitis. Neurology. 2007;68(16 Suppl 2): S23–36.
- Dale RC, Brilot F, Banwell B. Pediatric central nervous system inflammatory demyelination: acute disseminated encephalomyelitis, clinically isolated syndromes, neuromyelitis optica, and multiple sclerosis. Curr Opin Neurol. 2009;22(3):233–40.

28. You are seeing a 16-year-old boy in the ED with a history of headache, difficulty walking and numbness and paresthesia's in both arms for the last 3 days. His family states he has also been increasingly confused and lethargic over the past 24 h. He has some mild upper respiratory viral infection 2 weeks ago, otherwise his past medical history is unremarkable. He is difficult to arouse and unable to follow commands when you examined him. He has spastic paraparesis of both legs, brisk deep tendon reflexes and up going toes bilaterally. He has a generalized tonic-clonic seizure lasting 5 min immediately after you finished his exam. Head CT is normal. CSF analysis shows 50 white blood cells with a protein level of 95 ug/dL. Brain MRI is shown. You started him on 5 days of high dose intravenous solumedrol. A follow up MRI is performed 4 weeks later, at which point he has fully recovered back to normal.

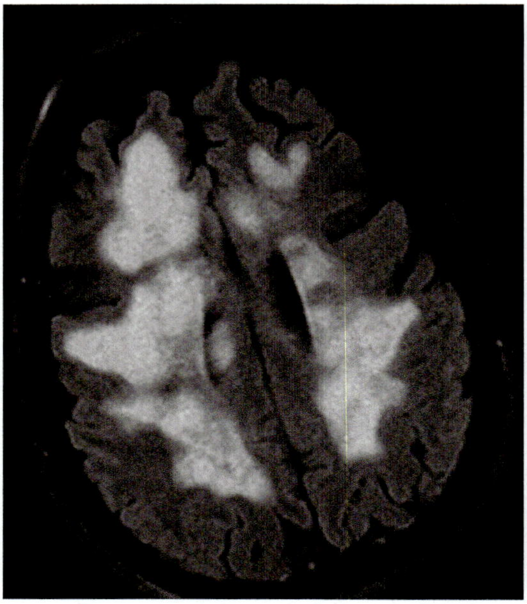

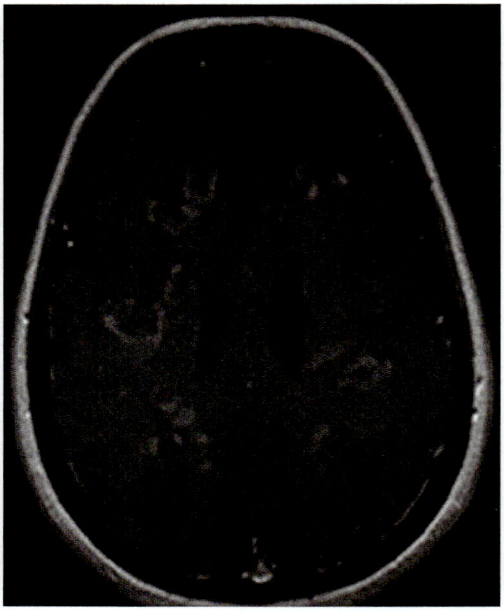

Figs. 5.18 and 5.19 ADEM, white matter changes on MRI. American Academy of Neurology Institute, produced by permission

What is the most likely diagnosis for this patient?

A. Acute Disseminated Encephalomyelitis
B. Adrenoleukodystrophy
C. Metachromatic leukodystrophy
D. Multiple sclerosis
E. Progressive multifocal leukoencephalopathy (PML)

Correct Answer is: A

The patient manifests clinical features of upper motor type weakness and encephalopathy. Additionally, noted are non-contrast enhancing diffuse confluent periventricual white matter lesions on MRI. Given the acute/sub-acute onset, acute disseminated encephalomyelitis (ADEM) should be strongly considered. There is no one diagnostic test to substantiate the diagnosis, however, and the patients clinical and radiographic examination must be followed closely to ensure marked improvement if not resolution has occurred. This condition is often "provoked" by a preceding illness or immunization, and is often treatable with steroids or intravenous immune globulin (IVIG). It is typically a monophasic illness, although the consensus criteria by the Pediatric Multiple Sclerosis Study Group allows for recurrence of symptoms within 3 months of the initial illness. The lesions on the MRI typically resolve on follow up imaging after recovery.

The patient does not present with the necessary dissemination in time criteria (though dissemination in space may be present if enough of the neuroaxis is imaged) for a diagnosis of multiple sclerosis. Additionally, the presence of such degree of encephalopathy, including a seizure, would be extremely unusual for a presentation of multiple sclerosis.

A leukodystrophy would not be expected to have such an acute onset (though this has rarely been reported), nor would near complete resolution of the radiographic features be expected with these progressive and degerative disorders of cerebral white matter.

PML (due to proposed reactivation of the JC virus in the central nervous system) would not be expected to occur in a young, healthy, immune-competent patient, nor would the lesions be expected to resolve so quickly.

Suggested Reading

- Wingerchuk D, Weinshenker B. Acute disseminated encephalomyelitis, transverse myelitis, and neuromyelitis optica. Continuum Lifelong Learning Neurol. 2013;19(4):944.
- Rezai MS, et al. Acute disseminated encephalomyelitis: a case series and review of literatures. J Pediatr Rev. 2013;1(2):88.

29. You are re-evaluating an 18-year-old female for peripheral demyelinating neuropathy, who you saw her 6 weeks in the hospital. 2 weeks ago, she started to have progressive weakness and paresthesias in the distal portions of her both lower extremities. CSF had been done and revealed no cells with an elevated protein level. You diagnosed her with an acquired demyelinating polyradiculoneuropathy, treated and responded to intravenous immunoglobulin and a diagnosis of Guillain-Barre syndrome on discharge. She improved clinically after discharge 4 weeks ago, but not fully. In the last 2 weeks she has an increase in her paresthesias and weakness in her lower legs. When you examined her today, she has a new mild weakness in her upper extremities and areflexia throughout all limbs. Her EMG showed a multifocal disturbance of conduction velocity.

What is her diagnosis?

A. Recurrent Guillain-Barre syndrome
B. Chronic demyelinating polyradiculoneuropathy
C. Charcot-Marie-Tooth Disease 1
D. Adult form of metachromatic leukodystrophy

Correct Answer is: B

Guillain-Barre is the acute form of acquired demyelinating polyradiculoneuropathy and the chronic inflammatory demyelinating polyradiculoneuropathy is the chronic form. In both forms, EMG and NCV findings show evidence of "patchy" or multifocal abnormalities in conduction velocity and elevated spinal fluid protein.

Mandatory diagnostic criteria are; 1) progressive or relapsing motor and sensory dysfunction of more than one limb, developing over a minimum of 8 weeks and 2) areflexia or hyporeflexia usually affecting all limbs.

Recurrent Guillain-Barre syndrome is rare and is estimated to occur in only 1–3% of the cases.

Charcot-Marie-Tooth 1 (CMT1), also referred to as hereditary motor and sensory neuropathy type I (HMSN1), is a demyelinating neuropathy that typically begins in the second decade of life and progresses gradually throughout the patient's life. The distal nerves in legs are affected first causing weakness and foot drop. A uniform slowing of conduction velocity characterizes CMT1.

Metachromatic leukodystrophy is an inherited disorder of myelin metabolism and is caused by a deficiency of the enzyme arylsulfatase A. In the childhood form segmental demyelination occurs in peripheral nerves and cell death in central oligodendroglia cells. The adult form accounts for about 20% of affected individuals and typically begins in the teenage years with psychiatric symptoms and eventually cognitive decline.

Suggested Reading

- Sung JY, Tani J, Park SB, Kiernan MC, Lin CSY. Early identification of 'acute onset chronic inflammatory demyelinating polyneuropathy. Brain. 2014;137(8):2155–63.

30. You are evaluating a 10-year-old girl in the hospital because of progressive weakness. 1 week ago, she started to complain of tingling and muscle cramping in her right foot and right lower leg. She became "clumsy" 2 days later and last night she was unable to walk up the stairs and she has to be carried. Today, she woke up and was unable to stand. On your examination, she had flaccid paralysis, impaired sensation and areflexia in her lower legs, and a left arm drift on arm extension and left-hand weakness. She has a history of "cold" 2 weeks ago.

What is the most likely diagnosis?

A. Myasthenia gravis
B. Acute demyelinating polyradiculoneuropathy
C. Polio secondary to immunization
D. Heavy metal neuropathy

Correct Answer is: B

Guillain-Barre syndrome (acute demyelinating polyradiculoneuropathy), is an acute monophasic demyelinating neuropathy. Majority of patients have an antecedent viral infection. An abnormal immune response generates a response targeting peripheral nerve antigens. Insidious sensory symptoms predate the onset of motor weakness.

Myasthenia gravis does not have sensory symptoms and the presentation is of generalized weakness.

Polio symptoms following immunization is rare but can occur. The poliovirus attacks the anterior horn cells exclusively and there are not sensory disturbances. In addition, the acellular polio vaccine is typically administered

as part of the DPT immunizations in younger childhood.

Heavy metal neuropathy is typically more gradual and acute presentations are associated with GI and systemic symptoms such as nausea, vomiting, renal failure or pneumonitis.

Suggested Reading

Yuki N, Hartung HP. Guillain-Barre syndrome. N Engl J Med. 2012;366(24):2294–304.

31. Which bacterial infection is most commonly associated with Guillain-Barre syndrome?
    A. Staphylococcus aureus
    B. Streptococcus pneumoniae
    C. Enterococci
    D. Campylobacter jejuni
    E. Listeria monocytogenes

Correct Answer is: D
Majority of Guillain-Barre syndrome (GBS) patients have a predated infection, surgery, or vaccination within the month prior to the onset of symptoms.

Campylobacter jejuni is the most common bacterial infection associated with GBS. Estimates vary, with C. jejuni found in 17–42% of patients with GBS. It is specifically associated with the axonal variant, acute motor axonal neuropathy (AMAN), with C. jejuni infections evident in up to 76% of such patients.

Mycoplasma pneumonia is often seen in children with GBS. GBS has also been linked to Hemophilus influenzae. Viral infections associated with GBS include cytomegalovirus, Epstein-Barr virus, varicella zoster, hepatitis A, hepatitis B, and HIV.

Isolated cases have been associated with vaccinations (e.g. influenza, tetanus, diphtheria, rabies, and oral polio) and drugs (e.g. heroin, streptokinase). The risk of GBS with influenza vaccination is approximately 1:1,000,000.

Suggested Reading

Bosch EP, Smith BE. Disorders of peripheral nerves. In: Bradley WG, Daroff RB, Fenichel GM, jankovic J, editors. Neurology in clinical practice. 4th ed. Elsevier, Inc.; 2004. p. 2299–401.

32. You are seeing a 14-year-old girl in the hospital, who developed headache, fever, visual blurring, trouble walking, and paresthesias of her limbs 2 days ago after she had a mild upper respiratory tract infection 2 weeks ago. Her MRI is shown below. On examination, she has bilateral papillitis, brisk reflexes with some limb ataxia, and up-going toes. She is confused and febrile. CSF shows a mild lymphocytic pleocytosis and negative oligoclonal banding.
    How is this related to multiple sclerosis?
    A. It appears to be a separate neuroimmunologic disorder
    B. It usually transitions into multiple sclerosis
    C. It never transitions into multiple sclerosis
    D. It is the pediatric equivalent of multiple sclerosis
    E. It is the same as multiple sclerosis

Correct Answer is: A
The clinical and radiological presentation is most consistent with acute disseminated encephalomyelitis (ADEM). ADEM is usually a monophasic syndrome usually predated by an infection or vaccination. It is a multifocal demyelinating syndrome with large lesions that can be peripheral and may involve the basal ganglia. CSF may show a pleocytosis, but usually does not show oligoclonal bands. Patients are often febrile and encephalopathic. It may leave residual deficits.

First-line treatment for ADEM is intravenous methylprednisolone. All treatment recommendations are anecdotal.

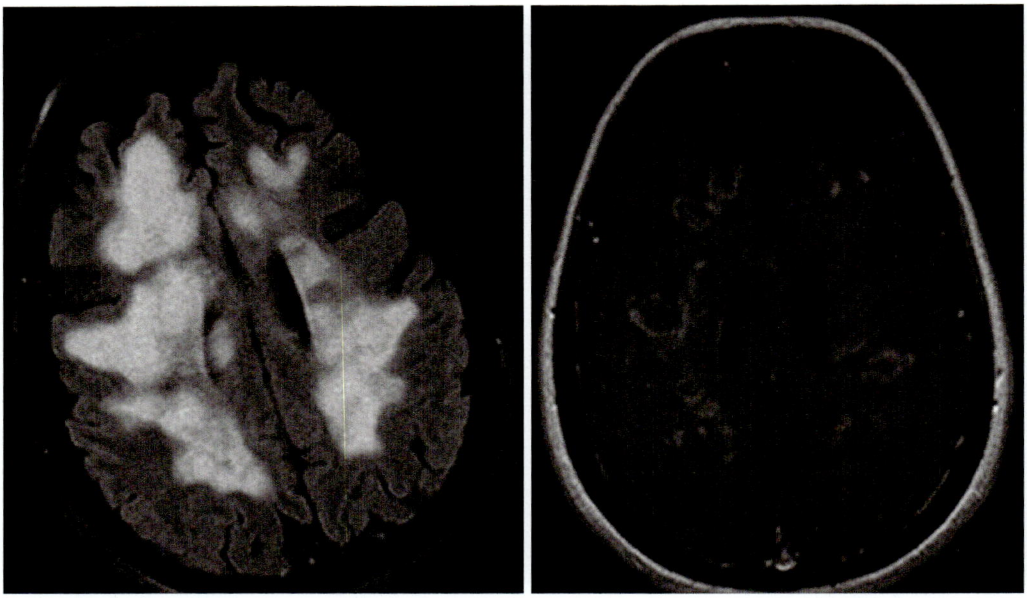

Figs. 5.20 and 5.21 ADEM on MRI. MRI showing white matter changes in (ADEM) disease. American Academy of Neurology Institute, produced by permission

Treatment consists of initial intravenous methylprednisolone and if this fails, trial of plasmapheresis. There is no indication for antibacterial or antiviral agents.

Suggested Reading

Tenembaum 5, Chitnis T, Nessj, et al. ADEM. Neurology. 2007; 68:523–536.

33. You are seeing a 14-year-old girl with a history of headache, altered mental status, inability to move her legs, and urinary incontinence. She had fever and cough 1 week ago. When you examined her, she was confused, had no meningeal signs, and had a flaccid paraplegia with areflexia and sensory loss below her waist. You ordered CSF analysis which shows 40 WBCs/mm3 (normal up to 5 lymphocytes/mm3) with lymphocytic predominance, a protein level of 70 mg/dl (normal up to 45 mg/dl) with normal glucose, and high immunoglobulin G index. MRI of the brain shows symmetric subcortical white matter lesions, and MRI of the spine shows an expanding intramedullary lesion between T5 and T10 with gadolinium enhancement.

What is the most likely diagnosis?

A. Multiple sclerosis
B. Acute disseminated encephalomyelitis
C. Neuromyelitis optica
D. Idiopathic transverse myelitis
E. Bacterial meningitis

Correct Answer is: B

The clinical presentation of an acute neurologic disorder followed a recent febrile illness is indicative of an inflammatory myelopathy and encephalopathy. At presentation, the illness was monophasic, with symmetric involvement of cerebral white matter and simultaneous spinal cord involvement.

CSF findings support an inflammatory disorder. The most likely explanation for her clinical picture is acute disseminated encephalomyelitis (ADEM).

ADEM is an inflammatory demyelinating disorder of childhood in which there is a monophasic immunologic reaction to a viral illness. Patients have an encephalopathy, with clear white matter changes on MRI and inflammatory markers in the CSF. Occasionally, the spinal cord is also affected with features of a transverse myelitis, in which the lesion affects more than three segments of the spinal cord. The treatment is intravenous steroids in high doses.

Encephalopathy is not a feature of neuromyelitis optica; the patient may have some white matter lesions, but in contrast to ADEM, they are not symmetric or confluent.

Multiple sclerosis is an inflammatory demyelinating disorder that presents with a relapsing and remitting or a progressive course. When it affects the spinal cord, the lesions are usually in short segments, not like in this case. Acute encephalopathy is not common in multiple sclerosis.

The diagnosis of idiopathic transverse myelitis is made when the patient has a transverse myelitis with no other explanation, and usually without other features, which is not the case here.

The clinical, imaging, and CSF findings do not correlate with bacterial meningitis.

34. Which of the following would be a suspected diagnosis in the study shown below?
   - A. Amyotrophic lateral sclerosis (ALS)
   - B. Chronic Inflammatory Demyelinating Polyneuropathy (CIDP)
   - C. Brachial plexus injury

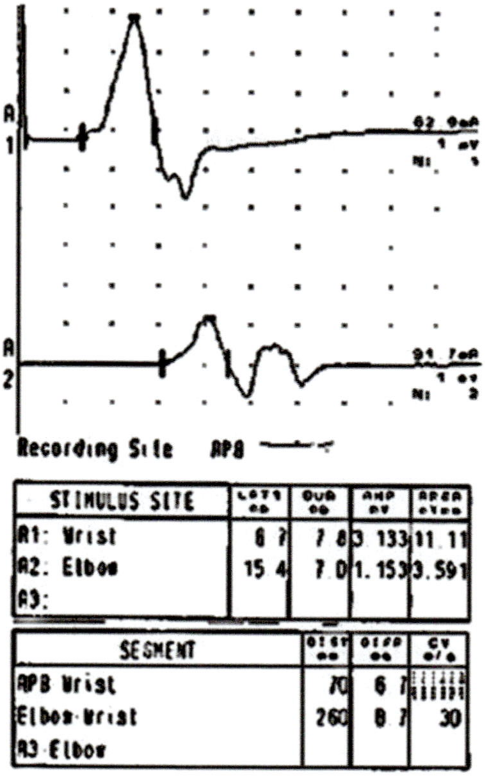

Fig. 5.22 EMG showing findings of (CIDP). MRI showing white matter changes in ADEM disorder. By permission from J Phys Ther Sci. 2013 Oct; 25(10)

Correct Answer is: B

The EMG shows Conduction block, prolonged distal latencies, temporal dispersion of compound muscle action potential, and slowed conduction have shown on the EMG. This is consistent with Chronic Inflammatory Demyelinating Polyneuropathy (CIDP).

Chronic inflammatory demyelinating polyradiculoneuropathy usually starts insidiously and evolves in either in a slowly progressive (<60%) or relapsing process, with some level of recovery between recurrences. Presenting symptoms include motor weakness (most common), and some have sensory and other symptoms such as autonomic complaints.

Most literature agrees on a minimum duration of 8 weeks to diagnose CIDP.80% of CIDP patients have elevated protein in the CSF, and EMG is used to determine the presence of demyelinating disease.

35. Acute disseminated encephalomyelitis (ADEM) differs from multiple sclerosis (MS) in that:
   A. There is a lack of oligoclonal bands in the cerebrospinal fluid of patients with ADEM Cerebrospinal fluid immunoglobulin levels are typically normal in ADEM
   B. Episodes of ADEM do not usually recur
   C. The development of ADEM has been linked to recent vaccination
   D. All of the above

Correct Answer is: D
ADEM is an acute, monophasic, demyelinating process, often predated by recent viral infections or vaccinations. It manifests as perivascular inflammation, edema, and demyelination of the CNS, with the rapid onset of focal or multifocal neurologic deficits.

The abrupt onset of simultaneous bilateral optic neuritis, impaired consciousness, meningismus, loss of deep tendon reflexes with intact abdominal reflexes and a positive Babinski sign, elevated temperature, seizures, and limb pain are the characteristic symptoms. Symptoms may be preceded by a prodromal of fever, malaise, and myalgias for several days.

ADEM differs from MS in that:

- **Patients recover more rapidly from ADEM, in some cases within days.**
- **Recovery is more complete from ADEM, with total recovery in approximately 50–70% of patients.**
- **In contrast to MS, follow-up MRI in several weeks demonstrates at least partial resolution of ADEM lesions, without the formation of new lesions.**
- **Episodes of ADEM do not usually recur.**
- **There is a lack of oligoclonal bands in the cerebrospinal fluid of patients with ADEM.**
- **Cerebrospinal fluid immunoglobulin levels are typically normal in ADEM.**
- **The development of ADEM has been linked to recent vaccination and a variety of infections.**
- **ADEM may be treated with steroids, immunomodulatory medications, and plasmapheresis.**

Suggested Reading

- Olek MJ, Dawson MJ. Multiple sclerosis and other inflammatory demyelinating diseases of the central nervous system. In: Bradley WG, Daroff RB, Fenichel GM, Jankovic J, editors. Neurology in clinical practice. 4th ed. Elsevier, Inc.; 2004. p. 1631–64.

36. You are seeing a 6-year-old boy presents with confusion and left sided weakness. On exam he has hyperreflexia on the left side and the patient being difficult to arouse. Brain MRI showed diffuse white matter lesions.
   What is the next step in evaluation and management?
   A. Lumbar puncture
   B. Methylprednisolone 20 mg/kg/d for 5 days
   C. IVIG 2 g/kg spread out between 2–5 days
   D. MRI of the cervical and thoracic spine
   E. Brain Biopsy

Correct Answer is: A
The clinical and radiological picture is most consistent with a diagnosis of acute disseminated encephalomyelitis. An infectious cause should be ruled out first so a lumbar puncture should be done to exclude this etiology. Cervical and thoracic spine MRI can also be done, but lumbar puncture should be performed first. If no infectious etiology is noted, treatment with IV methylprednisolone should be started. IVIG is considered a second line therapy.

Suggested Reading

- Chitnis T. Pediatric demyelinating disease. Continuum (Minneap Minn). 2013;19(4 Multiple Sclerosis):1023–45.

Developmental Disorders

Y. M. Awaad, *Absolute Pediatric Neurology*, https://doi.org/10.1007/978-3-319-78801-2_6

6

1. An 8 year old Duchenne Muscular Dystrophy boy in the office for a follow up visit with his family. The family showed up their concern that the child is having difficulty with academics in the 3rd grade. His difficulty is in all subjects. The family would like to know whether there can be cognitive involvement in a child with DMD.

What will be your response?

A. Intellectual disability is common in all children with DMD
B. Cognitive involvement is common in DMD
C. DMD children do not present with Attention Deficit Hyperactivity Disorder
D. The mean IQ in children with DMD is 60
E. Delayed language development is uncommon

Correct Answer is: B

Cognitive involvement is common in DMD. 30% DMD patients have intellectual disability. Eighty five is the average patient's IQ, one standard deviation below the mean. Performance IQ is less affected than Verbal IQ, and delayed language development is common.

The prevalence of comorbid neurodevelopmental /psychiatric disorders is more prevalent in DMD: 10–15% having attention deficit hyperactivity disorder, 3–6% having Autism spectrum Disorder, and 5% having obsessive compulsive disorder.

Suggested Reading

- Muscle disease. Continuum. 2013;19(6).

2. A 16-year-old male has been evaluated by you. He has been receiving special education services throughout his school years, currently maintained in a self-contained classroom. You reviewed his school records, psychological testing performed 3 years ago, his full scale IQ was 62. A Vineland Adaptive Behavioral Scales-II (VABS-II) found "Moderately Low" scores for most domains. On examination, head circumference at the 10th percentile, and mild speech and motor dyspraxia. Deep tendon reflexes are 3+ and symmetric, and he is mildly hypotonic throughout. The patient is conversant, and describes to you his favorite sport show. There are no abnormal movements noted.

In addition to the underlying neurological diagnoses, what is the most appropriate DSM-5 diagnosis?

A. Autism Spectrum Disorder
B. Mental Retardation-Mild
C. Intellectual Disability-Mild
D. Childhood-onset fluency disorder
E. Specific Learning Disorder

Correct Answer is: C

As a result of federal statute 111–256 ("Rosa's Law"), "intellectual disability" has replaced "mental retardation" in the DSM-5. In addition, the DSM-5 has emphasized the need to demonstrate deficient adaptive skills rather than only IQ when diagnosing intellectual disability.

Suggested Reading

- Greenspan S, Woods GW. Intellectual disability as a disorder of reasoning and judgement: the gradual move away from intelligence quotient-ceilings. Curr Opin Psychiatry. 2014;27(2):110–6. ► https://doi.org/10.1097/YCO.0000000000000037.
- Harris JC: New terminology for mental retardation in DSM-5 and ICD-11. Curr Opin Psychiatry. 2013;26:260–62. ► https://doi.org/10.1097/YCO.0b013e32835fd6fb.
- Papazoglou A, Jacobson LA, McCabe M, Kaufmann W, Zabel TA. To ID or not to ID? Changes in classification rates of

intellectual disability Using DSM-5. Intellect Dev Disabil. 2014;52(3):165–74. ▶ https://doi.org/10.1352/1934-9556-52.3.165.
- Public Law. 111–256, §2(b) (2), 5 Oct 2010, 124 Stat. 2643 (Rosa's Law).

3. Which of the following syndromes are typically associated with an intellectual disability?
   A. Fragile X syndrome
   B. Rett Syndrome
   C. de Morsier's syndrome
   D. Treacher Collins Syndrome

Correct Answer is: A, B, and C
Fragile X is the leading inherited cause of intellectual disability in boys. Rett syndrome is a common X-linked cause of syndromic intellectual disability. Intellectual disability is a common finding in de Morsier's syndrome (septo-optic dysplasia) and can occur in 50% of the patients.

Treacher Collins Syndrome is a syndrome involving the development of the facial bones. Those affected have normal intelligence.

Suggested Reading

- Mefford, H. et al. Genomics, intellectual disability, and autism. N Engl J Med. 2012;366:733–43.
- Signorini et al. Septo-optic dysplasia in childhood: the neurological, cognitive and neuro-ophthalmological perspective. Dev Med Child Neurol. 2012;54(11):1018–24. ▶ https://doi.org/10.1111/j.1469-8749.2012.04404.x. Epub 2012 Aug 27.
- Treacher Collins syndrome. ▶ http://ghr.nlm.nih.gov/condition/treacher-collins-syndrome.

4. A 10-year-old female was evaluated in your office with a previous diagnosis of Autism Spectrum Disorder-Moderate/Severe (under DSM-IV, Pervasive Developmental Disorder-Autistic Disorder) associated with no expressive language and impaired receptive language abilities, intellectual disability, and epilepsy, with focal onset seizures with evolution to bilateral convulsive seizures. Her mother mentioned that the child has occasional episodes of sudden and explosive aggression associated with an identifiable antecedent, such as transitioning away from a preferred activity. Overall, the patient has displayed neurodevelopmental regression. In spite of receiving lamotrigine, her seizures occurring more than once monthly. She was on Valproic acid 5 years ago but she had elevations in liver enzymes and she had to stop of the medication. On examination, she has ataxia and occasional myoclonic movements.
   Which of the following tests is most likely to provide a definitive biological diagnosis?
   A. Neuronal Ceroid Lipofuscinosis (NCL) testing
   B. Random lactate level
   C. Electromyography and nerve conduction velocities
   D. Mitochondrial genome sequencing, deletion detection, and heteroplasmy analysis, and exome DNA sequencing of nuclear mitochondrial genes
   E. Comparative Genomic Hybridization Microarray analysis
   F. Karyotype with molecular Fragile X analysis

Correct Answer is: C
The clinical presentation indicates a mitochondrial disorder. Mitochondrial disorders can presented with non-mitochondrial disorders symptoms and signs. The history of autism, developmental regression, intellectual disability, intractable epilepsy, valproate liver toxic-

ity associated with myoclonus and ataxia is highly suggestive of a mitochondrial disorder involving pathological gene variations of POLG.

Classically, mitochondrial phenotypes can include various combinations of neurodevelopmental delay or regression, seizures/epilepsy, ptosis/external ophthalmoplegia, hearing loss, cardiomyopathy or conduction defects, hepatopathy, myopathy, neuropathy, movement disorder/ataxia, and/or progressive optic atrophy or retinitis pigmentosa. It is difficult to diagnosis a mitochondrial disorder, also neuroimaging, laboratory and tissue biochemical studies often are non-diagnostic. However, the identification of mitochondrial disorders has advanced along with the growth in detection of mitochondrial regulatory genes, and the growing availability of comparative genomic hybridization microarray analysis, targeted DNA exome sequencing and enzymology.

6

Suggested Reading

- Cohen BH, Chinnery PF, Copeland WC. POLG-related disorders. In: Pagon RA, Adam MP, Ardinger HH, et al. editors. GeneReviews [Internet]; Seattle: University of Washington, Seattle; 1993–2014. Initial Posting: March 16, 2010; Last Update: Oct 11, 2012.
- Cohen BH, Naviaux RK. The clinical diagnosis of POLG disease and other mitochondrial DNA depletion disorders. Methods 2010;51:364–73.
- Legido A, Jethva R, Goldenthal MJ. Mitochondrial dysfunction in autism. Semin Pediatr Neurol. 2013;20:163–75.
- Lu JT, Campeau PM, Lee BH. Genotype-phenotype correlation-Promiscuity in the era of next-generation sequencing. N Engl M Med. 2014;371:593–96.
- Parikh S, Goldstein A, Koenig MK, et al. Practice patterns of mitochondrial disease physicians in North America. Part 1: Diagnostic and clinical challenges. Mitochondriaon. 2014;14:26–33. ► https://doi.org/10.1016/j.mito.2013.07.116. Epub 2013 Jul 26.
- Srivastava S, Cohen JS, Vernon H, Barañano K, McClellan R, Jamal L, Naidu S, Fatemi A. Clinical Whole Exome Sequencing In Child Neurology Practice. Ann Neurol. 2014;76:473–83. ► https://doi.org/10.1002/ana.24251. [Epub 2014 Aug 30].

5. You were called to evaluate a 6-year-old boy with Autism who was admitted to the hospital for gait abnormality. His family reported that he has refused to walk for several days. He also is more irritable. He was eating his typical diet of French fries, hamburger patty and artificially flavored water. On examination, he is very thin. His gums start bleeding after you look into his mouth. Also he has bruising on lower legs and his buttocks. His left leg is tender to palpation. CBC was ordered which showed anemia. An XRAY of his lower legs reveal ground glass osteopenia. **What is the most likely etiology for the above symptoms?**
   A. Lyme disease
   B. Vitamin C deficiency
   C. Celiac disease
   D. Lead poisoning
   E. Non accidental trauma

Correct Answer is: B

This a clinical presentation of scurvy. It is an ancient disease that has become more common in developmentally delayed children with restricted diets. Nowadays Scurvy is usually found among the elderly, the poor, alcoholics, and those restricted to

macrobiotic diets or other diets that contain < 10 mg/day of vitamin C. Clinical presentations of scurvy are small hemorrhages, abnormal mitochondrial metabolism, and abnormal collagen synthesis and may manifest as bleeding gums and hemarthroses, arthralgias, malaise, and weakness.

In reviewing the literatures, 23 case reports of scurvy in children with behaviorally restricted diets, including 2 autistic children and another with an unspecified behavioral problem, 1 with trisomy 21, 1 with static encephalopathy after pertussis-associated encephalitis, 2 with cerebral palsy, 4 with mental retardation, and 5 with global developmental delay; 7 otherwise reportedly normal children, including 1 morbidly obese teenager and another with a pathologic grief reaction, had scurvy in association with unusual diets and isolated food-avoidant behaviors.

Suggested Reading

- Noble, JM, et al. Scurvy and rickets masked by chronic neurologic illness: revisiting psychologic malnutrition. Pediatrics. 2007;119(3):e783–90.

6. Which medication from the list below has been approved by the FDA to treat an autistic child having "irritability"?
   A. Aripriprazole
   B. Clonidine
   C. Quetiapine
   D. Methylphenidate
   E. Oxcarbazepine

Correct Answer is: A

In two double blind, placebo controlled studies, Aripiprazole was found to be efficacious, safe and well tolerated in long-term extension studies. However, there are many reports indicating poorer responses in the management of aggression, hyperactivity, impulsivity, and self-injurious behaviors. Risperidone is the only other neuroleptic specifically FDA approved for use in autism spectrum disorders.

The other medications can be useful in the treatment of ASD, but none have been FDA approved.

It is important to determine if there is a biological cause or contributor to the adverse behavior before using medications for maladaptive behaviors in ASD children. Functional behavior analysis (FBA) has to be done to determine if there is an identifiable functional cause maintaining maladaptive behaviors (e.g. attention, escape from demands) or if the behavior is automatically maintained (i.e. biologically driven). The assessment and treatment team for those patients with maladaptive behavior patterns should include behavioral specialists who can perform FBAs. If a biological cause or contributor to maladaptive behavior is identified (for example, a tooth abscess), treatment should be directed to that source. If the behavior is determined to be mainly functional, behavioral management (i.e. applied behavior analysis and related methods) should be instituted and the response monitored. If behavioral interventions are not enough to control the behavior, medications can be added. Alpha-2 adrenergic agonists, psychostimulants, antiepileptic drugs, anxiolytics/antidepressants, and beta blockers can be useful in select patients with maladaptive behavior patterns, although not approved for ADS. Other medication classes or nutritional supplements may be indicated if specific ion channelopathy or mitochondrial disorder/dysfunction, have been identified as the cause.

6

Suggested Reading

- Marcus RN, Owen R, Manos G, et al. Safety and tolerability of aripiprazole for irritability in pediatric patients with autistic disorder: a 52-week, open-label, multicenter study. J Clin Psychiatry. 2011;72:1270–76.
- Minshawi NF, Hurwitz S, Morriss D, McDougle CJ. Multidisciplinary assessment and treatment of self-injurious behavior in autism spectrum disorder and intellectual disability: Integration of psychological and biological theory and approach. J Autism Dev Disord. 2014. [Epub ahead of print].
- Mintz M, Allesandri M, Curatolo P. Treatment approaches for autistic spectrum disorders. In: Tuchman R, Rapin I, editors. Autism: A neurological disorder of early brain development, International Child Neurology Association. London: Mac Keith Press; 2006. p. 281–307.

7. A 22 months child came with his mother because he is not walking yet. On your examination, he is babbling only vowel sounds, has a raking grasp, does not have a pincer grasp, and sits up but does not crawl. He cannot build a tower of two blocks. His brain MRI is normal.
Which genetic test has the highest diagnostic yield in a child with unexplained global developmental delay/intellectual disability?
   - A. MECP2
   - B. Karyotype
   - C. Current generation oligonucleotide-based chromosome microarray
   - D. Fragile X
   - E. FISH

Correct Answer is: C
The clinical presentation is for a global developmental delays. If the child is below the age of 6 has delays in at least two domains (speech/language, social, fine motor or gross motor) which are 2 SD below the mean in comparison to their age related peers, he/she will be considered having global developmental delays. It that Genetic testing is recommended to be done in this case. Microarray is the genetic test with the highest diagnostic yield in the child with unexplained GDD/ID. Karyotyping and FISH testing have a lower sensitivity. Fragile X may also be considered in a male with GDD/ID. MECP2 may also be considered in a female with GDD.

Suggested Reading

- Michelson DJ et al. Evidence report: genetic and metabolic testing on children with global developmental delays: Report of the Quality Standards Subcommittee of the American Academy of Neurology and the Practice Committee of the Child Neurology Society. Neurology. 2011;77:1629–35.

8. Angelman syndrome (AS) is a neurodevelopmental disorder characterized by severe mental retardation, absent speech, ataxia, sociable affect, and dysmorphic facial features.
If genetic testing for the maternal deletion in the 15q11.2-q13 critical region was negative, what genetic test should be considered next?
   - A. FMR
   - B. UBE3A
   - C. ARX
   - D. LIS
   - E. TSC

Correct Answer is: B
Angelman syndrome is a neurodevelopmental disorder characterized by mental retardation, movement or balance disorder, typical abnormal behaviors, and severe limitations in speech and language. Most cases are caused

by absence of a maternal contribution to the imprinted region on chromosome 15q11-q13. Approximately 70% of AS cases result from de novo maternal deletions involving chromosome 15q11.2-q13; approximately 2% result from paternal uniparental disomy of 15q11.2-q13; and 2 to 3% result from imprinting defects. A subset of the remaining 25% is caused by mutations in the gene encoding the ubiquitin-protein ligase E3A gene (UBE3A). Several patients with a clinical diagnosis of Angelman-like syndrome have been reported with mutations in the MECP2 gene.

Suggested Reading

- ▶ www.omim.org/entry105830.

9. You have admitted your 6-year-old patient with Autism to the hospital due to gait abnormality. His parents state that he has refused to walk for several days. He also is more irritable. His parents state that he has not been eating very much. In fact, his parents state for the past several months his food aversion has worsened; he only eats chicken nuggets and drinks only water. On examination you note he is very thin. His gums start bleeding after you look into his mouth. You also note bruising on lower legs and his buttocks. His right leg is tender to palpation. You order a CBC which revealed anemia. A BMP was negative. An XRAY of his lower legs reveal ground glass osteopenia.

   A deficiency in which Vitamin should be considered in this child with restricted intake of foods?

   A. Vitamin A
   B. Vitamin B
   C. Vitamin C
   D. Vitamin D
   E. Vitamin E

Correct Answer is: C

This a clinical presentation of scurvy. It is an ancient disease that has become more common in developmentally delayed children with restricted diets. Nowadays Scurvy is usually found among the elderly, the poor, alcoholics, and those restricted to macrobiotic diets or other diets that contain < 10 mg/day of vitamin C. Clinical presentations of scurvy are small hemorrhages, abnormal mitochondrial metabolism, and abnormal collagen synthesis and may manifest as bleeding gums and hemarthroses, arthralgias, malaise, and weakness.

In reviewing the literatures, 23 case reports of scurvy in children with behaviorally restricted diets, including 2 autistic children and another with an unspecified behavioral problem, 1 with trisomy 21, 1 with static encephalopathy after pertussis-associated encephalitis, 2 with cerebral palsy, 4 with mental retardation, and 5 with global developmental delay; 7 otherwise reportedly normal children, including 1 morbidly obese teenager and another with a pathologic grief reaction, had scurvy in association with unusual diets and isolated food-avoidant behaviors.

Suggested Reading

- Noble, JM, et al. Scurvy and rickets masked by chronic neurologic illness: revisiting psychologic malnutrition. Pediatrics. 2007;119(3):e783–90.

10. Parents of a 7-year-old boy with Duchenne Muscular Dystrophy bring their child in for a follow up visit. They are concerned that their child is having difficulty with academics in the 2nd grade. He is having difficulty with all subjects. The teacher is refusing to recommend psychoeducational testing at this time because many children in her class are having difficulty

and he is not failing any subjects. The parents would like your opinion on whether there can be cognitive involvement in a child with DMD.

What would be the proper response?

A. Cognitive involvement is uncommon in DMD
B. All children with DMD have intellectual disability
C. Attention Deficit Hyperactivity Disorder is prevalent in DMD
D. The mean IQ in children with DMD is 100
E. Delayed language development is uncommon

6

Correct Answer is: C
Cognitive involvement is common in DMD. Of patients with DMD, 30% have intellectual disability. The average patient's IQ is 85, one standard deviation below the mean. Verbal IQ is more affected than performance IQ, and delayed language development is common. There is a prevalence of comorbid neurodevelopmental /psychiatric disorders is more prevalent in DMD: Attention deficit hyperactivity disorder is 10–15%, Autism spectrum Disorder 3–6%, and obsessive compulsive disorder is 5%.

Suggested Reading

- Muscle disease. Continuum. 2013;19(6).

11. An 18-year-old female came for her appointment, she mentioned that she is not pregnant, but she has a concern about her prescribed medications effect on the fetus if she got pregnant. She takes phenytoin for epilepsy. Her psychiatrist has prescribed Valproic acid but has added lithium for severe bipolar disorder. She also states that her dermatologist is considering treating her severe acne with isotretinoin. (Accutane).

Which medication does not increase the risk of intellectual disability in utero exposure?

A. Valproic acid
B. Phenytoin
C. Isotretinoin
D. Lithium
E. All of the medications increase the risk of intellectual disability in the fetus

Correct Answer is: D
Fetus exposure to Phenytoin can lead to the fetal hydantoin syndrome, which is consisting of facial dysmorphism, cleft lip and palate, cardiac defects, digital hypoplasia, and nail dysplasia. IQ points could be decreased by Phenytoin exposure. Neural tube defects, Autism and intellectual disability have been reported with Valproic acid exposure. Isotretinoin has been shown to cause microcephaly, hydrocephalus and intellectual disability. Lithium has been shown to cause Ebstein anomaly but not an intellectual disability.

Suggested Reading

- Boyle RJ. Effects of certain prenatal drugs on the fetus and newborn. Pediatr Rev. 2002;23:17–24.
- American Academy of Pediatrics Committee on Drugs. Use of Psychoactive Medication during Pregnancy and Possible Effects on the Fetus and Newborn. Pediatrics 2000;105(4):880–7.
- Meador KJ. Cognitive/behavioral teratogenetic effects of antiepileptic drugs. Epilepsy Behav. 2007;11(3): 292–302.

12. Epilepsy syndromes can present in infancy and childhood with co morbid intellectual disability. Genetic defects have been identified in several syndromes.

Which epilepsy syndrome-gene defect pair is incorrect?

A. Severe myoclonic epilepsy of childhood (SMEI) - SCN1A
B. X-linked West Syndrome – ARX
C. Rett syndrome variant with intractable epilepsy – CDKL5
D. Glut1 deficiency – SLC2A1
E. Early Infantile Epileptic Encephalopathy With Suppression-burst - MECP2

Correct Answer is: E

Many of distinct clinical syndromes of pediatric genetic epilepsy have been described and linked to specific gene defects. Phenotypes may include, in addition to epilepsy, variable degrees of intellectual disability, elements of autism spectrum disorders, other psychiatric disorders, and motor impairment.

Severe myoclonic epilepsy of infancy (SMEI) is characterized by early-onset generalized febrile seizures, followed by very frequent afebrile generalized tonic–clonic seizures (GTCS), myoclonic seizures, absences and focal seizures, with arrest of psychomotor development, intellectual disability and motor impairment. Encode Sodium channel subunits, in particular SCN1A, is the suspected gene in this case, which is mutated in 61–87% of SMEI.

West syndrome is a common severe infantile epileptic syndrome characterized by typical brief tonic spasms, a profoundly abnormal electroencephalography pattern called hypsarrhythmia, and intellectual disability. Early infantile epileptic encephalopathy with suppression-burst (EIEE) is the earliest infantile epileptic syndrome, often evolving to West syndrome. Mutations in the X chromosome genes ARX and CDKL5 are found in some X-linked West syndrome cases (ISSX1 and ISSX2). ARX (Aristaless-related homeobox) is a transcription factor involved in brain development. It is frequently mutated in a spectrum of X chromosome-linked phenotypes characterized by intellectual disability as their cardinal feature.

CDKL5 mutations are associated with West syndrome, intellectual disability, and ASD, and also with a Rett syndrome variant that is characterized by infantile spasms and intractable seizures occurring before the appearance of the typical features of Rett syndrome (Hanefeld variant).

Altered glucose transport to the brain due to mutations in the GLUT1 transporter gene SLC2A1 causes epilepsy of variable severity and comorbidities. Classic GLUT1 deficiency is associated with very low cerebrospinal fluid (CSF) glucose concentrations and causes a severe early-onset (<1 year of age) metabolic encephalopathy characterized by movement disorders, epilepsy, and mental retardation, typically associated with de novoSLC2A1 mutations.

Suggested Reading

- Pandolfo, M. Pediatric epilepsy genetics. Curr Opin Neurol. 2013;26(2):137–45.

13. A 15-month-old boy migrated with his family from Eastern Europe is evaluated for microcephaly and developmental delay. He has 2 other maternal siblings (with different fathers) who both have mild mental retardation, microcephaly, and delay in linguistic development, congenital heart defects and severe growth retardation. The mother was "vegetarian" as a child but currently does not practice any dietary restrictions. She barely graduated high school and has

difficulty remembering appointments and paying bills.

What is the likely explanation for this child's condition?

A. Maternal phenylketonuria
B. Infantile autism
C. Leigh's disease
D. Chromosome disorder
E. Urea cycle disorder

Correct Answer is: A
Phenylketonuria (PKU) is an autosomal recessive disorder of amino acid metabolism affecting approximately 1/5000–10,000 infants in North America. It is most often due to deficiency of the enzyme phenylalanine hydroxylase which causes the accumulation of harmful metabolites, including phenylketones. If untreated, PKU leads to mental retardation, seizures, psychoses, eczema and a distinctive "mousy" odor. Pregnant PKU women who are not following dietary restrictions are at risk of delivering infants with the effects of untreated maternal PKU and may also be at risk of developing neurologic symptoms themselves if they don't maintain lifelong dietary restrictions. Mental retardation, microcephaly, intrauterine growth retardation, and congenital heart defects are the characteristic features of maternal PKU syndrome. The risk for these defects is increased with maternal plasma phenylalanine levels > 20 mg/dL).

6

Suggested Reading

- Bouchlariotou S, Tsikouras P, Maroulis G. Undiagnosed maternal phenylketonuria: own clinical experience and literature review. J Matern Fetal Neonatal Med. 2009;22(10):943–8.

14. A 5-year-old-boy has been in preschool for 2 years. The teachers mentioned to the mother that he is slower compared to the rest of his classmates and that he may need an extra year of preschool. The family is wondering if he is ready for Kindergarten this coming school year. His physical and neurological exam are normal.

What is your next step in management?

A. EEG
B. Standardized neurocognitive testing
C. Head MRI
D. Observe
E. Atypical antipsychotic medication

Correct Answer is: B
A child with a history of developmental delay is at risk for learning disabilities or mental retardation. Mental retardation is defined as "significantly sub-average general intellectual functioning with an intelligence quotient score (IQ) of < 70, existing concurrently with deficits in adaptive behavior and manifested during the developmental period, which adversely affects a child's educational performance". Stanford Binet Intelligence Scales-Fifth Edition (SB5), Wechsler Intelligence Scales for children, Wechsler Individual Achievement tests and, Mullen scales of early learning and Wide Range Test for Achievement are the cognitive testing can be used for evaluation. Because the concurrent difficulties in adaptive behavior. The common questionnaires for an adaptive behavior include Vineland scales can identify these children at risk for these disorders and to guide the school, clinicians and families with regards to his educational needs in school. AAN guidelines for the assessment of the child with developmental delay might also include MRI and genetic testing.

Suggested Reading

American Psychiatric Association. Diagnostic and statistical manual of mental disorders, 4th ed. Washington DC; 1994.

15. A 5-year-old Caucasian boy in your office for evaluation of developmental delay. He was born at full-term after an unremarkable pregnancy but stayed in the regular nursery for 2 days secondary to problems with feeding and jaundice. He was 7 lbs. 8 oz. (25–50%ile) and his length was 22 in. (> 95%ile). On examination, he is tall and macrocephalic (both > 97th percentile) with mildly dysmorphic facial features, including a high, broad forehead, down-slanting palpebral fissures, and a pointed chin. His has an enlarged hands and feet. His neurologic examination is non-focal. There are no family history of similar affected cases.

Which genetic test is most likely to yield a positive result?

A. Chromosome microarray
B. FISH for chromosome 22q11 deletion
C. Karyotype
D. Methylation analysis of chromosome 15q
E. Nuclear receptor SET domain containing protein-1 (NSD1 testing)

Correct Answer is: E
Sotos syndrome (cerebral gigantism), is a genetic condition that affects 1: 10,000 to 1: 50,000 individuals. The syndrome is characterized by prenatal and postnatal overgrowth, macrocephaly, and characteristic facial features—specifically a high anterior hair line; frontotemporal hair sparsity, a long, thin face; frontal bossing; down slanting palpebral fissures; and a prominent mandible. Advanced bone age is common but is not a universal finding. Neurologic hallmarks include hypotonia and global developmental delay, with most affected adults exhibiting mild intellectual disability. Sotos syndrome can be caused by either intragenic truncating mutations or microdeletions that result in haplo insufficiency of the nuclear receptor binding SET domain protein 1 (NSD1), located on chromosome 5q35.3. Intragenic mutations account for more than 80% of cases in European-origin white patients, where's microdeletions occur with a higher incidence in the Japanese population. The majority of cases are sporadic, though autosomal dominant pedigrees have been reported.

Suggested Reading

Leventopoulos G, et al. A clinical study of Sotos syndrome patients with review of the literature. Pediatr Neurol. 2009;40:357–64.

16. A 5-year-old boy evaluated by you for language delay. The mother reported that he said his first words at 23 months, but his motor development was on target. He has trouble understanding instructions in his preschool class, but his mother reports that he is able to hear loud speech even when there is significant background noise, such as a birthday party.

What is the reason for his speech delay?

A. Mild language disorder
B. Sensorineural hearing loss
C. Conductive hearing loss
D. No delays, speech and hearing is within normal variations.

Correct answer is: C
Speech delay is the most common symptom of hearing impairment in young children. Normally majority

of children use their first words by 16 months and after 21 months, this is considered a delay. External or middle ear problems can cause conductive hearing impairment. The deficient in conductive hearing impairment is Loss of amplification is the deficient in conductive hearing impairment, and therefore these children are able to hear loud speech in a noisy background better than soft speech in a quiet background.

The history suggests a hearing disorder. If the hearing was tested and normal, formal testing would be required to diagnose a language disorder.

Children with sensorineural hearing impairment have difficulty discriminating speech in the presence of background noise.

6

Suggested Reading

Smith RJ, Shearer AE, Hildebrand MS, Van Camp G. 2014. Deafness and hereditary hearing loss overview.

17. Which of the following drugs was shown to decrease the IQ of children born to mothers taking anticonvulsant medication?
    A. Levetiracetam
    B. Phenobarbital
    C. Valproic acid
    D. Carbamazepine
    E. Primidone

Correct Answer is: C

In 2013 the FDA issued a warning regarding valproate sodium (valproic acid, and divalproex sodium), if was taken during pregnancy. The Neurodevelopmental Effects of Antiepileptic Drugs (NEAD) study, showed that children exposed to valproate products in utero had decreased IQs at age 6 years compared to children exposed to carbamazepine, lamotrigine, and phenytoin, by a mean of 8–11 points. The FDA stated that:

Valproate is contraindicated for the prevention of migraine headaches in the setting of pregnancy, labeled category X ("the risk of use in pregnant women clearly outweighs any possible benefit of the drug").

Valproate should only be prescribed if other medications are not effective or otherwise unacceptable when treating epilepsy or bipolar disorder. In these settings, the drug is considered category D ("the potential benefit of the drug in pregnant women may be acceptable despite its potential risks," with human data suggesting risk to the fetus). In women who are of childbearing age but not pregnant, valproate should not be taken unless essential, and if prescribed, should be used with birth control.

On the other hand, women having epilepsy who become pregnant while on valproate should not abruptly discontinue the medication, and they have to discuss the treatment plan with their physicians.

Suggested Reading

Meador KJ, et al. Fetal antiepileptic drug exposure and cognitive outcomes at age 6 years (NEAD study): a prospective observational study. Lancet Neurol. 2013;12(3):244–52.

18. A 15-year-old boy has a known history of intellectual disability with a family history (brother and two maternal cousins) with intellectual disability as well. On examination, he has an elongated face, with a high forehead and elongated jaw, and protuberant ears. His testes are enlarged.

Which statement is incorrect regarding the most likely diagnosis in this boy?

A. It is the most common inherited form of intellectual disability
B. Females may be affected, although to a lesser degree
C. It results from expansion of the CGG repeat in the familial intellectual disability 1 gene on chromosome X
D. A family history of intellectual disability may be present, but not necessarily
E. Severe intellectual disability is invariably present

Correct Answer is: E
Intellectual disability has too many causes. Fragile X syndrome is the most common inherited form of intellectual disability. There is an expansion of the CGG repeat in the familial intellectual disability 1 gene on chromosome X. The function of this gene is yet to be fully understood. Because this gene is on the X chromosome, and because random X inactivation (lyonization) occurs in females, females are less often and less severely affected. Clinical manifestations in males include an elongated face, with a high forehead and elongated jaw, and protuberant ears and enlarged testes. Intellectual disability will range from mild and subtle to severe. A family history of intellectual disability in males may be present. Other neurologic manifestations may occur in adults with a permutation.

Suggested Reading

Comprehensive review in clinical neurology: a multiple-choice question book for the Wards and Boards ©2011 Wolters Kluwer Health Lippincott Williams & Wilkins. All rights reserved.

19. Which of the following statements regarding acquired intellectual disability are incorrect?
    A. Congenital infections such as cytomegalovirus or rubella are associated with intellectual disability
    B. Intellectual disability has been associated with exposure to radiation during the first trimester
    C. In utero exposure to AEDs can lead to varying degrees of intellectual disability and other CNS abnormalities
    D. Maternal alcohol intake is a common cause of acquired intellectual disability
    E. In utero exposure to alcohol does not lead to abnormalities outside of the CNS

Correct Answer is: E
Fetus exposed alcohol in utero can have a congenital heart disease. There are a myriad of established or suspected exposures associated with intellectual disability. Congenital cytomegalovirus and rubella lead to intellectual disability with a variety of other manifestations such as congenital blindness and periventricular calcifications. Exposure to radiation during the first trimester of pregnancy have also been associated with intellectual disability. Malnutrition during the first few months of life can lead to reversible cognitive delay. Maternal intake of alcohol, antiepileptics, vitamin A, and thalidomide are also associated with various nervous system and systemic malformations as well as intellectual disability. Maternal alcohol intake is a common cause of acquired (non-genetic) intellectual disability. Other manifestations of fetal alcohol syndrome include behavioral problems such as hyperactivity, microcephaly, short palpebral fissure (a short distance between the inner and outer canthi of the

eyes), presence of epicanthal folds, and hypoplasia of the maxilla, micrognathia, and thin upper lip with flattened philtrum, and congenital heart disease.

20. A 15-year-old boy has significant schoolwork problems mainly in reading. Evaluation shows that he reads below the 10th percentile for his age, however his IQ is measured to be 100. **What is your most likely diagnosis?**
    - A. Specific learning disorder
    - B. Mild intellectual disability
    - C. ADHD
    - D. Vision problems
    - E. Social communication disorder

Correct Answer is: A
DSM-5 diagnosis of specific learning disorder combines the DSM-IV diagnoses of reading disorder, mathematics disorder, disorder of written expression, and learning disorder not otherwise specified.

Specific learning disorder in the DSM-5 is defined as "A neurodevelopmental disorder of biological origin manifested in learning difficulty and problems in acquiring academic skills markedly below age level and manifested in the early school years, lasting for at least 6 months; not attributed to intellectual disabilities, developmental disorders, or neurological or motor disorders".

You can then specify if it is either: With impairment in reading, with impairment in written expression, or with impairment in mathematics. Also, Mild, Moderate, or Severe.

6

Eating Disorders

Y. M. Awaad, *Absolute Pediatric Neurology*, https://doi.org/10.1007/978-3-319-78801-2_7

1. An 18-year-old woman is referred to her college's health counselor after a pharmacist detects several unusual prescriptions for laxatives purchased by the patient. Her body mass index had been in the range of 23–24 since adolescence (normal 18.5–24.9). The patient admits to an intense fear of being fat for years, wishing to be thinner. She reported trying not to eat, but then gets so hungry that several times a week she would binge for hours, would subsequently feel guilty, and would take 30–40 pills of laxatives at once.

What is the most likely diagnosis in this patient?

A. Bulimia nervosa
B. Anorexia nervosa, restricting type
C. Anorexia nervosa, binge eating/purging type
D. Eating disorder not otherwise specified
E. Impulse control disorder

7

Correct Answer is: A

Patients suffering from bulimia nervosa binge eat over a discrete period of time at least twice a week for 3 months, they lose over the extent of food intake during that time period, followed by compensatory behaviors to prevent weight gain such as excessive exercise, induction of emesis or misuse of laxatives, diuretics, or other medications. Treatment of bulimia nervosa involves Psychotherapy combined in some cases with SSRI is the treatment of choice in this case. Bulimia nervosa is commonly associated with borderline personality disorder as comorbidity.

In patients with eating disorder not otherwise specified, patients may avoid food, binge with or without purging or participating excessively in exercise, and partake in other methods of minimizing weight loss, but the patient's weight is maintained within the normal range, the episodes of binging occur less than twice per week for 3 months, and menstruation remains regular. The binge eating form of eating disorder not otherwise specified is the most common eating disorder, followed by bulimia and anorexia nervosa. Teenage years is peak onset of eating disorders, though they may begin at any age. Eating disorders are more common in females than in males, with a 3:1 ratio, however males are likely underdiagnosed. The pathophysiology relates to be both environmental and genetic factors; there is a 50–80% concordance rate among monozygotic twins. Comorbid mood, anxiety, and personality disorders are common among patients with eating disorders.

Suggested Reading

- Comprehensive review in clinical neurology: a multiple choice question book for the wards and boards ©2011 Wolters Kluwer Health Lippincott Williams & Wilkins. All rights reserved.

Epilepsy 1

Y. M. Awaad, *Absolute Pediatric Neurology*, https://doi.org/10.1007/978-3-319-78801-2_8

1. A 10-year-old boy is brought by his family because of frequent episodes of drooping of the right or left side of his mouth that last 1–3 min each. He is completely awake and alert during the episodes, but has difficulty talking. He said to you that I am embarrassed by them because "Spit drips out of the drooping side of my mouth." He had one nocturnal seizure 6 months ago, and no work up has been done. He has unremarkable history and physical exam. He is otherwise a healthy boy who does quite well in school.

   You decide to get an EEG. A tracing from it is below:

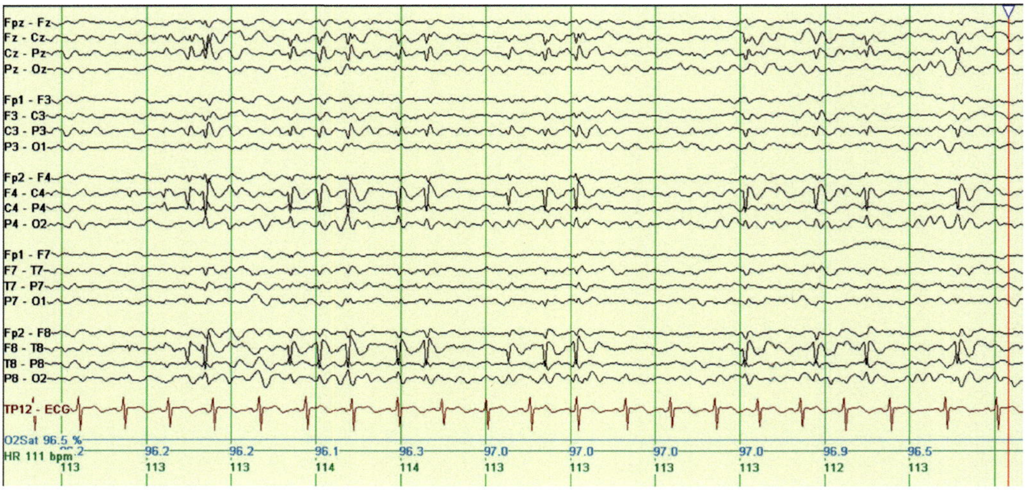

Fig. 8.1 EEG shows Centro-temporal spike. With a permission from ► ILAE.org, Diagnostic Manual, and ► EpilepsyDiagnosis.org

What are you going to tell the family?

A. He has a facial tic.
B. The seizure and the mouth drooping are unrelated.
C. He needs to have a video EEG to capture an episode.
D. He has a form of epilepsy that he is likely to outgrow.
E. He needs to take ethosuximide.

Correct Answer is: D

Benign Epilepsy with Centro-Temporal Spikes (BECTS- Benign Rolandic Epilepsy), it is very common in clinical practice, accounting for 13–23% of all cases of epilepsy during childhood. Patients are usually otherwise normal, and the most common seizure occurs shortly after going to sleep, with focal motor activity affecting the face and tongue, resulting in dysarthria or drooling. There is no loss of consciousness (simple partial seizure). EEG shows Centro-temporal spike, often with a surface dipole in which the spike is surface-negative in the Centro-temporal region, and surface-positive over the frontal region. It has a favorable prognosis, and seizures usually remit around puberty. However, atypical forms of BECTS are also recognized.

Suggested Reading

- Guerrini R, Pellacani S. Benign childhood focal epilepsies. Epilepsia. 2012;53 Suppl 4:9–18.
- Hughes JR. Benign epilepsy of childhood with centro-temporal spikes (BECTS): to treat or not to treat, that is the question. Epilepsy Behav. 2010;19(3):197–203.

2. A 7-year-old female recently stared to have spells for 5–10 s multiple times per day, both mother and teachers noted them, with behavioral inattention and activity arrest. No other seizures or spell have been reported. She is an excellent student, at or above grade level academically, and is otherwise medically well. A 10 s page from her outpatient EEG is shown.

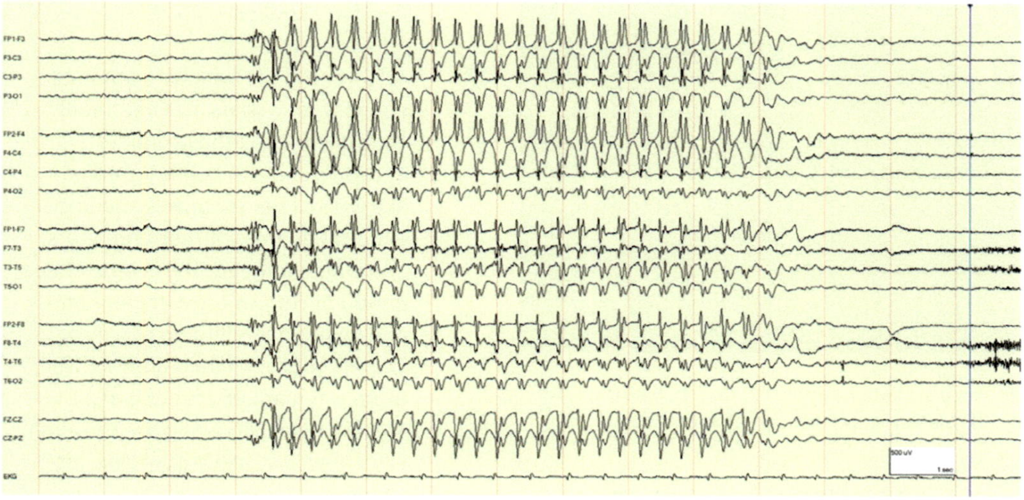

Fig. 8.2 With a permission from ▶ ILAE.org, Diagnostic Manual, and ▶ EpilepsyDiagnosis.org

What is your diagnosis?

A. Juvenile myoclonic epilepsy
B. Benign epilepsy with centrotemporal spikes
C. Localization-related epilepsy with complex partial seizures
D. Panayiotopoulos Syndrome
E. Childhood Absence Epilepsy

Correct Answer is: E
Childhood Absence Epilepsy (CAE) is very common in clinical practice. The peak age for presentation is 6–7 years. Seizures are usually frequent, have short duration with abrupt onset and resolution, and lack post-ictal confusion. The seizures are commonly provoked by hyperventilation, which is a useful maneuver for revealing the correct diagnosis during both the bedside exam and the EEG. Abundant focal inter-ictal EEG spikes are not expected, although fragmentary forms of the generalized spike-wave discharges may be seen, particularly during sleep.

Suggested Reading

Sadleir LG, Farrell K, Smith S, et al. Electroclinical features of absence seizures in childhood absence epilepsy. Neurology. 2006; 67:413–8.

3. A 6-month-old girl is brought to the ED for excessive fussiness and colicky behavior. On exam, she has repetitive clusters of stereotyped flexion movements of the trunk, associated with a cry. Her EEG shows hypsarrhythmia. A few flexion movements are captured and are associated with a generalized slow wave followed by an electrodecrement. She has several scattered hypo-pigmented spots on the trunk and extremities. A brain MRI scan is shown.

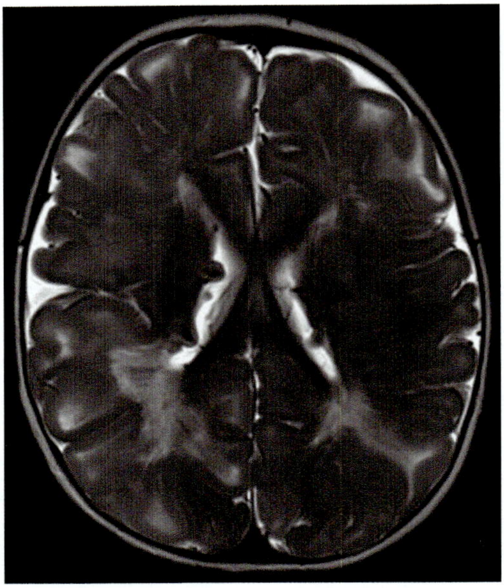

Fig. 8.3 With a permission from ► ILAE.org, Diagnostic Manual, and ► EpilepsyDiagnosis.org

What is the best treatment option?

A. Valproic acid
B. Felbamate
C. Ralfinamide
D. Pyridoxine
E. Vigabatrin

Correct Answer is: E

Vigabatrin (VGB) is a structural analogue of the inhibitory neurotransmitter gamma-aminobutyric acid (GABA) and irreversibly inhibits the GABA degradative enzyme GABA-transaminase (GABA-T), thus increasing brain levels of GABA. VGB is very effective against infantile spasms associated with tuberous sclerosis complex (TSC), and it is the first-choice drug of in this case based on many reports. One of VGB side effects is peripheral visual field defects (VFDs), which varies depending on age and degree of exposure to the medication. The prevalence in children is estimated at 15% and retinal defects in infants range from 15% to 31%. Cognitive, age-appropriate visual field testing is required at baseline and should be repeated at regular intervals in patients who are on long-term therapy.

Suggested Reading

- Hancock EC, Osborne JP, Edwards SW. Treatment of infantile spasms. Cochrane Database Syst Rev. 2008;8(4):CD001770.
- Willmore LJ, Abelson MB, Ben-Menachem E, Pellock JM, Shields WD. Vigabatrin: 2008 update. Epilepsia. 2009;50(2):163–73.

4. A 15-year-old female with absence epilepsy for 3 years, has been well controlled with ethosuximide. Recently, she fells quick, lightning-like jerks of her shoulders and upper extremities, in early morning hours and when fatigued. They come after a period of clumsiness with her hands and involuntary flinging of writing implements or kitchen utensils. Her exam is remarkable for BMI of 28. The interictal EEG is shown. The ictal EEG shows 10–16-Hz polyspike discharges.

Which of the following anticonvulsant medications is the best treatment option?

A. Carbamazepine
B. Levetiracetam
C. Phenytoin
D. Pregabalin
E. Valproic acid

Correct Answer is: B

Many anticonvulsants used in juvenile myoclonic epilepsy (JME). The primary agents are valproic acid, lamotrigine and levetiracetam. Carbamazepine, phenytoin, pregabalin, and oxcarbazepine are limited spectrum agents useful only in the adjunctive treatment of partial-onset seizures. Due to concerns regarding weight gain, hyperinsulinemia and an increased risk of hyper-androgenism, valproic acid is now commonly avoided in female patients. In males, all 3 medications are safe and used successfully. Levetiracetam is the only drug has FDA-approved indication for the adjunctive treatment of JME in patients 12 years and older.

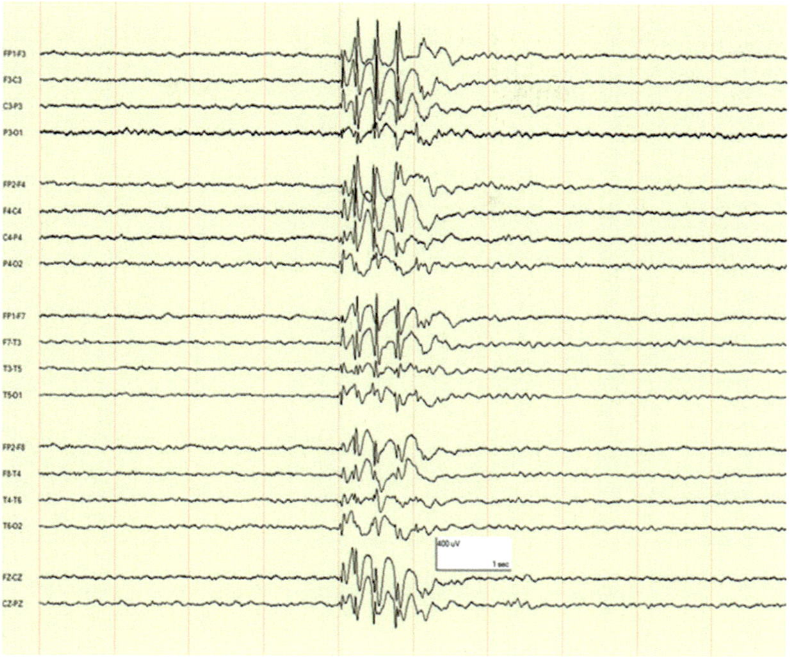

Fig. 8.4 With a permission from ► ILAE.org, Diagnostic Manual, and ► EpilepsyDiagnosis.org

Suggested Reading

- Welty TE. Juvenile myoclonic epilepsy: epidemiology, pathophysiology, and management. Paediatr Drugs. 2006; 8(5):303–10.
- Verrotti A, Manco R, di Marco G, Chiarelli F, Franzoni E. The treatment of juvenile myoclonic epilepsy. Expert Rev. Neurother. 2006;6(6):847–54.

5. A 3-year-old developmentally delayed boy has multiple paroxysmal events for few months. He was diagnosed with infantile spasms at 5 months of age, and had a complete responder to ACTH. He did not have any further seizures after he was weaned off until 6 months ago. Family reports nocturnal events involving whole-body stiffening, and while awake he has multiple brief periods of altered awareness with eyelid fluttering, eye rolling and head nodding. He also has quick jerking movements of his extremities. The scariest events are "falling seizures" during which he suddenly loses muscle tone and falls to the ground. He has broken a few teeth and sustained scalp contusions and lacerations which have required sutures. His EEG shows diffuse background slowing, as well as multifocal and generalized slow spike-wave discharges occurring at a frequency of 1.5–2.5 Hz.

What is the best treatment option at this time?

A. Phenobarbital
B. Carbamazepine
C. Oxcarbazepine
D. Topiramate
E. Felbamate

Correct Answer is: D

Lennox-Gastaut syndrome is refractory to medical treatment, but better seizure control has been achieved by the newer generation broad-spectrum medications. Topiramate and felbamate are good options, but felbamate is not a first-line medication because its side effects. Rufinamide and clobazam were recently approved for this condition. There are a number of effective non-pharmacological

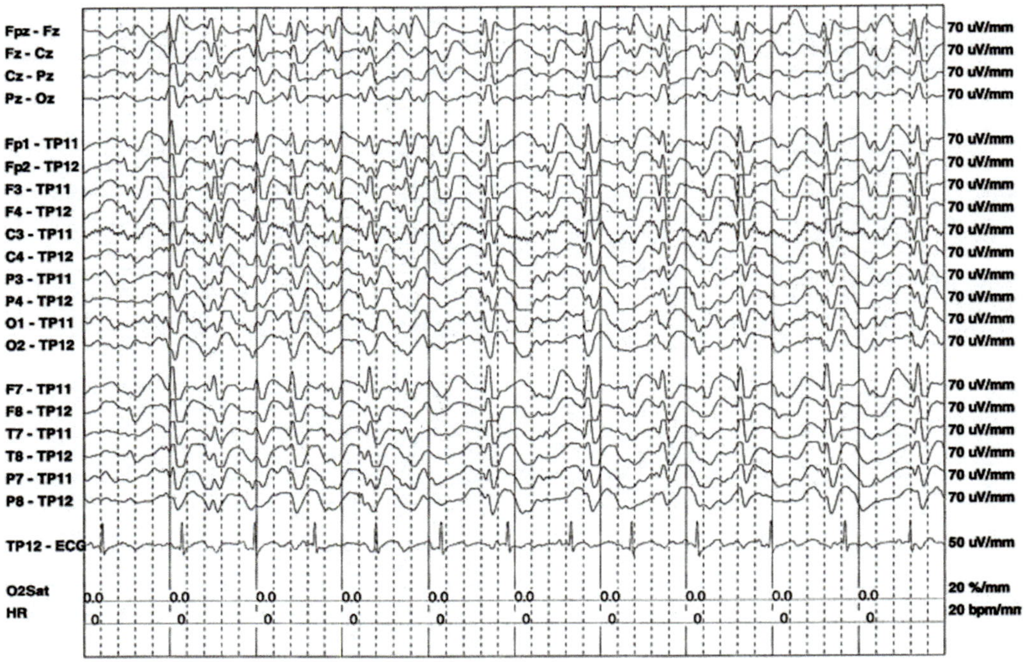

Fig. 8.5 Slow spike-wave IED typical of the Lennox-Gastaut syndrome. Also note the associated underlying background slowing, indicative of generalized cerebral dysfunction and an epileptic encephalopathy. Ipsilateral ear referential montage. (Figure courtesy of Jeffrey W. Britton, MD Electroencephalography (EEG): An Introductory Text and Atlas of Normal and Abnormal Findings in Adults, Children, and Infants ISBN: 978-0-9979756-0-4, Copyright c2016 by American Epilepsy Society, 135 S. LaSalle St., Suite 2850, Chicago, IL 60603)

options, including the ketogenic diet, VNS and corpus callosotomy. Finally, immunomodulation with IVIG or steroids can be helpful in some patients. In summary, most successful treatment strategies appear to involve combination pharmacological and non-pharmacological therapies which may provide complementary benefits.

Suggested Reading

- Arzimanoglou A, French J, Blume WT, Cross JH, Ernst JP, Feucht M, Genton P, Guerrini R, Kluger G, Pellock JM, Perucca E, Wheless JW. Lennox-Gastaut syndrome: a consensus approach on diagnosis, assessment, management, and trial methodology. Lancet Neurol. 2009; 8(1):82–93.

6. The family of an 8-year-old boy reports that their son is having a night events. They describe the event as a rhythmic jerking of the left side of the face, with drooling and dysarthria. The boy is fully alert and understand and following their instructions. He has a normal exam and doing well in school. His routine EEG is shown

What is the child's prognosis?

A. Controlled, but lifelong, epilepsy
B. Worsening myoclonus, ataxia, and dementia
C. Worsening myoclonus and ataxia, but without dementia
D. Disappearance of seizures and EEG abnormalities by mid-teens
E. Progressive aphasia

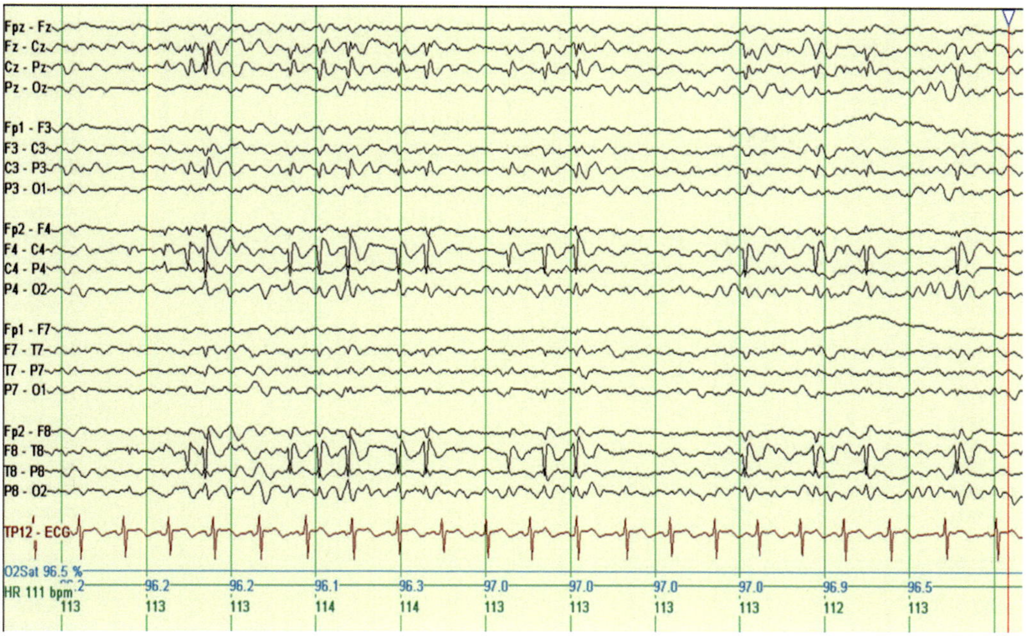

Fig. 8.6 With a permission from ► ILAE.org, Diagnostic Manual, and ► EpilepsyDiagnosis.org

Correct Answer is: D

Benign Rolandic Epilepsy (Benign Epilepsy with Centro-Temporal Spikes (BECTS) is a very common childhood seizure (13–23%). Children are normal, and the seizure occurs shortly after going to sleep. There is a focal motor activity affecting the face and tongue, resulting in dysarthria or drooling. There is no loss of consciousness. EEG shows Centro-temporal spike, often with a surface dipole in which the spike is surface-negative in the Centro-temporal region, and surface-positive over the frontal region. Prognosis is favorable, and seizures usually remit around puberty. Atypical forms of BECTS have been reported.

Suggested Reading

- Bouma PAD, Bovenkerk AC, Westendorp RGJ, Brouwer OF. The course of benign partial epilepsy of childhood with centrotemporal spikes: a meta-analysis. Neurology 1997.

7. A 5-year-old boy, who had a hypoxic ischemic encephalopathy complication at birth. He starts having generalized tonic-clonic seizures for 1 year. Recently, he starts having generalized tonic seizures at night, drops, and staring episodes during daytime. EEG is shown.

What is the most likely diagnosis?

A. Benign familial infantile seizures
B. Childhood absence epilepsy
C. Dravet syndrome
D. Lennox-Gastaut syndrome
E. West syndrome

Correct Answer is: D

EEG is characteristic of Lennox-Gastaut syndrome with slow sharp and slow wave complexes of 1.5–2 Hz. This is different than EEG with faster frequency seen in primary generalized epilepsy, like childhood or juvenile absence epilepsy. Also, the clinical scenario is consistent with Lennox-Gastaut syndrome. There are different

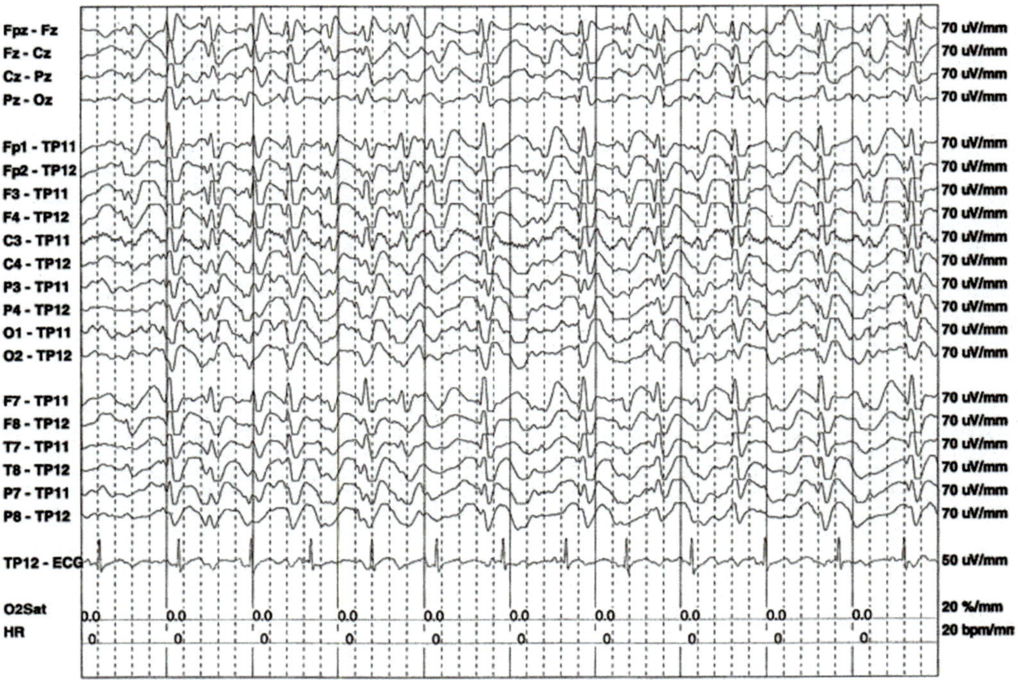

Fig. 8.7 Slow spike-wave IED typical of the Lennox-Gastaut syndrome. Also note the associated underlying background slowing, indicative of generalized cerebral dysfunction and an epileptic encephalopathy. Ipsilateral ear referential montage. Copyright 2013. Mayo Foundation for Medical Education and Research. All rights reserved. (Figure courtesy of Jeffrey W. Britton, MD Electroencephalography (EEG): An Introductory Text and Atlas of Normal and Abnormal Findings in Adults, Children, and Infants ISBN: 978-0-9979756-0-4, Copyright c2016 by American Epilepsy Society, 135 S. LaSalle St., Suite 2850, Chicago, IL 60603)

generalized seizure types (generalized tonic-clonic, generalized tonic and drop attacks, and probably atypical absence), and the EEG shows the characteristic diffuse slow spike-and-wave complexes (less than 2.5 Hz).

Suggested Reading

- VanStraten AF, Ng YT. Update on the management of Lennox-Gastaut syndrome. Pediatr Neurol 2012;47(3):153–61.
- Trevathan E. Infantile spasms in Lennox-Gastaut syndrome. J Child Neurol 2012;17(Suppl 2):2S9–22.

8. The mother of a 6-year-old boy rushed to her son room after she heard her son calling her after he went to sleep. She witnesses him having twitching of his left side of his face and he was drooling and his speech was not clear. Also, she noticed some twitching of his left hand. He is a healthy and excellent student. His EEG is shown.

What is the most likely diagnosis?

A. benign epilepsy with centrotemporal spikes (BECTS)
B. early onset benign childhood occipital epilepsy (Panayiotopoulos type)
C. epilepsy with myoclonic absences
D. late onset childhood occipital epilepsy (Gastaut type)
E. Lennox-Gastaut syndrome

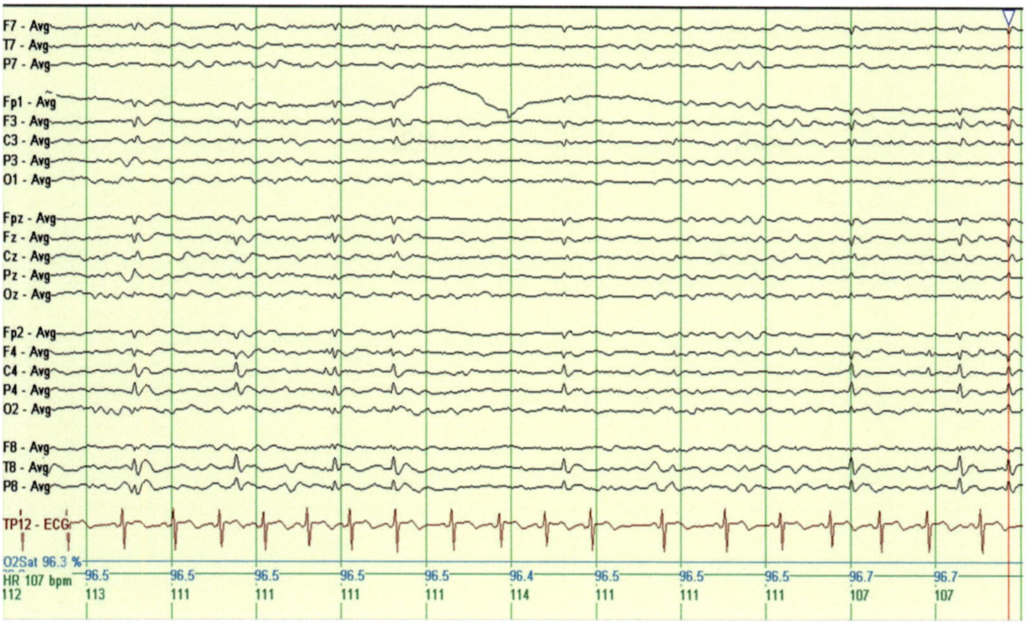

Fig. 8.8 With a permission from ► ILAE.org, Diagnostic Manual, and ► EpilepsyDiagnosis.org

Correct Answer is: A
The history and EEG are characteristic of benign childhood epilepsy with Centro temporal spikes (BECTS). The EEG shows central and temporal epileptiform discharges with a normal background (these may be bilateral, synchronous or asynchronous; often with horizontal dipole). This seizure is the most common partial epilepsy of childhood (2/3 of all idiopathic focal epilepsies in childhood). It occurs between 5 and 8 years of age. Usually, it is focal motor seizures, unilateral involving the face, the oropharyngeal muscles, and upper extremities. It occurs often during sleep; and less than 25% occurs during wakefulness. Treatment is not necessary because patients usually will have 1–2 seizures, and prognosis is excellent.

Suggested Reading

- Guerrini R, Pellacani S. Benign childhood focal epilepsies. Epilepsia 2012;53(Suppl 4):9–18.

9. A 6-year-old female wakes up after she went into her sleep. She vomited and was able to answer her family. Few minutes later she has forced eye deviation to the left but she was responsive. Then she closed her eyes, became unresponsive, and had a generalized convulsion. She then was postictal for few minutes. Her EEG is shown.
What is her most likely diagnosis?
A. benign familial infantile seizures
B. early-onset benign childhood occipital epilepsy (Panayiotopoulos type)
C. Landau-Kleffner syndrome
D. mesial temporal lobe epilepsy with hippocampal sclerosis
E. migrating partial seizures of infancy

Correct Answer is: B
EEG is classic for Panayiotopoulos type (early onset benign childhood occipital epilepsy). The EEG has occipital spikes, which can be either bilateral or unilateral.

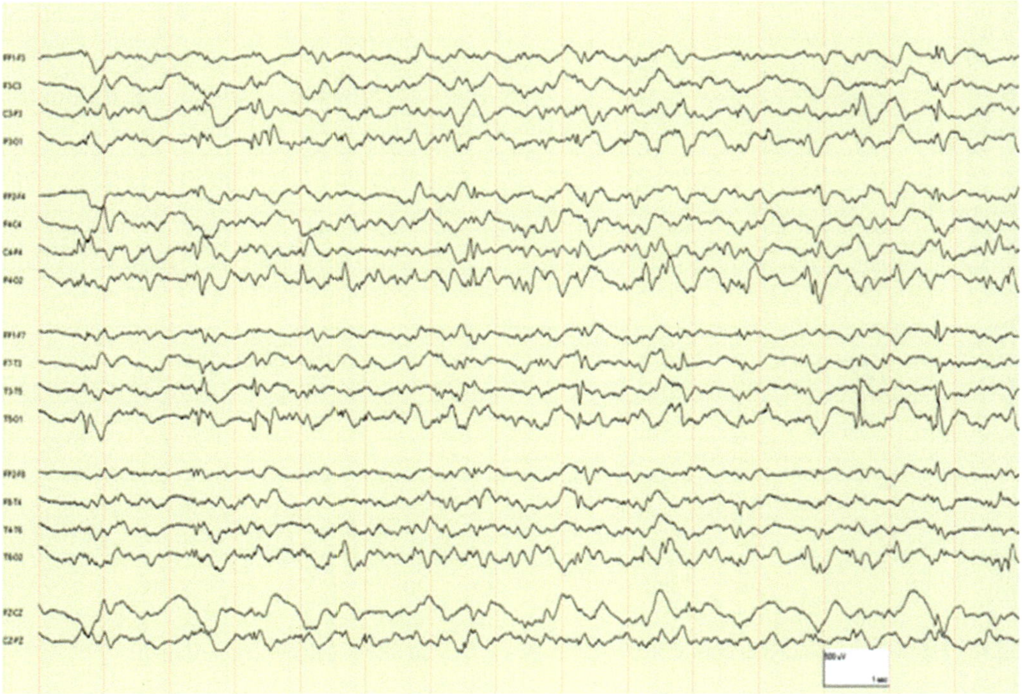

Fig. 8.9 With a permission from ► ILAE.org, Diagnostic Manual, and ► EpilepsyDiagnosis.org

The occipital spikes can be seen with eye closure, or with fixation and central vision are eliminated. The spikes are often reactive and decrease in frequency when the eyes are open. The clinical manifestations are autonomic and behavioral disturbances, vomiting, deviation of the eyes, and often impairment of consciousness that progresses to convulsions. Duration is usually long. It is 28% of all benign childhood partial seizures. Prognosis is excellent, it occurs as some single or infrequent seizures that subside within 1–2 years. Onset is between 2 and 12 years, with a median of 5 years.

Suggested Reading

- Panayiotopoulos CP. Benign childhood epileptic syndrome with occipital spikes: new classification proposed by the Internal League Against Epilepsy. J Child Neurol 2000;15(8):648–52.

10. A 5-year-old male with long events of vomiting, unresponsiveness, loss of tone, eye deviation, and face flushing. He has a normal development history and a normal. His interictal EEG shows a normal background and focal occipital sharp wave discharges which happened more during his sleep.

What is the most likely diagnosis?

A. Angelman syndrome
B. Doose syndrome
C. Landau-Kleffner syndrome
D. Lennox-Gastaut syndrome
E. Panayiotopoulos syndrome

Correct Answer is: E

This is a clinical presentation of Panayiotopoulos syndrome, a benign childhood seizure disorder with a good prognosis. Angelman syndrome is a genetic epilepsy with onset in the infantile period.

Doose syndrome, also known as epilepsy with myoclonic atonic seizures, with onset in the infantile period, is characterized by myoclonic, atonic, atypical absence, and bilateral convulsions. Landau-Kleffner syndrome is a childhood onset epileptic encephalopathy characterized by aphasia with continuous epileptiform discharges during sleep. Lennox-Gastaut syndrome is a severe epileptic encephalopathy with multiple seizure types, intellectual disability, and slow spike-and-wave on EEG.

Suggested Reading

- Ferrie C, Caraballo R, Covanis A, et al. Panayiotopoulos syndrome: a consensus view. Dev Med Child Neurol. 2006;48(3):236240.

11. A 7-month-old boy was diagnosed by his PCP with colic at age 5 months. He has spells of waist flexion and arms extension. They are brief, 1–2 s, and occur in clusters; mainly upon wakening from a nap, or during transitions from sleep to wake, or wake to sleep. The mother had uncomplicated pregnancy and he is a healthy child. His EEG is shown.

What is the most likely diagnosis?

A. benign familial infantile seizures
B. benign familial neonatal seizures
C. early myoclonic encephalopathy (EME)
D. migrating partial seizures of infancy
E. West syndrome

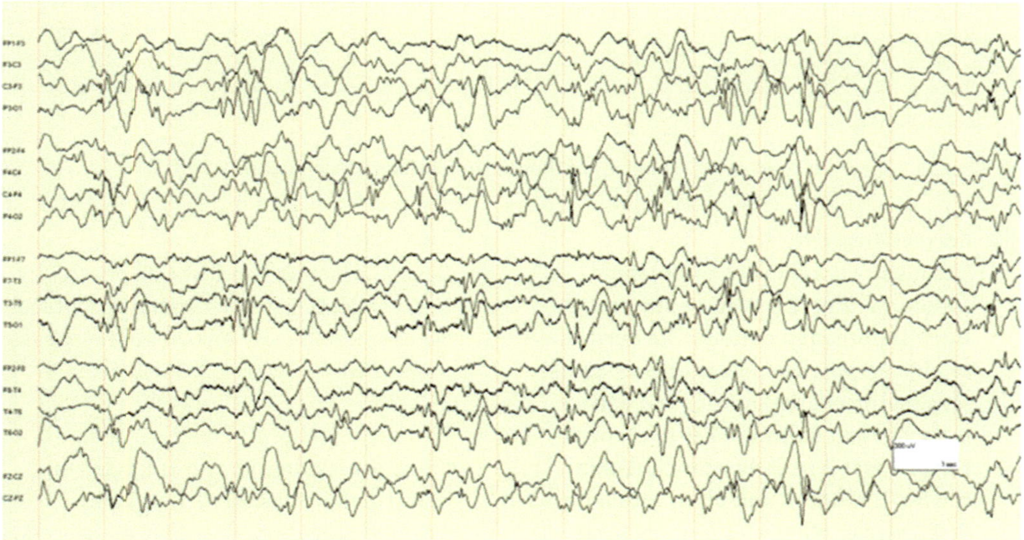

Fig. 8.10 With a permission from ▶ ILAE.org, Diagnostic Manual, and ▶ EpilepsyDiagnosis.org

Correct Answer is: E

This inter-ictal EEG shows chaotic non-rhythmic disorganized high-voltage spike and slow wave activity which is consistent with hypsarrhythmia. The spike and slow waves are varied from moment to moment in duration and location. The background is often greater than 300 microvolts. The hypsarrhythmic usually occur during non-REM sleep.

Suggested Reading

- Pellock JM, Hrachovy R, Shinnar S, et al. Infantile spasms: a US consensus report. Epilepsia 2010;51(10):2175–89.
- Kossoff EH. Infantile spasms. Neurologist 2010;15(2):69–75.

12. A 2-week old baby boy is brought to the ED by his mother because his seizures. The seizures are lasting for

5–10 s, many time a day, come in clusters of stiffening of all extremities. His labs are normal. Head CT is also normal. He has a normal birth history with Apgar scores of 9 and 9, at 1 and 5 min respectively. His EEG is shown.

What is the most likely diagnosis?

A. benign familial neonatal seizures
B. Dravet syndrome
C. infantile spasms
D. migrating partial seizures of infancy
E. Ohtahara syndrome

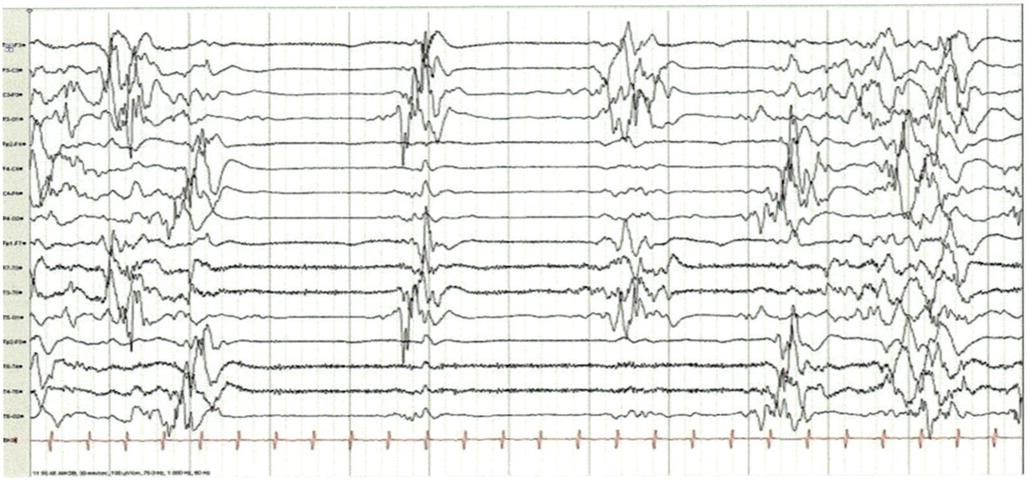

Fig. 8.11 American Academy of Neurology Institute. (Reproduced with permission)

8

Correct Answer is: E
The history is indicative of Ohtahara syndrome. The EEG shows a symmetric burst suppression pattern. The bursts are of high amplitude spikes and poly-spikes (symmetric or asymmetric). The pattern is unchanged during wakefulness and sleep. Onset is in early infancy, within the first 3 months, and often within the first 2 weeks. Manifestations are tonic spasms (generalized or lateralized), can occur both singly or in clusters, and are independent of sleep cycle. Tonic spasms typically last up to 10 s and can occur hundreds of times per day. Structural brain malformations or metabolic or genetic conditions could be the underling etiology, and in some no etiology is found. Genetic conditions which should be looked for include Abnormalities of the *ARX* and *STXBP1*, among others. Treatment is often not successful.

Suggested Reading

- Beal JC, Cherian K, Moshe SO. Early-onset epileptic encephalopathies: Ohtahara syndrome and early myoclonic encephalothopy. Pediatr Neurol. 2012;47(5):317–23.
- Pavone P, Spalice A, Polizzi A, et al. Ohtahara syndrome with emphasis on recent genetic discovery. Brain Dev. 2012;34(6):459–68.

13. An 8-year-old boy with multiple seizure types came to your office for an evaluation. His seizures started as a neonate; he would grimace his face with altered consciousness. Then he starts to have complex partial seizures, drop attacks, and generalized tonic-clonic seizures. He has behavioral difficulties and developmental delay. MRI of the brain is shown.

What is his most likely diagnosis?

A. epilepsy with myoclonic absences
B. seizures with hypothalamic hamartoma
C. Lennox-Gastaut syndrome
D. mesial temporal lobe epilepsy with hippocampal sclerosis
E. Rasmussen syndrome

Fig. 8.12 With a permission from ► ILAE.org, Diagnostic Manual, and ► EpilepsyDiagnosis.org

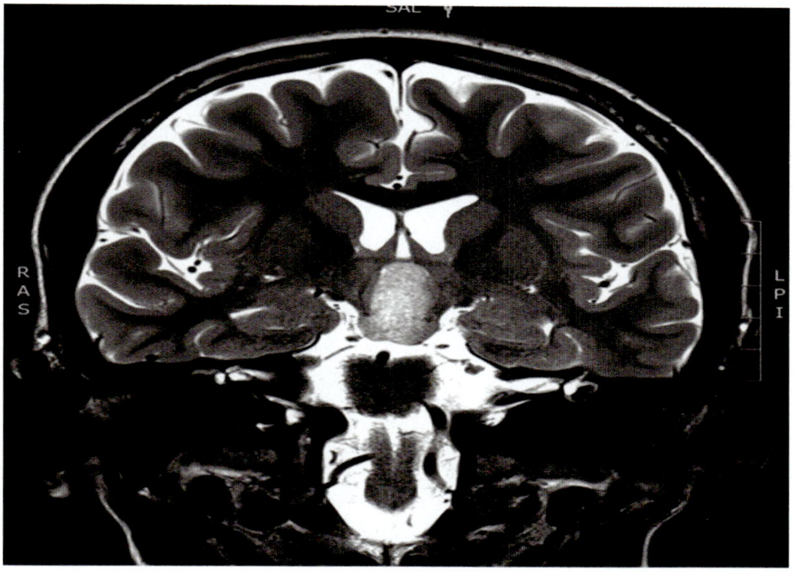

Correct Answer is: B
MRI shows left hypothalamic hamartoma. Hypothalamic hamartoma is hyper-intense relative to the cortical and deep grey matter on the T2-weighted image. The clinical history confirms the diagnosis, gelastic episodes (facial grimace) beginning in infancy, later development of other seizure types as children get older, typically associated with behavior difficulties and an epileptic encephalopathy.

Suggested Reading

- Mittal S, Mittal M, Montes JL, et al. Hypothalamic hamartomas Part 1. Clinical, neuroimaging, and neurophysiological characteristics. Neurosurg Focus. 2013;34(6):E-6.
- Mittal S, Mittal M, Montes JL, et al. Hypothalamic hamartomas Part 2. Surgical considerations and outcomes. Neurosurg Focus. 2013;34(6):E-7.

14. You are evaluating a 7-year-old boy for staring episodes. His teacher told his parents that she has witnessed many spells of staring off space for 5–10 s and the child cannot remember what happened. He has no change in his tone and no associated motor activity. On one occasion, the class was leaving the classroom; the child stood up to leave, but did not. He then asked the teacher what they were supposed to be doing. His EEG is shown.

What is the best treatment?

A. oxcarbazepine
B. methylphenidate
C. lamotrigine
D. ethosuximide
E. valproic acid

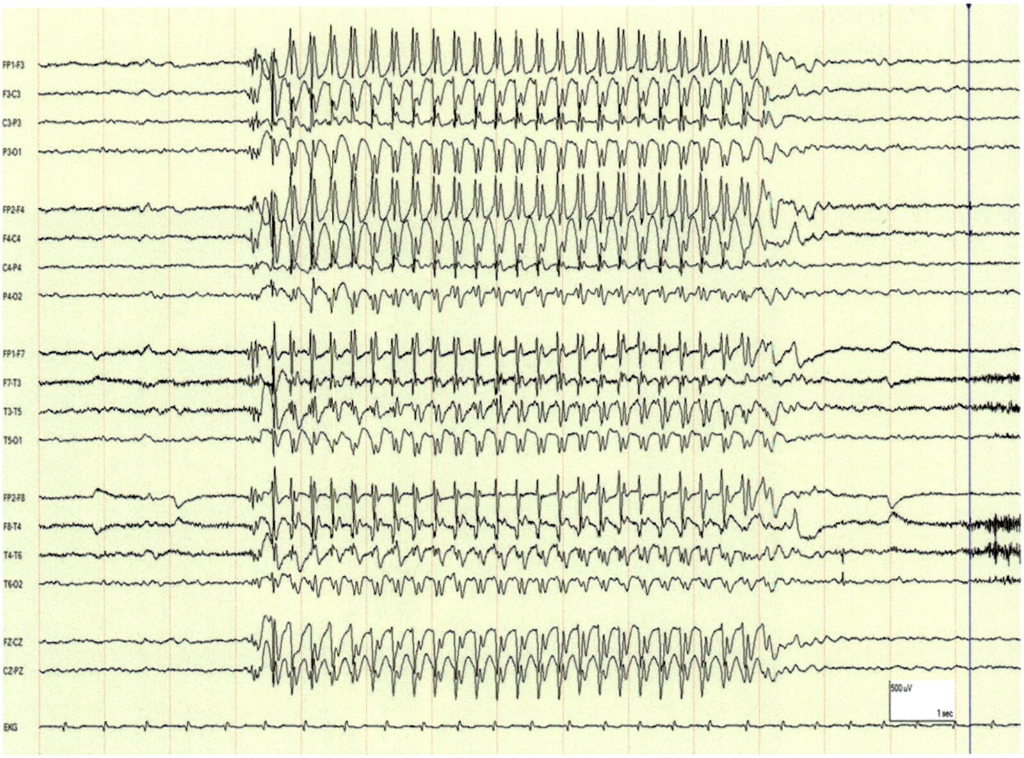

Fig. 8.13 With a permission from ► ILAE.org, Diagnostic Manual, and ► EpilepsyDiagnosis.org

8

Correct Answer is: D
Absence seizures is a childhood disorder, starts between 4 and 10 years and the peak onset is between 5 and 7 years, and usually begin. Childhood absence epilepsy is more common in girls than boys. It is frequent during daytime. Manifestations are loss of awareness, unresponsiveness, and behavioral arrest. Most children have a complete cessation of activity, but a few can continue activities in an altered fashion. The classic I EEG shows bilateral symmetric rhythm discharges 3 Hz (spike and slow wave complexes) with sudden onset and offset. Juvenile absence epilepsy typically occurs in older children and is associated with generalized tonic-clonic seizures. Patients with epilepsy, with generalized tonic-clonic seizures alone, do not have absence seizures. Treatment of choice is ethosuximide. Lamotrigine is less effective, and valproic acid causes more cognitive side effects. Oxcarbamazepine is not effective for absence and can make it worse. His attention problems are related to his seizures, so methylphenidate would not be appropriate.

Suggested Reading

- Matricardi S, Verrotti A, Chiarelli F, et al. Current advances in childhood absence epilepsy. Pediatr Neurol. 2014;50(30):205–12.
- Glauser TA, Cnaan A, Shinnar S, et al. Ethosuximide valproic acid and lamotrigine in childhood absence epilepsy. N Engl J Med. 2010;362(9):790–9.

15. A 14-year-old girl has her first generalized tonic-clonic seizure while she was taking a shower.

She has bilateral arm jerks before her seizure, she has similar jerks after awakening when she is sleep deprived. She has no episodes of staring or unresponsiveness. She has a normal neurologic examination and head CT. EEG before treatment is shown.

What is the most appropriate for first-line therapy?

A. carbamazepine
B. levetiracetam
C. patient does not require AED therapy
D. phenytoin
E. valproate

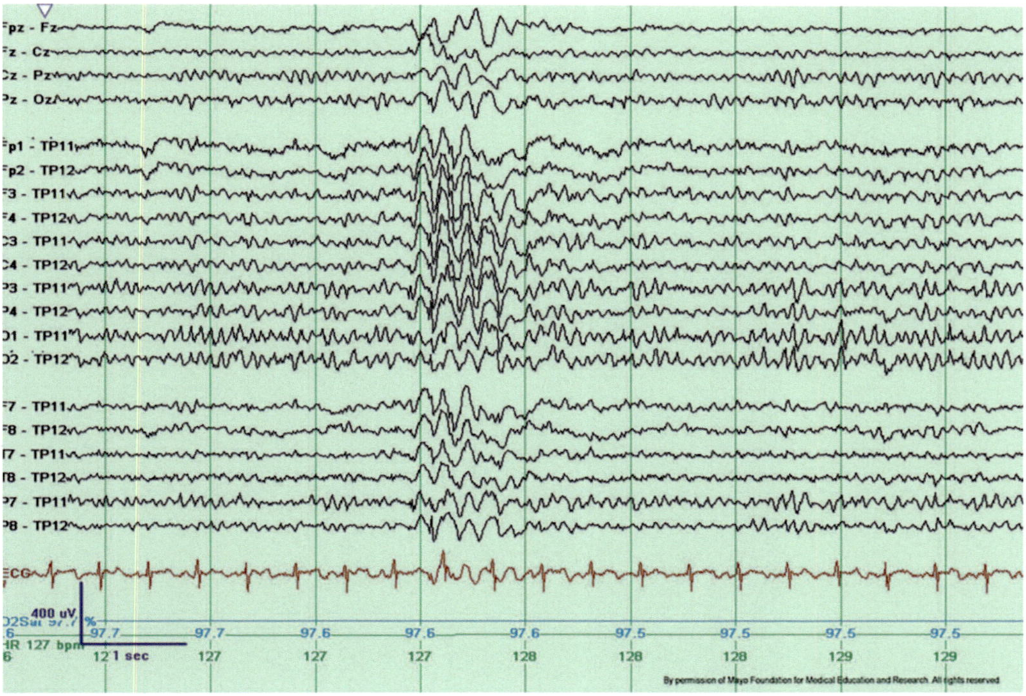

Fig. 8.14 Atypical generalized spike-wave IED. This IED is most commonly seen in children with juvenile absence or myoclonic epilepsy syndromes. The discharges are induced by the activating procedure of photic stimulation, representative of a so-called photo paroxysmal response, which often occurs in those with primary idiopathic generalized epilepsy syndromes. Copyright 2013. Mayo Foundation for Medical Education and Research. All rights reserved. (Figure courtesy of Jeffrey W. Britton, MDElectroencephalography (EEG): An Introductory Text and Atlas of Normal and Abnormal Findings in Adults, Children, and Infants ISBN: 978–0–9,979,756-0-4, Copyright c2016 by American Epilepsy Society, 135 S. LaSalle St., Suite 2850, Chicago, IL 60603)

Correct Answer is: B

The clinical history and EEG are typical of juvenile myoclonic epilepsy (JME). Valproate and levetiracetam both are effective medications for JME, but because the risk of birth defects and impact on fetal cognitive development valproate should not be first- (or second-) line therapy for a young woman (it would be quite appropriate for a young man). Carbamazepine and phenytoin are not broad-spectrum agents and would not be a first choice for treatment of this primary generalized (or genetic in the new classification) epilepsy. While sleep deprivation and alcohol can be provocative for the seizures of JME, this teenager is undoubtedly going to be sleep deprived in the future, so

therapy at this time is indicated. In addition, patients with JME have a high likelihood of recurrent seizures without treatment.

Suggested Reading

- Noachtar S, Andermann E, Mewisch P, et al. Levetiracetam for the treatment of idiopathic generalized epilepsy with myoclonic seizures. Neurology. 2008;70:607–16.

16. A 16-year-old boy with some medically resistant complex partial seizures. He started to have seizures at 10 years of age, he had some seizure-free intervals for 5–6 months. He was tried on arbamazepine, levetiracetam, topiramate, pregabalin, and zonisamide. His seizures are staring off space and left-hand automatisms, sometimes lip smacking. They are 40 s in duration; then, 3–4 min later his language function returns to baseline. Some typical events are captured on video EEG monitoring, showed left temporal lobe ictal activity. Neuropsychological evaluation was done and revealed remarkable impairment in naming and verbal memory, with intact other cognitive abilities. His MRI is shown.

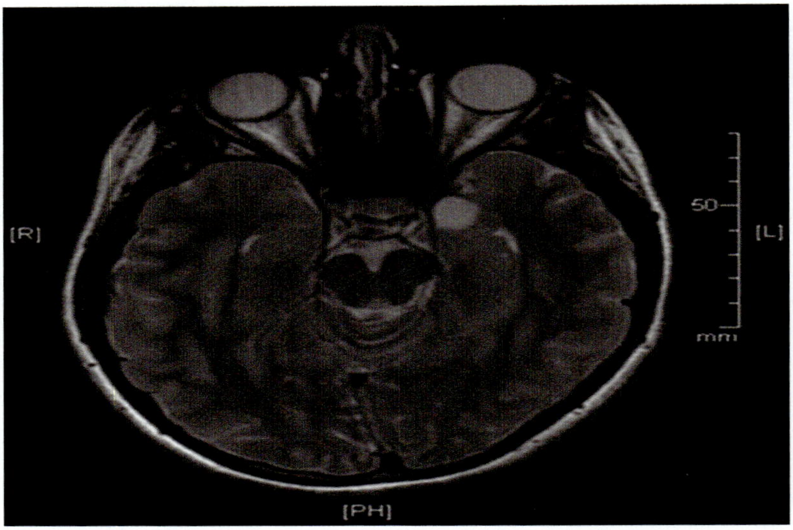

Fig. 8.15 American Academy of Neurology Institute. (Reproduced with permission)

What is the best next step in his management?

A. obtain a magnetoencephalogram
B. obtain PET of the brain
C. perform additional video EEG monitoring with intracranial electrodes
D. refer the patient for a clinical trial of a novel antiepileptic drug
E. resect the left anterial mesial temporal lobe

Correct Answer is: E
The patient has a drug resistant left temporal lobe epilepsy, with an abnormal MRI and a confirmatory EEG. Neuropsychological evaluation confirms the left temporal lobe dysfunction. He is a perfect candidate for anterial temporal resection and most probably he will respond fully to antiepileptic medications. Magnetoencephalogram can be helpful, particularly when the MRI is nonlesional; however, it is not necessary prior to surgery. As documented in the AAN 2003 Practice Parameter, the benefits of anterial mesial temporal lobe resection are greater than continuing treatment with antiepileptic medications, and the risks are comparable.

Suggested Reading

- Engle J, Wiebe S, French J, et al. Practice Parameter: temporal lobe and localized neocortical resections for epilepsy. Report of the Quality Standards Subcommittee of the American Academy of Neurology, in Association with the American Epilepsy Society and the American Association of Neurological Surgeons. Neurology. 2003;60(4):538–47.

17. EEG of a 10-year-old boy with staring spells (IOS = left eye lead; IOD = right eye lead), shows a response to intermittent photic stimulation marked by the tick marks at the bottom of the tracing.
What is the best explanation to this response?
A. abnormal posterior spiking
B. asymmetrical driving
C. driven eye blinks
D. prominent, but normal, occipital driving
E. spike-waves

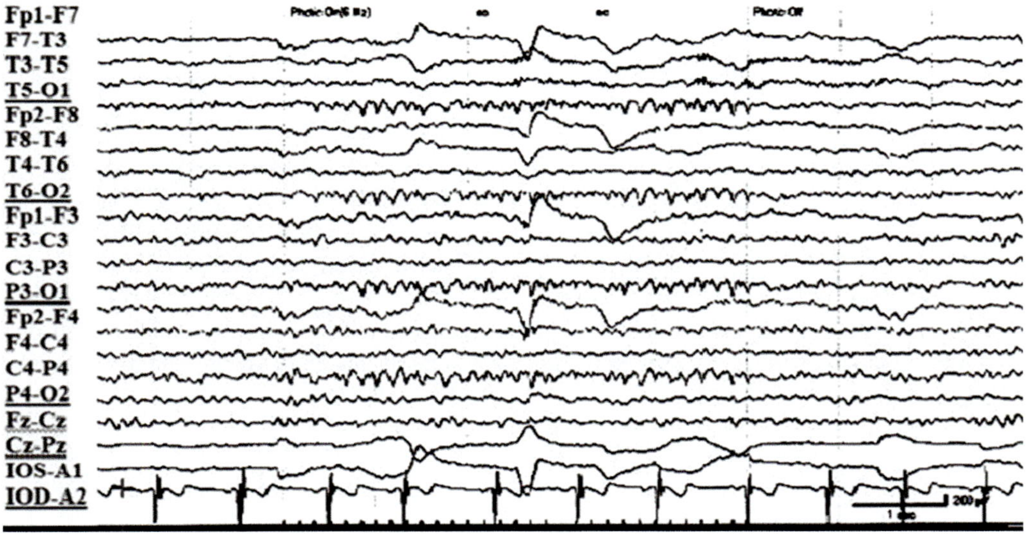

Fig. 8.16 American Academy of Neurology Institute. (Reproduced with permission)

Correct Answer is: D
The tick marks at the bottom of the tracing mark the time of light flashes during intermittent photic stimulation (IPS). Photic responses are abnormal when they produce spikes that outlast the stimuli or spread far anteriorly, seizures, slowing or marked asymmetry. Posterior spikes not outlasting the flashes can be normal.

Suggested Reading

- Trenite DG, Binnie CD, Harding GF, et al. Medical technology assessment photic stimulation–standardization of screening methods. Neurophysiol Clin. 1999;29(4):318–24.

18. An EEG was ordered on an 18-year-old female to rule out encephalopathy. She was diagnosed with lupus, steroid psychosis, and bizarre behavior.
The frontal leads rhythmical activity indicates the following activities?
A. delta activity from the brain
B. eye movements
C. phantom spike waves
D. possible frontal seizure
E. spike-wave activity

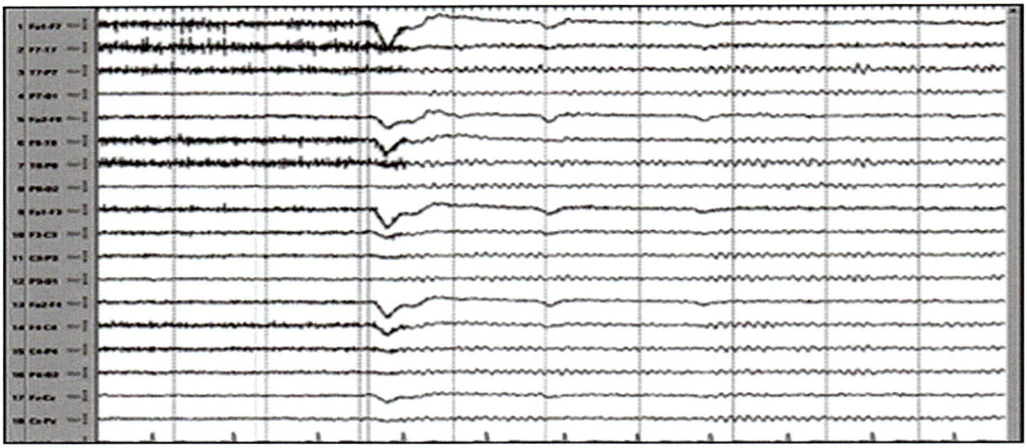

Fig. 8.17 Eye movement artifact. Electroencephalography (EEG): An Introductory Text and Atlas of Normal and Abnormal Findings in Adults, Children, and Infants ISBN: 978-0-9979756-0-4, Copyright c2016 by American Epilepsy Society, 135 S. LaSalle St., Suite 2850, Chicago, IL 60603

8

Correct Answer is: B
The fronto-polar leads show rhythmical slow waves, in this instance with little distribution to other leads. Leads below the eye (IOS, IOD) are out of phase with Fp1 and Fp2, documenting that these are vertical eye movements, likely resulting from partial blinking called eye flutter. Potentials from the frontal lobe would be in phase with electrodes above and below the eyes.

Suggested Reading

- Croft RJ, Barry RJ. Removal of ocular artifact from the EEG: a review. Neurophysiol Clin. 2000;30(1):5–19.

19. A 16 month--old boy presents with a history of infantile spasms. He is taken valproic acid and he was on ACTH before. His EEG (IOS = left eye lead; IOD = right eye lead) indicate which of the following diagnoses?
    A. herpes simplex encephalitis
    B. hypsarrhythmia
    C. low voltage
    D. simple partial seizures
    E. status epilepticus

Correct Answer is: B
The EEG has a very high voltage (200 μV calibration), as opposed to the more typical 50 μV calibration. The EEG shows all the features of hypsarrhythmia: multifocal spikes, diffuse slowing, periods of relative flattening of the background ("burst-suppression-like"). Hypsarrhythmia can be seen in infantile spasms and West syndrome. Herpes simplex would likely produce focal temporal epileptiform patterns.

Suggested Reading

- Kramer U, Sue WC, Mikati MA. Hypsarrhythmia: frequency of variant patterns and correlation with etiology and outcome. Neurology. 1997;48(1):197–203.

20. A 1-day-old full term infant has been evaluated to rule out seizure. The infant had distress at birth, a nuchal cord, and low Apgar scores; and now has occasional respiratory pauses and right leg tremors. EEG tracing is shown (IOS = left eye lead; IOD = right eye lead).
    What is the most likely diagnosis?
    A. encoche frontalis
    B. interictal spikes
    C. rhythmic artifact
    D. right temporal electroencephalographic seizure
    E. tracé alternant

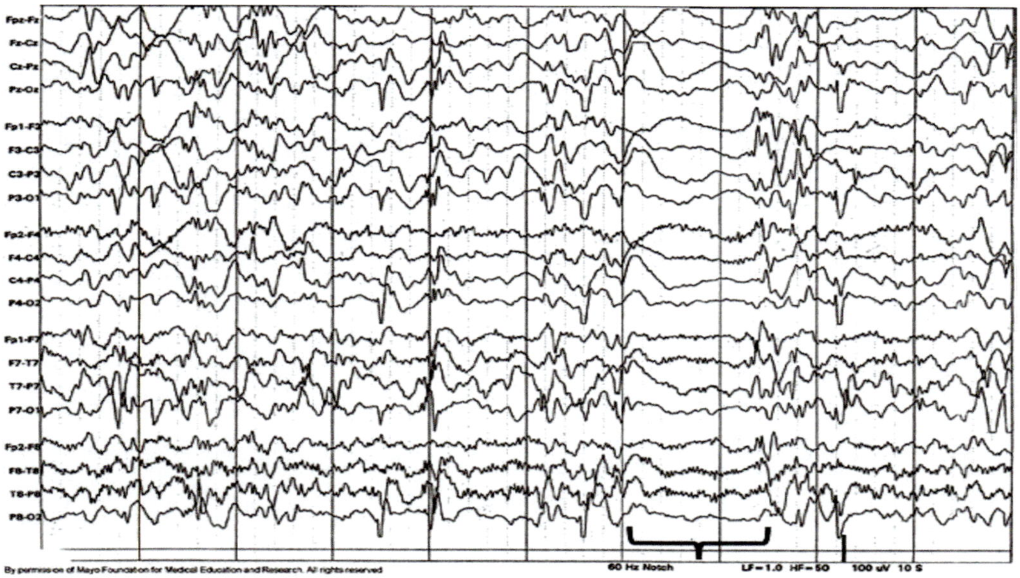

Fig. 8.18 Hypsarrhythmic EEG pattern in an infant with West syndrome. EEG of an 8-month-old infant with infantile spasms and developmental regression. An ictal electrodecremental response (black brackets) is seen during an epileptic spasm. Copyright 2013. Mayo Foundation for Medical Education and Research. All rights reserved. (Figure courtesy of Jeffrey W. Britton, MD. Electroencephalography (EEG): An Introductory Text and Atlas of Normal and Abnormal Findings in Adults, Children, and Infants ISBN: 978-0-9979756-0-4, Copyright c2016 by American Epilepsy Society, 135 S. LaSalle St., Suite 2850, Chicago, IL 60603)

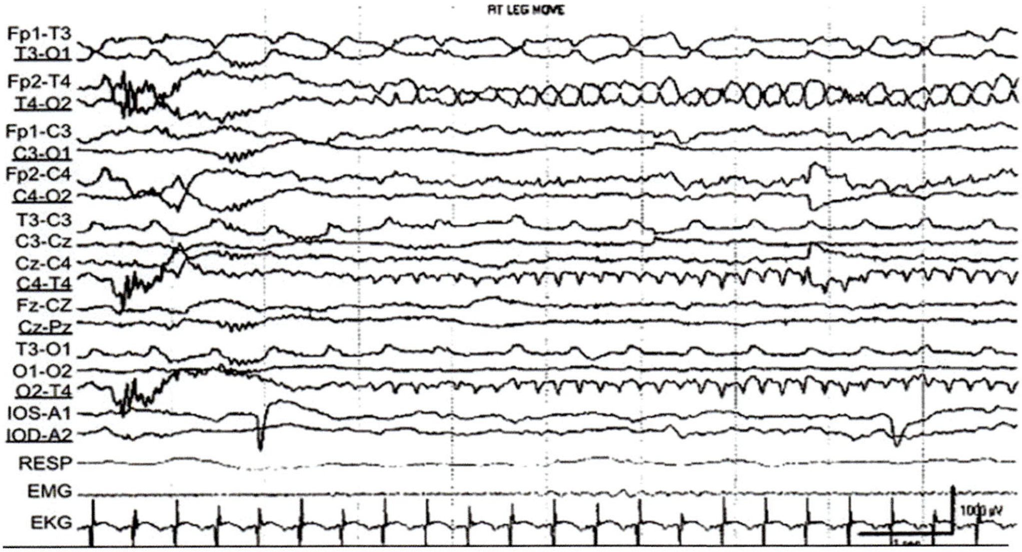

Fig. 8.19 American Academy of Neurology Institute, produced by permission

Correct Answer is: D

The EEG shows a localized rhythmical 4/second to 5/second spikes occur at T4. EEG of an older child or an adult, activity would not be expected to be so localized; but in a neonatal brain, with wider spaced electrodes, limited myelination and reduced connectivity, ictal events can remain

restricted to one or a few electrodes. Any focal, rhythmic evolving event in a neonatal EEG should be considered suspicious for ictal activity, unless it is an obvious artifact.

Suggested Reading

- Abend NS, Wusthoff CJ. Neonatal seizures and status epilepticus. J Clin Neurophysiol. 2012;29(5):441–8.

21. A 6-year-old boy has a history of 2-month of staring and unresponsive episodes lasting up to 20 s, multiple times per day. No treatment was given. In her EEG shown, (IOS = left eye lead; IOD = right eye lead).

What do you see during hyperventilation?

A. asymmetrical slowing
B. eye flutter artifact
C. generalized spike-waves
D. left temporal and parietal sharp waves
E. normal response

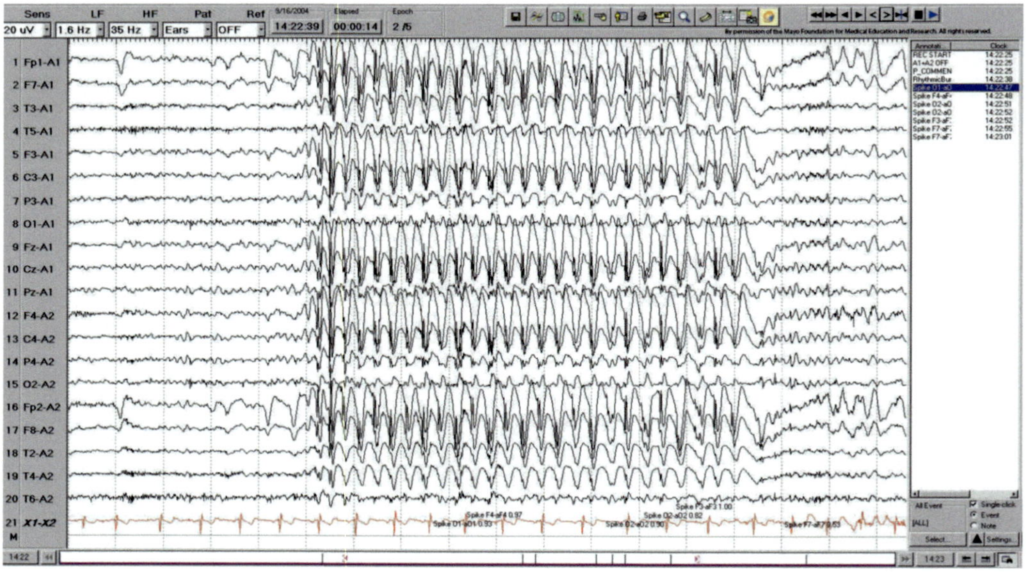

Fig. 8.20 Absence seizure. During an absence seizure, the typical ictal EEG pattern is an extension of the interictal pattern (i.e., 3-Hz generalized spike-wave of a prolonged duration, with usual clinical accompaniments of staring with behavioral arrest, or with variable accompaniment by oral and manual automatisms such as blinking, lip smacking, or hand-fumbling movements. (Figure courtesy of Erik K. St. Louis, MD Electroencephalography (EEG): An Introductory Text and Atlas of Normal and Abnormal Findings in Adults, Children, and Infants ISBN: 978-0-9979756-0-4, Copyright c2016 by American Epilepsy Society, 135 S. LaSalle St., Suite 2850, Chicago, IL 60603)

Correct Answer is: C

Hyperventilation produced early diffuse slowing, followed by a sudden 3/second to 4/second generalized spike-wave discharge with bilateral frontocentral maximum. This pattern is associated with primary generalized epilepsy, such as childhood absence epilepsy.

Suggested Reading

- Hughes JR. Absence seizures: a review of recent reports with new concepts. Epilepsy Behav. 2009;15(4):404–12.

22. A 2-month-old baby boy has a history of multiple clonic seizures in the past 24 h. He was delivered vaginally at full term

pregnancy. The mother had gestational diabetes, controlled with diet and insulin. On day one, he had feeding problems and required nasogastric feeding for several days. Otherwise he is healthy. Family history is negative of seizures. On examination, his head size is below 5rd percentile, mild hypotelorism, and a depressed nasal bridge. Neurologically, he is alert and has brief visual regard but does not track objects. He has hypotonic, with brisk reflexes bilaterally. You started him on phenobarbital and he became seizure-free 24 h later. His brain coronal MRI is shown.

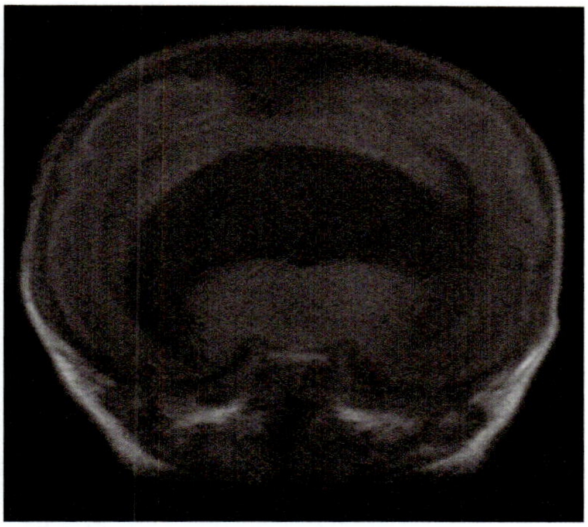

Fig. 8.21 American Academy of Neurology Institute. (Produced by permission)

Which of the following laboratory findings is most likely associated with this abnormality?

A. elevated ratio of very long-chain fatty acids
B. elevated serum lactate
C. hypernatremia
D. hyperthyroidism
E. hypocalcemia

Correct Answer is: C
The MRI shows incomplete telencephalic cleavage consistent with a diagnosis of holoprosencephaly (HPE). There are both environmental and genetic factors, which result in the fetal cerebral hemispheres, and often diencephalon, fail to separate to varying degrees. Facial malformations are common, and include mild facial deformities, such as hypotelorism and a flat nasal bridge, to the more severe cyclopia (a single midline eye) and a proboscis (a rudimentary single nostril nose above the eye). The condition varies from the most severe alobar form (complete failure of hemisphere and diencephalic cleavage), to the mildest interhemispheric variant (where most of the hemisphere is cleavage normal, and only the most inferior portions of the diencephalon and/or corpus callosum are malformed).

All types include microcephaly, developmental delay, and seizures forms as some common features (though most prevalent in the alobar forms.) Endocrine dysfunction secondary to subtle malformation of the hypothalamic/pituitary axis is very common, with diabetes insipidus (and associated hypernatremia) being the most common, occurring in up to 68% of cases. Growth hormone deficiency, hypothyroidism, and hypocortisolism are less common features. Alobar forms commonly lead to progressive hydrocephalus, through an associated midline dorsal cyst, which develops due to impaired egress of spinal fluid from the third ventricle related to blockage from a malformed surrounding fused diencephalon. VP shunting is common, and serial head circumferences should be followed closely.

The sonic hedgehog (SHH) protein plays an integral role in this normal cleavage process, and seems to be the pathway susceptible to environmental and genetic influences leading to the malformation. Maternal diabetes appears to be the strongest environmental factor, with an incidence of HPE of up to 1% (100 times the

risk in the general population). A distinct chromosomal abnormality is identified in 30–50% of cases, and HPE can be part of larger genetic syndromes, such as Smith-Lemli-Opitz. Other malformations of cortical development can be present as well, most commonly grey matter heterotopias.Based on the severity of the malformation, developmental and feeding ability vary, with alobar forms usually being entirely dependent on others for care, including frequent need for gastrostomy tube feeding and failure to sit or walk independently. Lobar forms may develop independent ambulatory skills and functional use of hands and typically feed exclusively by mouth. Life span is decreased, inversely related to the degree of malformation, though even alobar forms can survive (with appropriate attention to feeding safety, seizure control, prevention of fatal hydrocephalus and management of endocrine abnormalities) for up to 15 years.

8

Suggested Reading

Swaiman K, Ashwal S, Ferriero D, Schor N, editors. Swaiman's pediatric neurology: principles and practice. 5th ed. Philadelphia: Elsevier Saunders, 2012; 145–50.

23. A 6-year-old female came to the office with a history of frequent seizures. She has been having seizures since her first year of life, the mother called them "spasms." Her seizures stopped with treatment; however, she started having different seizures over the past several years. She has multiple seizures per day, despite she is on topiramate, levetiracetam, and clonazepam. Her spells are, stares unresponsively for 10–20 s, head drop and brief tonic stiffening of her extremities. She is a healthy girl, but she has severe developmental delay, and she is completely dependent on her mother for her daily living activities. She can sit and crawls, but cannot walk; she makes eye contact and babbles, but has no speech. Her EEG is shown.
    Which of the following epilepsy syndromes is most likely?
    A. absence epilepsy with eyelid myoclonia
    B. benign centrotemporal epilepsy
    C. Landau-Kleffner syndrome
    D. Lennox-Gastaut syndrome
    E. Panayiotopoulos syndrome

Correct Answer is: D
All children with epilepsy should be categorized into epilepsy syndromes, if possible. These syndromes carry specific information about age of onset, seizure types, associated neurocognitive issues, and etiologic origin; they provide information regarding long-term outcome from a seizure control/resolution and eventual cognitive/quality of life standpoint. There are different epilepsy syndromes for different age children, with onset in the neonatal, infantile, childhood, and adolescent age groups. These syndromes can otherwise be subdivided into focal or generalized epilepsies and idiopathic (primary) versus symptomatic (secondary) epilepsies, with symptomatic cases having a known or presumed underlying associated brain dysfunction, such as developmental delay. Other references may refer to "benign" and "catastrophic" epilepsies, usually referring to both ease of seizure control and eventual cognitive outcome.The case presented here entails intractable epilepsy and significant developmental delay, indicating a symptomatic or catastrophic epilepsy. Of the options, only Landau-Kleffner syndrome or Lennox-Gastaut syndrome would fit this description. Absence epilepsy with eyelid myoclonia (Jeavon's syndrome), benign centrotemporal (Rolandic) epilepsy, and Panayiotopoulos syndrome are well defined idiopathic epilepsies of childhood, none of which are associated with developmental delay.

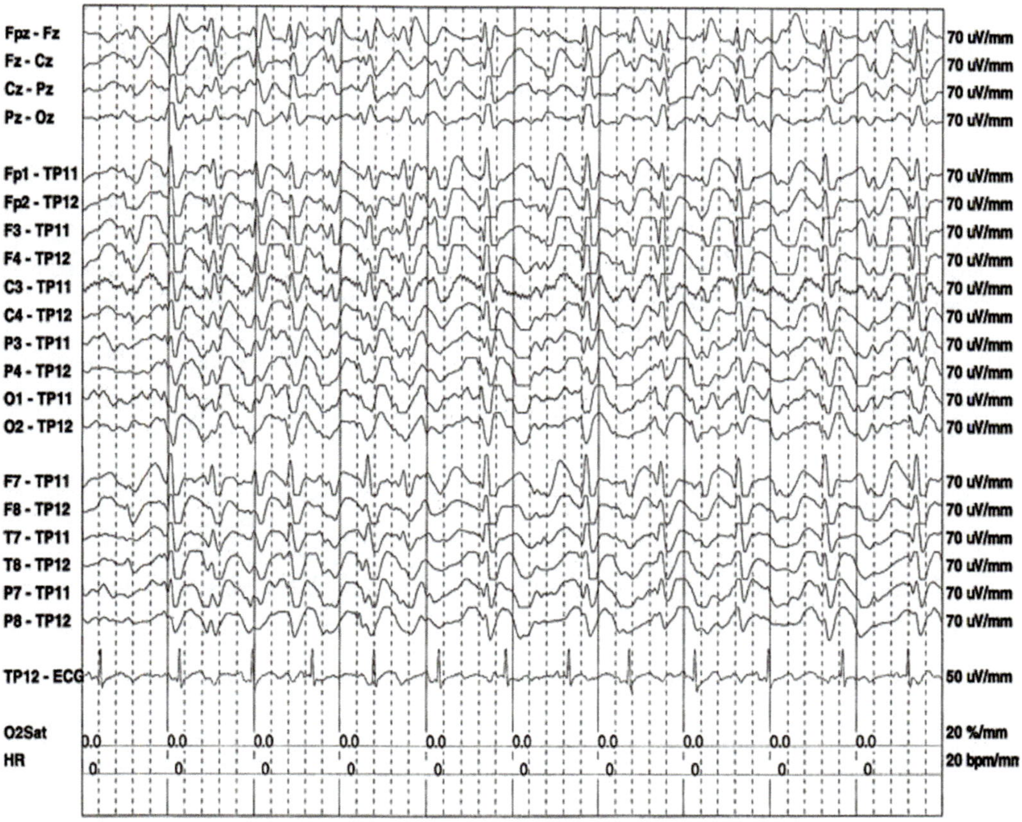

Fig. 8.22 Slow spike-wave IED typical of the Lennox-Gastaut syndrome. Also note the associated underlying background slowing, indicative of generalized cerebral dysfunction and an epileptic encephalopathy. Ipsilateral ear referential montage. Copyright 2013. Mayo Foundation for Medical Education and Research. All rights reserved. (Figure courtesy of Jeffrey W. Britton, MDElectroencephalography (EEG): An Introductory Text and Atlas of Normal and Abnormal Findings in Adults, Children, and InfantsISBN: 978-0-9979756-0-4, Copyright c2016 by American Epilepsy Society, 135 S. LaSalle St., Suite 2850, Chicago, IL 60603)

Lennox-Gastaut syndrome is classically defined by a triad consisting of: (1) multiple seizure types, to include tonic, atonic, myoclonic and atypical absence, (2) an interictal EEG pattern, similar to the figure, showing generalized 1.5–2.5 Hz slow spike-and-wave complexes on an abnormally slow background, and (3) cognitive dysfunction. A majority of cases have pre-existing structural causes, either from perinatal distress, malformations of cortical development, or other neurocutaneous, genetic, or metabolic disorders. In these cases, infantile spasms often predate evolution into this syndrome. The seizures themselves are often intractable and may require other nonpharmacologic therapies such at the ketogenic diet, vagal nerve stimulator, or even corpus callosotomy for refractory atonic seizures.

Landau-Kleffner syndrome (LKS), (and the related electrical status epilepticus in sleep or ESES), typically presents with normal initial development, followed by a period of regression with language, or more global regression. Associated seizures typically predate the onset of regression, though can occasionally start concurrently. The seizures themselves in LKS typically have onset from the temporal region, and usually manifest as nocturnal hemiclonic seizures. Treatment of the seizures

themselves is not very difficult, though improvement of the diffuse electrical status pattern often requires adjunctive therapy with corticosteroids, high dose nocturnal benzodiazepines, and even IVIG. Occasionally, standard anticonvulsants such as valproic acid or levetiracetam can also lead to improvement (and rarely resolution) of this pattern. Aggressive treatment early in the course is required to prevent permanent language dysfunction.

Suggested Reading

- Wirrell E, Nickels KC. Pediatric epilepsy syndromes. Continuum Lifelong Learning Neurol 2010;16(3):57–82.

24. A 7-year-old female has some attention problems, and poor school performance. Her teacher and parents have noted multiple events of staring off space and eye blinking lasting 10–20 s. She has multiple events per day. She does not respond for calling her name during the events and seems "in her own world." She has trouble sleeping at night and she wakes up screaming. Her EEG is shown. Her PCP started her on methylphenidate for presumed ADHD, but continues to have events.

What is your next step in her management?

A. change medication to ethosuximide
B. change methylphenidate to mixed amphetamine salts
C. perform brain MRI
D. perform polysomnogram
E. refer for neuropsychiatric evaluation

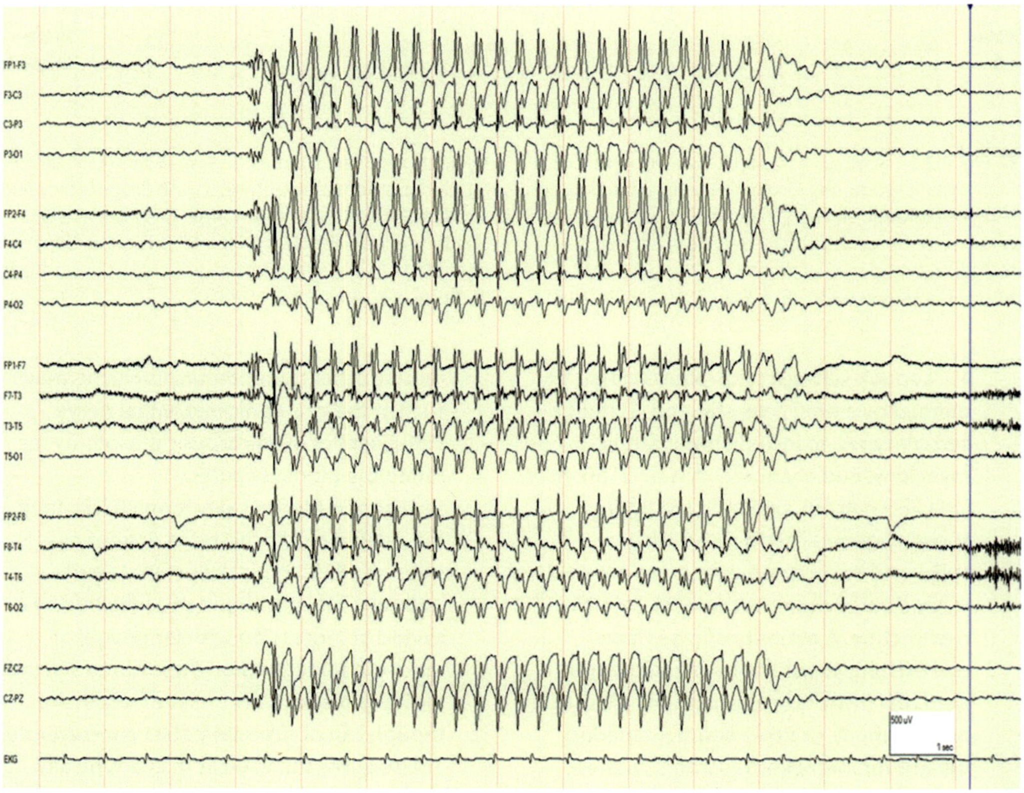

Fig. 8.23 With a permission from ▶ ILAE.org, Diagnostic Manual, and ▶ EpilepsyDiagnosis.org

Correct Answer is: A
The history is indicative of absence epilepsy. EEG shows a 3 Hz generalized spike-and-slow wave rhythm, classic for absence epilepsy. Patients will have many daily spells of brief staring and eye blinking, without postictal confusion. Because of her age, she has childhood absence epilepsy, which has a peak age of onset of 5–8 years. Juvenile absence epilepsy has onset at 10–12 years of age. The first-choice medication for childhood absence epilepsy is ethosuximide. Alternative choices are valproic acid and lamotrigine. On the other hand, oxcarbazepine, carbamazepine, tiagabine, gabapentin, and vigabatrin worsen the condition. Usually, childhood absence epilepsy is a transient disorder, but some patients will develop myoclonic and tonic-clonic seizures and are diagnosed then with juvenile myoclonic epilepsy.

The juvenile absence epilepsy is not as benign, with seizures typically persisting into adulthood, and these patients are also at higher risk of having generalized tonic-clonic seizures as well, although usually few in number. Methylphenidate and mixed amphetamine salts (Adderall) are useful for ADHD, but are ineffective for absence seizures. Brain MRI is not indicated for absence seizure evaluation. Polysomnogram might be indicated for further evaluation of the sleep disturbance, but is not the best next step in her management. Neuropsychiatric evaluation would be indicated if scholastic difficulties persist despite adequate treatment of the absence seizures.

Suggested Reading

- Glauser TA, Loddenkemper T. Management of childhood epilepsy. Continuum Lifelong Learning Neurol. 2013;19(3):656–81.
- Glauser TA, Cnaan A, Shinnar S, et al. Ethosuximide, valproic acid, and lamotrigine in childhood absence epilepsy. N Engl J Med. 2010;362:790–9.

25. An 8-year-old healthy boy had a seizure last night. His mother reports that he was asleep in the back seat of the car when she saw him having stiffening and shaking of his limbs, twitching of his face and upward deviation of his eyes. The event lasted approximately 30 s, and he was sleepy afterwards. His examination is normal. EEG is shown.

What is your diagnosis?

A. benign epilepsy with centrotemporal spikes
B. frontal lobe epilepsy
C. idiopathic generalized epilepsy
D. Panayiotopoulos syndrome
E. temporal lobe epilepsy

Correct Answer is: A
The EEG shows benign childhood epilepsy with centrotemporal spikes (BECTS). The location of the epileptiform discharges (central and temporal) and morphology (polyphasic dipole tangential to the Rolandic region) are characteristic. BECTS is the most common partial epilepsy of childhood, accounting for approximately 2/3 of all idiopathic focal epilepsies of childhood. The onset is 5–8 years of age. Focal motor seizures are the most common seizure type and are often unilateral, involving the face, oropharynx and upper extremity. The seizures most often occur during sleep; fewer than 25% of the seizures occur during wakefulness. Treatment can be delayed because many patients will not have more than 1–2, and remission of the epilepsy is expected.

Suggested Reading

- Bergqvist CA. Idiopathic pediatric epilepsy syndromes. Continuum Lifelong Learning Neurol. 2007;13(4):106–20.

26. A 17-year-old male collapsed to the ground at school. He denies any loss of consciousness. He reported having some jerking movements of his

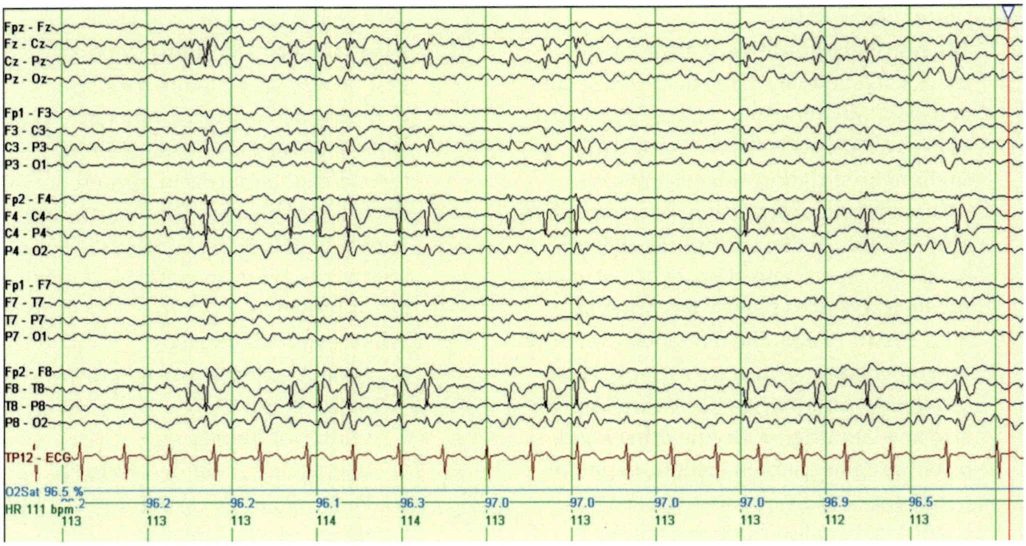

8

Fig. 8.24 With a permission from ► ILAE.org, Diagnostic Manual, and ► EpilepsyDiagnosis.org

arms that morning after staying up studding late the night before. He has those jerky movements of his arms for several years, usually in the morning. He has a normal examination. EEG is shown.

What is the best treatment you can provide?

A. carbamazepine
B. clonazepam as needed
C. counsel patient to always get a full night's sleep
D. divalproex sodium
E. propranolol

Correct Answer is: D

The clinical history is consistent with myoclonic seizures and it is confirmed by the generalized 4–5 Hz spike-wave complexes and polyspikes on his EEG. He has no history of generalized tonic-clonic seizure, but he is at high risk for one and should be treated with an antiepileptic drug (AED). Divalproex sodium is very useful in this case and is often the preferred AED for men with generalized epilepsy. Other AEDs that may be used for this syndrome include levetiracetam, zonisamide, topiramate and lamotrigine.

Carbamazepine may worsen generalized epilepsies, particularly myoclonic and absence types. Propranolol is not an antiseizure medication. Although sleep deprivation is a known seizure trigger for patients with myoclonic epilepsy and avoidance of sleep deprivation should be recommended, this would not be adequate as a single best treatment. Likewise, clonazepam as needed might be helpful for patients with a tendency toward sustained seizure clusters, but would not be the best single treatment.

Suggested Reading

Rudzinski LA, Shih JJ. Classification of seizures and epilepsy syndromes. Continuum Lifelong Learning Neurol. 2010;16(3):15–35.

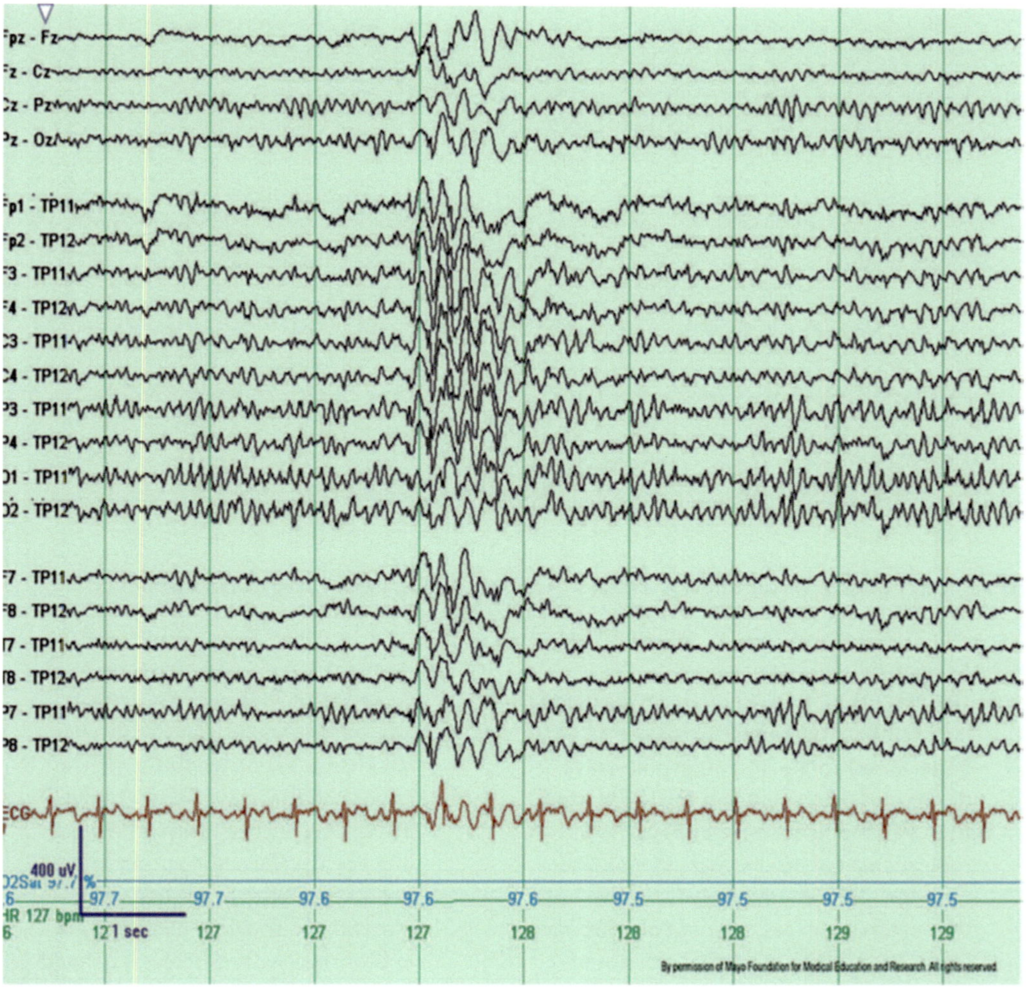

Fig. 8.25 Atypical generalized spike-wave IED. This IED is most commonly seen in children with juvenile absence or myoclonic epilepsy syndromes. The discharges are induced by the activating procedure of photic stimulation, representative of a so-called photo paroxysmal response, which often occurs in those with primary idiopathic generalized epilepsy syndromes. Copyright 2013. Mayo Foundation for Medical Education and Research. All rights reserved. (Figure courtesy of Jeffrey W. Britton, MDElectroencephalography (EEG): An Introductory Text and Atlas of Normal and Abnormal Findings in Adults, Children, and InfantsISBN: 978-0-9979756-0-4, Copyright c2016 by American Epilepsy Society, 135 S. LaSalle St., Suite 2850, Chicago, IL 60603)

27. A 14-year-old male has episodes of staring off space and Lip-smacking for 3 months. Past medical history is remarkable of attention deficit hyperactivity disorder (ADHD) and a family history of epilepsy. He is on atomoxetine. He has a normal examination. EEG is shown.

What is your diagnosis?

A. behavioral manifestations of ADHD
B. childhood absence epilepsy
C. frontal lobe epilepsy
D. juvenile absence epilepsy
E. medication side effects

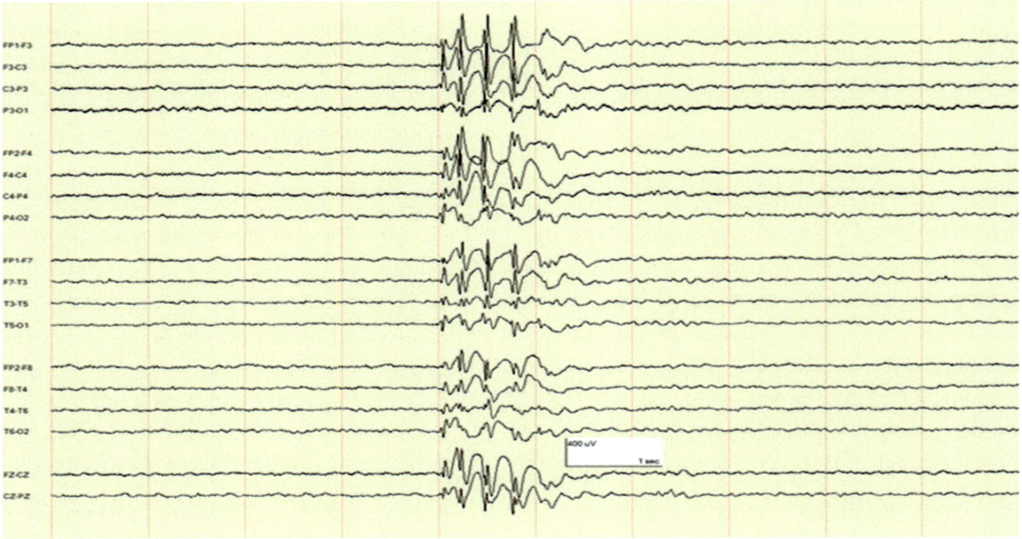

Fig. 8.26 With a permission from ► ILAE.org, Diagnostic Manual, and ► EpilepsyDiagnosis.org

Correct Answer is: D

The EEG is typical of juvenile absence epilepsy (JAE) with the characteristic 3.5–4 Hz generalized spike- and polyspike-wave discharges. The age onset for JAE is later than childhood absence epilepsy, with typical onset at 10–16 years of age. The absence seizure semiology is similar, but the seizures are less frequent and longer in duration, with a higher incidence of absence status and occasional generalized tonic-clonic seizures. Rarely, they have remission. The best treatment options are valproic acid and lamotrigine, which are effective for both absence and tonic-clonic seizures.

Suggested Reading

- Wirrell E, Nickels KC. Pediatric epilepsy syndromes. Continuum Lifelong Learning Neurol 2010;16(3):57–85.

28. A previously healthy 5-month-old boy started to have an abnormal twitching of his arms and legs for the past 3 weeks. The family brought a video EEG, showed a repetitive symmetric flexion of his both arms and head, lasting up to 5 s each and repeating every 5–10 s for 15 min. He will cry and be fussy in between the events. The events occur in cluster around sleep-wake transitions. Recently he showed mild delays in motor skills with worsening of head control and less vocal output since these movements started. He has a normal general examination, but the neurologic examination shows only mildly decreased truncal tone. EEG is shown.

What is the most appropriate diagnosis?

A. benign myoclonic epilepsy of infancy
B. benign sleep myoclonus of infancy
C. infantile spasms
D. Lennox Gastaut syndrome
E. Sandifer syndrome

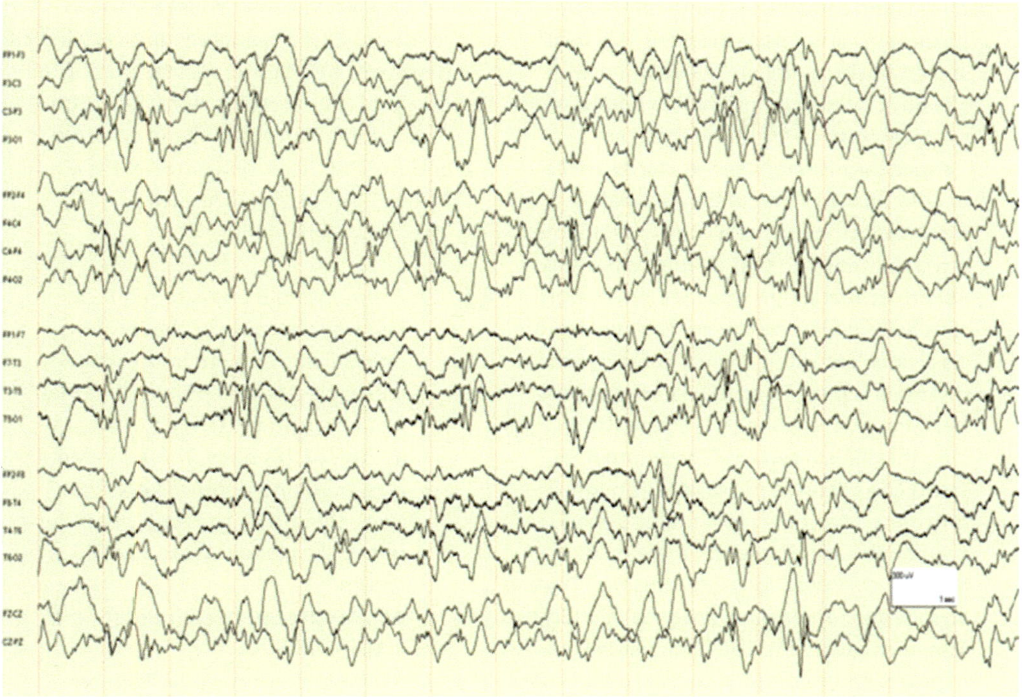

Fig. 8.27 With a permission from ▶ ILAE.org, Diagnostic Manual, and ▶ EpilepsyDiagnosis.org

Correct Answer is: C

The EEG pictured shows a very chaotic and disorganized background, with a mixture of very high amplitudes, and multifocal and generalized spike and sharp complexes. Additionally, noted is a brief 1-s segment of suppression of background, referred to as "electrodecrement." This pattern comprises hypsarrhythmia, the EEG pattern typical for infantile spasms (and one of the key features of the triad of the initial description of West syndrome). The disorganized EEG background belies the prominent encephalopathy seen in these patients. Although the myoclonic seizures of benign myoclonic epilepsy of infancy sometimes resemble an epileptic spasm, the interictal EEG background for this epilepsy syndrome is normal for age and would not be confused with Hypsarrhythmia. Benign sleep myoclonus of infancy and Sandifer syndrome are nonepileptic paroxysmal events. They are commonly noted in young infants and sometimes mistaken for seizures or infantile spasms, though they would not be associated with any EEG abnormalities. Lennox Gastaut syndrome (LGS) is another type of epileptic encephalopathy in which patients have several seizure types (including tonic, myoclonic, tonic-clonic, atypical absence, and partial) along with cognitive impairment and typically occurs in children older than 2 years of age. Infantile spasms typically present in the 4- to 9-month-old child, often with preceding developmental delay, though occasionally in a previously normal infant. They typically appear as clusters of flexor or extensor movements of the limbs, often with a quick myoclonic

phase (and sometimes a very brief tonic phase lasting no more than 1–2 s). If in a seated position, the child also will usually have head and neck atonia and lose postural control. Although these are frequently misdiagnosed as startle spells or colic (due to some of the associated fussiness during clusters), the movements are classic enough that diagnosis is often able to be made by a qualified neurologist simply from viewing the spells in person or on a video recording. Whether full hypsarrhythmia is present on EEG or not, current best practice recommends attempts to stop the clinical spasms (and improve the EEG) as soon as possible. Although outcome is typically most highly dependent on the specific cause, there is some thought that duration of spasms may have an independent inverse prognostic effect? Common causes include birth related hypoxic-ischemic injury, cortical malformations, genetic and metabolic disorders, neurocutaneous syndromes (especially tuberous sclerosis) and congenital infections. Treatment is typically with some type of steroid therapy (ACTH versus prednisone), though agents such as vigabatrin have been particularly effective for spasms secondary to tuberous sclerosis. Other more traditional anticonvulsant therapies or pyridoxine have been tried, though often with poor overall success (except in the setting of true pyridoxine dependent epilepsy.) The spasms usually go into remission with, or without treatment, over time; though the risk for ongoing developmental delay and other seizure types remains high.

8

Suggested Reading

- Wirrell E, Nickels KC. Pediatric epilepsy syndromes. Continuum Lifelong Learning Neurol. 2010;16(3):70–5.
- Go CY, Mackay MT, Weiss SK, et al. Evidence-based guideline update: Medical treatment of infantile spasms. Report of the Guideline Development Subcommittee of the American Academy of Neurology and the Practice Committee of the Child Neurology Society. Neurology. 2012;78(24):1974–80.

29. A 6-month-old boy is brought by his family because of clusters of unusual movements. In the office you witnessed an episode of sudden head drop and extension of his arms in front of this body. These tend to cluster around sleep-wake transitions, though he has clearly had clusters while already awake. His EEG is shown.

What is the best treatment for this young child?

A. Adrenocorticotropic hormone
B. Diazepam
C. Phenobarbital
D. Reassurance only, he has benign myoclonus of infancy
E. Vigabatrin

Correct Answer is: A

This a typical clinical history and EEG findings of infantile spasms. The EEG shows hypsarrhythmia, with a very high-amplitude and disorganized background with both generalized spike and slow bursts and multifocal discharges. The EEG of the benign myoclonus of infancy, EEG is normal, and the spells would be aborted by waking the child up. Adrenocorticotropic hormone (ACTH) is the first line therapy for infantile spasms not associated with tuberous sclerosis. Vigabatrin is used in children with infantile spasms associated with tuberous sclerosis. Phenobarbital is not a first line treatment modality.

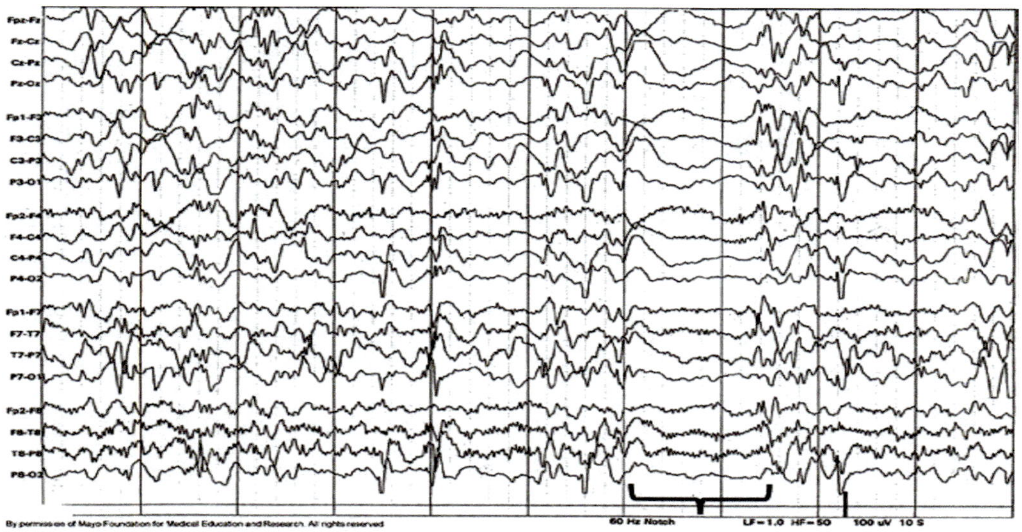

Fig. 8.28 Hypsarrhythmic EEG pattern in an infant with West syndrome. EEG of an 8-month-old infant with infantile spasms and developmental regression. An ictal electrodecremental response (black brackets) is seen during an epileptic spasm. Copyright 2013. Mayo Foundation for Medical Education and Research. All rights reserved. (Figure courtesy of Jeffrey W. Britton, MD Electroencephalography (EEG): An Introductory Text and Atlas of Normal and Abnormal Findings in Adults, Children, and Infants ISBN: 978-0-9979756-0-4, Copyright c2016 by American Epilepsy Society, 135 S. LaSalle St., Suite 2850, Chicago, IL 60603)

Benzodiazepines such as diazepam can be used in conjunction with other agents for refractory spasms, but would not be used as a first-line agent.

Suggested Reading

- Arya R, Shinnar S, Glauser TA. Corticosteroids for the treatment of infantile spasms: a systematic review. J Child Neurol. 2012;27(10):1284–8.

30. A 10-year-old female in your office for an evaluation because she has a school difficulty. Her teachers noted that she frequently stare off space with twitching movements in her face. These episodes happen every time she blows balloons. Her EEG is shown.

What is the most likely diagnosis?

A. Childhood absence epilepsy
B. Frontal lobe epilepsy
C. Juvenile myoclonic epilepsy
D. Panayiotopoulos syndrome
E. Reflex epilepsy

Correct Answer is: A

The EEG shows the classic 3-Hz generalized spike-wave discharges of the childhood absence epilepsy (CAE). The disorder starts between 4 and 10 years of age. The seizures are brief, lasting less than 10 , and may occur up to hundreds of times a day. Automatisms and brief clonic jerks can be seen during absence seizures. The seizures can be provoked by hyperventilation in approximately 90% of children.

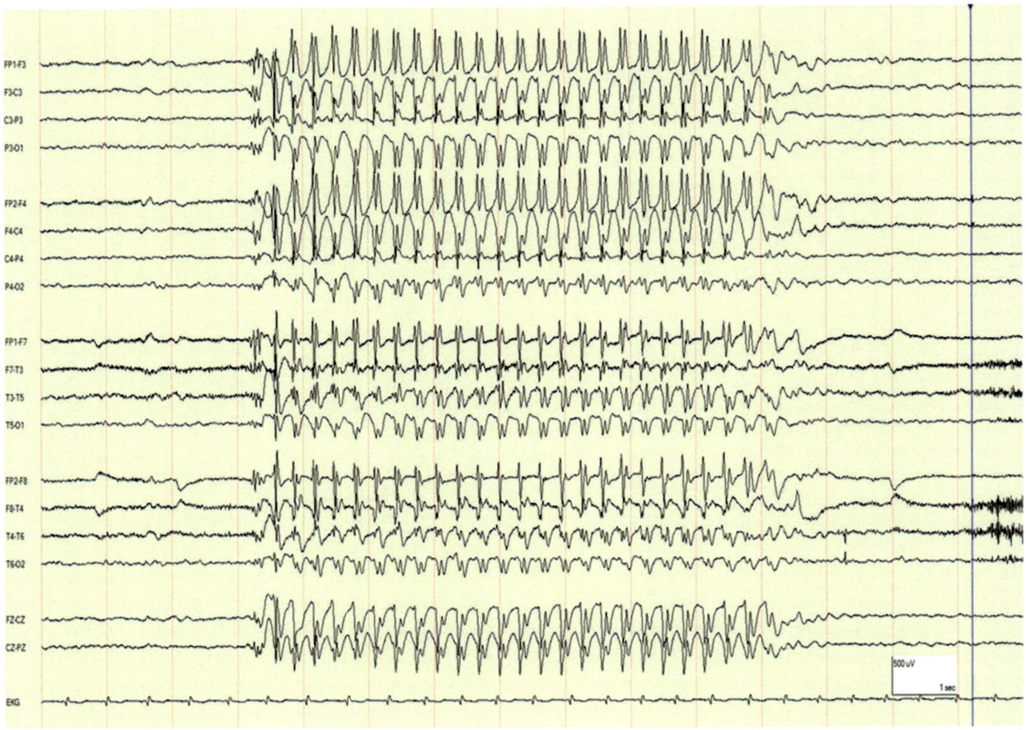

Fig. 8.29 With a permission from ► ILAE.org, Diagnostic Manual, and ► EpilepsyDiagnosis.org

Suggested Reading

- ► http://journals.lww.com/continuum/Fulltext/2010/06000/PEDIATRIC_EPILEPSY_SYNDROMES.6.aspx.

31. An 18-year-old female repots episodes of time lapses for few years. The time lapses usually occur while is driving her car or jogging in the park, especially if the sun is flickering through the trees. She also reports that she is clumsy in the morning and will sometimes give up on braiding her hair since she keeps dropping her brush. Her EEG is shown.

What is your diagnosis?

A. Childhood absence epilepsy
B. Frontal lobe epilepsy
C. Juvenile absence epilepsy
D. Juvenile myoclonic epilepsy
E. Progressive myoclonic epilepsy

Correct Answer is: D

She is severing of photosensitive seizures and episodes of myoclonus, which is typical of juvenile myoclonic epilepsy. The EEG shows generalized fast poly-spike wave discharges which is consistent with JME. JME is a common epilepsy syndrome (4–10% of all patients with epilepsy). It starts between 12 and 18 years of age. Children often have months to years of episodes of myoclonus and absence seizures. Routine EEG is usually abnormal in most children with JME and shows 4– 6-Hz generalized spike and poly-spike wave discharges. Focal discharges may also be present. Photosensitivity is present in 50–75% of people with JME. Neither childhood or juvenile absence epilepsy have prominent myoclonus, nor do the bursts of generalized epileptiform activity occur classically at 3–4 Hz. There are several forms of progressive myoclonus

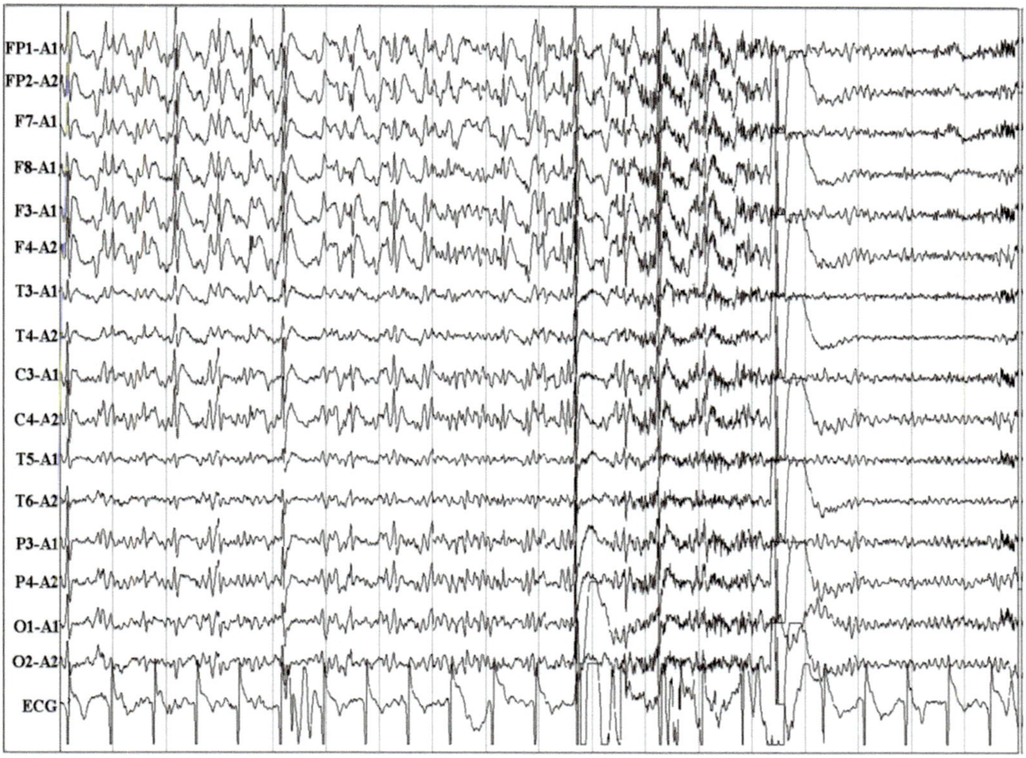

Fig. 8.30 Myoclonic seizure in a patient with JME. The patient had a generalized axial myoclonic jerk during second 14, which coincided with the generalized spike-wave discharge and electrodecremental pattern seen on EEG. Copyright 2013. Mayo Foundation for Medical Education and Research. All rights reserved. (Figure courtesy of Erik K. St. Louis, MDElectroencephalography (EEG): An Introductory Text and Atlas of Normal and Abnormal Findings in Adults, Children, and Infants ISBN: 978-0-9979756-0-4, Copyright c2016 by American Epilepsy Society, 135 S. LaSalle St., Suite 2850, Chicago, IL 60603)

epilepsy, typically with myoclonus and some prominent cognitive regression or visual loss. Frontal lobe epilepsy would be expected to have frontally-based focal epileptiform discharges (though interictal EEG is often normal), without absence or myoclonic seizure types.

Suggested Reading

- ► http://journals.lww.com/continuum/Fulltext/2010/06000/PEDIATRIC_EPILEPSY_SYNDROMES.6.aspx.

32. A 6-year-old female starts to have a language regression in the last 5 months. She stated to have few brief focal seizures, involving the left or right side of the face 2 years ago. Initial EEG showed bilaterally independent triphasic sharp and slow complexes. Her pediatrician started her on carbamazepine, with good control of her seizures until 5 months ago, in conjunction with her regressed language skills. A repeat EEG is ordered, with a segment of her sleep recording attached here.
What is the most appropriate diagnosis for this patient?
A. Landau-Kleffner syndrome
B. Lennox-Gastaut syndrome
C. Pervasive developmental disorder
D. Rett syndrome
E. Rolandic epilepsy

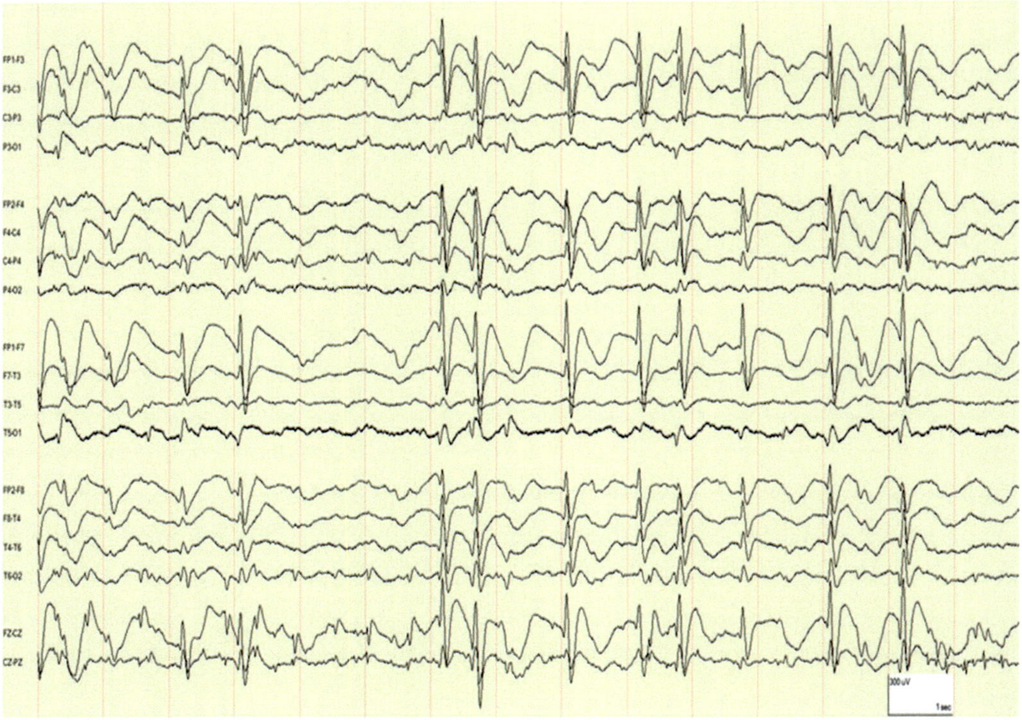

Fig. 8.31 With a permission from ▶ ILAE.org, Diagnostic Manual, and ▶ EpilepsyDiagnosis.org

Correct Answer is: A

The EEG shows continuous generalized spike and slow wave discharges seen in sleep. Language regression with severe sleep-activated epileptiform EEG is consistent with Landau-Kleffner syndrome, which has also been termed acquired epileptiform aphasia. Classically those children have normal development until sometime between the ages of 2–5, when expressive and even receptive language skills regress. Clinical seizures typically occur prior to, or early on in the course of the regression, though in some cases the seizures may occur later. Often, the initial EEG can have features of rolandic epilepsy, and worsen with treatment with traditional sodium channel blocking agents such as carbamazepine or oxcarbazepine. Although epileptiform discharges in Rolandic epilepsy increased in sleep, they do not generalize as seen in Landau-Kleffner syndrome. Treatment of Landau-Kleffner involves use of broader spectrum anticonvulsants such as valproic acid, levetiracetam or lamotrigine. Use of high dose nightly benzodiazepines or even oral steroid treatment can also be helpful in many cases. A normal development during the first 5 years of life is not compatible with pervasive developmental disorder or Rett syndrome. Lennox-Gastaut syndrome is characterized by multiple generalized seizure types, cognitive dysfunction, and EEG showing diffuse slow spike-and-wave complexes. Again, most patients with an eventual diagnosis of this epilepsy syndrome are never developmentally normal.

33. A 6-year-old female complains of occasional staring spells for the last 3 months. She has multiple spells a day and last about 10 s. Occasionally they are accompanied by eyelid fluttering. Also, she has trouble paying attention in the classroom. Her medical history is unremarkable and her examination is normal. Her EEG is shown.

What is best medications to be used first?

A. carbamazepine
B. ethosuximide
C. lamotrigine
D. methylphenidate
E. valproic aid

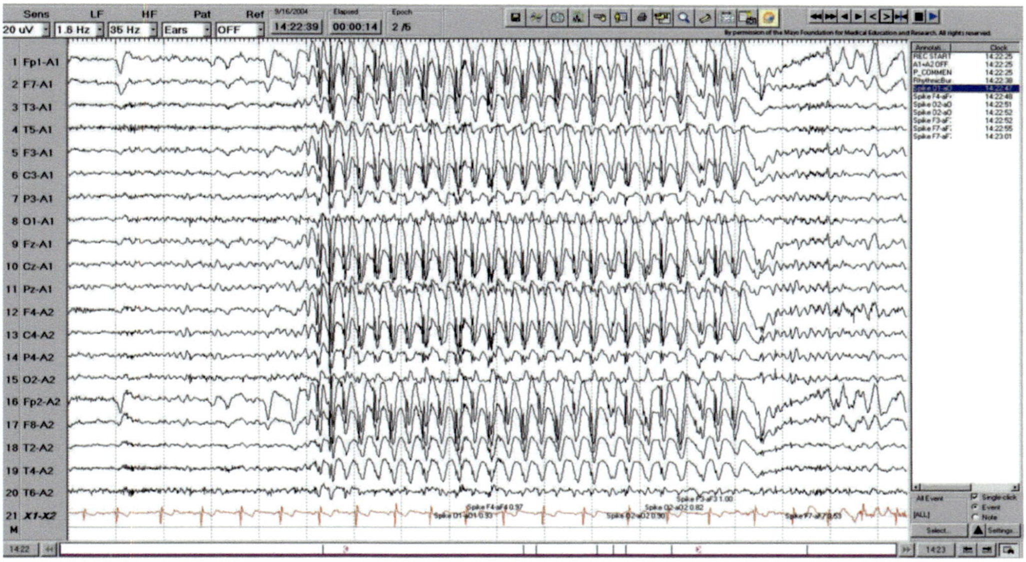

Fig. 8.32 Absence seizure. During an absence seizure, the typical ictal EEG pattern is an extension of the interictal pattern (i.e., 3-Hz generalized spike-wave of a prolonged duration, with usual clinical accompaniments of staring with behavioral arrest, or with variable accompaniment by oral and manual automatisms such as blinking, lip smacking, or hand-fumbling movements. Copyright 2013. Mayo Foundation for Medical Education and Research. All rights reserved. (Figure courtesy of Erik K. St. Louis, MD Electroencephalography (EEG): An Introductory Text and Atlas of Normal and Abnormal Findings in Adults, Children, and Infants ISBN: 978-0-9979756-0-4, Copyright c2016 by American Epilepsy Society, 135 S. LaSalle St., Suite 2850, Chicago, IL 60603)

Correct Answer is: B
The clinical presentation is consistent with a diagnosis of childhood absence epilepsy and supported with the EEG showing the 3 Hz spike-wave discharges. Ethosuximide, lamotrigine and valproic acid can all be used to treat this syndrome, but ethosuximide has been shown to be more effective than lamotrigine and associated with less side effects compared to valproic acid. Carbamazepine may worsen absence seizures and is contraindicated in this situation. Her attentional problems may be due to uncontrolled seizure activity and methylphenidate is not indicated at this time.

Suggested Reading

- Glauser, TA, Cnaan A, Shinnar S, et al. Ethosuximide, valproic acid and lamotrigine in childhood absence epilepsy. N Engl J Med 2010;362(9):790–9.

34. An 18-year-old female with right temporal lobe epilepsy has her first healthy baby. She is planning to breastfeed her baby but she does not know the risks of her anti- seizure medications on her baby. She had no seizures during her pregnancy and is currently on levetiracetam and carbamazepine.

Based on evidence-based medicine which of the following statements is most accurate regarding breastfeeding in this situation?

A. carbamazepine and levetiracetam both cross the placenta so further exposure via breastmilk would not contraindicate breastfeeding
B. risks are clearly defined and she should not breastfeed
C. risks are unknown and it is better not to breastfeed
D. she can breastfeed, but should expect increased fussiness and lethargy in the infant
E. transference of carbamazepine into the breast milk is much greater than levetiracetam

Correct Answer is: A
There are no controlled studies comparing symptomatic effects from AEDs in infant's breast fed by women with epilepsy. At this point the clinical consequences for the newborn ingesting AEDs via breast milk are unknown. Phenobarbital, primidone, phenytoin, carbamazepine, levetiracetam, gabapentin, lamotrigine, oxcarbazepine and topiramate cross the placenta and may be factored into the clinical decision making. Studies have shown significant penetration of levetiracetam into breast milk (as well as gabapentin, lamotrigine, topiramate and primidone). Valproate, phenobarbital, carbamazepine and phenytoin do not significantly penetrate into the breast milk.

Suggested Reading

- Harden CL, Pennell BP, Koppel BS, et al. Practice Parameter update: Management issues for women with epilepsy—focus on pregnancy (an evidence-based review): Vitamin K, folic acid, blood levels and breastfeeding. Neurology 2009;73:142–149.

35. A mother of 6-year-old boy said that her son has a weekly event of drooling and movements of his mouth while sleeping for the past 2 months. He has a history of sleep walking but does not sleepwalk during these episodes. There is a family history of his father and paternal uncle had childhood epilepsy and his maternal uncle has Tourette syndrome. He has a normal examination and developmental milestones. EEG is shown.
Which of the following is the most accurate statement regarding this patient?

A. diagnosis is Panayiotopoulos syndrome
B. diagnosis is benign Rolandic epilepsy
C. First-line treatment is low dose clonazepam before bedtime
D. genetic testing for autosomal dominant frontal lobe epilepsy is indicated
E. polysomnogram with full montage EEG during one of the episodes is necessary for accurate diagnosis

Correct Answer is: B
The EEG shows benign childhood epilepsy with centrotemporal spikes (BECTS). The location of the epileptiform discharges (central and temporal) and morphology (polyphasic dipole tangential to the Rolandic region) are characteristic. BECTS is the most common partial epilepsy of childhood, accounting for approximately 2/3 of all idiopathic focal epilepsies of childhood. The onset is 5–8 years of age. Focal motor seizures are the most common seizure type and are often unilateral, involving the face, oropharynx and upper extremity. The seizures most often occur during sleep; fewer than 25% of the seizures occur during wakefulness. Treatment can be delayed because many patients will not have more than 1–2, and remission of the epilepsy is expected.

Suggested Reading

- Bergqvist CA. Idiopathic pediatric epilepsy syndromes. Continuum Lifelong Learning Neurol 2007;13(4):106–20.

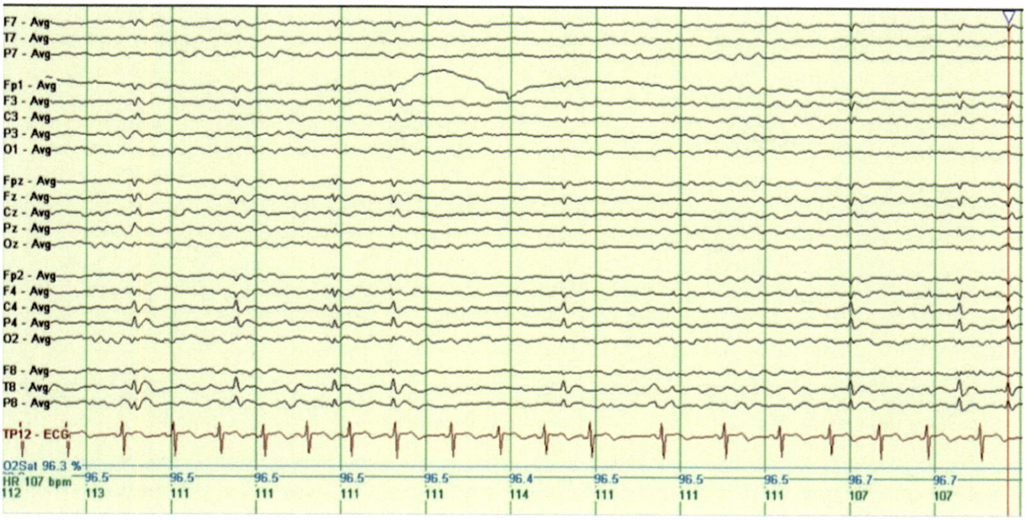

Fig. 8.33 With a permission from ▸ ILAE.org, Diagnostic Manual, and ▸ EpilepsyDiagnosis.org

36. A family of 5-month-old girl brought her because of recurrent episodes of abnormal movements, occur at sleep-wake transitions over the last 6 weeks. She has some mild gross motor milestones delay and she has been less active and visually attentive over the past 4 weeks. You reviewed a video recording brought by the family, shows a brief cluster episode of 3-second of head drop, arm and leg flexion associated with fussiness in between. The spells are not rhythmic, but are recurrent and stereotyped. Her general examination is normal, but her neurological exam showed poor ocular tracking, hypotonia in the neck and truncal muscles, with slightly brisk deep tendon reflexes. Brain MRI is normal. Her EEG is shown. **Which of the following statements is true regarding the treatment of this patient's condition according to a recent updated evidenced-based guideline from the American Academy of Neurology and the Child Neurology Society?**

A. high dose ACTH (150 IU/m2 qD) has clearly been shown to be superior compared to lower dosing regimens (20–30 IU qD)
B. this condition typically resolves without treatment by 2 years of age; therefore, patients should be spared the high likelihood of corticosteroid induced side effects and should only be treated if they develop other types of seizures
C. oral prednisone is more efficacious than injectable preparations of steroid treatment
D. pyridoxine (vitamin B_6) has been shown to be effective in the treatment of most patients with this condition
E. vigabatrin may be as effective as corticosteroids in the treatment of children with this condition, especially in symptomatic cases associated with tuberous sclerosis

Correct Answer is: E
Infantile spasms are a well-known age dependent seizure manifestation most often occurring in infants 4–12 months of age. Considered one of the earliest epileptic encephalopathies, developmental regression commonly occurs due to the

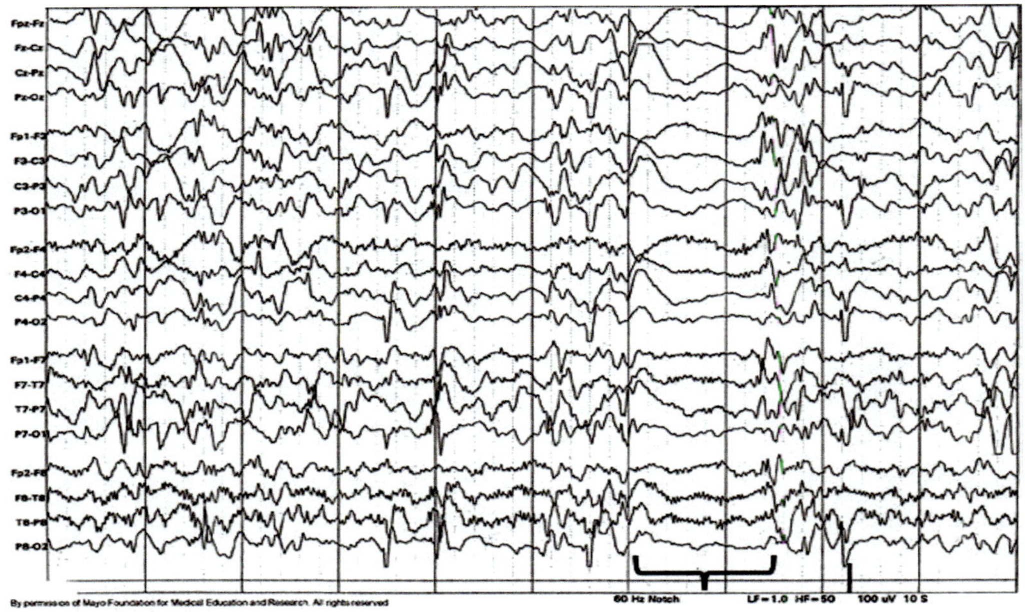

Fig. 8.34 Hypsarrhythmic EEG pattern in an infant with West syndrome. EEG of an 8-month-old infant with infantile spasms and developmental regression. An ictal electrodecremental response (black brackets) is seen during an epileptic spasm. Copyright 2013. Mayo Foundation for Medical Education and Research. All rights reserved. (Figure courtesy of Jeffrey W. Britton, MD Electroencephalography (EEG): An Introductory Text and Atlas of Normal and Abnormal Findings in Adults, Children, and Infants ISBN: 978-0-9979756-0-4, Copyright c2016 by American Epilepsy Society, 135 S. LaSalle St., Suite 2850, Chicago, IL 60603)

consistently abnormal EEG manifesting extremely high amplitude focal and generalized bursts of sharply contoured and spike activity, often intermixed with an electro-decremental response and disorganized background. Although the causes of infantile spasms are diverse, the clinical and electrographic features remain quite consistent. The events can be quite subtle at onset and often escape diagnosis for weeks to months. During this period of time there can also be loss of previously acquired milestones such as loss of head or trunk control, language abilities or visual attention. Although limited natural history studies show a spontaneous remission rate of spasms in up to 30% of cases, it has traditionally been accepted that prompt recognition and treatment of the spasms, as well as normalization of the EEG offers the best potential for long-term cognitive outcomes. The outcome, however, remains highly dependent on the etiology, with symptomatic causes (prior brain injury, CNS malformations, chromosomal and metabolic disorders) having a much higher risk of long-term intellectual disability and intractable epilepsy than the idiopathic cases. Even this last group, however, has nearly a 50–75% risk of long-term neurologic disability. Although practices vary greatly worldwide, corticosteroid treatment remains the mainstay for the majority of patients treated in developed countries. The recent 2012 updated guidelines from the AAN mention that amongst the steroid treatment options, injectable ACTH appears to have the best evidence,

though lower end dosing appears to be a very reasonable option. There was insufficient evidence to recommend using alternative oral or intravenous preparations as being as effective as ACTH for short-term treatment of spasms, though clearly individual case series have shown these agents to be potentially effective. Vigabatrin has also been recommended as a potential treatment, especially in the setting of symptomatic spasms associated with tuberous sclerosis. The evidence from the guideline suggests that ACTH may be more effective when considering all etiologic conditions. Although used as either initial therapy or as adjunctive treatment for refractory infantile spasms there remains insufficient evidence to recommend other therapies such as valproic acid, pyridoxine, levetiracetam, zonisamide, topiramate and the ketogenic diet.

Suggested Reading

- Go CY, MacKay MT, Weiss SK, et al. Evidence-based guideline update: Medical treatment of infantile spasms. Report of the Guideline Development Subcommittee of the American Academy of Neurology and the Practice Committee of the Child Neuro.

37. Spike and wave seizure-detection software has flagged this portion of an EEG recording.
 What is the most likely diagnosis?
 A. electrode pop artifact
 B. filtering artifact
 C. left parietal spike-and-wave discharge
 D. right parietal spike-and-wave discharge
 E. sneeze artifact

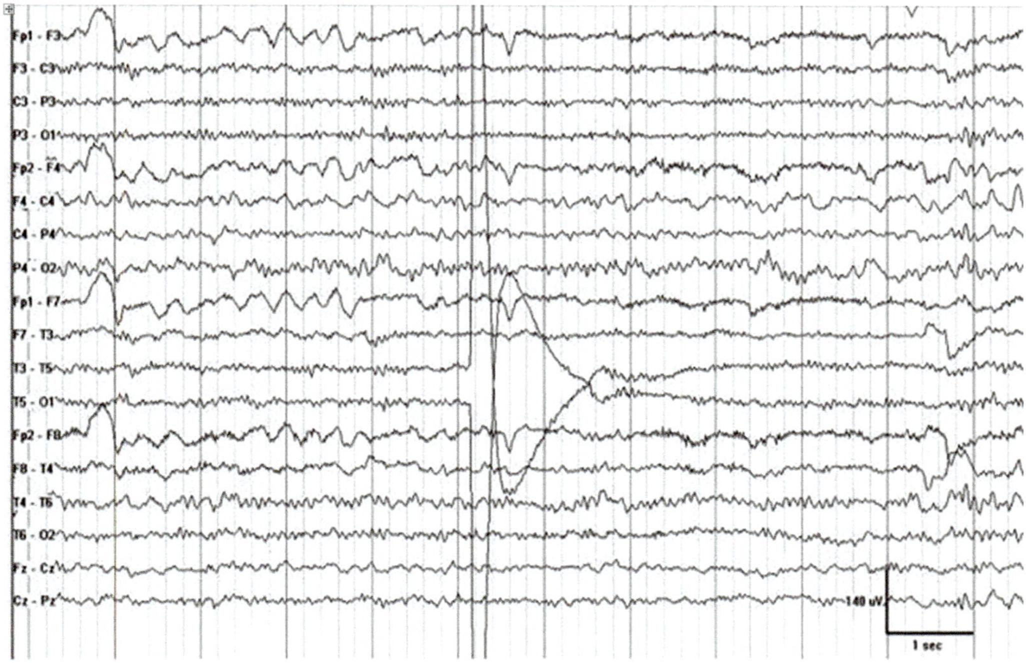

Fig. 8.35 American Academy of Neurology Institute, produced by permission

Correct Answer is: A
Any unusual waveform that is confined to a single or common electrode, as in this tracing at T5, must be considered artifactual. Note the sudden high amplitude deflection that involves only a single electrode. Epileptiform spike-and-wave discharges would be expected to demonstrate a phase reversal with involvement of adjacent electrodes. A sneeze, or other generalized bodily movement, would introduce generalized artifact. The deflection is not due to an incorrect filter setting since it affects only one electrode.

Suggested Reading

- Ebersole JS, Pedley TA. Current practice of clinical electroencephalography. 3rd ed. Philadelphia: Wolters Kluwer; 2003. 180 p. 282–3.

38. The EEG tracing shown is typical for which diagnoses?
   A. benign myoclonus of childhood
   B. childhood absence epilepsy
   C. infantile spasms (epileptic spasms)
   D. juvenile myoclonic epilepsy
   E. Landau-Kleffner syndrome

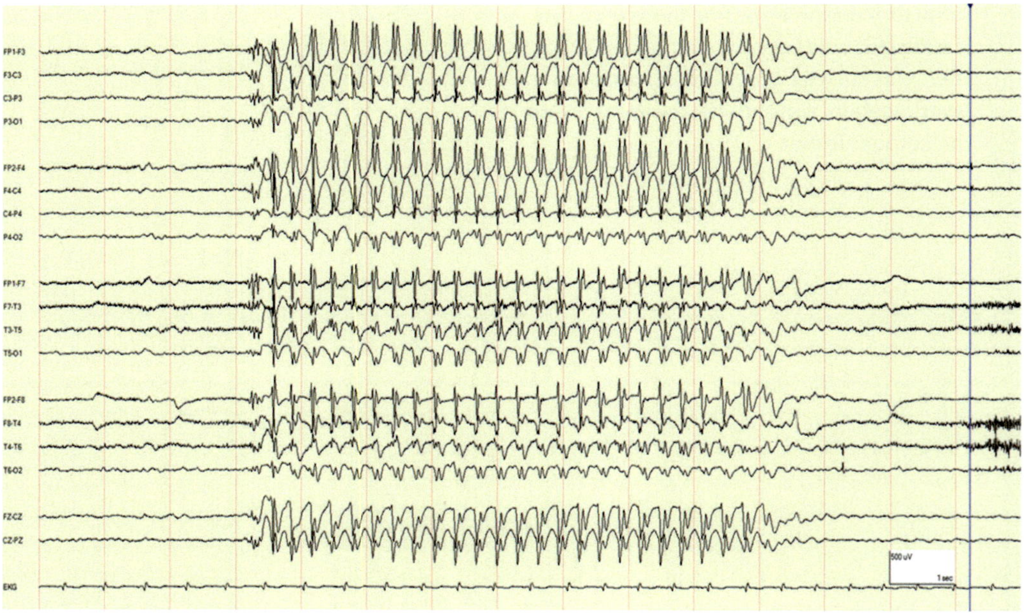

Fig. 8.36 With a permission from ▸ ILAE.org, Diagnostic Manual, and ▸ EpilepsyDiagnosis.org

Correct Answer is: C
The EEG shows hypsarrhythmia, which is characterized by a chaotic, high amplitude, asynchronous background. Generalized spike-wave activity, periods of focal or generalized voltage attenuation or focal spike-wave activity may be present in the recording. Hypsarrhythmia is associated with infantile spasms (epileptic spasms), which typically have an age of onset of 4–7 months old.

Suggested Reading

- Ebersole JS, Pedley TA, editors. Current practice of clinical electroencephalography. 3rd ed. Philadelphia: Lippincott, Williams & Wilkins; 2003.

39. A 6 -year-old female complains of spells characterized by staring, eye flutter, and unresponsiveness lasting 5–10 s. Her EEG is shown.
What is the most likely diagnosis?
   A. benign rolandic epilepsy of childhood
   B. childhood absence epilepsy
   C. juvenile absence epilepsy
   D. juvenile myoclonic epilepsy
   E. Lennox-Gastaut syndrome

Correct Answer is: B
The clinical scenario indicates absence seizures. The EEG shows a 3 Hz generalized spike-wave pattern, which is classic for absence seizures. Childhood absence epilepsy begins before age 8.

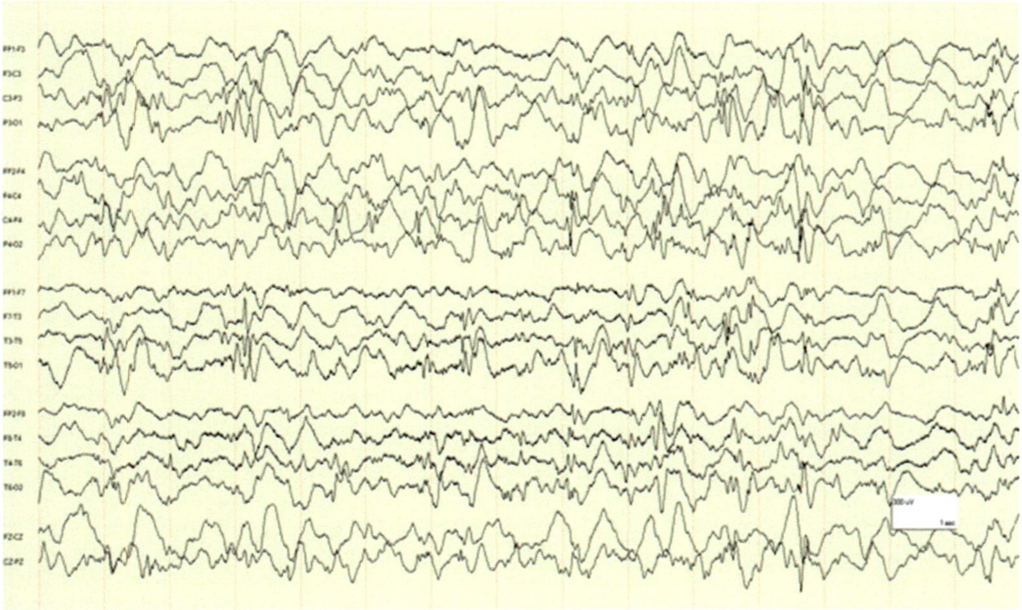

Fig. 8.37 With a permission from ▶ ILAE.org, Diagnostic Manual, and ▶ EpilepsyDiagnosis.org

Suggested Reading

- Rudzinski LA, Shih JJ. The classification of seizures and epilepsy syndromes. Continuum Lifelong Learning Neurol. 2010;16(3):15–35.

40. The EEG tracing shown demonstrates which of the following findings?
   A. cerebral sharp waves
   B. electrocardiogram artifact
   C. periodic lateralized epileptiform discharges
   D. periodic spike-wave discharges
   E. pseudoperiodic lateralized epileptiform discharges

Correct Answer is: B
The electrocardiogram (EKG) shown was recorded at the scalp and represents a far field potential, most often seen in referential montages. Note that the sharply contoured waveforms are uniform across the cerebral hemisphere and are time locked with the R-R intervals in the EKG tracing at the bottom of the image. EKG artifact can mimic cerebral sharp waves or spikes and are distinguished from them by the distribution and timing.

Suggested Reading

- Ebersole JS, Pedley TA. Current practice of clinical electroencephalography. 3rd ed. Philadelphia: Wolters Kluwer; 2003. p. 275–6.

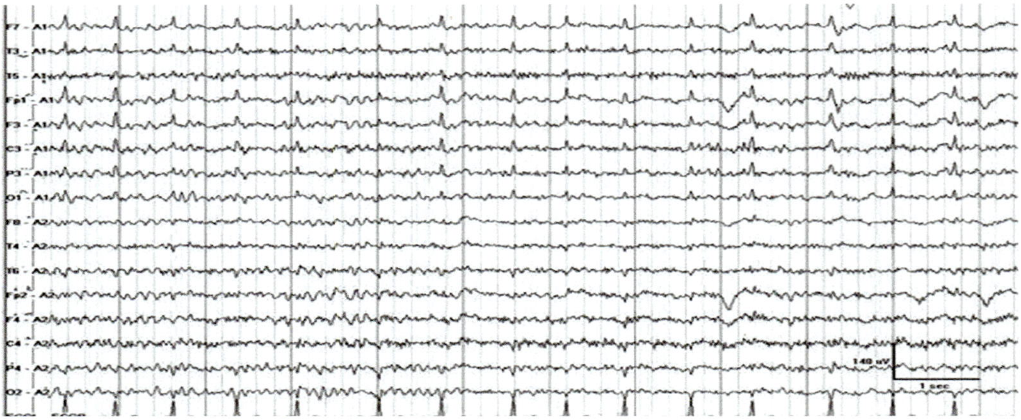

Fig. 8.38 American Academy of Neurology Institute, produced by permission

41. In a 2-week-old full term neonate, the trace alternant pattern is seen during which of the following states?
    - A. active sleep
    - B. quiet sleep
    - C. tonic seizures
    - D. transition from active sleep to wakefulness
    - E. wakefulness

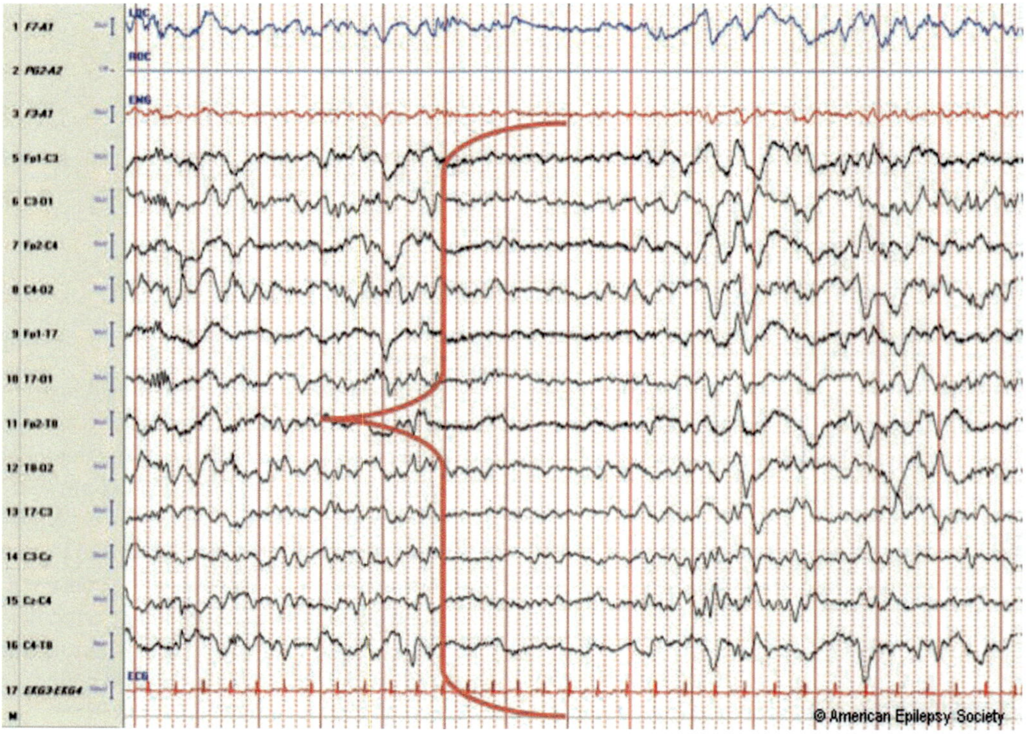

Fig. 8.39 Trace alternant. This is a neonatal EEG sample of a 25-day-old girl born at 39 weeks GA. The sample shows a segment of quiet sleep with trace alternant. (Figure courtesy of Elia M. Pestana-Knight, MD, Cleveland Clinic Foundation Electroencephalography (EEG): An Introductory Text and Atlas of Normal and Abnormal Findings in Adults, Children, and Infants ISBN: 978-0-9979756-0-4, Copyright c2016 by American Epilepsy Society, 135 S. LaSalle St., Suite 2850, Chicago, IL 60603)

Correct Answer is: B
In the term or immediate post-term neonate, the trace alternant pattern is a normal sleep pattern present only in quiet sleep.

Suggested Reading

- Ebersole JS, Pedley TA, editors. Current practice of clinical electroencephalography. 3rd ed. Philadelpia: Lippincott Williams & Wilkins, 2003. p. 183–5.

42. The tracing shown represents which of the following?
    A. 6 Hz spike-and-wave
    B. sleep spindles
    C. small sharp spikes
    D. temporal intermittent rhythmic delta activity (TIRDA)
    E. wicket waves

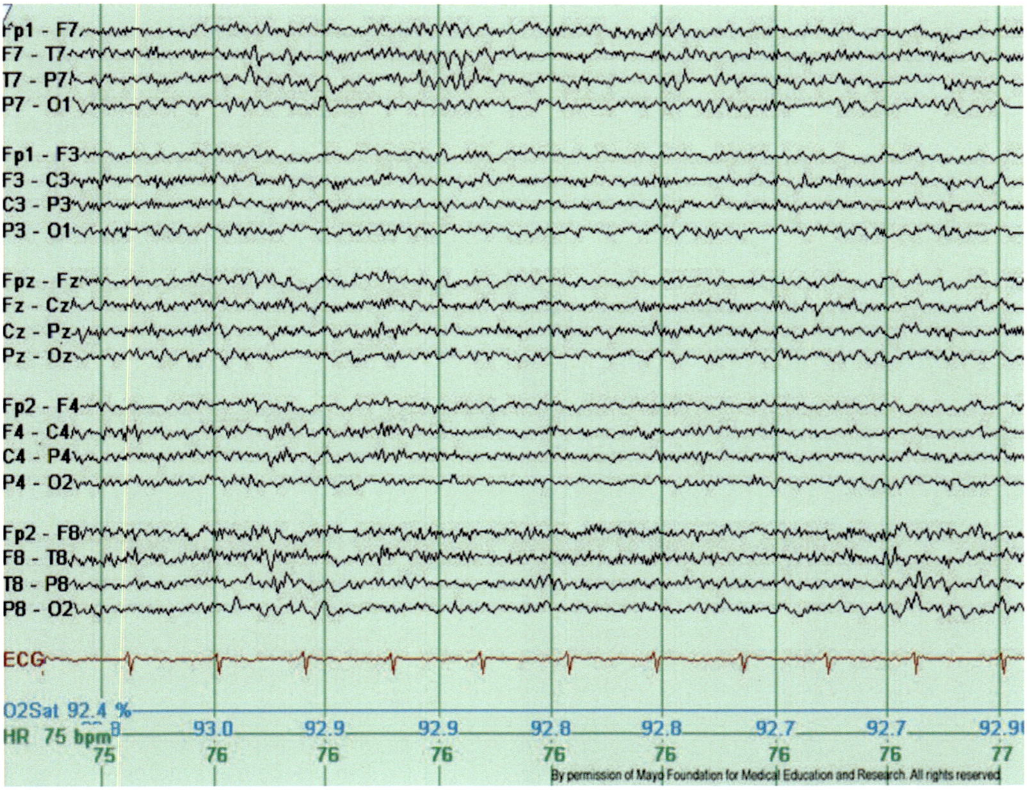

Fig. 8.40 Typical wicket waves. Note the arciform appearance, lack of after-going slow wave, and lack of background disruption or disturbance. The wicket waves are seen in the left temporal region with phase-reversal at T7 in seconds 3 and 4 of the tracing, longitudinal bipolar montage. Copyright 2013. Mayo Foundation for Medical Education and Research. All rights reserved. (Figure courtesy of Jeffrey W. Britton, MD.Electroencephalography (EEG): An Introductory Text and Atlas of Normal and Abnormal Findings in Adults, Children, and Infants ISBN: 978-0-9979756-0-4, Copyright c2016 by American Epilepsy Society, 135 S. LaSalle St., Suite 2850, Chicago, IL 60603)

Correct Answer is: E
Wicket waves are a benign variant often seen during drowsiness and light sleep in adults. It is one of the benign variants most commonly mistaken for epileptiform discharges. They are typically mid-temporal, 5–11 Hz, and typically occur in bursts. There is no focal slowing or slow wave component.

Suggested Reading

- Tatum WO, Husain AM, Benbadis SR, Kaplan PW. Normal adult EEG and patterns of uncertain significance. J Clin Neurophysiol. 2006;23:194–207.

43. A 7-year-old female came for an evaluation for her inappropriate and uncontrollable laughing spells for 2 years. She has features of precocious puberty. Video/EEG monitoring was ordered and captured multiple laughing fits. During laughing, the ictal EEG showed a diffuse suppression of background rhythm; MRI is shown.
    What is the etiology of her events?
    A. cordoma
    B. frontal lobe epilepsy
    C. hypothalamic hamartoma
    D. psychogenic
    E. skull base meningioma

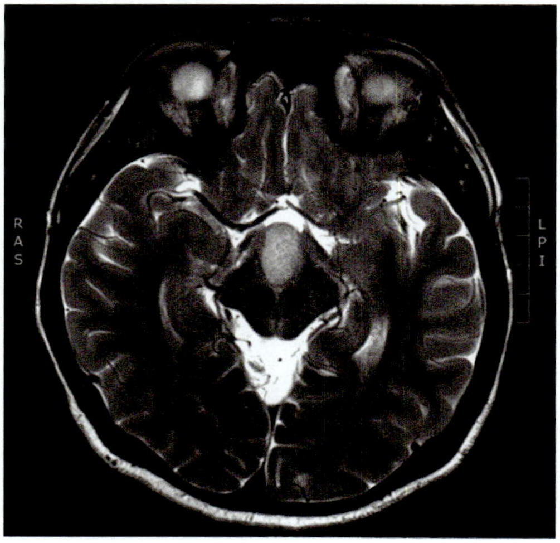

Fig. 8.41 With a permission from ► ILAE.org, Diagnostic Manual, and ► EpilepsyDiagnosis.org

Correct Answer is: C
The clinical and radiographic features are of the syndrome of hypothalamic hamartoma with epilepsy. This diagnosis is often quite devastating, with varying degrees of mental retardation and, often, multiple seizure types that are often refractory, including the well described gelastic seizures (associated with ictal laughter). Gelastic seizures are particularly associated with hypothalamic lesions, which may project seizure discharges to various parts of the cortex, but it can be seen in cortical epilepsy. In fact, it may be very challenging to demonstrate clear ictal evolution during a scalp EEG recording (as noted in the case above, where only diffuse suppression of the waking background is noted), depth electrodes may be required to better characterize the ictal pattern. Surgery in the vicinity of the hypothalamus is very hazardous as it can be very disruptive of many critical neuroendocrine pathways, though more selective radiosurgery offers promise of a slightly safer intervention strategy

Suggested Reading

- Berkovic SF, Azrimanoglou A, Kuzniecky R, et al. Hypothalamic hamartoma and seizures: a treatable epileptic encephalopathy. Epilepsia. 2003;44(7):969–73.

44. A 5-year-old female with a history of occasional spells of lip and right hand clonic movements for few seconds and she cannot talk during those spells and accompanied with drooling as well. Her medical history is unremarkable. She is a good student with no learning difficulties. Her brain MRI is normal. Her EEG is shown.
    What is your diagnosis?
    A. Benign Rolandic epilepsy
    B. Landau-Kleffner syndrome
    C. Panayiotopoulos syndrome
    D. Rett syndrome
    E. Right mesial temporal sclerosis

Correct Answer is: A
The EEG shows benign childhood epilepsy with centrotemporal spikes (BECTS). The location of the epileptiform discharges (central and temporal) and morphology (polyphasic dipole tangential to the rolandic region) are characteristic. BECTS is the most common partial epilepsy of

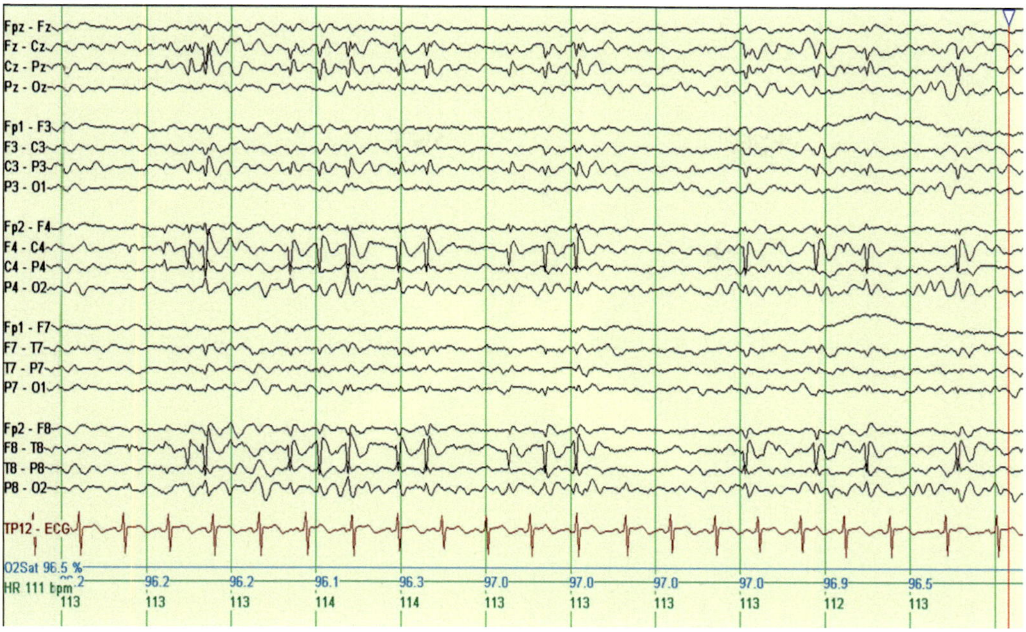

Fig. 8.42 With a permission from ► ILAE.org, Diagnostic Manual, and ► EpilepsyDiagnosis.org

childhood, accounting for approximately 2/3 of all idiopathic focal epilepsies of childhood. The onset is 5–8 years of age. Focal motor seizures are the most common seizure type and are often unilateral, involving the face, oropharynx and upper extremity. The seizures most often occur during sleep; fewer than 25% of the seizures occur during wakefulness. Treatment can be delayed because many patients will not have more than 1 to 2, and remission of the epilepsy is expected.

Panayiotopoulos syndrome is a benign occipital onset epilepsy in early childhood, with interictal discharges in the posterior brain regions and clinical semiology of ictal vomiting, and eye version with complex partial or secondary generalized seizures. Landau-Kleffner syndrome is one of the pediatric epileptic encephalopathies, where dramatic language regression accompanies seizures, and an EEG that shows nearly continuous epileptiform activity in slow wave sleep.

Rett syndrome would not be suggested in a typically developing child and a normal MRI and bilaterally independent discharges would not suggest a diagnosis of right sided mesial temporal sclerosis.

Suggested Reading

Wirrell E, Nickels K. Pediatric epilepsy syndromes. Continuum: Lifelong Learning Neurol. 2010;16(3): 57–85.

45. A previously healthy 8-month old infant boy came with his mother to see you for recurrent clusters of sudden flexion at the trunk and neck with arms extension spells. They last for 1–2 s and occur in multiple times a day. They have increased in frequency in the last month and he starts to struggle to sit up and does not babble as often. EEG and MRI are shown.
What is the most likely etiology?
A. Tuberous sclerosis
B. Down Syndrome
C. Trauma
D. Mitochondrial disease
E. Infection

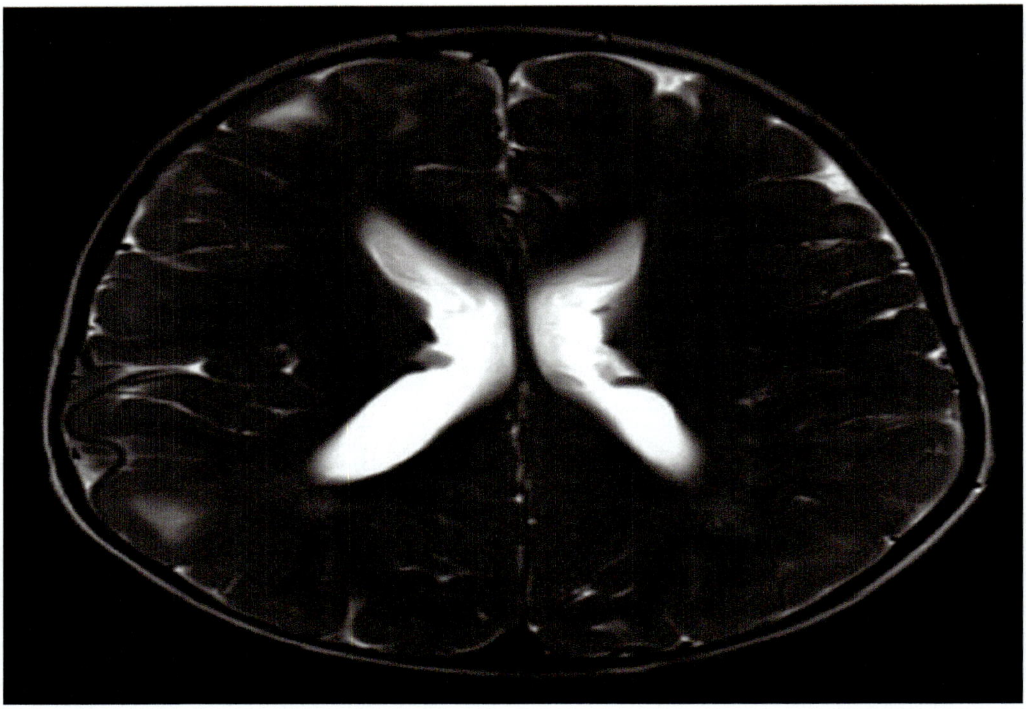

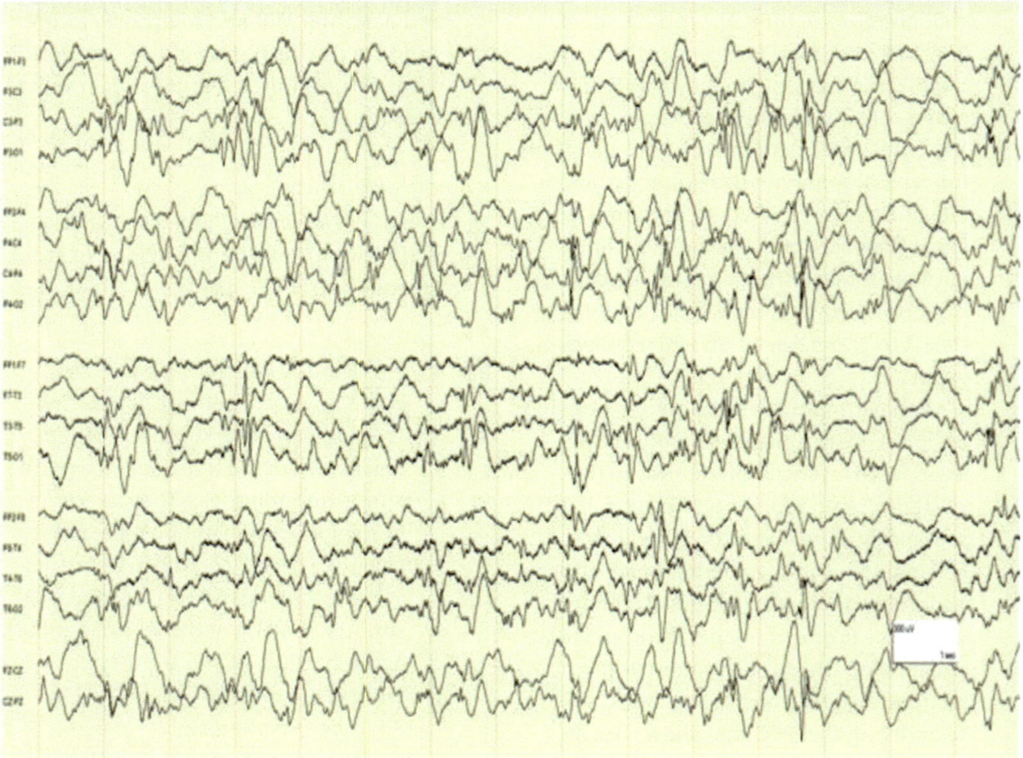

Figs. 8.43 and 8.44 With a permission from ► ILAE.org, Diagnostic Manual, and ► EpilepsyDiagnosis.org

Correct Answer is: A
This is a case of infantile spasms, which can have many different etiologies. The EEG shows slow disorganized background and continuous high amplitude polymorphic generalized slowing and multifocal spikes which is consistent hypsarrhythmia. West syndrome is the triad of infantile spasms, hypsarrhythmia and developmental delay. West syndrome has many different etiologies as well. Approximately 70% of patients with West syndrome have abnormal MRI findings. The most common etiology is tuberous sclerosis as seen in this MRI. The MRI shows multiple focal areas of broadened gyri, blurring of the gray-white junction and increased signal in the subcortical white matter typical of cortical tubers. There are also subependymal nodules consistent with sub-ependymal hamartomas.

Suggested Reading

- ► http://journals.lww.com/continuum/Fulltext/2015/04000/BenignBrainTumorsandTumorsAssociatedWith.12.aspx.

46. A 7 y7-year-oldy just moved with his family to your area. His family brought a previous CT to the visit (see figure).
    Which of the following features, if present, would be most specific in making a definitive diagnosis?
    A. Autosomal recessive inheritance pattern
    B. Facial capillary malformation
    C. Failure to meet developmental milestones in the first few months of life
    D. Retinal astrocytoma on dilated eye exam
    E. Seizures in the first year of life

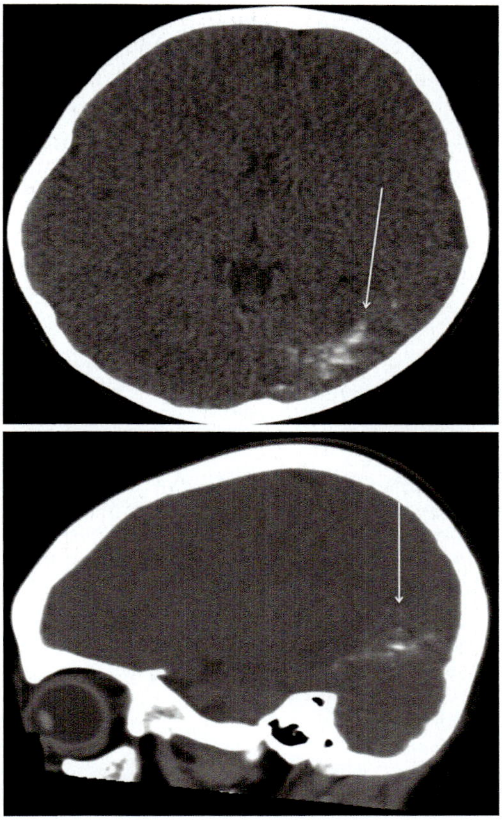

Figs. 8.45 and 8.46 With a permission from ► ILAE.org, Diagnostic Manual, and ► EpilepsyDiagnosis.org

Correct Answer is: B
The MRI shows right parieto-occipital pial enhancement, gyral calcifications, and atrophy consistent with leptomeningeal capillary-venous malformation. The presence of facial capillary malformation (a port wine stain) in the 1st or 2nd division of the trigeminal nerve in this setting would be diagnostic of Sturge-Weber syndrome (SWS). This neuro-cutaneous finding is typically ipsilateral to the cerebral vascular malformation. An autosomal dominant inheritance pattern would be atypical. SWS, although congenital, is a sporadic disease and so unlikely to occur in siblings or offspring of affected individuals.

Glaucoma is a common but inconsistent feature of SWS, occurring in 30–70% of patients with SWS. Glaucoma may be congenital or develop later in life. In the rare patient without facial capillary malformation, the presence of glaucoma

and typical MRI pattern is highly suggestive of SWS. Retinal astrocytoma is seen in patients with tuberous sclerosis, not SWS.

Though seizures and developmental delay occur commonly in patients with SWS, (with 95% having developed seizures by age five), neither are specific to SWS and may occur in a multitude of congenital and developmental diseases.

Suggested Reading

- Thomas-Sohl KA, Vaslow DF, Maria BL. Sturge-Weber syndrome: a review. Pediatr Neurol. 2004;30(5):303–10.

47. The tracing shown is recorded initially while the patient is reading. Beside the eye closure. What another wave is presented here?

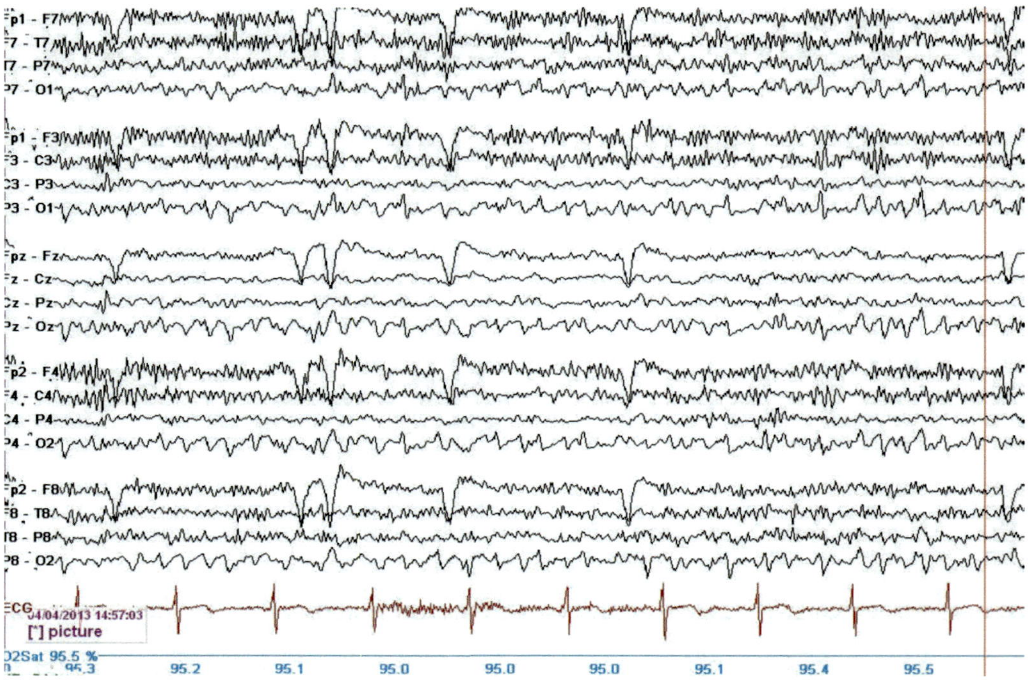

Fig. 8.47 Lambda waves. Lambda waves over posterior head regions, elicited by complex pattern viewing. Note the surface positive waveforms over both occipital regions. Longitudinal bipolar montage. Copyright 2013. Mayo Foundation for Medical Education and Research. All rights reserved. (Figure courtesy of Jeffrey W. Britton, MDElectroencephalography (EEG): An Introductory Text and Atlas of Normal and Abnormal Findings in Adults, Children, and Infants ISBN: 978-0-9,979,756-0-4, Copyright c2016 by American Epilepsy Society, 135 S. LaSalle St., Suite 2850, Chicago, IL 60603)

A. benign lambda waves
B. benign small sharp spikes
C. benign vertex waves ("V waves")
D. epileptiform lambda waves
E. epileptiform sharp waves

Correct Answer is: A
Although sharply contoured, lambda waves are a normal finding and occur in occipital leads when the subject is scanning with rapid saccadic eye movements

such as during reading. They are surface positive and occur bilaterally. They can be asymmetric and easily misinterpreted as epileptiform discharges. They are not associated with epilepsy, and they do not occur over the vertex. They can be abolished by closing the eyes or eliminating the visual stimulus producing them.

Suggested Reading

- Tatum WO, Husain AM, Benbadis SR, Kaplan PW. Normal adult EEG and patterns of uncertain significance. J Clin Neurophysiol. 2006;23:194–207.

Epilepsy 2

Y. M. Awaad, *Absolute Pediatric Neurology*, https://doi.org/10.1007/978-3-319-78801-2_9

1. You have been consulted on an actively seizing 16-month-old boy brought to the ED with a fever of 104 °f. He has been seizing for approximately 30 min despite his family gave him 0.5 mg/kg diazepam rectally prior to the arrival of EMS and he received another 0.3 mg/kg diazepam intravenously upon arrival to the ED. The seizure ultimately stopped after he was given a 20 mg/kg load of intravenous phenobarbital. Past medical history is remarkable for a prior self-limited febrile seizure at age 12 months, and a paternal cousin with a febrile seizures in. He has a normal developmental milestone.

Which statement below is correct?

A. At the time of discharge, this child should be sent home with rectal diazepam due to a high risk of developing recurrent febrile status epilepticus.
B. Due to the risk of respiratory suppression with the combination of benzodiazepines and barbiturates, intravenous fosphenytoin should have been used to break the seizure as opposed to intravenous phenobarbital.
C. An EEG should be performed due to this child's increased risk of developing epilepsy.
D. The parents of this child should be counseled about seizure management as this patient has an approximately 30% risk of febrile seizure recurrence.
E. This child should be sent home on maintenance phenobarbital due to his increased risk of neurological morbidity due to his febrile status epilepticus.

Correct Answer is: D
There is no increased risk of death or neurological morbidity in neurologically and developmentally normal children with febrile status epilepticus compared to children with simple febrile seizures. Also, there is no increased risk for epilepsy or for recurrent febrile seizures or febrile status epilepticus. On the other hand, children with preexisting neurological deficits have a much higher risk of recurrent febrile status epilepticus and rescue medicine should be considered. It has also been shown that intravenous phenytoin is much less effective in aborting status epilepticus than intravenous phenobarbital.

Suggested Reading

- Ismail S, Levy A, Tikkanen H, et al. Lack of efficacy of phenytoin in children presenting with febrile status epilepticus. Am J Emerg Med. 2012;30(9):2000–4.
- Maytal J, Shinnar S. Febrile status epilepticus. Pediatrics. 1990;86(4):611–6.

2. A 4-year-old girl came with her adoptive mother for evaluation of frequent brief episodes of shaking-type movements affecting her limbs and trunk and often causing falls. There is no loss of consciousness with these episodes and no apparent aura or post-ictal state following. They occur multiple times per day and they are a couple of seconds in duration, though longer episodes have also been recorded. On examination, she has normal tone, plantar flexor responses, and easily elicitable DTR's. There was no tremor or ataxia. There were no involuntary movements seen.

The next step in her diagnostic evaluation should be:

A. Trial of low-dose carbamazepine
B. Overnight video EEG to get an ictal recording
C. Asking the father to record the events on home video
D. Answers B and C
E. Any of the above (A, B, or C)

Correct Answer is: E

The clinical presentation looks like a paroxysmal movement disorder that was not directly witnessed in the office, with an essentially normal neurological examination. Paroxysmal events may include seizures, migraine, Channelopathies, behavioral, or involuntary movements. Because the short duration of these patients' events, an ictal EEG recording may be helpful for eliminating seizures. Video clips brought by the family of their children when they are having an event can be extremely useful. The neurologist will be able to actually see the details of the events in "real time" instead of just creating a mental image of the event from the family's history. Given the age of onset and details of her spells, it is highly likely that she has paroxysmal kinesiogenic choreoathetosis. So forth, a diagnostic trial of low dose carbamazepine (other anticonvulsants have also been successfully used) is also a reasonable approach. Autosomal dominant familial paroxysmal choreoathetosis has been linked in many families to mutations in the PRRT2 gene on chromosome 16q11.2-q12.1. The disorder is autosomal dominant with variable penetrance. As this child was adopted, her family history, which may also be helpful with defining the cause of the movement disorder, was unknown.

Suggested Reading

- Bhatia KP. Familial (idiopathic) paroxysmal dyskinesias. Semm Neurol. 2001;21:69–74.
- Erro R, Sheerin UM, Bhatia KP. Paroxysmal dyskinesias revisited: a review of 500 genetically proven cases and a new classification. Mov Disord. 2014;29(9):1108–16.

3. You have been consulted on a full term 10 days old male infant in the NICU, who has multiple refractory focal motor and tonic seizures. He is receiving intravenous phenobarbital and levetiracetam with high therapeutic levels and oral pyridoxine at 30/mg/kg/day QID. To protect the child against central apnea, the child is also receiving oral caffeine. Yet despite these interventions, the infant is still having multiple daily seizures often associated with oxygen desaturations. The neonatologists ordered a brain MRI which is normal as well as a lumbar puncture with 12 WBC's, protein of 60 mg/dl, glucose of 42 mg/dl with a serum glucose of 80 mg/dl. Gram stain and cultures are both negative. The child is receiving ampicillin, cefotaxime and acyclovir as prophylaxis for a possible CNS infection and the child's newborn screen results are normal. You are considering glucose transporter deficiency and are considering initiation of the ketogenic diet. **What other interventions should be undertaken to help control this patient's epilepsy?**

   A. Add intravenous Valproic acid.
   B. Discontinue the levetiracetam.
   C. Discontinue the phenobarbital and caffeine.
   D. Increase the serum glucose concentration by using 15% dextrose intravenous fluids to overcome the relatively low CSF glucose concentrations.
   E. Perform another lumbar puncture to measure CSF and concurrent glucose levels since the first results were borderline.

Correct Answer is: C

The clinical presentation meets diagnostic criteria for glucose transporter deficiency with a CSF glucose of 42 mg/dl. In 90% of patients with Glucosec-1 transporter deficiency (GluT1DS) CSF glucose concentrations is below 40 mg/dl, the other 10% have glucose concentrations between 40 and 60 mg/dl. Also,

while this patient's CSF/serum ratio is 0.51 and above the typical cut-off value of less than 0.4, total CSF glucose concentrations have been found to be more reliable in diagnosing GluT1DS than just the ratio. The ketogenic diet is the treatment of choice for patients with GluT1DS as the result is to create ketone bodies that use a different transporter system to cross the blood-brain-barrier and provide an alternative energy source for neurons. Medications such as barbiturates, Valproic acid, benzodiazepines and methylxanthines should be avoided in patients with GluT1DS as they tend to competitively inhibit the brain glucose transporter.

Suggested Reading

- De Giorgis V, Veggiotti P. GLUT1 deficiency syndrome 2013: current state of the art. Seizure. 2013;22(10):803–11. ► https://doi.org/10.1016/j.seizure.2013.07.003. Epub 2013 Jul 26. Review.
- Wang D, Pascual JM, DeVivo D. Glucose Transporter Type 1 Deficiency Syndrome. In: Pagon RA, Adam MP, Ardinger HH, Bird TD, Dolan CR, Fong CT, Smith RJH, Stephens K, editors. GeneReviews® [Internet]. Seattle: University of Washington, Seattle; 1993–2014. 2002 Jul 30 [updated 2012 Aug 09].

9

4. A 17-year-old female came to your office with a history of migraine headaches and epilepsy. She was diagnosed with generalized anxiety disorder and has been taking paroxetine 40 mg per day for the past 9 months which has helped with her symptoms. Currently she has daily migraine headaches. She had her second convulsive seizure 3 months ago. Her PCP prescribed topiramate, 50 mg once a day, 2 weeks ago in an attempt to treat both her epilepsy and migraine headaches while the patient was waiting for a neurology appointment. One day before her scheduled office visit with you, she developed one of her usual headaches associated with blurry vision as well as severe nausea. On examination, the patient's visual acuity is 20/200 OU at 20 feet and 20/40 OU at near. Fundoscopic examination and her extraocular movements are normal. The rest of her neurological examination is normal.

At this time, the best course of action should be to:

A. Add acetazolamide to the topiramate to treat presumptive benign intracranial hypertension without papilledema.
B. Increase the topiramate to 100 mg twice a day to get her in the therapeutic range for epilepsy.
C. Schedule her for an outpatient optometrist visit to evaluate her for glasses.
D. Immediately discontinue the topiramate and arrange for an urgent ophthalmology consultation through the emergency room.
E. Given her past psychiatric history, diagnose her with conversion disorder and schedule her for an outpatient psychology evaluation.

Correct Answer is: D

The clinical scenario is of bilateral acute angle closure glaucoma (AACG). This idiosyncratic side effect of topiramate usually occurs around 2 weeks after starting the medication. The mechanism of action is believed to be secondary to ciliary body edema which then results in anterior displacement of the iris and closure of the anterior chamber angle of the eye. Symptoms are blurred vision and myopia with or without ocular pain and/or conjunctival injection. SSRI's given concurrently with topiramate,

may help precipitate (AACG) by adding an element of pupillary block. The first step to treat AACG is the immediate discontinuation of the topiramate and in some cases, the addition of cycloplegia (atropine drops) and intravenous methylprednisone.

Suggested Reading

- Boentert M, Aretz H, Ludemann P. Acute myopia and angle closure glaucoma induced by topiramate. Neurology 2003;61(9):1306.
- Rhee DJ, Goldberg MJ, Parish RK. Bilateral angle closure glaucoma and ciliary body swelling from topiramate. Arch Opthalmol. 2001;119(11):1721–3.

5. You are evaluating a developmentally normal 14-year-old female in the ED who was found by her mother earlier that morning to be convulsing for approximately 3 min. She returned to her baseline after being sleep and ataxic for 1 h after the seizure. There is no family history of epilepsy. She reports that she has not been allowed to drive to school for the last 3 months due to frequent whole-body jerks that seem to be triggered by flickering morning sunshine. Her EEG performed in the ED shows a normal background with rare occipital sharp waves. During photic stimulation, occipital paroxysms of high voltage spike and polyspike complexes are seen as well as more generalized polyspike and wave discharges.
The best management strategy at this point is:
   A. Load her with phenobarbital until the occipital epileptiform discharges abate.
   B. Do not start anticonvulsants since she has had only one seizure and her risk for recurrence is low.
   C. Allow her to drive under the condition that she wears sunglasses.
   D. Order visual evoked potentials to look for optic pathway electrical conductance problems.
   E. Start her on sodium valproate with 4 mg of folic acid and counsel her about pregnancy risks.

Correct Answer is: E
Idiopathic photosensitive occipital lobe epilepsies show hallmark EEG findings of occipital epileptiform discharges and photosensitivity. They are classified as either focal or generalized depending on the semiology of the seizures. Seizure types may include multicolored visual hallucinations with associated blindness, autonomic symptoms such as retching and ictal vomiting, myoclonic jerks, absence seizures and generalized convulsive seizures. Watching video games or flickering lights can trigger these seizures. EEG may show occipital paroxysms of spikes or polyspikes or more generalized photoparoxysmal responses. Given this patient's generalized photoparoxysmal discharges and her history of photic-induced myoclonic seizures, it would be wise to start her on a broad-spectrum anticonvulsant and restrict her driving privileges until she remains seizure-free and myoclonic jerk-free for 6 months. Polarized sunglasses may be useful for patients with photic-induced seizures.

Suggested Reading

- Guerrini R, Dravet C, Genton P, et al. Idiopathic photosensitive occipital lobe epilepsy. Epilepsia. 1995;36:883–91.
- Panayiotopoulos CP. Benign childhood partial seizures and related epileptic syndromes. London:John Libby and Company Ltd.; 1999.

6. What is the correct statement about Panayiotopoulos syndrome?
   A. Seizures are frequent
   B. There is focal slowing consistently over one area
   C. Head imaging is required to make the diagnosis
   D. Autonomic features are required for the diagnosis

Correct Answer is: D
The onset of Panayiotopoulos syndrome is usually in the early childhood of autonomic seizures that are often prolonged. The EEG commonly shows high amplitude focal spikes and may be activated by sleep. Seizures are infrequent in most patients, with 25% only having a single seizure (which may be autonomic status epilepticus) and 50% having six seizures or less. Seizures are self-limiting with remission typically within a few years from onset.

10% of patients have a normal single routine EEG. Multifocal high voltage repetitive spikes or sharp and slow-waves are seen in 90% of patients, these often are present in different focal areas on sequential EEGs. All focal brain regions may be affected but posterior regions is commonly affected, with occipital spikes seen on EEG in 60% of patients. Low voltage spikes and generalized discharges may be seen in a minority of cases.

Focal slowing consistently over one area is not seen; therefore, if present consider structural brain abnormality.

Neuroimaging is usually normal. If the diagnosis of Panayiotopoulos syndrome has been made and there are no atypical features, neuroimaging is not necessary.

The mandatory seizure type for this syndrome is the presence of seizures with prominent autonomic features mainly emetic (nausea, retching, vomiting) but pupillary (mydriasis), circulatory (pallor, cyanosis), thermoregulatory and cardiorespiratory (heart and respiratory rate disturbances) changes also occur.

Suggested Reading

- International League Against Epilepsy.
- ► https://www.epilepsydiagnosis.org/syndrome/panayiotopoulos-overview.html.

7. A 6-year-old boy with autistic behaviors came for an evaluation. He has a normal developmental history, his difficulties started around 4 years of age when he stopped responding to his name being called. Eventually he developed severe global aphasia with mutism as well as hyperactive and aggressive behavior. He has no history of seizure. He is on a combination of risperidone and clonidine which do not seem to be very helpful in controlling his behavior. His sedated EEG shows multifocal and bisynchronous posterior temporal sharp and slow wave complexes that activate during sleep.
   The next step in his management should be to:
   A. Obtain a high-resolution MRI of the brain.
   B. Start oxcarbazepine to treat the interictal epileptiform discharges.
   C. Add a stimulant medication to help control his hyperactivity.
   D. Start the child on high-dose ACTH therapy.
   E. Consider a trial of sodium valproate and/or clobazam therapy.

Correct Answer is: E
The clinical history of subacute regression in speech and language, including acquired auditory agnosia, after 3 years of age with previously normal social and language development is strongly suggestive of Landau-Kleffner syndrome. LKS is much less common than autistic spectrum disorders which begin prior

to 3 years of age with delayed development of language and social skills. 75% patients with LKS experiences seizures; generally frontal lobe complex partial seizures or secondarily generalized convulsive, but 25% never have any seizures. Interictal EEG in the awake state may be normal or show posterior temporal epileptiform discharges that may be bisynchronous or multifocal. The discharges increase in frequency during sleep. Slow wave sleep is not necessary to obtain a diagnosis of LKS, although it is necessary to diagnose epilepsy with continuous spike and waves during slow wave sleep. First-line agents such as sodium valproate, benzodiazepines, or ethosuximide should be used first in the treatment of LKS, but they are often not effective in improving language and cognitive functioning. Second line treatment is high dose oral steroids for at least 3 months or a trial of ACTH. The monitoring of any treatment modality should include serial neurocognitive testing as well as awake and sleep EEG.

Suggested Reading

- Lerman P, Lerman-Sagie T, Kivity, S. Effect of early corticosteroid therapy for Landau-Kleffner Syndrome. Dev Med Child Neuro. 1991;33(3): 257–60.
- Smith M, Hoeppner TJ. Epileptic encephalopathy of late childhood: Landau-Kleffner syndrome and the syndrome of continuous spikes and waves during slow-wave sleep. J Clin Neurophysiol. 2003;20(6):462–72.

8. Epilepsy syndromes can present in infancy and childhood with comorbid intellectual disability. Genetic defects have been identified in several syndromes.
   Which epilepsy syndrome-gene defect pair is incorrect?
   A. Severe myoclonic epilepsy of childhood (SMEI) – SLC21A
   B. X-linked West Syndrome – ARX
   C. Rett syndrome variant with intractable epilepsy – CDKL5
   D. Glut1 deficiency – SCN1A
   E. A and D

Correct Answer is: E
A number of distinct clinical syndromes of pediatric genetic epilepsy have been described and linked to specific gene defects. Phenotypes may include, in addition to epilepsy, variable degrees of intellectual disability, elements of autism spectrum disorders, other psychiatric disorders, and motor impairment.

Severe myoclonic epilepsy of infancy (SMEI) is characterized by early-onset generalized febrile seizures, followed by very frequent afebrile generalized tonic–clonic seizures (GTCS), myoclonic seizures, absences and focal seizures, with stagnation of psychomotor development, intellectual disability and motor impairment. The main genes involved in these conditions encode sodium channel subunits, in particular *SCN1A*, which is mutated in 61–87% of SMEI.

West syndrome is a common severe infantile epileptic syndrome characterized by typical brief tonic spasms, a profoundly abnormal electroencephalography pattern called hypsarrhythmia, and intellectual disability. Early infantile epileptic encephalopathy with suppression-burst (EIEE) is the earliest infantile epileptic syndrome, often evolving to West syndrome. Mutations in the X chromosome genes *ARX* and *CDKL5* are found in some X-linked West syndrome cases (ISSX1 and ISSX2). ARX (Aristaless-related homeobox) is a transcription factor involved in brain development. It is frequently mutated in a spectrum of X chromosome-linked phenotypes characterized by intellectual disability as their cardinal feature.

CDKL5 mutations are associated with West syndrome, intellectual disability,

and ASD, and also with a Rett syndrome variant that is characterized by infantile spasms and intractable seizures occurring before the appearance of the typical features of Rett syndrome (Hanefeld variant).

Altered glucose transport to the brain due to mutations in the GLUT1 transporter gene *SLC2A1* causes epilepsy of variable severity and comorbidities. Classic GLUT1 deficiency is associated with very low cerebrospinal fluid (CSF) glucose concentrations and causes a severe early-onset (<1 year of age) metabolic encephalopathy characterized by movement disorders, epilepsy, and mental retardation, typically associated with *de novoSLC2A1* mutations.

9

Suggested Reading

- Pandolfo M. Pediatric epilepsy genetics. Curr Opin Neurol. 2013;26(2):137–45.

9. What is the wrong match of the following pathological membrane Channelopathies?
   A. Benign Familial Neonatal Seizures and KCNQ2α
   B. Autosomal Dominant Juvenile Myoclonic Epilepsy and CACNA1A
   C. Severe Myoclonic Epilepsy and SCN1A
   D. Autosomal Dominant Nocturnal Frontal Lobe Epilepsy and CHRNA4
   E. Migrating Partial Seizures of Infancy and KCNT1

Correct Answer is: D

Benign familial neonatal seizures (BNFS) is an autosomal dominant epileptic seizure that presents on the second or third day of life in otherwise healthy term infants. The seizures are brief but may occur multiple times per day. They are tonic seizures with associated autonomic features. KCNQ2α and KCNQ3α are both potassium channels that modulate the M-current, a low-threshold K^+ current modified by muscarinic receptors.

Juvenile myoclonic epilepsy (JME) is a myoclonic seizure and primarily generalized convulsive seizures which usually occur in the early morning hours. It occurs in adolescence or early adulthood and most patients do not attain remission. Usually JME is sporadic inheritance, though many patients with an autosomal dominant pattern of inheritance have been found to have mutations of the gene encoding the α-1 subunit of the $GABA_A$ channel (GABRA1). CACNA1A is the alpha subunit of the neuronal calcium channel. Mutations of the CACNA1A gene result in familial hemiplegic migraine, spinocerebellar ataxia type 6 and episodic ataxia.

Dravet syndrome (Severe myoclonic epilepsy of infancy "SMEI") starts within the first year of life with prolonged or focal convulsive febrile seizures followed later by myoclonic, atypical absence, and complex partial and generalized convulsive seizures. The seizures are refractory to medication and associated with a severe epileptic encephalopathy and ataxia. SCN1A encodes for α subunit of the voltage-gated sodium channel $N_{AV}1.1$ which allows for fast Na^+ influx within the dendrites of neurons.

Autosomal dominant nocturnal frontal lobe epilepsy (ADNFLE) usually occurs in late childhood with nocturnal frontal lobe seizures. The seizures often have dystonic or hyperkinetic qualities, are of abrupt onset, and are generally not associated with any post-ictal state. CHRNA4 and CHRNB2 are nicotinic, pre-synaptic, acetylcholine receptors. As a non-selective cation channel, these receptors modulate the release of neurotransmitters due to an overall depolarization of the neuronal membrane due to an influx of Na^+ ions which is greater than the outflow of K^+ ions.

Migrating partial seizures of infancy (MPSI) usually occurs within the first 10 months of life with refractory focal migrating motor seizures, epileptic encephalopathy and loss of previously attained developmental milestones. The KCNT1 gene encodes the pore-forming alpha subunit of a sodium-activated potassium channel. Mutations in the gene result in a gain of function for the channel which may be at least partially blocked by quinidine.

Suggested Reading

- Alfred G. Inherited Channelopathies associated with epilepsy. Epilepsy Curr. 2004;4(2):65–70.
- Kullman D. The neuronal channelopathies. Brain. 2002;125(6):1177–95.

10. A 6-year-old boy came for a second opinion regarding his seizures management. He was diagnosed with Childhood Absence Epilepsy. He is taking ethosuximide 500 mg po qAM and 750 mg po qHS (39 mg/kg/day). He has a fair control of his absence seizures. His mother reports that he has been falling a lot lately. You witnessed a couple of brief head drops and bilateral upper extremity shoulder jerks. His EEG 1 year ago showed a normal awake background with periods of 3 per second, frontally dominant, generalized spike and slow wave discharges lasting 1–20 s in duration and activated by hyperventilation. Also, his Brain MRI a year ago was normal. His developmental milestones are normal. His neurological examination is normal.

    The most appropriate medication adjustment should be to:

    A. Add vigabatrin to his current dose of ethosuximide.
    B. Taper off his ethosuximide and replace it with topiramate.
    C. Taper off his ethosuximide and start him on lamotrigine.
    D. Taper off his ethosuximide and start sodium valproate.
    E. Order an overnight video EEG to capture epochs of slow wave sleep.

Correct Answer is: D

This child in the case starts to have astatic seizures in addition to his absence seizures. The term "astatic" is not necessarily synonymous with "atonic". Astatic seizures refer to either atonic, myoclonic or brief tonic seizures that can cause loss of erect posture. The patient has both atonic (head drops) and myoclonic (shoulder jerks) which noticed by you. As a result, he now has absence seizures, myoclonic seizures and atonic seizures. He is also neurologically and developmentally normal with a normal MRI of the brain. As such he meets criteria for Doose syndrome or myoclonic-astatic epilepsy. A slow wave sleep seen on an overnight EEG is not necessary to order because this diagnosis can be made clinically or by performing a routine awake EEG to show that astatic and myoclonic jerks have an electrical origin with polyspike and slow wave discharges correlating with myoclonic jerks and atonic seizures. Valproate acid is a broader spectrum anti-seizure medication which can cover all three seizure types better than ethosuximide. Ethosuximide may be useful adjunctively if he begins to experience an increase in his absence seizures. Vigabatrin, phenytoin, carbamazepine, and oxcarbazepine should be avoided as these medications may increase absence seizures. Lamotrigine may exacerbate myoclonic seizures. Topiramate may not be terribly effective for absence seizures.

Suggested Reading

- Doose H, Gerken H, Leonhardt T, et al. Centrencephalic myoclonic-astatic petit mal. Clinical and genetic investigation. Neuropadiatrie. 1970;2:59–78.
- Kelley S, Kossoff E. Doose syndrome (myoclonic-astatic epilepsy): 40 years of progress. Dev Med Child Neuro. 2010;52(11):988–93.

11. You are seeing a previously healthy 8-month-old girl in the PICU who is having nearly continuous seizures despite being loaded with phenobarbital, levetiracetam and fosphenytoin as well as being placed on a continuous midazolam drip. Her seizures are rapidly migrating focal clonic and asymmetric tonic seizures with EEG findings of focal onset rhythmic sharp and slow wave discharges that suddenly start and evolve from different areas of the cortex. She reached all of her developmental milestones on time and her seizures began 4 weeks before admission. Another neurologist started her on levetiracetam which has not been effective in controlling her seizures. She has had an extensive diagnostic work up including a brain MRI, analysis of serum amino acids, urine organic acids, serum acylcarnitine profile, serum very long chain fatty acids, serum ammonia, serum biotinidase activity, smf CSF analysis of neurotransmitters, amino acids, and glucose levels. All tests were normal. She has been given trials of pyridoxal phosphate and folinic acid and was recently initiated on the ketogenic diet but no improvement. A genetic analysis including chromosomal microarray analysis has been normal. **What is your next step in evaluating her?**

 A. Diagnostic muscle biopsy.
 B. Serum and urine studies for disorders of creatinine synthesis.
 C. Chromosomal microarray analysis of her parents.
 D. Genetic analysis for Channelopathies causing infantile epileptic encephalopathies.
 E. Lysosomal storage disorders battery.

Correct Answer is: D
This is a case of Partial Migrating Seizures of Infancy (MPSI) based on the clinical course and EEG correlate. This disorder usually occurs in the first 10 months of life with refractory focal migrating motor seizures, epileptic encephalopathy and loss of previously attained developmental milestones. The etiology of MPSI has been attributed to a variety of genetic channelopathies including (but not limited to) mutations in the genes SCN1A, SCN1B, SLC25A22, and KCNT1. The latter gene encodes for the pore-forming alpha subunit of a sodium activated potassium channel which is highly expressed in neurons and cardiomyocytes. Patients with MPSI due to heterozygous mutations in the KCNT1 gene have all shown gain of function mutations resulting in constitutive activation of the channel. Treatment with quinidine has been successful in significantly reducing seizure frequency in some patients with KCNT1 gain of function mutations but not necessarily with improving their developmental outcomes.

Suggested Reading

- Bearden D, Strong A, Ehnot J, et al. Targeted treatment of migrating partial seizures of infancy with quinidine. Ann Neurol. 2014;76:457–61.
- Coppola G, Plouin P, Chiron C, et al. Migrating partial seizures in infancy: a malignant disorder with developmental arrest. Epilepsia. 1995;36:1017–24.

9

12. A 13-year-old boy with medically-refractory convulsive seizures came to your office for an evaluation. He has a history of febrile convulsions beginning at age 9 months and continuing through 10 years of age. He has a family history of febrile seizures, his mother and maternal aunt, as well as refractory epilepsy with developmental delay in his maternal aunt's 7-year-old son. He has been having 3 to 5 generalized unprovoked convulsive seizures weekly. He has recently started having myoclonic seizures over the past 4 months since lamotrigine (100 mg/kg/day) was introduced. He also on topiramate (12 mg/kg/day) and phenobarbital (4 mg/kg/day). He was previously an honor roll student in school but over the past year he has shown declining grades and difficulties with his behavior at school.
Which of the following is unlikely to be true of this patient's medical care?
   A. He likely has a mutation of the genes encoding for SCN1A, SCN1B, SCN2A, or GABRG2.
   B. An increase in the dose of his lamotrigine is likely to improve his epilepsy control.
   C. The use of sodium valproate is relatively contraindicated for use in this patient.
   D. His prognosis for seizure control and cognitive outcome is questionable at this point.

Correct Answer is: C
Febrile seizures beyond age 6 years indicates "Febrile Seizures +" categorization. GEFS+ is a spectrum of epileptic syndromes that include recurrent febrile seizures at the mildest end of the spectrum. More severe manifestations include Intractable Childhood Epilepsy with Generalized Tonic Clonic seizures (ICEGTC) to Severe Myoclonic Epilepsy of Infancy or Childhood (Dravet syndrome). Many patients with GEFS+ have a multigenerational family history of febrile seizures or other more malignant epilepsy syndromes. Patients on the more severe end of the GEFS+ syndrome generally have more intractable generalized seizure types, such as myoclonic, absence, and/or atonic seizures and their long-term neurological prognosis for seizure control and cognitive outcome is poor. Patients with GEFS+, especially at the more severe end of the spectrum should avoid using carbamazepine, lamotrigine, or vigabatrin as these medications may worsen seizures, especially myoclonic seizure. Benzodiazepines, stiripentol, topiramate, ethosuximide, and sodium valproate are preferred medications for use in patients with GEFS+.

Suggested Reading

- Fujiwara T. Clinical spectrum of mutations in SCN1A gene: severe myoclonic epilepsy in infancy and related epilepsies. Epilepsy Res. 2006;70(Suppl 1):S223–30.
- Scheffer JE, Berkovic SF. Generalized epilepsy with febrile seizures plus: a genetic disorder with heterogeneous clinical phenotypes. Brain. 1997;120: 479–90.

13. A full-term newborn was being discharged on day 2 of life when his mother observed staring followed by chewing and then bilateral limb jerking. His nurse witnessed the end of the event in which the baby had rhythmic clonic activity of both upper extremities and face lasting approximately 20 s. The whole event lasted 2 min. He had been born uneventfully with Apgar scores of 9/10. His blood lab work and head ultrasound immediately following the episode

were unremarkable. An interictal EEG shows normal active and quiet sleep with a normal state change. He has family of a father who had neonatal seizures which resolved by 2 months of age.

What is the underlying pathophysiological mechanism for his condition?

A. Unknown
B. Acetylcholine receptor abnormality
C. Sodium channel abnormality
D. Potassium channel abnormality
E. Glutamate metabolism abnormality

Correct Answer is: D

Benign familial neonatal convulsions (BFNC) is a well-known cause for neonatal seizures and the diagnosis is made by the family history of similar events in an infant with no risk factors for neonatal seizures and a normal interictal EEG. The syndrome occurs in 14.4 per 100,000 live births. It is an autosomal dominant inheritance with penetration of 85 percent. BFNC is one of several epileptic disorders characterized as a channelopathy. The two major genes identified in this condition are both voltage-gated potassium channels (KCNQ2, KCNQ3) that are responsible for the M-current. This current is a slowly repolarizing current that is responsible for modulating neuronal bursting by hyperpolarizing the cell membrane. In mice disruption of kcnq2 is lethal and only a 25% disruption of the M-current in humans is sufficient to produce BFNC (making the mutation of a single allele potentially pathologic and explaining the dominant mode of inheritance). Clinical features of BFNC are characterized by focal or multifocal clonic or tonic seizures, a family history of neonatal seizures, and no other neurologic abnormalities. The onset of seizures typically occurs within a few days to 1 week of life, although there is some variability in age at onset. Seizures are usually brief, but recurrence may occur until age 2–3 months, when spontaneous resolution typically occurs. The interictal EEG is usually normal. The treatment for benign familial neonatal convulsions is similar to that for other neonatal seizures.

9

Suggested Reading

- Mulley JC, Scheffer IE, Harkin LA, Berkovic SF, Dibbens LM. Susceptibility genes for complex epilepsy. Hum Mol Genet. 2005;14:R243–49.

14. A family of 9-year-old girl complaining that their daughter has multiple stereotyped episodes each week. She reports that, "I see a funny shape in front of my eyes" with each of these episodes. Then the room feels like it tilts to the side for a little while. Then I get sick to my stomach and feel dizzy. Sometimes it only lasts a few minutes. But if it lasts longer somewhere when I can lie down and go to sleep, I can make it go away." As a child she had benign infantile episodic head tilt from 2 to 6 months of age. She has a very strong family history of migraine, her mother, sister, and maternal grandmother. Her neurological examination is normal, including response to Hallpike maneuver. During a particularly long episode, she had a 30-min "awake only" EEG, and it was normal.

Due to the frequency of episodes:

A. Give her a dose of sumatriptan when her next episode starts.
B. Consideration of a preventative medication such as nortriptyline.
C. Send her to an ENT surgeon to get tubes put into her ears.
D. Get an MRI scan with particular attention to her posterior fossa.
E. Send her to a physical therapist for vestibular conditioning.

Correct Answer is: B
Those episodes have the time course and accompanying and attenuating features of migraine equivalents. She can make them go away with sleep. The sensory distortions are accompanied by nausea. She has a past medical history of benign intermittent infantile torticollis. She has a positive family history for migraine and a negative awake EEG. She is getting episodes frequently, so prophylactic treatment is advised.

Suggested Reading

- Dooley JM, Augustine HF, Gordon KE, Brna PM, Westby E. Alice in wonderland and other migraine associated phenomena-evolution over 30 years after headache diagnosis. Pediatr Neurol. 2014;51(3): 321–3.

15. A 6-year-old boy came to the office with his parents because they have a concern about his recent nocturnal episodes. He sleeps at his regular time, but at around midnight two or three nights per week, he will scream and cry as if frightened. When they go to see him, they find him sitting upright with his eyes wide open, but they cannot confer him or get him to calm down. It is as if he does not hear them at all. Eventually, he goes back down and go back to sleep. He is not incontinent during these episodes and does not have abnormal movements of his limbs or eyes. He does not remember the event the following morning. His past medical history, family history, and physical examination are unremarkable.
What can you tell his parents?
    A. The boy should have a video EEG as soon as possible.
    B. The boy is likely to outgrow these episodes.
    C. You are asking Child Protective Services to take the boy out of their custody.
    D. You would like the family to be seen by a psychiatrist.
    E. The boy needs to be treated with zolpidem.

Correct Answer is: B
This is the clinical presentation of a night terrors which occurs in young preschool and school age children. They are characterized by appearing to be awake but not being aware of surroundings or others in them. Screaming, fearfulness, excited babbling, and crying are characteristic as well. They are very frightening for the family, but the child is not aware they occurred the following morning. They typically remit before age 10 years. Reassurance of the family is the only thing usually needed.

Suggested Reading

- Carter KA, Hathaway NE, Lettieri CF. Common sleep disorders in children. Am Fam Physician. 2014;89(5):368–77.
- Haupt M, Sheldon SH, Loghmanee D. Just a scary dream? A brief review of sleep terrors, nightmares, and rapid eye movement sleep behavior disorder. Pediatr Ann. 2013;42(10):211–6.

16. A mother of an 8-month-old child reports a recurrent event of flaccid paralysis of one side of the body, or the other, with complete recovery of motor function between individual events. The child has no previous history of medical problems or developmental concerns, and there is no family history of similar condition. Every event lasts for approximately 4 h, and do not seem to be distressing to the child. The mother reports that some of the events seem to be precipitated by a bath or sudden change in environmental temperature. He does not lose consciousness during the spell. Brain MRI and MR angiography are normal. Video-EEG was ordered and captured one event,

showing EEG slowing over the cerebral hemisphere contralateral to the weakness, but no epileptiform abnormalities.
What is the correct diagnosis for this patient?
A. Multiple sclerosis, relapsing and remitting type
B. Temporal lobe epilepsy
C. Transient ischemic attack
D. Alternating hemiplegia of childhood
E. Segawa disease

Correct Answer is: D
Alternating hemiplegia of childhood is a rare disorder which occurs in perhaps 1 in 1000,000 births. The majority of patients present with first symptoms during infancy or even in the newborn period. The pathogenesis of unknown, although some clinical features are shared with conditions such as migraine and mitochondrial disorders (mitochondrial encephalopathy with lactic acidosis and stroke-like episodes [MELAS]). Large vessel occlusion or vasospasm appears to be an unlikely mechanism.

9

Suggested Reading

- Sweney MT, Silver K, Gerard-Blanluet M, et al. Alternating hemiplegia of childhood: early characteristics and evolution of a neurodevelopmental syndrome. Pediatrics. 2009;123:e534–41.

17. A 16-year-old boy came to your office because of episodes of loss of consciousness. He had 4 of such events in the last 6 months. His mother witnessed one of the event. She was in another room and when she heard a loud thud. She ran into the room into which her son had just walked from outside and found him limp and unconscious on the floor. He remained unconscious with rapid, non-rhythmic eye flutter for 3–4 min, and then awakened but was confused and sleepy for almost an hour afterwards. The boy does not remember the episodes, but remembers dropping cups and feeling clumsier prior to the episodes. The feeling of clumsiness occurs more upon awakening. Family history is unremarkable of epilepsy or seizures. His past medical history is negative. He has normal general and neurological examinations.
His EEG is most likely to show:
A. Generalized 6 Hz polyspike discharges on a slow background.
B. No discharges on a normal background.
C. Generalized 4–5 Hz spike-and-wave discharges on a normal background.
D. Lateralized 6 Hz polyspike discharges on a normal background.
E. Decremental beta discharges on a slow background.

Correct Answer is: C
This is a presentation of juvenile myoclonic epilepsy, likely sometimes triggered by bright light (e.g., being outside in the sun). He has normal cognitive function and not likely to have background slowing on his interictal EEG. But discharges are common interictally in patients with this syndrome. It runs in families and at least one gene responsible for the syndrome is inherited as an autosomal dominant trait, it is not surprising that his family history is negative, as the inheritance patterns of other associated genes and the genetics of the disorder in many patients are not understood.

Suggested Reading

- Panayiotopoulos CP, Obeid T, Tahan AR. Juvenile myoclonic epilepsy: a 5-year prospective study. Epilepsia. 1994;35(2):285–96.

18. A mother of a 14-year-old boy has witnessed recent paroxysmal events of her son shortly after he is transitioning to sleep at night. He has no significant academic or behavioral problems. Brain MRI was normal, but video-EEG seizure monitoring showed a subtle but consistent ictal pattern over the frontal head regions at the time of the spells. He has a family history of nocturnal seizures in an older brother and maternal uncle.

Which of the following is the most accurate description of the seizures expected in this patient?

A. Unresponsive staring, with chewing movements of the mouth, and non-purposeful fumbling movements of the hands
B. Sudden rage behaviors, with directed violence, after minor frustration
C. Sudden, shock-like contractions of head, neck, and both arms
D. Brief paroxysmal events during sleep with thrashing and yelling
E. Throbbing headaches associated with vomiting

Correct Answer is: D

Autosomal Dominant Nocturnal Frontal Lobe Epilepsy (ADNFLE) has been associated with gain-of-function mutations in genes encoding subunits of the neuronal nicotinic acetylcholine receptors (nAChRs) in some affected families. The seizures are frequent, brief, usually nocturnal, and may involve unusual motor features with posturing or thrashing with intact awareness. Muscle and movement artifact make the ictal changes on the EEG difficult to define, and onset of seizure activity from mesial frontal or orbitofrontal regions. Most patients respond well to conventional antiepilepsy drug (AED) therapy.

Suggested Reading

- Ryvlin P, Rheims S, Risse G. Nocturnal frontal lobe epilepsy. Epilepsia. 2006;47(Suppl 2):83–6.

19. A 5-year-old female has a spell of sudden confusion and became pale. 10 min later she began to vomit repeatedly, and she was unresponsive when she arrived to the ED, with tonic eye deviation to her left side. An intravenous dose of lorazepam was given and all her symptoms were resolved. She has a normal brain MRI, and EEG showed independent focal spikes over the occipital head regions bilaterally. The family reported that she had similar but slightly briefer spells 6 months ago, which was attributed to food poisoning.

What is your diagnosis?

A. Lennox-Gastaut syndrome
B. Cyclic vomiting
C. Panayiotopoulos syndrome
D. Benign Rolandic epilepsy
E. Landau-Kleffner syndrome

Correct Answer is: C

Initially reported by Panayiotopoulos as a distinct clinical entity in 1989, this syndrome is now recognized by the International League Against Epilepsy (ILAE) as Early-Onset Benign Childhood Seizures with Occipital Spikes. It is an increasingly recognized syndrome, notable for mimicking other paroxysmal or acute disorders, such as syncope, gastroenteritis, or toxic ingestion. Autonomic symptoms such as pallor, mydriasis, and tachycardia are common. Individual seizures are usually at least 5 min in duration, and status epilepticus is common. However, seizures tend to be relatively infrequent, and remit for many affected patients.

Suggested Reading

- Covanis A. Panayiotopoulos syndrome: a benign childhood autonomic epilepsy frequently imitating encephalitis, syncope, migraine, sleep disorder, or gastroenteritis. Pediatrics. 2006;118:e1237–43.

20. A 2-year-old boy was admitted to a local ED with multiple seizures of either whole body jerks or rhythmic shaking of the extremities, often involving only one side. He has normal perinatal history, but he had a history of recurrent febrile seizures beginning at 6 months of age, 2 of which were prolonged and required high-dose of pentobarbital. He has a normal early developmental history but recently his language skills have lagged behind compared to other children the same age. His EEG shows abundant generalized spike-waves and polyspike waves with diffuse background slowing. Brain MRI scan is normal.

    What is the most likely diagnosis?

    A. Benign myoclonic epilepsy of infancy
    B. Dravet syndrome
    C. Lennox-Gastaut syndrome
    D. Doose syndrome
    E. Generalized epilepsy with febrile seizures plus

Correct Answer is: B

This is the clinical presentation of Dravet syndrome, also known as severe myoclonic epilepsy of infancy. Children have normal development before the onset of seizures. Usually, it occurs in the first year of life with febrile convulsions, often with unilateral features. Later, they can have other seizure types which include generalized clonic, tonic-clonic, absence, and myoclonic seizures, or unilateral hemiclonic and/or complex partial seizures. The occurrence of status epilepticus is frequent. Psychomotor retardation is usually observed during the second year after the onset of seizures. Ataxia and corticospinal tract signs as progressive neurologic deficits develop subsequently. Diagnosis of Dravet syndrome is based on electroclinical features, and the majority of affected patients have demonstrable mutations in the SCN1A gene which encodes the alpha subunit of a voltage-gated sodium channel.

Suggested Reading

- Dravet C, Bureau M, Oguni H, Fukuyama Y, Cokar O. Severe myoclonic epilepsy in infancy: Dravet syndrome. Adv Neurol. 2005;95:71–102.

21. You are evaluating a 10-month-old girl for her extreme irritability, failure to thrive, vomiting, and possible seizures. She was full term, birth weight 3.8 kg, with fetal distress during labor and associated with uterine rupture and placental abruption. She was delivered by emergency caesarean section. She had significant hypoxic-ischemic encephalopathy with severe metabolic acidosis and neonatal depression. There were no seizures. Her development was very slow, with signs of increased tone, and microcephaly. Over the past 3 months she has been vomiting several times daily, with increased irritability, and poor weight gain. In the last 2 weeks she has also developed peculiar spells, with tonic extension of the neck and back, while turning the head forcefully to the right side and crying as if in pain. These events may last for 20 min. Her EEG showed a mild degree of generalized slowing, but no epileptiform abnormality.

    Which of the following is the most likely explanation for these spells?

    A. Frontal lobe seizures
    B. Infantile spasms

C. Pallid breath-holding spells
D. Sandifer syndrome
E. Increased intracranial pressure

Correct Answer is: D
Sandifer syndrome is secondary to gastro-esophageal reflux disease (GERD) and it results from irritability and discomfort associated with reflux esophagitis. The symptoms are episodic dystonic posturing with torticollis, usually with crying or other signs of distress. It is more likely to occur in children with pre-existing neurological abnormalities, who are at increased risk for GERD, but it can occur in normal children with severe untreated reflux. Many of these children have epilepsy, and the events of Sandifer syndrome may be mistaken for epileptic seizure events. Identifying the correct diagnosis is important, as anti-reflux therapy may be dramatically effective.

Suggested Reading

Kabakus N, Kurt A. Sandifer syndrome: a continuing problem of misdiagnosis. In: Pediatrics International 2006;48:622–25.

22. A family of a 10-year-old boy is seeking a second opinion for their son's treatment-resistant epilepsy. He has the diagnosed of Lennox-Gastaut syndrome in the last 7 years of age, although prior studies have not identified a specific underlying etiology. He has multiple brief tonic seizures per day. These occur suddenly and unexpectedly, and often lead to falls, resulting in injuries to the head and face. He wears a helmet when he is outside the home to protect him of physical injury associated with these drop seizures. He also has frequent absence seizures, and sometimes generalized tonic-clonic seizures. His developmental quotient (DQ) is 45.

Which of the following EEG patterns is most likely to be observed in this patient?

A. Generalized 1.5–2.5 spike-wave
B. Generalized 3 Hz spike-wave
C. Generalized 5–6 Hz spike-wave
D. Normal awake EEG background
E. Unilateral temporal lobe epileptiform discharges

Correct Answer is: A
Lennox-Gastaut Syndrome (LGS) diagnosis is based upon three elements: (1) refractory epilepsy with multiple seizure types (usually including tonic, atonic, and atypical absence, in addition to others), (2) mental retardation, and (3) a characteristic EEG pattern, consisting of generalized "slow spike-wave", typically at 1.5–2.5 Hz, superimposed upon a slow and disorganized awake background. On the other hand, infantile spasms is an epileptic syndrome with multiple etiologies, including structural, metabolic, and genetic causes. A large subgroup is cryptogenic, without a definite identified etiology. Seizures are usually treatment-resistant. Those patients can be treated with alternative treatments such as ketogenic diet, vagus nerve stimulation, or corpus callosotomy (the latter may be particularly beneficial for those with frequent drop attacks leading to physical injury). Generalized 3 Hz spike-wave is usually associated with Childhood Absence Epilepsy (CAE), and "rapid" 5–6 Hz spike-wave is more likely to be associated with Juvenile Myoclonic Epilepsy (JME).

Suggested Reading

Arzimanoglou A, French J, Blume WT, Cross JH, Ernst JP, Feucht M, Genton P, Guerrini R, Kluger G, Pellock JM, Perucca E, Wheless JW. Lennox-Gastaut syndrome: a consensus approach on diagnosis, assessment, management, and trial methodology. Lancet Neurol. 2009;8:82–93.

23. A 1-week-old girl is seen for unusual jerking movements during sleep. She was a full-term gestation, with no complication during pregnancy and delivery. She was discharged home after 1 day without recognized problems. She seems otherwise healthy and alert to her parents. However, for the last 3 days, shortly after she goes to sleep she develops repetitive, arrhythmical jerks of both arms, sometimes stronger on one side of the body or the other. They are 2 min in duration then they disappear. They do not awaken her. These can sometimes be provoked by touching her or picking her up while asleep, but she does not have them while she is awake. No family history of similar condition. She has a normal awake exam, with normal findings for her age. Her routine EEG is normal, while awake and during sleep, although no clinical events occurred during the EEG study.
What is the single best treatment choice for this patient?
A. Adrenocorticotropin hormone (ACTH) injections daily
B. Diazepam rectal gel given at the times of the events
C. Phenobarbital given orally
D. Pyridoxine intravenous trial
E. Re-assurance and continued observation

Correct Answer is: E
Benign Neonatal Sleep Myoclonus is probably under-diagnosed relative to its true incidence in the population. It occurs exclusively during sleep. Myoclonus may occur in any sleep stage, but they are reportedly less common during active sleep. Usually, they occur during the first 2 weeks of life, and disappear within 3–6 months. The jerks are often bilateral, affect the arms more than the legs or the face, and are irregularly repetitive. They are less than a minute in most patients, but can be longer, lasting up to 30 min or even an hour if the child is not awakened. The EEG is normal between and during the spells. If the diagnosis is correct, a normal neurological and developmental outcome is expected. Anti-epilepsy drugs (AEDs) are not advised, and have been reported to worsen some patients with this condition.

Suggested Reading

- Maurer VO, Rizzi M, Bianchetti MG, Ramelli GP. Benign neonatal sleep myoclonus: a review of the literature. Pediatrics. 2010;125:e919–24.

24. A 9-month-old girl starts having infantile spasms. She has a slower development than her older siblings at the same age, but she had not undergone evaluation. On examination, she has multiple hypopigmented macules. Brain MR shows many small subependymal nodules, and several high signal abnormalities in the subcortical white matter consistent with cortical tubers. An echocardiogram shows a right intraventricular rhabdomyoma. A mutation in the TSC2 gene supports the clinical diagnosis. Different treatment options have been discussed with the family. After informed consent, they are eager to begin therapy with oral vigabatrin.
For which of the following side effect should this patient be regularly assessed?
A. Gastrointestinal bleeding
B. Glucose intolerance
C. Hypertension
D. Increased risk of serious infection
E. Permanent loss of peripheral vision

Correct Answer is: E

Vigabatrin was approved for the treatment of infantile spasms (IS) between the ages of 1 month and 2 years by the United States Food and Drug Administration (US FDA) in August 2009. Vigabatrin works by binding irreversibly to and thereby inhibiting the function of GABA-transaminase, the enzyme responsible for breaking down GABA at synaptic junctions. Vigabatrin results in increased brain levels of GABA, the major inhibitory neurotransmitter in mammalian brain. However, vigabatrin is also associated with an increased risk for permanent changes in vision in up to 30% of adult patients, usually with asymptomatic concentric visual field loss. Monitoring children for these changes is difficult, although ocular coherence tomography (OCT) appears to be a promising technology. The other adverse events listed above are more likely to occur with intramuscular adrenocorticotropin hormone (ACTH) therapy.

Suggested Reading

- Lawthom C, Smith PEM, Wild JM. Nasal retinal nerve fiber layer attenuation: a biomarker for vigabatrin toxicity. Ophthalmology. 2009;116:565–71.

25. A 14-month-old boy is evaluated for the recent onset of spells which are triggered by minor head injury or impact. Recently, he tripped on the carpet and striking his head against living room furniture, leading to a spell where he seemed to be upset and in pain, but unable to take his next breath. He was very pale. As the event progressed, he lost consciousness, associated with rolling up of the eyes, and generalized opisthotonic posturing. He remained rigid for several seconds, and then relaxed, with return of his breathing and color to normal. He regained consciousness quickly, but seemed tired and behaviorally subdued. He was a full-term gestation, and had a negative medical history, and normal development for age. There is no family history for epilepsy or similar events. He has a normal examination.

What is the most likely diagnosis?

A. Cataplexy
B. Complicated migraine
C. Pallid breath-holding spell
D. Post-traumatic seizures
E. Anoxic seizures

Correct Answer is: C

Breath-holding spells (BHS) are involuntary, non-epileptic paroxysmal events that are provoked by an external circumstance. Pallid BHS (associated by a pale appearance) are usually provoked by pain, often involving the head or scalp, whereas cyanotic BHS are more likely to be provoked by some emotional upset (such as an older sibling taking a toy). Most BHS tend to have one subtype or the other, although 20% of patients can have both. The pathophysiology is not well-understood, although there is circumstantial evidence for autonomic nervous system dysregulation in a significantly higher percentage of BHS patients compared to normal age-matched controls. The events occur at the end of the expiratory phase (rather than at the end of the inspiratory phase). Iron-deficiency anemia is higher than otherwise expected in children with BHS. Anti-epilepsy drugs (AEDs) are not effective for treatment.

Suggested Reading

- DiMario FJ. Prospective study of children with cyanotic and pallid breath-holding spells. Pediatrics 2001;107:265–69.

26. An 18-year-old female was admitted to the ED because she has a new-onset generalized tonic clonic seizure this morning, which lasted about 4 min. She has been diagnosed with an acute intermittent porphyria at 13 years of age. Her classic attack has previously included abdominal pain with nausea and vomiting as well as numbness in her legs. She has a remarkable family for porphyria in her mother and sister. On neurological examination, she has mild proximal weakness in all limbs and decreased tendon reflexes.
Which of the following antiepileptic medication would be safe to use if prophylactic medication is required?
   A. Carbamazepine
   B. Gabapentin/Keppra
   C. Lamotrigine
   D. Phenobarbital
   E. Valproic acid

9

Correct Answer is: B
Acute intermittent porphyria is an autosomal dominant disorder, and results from partial deficiency of porphobilinogen deaminase enzyme. Classic presentation is with an acute abdomen, but the neurological symptoms can include peripheral neuropathy, respiratory paralysis, seizures and loss of consciousness. You have to be aware of that the use of enzyme-inducing antiepileptic drugs can cause worsening of seizures, which can be fatal. Carbamazepine, clonazepam and other benzodiazepines, lamotrigine, phenytoin, sodium valproate, barbiturates including primidone, topiramate, and tiagabine can worsen and exacerbate porphyria or affect metabolism of porphyrins. The incidence of the disease may be underestimated, so high clinical suspicion is warranted.

Suggested Reading

- Kochar et al. Acute intermittent porphyria presenting with neurological emergency: Review of six cases. Neurology India. 2007. 55(4):413–5.
- Solinas et al. Neurological complications of porphyria. J Clin Neurosci. 2008;15(3):263–8.

27. A 5-month-old girl was born at 38 weeks gestation with microcephaly, petechiae, and hepatosplenomegaly. Upon her pediatrician as a newborn, she had intracranial calcifications and sensorineural hearing loss, and he diagnosed her with congenital cytomegalovirus (CMV) infection. There weeks ago, she developed body jerks, with sudden, forceful flexion of the head and neck, torso, and arms, occurring in clusters, more likely upon awakening from sleep. She cries briefly between each jerk, which are 4–6 s apart. The clusters last up to 3 min in duration, although some are shorter. Now those clusters are occurring daily. The EEG pattern you are going see with this new symptom is:
   A. Burst-suppression background
   B. Hypsarrhythmia
   C. Photo paroxysmal occipital discharges
   D. Spike transients over the right temporal head region
   E. 3-Hz generalized spike-wave discharges

Correct Answer is: B
The presentation of the infantile spasms (IS) includes clusters of myoclonic/tonic spasms, each cluster can last up to several minutes in duration, and more likely to occur with sleep-wake transitions. They usually begin between 4 and 12 months of age, although older children may also have clusters of epi-

leptic spasms. Many children with IS have pre-existing neurological symptoms. The list of etiologies for IS is very long, including structural, metabolic, and genetic causes. 10% of IS patients have a favorable prognosis, but the outcome for the majority includes at least a mild degree of developmental abnormality and the later appearance of other seizure types. Hypsarrhythmia (or one of its several "modified" forms, or variants) is the EEG pattern most likely to be seen in IS patients, although the absence of hypsarrhythmia does not exclude the clinical diagnosis.

Suggested Reading

- Zupanc ML. Clinical evaluation and diagnosis of severe epilepsy syndromes of early childhood. J Child Neurol. 2009;24(Suppl 8):6S–14S.

28. A 17-month-old boy came to the ED after a 5-min generalized tonic-clonic convulsion in association with high fever at home. His parents report that he was not, but he was very hot to the touch when the seizure occurred. In ED he has a temperature of 103.8° rectally. On exam, he has otitis media, after he was given acetaminophen, he became happy and playful as his baseline. His prior history is notable for birth at term gestation, and subsequent normal development. His family history is remarkable of his mother who she had three seizures with high fever when she was an infant.
What is your next step in management?
    A. Intravenous loading dose of phenobarbital followed by oral treatment
    B. Lumbar puncture for CSF examination
    C. EEG to be scheduled later as an outpatient
    D. Reassurance and anticipatory guidance
    E. Admission to the hospital for further evaluation and observation

Correct Answer is: D
Benign febrile convulsions occur in 2–5% of the normal population of infants, typically between the ages of 6 months and 3 years. Maximal incidence is at 18–20 months of age. Simple febrile seizures last less than 15 min, without focal or lateralizing features with ictal semiology, and do not recur within the same 24-h time period.
For those children over 18 months of age without previously recognized neurological symptoms or signs, the evaluation should be limited to a careful history and physical examination. If this is reassuring (including the absence of meningeal signs suggesting an acute neurological infection), then routine laboratory tests, EEG, brain imaging, and lumbar puncture are not recommended, and hospital admission is not necessary. Families should be educated, however, about the expected natural history of benign febrile seizures, and indications for medical intervention if febrile seizures should occur in the future.

Suggested Reading

- Capovilla G, Mastrangelo M, Romeo A, Vigevano F. Recommendations for the management of "febrile seizures". Epilepsia. 2009;50(Suppl 1):2–6.

29. A 4-day-old baby was admitted to the Emergency Department for suspected seizures. His mother has no problems during her pregnancy, and she delivered him at term via uncomplicated vaginal delivery. He went home with his mother after 1 day. He has normal feeding pattern and seemed

otherwise well, but had 3 episodes of unresponsiveness, stiffening, tonic eye deviation, and cyanosis. Every episode was less than a minute, and he seemed to recover quickly. He has a family history of similar episodes in his mother and other maternal relatives. In the emergency department he is awake and has a normal vital signs and intact examination.

What is your most likely diagnosis?

A. Benign familial neonatal convulsions
B. Encephalitis with herpes simplex virus
C. Ischemic stroke in the middle cerebral artery
D. Methylmalonic aciduria
E. Pyridoxine dependency

9

Correct Answer is: A

Newborns with Benign Familial Neonatal Convulsions (BFNC) typically begin to have seizures on the third day of life. Those seizures are brief, and are associated with limited post-ictal manifestations, but they may be repetitive. This condition is one explanation for "well-baby seizures". CNS infection, metabolic perturbations or consequences of trauma must be considered and excluded. Seizures usually permanently remit in 1–3 months, without residual neurological or developmental impairment. However, 10–20% of patients may have seizures later in life. BFNC have been associated with loss-of-function mutations in KCNQ2 and KCNQ3 genes, which express neuronal voltage-dependent potassium channel subunits Kv7.2 and Kv7.3, respectively.

Suggested Reading

- Rosen GM, Rosales TO, Connolly M, Anderson VE, Leppert M. Seizure characteristics in chromosome 20 benign familial neonatal convulsions. Neurology. 1993;43:1355–60.

30. A 6-year-old female came to the ED because she has for two recent nocturnal spells. The family found her in the early morning in her room having retching behavior, followed by several bouts of vomiting. She was pale, disoriented, and unable to coherently respond to her family. 10 min later, she started to have subtle clonic jerking to her right side, including face, neck and arm, lasting another 8 min. Her evaluation in the ED was unrevealing, including head CT imaging. A month later, she had a second identical spell in her sleep. She has a normal neurological examination, and a normal development for her age. She has negative family history of epilepsy. You ordered an EEG, shows normal background, but also frequent spikes from the left occipital head region, which appeared to suppress with eye opening. During sleep, spikes were more frequent, and appeared independently from both the right and left occipital regions.

What is your diagnosis?

A. Benign Rolandic epilepsy of childhood
B. Migraine with aura
C. Obstructive sleep apnea
D. Panayiotopoulos syndrome
E. Rasmussen syndrome

Correct Answer is: D.

Beginning in 1988, and in subsequent reports, Panayiotopoulos has described this benign epilepsy syndrome, characterized by infrequent but nevertheless often prolonged seizure events, usually nocturnal, dominated by autonomic symptoms, including pallor, nausea, retching and vomiting, sometimes associated with confusion and occasionally concluding in a focal clonic seizure event. EEG is characterized by interictal spikes located most likely over the occipital regions, but can be observed

over other areas as well. Approximately only 10% of patients report visual symptoms. Because of these features, now confirmed by multiple reports, it has been proposed that Panayiotopoulos syndrome should be classified as an autonomic epilepsy, rather than as an occipital epilepsy. Most patients have only a few seizures, and do not require daily anti-epilepsy drug (AED) therapy. The prognosis is always good.

Suggested Reading

- Covanis A. Panayiotopoulos syndrome: a benign childhood autonomic epilepsy frequently imitating encephalitis, syncope, migraine, sleep disorder, or gastroenteritis. Pediatrics. 2006;118:e1237–43.

31. You are evaluating a 2-week-old boy with congenital heart disease for possible seizures. He is a full-term baby. He became hypotensive shortly after birth. While he was at NICU, an evaluation was done which determined that he has an interrupted aortic arch, and has been dependent upon a prostaglandin infusion to maintain systemic blood flow through the ductus arteriosus. On general exam, he has dysmorphic features with micrognathia and low-set ears. He has been irritable since birth and he have repeated events involving clonic jerking of the extremities for 24 h, usually on the left side, although the nursing staff also documents right-sided clonic events as well. Serum calcium is abnormally low (ionized calcium 2.8 mg/dl, normal range 4.1–5.2 mg/dl). CT head is normal, but the EEG is markedly abnormal, with low amplitude irregular slowing, and high amplitude multifocal independent spikes. He has been on intravenous administration of calcium gluconate and phenobarbital.

    What is your most likely diagnosis?
    A. DiGeorge syndrome (chromosome 22q11.2 deletion syndrome)
    B. Down syndrome (trisomy 21)
    C. Group B streptococcal sepsis and meningitis
    D. Propionic aciduria
    E. Prenatal hypoxic-ischemic brain injury

Correct Answer is: A
In the 1960's and 1970's, neonatal hypocalcemia (and seizures) were commonly encountered as an unintended result of high phosphate levels in cow's milk-derived infant formulas. In current clinical practice, neonatal hypocalcemic seizures are uncommon, and usually result from deficiency of parathyroid hormone due to hypoplasia of the parathyroid glands. This is often associated with various forms of congenital heart disease including the cardiac outflow tract malformations associated with DiGeorge syndrome (chromosome 22q11.2 syndrome). Treatment consists of restoring physiological levels of calcium. It should be recognized that the seizures and encephalopathy associated with hypocalcemia may take several days to resolve after normal calcium levels have been achieved.

Suggested Reading

- Kossof EH, Silvia MT, Maret A, Carakushansky M, Vining EPG. Neonatal hypocalcemic seizures: case report and literature review. J Child Neurol. 2002;17:238–41.

32. A 25-month-old female is being evaluated for unexplained spells. She developed normally until episodes of unusual eye movements were noted around 4 months of age, consisting of nystagmus, sometimes affecting only one eye. She never has an alteration

of consciousness. At 8 months of age she developed episodes of flaccid weakness, affecting one side of the body or the other. These events occurred only while awake, and were sometimes provoked by bathing. Weakness would last for several hours before recovery to baseline. If she goes to sleep after the onset of the episode, she would always awaken without the unilateral weakness. Therapeutic trials of medications for epilepsy and migraine have proven ineffective. On physical examination, she is poorly socialized and has only a few words. She appears to be clumsy and mildly ataxic, despite the fact that she is on no medications at this time. Her eye movements are normal. She was mildly hypotonic, but showed no lateralizing features on her motor exam.

What is your most likely diagnosis?

A. Alternating hemiplegia of childhood
B. Hypokalemic periodic paralysis
C. Mitochondrial encephalopathy with lactic acidosis and stroke-like syndrome
D. Narcolepsy with cataplexy
E. Simple partial epilepsy

Correct Answer is: A

Alternating hemiplegia of childhood (AHC) is a rare disorder with very specific symptomatology. The correct diagnosis is usually delayed for several years relative to the onset of first symptoms. AHC is in some ways an inadequate descriptive name for the syndrome: (1) the first symptoms are usually episodes of abnormal eye movements, occurring in early infancy, (2) unilateral flaccid hemiplegia occurring independently on each side is the classic expectation, but many patients have simultaneous involvement of both sides of the body for at least some events (double hemiplegia), with episodes characterized by quadriplegia, dysphagia, dysarthria, and possibly respiratory compromise, (3) some episodes may consist of unilateral dystonia, rather than flaccid weakness, and (4) virtually all patients develop persisting co-morbid symptoms in between hemiplegic episodes, with developmental delay, ataxia, and/or epilepsy. Sleep predictably relieves the hemiplegic episodes, and induction of sleep is the most effective way of acutely treating an event. Flunarizine can be effective in some patients to reduce the frequency and severity of attacks.

Suggested Reading

- Sweney MT, Silver K, Gerard-Blanluet M, Pedespan JM, Renault F, Arzimanoglou A, Schlesinger-Massart M, Lewelt AJ, Reyna SP, Swoboda KJ. Alternating hemiplagia of childhood: early characteristics and evolution of a neurodevelopmental syndrome. Pediatrics. 2009;123: e534–41.

33. A 5-year-old girl has been evaluated for several acute episodes of unsteadiness and difficulty walking lasting for few minutes. The family describes the child as appearing pale and "sickly", and with unusually fussy behavior. The young girl was awake and interactive with the family during these spells, and she wanted to be held closely. When the family encouraged her to walk, she had a wide-based wobbly gait. Additionally, they noted unusual jerking movements of the eyes to the sides. Afterwards, she would generally fall asleep and upon awakening was back to baseline. There were no previous illnesses or symptoms, and no family history of seizures or epilepsy.

What is your most likely diagnosis?

A. Drug intoxication
B. Benign paroxysmal vertigo

C. Acute post-infectious cerebellitis
D. Neuroblastoma, with opsoclonus-myoclonus
E. Complex partial seizure

Correct Answer is: B
Benign paroxysmal vertigo is thought to be a migraine variant and occurs usually in toddlers or young children who have family history of migraine. Nystagmus or vomiting can occur, and in older children, unilateral throbbing headache may be present. The attacks are generally brief, last from a few minutes to several hours, and they often resolve with sleep. Between attacks, the child is perfectly normal. These episodes are benign, have a favorable prognosis, and no treatment is needed. Despite the prevailing view that BPV is a migraine variant, there is no strong evidence that these events presage the development of typical migraine in adolescence or early adulthood.

Suggested Reading

- Drigo P, Carli G, Laverda AM. Benign paroxysmal vertigo of childhood. Brain Dev. 2001;23(1):38–41.
- Al-Twaijri WA, Shevell MI. Pediatric migraine equivalents: occurrence and clinical features in practice. Pediatr Neurol. 2002;26(5):365–8.

34. A previously healthy 1-month-old boy was admitted to the ED 2 h ago, he is in generalized status epilepticus which began 30 min prior to arrival. ED physician intubated him and gave him phenobarbital 20 mg/kg and fosphenytoin 20 mg/kg.which stopped the convulsion after an hour. 1 week ago, he started to vomit and to be irritable. He has also been noted to have intermittent twitching of the limbs since birth. He is afebrile, comatose, with a flat anterior fontanelle. Lab work including CRP showed no sign of acute infection. Head CT and lumbar puncture were normal. His EEG shows on-going generalized epileptiform ictal activity despite cessation of overt clinical seizures.
What is your next step in management?
A. MRI brain scan
B. High-dose pentobarbital
C. Pyridoxine 100 mg IV
D. Ganciclovir 6 mg/Kg IV every 4 h
E. Ativan 1 mg/Kg IV

Correct Answer is: C
Patient having status epilepticus without any obvious cause at 1 month with a history of irritability, suggestive of an encephalopathy. This patient has normal general lab, CSF and CT scan, he is in the category of neonatal epileptic encephalopathy. A trial of IV pyridoxine is warranted in all children with status of unknown etiology as pyridoxine dependency is a treatable cause of epilepsy in children less than 3 years of age. Pyridoxine dependency (PD) is an autosomal recessive and recent discovery of mutations in families with the condition involving the gene ALDH7A1 (antiquitin) is making this a rapidly changing field. PD is currently a clinical diagnosis that depends on the response to pharmacological doses of pyridoxine (Vitamin B6) with cessation of clinical and electrographic seizures. 100 mg of IV pyridoxine with EEG monitoring is recommended by many authors. The paroxysmal activity (both clinical and/or electrographic) should cease. If there is no positive result, a trial of pyridoxal phosphate is warranted. If other AEDs have been used to treat the seizures (this is likely as pyridoxine-dependent seizures are usually intractable) then after a time the other AEDs need to be withdrawn. If the seizures remain controlled on daily oral pyridoxine (at 15 mg/Kg) then a

trial without pyridoxine, which results in recurrence of the seizures which are again quickly controlled by oral pyridoxine, confirms the diagnosis. Pyridoxine should then be continued for life. A DNA diagnosis should be pursued. Pyridoxine dependency is a different disorder than the pyridoxine-deficiency which is an acquired condition that occurs in neonates as a result of a deficient diet usually associated with powdered goat's milk diet.

Suggested Reading

- Basura GJ, Hagland SP, Wiltse AM and Gospe SM. Clinical features and the management of pyridoxine-dependent and pyridoxine-responsive seizures: review of 63 North American cases submitted to a patient registry. Eur J Pediatr. 2008 [Epub ahead of print]. PMID: 18762976.

9

35. An 11-month-old baby boy presents with febrile hemi-clonic status epilepticus. He is treated acutely. Two months later, he has another episode of febrile hemi-clonic status epilepticus involving the other side of his body. He then begins having apparent absence seizures, focal motor seizures, and generalized tonic-clonic seizures associated with illnesses. The parents note stagnation of his psychomotor development. MRI of the brain is normal. Genetic studies disclose an abnormality in the SCN1A gene.
What is his most likely diagnosis?
A. Dravet syndrome
B. epilepsy with myoclonic absences
C. Lennox-Gastaut syndrome
D. migrating partial seizures of infancy
E. West syndrome

Correct Answer is: A
The patient history is consistent with Dravet syndrome, a distinct epilepsy syndrome that begins in infancy with onset of febrile hemi-clonic status epilepticus and evolves to a pattern of multiple seizure types, including focal motor, myoclonic, absence, and generalized tonic-clonic seizures associated with marked slowing or stagnation of development often accompanied by behavioral disturbances. Metabolic investigations are normal. EEG may show generalized spike and slow wave complexes and a photoparoxysmal response. Many patients have a characteristic defect in the SCN1A gene which encodes the alpha one subunit of the neuronal sodium channel.

Suggested Reading

- Petrelli C, Passamonti C, Cesaroni E, et al. Early clinical features in Dravet Syndrome patients with and without SCN1A. Epilepsy. 2012;99(1–2):21–7.
- Brunklaus A, Ellis R, Reavey E, et al. Prognostic, clinical and demographic features in SCN1A mutation – positive Dravet syndrome. Brain. 2012; 135(Pt 8):2329–36.

36. An 8-month-old boy has seizures, characterized by stiffening of arms and legs, lasting 15–20 s.
What is the most likely seizure type?
A. absence seizure
B. focal seizure
C. infantile spasms
D. myoclonic seizure
E. tonic seizure

Correct Answer is: E
The seizure description is most consistent with a tonic seizure. No focality with tonic seizure. Absence seizures would be atypical in a 10-month-old. The duration of the stiffening is too prolonged for infantile spasms or myoclonic seizures, and did not include flexion component.

Suggested Reading

- Berg AT, Berkovic SF, Brodie MJ, et al. Revised terminology and concepts for organization of seizures and epilepsies: report of the ILAE Commission on Classification and Terminology, 2005–2009. Epilepsia. 2010;51:676–85.

37. A 7-year-old boy with a history of treatment-resistant epilepsy with multiple seizure types, secondary to perinatal hypoxic-ischemic encephalopathy. This resulted in severe cognitive and motor impairment. He had multifocal electrographic seizures during the first week of life that resolved with phenobarbital. At 6 months of age he developed infantile spasms that were initially responsive to treatment with adrenocorticotrophin hormones. His seizures recurred, characterized by brief stiffening, drops, and episodes of unresponsiveness. He has been having daily seizures despite multiple medications.

What is the most likely diagnosis?

A. Angelman syndrome
B. Doose syndrome
C. Landau-Kleffner syndrome
D. Lennox-Gastaut syndrome
E. West syndrome

Correct Answer is: D

The clinical presentation indicates Lennox-Gastaut syndrome. Infantile spasms may follow perinatal hypoxic-ischemic encephalopathy and subsequently evolve into Lennox-Gastaut syndrome. The onset and evolution from West syndrome to Lennox-Gastaut syndrome are the key clinical features to differentiate from the other choices. Angelman syndrome is a genetic epilepsy which occurs during infancy. Doose syndrome, also known as epilepsy with myoclonic atonic seizures, Doose and other epilepsy syndrome occur during infancy are characterized by myoclonic, atonic, atypical absence, and bilateral convulsions. Landau-Kleffner syndrome is a childhood-onset epileptic encephalopathy characterized by aphasia with continuous epileptiform discharges during sleep.

Suggested Reading

- Berg AT, Berkovic SF, Brodie MJ, et al. Revised terminology and concepts for organization of seizures and epilepsies: report of the ILAE Commission on Classification and Terminology, 2005–2009. Epilepsia. 2010;51:676–85.

38. A 4-year-old boy has been evaluated for frequent head jerks, staring spells, and infrequent bilateral convulsions. He has a happy demeanor, but suffers global developmental delay with ataxia. His examination shows a nonverbal child with diffuse hypotonia, and jerking movements which include hand flapping and tremor. His brain MRI is normal. Interictal EEG shows intermittent bursts of diffuse polymorphic delta activity, with admixed sharp wave discharges, giving it a "notched" appearance.

What is your most likely diagnosis?

A. Angelman syndrome
B. Doose syndrome
C. Landau-Kleffner syndrome
D. Lennox-Gastaut syndrome
E. West syndrome

Correct Answer is: A

The patient has Angelman syndrome, a genetic epilepsy occurs in the infantile period. Typically, patients have developmental delay, seizure onset usually before age 3 years, happy demeanor, ataxia with hand flapping movements, and EEG with characteristic pattern with large amplitude slow-spike waves. West

syndrome is a severe infantile-onset epileptic encephalopathy characterized by a triad of infantile spasms, hypsarrhythmia on EEG, and development regression. Doose syndrome, also known as myoclonic astatic epilepsy (myoclonic seizure followed immediately by an atonic seizure), which occurs in the infantile period and is characterized by myoclonic, atonic, atypical absence, and bilateral convulsions; EEG shows regular and irregular bilaterally synchronous 2- to 3-Hz spike-waves and polyspike patterns with a 4–7-Hz background. Landau-Kleffner syndrome is a childhood-onset epileptic encephalopathy characterized by aphasia with continuous epileptiform discharges during sleep. Lennox-Gastaut syndrome is a severe epileptic encephalopathy with multiple seizure types, intellectual disability, and slow spike-and-wave on EEG.

9

Suggested Reading

- Valente KD, Koiffmann CP, Fridman C, et al. Epilepsy in patients with Angelman syndrome caused by deletion of the chromosome 15q11–13. Arch Neurol. 2006; 63(1):122–8.

39. A 10-year-old boy has a history of three nocturnal seizures associated with left-sided facial, mouth and tongue paresthesias and twitching of the left side of his face with associated hypersalivation. He had one secondarily generalized tonic-clonic seizure followed one of his regular seizure. Brain MRI scan is unremarkable.
Which of the following interictal EEG features is most likely?
   A. 1 Hz to 2 Hz generalized spike-and-wave discharges
   B. 4 Hz to 5 Hz generalized polyspike-and-wave discharges
   C. bilateral centrotemporal spikes
   D. bilateral occipital sharp waves
   E. generalized paroxysmal fast activity

Correct Answer is: C
The clinical scenario is consistent with a diagnosis of benign epilepsy with centrotemporal spikes (BECTs, also known as benign rolandic epilepsy.) Typically, seizures in this condition begin between the ages of 3–13 (peaking between ages 8 and 12) and are associated with unilateral facial sensorimotor symptoms, hypersalivation, speech arrest, and/or oropharyngeal symptom. 50% of patients can have secondarily generalize seizures. Interictal EEG shows high amplitude central spikes, often with shifting laterality. Seizures typically resolve by age 18.

Suggested Reading

- Guerrini R, Pellacani S. Benign childhood focal epilepsies. Epilepsia. 2012; 53(Suppl 4):9–18.

40. A 7-month-old girl develops spells of sudden bending forwards, and then her arms and legs stiffen and extend. She can lift her head without support, and she has a social smile; however, she is not able to sit without support or turn from her back onto her stomach.
What is the most likely interictal EEG features?
   A. 3 Hz generalized spike-and-wave discharges
   B. asymmetric beta activity
   C. hypsarrhythmia
   D. suppression-burst pattern
   E. temporal sharp waves

Correct Answer is: C.
The clinical description is most consistent with a diagnosis of West syndrome. The spells the infant is experiencing are most consistent with infantile spasms. West syndrome is characterized by developmental delay, hypsarrhythmia on EEG, and infantile spasms.

Suggested Reading

- Hrachovy RA, Frost JD Jr. Infantile epileptic encephalopathy with hypsarrhythmia (infantile spasms/West syndrome). J Clin Neurophysiol. 2003;20(6):408–25

41. A 12-year-old boy with normal development presents with new-onset epilepsy with focal seizures. His seizures are characterized by a rising sensation, followed by unresponsiveness and lip smacking for several minutes. He has 2–3 seizures per month despite appropriate anticonvulsant.
Which of the following conditions is most likely to be present in his medical history?
A. brain tumor
B. family history of epilepsy
C. febrile status epilepticus
D. hypoxic-ischemic encephalopathy
E. traumatic brain injury

Correct Answer is: C
The clinical history indicates temporal lobe epilepsy which may be secondary to mesial temporal sclerosis following an episode of febrile status epilepticus during childhood. Although the other options are risk factors for epilepsy, the age of onset would be most consistent with this specific clinical scenario.

Suggested Reading

- Hesdorffer DC, Shinnar S, Lewis DV, et al. FEBSTAT study team. Design and phenomenology of the FEBSTAT study. Epilepsia. 2012; 53:1471–80.

42. A 7-year-old boy has intractable epilepsy with multiple seizure types, and a progressive encephalopathy. He started to have seizures at 2 years old and initially characterized by a behavioral arrest, eye deviation, tachycardia, and facial flushing. He also had brief stiffening episodes in sleep and frequently exhibited inappropriate laughter.
What can you find on his MRI?
A. focal cortical dysplasia in the right frontal lobe
B. hypothalamic hamartoma
C. mesial temporal sclerosis
D. normal MRI of the brain
E. perinatal right MCA infarct

Correct Answer is: B
This patient's presentation is most consistent with gelastic, tonic, and focal seizures secondary to hypothalamic hamartoma. Although other structural causes of epilepsy may manifest with similar focal seizures, the inappropriate laughter is most commonly associated with this localization.

Suggested Reading

- Berkovic SF, Arzimanoglou A, Kuzniecky R, et al. Hypothalamic hamartoma and seizures: a treatable epileptic encephalopathy. Epilepsia. 2003;44:969–73.

43. A 10-month-old boy with normal development has a history of prolonged alternating hemiconvulsive seizures, usually associated with fever and/or illness. Seizure began 1 day after his 4-month vaccinations. He has 2–3 seizures per month despite two anticonvulsants, and seem to worsen with carbamazepine.
What is your the most likely diagnosis?
A. atypical febrile seizures
B. complex febrile seizures
C. Dravet syndrome
D. infantile spasms
E. simple febrile seizures

Correct Answer is: C
This patient is most likely has Dravet syndrome. Development is typically normal very early in the course with later deterioration. Febrile seizures,

either simple or atypical, are usually not so frequent, are usually do not require prophylactic antiepileptic medications, and are not considered a diagnosis of epilepsy. The clinical presentation is not consistent with infantile spasms, which are clusters of quick jerks that are typically associated with developmental regression and an EEG background of hypsarrhythmia.

Suggested Reading

- Berg AT, Berkovic SF, Brodie MJ, et al. Revised terminology and concepts for organization of seizures and epilepsies: report of the ILAE Commission on Classification and Terminology, 2005–2009. Epilepsia. 2010; 51:676–85.

9

44. An 18-year-old girl with complex partial seizures that have been well controlled for the last 3 years. In the past 2 years, she was taken lamotrigine and a combination type oral contraceptive. She takes lamotrigine 300 mg tablets twice daily. She has not had any seizures for 3 years and has regular menses. She came to you because she recently stopped taking her oral contraceptive medication, and approximately 1 week later had intermittent nausea with vomiting, and she became ataxic.
What is your next step in her management?
A. lower her lamotrigine dose to 200 mg twice daily
B. obtain MRI of the brain to exclude space occupying lesion
C. obtain urine toxicology
D. perform a lumbar puncture
E. perform a serum pregnancy test

Correct Answer is: A
Oral contraceptives induce the metabolism of lamotrigine by inducing uridine diphosphate glucuronosyltransferase (UGT), which is a major root of elimination for lamotrigine. If the oral contraceptive pill is withdrawn, then deinduction of the lamotrigine metabolism occurs quickly, typically within days and maximally by 1 week. This results in increased serum levels of lamotrigine, with typical symptoms of medication toxicity such as nausea, vomiting, and ataxia. This is best managed by lowering the dose of lamotrigine; the symptoms should abate within a couple of days.

Suggested Reading

- Christiansen J, Petrenaite V, Atterman J, et al. Oral contraceptives induce lamotrigine metabolism: Evidence from a double-blind, placebo-controlled trial. Epilepsia. 2007;48(3):484–9.

45. A 6-year-old boy has been having myoclonic, myoclonic-atonic, and atonic seizures. He has early normal development. His seizures have not responded adequately to treatment with levetiracetam, valproate, clobazam, lamotrigine, or topiramate. He is diagnosed with epilepsy with myoclonic-atonic seizures.
What is the best next step in his management?
A. ketogenic diet
B. obtain a magnetoencephalogram
C. refer the patient for a clinical trial of a novel antiepileptic drug
D. responsive neurostimulation
E. video EEG monitoring with intercranial electrodes

Correct Answer is: A
The patient has myoclonic-atonic seizures. This is an epilepsy syndrome occurs in childhood between the ages of 7 months and 6 years. Normal development is expected. The ketogenic diet has been shown to be effective in several series of patients with myoclonic-atonic epilepsy. Ketogenic diet in the treatment of myoclonic-atonic

epilepsy is very effective if used early in the course of treatment. Given the failure of multiple medications in this child, this would be the next best step in management.

Suggested Reading

- Nangia S, Carbaloo RH, Kang HC, et al. Is the Ketogenic diet effective in specific epilepsy syndromes?. Epilepsy Res. 2012;100(3):252–7.

46. The implementation of the ketogenic diet can prove harmful in which of the following conditions associated with epilepsy?
    - A. glucose transporter type 1 (Glut1) deficiency
    - B. myoclonic astatic epilepsy
    - C. pyruvate carboxylase deficiency
    - D. pyruvate dehydrogenase (E1) deficiency
    - E. tuberous sclerosis related Lennox-Gastaut syndrome

Correct Answer is: C

The ketogenic diet is safe and effective in management of epilepsy associated with glucose transporter type 1 (Glut1) deficiency, pyruvate dehydrogenase (E1) deficiency, infantile spasms, myoclonic astatic epilepsy, and severe myoclonic epilepsy of infancy, tuberous sclerosis complex, Lennox-Gastaut syndrome and Rett syndrome. On the other hand, the ketogenic diet is contraindicated in pyruvate carboxylase deficiency, primary carnitine deficiency, carnitine palmitoyl transferase I and II deficiencies, carnitine translocase deficiency, beta-oxidation defects and porphyria.

Suggested Reading

- Lee RR, Kossoff EH. Dietary treatments for epilepsy: management guidelines for the general practitioner. Epilepsy Behav. 2011;21(2):115–21.

47. The family of a 6-month-old boy reports clusters of brief neck flexion and arm extension and developmental regression. His EEG shows a chaotic high-voltage background, polymorphic delta activity with admixed multifocal spike-wave discharges and electrodecrements. His birth, past medical history, and family history were unremarkable. He has no hypopigmented macules on examination. MRI brain is normal. Standard metabolic evaluation of CSF, serum, and urine is unrevealing. He was diagnosed with West syndrome and treated with adrenocorticotropic hormone. The parents reported clinical cessation of infantile spasms within 1 week. **What is the recommended EEG type and time of testing from the time treatment was initiated?**
    - A. 1-h routine EEG after 2 months
    - B. 1-h routine EEG after 2 weeks
    - C. 1-h routine EEG after 4 weeks
    - D. 24-h inpatient video EEG after 2 months
    - E. 24-h inpatient video EEG after 2 weeks

Correct Answer is: E

The recommendation form the 2010 US consensus report is short duration therapy with a first-line treatment (ACTH or vigabatrin) and timely EEG evaluation of treatment effectiveness. The patient has been improved clinically on ACTH, so a 24-h inpatient video EEG is recommended after 2 weeks of treatment to evaluate for subtle persistent infantile spasms. If difficult infantile spasms or hypsarrhythmia are detected, then prompt treatment modification may still be needed.

Suggested Reading

- Pellock JM, Hrachovy R, Shinnar S, et al. Infantile spasms: a U.S. consensus report. Epilepsia. 2010;51:2175–89.

48. What is the mechanism of action of vigabatrin?
    A. activation of GABA-B receptors
    B. allosteric binding to GABA-A receptors
    C. increasing GABA synthesis
    D. inhibiting neuronal and glial reuptake of GABA
    E. inhibition of GABA transaminase

Correct Answer is: E
Vigabatrin is an irreversible inhibitor of GABA transaminase, and its antiepileptic effects are based on inhibition of metabolic breakdown of GABA. Phenobarbital and benzodiazepines bind to GABA-A receptors; tiagabine inhibits neuronal and glial reuptake of GABA; baclofen (not an AED) activates GABA-B receptors; valproic acid is thought to possibly increase GABA synthesis, among other actions.

9

Suggested Reading

- Browne TR, Holmes GL. Handbook of epilepsy. 4th ed. Philadelphia: Lippincott: Williams & Wilkins; 2008.

49. Which of the following statements is most true about the management of status epilepticus?
    A. among the anesthetic agents, intravenous midazolam has the lowest rates of breakthrough seizures
    B. intramuscular midazolam has inferior efficacy compared to intravenous lorazepam
    C. intravenous diazepam has longer lasting anticonvulsant activity than lorazepam
    D. intravenous lorazepam has more rapid onset than diazepam
    E. there is a time-dependent efficacy of first-line agents

Correct Answer is: E
Treatment of status epilepticus is initiated with benzodiazepines. Because of greater lipid solubility, diazepam has a more rapid onset of action. On the other hand, lorazepam has a longer lasting anticonvulsant activity with less respiratory side effects due to smaller volume distribution. As shown in the Rapid Anticonvulsant Medication Prior to Arrival Trial (RAMPART) study, intramuscular midazolam was noninferior by a margin of 10% to that of intravenous lorazepam in patients treated by paramedics for status epilepticus and had comparable safety. All these first-line agents act on a subset of benzodiazepine-sensitive GABAA receptors, whose reduction in surface expression during status epilepticus parallels their time-dependent efficacy. In systematic review of prior studies for treatment of refractory status epilepticus, pentobarbital was associated with the lowest rates of acute failure and withdrawal seizures, but the highest rates of systemic hypotension requiring pressors.

Suggested Reading

- Treiman DM. The role of benzodiazepines in the management of status epilepticus. Neurology. 1990;40(5 Suppl 2):32–42. Review.
- Claassen J, Jirsch LJ, Emerson RG. Treatment of refractory status epilepticus with pentobarbital, propofol, or midazolam: a systematic review. Epilepsia. 2002;43(2):146–53. Review.
- Goodkin HP, Joshi S, Mtchedlishvili Z, et al. Subunit-specific trafficking of GABA(A) receptors during status epilepticus. J Neurosci. 2008;28(10):2527–38.
- Silbergleit R, Lowenstein D, Durkalski V, Conwit R; NETT Investigators. Lessons

from the RAMPART study--and which is the best route of administration of benzodiazepines in status epilepticus. Epilepsia. 2013;54(Suppl 6):74–7.
- Browne TR. The pharmacokinetics of agents used to treat status epilepticus. Neurology. 1990;40(5 Suppl 2):28–32. Review.

50. A focal disconnection surgical procedure would be favored over a resective procedure with which of the following conditions?
   A. Hemimegalencephaly
   B. Cortical dysplasia
   C. Rasmussen encephalitis
   D. Sturge-Weber syndrome
   E. Landau-Kleffner syndrome

Correct Answer is: E
Rasmussen encephalitis, hemimegalencephaly, Sturge-Weber syndrome and cortical dysplasias are commonly associated with refractory epilepsy that can be surgically curable with a radical resection such as a modified hemispherectomy. Landau-Kleffner on the other hand is a form of acquired epileptic aphasia arising from the posterior temporal region of the dominant hemisphere and is either treated with medications or with disconnection surgical procedures, such as multiple subpial transections, aiming to preserve the eloquent cortex in that region.

Suggested Reading

- Gonzalez-Martinez JA, Gupta A, Gidal B, et al. Hemispherectomies, hemispherotomies and other hemispheric disconnections. In: Wyllie E, Cascino G, Gidal B, editors. Wyllie's treatment of epilepsy: principles and practice. Philadelphia: Lippincott Williams & Wilkins; 2011.
- Smith MC, Byrne R, Kanner AM, et al. Corpus callosotomy and multiple subpial transection. In: Wyllie E, Cascino G, Gidal B, editors. Wyllie's treatment of epilepsy: principles and practice. Philadelphia: Lippincott Williams & Wilkins; 2011.

51. Which cardiac conduction abnormality has been reported with rufinamide?
   A. prolonged PR interval
   B. prolonged QT interval
   C. right bundle branch block
   D. shortened PR interval
   E. shortened QT interval

Correct Answer is: E
Rufinamide has been reported to shorten the QT interval, and is contraindicated in patients with short QT interval. It has been advised to obtain a baseline EKG prior to initiating therapy with rufinamide.

Suggested Reading

- Spanaki MV, Barkley GL. An overview of third-generation antiseizure drugs: Clobazam, lacosamide, rufinamide and vigabatrin. Neurol Clin Pract. 2012;2: 236–41.

52. Which of the following sporting activities is classified as low risk for persons with epilepsy?
   A. baseball
   B. scuba diving
   C. gymnastics
   D. hockey
   E. soccer

Correct Answer is: A.
Sports activities for an epilepsy patient should be decided on an individual basis. Scuba diving, hang gliding, boxing, and hockey are classified as a

high-risk activity. On the other hand, football, soccer, basketball, gymnastics, horseback riding are moderate risk activities, but golf, bowling, ping-pong and baseball are low risk activities.

Suggested Reading

- ILAE Commission report. Restrictions for children with epilepsy. Commission of Pediatrics of the ILAE. International League Against Epilepsy. Epilepsia. 1997;38(9):1054–6.
- Drazkowski JF, Sirven JI. Driving and social issues in epilepsy. In: Wyllie E, Cascino G, Gidal B, editors. Wyllie's treatment of epilepsy: principles and practice. Philadelphia: Lippincott Williams & Wilkins; 2011.
- Mesad SM. Epilepsy and the athlete. In: Jordan BD, Tsairis P, Warren R, editors. Sport neurology. 2nd ed. Philadelphia: Raven Press; 1998.

53. A 14-year-old male has been evaluated for nocturnal seizures. His birth and past medical history are unremarkable. There is a family history nocturnal seizure in his father that began in adolescence, are well controlled, and persisted into adulthood. The boy's seizures happened exclusively in sleep, are brief (lasting less than 30 s), and characterized by sudden eye opening, head raising or sitting up in bed, often with a frightened expression, and sometimes vocalization. His interictal awake and drowsy EEG is normal. Genetic studies are performed, showing a mutation in the *CHRNA4* gene coding the alpha subunit of the neuronal nicotinic acetylcholine receptor (nAChR).
What is your most likely diagnosis?
    A. autosomal dominant nocturnal frontal lobe epilepsy (ADNFLE)
    B. familial focal epilepsy with variable foci
    C. gelastic seizures
    D. juvenile absence epilepsy
    E. mesial temporal lobe epilepsy with hippocampal sclerosis

Correct Answer is: A
The clinical presentation of this patient would be consistent with frontal lobe epilepsy. Given the almost exclusive nocturnal events, family history, and description, this would make autosomal dominant nocturnal frontal lobe epilepsy likely. The genetic studies performed confirmed the classic chromosomal abnormality associated with this condition.

Suggested Reading

- Combi R, Dalpra L, Tenchini ML, Ferini-Strambi L. Autosomal dominant nocturnal frontal lobe epilepsy – A critical overview. J Neurol. 2004;251(8):923–34.
- Oldani A, Zucconi M, Asselta R, et al. Autosomal dominant nocturnal frontal lobe epilepsy--A video-polysomnographic and genetic appraisal of forty patients and delineation of the epileptic syndrome. Brain. 1998;121(Pt 2): 205–23.

54. Blue discoloration of the skin and retinas has been associated with use of which of the following antiepileptic medications?
    A. eslicarbazepine
    B. ezogabine
    C. lacosamide
    D. perampanel
    E. rufinamide

Correct Answer is: B.
Prolonged use of ezogabine (also known as retigabine) has been associated with a bluish discoloration of lips, fingernails and skin, as well as bluish discoloration of the retina.

Suggested Reading

- Faulkner MA, Burke RA. Safety profile of two novel antiepileptic agents approved for the treatment of refractory partial seizures: ezogabine (retigabine) and perampanel. Expert Opin Drug Saf. 2013;12:847–55.
- FDA safety warning.

55. An 18-year-old male came for evaluation of medically resistant, idiopathic complex partial seizures. He started to have his seizures in his adolescence; brain MRI is normal. His physical and neurologic exams are normal. He failed pregabalin, carbamazepine, gabapentin, and valproate. His current medication is valproate. The seizures occur in the day time and in sleep, but more often in sleep and are characterized by awakening, staring off, automatisms and nonresponsiveness for up to 90 s. Approximately 25% go on to secondary generalized tonic-clonic activity. He has a significant history of snoring at night and excessive daytime sleepiness for the last 2 years. **What is the best next step in his management?**
    A. addition of perampanel to the patient's drug regimen
    B. counsel the patient on weight loss
    C. obtain a sleep study
    D. refer the patient for a clinical trial of a novel antiepileptic drug
    E. vagus nerve stimulation therapy

Correct Answer is: C
People with epilepsy frequently report day time sleepiness and poor quality of sleep. Patients with excessive day time sleepiness have significantly lower quality of life scores. The association between obstructive sleep apnea and epilepsy has been known for years. Obstructive sleep apnea is common in men who are overweight. Seizure control will improve significantly after the treatment of the obstructive sleep apnea with continuous positive airway pressure (CPAP). In patients who are overweight and have a history of snoring and excessive daytime sleepiness, a sleep study would be the next best strategy in their management. If the study shows evidence of obstructive sleep apnea, treatment with CPAP could improve the patient's seizure control, excessive daytime sleepiness, and quality of life before further interventions are performed. All the antiepileptic medications he used can increase weight. If the patient is overweight, changing to an antiepileptic medication not associated with weight gain should be considered, as obesity can contribute to sleep apnea.

Suggested Reading

- Derry CP, Duncan S. Sleep and epilepsy. Epilepsy Behav. 2013;26(3):394–404.
- Mallow BA, Fromes GA, Aldrich MS. Usefulness of polysomnography in epilepsy patients. Neurology. 1997;48(5):1389–94.

56. Medical management would be favored over surgical evaluation in which of the following cases of refractory epilepsy?
    A. a 9-month-old boy presents with refractory infantile spasms in the context of multifocal tubers on MRI and TSC1 mutation on genetic testing
    B. a 15-year-old boy presents with refractory nocturnal frontal lobe seizures in the context of normal MRI and presence of CHRNA4 mutation on genetic testing
    C. a 20-year-old woman presents with refractory generalized convulsions in sleep, in the context of right frontal lobe dysplasia on MRI and 15q14 chromosome mutation on genetic testing

D. a 25-year-old man presents with refractory complex partial seizures in the context of cavernous malformations in the left temporal pole and the right frontal lobes and CCM2 mutation on genetic testing
E. a 30-year-old woman presents with refractory complex partial seizures in the context of right mesial temporal sclerosis on MRI and GABRA1 mutation on genetic testing

Correct Answer is: B
Autosomal dominant nocturnal frontal lobe epilepsy is an inherited genetic condition due to widespread dysfunction in the nicotinic acetylcholine receptors and would therefore not be surgically remediable. The other conditions listed could still demonstrate potentially focal epileptogenicity, and thus merit presurgical evaluation.

9

Suggested Reading

- Steinlein OK, Kaneko S, Hirose S. Nicotinic acetylcholine receptor mutations. In: Noebels JL, Avoli M, Rogawski MA, et al. editors. Jasper's basic mechanisms of the epilepsies. 4th ed. Bethesda: National Center for Biotechnology Information (US); 2012.
- Loddenkemper T, Cosmo G, Kotagal P, et al. Epilepsy surgery in children with electrical status epilepticus in sleep. Neurosurgery. 2009;64(2):328–37.
- Jeha LE, Morris HH, Burgess RC. Coexistence of focal and idiopathic generalized epilepsy in the same patient population. Seizure. 2006;15(1):28–34.
- Bernasconi A, Bernasconi N, Bernhardt BC, Schrader D. Advances in MRI for 'cryptogenic' epilepsies. Nat Rev Neurol. 2011;7(2):99–108.
- Michelucci R, Pasini E, Riquzzi P, et al. Genetics of epilepsy and relevance to current practice. Curr Neurol Neurosci Rep. 2012;12(4):445–55.
- Dashti SR1, Hoffer A, Hu YC, Selman WR. Molecular genetics of familial cerebral cavernous malformations. Neurosurg Focus. 21(1):e2.

57. An 18-year-old female with idiopathic complex partial seizures. She has been seizure-free for years on 400 mg carbamazepine twice daily. One month ago, her primary care physician added fluoxetine because of her mood disorder. She is complaining of diplopia, nausea, and gait and balance difficulties.
What is the best next step in her management?
A. discontinue fluoxetine and replace it with fluvoxamine
B. discontinue fluoxetine and replace it with citalopram
C. obtain a urine toxicology study
D. obtain an MRI of the brain
E. send her to laboratory for a serum sodium level

Correct Answer is: B
Carbamazepine is metabolized extensively through the P450 CYP3A4 enzyme system. Medications used to influence mood may affect this metabolism. Both fluoxetine and fluvoxamine inhibit metabolism of the CYP3A4 isoenzyme, resulting in increasing carbamazepine levels significantly. This medication interaction can produce the symptoms of carbamazepine toxicity, namely diplopia, ataxia, and gastrointestinal upset. If a medication is needed for mood disorder, both citalopram and escitalopram have no effect on the CYP450 system and would not have an interaction. Either of these medications would be a good alternative for this patient. The urine toxicology test is likely to be negative given the history.

Carbamazepine can produce hyponatremia, but the sudden onset of her symptom after years of treatment would be unlikely due to hyponatremia.

Suggested Reading

- Mula M. Anticonvulsant--antidepressant pharmacokinetic drug interactions: the role of the CYP450 system in psychopharmacology. Curr Drug Metab. 2008;9(8):730–7.
- Spina E, Santoro V, D'Arrigio C. Clinically relevant pharmacokinetic drug interactions with second-generation antidepressants: an update. Clin Ther. 2008;30(7):1206–27.

58. Which of the following patients carries the highest chances of becoming seizure free?
    A. an 8-year-old boy with benign childhood epilepsy with centrotemporal spikes
    B. an 11-year old boy with benign childhood epilepsy with occipital spikes
    C. a 12-year-old girl with juvenile absence epilepsy
    D. a 20-year-old woman with juvenile myoclonic epilepsy
    E. a 35-year-old man with lesional mesial temporal lobe epilepsy

Correct Answer is: A

In benign childhood epilepsy with centrotemporal spikes (Rolandic epilepsy), remission occurs almost universally by adolescence and treatment during symptomatic period is controversial; 1% of patients develop refractory seizures into adulthood. In benign childhood occipital epilepsy of Gastaut type, the remission rates are much than Rolandic epilepsy. In childhood absence epilepsy, spontaneous remission occurs in 65% to 70% of patients during adolescence. In juvenile absence epilepsy, seizures may persist for many years, but the prognosis is usually good and response to treatment is excellent. Similarly, in juvenile myoclonic epilepsy, response to treatment is good in 85% of patients, but it is a lifelong treatment. On the other hand, patients with hippocampal sclerosis are likely to be intractable in about 90% of cases.

Suggested Reading

- Bergqvist C. Idiopathic pediatric epilepsy syndromes. Continuum Lifelong Learn Neurol. 2007;13(4):106–20.
- D'Argenzio L, Cross JH. Hippocampal sclerosis and dual pathology. In: Wyllie E, Cascino G, Gidal B, editors. Wyllie's treatment of epilepsy: principles and practice. Philadelphia: Lippincott Williams & Wilkins; 2011.

59. The predominant site of action of the new antiepileptic (antiseizure) medication perampanel is on:
    A. AMPA receptors
    B. NMDA receptors
    C. postsynaptic GABA receptors
    D. presynaptic SV2A receptors
    E. voltage-dependent sodium channels

Correct Answer is: A

Perampanel is a selective noncompetitive antagonist of AMPA receptors, a major subtype of excitatory amino acid receptors activated by glutamate. It has no other known major mechanism of action. Benzodiazepines and barbiturates act on GABA receptors, while phenytoin, carbamazepine, and lamotrigine are voltage-dependent sodium channels. Levetiracetam acts on SV2A receptors to modulate neuronal activity. Ketamine blocks NMDA receptors, but there are no chronic oral seizure medications that act on this

excitatory amino acid receptor; actions at this site cause a variety of major side effects, predominantly psychological and sedative.

Suggested Reading

- Rogawski MA. AMPA Receptors as a molecular target in epilepsy therapy. Acta Neurol Scand Suppl. 2013;(197):9–18.

60. A 5-year-old boy has known epilepsy with multiple seizure types and mild developmental delay. Seizure started at 5 months of age, with focal seizures characterized by staring, and cyanosis. His EEG showed multifocal spike-wave discharges. Seizures were refractory to initial anticonvulsant trials. He developed new seizure types including atypical absence, myoclonic, and tonic-clonic, with generalized epileptiform discharges on EEG. Seizures were completely controlled with the introduction of the ketogenic diet.
Mutation of which of the following genes would confirm the diagnosis?
A. *SLC2A1*
B. *SCN1A*
C. *KCNQ2*
D. *KCNT1*
E. *ALDH7A1*

9

Correct Answer is: A.
The clinical presentation indicates glucose transporter type I deficiency syndrome (GLUT1-DS) that is characterized by infantile onset of seizures that are refractory to anticonvulsants, and the development of generalized seizures in early childhood. GLUT1-DS is known as "De Vivo disease" and diagnosed with careful CSF glucose concentration measurements. *SLC2A1* gene mutation is known to cause GLUT1-DS; and testing can confirm the clinical suspicion. *SCN1A* is associated with Dravet syndrome. *KCNQ2* is associated with benign familial neonatal convulsions, and mutations in the KCNQ2 gene can also result in a more severe disorder with early-onset epileptic encephalopathy. *KCNT1* associated with migrating partial seizures of infancy. *ALDH7A1* is associated with pyridoxine-dependent epilepsy.

Suggested Reading

- De Vivo DC, Trifiletti RR, Jacobson RI, et al. Defective glucose transport across the blood-brain barrier as a cause of persistent hypoglycorrhachia, seizures, and developmental delay. N Engl J Med. 1991;325:703–9.

61. An 8-month-old male infant develops seizures 2 days after receiving a vaccine for *Haemophilus influenza*. Initially, his seizures are relatively infrequent clonic seizures. At the age of 10 months, he started to have frequent, prolonged myoclonic seizures. He also has infrequent absence seizures. He subsequently develops two episodes of refractory status epilepticus. His interictal EEG shows generalized polyspike-and-wave and spike-and-wave discharges of 1.5–2 Hz.
Screening for mutations in which of the following genes is most likely to reveal the etiology of this child's epilepsy?
A. *CHRNA4*
B. *EPM1*
C. *EPM2A*
D. *SCN1A*
E. *TSC1*

Correct Answer is: D
This child has severe myoclonic epilepsy of infancy, also known as Dravet syndrome. 75% of Dravet syndrome cases are secondary of mutations to the *SCN1A* gene. Fever or vaccination can trigger the seizures in 30% to 40% of

infants with severe myoclonic epilepsy. Initial seizures are relatively infrequent clonic or tonic-clonic seizures. However, affected individuals subsequently developed abundant severe, prolonged myoclonic seizures, as well as absence seizures and focal motor seizures. Frequent episodes of status epilepticus are not uncommon in this condition. Mutations in *CHRNA4* are typically seen in individuals with nocturnal frontal lobe epilepsy. Mutations in *EPM1* and *EPM2A* lead to Unverricht-Lundborg and Lafora body disease, respectively, which are two forms of progressive myoclonic epilepsy that affect children and teenagers. Mutations in *TSC1* lead to tuberous sclerosis.

Suggested Reading

- Marini C, Scheffer IE, Nabbout R, et al. The genetics of Dravet syndrome. Epilepsia. 2011;52.

62. Sudden unexplained death in epilepsy (SUDEP) is best characterized by which of the following factors?
    - A. may be associated with profound and prolonged postictal EEG suppressions
    - B. more common in patients with refractory atonic seizures
    - C. more frequent in children
    - D. occurs from status epilepticus
    - E. risk may be increased in patients on selective serotonin reuptake inhibitors (SSRIs)

Correct Answer is: A

Sudden unexplained death in epilepsy (SUDEP) is defined as unexpected, witnessed or unwitnessed, nontraumatic and nondrowning deaths in patients with epilepsy, with or without evidence of a seizure and excluding documented status epilepticus. Postmortem examination does not reveal a toxicologic or anatomic cause of death and is rare in patients with new-onset epilepsy and in patients in remission. Incidence is about 0.35 cases/1000 person-years in population-based incidence cohort of epilepsy. Incidence is considerably higher in patients with chronic epilepsy, 1–2/1000 person-years, and highest with severe, refractory seizures, 3–9/1000. The highest rates occur from 20 to 40 years. Refractory epilepsy with convulsive seizures and onset at an early age, as well as long duration and polytherapy are other reported risk factors. Some studies suggest that postictal generalized electroencephalography suppression greater than 20 s following generalized convulsions is a risk factor for SUDEP, but this contention as an independent risk factor, as opposed to an epiphenomenon, is still debated. Similarly, some animal and human data have suggested that SSRIs are associated with reduced likelihood of ictal oxygen desaturation in patients with partial seizures.

Suggested Reading

- Tomson T, Walczak T, Sillanpaa M, Sander JW. Sudden unexpected death in epilepsy: a review of incidence and risk factors. Epilepsia. 2005;46(Suppl 11):54–61.
- Bateman LM et al. Serotonin reuptake inhibitors are associated with reduced severity of ictal hypoxemia in medically refractory partial epilepsy. Epilepsia. 2010;51(10):2211–4.
- Lhatoo SD, Faulkner HJ, Dembny K, et al. An electroclinical case-control study of sudden unexpected death in epilepsy. Ann Neurol. 2010;68(6):787–96.

63. You are requested to evaluate a 3-day-old boy, who is irritable with poor feeding. He is having multiple focal seizures characterized by apnea and clonic jerking. His mother had no complication during pregnancy and delivery. He has no family history

of epilepsy. MRI brain is normal.
The interictal EEG background is excessively discontinuous for stated postconceptional age. He was refractory to phenobarbital, but seizures were subsided with a trial of oral pyridoxine.
Which gene is the most likely responsible for his seizures?

A. *ALDH7A1*
B. *KCNQ2*
C. *KCNT1*
D. *SCN1A*
E. *SLC2A1*

Correct Answer is: A
The clinical history is most consistent with pyridoxine-dependent epilepsy, caused by mutations in *ALDH7A1*. Dravet syndrome is usually secondary to mutations in the *SCN1A* gene. In the past, *KCNQ2* was associated only with benign familial neonatal convulsions, but recently different mutations are responsible for previously undiagnosed cases of Ohtahara syndrome. *SLC2A1* is the only gene in which mutations are known to cause GLUT1-DS and testing can confirm the clinical suspicion. *KCNT1* is the causative gene for the migrating partial seizures of infancy.

9

Suggested Reading

- Gospe SM. Pyridoxine-dependent epilepsy. In: Pagon RA, Adam MP, Ardinger HH, et al. editors. GeneReviews® [Internet]. Seattle: University of Washington, Seattle; 1993–2014.

64. A 12-year-old boy is evaluated for his history of hyperkinetic nocturnal events, sometimes with tonic or dystonic features. They are stereotyped, often cluster and may have relatively preserved consciousness. His family history showed a similar disorder in his father and older sister. He had a video-EEG monitoring that showed nocturnal partial seizures, possibly from the frontal lobe. His seizures have been totally controlled with carbamazepine.
This is associated with a genetic mutation that encodes for which of the following areas?

A. NMDA receptor
B. one of the voltage-gated potassium channels
C. SCN1A sodium channel
D. subunit of the GABA-A receptor
E. subunit of the nicotinic acetylcholine receptor

Correct Answer is: E
The clinical scenario is consistent with autosomal dominant nocturnal frontal lobe epilepsy (ADNFLE)--a disorder that produces brief, often multiple nocturnal frontal lobe seizures during slow wave sleep. This is an autosomal dominant disorder with70% to 80% penetrance, and it is associated with a mutation in the gene *CHRNA4*, encoding the alpha 4 subunit of a neuronal nicotinic acetylcholine receptor (nAchR). This was the first ion channel mutation found in an inherited form of epilepsy. How this mutation produces epilepsy is still unknown.

Suggested Reading

- Steinlein OK, Mulley JC, Propping P et al. A missense mutation in the neuronal nicotinic acetylcholine receptor apha 4 subunit is associated with autosomal dominant nocturnal frontal lobe epilepsy. Nat Genet 1995;11:201–3.
- Guerrini R, Marini M, Mantegazza M. Genetic epilepsy syndromes without structural brain abnormalities: clinical features and experimental models. Neurotherapeutics. 2014;11:269–85.

65. A 4-day-old boy with normal birth history has tonic seizures, characterized by stiffening and apnea. His interictal EEG shows burst suppression. Pyridoxine trial was ineffective. MRI

brain was normal. CSF, serum, and urine tests results were negative. His seizures remain refractory to multiple anticonvulsant trials, but gradually decrease in frequency at 2 years old. He has severe cognitive and motor impairments without progression.

Which gene mutation will most likely confirm the diagnosis?

A. *ALDH7A1*
B. *KCNQ2*
C. *KCNT1*
D. *SCN1A*
E. *SLC2A1*

Correct Answer is: B.
KCNQ2 **was previously associated only with benign familial neonatal convulsions. Different mutations were recently found with previously undiagnosed cases of Ohtahara syndrome.** ***SLC2A1*** **is the only gene in which mutations are known to cause GLUT1-DS and has been associated with early onset seizures (e.g., absence).** ***SCN1A*** **is associated with Dravet syndrome.** ***KCNT1*** **is associated with migrating partial seizures of infancy.** ***ALDH7A1*** **is associated with pyridoxine dependent epilepsy.**

Suggested Reading

- Weckhuysen S, Ivanovic V, Hendrickx R, et al. on behalf of the KCNQ2 Study Group. Extending the <em>KCNQ2</em> encephalopathy spectrum.

66. A 2-day-old baby has a routine EEG in the nursery because he has intermittent episodes of apnea. He was born by vaginal delivery after uncomplicated pregnancy at 39 weeks gestation. Family history is negative for epilepsy. The infant is otherwise healthy, vigorous, and feeding well. He has normal exam. The EEG showed quiet sleep that was clinically characterized by closed eyes and little movement. The EEG background activity shows predominantly asynchronous bursts of medium to high voltage delta activity of approximately 3–5 s duration alternating with 1–2 s of interburst periods of 25 μV to 50 μV, mixed theta and delta activity.

What is the EEG pattern consistent with?

A. activité moyenne
B. burst suppression
C. theta pointu alternant
D. tracé alternant
E. tracé discontinu

Correct Answer is: D
This is the normal trace alternant EEG pattern, which is the normal quiet sleep background for a term neonate. Trace discontinu is another normal sleep background seen in preterm neonates which is more discontinuous, as the name implies. Activité moyenne is the normal wake background in a term neonate and characterized by continuous mixed frequency activity. Burst suppression is a severely abnormal background characterized by invariant bursts and prolonged low-voltage interburst intervals. Theta pointu alternant is characterized by runs of unilateral alternating theta activity in admixed sharp waves; this pattern is nonspecific and is an interictal finding that may be seen associated with multiple causes of neonatal seizures.

Suggested Reading

- Tsuchida TN, Wusthoff CJ, Shellhaas RA, et al. American Clinical Neurophysiology Society Critical Care Monitoring Committee.
- American clinical neurophysiology society standardized EEG terminology and categorization for the description of continuous EEG monitoring in neonates: report of the American Clinical Neurophysiology Society critical care monitoring committee. J Clin Neurophysiol. 2013; 30:161–73.

67. To apply for the social security administration disability benefits in relation to epilepsy, the presence of which of the following factors would be sufficient?
  A. Three daytime nonconvulsive seizures per month, which interfere with awareness
  B. history of prior employment
  C. nocturnal convulsions without prolonged postictal confusion
  D. One convulsive seizure every 2 months
  E. significant comorbid conditions

Correct Answer is: E
Regardless of prior employment, consideration of social security administration disability benefits can be given in patients with epilepsy if they have one of the following: (1) at least four partial seizures per month that are of sufficient severity to cause clouding of consciousness or significant impairment of daytime activities (2) at least one daytime convulsive seizure per month (3) predominantly nocturnal convulsive seizures with aftereffects that persist during the day, or (4) significant neuropsychiatric or medical comorbidities exist. The treating physician usually is asked to submit a medical documentation and opinion on the disability claim and can therefore function as an advocate for the patient by helping to ensure that they are fairly considered for employment or benefits.

Suggested Reading

- Social Security website [accessed May 2014].
- Drazkowski JF, Cascino G, Gidal BE, et al. Driving and social issues in epilepsy. In: Wyllie E, Cascino G, Gidal BF, editors. Wyllie's treatment of epilepsy: principles and practice. Philadelphia: Lippincott Williams & Wilkins; 2011.

9

68. 3-year-old girl came to the ED by EMS after she abruptly became limp and exhibited shaking of her arms and legs in her daycare. While she was playing with other children, she fell down, cried briefly, and then she lost her conciseness. In the ambulance, she woke up, started crying for her mother. She has normal general and neurologic examinations. Her mother reports that she had previous 3 such episode and all of them have been provoked by minor injuries. Her EKG was normal after the first episode. **What is your next step in her management?**
  A. perform a 1-week cardiac event monitor
  B. perform MRI of the brain
  C. perform routine electroencephalogram (EEG)
  D. prescribe levetiracetam
  E. reassurance

Correct Answer is: E
Pediatric neurologists always have a lot of paroxysmal spells referrals. Usually, the concern is about possible seizure. Typically, the pediatric neurologist does not witness the event and children are normal between events, so the neurologic examination is of limited benefit. A full detailed history is the way to figure out the nature of the spell and determining whether further evaluation or treatment is needed. Video recording by caregivers is off utmost importance. The patient spells are triggered by minor injuries and probably represent a vasovagal attack (pallid breath-holding spells.) Other children cry vigorously and get "caught" in the exhalation phase of breathing. In this case, their face becoming deep red, their bodies often becoming rigid, they lose consciousness; and then they begin breathing again (cyanotic breath-holding spells). Children with these spells

require no further testing or treatment, only parental reassurance.Different types of paroxysmal non-epileptic spells come different ages. In infancy, it is quite common for the immature cortex to fail to inhibit unwanted, or undesired, movements. These can occur in wakefulness, in the case of clonus, which is not always a sign of pathology in a young infant; or during sleep, as in the setting of benign sleep myoclonus of infancy. On the other hand, gastroesophageal reflux can cause an unwanted movements, sometimes associated with color changes, which can trigger laryngospasm and affect breathing--leading to dystonic posturing. During the toddler years, breath-holding spells and infantile gratification disorders are common; and they often mark the onset of the sleep parasomnias, such as night terrors. Breath-holding spells in particular can often mimic seizures; breathing is affected, often followed by loss of postural tone and then abnormal movements (similar to those associated with syncope.) Color change, either pallor or cyanosis, occurs. A history of consistent provocation of the spells, by anger or pain, should raise suspicion.Older children can have continued sleep related events (parasomnias, periodic limb movements in sleep, confusion arousals) which can be mistaken as seizures. Tic disorders typically begin in childhood and the history of willful control, which can help distinguish tics from simple partial seizures, is often lacking in young children. Syncope causes collapse, often with a series of associated myoclonic limb movements, which lead to a wrong seizure diagnosis. Other causes of transiently altered awareness that can mimic absence or complex partial seizures include hypersomnia from multiple causes, including narcolepsy and obstructive sleep apnea, attention deficit disorders, simple daydreaming, and complex migraine headaches. Children with developmental delay and autism of all ages commonly have periods of disengagement, or other stereotyped movements. For all of these conditions, a detailed history is the most important aspect of evaluation.

? 69. A 6-month-old girl is admitted to the hospital for a cluster of seizures. Her seizures are typically last 1–2 min and associated with sudden behavioral arrest, followed by clonic activity of her extremities. She has been having those seizures for the last month; however, they were shorter and only one every few days, until the day of admission. She became less interactive, especially with visual attention over the past 2 weeks. She is not sick, has no fever or upper respiratory symptoms. Her head circumference at the 10th percentile, with height and weight at the 25th percentile. She does not have any dysmorphic features or neurocutaneous lesions are seen. She is alert, has normal visual regard, conjugate tracking, and normal sucking abilities. She has mild decrease in the truncal and extremity tone, but tendon reflexes are normal. She does not make any attempts to reach or bear weight in sitting or standing. Her brain MRI is normal. EEG shows interictal sharp waves from both sides of the brain, and during a seizure shows ictal epileptiform patterns arising from the left central region. Her serum sodium is142; glucose 75; calcium of 9.2; and magnesium of 2.2. Seizures are resistant to treatment with phenobarbital, levetiracetam, and carbamazepine. Further evaluation includes a lumbar puncture which reveals 1 WBC; 0 RBC; glucose 30 mg/dL; and protein 20 mg/dL.

What is the most likely diagnosis?
A. cerebral folate deficiency
B. glucose-1-transporter deficiency
C. pyridoxine dependent epilepsy
D. severe myoclonic epilepsy of infancy
E. tuberous sclerosis complex

Correct Answer is: B
The child has a history of intractable infantile-onset epilepsy, of multifocal origin, and delayed development. Differential diagnosis is extensive, including pre- and perinatal insult, malformations of cortical development, neurocutaneous disorders (including tuberous sclerosis), and inborn errors of metabolism, chromosomal deletion/duplication syndromes, vitamin/cofactor responsive seizures, and the symptomatic generalized epilepsy syndromes of childhood.Our efforts have to be focused on treatable causes of refractory epilepsy in infants and young children. Until recently, empiric trials of vitamins/cofactors such as pyridoxine, pyridoxal phosphate (the active metabolite of pyridoxine) and folinic acid were given for vitamin B_6 dependency conditions, but now these disorders are diagnosed by urine/blood/CSF metabolite studies or genetic testing. Each one of these disorders can be partially responsive to conventional antiepileptic therapies, though complete seizure control is not achieved until the appropriate cofactor is supplemented in the diet.Both cerebral folate deficiency and glucose-1-transporter deficiency (GLUT-1) are diagnosed chiefly by examination of the spinal fluid (though confirmatory genetic sequencing tests are available for both.) Cerebral folate deficiency has a wide spectrum of neurologic presentations, including seizures, and tends to respond at least partially to use of folinic acid.Glucose-1-transporter deficiency (GLUT-1), due to a mutation in the SLC2A1 gene region on chromosome 1, leads to inability to efficiently transport glucose across the blood-brain barrier. The hallmark laboratory finding in such patients is a low cerebrospinal fluid glucose level (with over 90% of patients having values less than 40 mg/dL). When collected fasting, with a paired serum glucose level, there is also a low CSF/blood glucose ratio of less than 0.4 (with normal being over 0.5). Although typically presenting with seizures prior to the age of 2, there are several other variants, including intermittent dystonia, choreoathetosis, and ataxia. The disease occurs as a de novo mutation in 90% of cases, with the remaining 10% inherited in an autosomal dominant fashion.Treatment is centered on utilization of ketones bodies as an alternative source of energy for the brain, and when instituted promptly, the ketogenic diet can lead to full control of seizures, and even prevention of the intellectual disability and microcephaly which result from chronically low brain glucose levels. Although all of the other options can lead to refractory epilepsies in children, only GLUT-1 has the finding of a low cerebrospinal glucose level.

Suggested Reading

- Pagon RA, Adams MP, Bird TD, et al. editors. GeneReviews. Seattle: University of Washington, Seattle; 1993–2013.

70. A 17-year-old male hit his head after accidental fall followed by a 2 min generalized tonic-clonic seizure. In the ambulance, he came back to his baseline. He was evaluated at the ED and found no injuries. He has a normal brain CT. Serum toxicology was positive for cocaine. They kept him overnight for observation and the following morning had a normal neurologic examination and EEG.

Which of the following is the best recommendation regarding duration of antiepileptic drug therapy for this patient?

A. 0 days
B. 14 days
C. 6 months
D. 1 year
E. 2 years

Correct Answer is: A
7 days of antiepileptic drug (AED) prophylaxis is recommended after severe traumatic brain injury. However, in a mild injury, there is no definite consensus. This patient had an immediate provoked seizure and had no sequelae, therefore an AED is often not recommended. He also had two reasons for a provoked seizure, the head trauma with the fall and possible acute use of cocaine. In cases of a provoked seizure, AED prophylaxis is not generally recommended. In addition, even after a single nonprovoked seizure, AED prophylaxis is not generally used.

Suggested Reading

- Practice parameter: Antiepileptic drug prophylaxis in severe traumatic brain injury Report of the Quality Standards Subcommittee of the American Academy of Neurology

71. A 16-year-old male came for his seizure evaluation. His seizures started at 10 years of age. They only happen at night and involve hand clenching, rapid arm movements, and knee bending. He shouts and screams during the seizures. He was misdiagnosed of having nightmares, but seizures have stopped with the use of carbamazepine. He has a normal brain MRI and EEGs. His family history is remarkable of his father, paternal uncle, and paternal grandmother all have similar seizures.

An abnormality affecting which of the following cellular structures is most likely?

A. AMPA receptors
B. nicotinic acetylcholine receptors
C. potassium channels
D. sodium channels
E. T-type calcium channels

Correct Answer is: B
This family history and seizure semiology is consistent with autosomal dominant nocturnal frontal lobe epilepsy (ADNFLE). Those seizures are typically brief, tonic and hyperkinetic motor seizures occurring during the Non-REM sleep. Vocalizations are common. Usual onset is in childhood around 10 years of age. Bilateral frontal lobe epileptiform discharges are common during ictal EEG, but EEG is normal interictally. ADNFLE is secondary to mutations in the CHRNA4, CHRNB2, and CHRNA2 encoding subunits of the neuronal nicotinic acetylcholine receptor. Nicotine treatment seems to reduce seizure frequency in these patients.

Suggested Reading

- Chyung A, Ptacek LJ. Genetics of epilepsy. Continuum Lifelong Learn Neurol. 2005;11(2):79–94.
- Steinlein O, Mulley J, Propping P, et al. A missense mutation in the neuronal nicotinic acetylcholine receptor alpha 4 subunit is associated with autosomal dominant nocturnal frontal lobe epilepsy. Nat Genet.

72. A 5-year-old boy has been evaluated for episode of unresponsiveness. He awoke from sleep with vomiting, appeared pale, and had dilated pupils. He vomited for 15 min, then he suddenly became limp and unresponsive with eyes open and deviated up and to the left. 15 min later, he began to respond and complained

of a headache. His family reported 3 other episodes in the past 6 months of awakening from sleep and vomiting repeatedly, but he never became unresponsive with those spells. He has a normal neurologic examination in the ED.

Which of the following test results is most likely?

A. EEG showing occipital spikes
B. extreme somatosensory evoked potentials
C. genetic testing showing a point mutation in the CACNA1A gene
D. MRI showing pontine mass
E. serum test positive for antigliadin antibodies

Correct Answer is: A

Panayiotopoulos syndrome (early onset, benign focal epilepsy with occipital paroxysms) is a common focal epilepsy syndrome with a peak age of onset at 5 years. The typical seizures consist predominantly of autonomic symptoms, more often arise from sleep, and tend to be prolonged. A typical seizure is characterized by the child maintaining consciousness, complaining of feeling sick, and then turns pale and vomits. Other autonomic features may also be present such as cyanosis, mydriasis, incontinence, or hypersalivation. 20% of the seizures progress into unresponsiveness and loss of tone (ictal syncope). The seizures may last from 30 min to several hours. The interictal EEG shows multifocal, occipitally predominant, spike- and slow waves accentuated by sleep.

9

Suggested Reading

- Bergqvist C. Idiopathic pediatric epilepsy syndromes. Continuum Lifelong Learn Neurol 2007;13(4):106.

73. An 18-year-old female was admitted to the ED after a witnessed generalized tonic-clonic seizure at home. When she woke up. She was disoriented, but then able to provide a history of depression and one other GTC seizure in the past, as well as morning episodes of arm jerking and dropping objects. She takes citalopram and her PCP increased her dose recently to 80 mg daily. Her EEG in the ED shows bilateral theta slowing and occasional frontal intermittent rhythmic delta activity.

What is her seizure etiology?

A. cerebral vasospasm
B. increased intracranial pressure
C. juvenile myoclonic epilepsy
D. serotonin syndrome
E. sleep deprivation

Correct Answer is: C

The clinical scenario of morning myoclonus and a generalized tonic-clonic seizure is indicative of juvenile myoclonic epilepsy. A postictal EEG may show interictal 4 Hz to 6 Hz generalized spike-wave and polyspikes, but could be normal or show postictal slowing. Postictal slowing may consist of generalized theta and delta slowing, as well as frontal intermittent rhythmic delta activity (FIRDA). Morning myoclonus is not typical of increased intracranial pressure. Serotonin syndrome is not typically associated with convulsions. Sleep deprivation can exacerbate seizures in individuals with epilepsy, but is not part of this history.

Suggested Reading

- Bergqvist C. Idiopathic pediatric epilepsy syndromes. Continuum Lifelong Learn Neurol. 2007;13(4):106–20.

74. An 18-year-old male, with Lennox-Gastaut syndrome, starts to have an increase in his seizures. Usually, he has 1 to 5 seizures a day consisting of body stiffening and head drop. Four

weeks ago, his seizures increased to up to 20 seizures a day, and he has fallen twice in the past week. It is not safe for him to walk unassisted because of the seizures. He is on rufinamide, levetiracetam, and zonisamide. He has tried multiple antiepileptic drugs in the past.

What do you recommend as a next step in his management?

A. add on perampanel
B. prescribe a wheelchair
C. prescribe gait belt
D. refer for a vagal nerve stimulator
E. refer for transcranial magnetic stimulation

Correct Answer is: D

Vagal nerve stimulation (VNS) is efficacious as well as the new antiepileptic drugs. A 2009 AAN Guideline concludes that "sufficient evidence exists to rank VNS for epilepsy as effective and safe, based on a preponderance of Class I evidence". A study by Lundgren et al. found among 6 children with Lennox-Gastaut syndrome, 5 sustained at least a 90% reduction of seizures. Transcranial magnetic stimulation and perampanel could be effective, but have less evidence for use in this situation. A wheelchair or gait belt would improve safety, but would not address the seizures increase.

Suggested Reading

- Fisher RS, Handforth A. Reassessment: Vagus nerve stimulation for epilepsy. Neurology. 1999;53:666.
- Lundgren J, Amark P, Blennow G, et al. Vagus nerve stimulation in 16 children with refractory epilepsy. Epilepsia. 1998;39:809–13.

75. A 15-month-old boy is brought by his parents because he had 3 febrile generalized tonic clonic seizures, each seizure lasted 30–45 min, one of which occurred the same day as he received vaccines. He has a family history of a brother had febrile seizures and now has 10–15 seizures a day, despite taking multiple antiepileptic drugs. His mother and maternal aunt had febrile seizures. His family would like to know more about the cause of his seizures.

This patient most likely has a mutation in the gene associated with which of the following cellular structures?

A. Calcium channel
B. GABA receptor
C. nicotinic acetylcholine receptor
D. potassium channel
E. sodium channel

Correct Answer is: E

Generalized epilepsy with febrile seizures plus (GEFS+) is an autosomal dominant epilepsy syndrome, with approximately 60% to 70% penetrance. Individuals can have multiple different phenotypes. Some patients have isolated simple febrile seizures and others may have refractory epilepsy with multiple seizure types and associated developmental compromise. The far end of the spectrum is Dravet syndrome (aka severe myoclonic epilepsy of infancy). The most common genetic mutations associated with this syndrome is in the sodium channel SCN1A (also implicated in severe myoclonic epilepsy of infancy).The patient in this vignette, and his brother, probably have Dravet syndrome, a severe infantile-onset epilepsy syndrome with a distinctive but complex electroclinical presentation. A healthy, developmentally normal infant present at around 6 months of age with convulsive status epilepticus, which may be hemiclonic or generalized; seizures may be triggered by fever, illness or vaccination. The infant typically has further episodes of status epilepticus every month or two, often triggered by fever. Other seizure types including

focal dyscognitive seizures, absence and myoclonic seizures develop between 1 and 4 years. Atonic drop attacks and episodes of nonconvulsive status may occur. Early development is normal, but slows in the second year. Developmental regression may occur, particularly with status epilepticus. EEG studies are initially normal, but after 2 years they show generalized spike-wave and polyspike-wave activity with multifocal discharges. Photosensitivity may be seen. Imaging is normal or shows nonspecific findings, such as atrophy.Dravet syndrome is associated with mutations of the gene encoding the alpha-1 subunit of the sodium channel, SCN1A, in more than 70% of patients. These include sequencing mutations and copy number variant anomalies; 90% of mutations arise de novo. PCDH19 mutational analysis is a second-tier test for girls with a Dravet-like picture who do not have SCN1A mutations. Outcome is poor, with intellectual disability in most patients and ongoing seizures. Intellectual impairment varies from severe in 50% patients, to moderate and mild intellectual disability each accounting for 25% cases. Rare patients have normal intellect. The long-term course involves ongoing, brief nocturnal convulsions and a characteristic deterioration in gait.

9

Suggested Reading

- Wirrell E, Nickels KC. Pediatric epilepsy syndromes. Continuum Lifelong Learn Neurol. 2010;16(3):57–85.
- Scheffer IE. Diagnosis and long-term course of Dravet syndrome. Eur J Paediatr Neurol. 2012;16(Suppl 1):S5–S8.

76. An 18-year-old female who was diagnosed with juvenile myoclonic epilepsy at 13 years of age, came for her routine follow-up visit. She has unwanted side effects from the following medications, topiramate, valproic acid, levetiracetam, lamotrigine, and zonisamide. The most recent side effect is weight gain of 13 kg on valproic acid.

She tried diet and exercising, but kept gaining weight, so she stopped taking her medication 1 week ago and had a tonic-clonic seizure 2 days ago. She is not interested in more treatment for her epilepsy as "the side effects of medication are worse than the seizures."

Which of the following approaches is most likely to lead to the best possible outcome and compliance with further treatment attempts?

A. agree to observe without any further medications, but notify the state motor vehicle department of her treatment noncompliance
B. continue valproic acid and tell her to go on a stricter diet and get more exercise
C. refer for psychiatric evaluation to determine competency
D. refer for surgical evaluation
E. review prior medication doses and side effects in detail, with a discussion of other non-medical treatment options, including vagal nerve stimulator or diet modifications

Correct Answer is: E

It is not easy to deal with teenage having chronic medical conditions, it is very important to respect their need for autonomy and for them to have a say in their own medical decision making. To determine if an adolescent has the ability to make medical decisions, it is crucial to understand their mental abilities and insight into their own medical illness. Including parents in the decision-making process is also crucial, though their opinions should not necessarily carry more weight than the teenager's.This girl has a lot of frustration regarding side effects;

therefore, specifically detailing the side effects of previous medications would be worthwhile. Highlighting the positive and negative effects for each specific dose, of each medication, would help designing a treatment plan using rational polytherapy. It would be important to discuss other adjunctive treatments (surgical and dietary) to achieve the goal of minimizing the effect of seizures on her quality of life; including safety, employability, and the ability to drive.If a teenager has an emotional, or cognitive disability, or not able to process information for medical decision making, consultation from mental health providers, and/or legal counsel, would be necessary to determine whether the patient is competent to assist in decision making. It seems clear that the patient presented here has reasonable concerns, so these steps are likely to be unnecessary.

Suggested Reading

- Rodgers-Neame N, Orlowski JP. Ethical perspectives in neurology. Continuum Lifelong Learn Neurol. 2009;15(6):203–6.

77. A family of a 3-year-old girl brought a video of one of their daughter recurrent episodes of loss of consciousness which occurred in the last 2 months. She was playing with a doll and her sister took the doll from her. She became angry and her face turns red and then cyanotic. She fell to her side and has several jerking movements. One minute later, she is alert and walking normally. She is otherwise well and has normal developmental milestones and a normal examination.
    Which of the following is the most likely diagnosis?
    A. Absence seizure
    B. Breath holding spell
    C. Cataplexy
    D. Psychogenic nonepileptic event
    E. Temporal lobe seizure

Correct Answer is: B
Children have 2 types of breath holding spells. Cyanotic breath-holding is usually provoked by anger or frustration. Pallid breath-holding spells are typically induced by pain, which results in excessive vagal tone leading to bradycardia or asystole. Although cataplexy and psychogenic nonepileptic events often have an emotional trigger, presentation at age 3 would be unusual. Absence and temporal lobe seizures are the 2 types of nonconvulsive seizures, presenting with episodes of behavioral arrest, not typically provoked by anger.

78. A 4-year-old boy came to your office because of he has episodes of recurrent nausea and vomiting and also, he appears pale. An empiric trial of ranitidine was not helpful, and upper endoscopy was performed and normal. Cyproheptadine and later amitryptiline were used to treat a presumed cyclic vomiting, but they were not either. You ordered an EEG after the family notices gaze deviation and speech arrest around the most recent event and shows multifocal spikes, with greatest prevalence in the right occipital region.
    What is your most likely diagnosis?
    A. Panayiotopoulos syndrome
    B. Reflex epilepsy
    C. Rolandic epilepsy
    D. Subacute sclerosing panencephalitis
    E. Temporal lobe epilepsy

Correct Answer is: A
It is very common to see occipital spikes in Panayiotopoulos Syndrome (early onset childhood benign occipital epilepsy). 80% of cases are associated with ictal vomiting. Nausea or retching may occur during or before the vomiting. Pallor is the most frequent autonomic manifestation. The autonomic

manifestations can be quite prolonged at times, and it might get confused with the cyclic vomiting. This autonomic status epilepticus can require use of rescue benzodiazepines. Although generalized convulsions are rare with this syndrome, often the initial autonomic phase can be followed by gaze deviation, speech arrest and confusion. As with many of the benign epilepsies of childhood, the spontaneous remission rate is quite high with this disorder.

Suggested Reading

- Panayiotopoulos CP. Benign childhood epileptic syndromes with occipital spikes: new classification proposed by the International League Against Epilepsy. J Child Neurol. 2000;15:548–52.
- Wirrell E, Nickels K. "Pediatric Epilepsy Syndromes," Continuum Lifelong Learn Neurol. 2010;16(3):57–85.

79. A 12-year-old boy with epilepsy is having monthly seizures at school. On several occasions, his anti-seizure medication level has been very low or undetectable. While in the hospital, on the same dose, his level is within a therapeutic range. His parents have taken him to a faith healer.
Which of the following is the best initial approach in communicating with the parents?
    A. Ask them to stay outside the room while you speak to the patient in private
    B. Determine what the parents know about epilepsy and what their concerns are
    C. Inform them that child protective services will be notified
    D. Set up a conference call and include the faith healer, school nurse and counselor
    E. Tell them you will no longer be able to care for the patient as he is at risk for SUDEP

Correct Answer is: B
Parents are able and have the right to make most treatment decisions for their children. But in this situation, the parents are not enforcing a medically necessary and clearly beneficial treatment with a favorable benefit-to-risk ratio and are acting counter to the child's best interests. An ethics consultation is helpful in situations that cannot be resolved with more communication and education. Parental non-compliance is often due to ignorance, anxiety or other stressors. An initial approach of determining the parent's knowledge and perspective will increase the possibility of a resolution.

Suggested Reading

- Menahem S, Halasz G. Parental non-compliance–a paediatric dilemma. A medical and psychodynamic perspective. Child Care Health Dev. 2000;26(1):61–72.

80. A 13-month-old female started to have her febrile seizures at 8 months of age. They are generalized convulsions lasting 2 min and occasionally precede her fever by several hours. She has now had five, the last of which was 2 days ago. She has normal development and physical examination. You are preparing to print out her discharge paperwork, when she states she is not leaving without some testing to find out why her daughter is having seizures. You are already 1 h behind schedule with three patient's waiting to be seen.
What is the best way to address the mother's concern?
    A. Begin treatment with levetiracetam to minimize any future seizures
    B. Demand that she leaves the office immediately, other testing in this case is a waste of resources

C. Perform an EEG to prove she does not have a tendency toward unprovoked seizures
D. Refer mom for counseling to address her obvious anxiety disorder
E. Suggest that a follow up appointment can be scheduled to talk some more about mom's concerns

Correct Answer is: E
A good prognosis is the norm for simple febrile seizures and they have less than 5% incidence of epilepsy even in children with multiple episodes. Febrile seizures are the most common seizure disorder in childhood and on average affect 2% to 5% of children between the ages of 6 and 60 months. Simple febrile seizures are defined as brief (<15-min) generalized seizures that occur once during a 24-h period in a febrile child and absence of preexisting neurologic abnormality. Despite they are very benign, seizures of any type or cause can cause a lot of fear and anxiousness in any parent. It is important to find out how to try and gently alleviate these concerns without ordering unnecessary tests or placing a child on medication that they do not need. If family reassureness is not successful, a polite referral to a colleague for another opinion, or offering assistance from a social worker or counselor could be considered, but again, typically with better communication strategies, this challenge can be resolved in the office.

81. A 14-year-old female has been evaluated of possible seizures. She has had two episodes in the last month. She will feel dizzy, then her vision will fade in both eyes, she cannot hear, then she passes out and falls to the ground. One event was witness by the mother, who said that her daughter was pale and there was jerking of her arms and legs for a few seconds. After about a minute she started to wake up and was able to stand and walk within 5 min. She does not have a significant past medical history except she feels lightheaded upon standing several times every day. She takes no medications. She has a family history of first degree relatives with both migraine and seizures. Her neurologic examination is normal.
Which of the following is the best next step in her management?
A. bedside orthostatic heart rate and blood pressure measurement
B. perform electroencephalogram
C. prolonged cardiac event monitoring
D. serum glucose
E. urine drug testing

Correct Answer is: A
This is a presyncope/syncope case. The myoclonic jerks which often occur during these episodes can mistakenly interpreted as seizures. A careful history is important to order further testing and treatment. The most important clues are the sequence of symptoms and presyncopal symptoms provide by standing up. The patient describes several core features consistent with neurally-mediated syncope including an aura of visual dimming and hearing loss with systemic pallor. The patient's frequent complaints of near syncope on standing should prompt careful assessment of orthostatic tolerance (or intolerance) and bedside measurement of blood pressure and heart rate should be checked in the supine, seated and standing positions. There are many reasons for syncope, but the most common is the vasovagal (also referred to as neurally mediated) syncope. The precise pathophysiology remains incompletely understood, but it is the most frequent cause of unexplained transient loss of consciousness.

This response can be triggered centrally (fear or anger), by other peripheral stimuli affecting mechanical and/or chemoreceptors (wearing of a stiff collared shirt, micturition, defecation and coughing), or by some "hemodynamic stressor" (abrupt standing, prolonged standing or relative dehydration). Abnormal motor movements with sudden and transient cerebral anoxia are commonly seen in syncope. Most are myoclonic in nature, but they can be tonic posturing or clonic activity. This so-called "convulsive syncope", seen in 40–90% of all syncopal events, contributing to the confusion of whether a true epileptic event occurred. When the history is consistent with syncope and despite these movements, EEG is not necessary. Syncope due to cardiac disease can arise either from an arrhythmia or some type of obstructive heart lesion (aortic stenosis). Red flags suggesting a potential cardiac etiology include lack of any aura, exertional syncope or a family history of sudden cardiac death or arrhythmia. 12-lead EKG is recommended, though other more detailed cardiac monitoring should be saved for atypical cases or patients with the above red flags. Other causes for syncope are variations in blood glucose regulation, toxic ingestion, iatrogenic (medication), primary autonomic failure (neurodegenerative disorders) and brainstem/ventricular masses (colloid cysts). It would be unlikely that a spot serum glucose would be diagnostic in this patient during the office visit when not experiencing symptoms, though a sample taken immediately during or after an event would not be unreasonable. A urine drug screen is not indicated as a first step in straightforward syncope.

Suggested Reading

- Drazkowski JF, Chung SS. Differential diagnosis of epilepsy. Continuum Lifelong Learn Neurol. 2010;16(3):36–56.

9

82. A 3-year-old boy is admitted to the ED when he became lethargic and fever of 39.4 °C. In the ED he has a generalized convulsive activity which does not stop spontaneously. He is a healthy child with no history of seizures. He met all of his developmental milestones and he is not taking any medications. There is a history of seizures in a distant cousin. He has been sick for the last 72 h with vomiting, cough, rhinorrhea and intermittent low-grade fevers. He received 2 doses of lorazepam (0.1 mg/kg each) and fosphenytoin (20 mg/kg), but the convulsive activity have not stopped and has been continued for 40 min. Beside all anticonvulsant medications to stop the seizure which of the following tests should be considered immediately in the care of this patient?

A. electroencephalogram
B. lumbar puncture
C. MRI of the brain
D. serum glucose
E. urine organic acid measurement

Correct Answer is: D

Status epilepticus (established) defined as seizure of 30 min or more, or two or more sequential seizures without full recovery of consciousness inbetween. The incidence in children has ranged from 10–58 / 100,000 per year ages 1–19 years, with the highest in under 1 year of age. Status epilepticus is a common occurrence in children with epilepsy and can also be the presenting manifestation of epilepsy; although increased recognition of nonconvulsive status epilepticus, especially in the intensive care setting, has developed in both pediatric and adult age patients. Status epilepticus can be divided into acute symptomatic cases (CNS infection, electrolyte disturbance, sepsis, hypoxia, trauma or intoxication), remote symptomatic cases (cortical malformation, prior traumatic

brain injury or insult, chromosomal disorders, inborn errors of metabolism) and idiopathic febrile status epilepticus. Diagnose of idiopathic febrile status epilepticus is challenging because no tests to confirm. Further testing must be done to exclude a direct infection of the CNS. Although a LP should be deferred until an imaging study has excluded a space occupying lesion with local mass effect. Antibiotics must be started empirically. Performing a lumbar puncture in children with status epilepticus without fever varies based on the clinical scenario and may be performed at the discretion of the treating physician. Identification of readily reversible acute symptomatic causes of status epilepticus such as hypoglycemia or electrolyte imbalance should always be a priority as there is a prompt treatment that may abort the event. Serum glucose in particular should be checked early in the course of a patient's seizure. Brain MRI and screening tests for inborn errors of metabolism are indicated when etiology cannot be established with initial testing. Serum anticonvulsant levels are strongly suggested in patients who are taking anticonvulsant medication. Serum and urine toxicology panels should be considered when no clear cause is identified by the history as up to 3.6% of cases of pediatric status epilepticus are associated with a toxic ingestion. EEG has multiple dications in the pediatric patient with status epilepticus including exclusion of nonconvulsive status in the recovery period from the convulsive seizure, appropriateness of response to more aggressive IV infusions for refractory status epilepticus, exclusion of pseudo status epilepticus and interictally to determine if there are focal or generalized abnormalities that may influence other diagnostic or treatment decisions. Assessment of glucose level is more important than EEG in this patient.

Suggested Reading

- Riviello JJ, Ashwal S, Hirtz D, et al. Practice parameter: Diagnostic assessment of the child with status epilepticus (an evidence-based review): Report of the Quality Standards Subcommittee of the American Academy of Neurology and the Practice Committee of the Child Neurology Society. Neurology. 2006;67:1542–50.

83. An 18-year-old man with a past medical history of depression and post-traumatic stress disorder came to the ED with his roommate. He witnesses multiple episodes of screaming and thrashing movements during the night. While in the emergency room he appears to be asleep and is witnessed to have an event consisting of yelling and moving all extremities in a desynchronized fashion. The movements last 40 s; then he stops moving suddenly and is fully awake and oriented. His examination, EEG and MRI are normal. Prolactin level measured 10 min after the event is normal.
What do you recommend as a next step?
    A. diagnose him with psychogenic nonepileptic seizures
    B. prescribe clonazepam
    C. recommend admission to an inpatient psychiatric unit
    D. refer for inpatient video-EEG monitoring
    E. refer for polysomnogram

Correct Answer is: D
This patient may have frontal lobe seizures, which occur in approximately 30% of patients with focal epilepsy. They are often mistaken as psychogenic nonepileptic seizures or parasomnias due to the bizarre clinical semiology. They are often hypermotor, brief and without postictal confusion. A normal prolactin level does not

rule out an epileptic seizure as it has a sensitivity of approximately 46% in complex partial seizures and 60% in generalized tonic-clonic seizures and is possibly less sensitive in frontal lobe seizures. Inpatient video-EEG monitoring is helpful in diagnosis. The EEG may be obscured by movement artifact but the clinical semiology can be recorded to allow for assessment of stereotyped events, which can be helpful in diagnosis.

Suggested Reading

- Rudzinski LA, Shih JJ. The classification of seizures and epilepsy syndromes. Continuum Lifelong Learn Neurol. 2010;16(3):15–35.
- Chen DK, So YT, Fisher, RS. Use of serum prolactin in diagnosing epileptic seizures. Report of the Therapeutics and Technology Assessment Subcommittee of the American Academy of Neurology. Neurology. 2005;65:668–75

84. A 16-year-old boy in the office with his mother for follow-up visit for his juvenile myoclonic epilepsy. He is carrying this diagnosis since he was 14 after his first generalized convulsive seizure. He still has a few clusters of myoclonic seizures in the early morning hours but no seizure of any type for the past 8 months. He is otherwise healthy without medical complications. He is taken only levetiracetam, 750 mg twice daily. His prior EEG's have shown generalized 4–6 Hz spike and polyspike and slow waves with some photosensitivity. He often forgets to take his medication, but he has not had any seizures and told his mother in the morning this must mean he does not need medication any more. In the office he and his mother begin a loud verbal disagreement and he leaves the room.

Which of the following treatment approaches may foster the best long-term compliance in this situation?

A. refer him to a psychiatrist for a possible mood disorder
B. speak with him alone, make sure he is not having any side effects of the medication and discuss the long-term risks and benefits of staying on medication for seizures, including safety with driving
C. tell him he will never outgrow his tendency for seizures and he better get used to taking medication
D. tell him it's OK to stop his medication but if he has a seizure he won't be able to drive for 6 months
E. tell his mother he is not yet of adult age and she needs to make him take his medication

Correct Answer is: B
Management of epilepsy can be complicated enough without adding medication noncompliance into play. Teenage patients in particular are often unhappy that they require medication on a daily basis to "be normal." They feel impenetrable and vulnerable at the same time and despite physical maturity sometimes do not have the cognitive or emotional maturity to take care of their own medical needs. The treating physician's duty is to ensure the best interests of the patient are being met regardless of emotional, cognitive or age-dependent limitations that may arise. Although a teenage patient may not be completely independent from a medical decision-making standpoint, it is essential that they understand the implications of their medical condition on their life and that they feel like they have an important voice in the ongoing management of their condition. In the above scenario a careful assessment of the patient's mental state, including how much insight the patient has of the possible risks of

medication noncompliance, is essential. There may be a very obvious reason the patient is not taking the medication as directed, such as untoward side effects. Having the patient "buy in" to the importance of medication compliance is always ideal, rather than forcing them to take the medication. If it becomes apparent, despite a constructive conversation, that compliance will continue to be an issue, safety measures especially regarding driving must be put into place, and the patient will have to understand these potential consequences of failing to take the medication as needed. Referral to an appropriate counselor may be of some benefit especially if there is still an issue adjusting to the diagnosis of a chronic disease.

Suggested Reading

- Rodgers-Neame NT, Orlowski JP. Ethical perspectives in neurology. Continuum. 2009;15(6):203–6.

85. A posterior dominant alpha rhythm of 9 Hz is usually reached by what age?
    - A. 10
    - B. 12
    - C. 14
    - D. 16
    - E. 18

Correct Answer is: A

By the age of 9, the mean alpha frequency is 9 Hz in 65% of controls.

Suggested Reading

- Ebersole JS, Pedley TA, editors. Current practice of clinical electroencephalography. 3rd ed. Philadelphia: Lippincott, Williams, & Wilkins; 2003. p. 102–3.

86. Which of the following characteristics of the mu rhythm is most accurate?
    - A. attenuated with contralateral hand movement
    - B. attenuated with eye opening
    - C. frequency of 6–7 Hz
    - D. maximal over the occipital region
    - E. most commonly observed in stage II sleep

Correct Answer is: A

The mu waveform occurs in the central regions in an awake patient and not in drowsiness, which can be markedly asymmetrical. It is usually in the alpha frequency range, with rounded positive aspects on one side and sharpened negative aspects on the other. It is not attenuated with eye opening, but will resolve with movement of the contralateral limb or even with the thought of such movement.

Suggested Reading

- Fisch B. Fisch and Spehlmann's EEG Primer. 3rd ed. Amsterdam: Elsevier; 1999.
- Niedermeyer E, Lopes da Silva F. Electroencephalography: basic principles, clinical applications, and related fields. 5th ed. Baltimore: Willliams & Wilkins; 2005.

87. After gently scrubbing EEG scalp electrodes, used on an HIV-positive patient in which there is no contact with blood, which of the following is the most appropriate cleaning method?
    - A. air dry
    - B. soak in distilled water
    - C. soak in hydrogen peroxide
    - D. soak in tap water
    - E. soak in tenofovir

Correct Answer is: C

There are no reported cases of HIV transmission via scalp EEG electrodes. Universal precautions are the standard of care for sterilization of EEG electrodes after use in patients who are HIV-positive, HIV-negative, or in whom HIV status is unknown. Tap or distilled water is inadequate for disinfection

purposes and antiretroviral medication is unnecessary, according to the Committee on Infectious Diseases. Electrodes should be soaked in a noncorrosive disinfectant solution such as hydrogen peroxide, glutaraldehyde, sodium hypochlorite, or a combination of isopropanol, 2-butoxyethanol, and benzethonium chloride.

Suggested Reading

- Report of the Committee on Infectious Diseases. J Clin Neurophysiol. 1994;11(1):128–32.
- Beltrami EM, Williams IT, Shapiro CN, Chamberland ME. Risk and management of blood-borne infections in health care workers. Clin Microbiol Rev. 2000;13:385–407.
- Kelen GD. Human immunodeficiency virus and the emergency department: risks and risk protection for health care providers. Ann Emerg Med. 1990;19:242–8.
- Center for Disease Control Recommendations for Prevention of HIV Transmission in Healthcare Settings. Published at: ► www.cdc.gov/mmwr/preview/mmwrhtml/00023587 [accessed 4-10-13].

88. A 4-year-old girl might have absence seizures because of multiple daily episodes of staring and decreased level of attention. 1-min hyperventilation was done during her EEG which was normal.

Which of the following facts about hyperventilation is most accurate?

A. considered a safe activating procedure for individuals of all age groups
B. 1 min is an adequate amount of time and should capture abnormal activity
C. requires rapid shallow breathing
D. should be performed for 15 min
E. should be performed for 5 min

Correct Answer is: E
Hyperventilation is most often used to activate the 3-per-second, spike-and-wave discharge of primary generalized epilepsy. In some patients, discharges are only seen during hyperventilation. The patient is asked to mouth-breathe deeply for 3 min; however, if there is suspicion of absence seizures, the patient should hyperventilate for 5 min. Generalized slowing of the background activity in the theta range is the normal response to hyperventilation. Absence of slowing is not abnormal and depends on effort, age, and time of hyperventilation. Hypoglycemia may increase slowing. Because hyperventilation may cause hypocapnia and alkalosis, vasospasm and impaired cerebral perfusion may occur; therefore, hyperventilation should not be performed in patients with cerebrovascular disease or intracranial hemorrhage.

Suggested Reading

- Misulis KE, Head TC. Essentials of clinical neurophysiology. 3rd ed. Philadelphia: Butterworth-Heinemann; 2003.

89. An 18-year-old male is unconscious and unresponsive to painful stimuli upon admission to the hospital after he had sustained head trauma while downhill skiing. On examination, there is no pupillary responses, corneal reflexes, oculocephalic reflexes, gag reflex, and spontaneous breathing. He has an EEG 4 h after admission as part of the clinical assessment for brain death, shows no detectable electrical activity.

What additional information is required before concluding that the EEG is consistent with brain death?

A. core temperature greater than 32 °C
B. electrocardiogram evidence of asystole

C. electrocardiogram evidence of bradycardia
D. systolic blood pressure less than 80 mm Hg
E. the patient has an advance directive

Correct Answer is: A
Exclusion of hypothermia (a core temperature greater than 32 °C) is a condition of the diagnosis of brain death by neurologic exam, and diagnosis of electrocerebral silence by EEG. The clinician should consider hypothermia in this case, especially since the patient was in a cold outdoor environment hour before the EEG. Whether an advance directive exists is irrelevant to the clinical diagnosis, although it would direct clinical decision making following the diagnosis. Cardiac arrest (asystole), bradycardia, or hypotension is not necessary for a diagnosis of brain death.

Suggested Reading

- Practice Parameters for determining brain death: (Summary Statement). Report of the Quality Standards Subcommittee of the American Academy of Neurology. Neurology. 1995;45:1012–4.

90. Spindle delta brushes are most commonly seen in infants of what age?
 A. premature
 B. full-term infants
 C. 2-month-old infants
 D. 4-month-old infants
 E. between full-term birth and 1 month old

Correct Answer is: A
Delta brushes are present from 29 weeks of conceptional age to 1-month post-term. Their peak expression is at 32–33 weeks of conceptional age.

Suggested Reading

- Torres F, Anderson C. The normal EEG in the human newborn. J Clin Neurophysiol. 1985;2(2):89–103.

91. An 18-year-old female with a history of sexual abuse is suspected of having psychogenic seizures. Long-term video EEG monitoring is performed, during which she exhibits hip thrusting and side-to-side flailing movements, which are not followed by a postictal period. She has a normal neurologic exam.
 Which of the following findings on EEG is considered a normal variant on EEG?
 A. lambda waves
 B. parietal sharp waves
 C. periodic lateralized epileptiform discharges
 D. rolandic spikes
 E. temporal sharp waves

Correct Answer is: A
Lambda waves are a normal finding on EEG and are seen on a waking record, when the subject is viewing a scene. These positive occipital waves are blocked by eye closure. Parietal sharp waves are often associated with versive head and eye movements or sensory seizures. Temporal sharp waves are often associated with partial complex and generalized tonic clonic seizures. Psychological complaints may be seen in individuals with temporal sharp waves. Although rolandic spikes may be seen in subjects without seizures, they are also seen in benign rolandic epilepsy. Periodic lateralized epileptiform discharges may be either unilateral or bilateral and are due to any destructive process. Common causes of PLEDs include anoxia, herpes simplex encephalitis, stroke, and tumor.

Suggested Reading

- Misulis KE, Head CH. Essentials of clinical neurophysiology. 3rd ed. Philadelphia: Butterworth-Heinemann; 2003.

92. A 16-year-old female came for an evaluation of spells characterized by thrashing movements of the arms, vocalizations, and rocking movements of the trunk and body. Each spell lasts about 30 s. She does not respond during the spell, but appropriately answers questions within 10 s after movement cessation. Over 50% of the spells occur in sleep.
    What is your diagnosis?
    A. frontal lobe seizures
    B. night terrors
    C. parietal lobe seizures
    D. psychogenic nonepileptic events (psychogenic seizures)
    E. temporal lobe seizures

9

Correct Answer is: A
Frontal lobe onset seizures are characterized by an abrupt onset of stereotyped hypermotor behavior and may include vocalizations, gestural or sexual automatisms, and bilateral leg automatisms consisting of pedaling or bicycling movements. Frontal lobe seizures often arise in sleep. In contrast, temporal lobe seizures are characterized by behavioral arrest and hypomotoric movements.

Suggested Reading

- Jobst BC, Siegel AM, Thadani VM, et al. Intractable seizures of frontal lobe origin: clinical characteristics, localizing signs, and results of surgery. Epilepsia. 2000;41(9):1139–52.

93. Compared to older children and adolescents, hyperventilation in young children tends to show maximal slowing in which of the following head regions?
    A. all head regions
    B. alternates between the anterior and central head regions
    C. anterior
    D. central
    E. posterior

Correct Answer is: E
Compared to older children and adolescents, hyperventilation-induced slow activity in young children is usually maximal over the posterior head region.

Suggested Reading

- Daube J. Clinical neurophysiology. 2nd ed. Oxford: Oxford University Press; 2002.

94. A 17-year-old boy complaining of spells characterized by a warm ascending sensation in the epigastrium, associated with a sensation of fear, followed by loss of contact with the environment and oromandibular automatisms. During a video EEG, his left hand continually rubs his leg and his right arm remains immobile and stiff. He has difficulty following commands during the seizure.
    Where is the location of the ictal discharge?
    A. left lateral temporal lobe
    B. left mesial frontal lobe
    C. left mesial temporal lobe
    D. left perirolandic region
    E. right lateral temporal lobe

Correct Answer is: C
Mesial temporal lobe epilepsy is one of the most common types of epilepsy referred for epilepsy surgery and is often refractory to antiepileptic drugs. The age of onset is between late childhoods to mid adolescence. Patients often had febrile convulsions in infancy or early childhood. Most patients report an aura. Common auras include an epigastric sensation (a rising sensation, butterflies, and nausea), fear, olfactory hallucinations, lightheadedness, and déjà vu. Complex partial seizure semiology may also consist of ipsilateral upper

extremity automatisms and ipsilateral early non-forced head turn. Contralateral dystonic posturing, Todd paralysis, and late forced head turn prior to secondary generalization can also be seen.

95. A 16-year-old male has a witnessed generalized tonic seizure early in the morning by his mother. His past medical history is unremarkable. He just came back from a trip to Europe and reports still feeling jet lagged, but otherwise well. He has a normal neurologic exam. Vital signs, labs, and CT of the head are normal. There is no history of head injury, drug, or alcohol abuse. He noticed that he is occasionally clumsy, especially in the morning. He spills his drink or drops items from his hands. Jerking movements of the head, neck, and upper extremities have also been noticed.

What are you going to see on his EEG?

A. 1.5–2.5 generalized spike-and-wave discharges predominantly in the frontal regions, superimposed on an abnormal slow background activity
B. frequent centrotemporal spikes
C. generalized 10–16 Hz polyspike discharges followed by slow waves
D. generalized 4–5 Hz spike-and-wave discharges
E. regular symmetrical 3 Hz spike-and-wave discharges with a normal background

Correct Answer is: C

The clinical scenario is suggestive of juvenile myoclonic epilepsy (JME), which accounts for 10% of all epilepsies. The normal neurologic exam and myoclonic movements in the morning are important findings. JME is an autosomal dominant trait, characterized by myoclonic tonic-clonic seizures that tend to occur in the morning in individuals between 12 and 18 years old. Generalized tonic-clonic seizures can also manifest after awakening and are triggered by sleep deprivation, alcohol, stress, and fatigue. The EEG recording is consistent with generalized 10–16 Hz polyspike discharges, followed by slow waves.In Lennox-Gastaut syndrome, EEG shows slow 1.5 to 2.5 generalized spike-and-wave discharges, predominantly in the frontal regions on an abnormal slow background. In benign childhood epilepsy with centrotemporal spikes, EEG shows biphasic high-voltage central temporal spikes, followed by slow waves and a normal background activity. Are patterns seen in childhood absence and juvenile absence epilepsy, EEG shows generalized 3- and 4.5–5 Hz spike-and-wave discharges with normal background activity respectively.

Suggested Reading

- Dodson WE, Pellock JM. Pediatric epilepsy: diagnosis and therapy. New York: Demos; 1993. p.171–81.
- Fenichel GM. Clinical pediatric neurology. 3rd ed. Philadelphia: WB Saunders; 1997. p. 28–31.
- Schmitz B, Saunder T, editors. Juvenile myoclonic epilepsy: the Janz syndrome. Wrightson Biomedical; 2000.
- Wyllie, E. The Treatment of epilepsy: principles and practice. Philadelphia: Lea and Febiger; 1993. p. 552–83.
- De Vivo DC. Early onset epilepsy. Continuum Lifelong Learn Neurol. 2000;6:94–113.
- Menkes JH, Sarnat HB. Paroxysmal disorders. In: Child neurology. 6th ed. Philadelphia: Lippincott Williams & Wilkins; 2000. p. 919–1026.

96. A 14-year-old boy presents with a history of perinatal asphyxia. His seizures are drop attacks, staring spells, myoclonic jerking and generalized tonic-clonic seizures. His IQ is 62. His EEG shows 1.5–2.0 Hz generalized spike-wave discharges as a baseline pattern.

What is the most likely diagnosis?

A. Baltic myoclonus
B. Lennox-Gastaut syndrome
C. myoclonic astatic epilepsy
D. Ohtahara syndrome
E. West syndrome

Correct Answer is: B
Lennox-Gastaut syndrome (LGS) is one of the epileptic encephalopathies. Usually, it starts before 8 years of age, with a peak age of onset between 3 and 5 years of age. Rarely, the disorder can present in early adulthood. The syndrome is characterized by a triad of multiple seizure types (tonic and atypical absence are the most common), slow spike-and-wave on EEG (1–2.5 Hz), and some degree of mental retardation.

9

Suggested Reading

- Rudzinski LA, Shih JJ. The classification of seizures and epilepsy syndromes. Continuum Lifelong Learn Neurol. 2010;16(3):15–35.

97. A 16-year-old female has a 3-year history of seizures, occur in the early morning and characterized by rapid jerks of her limbs and trunk. She has occasional generalized tonic-clonic seizures, which usually occur in the setting of sleep deprivation, or increased stress. She was initially on lamotrigine and then levetiracetam, but could not tolerate either drug.
What is the most appropriate next treatment option?

A. carbamazepine
B. gabapentin
C. phenytoin
D. valproic acid
E. zonisamide

Correct Answer is: E
The clinical presentation of juvenile myoclonic epilepsy, which is a primary generalized epilepsy. Broad spectrum antiepileptic medications are the treatment of choice. Narrow spectrum antiepileptic medications such as carbamazepine and gabapentin can exacerbate myoclonic seizures, as can phenytoin. Valproic acid should be avoided in women of childbearing age because of its potential for teratogenicity. Zonisamide is considered a second-line agent for treating myoclonic and generalized tonic-clonic seizures.

Suggested Reading

- Auvin S. Treatment of juvenile myoclonic epilepsy. CNS Neurosci Ther. 2008;14(3):227–33.

98. Photic stimulation (PS) is one of the activation methods used to enhance EEG changes, both normal and abnormal. PS is essentially done to evaluate responses that can occur in photosensitive seizures.
Which of the following factors is most accurate regarding PS?

A. normal results of PS include significantly asymmetric photic driving responses
B. occurrence of photoparoxysmal response in a seizure-free individual is common
C. photomyogenic response can be seen in hypercalcemia
D. photomyogenic response is an epileptic response to PS
E. photoparoxysmal response consists of generalized polyspike-wave alterations

Correct Answer is: E
Normal results of PS include symmetric photic driving. The photomyogenic response is an exaggerated nonepileptic motor response to PS and can be enhanced in hypocalcemia and withdrawal from sedatives. A photoparoxysmal response is frequently associated with juvenile myoclonic epilepsy, and it is a rare finding in a seizure-free individual (less than 2%).

Suggested Reading

- Schomer D, Lopes da Silva, editors. Niedermeyer's electroencephalography: basic principles, clinical applications, and related fields. Philadelphia: Lippincott Williams & Wilkins; 2011. p. 221–2

99. Activation methods are used to enhance EEG changes, both normal and abnormal. Which of the following statements is most accurate regarding hyperventilation (HV) activation procedure?
   A. buildup of slow waves after the end of HV (rebuildup) may be a diagnostic finding in moyamoya disease
   B. HV is rarely achieved in young children
   C. HV procedure is indicated in patients with acute stroke
   D. HV-induced slowing is always abnormal in adults
   E. HV-induced slowing is the result of increased cerebral blood flow

Correct Answer is: A

Buildup of slow waves after the end of HV (rebuildup) may be a diagnostic finding in moyamoya disease. Sickle cell disease and acute stroke are contraindications to HV. HV-induced slowing is the result of hypocapnic cerebral vasoconstriction with reduction of CBF. HV-induced slowing is normal unless it is significantly asymmetric or contains definite spikes. In young children, HV can be achieved by asking the child to blow on a pinwheel.

Suggested Reading

- Schomer D, Lopes da Silva FH, editors. Niedermeyer's electroencephalography: basic principles, clinical applications, and related fields. Philadelphia: Lippincott Williams & Wilkins; 2011. p. 216–217.

100. A 6-month-old baby girl is seen in the emergency room due to a seizure. The seizure involved left arm shaking and then generalized. It lasted 15 min. Her birth and delivery history are unremarkable. Her developmental milestones were on time. Her father had febrile seizures as a child. On examination, she smiles and coos, but does not reach with her left hand. She has signs of a left otitis media and is febrile.
   Which of the following is consistent with a simple febrile seizure in this patient?
   A. Age of the patient
   B. Family history
   C. Length of seizure
   D. Neurologic examination
   E. Seizure semiology

Correct Answer is: A

Febrile seizures are extremely common in the young child, with an age range of onset typically listed as 3 months to 6 years of age. Simple febrile seizures are characterized by seizures accompanied by fever that are generalized in onset, last less than 15 min, and do not occur more than once in 24 h. Febrile seizures are complex due to either longer duration, focal signs at onset, or recurrence within 24 h. Normal achievement of neurodevelopmental milestones and a normal neurologic exam are also typically required to classify the event as a febrile seizure. Prominent encephalopathy prior to or after the seizure should raise suspicion of a secondary cause such as a central nervous system infection and focal onset seizures with post-ictal hemiparesis may suggest a structural cause such as tumor, stroke or abscess. Although the genetics of febrile seizures is still not well known (other than for syndromes such as generalized epilepsy febrile seizures plus- GEFS+), a family history of such events is quite

commonly obtained, though not effective in differentiating between simple and complex febrile seizures.

Suggested Reading

- Waruiru C, Appleton R. Febrile seizures: a consensus of their significance, evaluation, and treatment. Consensus development conference of febrile seizures. National Institute of Health. Pediatrics.1980;66:1009–12.
- Shinnar S, Glauser TA. Febrile Seizures. J Child Neuro. 2002:17(1):s44–52.

101. A 10-year-old female has been evaluated for loss of consciousness. She was playing soccer for the first time this season, she has a sudden loss of consciousness with witnessed convulsions and urinary incontinence. After a few minutes she returns to her baseline of consciousness and reports no recall of any warning symptoms. She has a normal developmental history. Her father had a seizure in his 20 s after diving into cold water. A paternal uncle had childhood seizures and died while swimming as a teenager. She has a normal general medical and neurological examinations.
Which of the following is the most urgent diagnostic test?
A. 12-lead electrocardiogram
B. Transthoracic echocardiogram
C. Routine EEG
D. MRI brain
E. Tilt table test

9

Correct Answer is: A
This is a clinical presentation of exercise-induced syncope with convulsions. Her family history is indicative of autosomal dominant pattern of convulsions possibly induced by cold water immersion. This is most concerning for a congenital long QT syndrome and a 12-lead electrocardiogram (ECG) is essential for screening. If normal, the patient should have exercise testing or be referred to pediatric cardiology, as occasionally the initial resting EKG can be normal. Most patients with congenital long QT syndrome have a normal cardiac exam on echocardiography so this is not a high priority test in this population. A routine EEG may be warranted if the ECG is normal or the patient has recurrent episodes outside the setting of exercise. Typically, however, convulsions associated with long QT syndrome are due to anoxic seizures, and would not be likely to reveal any interictal abnormalities on EEG. Brain MRI is not indicated for congenital long QT syndrome but may be indicated if the patient is felt to have epilepsy rather than anoxic seizures. A tilt table test may be helpful is cases neurocardiogenic syncope due to orthostatic hypotension. Those patients typically do not have syncope during active phases of exercise.

Suggested Reading

- McLeod KA. Syncope in childhood. Arch Dis Child. 2003;88(4):350–3.

102. A 16-year-old female with juvenile myoclonic epilepsy is here for her annual check up. She has been seizure free for 1 year. She is on lamotrigine.
What are the current guidelines in her case?
A. There is no need to discuss contraception and pregnancy until she is older.
B. Annual counseling of how epilepsy and its treatment may affect contraception or pregnancy is recommended.
C. Before discussing contraception or pregnancy, you must obtain the permission of a parent or legal guardian.

D. Prophylactic use of an intrauterine device is recommended given the interaction of oral contraceptives and lamotrigine.
E. Pregnancy test should be done annually and prior to any changes in antiepileptic drug therapy.

Correct Answer is: B
One of the most important issues in epilepsy is "Counseling for Women of Childbearing Potential with Epilepsy", and it is one of the core quality measurables for caregivers of patients with epilepsy. All female epilepsy patients of childbearing potential (12 to 44 years old) should be counseled or referred for counseling for how epilepsy and its treatment may affect contraception OR pregnancy at least once yearly. Postmenopausal females, or those who are surgically sterile are excluded.

Parental presence or permission for this discussion is not mandated, nor pregnancy testing unless clinical concern is present. Lamotrigine does not lessen the effectiveness of oral contraceptive agents (unlike topiramate), though concomitant use of oral contraceptives can induce the metabolism of lamotrigine, resulting in lower serum levels. Typically, adjustments can be made in the dose of lamotrigine if this occurs, and would not necessitate another form of birth control, unless desired by the patient.

Suggested Reading

- Fountain NB, Van Ness PC, Bennett A, Absher J, et al. Quality improvement in neurology: Epilepsy Update Quality Measurement Set. Neurology. 2015; 84(14):1483–7.

103. A 5-month-old boy has been evaluated for a history of spasms. His family reports that he is very sensitive to any noise and reacts with an exaggerated startle response with muscle spasms involving the whole body. They also reported that symptoms will continue to recur each time the stimulation is repeated. It became very difficult for them to take care of him as he would become very stiff every time they will pick him up for change of diapers or to feed him. His muscle tone appears normal when lying in bed by himself.
What is the most likely diagnosis of this patient?
A. Serum anti-glutamic acid decarboxylase (GAD) antibodies will be positive.
B. EEG will show generalized 3 Hz spike and wave activity.
C. CSF will be positive for 14-3-3 protein.
D. Autosomal recessive inheritance is most common.
E. It involves mutation in the gene for alpha-1 subunit of the glycine receptor.

Correct Answer is: E
This is a typical presentation of exaggerated startle disease or hyperekplexia. The event in hyperekplexia is markedly exaggerated and does not habituate with repetition of the stimulus which differentiates it from normal infantile startle response. The child will massive flexion of the neck (severe enough to at times compromise the airway of the infant) and trunk with abduction and flexion of the arms. It can also result in tonic muscle spasms. Although these may resemble tonic seizures, the consistent ability to be provoked by a stimulus is atypical for seizures. An EEG will show only movement artifact during the spells. The condition most commonly is due to mutations in the glycine receptor alpha1-subunit (GLRA1) gene and inherited as an autosomal dominant trait (though autosomal recessive and x-linked inheri-

tance has been reported.) Mutations typically result in deficient production and activity of glycine (a major inhibitory neurotransmitter) in the central nervous system. Anti-GAD antibodies are negative in this case, it is positive in "stiff-person syndrome." CSF exam is typically normal in these patients (not consistently showing abnormal glycine levels). Though the condition can improve over time, benzodiazepines, such as clonazepam, provide effective symptomatic treatment for this condition.

Suggested Reading

- Espay A, Chen R. Myoclonus. Continuum Lifelong Learn Neurol. 2013;19(5):1264.
- Bode A, Lynch J. The impact of human hyperekplexia mutations on glycine receptor structure and function. Molecular Brain. 2014:7:2.

9

104. An 18-year-old male has focal epilepsy due to an intrauterine stroke. He denies any seizures since his last visit 6 months ago. He takes carbamazepine 400 mg bid, but read recently that it can lower testosterone levels and decided to take it only once a day. His serum level is undetectable. He is currently driving. **What is the most appropriate action by you?**
   A. Bring his parents into the examination room to discuss his risky behavior
   B. Report the patient to the Department of Motor Vehicles (DMV), so that his license can be temporarily suspended
   C. Request the patient sign a form that notifies him that he is at risk of death and driving is not recommended
   D. Prescribe testosterone in addition to carbamazepine to increase adherence to the treatment regimen
   E. Ask the patient to further discuss his thoughts on antiepileptic drug treatment and the risks of not taking the medication

Correct Answer is: E
Noncompliance is very common for different reasons and the patient's explanation and understanding of the risks should be thoroughly explored by the physician. The risk of having a seizure is very high, including while driving, and should be advised not to drive until he is compliant and the level is back to his therapeutic range. Honesty between the patient and the physician in a key principle in the management of patient's with epilepsy and is the reason that most states do not have a mandatory reporting law to the DMV after a seizure.

Suggested Reading

- Bacon D, Fisher RS, Morris JC, Rizzo M, Spanaki MV. American Academy of Neurology position statement on physician reporting of medical conditions that may affect driving competence. Neurology. 2007;68(15): 1174–7.

105. A 15-year-old male came to the office for a second opinion. He was diagnosed with epilepsy 8 months ago and is taking carbamazepine. He has had 6 seizures. Seizures occurred 1–2 h after waking from sleep, some early in the morning and some after awakening from a midday nap. No loss of consciousness and he did not have twitches of the hands have been reported by the patient or family or friends. He has no family history of epilepsy. He has a normal examination and MRI of the brain. EEG shows 3–4 Hz generalized spike wave discharges and photosensitivity. There are rare discharges with a left sided predominance.

What is your most accurate diagnosis?

A. Autosomal dominant nocturnal frontal lobe epilepsy (ADNFLE)
B. Epilepsy with grand mal seizures on awakening
C. Left frontal lobe epilepsy
D. Juvenile myoclonic epilepsy
E. Progressive myoclonic epilepsy

Correct Answer is: B

This is a clinical presentation of epilepsy with grand mal seizures upon awakening which is an idiopathic generalized epilepsy (IGE) syndrome characterized by generalized tonic clonic seizures occurring predominantly on awakening (independent of the time of day.) The EEG shows predominantly generalized spike and slow waves (though focal abnormalities can also be noted) and photosensitivity. This syndrome shares many features with the more common juvenile myoclonic epilepsy, including similar provoking features (sleep deprivation, alcohol use and bright flickering lights), though a formal diagnosis of JME would typically require either clinical absence or myoclonic events in addition to generalized tonic-clonic seizures. Treatment for both disorders is a broad spectrum agents such as lamotrigine, levetiracetam, sodium valproate, topiramate or zonisamide. Narrow spectrum sodium channel blocking agents such as carbamazepine would be relatively contraindicated.

Though frontal lobe seizures can occur during sleep-wake transitions, they most commonly occur out of sleep, and not 1–2 h after awakening. Additionally, although very rapidly generalizing discharges can be present on EEG, photosensitivity is rare. Without a suggestive family history, a diagnosis of ADNFLE would be hard to confidently make. The patient has not been identified to have myoclonic seizures, and has not have the typical progressive cognitive decline seen with the disorders leading to a progressive myoclonic epilepsy.

Suggested Reading

- Janz D. Epilepsy with grand mal on awakening and sleep-waking cycle. Clin Neurophysiol. 2000;111(S2):S103–10.
- Rudzinski LA, Shih JJ. The Classification of Seizures and Epilepsy Syndromes. Continuum 2010;16(3): 15–35.

106. A 16-month-old boy has an unprovoked generalized tonic clonic seizure (GTC). He has a history of 2 complex febrile seizures, they were prolonged unilateral convulsions (one right and one left-sided). Recently his mother has noted some jerking movements of his arms. This jerking occurred as increased clusters prior to onset of the GTC. Mom has also reported increased falls. You admitted the patient for evaluation and an EEG and brain MRI were ordered, both of which are normal. Forty-eight hours later, he is awake, but has some mild truncal ataxia on exam.

What gene abnormalities would best explain his condition?

A. CACNA1A
B. DMPK gene
C. KCNQ2
D. SCN1A
E. TSC1

Correct Answer is: D

Dravet syndrome is one of a genetic epileptic encephalopathy. In typical cases, unprovoked seizures begin in the first or second year of life in an otherwise healthy infant. However, recurrent spells of hemiconvulsive febrile status epilepticus in the first year of life may also herald the diagnosis. Also known as severe myoclonic epilepsy of infancy (SMEI), this naming is not in favor because a lot of cases are being identified without obvious myoclonic events. Development may be normal at the onset of seizures, though most patients will have very obvious delays in motor, language and cognitive development by 3–4 years

of age. Progressive ataxia has seen in this syndrome. Up to 80–90% of cases meeting clinical criteria of Dravet syndrome will have a mutation identified in the SCN1A gene region.

Mutations in the CACNA1A region lead to multiple phenotypes including sporadic and familial hemiplegic migraine, episodic ataxia and spinocerebellar ataxia, type 6. KCNQ2 mutations typically lead to benign familial neonatal convulsions, though a more aggressive phenotype with a severe epileptic encephalopathy has been described (though without myoclonic seizures or prolonged hemiconvlusive febrile status). TSC1 mutations lead to tuberous sclerosis, unlikely given the normal MRI scan in this patient and DMPK mutations are seen in myotonic dystrophy.

9

Suggested Reading

- Dravet C. The core Dravet syndrome phenotype. Epilepsia. 2011;52(s2):3–9.

107. A 9-year-old girl with Lennox-Gastaut syndrome came to your office for follow-up. She has been having daily seizures despite treatment with sodium valproate, clobazam and rufinamide. She would like to try cannabinoid oil but they don't live in a state where there is a legal prescription for the cannabinoid, it is available on the internet.
Which of the following statements is most ethically appropriate?
   - A. Cannabinoid oil use is unethical
   - B. The physician is obligated to report the parents to the Drug Enforcement Agency
   - C. In order to legally use cannabinoid oil, the patient must move to Colorado
   - D. The child should be referred to a social worker for an interdisciplinary approach
   - E. The mother should be encouraged to participate in a clinical trial

Correct Answer is: E
The patient may be better joined a structured clinical trial if he or she is interest in unproven medications or alternative treatments especially if a clinical trial is ongoing. There are many patients and parents who use alternative and unproven treatments. An open discussion of potential risks and benefits is important in these circumstances. Use of cannabinoid oil as a treatment for medically intractable epilepsy is not "unethical", though the efficacy and side effect profile has as of yet not been well studies through randomized clinical trials. Each year, additional states are passing legislature making the product legally obtainable if used for intractable patients and grown within state boundaries. Even when obtained through other methods, there is no requirement for the physician to report the patient or family to law enforcement officials.

Suggested Reading

- Gloss DS, Maa EH. Medical marijuana: between a plant and a hard place. Neurology. 2015; 5(4):281–4.

108. A 6-year-old boy has seizures that are associated with stroke-like episodes of cortical blindness, most likely has which type of metabolic disorder?
   - A. Glycogen storage
   - B. Lysosomal
   - C. Mitochondrial
   - D. Copper metaboli

Correct Answer is: C
Mitochondrial encephalopathy, lactic acidosis, and stroke-like episodes (MELAS) is a multisystem disorder which is associated with generalized tonic-clonic seizures, recurrent headaches, anorexia and recurrent vomiting. Occipital lobe seizures that often manifest as transient periods of blindness is a hallmark feature of this condition. The cumulative effects of the stroke like

episodes progressively impair motor abilities, vision and cognition.

Glycogen storage diseases are characterized by cellular build up of glycogen causing organ dysfunction. Affected newborns my developed generalized seizures as a result of hypoglycemia.

Lysosomal storage diseases are characterized by the cellular accumulation of intracellular products that cannot be broken down by lysosomal enzymes. Severe motor symptoms and cognitive deficits typically are present in infancy. Seizures are associated with some conditions. Wilson's disease is a disorder of copper metabolism resulting in copper accumulation and dysfunction in the liver and specific brain regions. Kayser-Fleisher rings are copper colored rings in the cornea; Neurological symptoms are not common in children.

Suggested Reading

- Munnich A, Rotig A, Chretien D, Cormier V, Bourgeron T, Bonnefont JP, Rustin P. Clinical presentation of mitochondrial disorders in childhood. J Inherit Metab Dis. 1996;19(4):521–7.

109. An 18-month-old healthy boy was admitted to the PICU after having a 2-min generalized tonic-clonic seizure in your office. He had a second prolonged seizure, he was loaded with phenobarbital. He is obtunded, but has non-focal examination. He has a normal general physical examination with stable vital signs with the exception of a temperature of 100.5 F. Two days ago, his PCP diagnosed him with strep throat and started him on amoxicillin. His mother reported the child was irritable and crying for many hours 1 day before your visit. His past medical history is unremarkable, he has a negative family history of seizures and his immunizations are up-todate.

What is the likely etiology of this child's seizures?

A. Meningococcemia
B. Group B streptococci
C. Whole cell pertussis vaccine
D. Acellular pertussis vaccine

Correct Answer is: C

Presentation of post-immunization encephalopathy due to whole cell pertussis vaccine includes seizures with or without fever occurring within 3 days of immunization and persistent, severe, inconsolable crying for 3 or more hours within 48 h of immunization. Dissemination of Neisseria meningitides presents with fever, headache, fatigue, muscle aches, nuchal rigidity and with subsequent signs of sepsis. The child in the vignette has normal vital signs and he has no associated characteristic rash. Seizures are not a common manifestation of meningitis. Group B streptococci is a common cause of sepsis in newborns and may progress to meningitis. Acellular pertussis vaccination is not associated with postimmunization encephalopathy and seizures.

Suggested Reading

- Patel MK, Patel TK, Tripathi CB. Diphtheria, pertussis (whooping cough), and tetanus vaccine induced recurrent seizures and acute encephalopathy in a pediatric patient: Possibly due to pertussis fraction. J Pharmacol Pharmacother. 2012;3(1):71.
- Barlow WE, Davis RL, Glasser JW, Rhodes PH, Thompson RS, Mullooly JP, Destefano F. The risk of seizures after receipt of whole-cell pertussis or measles, mumps, and rubella vaccine. N Engl J Med. 2001;345(9):656–61.

110. An 18-year-old male is referred to your practice because he has a medically refractory seizure. He has a complex partial seizure in which

he initially has an "out of body" type feeling, then he feels fearful, because he knows a seizure is coming on. He has been told that he will then start to stare, and at times makes a sound like he has been holding his breath, then lets out a cry/scream.

Occasionally, he had some generalized tonic clonic seizures after this. His MRI scan showing hippocampal atrophy, and was referred to you for confirmatory PET scan and further management of his seizures.

What is your diagnosis?

A. absence seizures
B. Auditory seizures
C. temporal lobe epilepsy
D. Kojenikow's syndrome
E. none of the above

9

Correct Answer is: C
Temporal lobe epilepsy is the most common form of focal epilepsy in adults. Absence seizures are generalized seizures. Auditory seizures, are not the most common form of focal epilepsy, and can form a subset of the temporal lobe epilepsies. Kojenikow's syndrome, is chronic progressive epilepsia partialis continua of childhood, and is fairly rare.

Suggested Reading

- Lee HW, Khoshbin S. "Seizure Disorders" Chapter 76, page 1045, Mass General Comprehensive Clinical Psychiatry.

111. A 15-year-old girl had the onset of seizures, which manifested as transient blindness. She later developed progressive resting and action myoclonus, with cognitive decline.

What is the most likely diagnosis is?

A. Unverricht-Lundborg disease
B. Myoclonic epilepsy with ragged red fibers
C. Mitochondrial encephalomyopathy, lactic acidosis, and stroke-like episodes
D. Lafora disease
E. Dentatorubral-pallidoluysian atrophy

Correct Answer is: D
Unverricht-Lundborg disease, myoclonic epilepsy with ragged red fibers (MERRF), mitochondrial encephalomyopathy, lactic acidosis, and stroke-like episodes (MELAS), Lafora disease, and dentatorubra l-pallidoluysian atrophy (DRPLA) are progressive myoclonus epilepsies. They started in childhood, consisting of myoclonus, generalized tonic-clonic seizures, and neurological deterioration. Lafora disease is distinct because it has partial visual seizures of occipital onset. Presentation includes visual hallucinations, and transient blindness or scotomas. Patients may also have generalized tonic-clonic seizures. In Lafora disease, patients develop resting and action myoclonus, with cognitive decline. Death typically occurs within several years of onset.

It is an autosomal recessive disorder, with mutations of the EPM2A or NHLRC1 genes. The EPM2A gene encodes laforin, a tyrosine kinase inhibitor. The NHLRC1 gene encodes the protein malin.

Suggested Reading

- Alduligan MS, Pearl PL. Electroencephalography in the metabolic epilepsies. In: Pearl P, editor. Inherited Metabolic Epilepsies. New York: Demos Medical; 2013. p. 39–68.
- Trescher WH, Lesser RP. The epilepsies. In: Bradley WG, Daroff RB, Fenichel GM, Jankovic J, editors. Neurology in clinical practice. 4th ed. Elsevier Inc.; 2004. p. 1953–92.

112. Which of the following is most likely to be associated with benign idiopathic neonatal seizures?

A. An APGAR score of less than 5
B. Birth prior to 35 weeks
C. Clonic or apneic seizures
D. Seizures continuing after infancy
E. Mutations affecting K potassium channel, voltage gated, subfamily Q, member 2 (KCNQ2)

Correct Answer is: C
Criteria for benign idiopathic neonatal seizures include child born after 39 weeks gestation, Apgar score of at least 9 at 5 min, no apparent etiology, and lack of seizures beyond the neonatal period, normal neurological development, the presence of a seizure free interval between the time of birth and the onset of seizures, and the presence of apneic or clonic seizures. These are also known as "fifth day fits" and prognosis is typically good. Apneic and clonic seizures, the latter occurring bilaterally or unilaterally, are typical and the presence of one or the other is suggested for a diagnosis of benign idiopathic neonatal seizures. Despite the fact that prognosis is good ultimately, up to 82% of infants may go into status epilepticus.

Per the proposed diagnostic criteria, an Apgar score of at least 9 at 5 min of life is required. Regardless of official diagnostic criteria, these seizures occur in healthy infants with a history of uncomplicated pregnancy and delivery.

Per the proposed criteria, birth after 39 weeks gestation is required for a diagnosis of benign idiopathic neonatal seizures. Again, even if the criteria are not strictly followed, benign idiopathic neonatal seizures occur after an uncomplicated pregnancy and delivery.

Cessation of seizures after the neonatal period is required for a diagnosis of idiopathic neonatal seizures per the proposed criteria. Even if the criteria are not followed strictly, continuation of seizures past the neonatal period is not a characteristic of this condition.

Mutations affecting potassium channel, voltage gated, subfamily Q, member 2 (KCNQ2) may underlie benign familial neonatal convulsions. Potassium channel, voltage gated, subfamily Q, member 3 (KCNQ3) is also implicated in this condition. Benign familial neonatal convulsions may present within days of birth and usually present within the first 2 months. Seizures observed in patients with this condition include tonic or clonic seizures which may be multifocal.

Suggested Reading

- Millichap JJ, Millichap JG. Clinical features and evaluation of febrile seizures. UpToDate, Nordli DR, Eichler AF (Ed), UpToDate, Waltham. Accessed on 1 Dec 2015.
- Abram HS. Febrile seizure. In: Tatum WO, Sirven JI, Cascino GD, ed. Epilepsy Case Studies. New York: Springer Science and Business Media; 2014. p. 13–16.
- Deivasumathy M, Hartman AL. Pediatric epilepsy syndromes. Neurologist. 2010;16(4):223–37.
- Park JT, Shahid AM, Jamoul A. Common pediatric epilepsy syndromes. Pediatr Ann. 2015;44(2):e30–5.
- Korff CM. Juvenile myoclonic epilepsy. UpToDate, Nordli DR, Eichler AF (Ed), UpToDate, Waltham. Accessed on 1 Dec 2015.
- Korff CM. Childhood absence epilepsy. UpToDate, NordIi DR, Eichler AF (Ed), UpToDate, Waltham. Accessed on 1 Dec 2015.

113. Which of the following mutations has not been associated with generalized epilepsy with febrile seizures plus (GEFS+)?
A. SCN1D
B. SCN1A
C. SCN1 B
D. SCN2A
E. GABRD

Correct Answer is: A
Generalized epilepsy with febrile seizures plus (GEFS+) is a familial syndrome and SCN1 D mutations are not a recognized etiology. In contrast to febrile seizures (FS), which occur most commonly between 6 months and 6 years of age, the phenotype of "febrile seizures plus" includes patients in whom FS continue past the defined upper limit of age. GEFS+ may also be associated with afebrile generalized tonic-clonic (GTC) seizures. One-third of patients have other seizure types as well. It has a complex pattern of inheritance, although initial genetic discoveries first identified an autosomal dominant familial pattern. Mutations of a number of ion channel genes have been identified in GEFS+ kindreds. These include sodium channel (SCN) subunits (SCN1A, SCN1 B, and SCN2A) and GABAA receptor subunit genes (GABRD and GABRG2). The result is increased sodium channel activity or impaired GABA activity, ultimately leading to increased cortical hyperexcitability. The most frequently reported mutation is SCN1A, which encodes the pore-forming A-subunit of the sodium channel and comprises four transmembrane domains. The EEG usually shows generalized spike-wave or polyspikes.

9

Suggested Reading

- Scheffer IE, Zhang YH, Jansen FE, et al. Dravet syndrome or genetic (generalized) epilepsy with febrile seizures plus? Brain Dev. 2009;31(5):394–400.
- Zucca C, Redaelli F, Epifanio R, et al. Cryptogenic epileptic syndromes related to SCN1A: twelve novel mutations identified. Arch Neurol. 2008;65(4):489–94.
- Comprehensive Review in Clinical Neurology: A Multiple-Choice Question Book for the Wards and Boards ©2011 Wolters Kluwer Health Lippincott Williams & Wilkins. All rights reserved.

114. A 3-month-old boy brought to the clinic by his mother. She noticed that sometimes when he is picked up, he stiffens up for several seconds. When he is put back down, he loosens up again. This happens all the time and she is concerned. He is "jumpy": even with slightly loud or unexpected noises. You suspected the diagnosis of hyperekplexia.
Which of the following statements is incorrect regarding hyperekplexia?
A. Some patients respond to benzodiazepines or sodium valproate
B. Mutations in the glycine receptor and presynaptic glycine transporter have been identified in familial hyperekplexia
C. Glycine is the inhibitory neurotransmitter at spinal interneurons, including Renshaw cells and Ia inhibitory interneurons
D. Hyperekplexia results from abnormal spinal Ia inhibitory interneuron reciprocal inhibition
E. Hyperekplexia is a startle-evoked epileptic seizure

Correct Answer is: E
Hyperekplexia is not epileptic, but it must be distinguished from startle evoked seizures. Hyperekplexia, or exaggerated startle, can manifest with sudden brief exaggerated startle reactions (blinking, flexion of the neck and trunk, abduction and flexion of the arms) or more prolonged tonic startle spasms. These sometimes occur secondary to minor stimuli and do not habituate. There are primary familial forms of hyperekplexia in which mutations in the glycine receptor and presynaptic glycine transporter have been identified. Glycine is the inhibitory neurotransmitter at spinal interneurons including Renshaw cells and Ia inhibitory interneurons, and abnormal spinal Ia inhibitory interneuron reciprocal

inhibition is thought to be the cause of startle in these cases. Secondary forms of exaggerated startle occur in a variety of brainstem disorders as well as in CreutzfeldtJakob disease and stiff person syndrome.

Suggested Reading

- Fahn S, Jankovic j. Principles and practice of movement disorders. Philadelphia: Elsevier; 2007.

115. A 15-year-old male with progressive cognitive decline and ataxia has a history of myoclonic epilepsy and multiple seizure types. EEG shows occipital region spikes and waves. You have done a skin biopsy, which showed periodic-acid-Schiff (PAS)-positive intracellular inclusions. **Which of the following is the most likely finding in this patient?**
    A. Mutation affecting cystatin
    B. Cherry red spot on fundoscopic examination
    C. Ragged red fibers on muscle biopsy
    D. EPM1 mutation
    E. EPM2 A mutation

Correct Answer is: E
The clinical presentation is indicative of Lafora body disease, which is an autosomal recessive disorder associated with a mutation in the gene EPM2A on chromosome 6q, encoding laforin, a ribosomal protein with undetermined function. It presents between 12 and 17 years of age. Patients usually have different seizures types, including myoclonus, atypical absences, atonic, complex partial, and occipital seizures with transient blindness and visual hallucinations. Patients can have dysarthria, ataxia, as well as emotional disturbance, and cognitive decline leading to dementia. EEG shows an evolution, with multiple spike-wave discharges at the beginning, but progressively over months or years, the background deteriorates and multifocal epileptiform abnormalities appear, mainly in the occipital regions, in addition to generalized bursts. Lafora bodies are PAS positive intracellular polyglucosan inclusion bodies found in neurons, cardiac muscle, skeletal muscle, hepatocytes, and sweat gland duct cells, making it possible to detect these bodies in skin biopsy specimens. Most patients die within 10 years of onset, and the treatment remains supportive.

Mutation in cystatin B and EPM1 mutation are seen in Unverricht Lundborg syndrome. Cherry red spot in a patient with progressive myoclonic epilepsy (PME) suggests sialidosis. Ragged red fibers on muscle biopsy are seen in myoclonic epilepsy with ragged red fibers.

Suggested Reading

- Delgado-Escueta AV, Ganesh S, Yamakawa K. Advances in the genetics of progressive myoclonus epilepsy. Am J Med Genet. 2001;106:129–38.
- Shahwan A, Farrel M, Delanty N. Progressive myoclonic epilepsies: a review of genetic and therapeutic aspects. Lancet Neural. 2005;4:239–48.
- Comprehensive Review in Clinical Neurology: A Multiple-Choice Question Book for the Wards and Boards ©2011 Wolters Kluwer Health Lippincott Williams & Wilkins. All rights reserved.

116. A 5-year-old girl has moderate intellectual disability came for her follow-up. She has history of intractable seizures and is on 4 different antiepileptic medications. On examination, she very small eyes with very poor vision. She has small philtrum, a flat nose with an upturned tip, large ears, and sparse eyebrows. Her brain MRI shows agenesis of corpus callosum.

Which one of the following is true regarding this condition?

A. This condition is inherited in autosomal dominant pattern
B. This condition is lethal in boys and occurs almost exclusively in females
C. Patient will slowly improve in her mental development to have normal IQ
D. Patient will have syringomyelia along with above features
E. This condition is inherited in autosomal recessive pattern

Correct Answer is: B
The clinical scenario is Aicardi syndrome. Aicardi syndrome is an X-linked dominant disorder and occurs almost exclusively in females. It has a triad. (1) Agenesis or dysgenesis of the corpus callosum. (2) Infantile spasms and epilepsy, and (3) Chorioretinal lacunae. Additional brain abnormalities include - asymmetry between hemispheres, polymicrogyria, cysts, microcephaly and hydrocephalus. Other ophthalmic abnormalities include - microphthalmia or coloboma, which can cause blindness. Facial features may include - small philtrum, a flat nose with an upturned tip, large ears, and sparse eyebrows. Other features include - small hands, scoliosis. They often have gastrointestinal problems such as constipation or diarrhea, gastroesophageal reflux, and difficulty feeding.

9

Suggested Reading

- Mowzoon N, Flemming KD. Neurology Board Review: an illustrated study guide. Rochester: Mayo Clinic Scientific, 2007. Print.

117. A third grade student was referred to you by her teacher with concerns that the student seems to "space out" frequently in her class. The teacher reports that the student has episodes "several times a day" when she is unable to respond to her name for a few seconds when the teacher calls on her, but then "snaps out of it" and can answer whatever questions are posed a few seconds later. The child claims that she does not heard the teacher calling her name initially. The teacher has a concern that the child might have ADHD. Also, her family have seen similar behavior at home, but felt that she was "going through a phase", as her parents have recently separated.
If this is a seizure, how would you classify it?

A. absence seizure, partial with impairment of consciousness only
B. absence seizure, general, with impairment of consciousness and mild clonic components
C. absence seizure, general, non-convulsive, with atonic components
D. absence seizure, general, with autonomic components
E. none of the above adequately describes this seizure, there is insufficient information

Correct Answer is: E
We do not have enough descriptions adequately describe this as a seizure. Further testing, and more history are needed. It might got confused with an absence seizure, but it could be due to other causes. However, absence seizures are generalized. While there is description of impairment of consciousness only, there is also no description of other symptoms. This question is not meant to be confusing, but to expose the student to the idea that seizures need to be diagnosed by a medical professional on the basis of observed

phenomena and concrete evidence.
In order to diagnose a seizure certain parameter must be reported, and not all of the details needed are mentioned in this case. A description of the eye movements, if any, a description of any clonic, atonic, or tonic movements present, any automatisms or autonomic phenomena would be needed in order to fully classify/describe an absence seizure. While this sounds like an absence seizure, with impairment of consciousness only we cannot be sure until more history is gathered and an episode observed by a medical professional. Other helpful tests would be an EEG, a brain MR, as well as basic blood work.

Suggested Reading

- Lee HW, Khoshbin S. "Seizure Disorders" Chapter 76, page 1042, Mass General Comprehensive Clinical Psychiatry.

118. A 14-year-old female had a generalized tonic clonic seizure. She had no alarming preceding aura and was associated with urinary incontinence and tongue biting. It lasted for 3 min and was followed by several hours of lethargy and confusion. Her mother reported that the patient has persistent difficulties in school. Her teachers have reported that she doesn't pay attention during class. The patient is also clumsy and frequently drops items, especially in the morning. **What is the most likely diagnosis?**
    A. juvenile absence epilepsy
    B. juvenile myoclonic epilepsy
    C. Late onset childhood occipital epilepsy
    D. Panayiotopoulos syndrome

Correct Answer is: B
This is a clinical presentation of juvenile myoclonic epilepsy. Usually, patients present with generalized tonic clonic seizures, but, on taking detailed history, a history of absence seizures (occurring in between 20% and 40% of patients) and myoclonic jerks may be elicited. Myoclonic jerks, often occurring in the morning, may be misinterpreted as clumsiness. Patients may fling items and drop things. The EEG shows 4 to 6 Hz polyspike and slow waves bilaterally. This condition is treated with valproate as a first line although women of child bearing age may choose to take lamotrigine. Levetiracetam and topiramate can be used as a second line treatment. Phenytoin, carbamazepine, and oxcarbazepine may cause increases in absence seizures and increased myoclonic jerks. Pregabalin, tiagabine, vigabatrin, and gabapentin may also increase seizure frequency in those with juvenile myoclonic epilepsy.

Patients with juvenile myoclonic epilepsy may have absence seizures; however, childhood absence epilepsy is a separate entity. Childhood absence epilepsy starts at 4 to10 years of age, they have a normal neurological development, and the presence of generalized rhythmic spikes or double spike wave discharges around 3 Hz. In addition, seizures should be brief, lasting between 4 and 20 s, and should occur frequently. The presence of other seizure types is one of the exclusion criteria.

Late onset childhood occipital epilepsy has also been referred to as late onset childhood epilepsy with occipital spikes or Gastaut type. Onset is often between 8 or 9 years of age and seizures are characterized by visual loss or hallucinations, sometimes with post ictal headache. Hemiclonic activity or generalized convulsions may also occur. EEG may show bursts of spike wave complexes in the occipital region.

Panayiotopoulos syndrome is also referred to as early onset benign occipital epilepsy. Age of onset is often between the ages of 3 and 6 years. Seizures are

characterized by emesis in up to 80% of patients. In about half of cases, these seizures may last up to a half hour. Other seizure manifestations include pallor, hypersalivation, and urinary incontinence all with preservation of consciousness. Gaze deviation may occur after episodes of emesis. Generalized convulsions, hemi convulsions, and visual hallucinations may also be observed.

Suggested Reading

- Millichap JJ, Millichap JG. Clinical features and evaluation of febrile seizures. UpToDate, NordIi DR, Eichler AF (Ed), UpToDate, Waltham. Accessed on 1 Dec 2015.
- Abram HS. Febrile seizure. In: Tatum WO, SirvenJI, Cascino GD, editors. Epilepsy case studies. New York: Springer Science and Business Media; 2014. p. 13–6.
- Deivasumathy M, Hartman AL. Pediatric epilepsy syndromes. Neurologist. 2010;16(4):223–37.
- ParkJT, Shahid AM, Jamoul A. Common pediatric epilepsy syndromes. Pediatr Ann. 2015; 44(2):e30–e35.
- Korff CM. Juvenile myoclonic epilepsy. UpToDate, Nordli DR, Eichler AF, editors. UpToDate, Waltham. Accessed on 1 Dec 2015.
- Korff CM. Childhood absence epilepsy. UpToDate, Nordli DR, Eichler AF, editors. UpToDate Waltham. Accessed on 1 Dec 2015.
- Moller RS, Heron SE, Larsen LH, Lim CX, Ricos, MG, Bayly MA, van Kempen MJ, Klinkenberg S, Andrews I, Kelley, K, Ronen GM, Callen D, McMahon JC, Yendle SC, Carvill GL, Mefford HC, Nabbout R, Nabbout R, Poduri A, Striano P, Baglietto MG, Zara F, Smith NJ. Pridmore C, Gardella E, Nikanorova M, Dahl HA, Gellert P, Scheffer IE, Guning, Kragh-Olsen B, Dibbens LM. Mutations in KCNT1 cause a spectrum of focal epilepsies. Epilepsia. 2015;56(9):e114–20.
- Nordi DR. Focal and multifocal seizures. In: Swaiman K, Ashwal S, Ferriera OM, Ferriero D, editors. Swaiman's pediatric neurology: principles and practice. 5th ed. Elsevier; 2012. p. 751–66.
- Nickels KC, Wirrell EC. Benign and malignant childhood epilepsies. In: Miller JW, Goodkin HP, editors. Epilepsy. Hoboken: Wiley; 2013. p. 147–58.
- Pandolfo M. Pediatric epilepsy genetics. Curr Opin Neurol. 2013;26:137–45.
- Hani AJ, Mikati HM, Mikati MA. Genetics of pediatric epilepsy. Pediatr Clin North Am. 2015;62(3):703–22.

119. A baby with epileptic encephalopathy has been evaluated for microcephaly and prominent developmental delay. His CSF analysis shows a glucose level of 30 mg/dl, whereas the level of serum glucose was 112 mg/dl. Other CSF tests are normal.
Which **of the following is correct regarding the most likely condition in this patient?**
  A. Brain MRI usually suggests the diagnosis
  B. It is caused by deficiency in the glucose transporter type 1
  C. Phenobarbital is the treatment of choice
  D. Ketogenic diet has been shown to be ineffective for seizure control
  E. It is inherited in an X-linked fashion

Correct Answer is: B
This is a case of a glucose transporter type 1 (GLUT-1) deficiency. The brain utilizes glucose as its primary source of energy. In fasting conditions, glycogen is depleted within minutes, and since amino acids and fat cannot be used for the production of energy in the brain, ketones become the alternative fuel. Glucose crosses the blood brain barrier facilitated by GLUT-1, which is a membrane-bound protein encoded by the

SLC2A 1 gene on chromosome 1p35–31.3. It is inherited as an autosomal dominant fashion and causes a defect in glucose transport across the blood-brain barrier and into brain cells, manifesting as an epileptic encephalopathy with infantile-onset seizures, developmental delay, microcephaly, and complex movement disorders. CSF glucose level is low with a normal serum glucose level, and other CSF studies are normal, excluding other causes of hypoglycorrhachia (such as CNS infection). EEG may show 2.5 to 4 Hz spikes and waves and the interictal EEG findings may improve with glucose. Neuroimaging shows no specific abnormalities. Later-onset forms with episodic movement disorders and ataxia, paroxysmal exertional dyskinesia, or early-onset atypical absence epilepsy have been described. A ketogenic diet should be started as soon as the diagnosis is suspected, since this treatment option improves seizure control and the abnormal movements; however, it is less effective for the psychomotor impairment.

Suggested Reading

- Comprehensive review in clinical neurology: a multiple-choice question book for the Wards and Boards ©2011 Wolters Kluwer Health Lippincott Williams & Wilkins. All rights reserved.

120. You are evaluating a newborn for seizures. His seizures are characterized by apneic spells associated with unilateral or bilateral clonic movements. Starting on day 5 of life he has been having multiple spells per day. He has a normal neurological exam in between seizures. His interictal EEG is normal.

Which of the following is the most likely diagnosis?

A. West syndrome
B. Benign neonatal seizures
C. Aicardi syndrome
D. Ohtahara syndrome
E. Benign myoclonic epilepsy of infancy

Correct Answer is: B

This is a presentation of benign neonatal seizures. In this syndrome, full-term, otherwise healthy, newborns develop seizures around day 5 of life (also referred to as "fifth day fits"), which are partial clonic seizures that may be unilateral and/or symmetric and may migrate to other regions of the body. They are frequently associated with apneic spells. The EEG is normal, but may demonstrate the "pointu alternant" pattern, characterized by discontinuous, asynchronous, unreactive activity with intermixed sharp waves. Patients are neurologically normal. No seizure treatment is need, and seizures resolve spontaneously by 4–6 weeks of age. Benign neonatal seizures and benign familial neonatal seizures should be diagnoses of exclusion, and workup to rule out symptomatic seizures is recommended. Benign familial neonatal seizures is an autosomal dominant disorder, characterized by seizures in the first few days of life, which resolve spontaneously within few weeks. Genetic linkage studies have mapped two disease loci, both associated with mutations in voltage-gated potassium channels, in the genes KCNQ2 on chromosome 20 and KCNQ3 on chromosome 8.

Suggested Reading

- Bradley WG, Daroff RB, Fenichel GM, et al. Neurology in Clinical Practice, 5th ed. Philadelphia: Elsevier; 2008.
- Browne TR, Holmes GL. Handbook of Epilepsy, 4th ed. Philadelphia: Lippincott Williams & Wilkins; 2008.
- Comprehensive review in clinical neurology: a multiple-choice question book for the Wards and Boards ©2011 Wolters Kluwer Health Lippincott Williams & Wilkins. All rights reserved.

121. A first-time mother brings her 9-day-old infant in with a chief complaint of seizures. The infant had an uncomplicated term delivery and has been well. Her infant has been and remains afebrile.
Which of the following is the most likely cause of this infant's seizures?
A. Hypokalemia
B. Hyponatremia
C. Hypocalcemia
D. Hypomagnesemia
E. Maple syrup urine disease

Correct Answer is: B
Hyponatremia is the most common cause of seizures in a well newborn without fever. Water intoxication is the most common cause of hyponatremia during infancy. Infants are unable to adequately concentrate urine so parents who dilute formula or give their infants tap water put their infants at risk.

Hypocalcemia is also a very common cause of seizures in the neonate, so serum calcium levels should be checked. In fact, all infants have a slight decline in serum calcium levels with a nadir at 24–48 h.

Symptomatic hypocalcemia is more common in infants of diabetic mothers, preterm infants, or infants with a history of anoxic encephalopathy.

Hypomagnesemia is not as common as hypocalcemia, but symptoms of hypomagnesemia mimic those of hypocalcemia and it is difficult to correct hypocalcemia if the serum magnesium is also low. Therefore, infants with seizures should have a comprehensive evaluation of their electrolytes.

Hypokalemia is uncommon in infancy and does not typically cause seizures.

Maple syrup urine disease is a rare disease resulting from the inability to catabolize branched chain amino acids. Infants typically present between 4 and 7 days of life with poor feeding, vomiting, or lethargy. Neurologic manifestations rapidly develop, such as alternating hypotonia and hypertonia, dystonia, seizures, and encephalopathy.

122. Myoclonic seizures (sudden, brief muscular contractions that occur singly or repetitively) are characteristically seen in what setting?
A. West syndrome
B. adolescents with gray matter disease
C. adults with viral encephalitis
D. adults with prion disease
E. all of the above
F. none of the above

Correct Answer is: E
All of the previous seizure disorders are characterized by a tendency of having myoclonic seizures. West Syndrome is characterized by childhood spasms, hypsarrhythmia on interictal EEG, and intellectual disability. The spasms may occur up to hundreds times per day. The cause of West syndrome is theorized to be organic brain dysfunction but the precise etiology is unknown. Gray matter diseases usually manifest as a neuronal dysfunction, and may occur from metabolic storage disease, such as (Tay-Sachs disease, Nieman-Pick disease, etc). Gray matter is where the neuronal dendrites and cell bodies are, so it makes sense that diseases which affect the neuron would cause seizures. Adults with viral encephalitis, such as that caused by HSV, HIV, and other viruses, can cause seizures. It is postulated that the viral infection makes changes to the neuron, and the neurons are unable to heal the changes caused, which results in abnormal functioning. Prion diseases, such as BSE, "mad cow disease", or Kuru, affect the proteins in the brain, but at present the exact mechanisms by which they operate is still under debate.

Suggested Reading

- Lee, HW, Khoshbin, S. "Seizure Disorders" Chapter 76, page 1044, Mass General Comprehensive Clinical Psychiatry.

123. An 18-year-old female was admitted to the emergency room after a generalized tonic clonic seizure that began focally in her right lower extremity. Although the seizure stopped within 1 min, there was persistent weakness of the right lower extremity lasting several hours. Further testing revealed a small arteriovenous malformation near the motor cortex. Focal weakness lasting for 24 h following a motor seizure is most likely attributable to which of the following?
    A. Intracerebral hemorrhage
    B. Subarachnoid hemorrhage
    C. Encephalitis
    D. Todd paralysis
    E. Hyponatremia

Correct Answer is: D

Weakness after seizure activity is evidence of a postictal paralysis, or Todd paralysis. Postictal weakness does not suggest bleeding or new areas of cerebrocortical damage, but imaging with CT scan is appropriate to exclude these possibilities. Postictal paralysis may last for many hours, or even days. The precise cause is unknown, but it appears to be caused by some kind of neuronal exhaustion occurring after frequent repetitive discharges. It may reflect depletion of glucose in the neurons in the epileptic focus.

124. What is the drug of choice for a 6-year-old girl that is symptomatic and is found to have 3 per second spike and wave complexes on her EEG?
    A. Valproic acid
    B. Ethosuximde
    C. Carbamazepine
    D. Lamotrigine

Correct Answer is: B

Ethosuximde controls absence seizes in about 80% of cases. In addition, the drug has a very safe side effect profile and is therefore the drug of choice in this seizure type. Valproic acid and lamotrigine are effective in about 60% of cases but have more serious potential side effects. Carbamazepine has been shown to aggregate absence seizures and worsen the condition. This can occur when the clinical presentation of absence seizures is mistaken for complex partial seizures, in which carbamazepine is chosen.

Suggested Reading

- Camfield P, Camfield C. Epileptic syndromes in childhood: clinical features, outcomes, and treatment. Epilepsia. 2002;43(Suppl 3):27–32.

125. Which of the following is the best treatment option for simple febrile seizures?
    A. IV lorazepam
    B. Rectal diazepam
    C. Supportive management
    D. Phenobarbital
    E. Intranasal midazolam

Correct Answer is: C

Supportive care is the best management choice for a simple febrile seizure (FS). It is estimated that about 3–5% of children aged 5 months to 5 years have simple FS. 90% occurs in the first 3 years of life. 1/3 of patients have at least one additional seizure. Risk factors of simple FS are family history of FS, prolonged neonatal ICU stay, developmental delay, and day care.

Incidence does not increase in proportion to increase in temperature. No risk factors are found in 50% of children with an FS. The risk of afebrile epilepsy after FS is increased in children with developmental delay, abnormal neurologic examination, complex FS, and a family history of

afebrile seizures. There is a < 5% risk that patients with a simple FS will develop epilepsy. It is estimated that approximately 15% of patients with epilepsy have a history of FS. Simple FS are characterized by the following: <15 min in duration, generalized seizure, and no focality, normal neurologically examination, no persistent deficits, and negative family history for seizures. Complex FS occur in approximately 20% of FS and are characterized by the following: >15 min in duration, focal features, abnormal neurologic examination, and seizure recurrence in < 24 h, postictal signs (Todd's paralysis), and are more likely to be due to meningitis, encephalitis, or an underlying seizure disorder. No need for prophylaxis medications, but can be considered for recurrent or prolonged seizures, afebrile seizures, after complex FS, and with an abnormal neurologic examination and developmental delay. Chronic prophylaxis commonly includes phenobarbital and valproic acid, whereas short-term prophylaxis could include diazepam and antipyretics, though definitive data on the use of antipyretics for the prevention of FS are lacking. Furthermore, the potential toxicities associated with available antiepileptic agents outweigh the relatively minor risks associated with simple FS. After reviewing the potential risks and benefits of available effective therapies for short- and long-term prophylaxis, the AAP concluded (in its clinical practice guideline on long-term management of children with FS) that neither continuous nor intermittent anticonvulsant therapy is recommended for children with one or more simple FS.

9

Suggested Reading

- Berg AT, Shinnar S. Complex febrile seizures. Epilepsia. 1996;37:126–33.
- Knudsen FU. Febrile seizures: treatment and prognosis. Epilepsia. 2000;41(1):2–9.
- Steering Committee on Quality Improvement and Management, Subcommittee on Febrile Seizures American Academy of Pediatrics.
- Febrile seizures: clinical practice guideline for the long-term management of the child with simple febrile seizures. Pediatrics. 2008;121:1281–6.
- Comprehensive review in clinical neurology: a multiple-choice question book for the Wards and Boards ©2011 Wolters Kluwer Health Lippincott Williams & Wilkins. All rights reserved.

126. Which infant with infantile spasms has the best prognosis?
    - A. An infant with tuberous sclerosis
    - B. An infant with cryptogenic infantile spasms
    - C. An infant who was premature
    - D. An infant with Sturge-Webber Syndrome
    - E. An infant with Maple-Syrup Urine Disease

Correct Answer is: B

Infantile spasms, or "drop attacks" are a form of seizure in which there is a sudden tonic contraction of the trunk and limbs that lasts a few seconds. Typically, there is developmental regression. They occur more common just before sleep or upon awakening, but they can occur at any time. They tend to occur in clusters. An EEG shows a hypsarrhythmia pattern, which is pathognomonic for this condition. Infants who develop infantile spasms often have an underlying condition, which may or may not have been previously diagnosed. Therefore, part of the workup includes an evaluation for an underlying issue; this would include a brain MRI and CT, genetic studies, a metabolic work-up, and a lumbar puncture. Tuberous sclerosis is the most common disorder associated with infantile spasms.

Treatment is with ACTH and antiepileptics, and the prognosis is poor, with a high likelihood of developmental delay and/or autism. Prognosis is often related to the underlying condition. Prognosis is best in the cryptogenic (or idiopathic) form, where there is no underlying disorder. Other positive prognostic indicators is age of diagnosis over the age of 4 months, short time from onset to treatment, and early response to treatment. Early intervention is imperative. All of the other answers are conditions that are found in patients with infantile spasms, and all carry a poor prognosis.

127. Levels of which of the following hormones is evidently used to evaluate recent seizure?
  A. TSH
  B. Prolactin
  C. ACTH
  D. GH

Correct Answer is: B
Serum prolactin levels are increased for 5–30 times, if measured within 20 min of generalized tonic clonic seizures. This level helps in excluding pseudoseizures in few patients.

Suggested Reading

- Sadock BJ, Sadock VA, Kaplan HI. Kaplan & Sadock's comprehensive textbook of psychiatry. Philadelphia: Lippincott Williams & Wilkins. Chapters 2.4;2005.

128. An 18-year-old male has refractory epilepsy. Which of the following conditions is a likely contradiction to epilepsy surgery in this patient?
  A. Grade 1 Astrocytoma
  B. Autism
  C. Primary generalized epilepsy
  D. Prior pacemaker placement for arrhythmia
  E. Frontal lobe seizures

Correct Answer is: A
Diagnosis of primary generalized epilepsy (PGE) is a contraindication in consideration of epilepsy surgery for refractory epilepsy. Best candidates will have a focal non-dominant hemisphere seizure focus who failed at least 2 or 3 antiepileptic agents. Other listed conditions are not contraindications for epilepsy surgery.

129. Which of the following anticonvulsants binds to synaptic vesicle protein SV2A?
  A. Levetiracetam
  B. Topiramate
  C. Lamotrigine
  D. Ethosuximide
  E. Perampanel

Correct Answer is: A
Levetiracetam binds to synaptic vesicle protein SV2A, which decreases calcium influx into the presynaptic terminal. The drug also blocks high voltage activated calcium channels and affects gamma aminobutyric acid (GABA) function. It is unclear, however, how these actions relate to its anticonvulsant effect.

Topiramate has multiple mechanisms of action, blocking sodium channels, calcium channels, kainate receptors, and a-amino-3-hydroxyl-5-methyl-4-isoxazole-proprionate (AMPA) glutamate receptors, while enhancing GABA activity.

Lamotrigine also has multiple mechanisms of action, blocking sodium channels and high voltage activated calcium channels.

Ethosuximide blocks thalamic T-type calcium channels, and likely inhibits sodium currents. Perampanel is a new anticonvulsant with a novel mechanism of action, acting as a non-competitive AMPA glutamate receptor antagonist.

Suggested Reading

- Stafstrom CE. Mechanisms of action of antiepileptic drugs: the search for synergy. Curr Opin Neurol. 23:157–63.

130. Which of the following is most likely to be true of benign focal epilepsy with central mid temporal spikes?
   A. Lifelong treatment with anti-epileptic medications is often necessary
   B. Seizures usually occur during the daytime while the child is awake
   C. Children with this disorder may complain of facial numbness or may be observed drooling
   D. EEG findings are used to determine whether to continue, discontinue, or start anti-epileptic medications

9

Correct Answer is: C
Benign focal epilepsy with centrotemporal spikes (benign rolandic epilepsy), accounts for 15% of childhood epilepsy. Usually, it starts around age of 7 and 9 years. Its name is based on typical EEG findings. There are diphasic or triphasic sharp waves occur in the mid temporal and central areas. Clinical manifestations include: speech arrest, hypersalivation, unilateral facial twitching, and paresthesias inside the mouth.

Treatment with anti-epileptic medications is often not necessary. Seizures usually occur at night and most patients have under 10 seizures total. Patients may enter remission after 2 to 4 years of onset of seizures. Most are in remission by age 16. Treatment is indicated in patients with frequent seizures, or in those with generalized seizures. 75% of seizures occur either during the night, or when the patient wakes. On EEG studies, epileptiform activity is more prominent during Non-REM sleep.

EEG activity typical of benign focal epilepsy with centrotemporal spikes may occur in individuals who do not have known seizures. Also, in patients who do have clinical and EEG findings characteristic of this form of epilepsy, the EEG abnormalities may persist even after the seizures have stopped. Thus, decisions on whether to start or stop anti-epileptic drugs are not based on EEG findings. As mentioned above, anti-epileptic medications are often not indicated at all.

Suggested Reading

- Millichap JJ, Millichap JG. Clinical features and evaluation of febrile seizures. UpToDate, Nordli DR, Eichler AF editors. UpToDate, Waltham. Accessed on 1 Dec 2015.
- Abram HS. Febrile seizure. In: Tatum WO, Sirven JI, Cascino GD, editors. Epilepsy case studies. New York: Springer Science and Business Media; 2014. p. 13–6.
- Deivasumathy M, Hartman AL. Pediatric epilepsy syndromes. Neurologist. 2010;16(4):223–74.
- Park JT, Shahid AM, Jamoul A. Common pediatric epilepsy syndromes. Pediatr Ann. 2015;44(2):e30–5.
- Korff CM. Juvenile myoclonic epilepsy. UpToDate, Nordli DR, Eichler AF editors. UpToDate, Waltham. Accessed on 1 Dec 2015.
- Korff CM. Childhood absence epilepsy. UpToDate, Nordli DR, Eichler AF editors. UpToDate, Waltham. Accessed on 1 Dec 2015.
- Hani AJ, Mikati HM, Mikati MA. Genetics of pediatric epilepsy. Pediatr Clin North Am. 2015;62(3):703–722. 12. Mizrah EM. Neonatal epileptic syndromes.
- Anderson GD. Pharmacopeia. In: Miller JW, Goodkin HP, editors. Epilepsy. Hoboken: Wiley; 2013. p. 126–38.
- Glaze DG. Clinical features and diagnosis of infantile spasms. UpToDate, Nordli DR, Eichler AF, editors. UpToDate, Waltham. Accessed on 5 Dec 2015.
- Glaze DG. Management and prognosis of infantile spasms. UpToDate, Nordli DR, Eichler AF editors, UpToDate, Waltham. Accessed on 5 Dec 2015.

- Glaze DG. Etiology and pathogenesis of infantile spasms. UpToDate, Nordli DR, Eichler AF editors. UpToDate, Waltham. Accessed on 5 December 2015.

131. A 6-year-old female came to the office with her mother who complains about her daughter declining school performance. Her teachers have complained to the mother that the child doesn't listen and tends to "stare off." You ordered an EEG which showed 3 Hertz spike and slow wave complexes.
What is the best next step in management?
A. The child should be started on phenytoin
B. The child should be started on tiagabine
C. The child should be started on carbamazepine
D. The child should be started on ethosuximide
E. The child should be started on phenobarbital

Correct Answer is: D
This is a clinical presentation of childhood absence epilepsy. Exclusion criteria include (1) the presence of other seizure types (2) eyelid, perioral, head, or limb myoclonias that are massive and sustained (3) sensory or visual seizure precipitants, and (4) either no impairment, or mild impairment, of consciousness during spike wave discharges, and (5) spike wave discharges lasting under 4 s on EEG. Inclusion criteria include.

normal neurological exam and normal development, (2) seizures lasting between 4 and 20 s occurring many times per day and (3) the presence of 3 Hz spike wave discharges. Ethosuximide is the first line medication. Valproate, lamotrigine, topiramate, benzodiazepines, and acetazolamide are also efficacious. Phenytoin is not effective in management of absence seizures and is thus not a first line therapy. Similarly, phenobarbital is not effective in the management of this seizure type. Tiagabine may worsen absence seizures, and is thus contraindicated. Carbamazepine, gabapentin, and vigabatrin are also contraindicated.

It is worthwhile to note that carbamazepine may worsen absence seizures, and it is contraindicated.

132. West's syndrome consists of the triad of:
A. infantile spasms, hydrocephalus, 3 Hz spike-wave
B. absence seizures, myoclonic seizures, 3 Hz spike-wave
C. myoclonic seizures, agenesis of the corpus callosum, hypsarrhythmi
D. infantile spasms, developmental arrest, hypsarrhythmia
E. absence seizures, developmental arrest, 4-6 Hz spike-wave

Correct Answer is: D
West's syndrome consists of: (1) Infantile spasms. Flexor spasms include flexion of the head, trunk, and lower extremities, with adduction of the upper extremities. Extensor spasms involve extension of the head and trunk, with abduction of the upper extremities. The infantile spasms typically occur in clusters during morning feedings. (2) Developmental arrest, beginning with or prior to the onset of infantile spasms. (3) Hypsarrhythmia on EEG. Up to 40% of cases have no identifiable etiology (cryptogenic), while the remaining cases may be due to cerebral dysgenesis, genetic or metabolic disorders, infections, anoxic injury, and head trauma. Onset is typically within the first year, most often between 3 and 7 months of age. Corticosteroids are first-line agents, but the prognosis remains poor.

Suggested Reading

- Trescher WH, Lesser RP. The epilepsies. In: Bradley WG, Daroff RB, Fenichel GM, Jankovicj, editors. Neurology in clinical practice. 4th ed. Elsevier, Inc.; 2004. p. 1953–92.

133. A 20-month-old girl has a generalized seizure lasting 5 min with fever of 39C. She has no significant past medical or family history. The patient recovered without any residual neurologic deficit. The family would like to know the risk of recurrence. **Which of the following is not a predictor of recurrence of febrile seizures (FS)?**
   - A. Family history of FS
   - B. Age younger than 18 months at the time of FS
   - C. Shorter duration of fever prior to FS
   - D. Lower peak temperature at the time of FS
   - E. Complex FS

9

Correct Answer is: E

This patient had a simple febrile seizure (FS). FS is defined as a seizure that occurs in association with a febrile illness in the absence of CNS infection or acute electrolyte imbalance in children without prior afebrile seizures. These occur commonly between 6 months and 5 years of age, with a peak incidence at 18 months. FS can be simple or complex. Most FS represent simple FS, that is, generalized, usually isolated, seizures of relatively brief duration lasting less than 15 min. Complex FS on the other hand are prolonged, lasting more than 15 min, have focal features, and may occur multiple times in the course of the same febrile illness, or within the same 24-h period. A prior history of a complex FS is a known risk factor for subsequent development of epilepsy, whereas a family history of FS does not increase the risk of subsequent epilepsy. Interestingly, a prior history of a complex FS has not been found to be associated with a higher risk for recurrence of FS. Risk factors to develop a first FS include a first- or second-degree relative with a history of FS, developmental delay, neonatal nursery stay for more than 30 days, and attendance of day care. Most patients will have only one FS without recurrence and without subsequent development of epilepsy. Recurrent FS may occur, especially in the presence of recognizable risk factors, which include a family history of FS, age younger than 18 months at the time of the first FS, lower peak temperature, and shorter duration of fever prior to the FS. Simple or complex FS carry similar risk of recurrence. The risk of developing epilepsy following a single simple FS is not substantially different than the risk in the general population. On the other hand, patients with complex FS may be at risk of developing epilepsy in the future. The risk is even higher when the complex FS was very prolonged in duration (i.e., febrile status epilepticus). Other risk factors to develop epilepsy include the presence of a neurodevelopmental abnormality and/or family history of epilepsy. Importantly, a family history of FS does not predispose the patient to subsequent development of epilepsy. The evaluation of patients with FS should be targeted at assessing the cause of the seizure and ruling out CNS infections or abnormalities. The exact pathophysiology of FS remains unclear. A relationship between prolonged FS and mesial temporal lobe sclerosis has been proposed; however, this association is controversial and has not conclusively been confirmed in prospective and population-based studies, which are ongoing. Long-term prophylaxis and AEDs are not indicated for FS, but can be considered in some cases, especially if a high risk of recurrence exists. In these

cases, phenobarbital or valproic acid can be considered on a case-by case basis. Short-term prophylaxis may also be needed in some cases, and should be focused on temperature control during febrile illness and use of benzodiazepines, such as rectal diazepam gel.

Suggested Reading

- Shinnar S, Glauser TA. Febrile Seizures. J Child Neural. 2002;17:S44–52.

134. Which of the following is most likely to be associated with epilepsy of infancy with migrating focal seizures?
    A. Potassium channel, voltage gated, subfamily Q, member 2 (KCNQ2)
    B. Sodium channel, voltage gated, type II, alpha subunit (SCN2A)
    C. Potassium channel, subfamily T, member 1 (KCNT1)
    D. Aristaless related Homeobox, X linked (ARX)
    E. Cholinergic receptor, neuronal nicotinic, alpha polypeptide 4 (CHRNA4)

Correct Answer is: C

Epilepsy of infancy with migrating focal seizures is characterized by onset prior to 6 months of age (with normal development until seizure onset) and the presence of focal motor seizures which ultimately become intractable and unresponsive to conventional anti epileptic medications. Psychomotor delay usually follows seizure onset.

Mutations in the potassium channel, subfamily T, member 1 (KCNT1) gene result in persistent channel activity, thereby lowering the seizure threshold. Other genes implicated in this disorder include solute carrier family 25 (mitochondrial carrier: glutamate), member 22 (SLC25A22) and phospholipase C, beta 1 (phosphoinositide-specific) (PLCB1).

Mutations in potassium channel, voltage gated, subfamily Q, member 2 (KCNQ2) are implicated in benign familial neonatal convulsions. A related gene-potassium channel, voltage gated, subfamily Q, member 3 (KCNQ3) is also implicated in this disorder. Benign familial neonatal convulsions are an autosomal dominant condition characterized by seizures which may start a few days after birth, often persisting for 6 weeks. If they do not occur within a few days of birth, seizures are usually present by 8 weeks of age, and may persist for up to 6 months. Seizures may be either generalized or focal and development is usually normal.

Mutations in sodium channel, voltage gated, type II, alpha subunit (SCN2A) are implicated in benign familial infantile seizures 3 and early infantile epileptic encephalopathy 11. Less commonly, this gene is implicated in severe myoclonic epilepsy of infancy, and generalized epilepsy with febrile seizures plus.

Mutations in aristaless related homeobox (ARX), which codes for a homeobox transcription factor, are implicated in early infantile epileptic encephalopathy 1. Cyclin dependent kinase-like 5 (CDKL5), solute carrier family 25, member 22 (SLC25A22}, syntaxin binding protein 1 (STXBP1), spectrin,alpha, nonerythrocytic 1 (SPTAN1}, sodium channel, voltage gated, type I, alpha subunit (SCN1A),sodium channel,voltage gated, type IX, alpha subunit (SCN9A),potassium channel,voltage gated, subfamily Q, member 2 (KCNQ2),cdc42 guanine nucleotide exchange factor 9 (ARHGEF9), protocadherin 19 (PCDH19), polynucleotide kinase 3-prime phosphatase (PNKP}, sodium channel,voltage gated, type II,alpha subunit (SCN2A}, phospholipase C, beta 1 (PLCB1),sodium channel,voltage gated, type VIII, alpha subunit (SCN8A), potassium channel, subfamily T, member 1 (KCNT1), ST3 beta-galacstoside alpha-2,3-sialyltransferase 3 (ST3GAL3),tre2- bub2-

cdc16- domain family, member 24 (TBC1024), guanine nucleotide binding protein,alpha-activating polypeptide O gene (GNA01),mouse seizure threshold 2 gene (SZT2),gamma-aminobutyri c acid (GABA) A receptor, alpha 1 (GABRA 1), phosphatidylinositol glycan,class A (PIGA), NECAP endocytosis-associated protein 1 (NECAP1), solute carrier family 35, member 2 (SLC35A2), dedicator of cytokinesis 7 (DOCK7), hyperpolarization activated cyclic nucleotide-gated potassium channel 1 (HCN1), solute carrier family 13, member 5 (SLC13A5), SLIT-ROBO rho GTP-ase activation protein 2 (SRGAP2), and MADs Box transcription enhancer factor 2, polypeptide C (MEF2C) are implicated in early infantile epileptic encephalopathy. This typically starts in infancy; patients may have tonic spasms, and burst suppression on EEG.

Cholinergic receptor, neuronal nicotinic, alpha polypeptide 4 (CHRNA4) is implicated in autosomal dominant nocturnal frontal lobe epilepsy 1. The product of this gene regulates nicotinic acetylcholine receptor GABAergic inhibition. Other genes implicated in autosomal dominant frontal lobe epilepsy include cholinergic receptor, nicotinic, beta 2 (Neuronal) (CHRNB2), cholinergic receptor, nicotinic, alpha 2 (neuronal) (CHRNA2), and potassium channel, subfamily T, member 1 (KCNT1).

Autosomal dominant nocturnal frontal lobe epilepsy typically starts in adolescence or late childhood and is characterized by predominately night time frontal lobe seizures.

135. A The mother of a 13-month-old boy brought him to the ER after she witness a jerky movement in his arms and legs. The event lasts 1 min and afterwards, the child seems tired and uninterested in his surroundings. The child has an upper respiratory tract infection and his temperature in the ER is 38 C. No family history of seizures. His CSF and brain MRI are normal.

Which of the following is associated with increased risk of future seizures?

A. No family history of epilepsy or febrile seizure
B. Age over 2 years
C. Long interval between onsets of fever to onset of seizure
D. Seizure duration more than 15 min

Correct Answer is: D

Febrile seizures are generally associated with temperature more than 38C in a child between 3 months and 6 years of age with (1) no central nervous system infection (2) no acute metabolic or systemic abnormalities and (3) no history of prior afebrile seizures. The child in this case has a simple febrile seizure. Simple febrile seizures last under 15 min with no seizure recurrence within 24 h are typically generalized and may be clonic, atonic, or tonic. Complex febrile seizures are characterized by duration more than 15 min, focal onset, recurrence within 24 h, or the presence of baseline neurological deficits. Risk factors for recurrent febrile seizures include age under 15 months, developmental delay, time spent in daycare, shorter time between fever onset and seizure, low grade fever at onset, and first degree relative with febrile seizures or another epilepsy type. In the absence of known risk factors, there is a 2.5% risk of epilepsy by the third decade. If there are multiple risk factors, the risk may be as high as 17%.

Family history of epilepsy or febrile seizures is associated with increased risk of future febrile seizure. A child with either a parent or sibling with febrile seizures has a risk 2 to 3 times higher of febrile seizure than that of a child with no family history.

Age under 15 months is associated with increased risk of future febrile seizures.

Shorter fever duration prior to onset of seizure is associated with increased risk of future seizures.

136. A mother of a 12-year-old girl with a history of febrile seizures brought her to your office, with a concern that her daughter had a generalized tonic clonic seizure in the absence of elevated temperature. The family history is remarkable of several family members including the child's biological father and sister have had febrile and afebrile seizures.
Which of the following is most likely true?
   A. The patient has a mutation affecting voltage gated KQT-like subfamily Q, member 2 (KCNQ2)
   B. The patient has a mutation affecting aristaless related homeobox (ARX)
   C. The patient has a mutation affecting sodium channel, voltage-gated, type I, alpha subunit (SCN1A)
   D. The patient has a mutation affecting Gamma-Aminobutyri c Acid (GABA) A receptor, alpha 1 (GABRA1).
   E. The patient has a mutation affecting chloride channel, voltage-sensitive 2) CLCN2.

Correct Answer is: C
The clinical presentation is indicative of generalized epilepsy febrile seizures plus (GEFS+). Patients with this condition may have febrile seizures initially, but both febrile and afebrile seizures persist past age 6. It is an autosomal dominant disorder, so there is often a known family history of febrile and afebrile seizures. Myoclonic, atonic, or absence seizures may be present in addition to tonic clonic seizures. Genes implicated in this disorder include sodium channel, voltage-gated, type I, alpha subunit (SCN1A), sodium channel, voltage gated, type I, beta (SCN1 B), gamma-aminobutyric acid (GABA) A receptor, gamma 2 (GABRG2), gamma-aminobutyric acid (GABA) A receptor, delta (GABRD), and sodium channel, voltage gated, type IX, alpha subunit (SCN9A). Mutation affecting voltage gated KQT-like subfamily Q, member 2 are implicated in benign familial neonatal seizures and in early infantile epileptic encephalopathy. Mutations affecting voltage gated KQT-like subfamily Q, member 3 (KCNQ3) may also cause benign familial neonatal seizures.

Mutations in aristaless related homeobox (ARX) may be seen in early infantile epileptic encephalopathy, and X linked lissencephaly.

Mutations affecting Gamma-Aminobutyric Acid (GABA) A receptor, alpha 1 (GABRA1) are thought to cause some forms of early infantile epileptic encephalopathy. Additionally, variations in this gene may increase one's susceptibility to juvenile myoclonic epilepsy.

Mutations affecting chloride channel, voltage-sensitive 2 (CLCN2) may increase one's susceptibility to juvenile absence epilepsy or juvenile myoclonic epilepsy.

137. A 5-month-old baby boy is brought to your office by his mother who is concerned about abnormal movements. She reports that the child seems to "jerk" briefly. She states that these episodes are becoming more frequent and she is concerned that the child is uncomfortable. You ordered an EEG which showed hypsarrhythmia. Brain MRI brain is normal. The mother wants to know what she can do to treat the condition.

Which of the following is the best initial therapy?
A. Vigabatrin
B. Valproic acid
C. Zonisamide
D. Adrenocorticotropic hormone (ACTH)
E. Topiramate

Correct Answer is: D
This a case of infantile spasms (IS). IS generally starts between 3 and 7 months of age. It is characterized by a brief (often lasting under 2 s) muscle contractions which may involve the extremities, trunk, and/or neck. Those contractions are followed by a tonic component lasting up to 10 s. There is considerable variation between patients and between seizures in a single patient. Extensor spasms are characterized by extension of the trunk and neck with either adduction or abduction of the legs and/ or arms. Flexer spasms may involve the neck, arms, legs, and/ or trunk. Mixed flexor extensor spasms may also occur as well. IS may occur with other conditions including Miller-Dieker syndrome, Aicardi syndrome, hemimegalencephaly, tuberous sclerosis complex, nevus linearis sebaceous, incontinentia pigmenti, Ito syndrome, and neurofibromatosis type I. Additionally, chromosomal abnormalities including trisomy 21 and 18q duplication may occur in association with IS. A number of genes have been identified which may play a causative role. Mutations in calcium/calmodulin-dependent serine protein kinase (CASK), ALG13, pyridoxamine-5′-phosphate oxidase (PNPO), adenylosuccinate lyase (ADSL), aristaless-related homeobox (ARX) gene syntaxin-binding protein 1 (STXBP1), and forkhead protein G1 (FOXG1) are associated with infantile spasms. Metabolic conditions associated with IS include Menkes disease, cytochrome C oxidase deficiency, pyridoxine deficiency, dihydropteridine reductase deficiency, histidinemia, and a number of disorders affecting the urea cycle. Syphilis, cytomegalovirus and toxoplasmosis are potential infectious etiologies and hypoxic ischemic encephalopathy is another potential underlying cause.

Cryptogenic IS may be diagnosed in a child with no other seizure type, a normal neurological exam, normal brain imaging, and normal development prior to symptom onset. The recommended first line therapy for this condition is ACTH, often given IM. Vigabatrin may also be given although ACTH is deemed preferential as per American Academy of Neurology (AAN) Guidelines.

Vigabatrin is not recommended as first line therapy for cryptogenic infantile spasms. However, in those with tuberous sclerosis this medication is particularly efficacious. Unfortunately, vigabatrin can cause visual loss, something difficult to monitor in infants. An initial ophthalmological exam is recommended with follow up every 3 months.

The benefits afforded by valproic acid are unclear although this has been used. Adequate clinical trials are lacking.

Zonisamide may be effective, although there is insufficient evidence to recommend this. Topiramate is also not recommended as first line. Nitrazepam, pyridoxine, IVIg, thyrotropin releasing hormone, levetiracetam and the ketogenic diet have also been considered as possible treatments. Again, there is insufficient evidence to recommend any of these treatments. ACTH remains first line.

138. Which of the following is typical of juvenile absence seizures?
A. Patients often have more than 100 seizures per day
B. The average age of onset is between 7 and 10 years

C. Patients usually do not need lifelong anti-epileptic drug treatment
D. Most patients eventually have generalized tonic clonic seizure

Correct Answer is: D
Juvenile absence epilepsy tends to present later than childhood absence epilepsy- starting between 10 and 16 years of age, as opposed to between 3 and 10 years of age. Up to 80% of patients with juvenile absence epilepsy may have a generalized tonic clonic seizure within 2 years of diagnosis. Variations in the chloride channel, voltage-sensitive 2 gene (CLCN2) and the G protein-coupled receptor kinase 1 gene (GRK1) are implicated in this disorder.

People with juvenile absence epilepsy may have up to 3 absence seizures per day, while those with child absence epilepsy may have between 25 and 50 seizures per day.

Most patients with juvenile absence epilepsy do require lifelong treatment with anti-epileptic medications. Medications used for this disorder include lamotrigine, valproate, topiramate, zonisamide, and levetiracetam.

139. Which of the following anti-epileptic medications works primarily through sodium channel inhibition?
A. Eslicarbazepine
B. Ethosuximide
C. Ezogabine
D. Phenobarbital
E. Diazepam

Correct Answer is: A
Eslicarbazepine is a voltage gated sodium channel blocker. This is approved for management of partial seizures (either with or without secondary generalization) in patients at least 6 months of age, although it is not approved as a monotherapy. Other medications that through inhibition of sodium channels include phenytoin and carbamazepine; the use of either medication blocks repetitive action potential firing. Rufinamide works by prolonging voltage dependent sodium channel inactivation. Similarly, lacosamide works on voltage gated sodium channels, enhancing slow inactivation. Felbamate inhibits voltage gated sodium channels and it blocks sodium and calcium conduction by binding to N-methyl-0-aspartate (NMDA) glutamate receptors. Lamotrigine works both through blockage of sodium channels and by inhibition of high threshold activated calcium channels.

Topiramate works through blockage of voltage activated sodium channels; this medication also acts at the kainate/alpha-amino-3 -hydroxy-5- methylisoxazole-4-proprioni c acid (AMPA) glutamate receptor subtype, decreasing glutamate mediated excitation. Topiramate also activates hyperpolarizing potassium conduction, enhances chloride current at GABAA receptors, and reduces high voltage activated calcium current amplitude.

This medication is also a carbonic anhydrase inhibitor. Oxcarbazepine stabilizes cell membranes through blockage of sodium, potassium, and calcium conduction. Zonisamide inhibits slow sodium channels, blocks T type calcium channels, and inhibits carbonic anhydrase. This also works on GABAA receptors through alteration of ligand biding. Valproate works through sodium channel inhibition and through attenuation of voltage sensitive calcium channels. This is also an NMDA receptor antagonist.

Ethosuximide works through attenuation of voltage sensitive calcium channels. This medication is indicating for the management of absence seizures in patients at least 3 years of age and is approved as a monotherapy.

Ezogabine works through activation of voltage gated potassium channels and also potentiates GABA evoked currents. This is indicated for management of partial seizures in patients at least 18 years of age and it is not approved as a monotherapy.

Phenobarbital works through enhancement of chloride currents mediated by GABAA receptors. This is approved as a monotherapy in patients of all ages.

Clonazepam works by enhancing chloride currents mediated by GABAA receptors. Clobazam, diazepam, and lorazepam have the same mechanism. Gabapentin decreases GABA turnover, thereby increasing GABA levels. This medication also inhibits monoamine neurotransmitter release and binds to L type calcium channels at the a2o subunit. Similarly, pregabalin inhibits voltage gated calcium channels at the a2o subunit. Vigabatrin increases GABA levels in the brain through inhibiting GABA transaminase irreversibly. Tiagabine also increases GABA levels, by blocking neuronal and glial GABA transporters. Stiripentol increases GABA release and enhances the activation of GABAA receptors. Perampanel works as an antagonist of the ionotropic AMPA glutamate receptor on post synaptic neurons, thereby reducing neuronal excitation. Levetiracetam binds to synaptic vesicle protein 2A and decreases influx of calcium through N type voltage sensitive calcium channels.

140. An 18-year-old female with idiopathic generalized epilepsy well controlled with moderate-dose lamotrigine has a sudden onset of multiple paroxysmal episodes unlike those previously experienced. Her family described a sudden startled look, followed by whole-body stiffening and arching in conjunction with "swimming" movements of the upper extremities and thrashing of the body. The spells last 30 s to 5 min in duration and are followed by somnolence and lack of recall for the event. There are no obvious medical precipitants, and serum levels of lamotrigine have been in the mid therapeutic range. An extended video-EEG is obtained, demonstrating occasional generalized polyphasic spike/wave discharges. One of the episodes described above occurs during the recording and is associated with muscle artifact, with resumption of normal waking patterns after the event ends.
Which of the following is the most appropriate next step in management?
   A. Replace lamotrigine with valproic acid
   B. Obtain psychiatry consultation
   C. Increase dose of lamotrigine
   D. Start diphenhydramine
   E. Obtain brain MRI

Correct Answer is: B
There are a constellation of evidence that strongly suggest psychogenic non-epileptic seizures, which is a form of conversion disorder. They are: Episodes are induced by stress, in certain settings, or by specific individuals. Seizures recur despite therapeutic antiepileptic drug levels. The ictus is of gradual onset and of unusually prolonged duration. There are thrashing/writhing movements, crying and/or screaming, pelvic thrusting, and rolling side-to-side. Movements are intermittent, arrhythmic, out-of-phase jerking, or with multiple periods of starting and stopping.There is no loss of consciousness despite bilateral movements, and a lack of incontinence or cyanosis. There is a lack of post-ictal confusion or lethargy. Presence of crying or shouting of obscenities. Eyes

will be closed, and patients will tend to resist having their eyes forced open.

The diagnosis of psychogenic seizures rests primarily on video-EEG documentation of the non-epileptic nature of the clinical episodes of concern. While considered the definitive diagnostic test, video-EEG testing does not have perfect sensitivity and specificity. Some non-lesional focal epilepsies may be missed. Also, there is a high co-morbidity between true epileptic seizures and psychogenic non-epileptic seizures (up to 30–40%), making it extremely difficult to ascertain what are or aren't true epileptic events in the usual clinical settings, and even in the context of an emergency department visit. The presentation of the diagnosis of psychogenic non-epileptic seizures must be made with great care and sensitivity. The possibility of sexual abuse should always be considered.

Suggested Reading

- Bodde NM, Brooks JL, Baker GA, Boon PA, Hendriksen JG, Aldenkamp AP. Psychogenic non-epileptic seizures – diagnostic issues: a critical review. Clin Neurol Neurosurg. 2009;111(1):1–9.
- LaFrance WC Jr. Psychogenic nonepileptic seizures. Curr Opin Neurol. 2008;21(2):195–201.

141. You are evaluating a 7-year-old girl for language difficulties. She was a product of a full-term uncomplicated pregnancy by normal spontaneous vaginal delivery. She walked at 10 months, said single words at 12 months, and combined words at 22 months. At age 5, her speech became progressively more telegraphic, and she began indicating her needs by pointing or by using sign language. She can follow simple commands. She has word-finding difficulties in spontaneous speech and on naming tasks and is unable to repeat short phrases. Otherwise the rest of her neurologic examination is normal. Formal audiometric testing is unremarkable. Her parents state that she occasionally stares off into space for 30 s to 1 min. She has never had a convulsive seizure, nor does she have a family history of epilepsy.

An EEG is most likely to show which of the following patterns?

A. Bilateral periodic epileptiform discharges (BiPEDs)
B. Continuous, diffuse, polymorphic theta and delta slowing
C. Hypsarrhythmia with periods of electrodecrement
D. Electrical status epilepticus in slow wave sleep
E. Normal waking and sleep

Correct Answer is: D

In 1957, William L. Landau and Frank R. Kleffner reported a "syndrome of acquired aphasia with convulsive disorder in children" and postulated that persistent convulsive discharges were causing a functional ablation of brain areas concerned with language. Since that time, it has become apparent that there are several epileptic encephalopathy syndromes of childhood that are characterized by deterioration of one or more cognitive functions with or without motor, behavioral, and/or psychomotor decline in association with an EEG that shows strong activation of epileptic activity during sleep. At this point, electrical status epilepticus of slow wave sleep (ESES) and continuous spikes and waves during slow wave sleep (CSWS) are considered synonymous terms, and Landau-Kleffner syndrome (LKS) a distinct presentation of ESES/CSWS in which acquired aphasia is the core symptom.

LKS typically presents with language disturbance in normally developing

children aged 3 and 8 years. Some have argued that the language disturbance is actually a verbal auditory agnosia (i.e. inability to comprehend spoken language in the absence of hearing difficulties). Over time, affected children experience a gradual deterioration in verbal comprehension and production, eventually leading to failure to respond to non-verbal sounds and mutism.

Seizure semiology varies, and 20–30% of patients do not exhibit clinical seizure activity at all. There is no clear relationship between the severity of the seizures and the severity of the language deficits. EEG shows predominantly bilateral posterior temporal spikes or spike-wave discharges that are activated by sleep. The clinical seizures are usually easy to control, with spontaneous resolution occurring in mid-adolescence. There are several treatment options, including corticosteroids, levetiracetam, benzodiazepines, and valproic acid. Language function improves when the active phase of spike-wave discharges resolves; however, if the aphasia begins in early childhood and/or persists for more than 1–2 years, long-term language deficits are almost universal.

Suggested Reading

- Smith MC, Hoeppner TJ. Epileptic encephalopathy of late childhood. J Clin Neurophysiol. 2003;20(6):462–72.
- Van Bogaert P, Paquier PF. Landau-Kleffner syndrome: 50 years after. Epilepsia. 2009;50(S7):1–2.

142. An 18-year-old pregnant female comes for evaluation of new onset epilepsy. She is concerned about the possibility of cognitive difficulties in her child if she is taking seizure medications.

You counsel her:

A. Her child's IQ may be lower with in utero exposure to divalproex monotherapy
B. Her child's IQ may be lower with in utero exposure to levetiracetam monotherapy
C. Her child's IQ may be lower with in utero exposure to lamotrigine monotherapy
D. Her child's IQ may be lower with in utero exposure to carbamazepine monotherapy
E. Her child IQ may be lower with in utero exposure to all anti-epileptic drugs

Correct Answer is: A

While divalproex's association with physical malformations following in utero exposure, the NEAD study's 6 year follow up report also demonstrated that children exposed to divalproex in utero are at risk for cognitive differences compared to children exposed to other anti-epileptic drugs. The difference ranged from 8–11 IQ points.

Suggested Reading

- Meador KJ, Baker GA, Browning N, Cohen MJ, Bromley RL, et al. Fetal antiepileptic drug exposure and cognitive outcomes at age 6 years (NEAD study): a prospective observational study. Lancet Neurol. 2013;12(3):244–52.

143. You are seeing a 17-year-old boy in the ED with a prolonged seizure lasting 45 min. ED team could not obtain an IV access.

What is the next best step in management?

A. Phenytoin 1000 mg intramuscular
B. Intubate the patient to secure the airway
C. Insert an internal jugular central line
D. Midazolam 10 mg intramuscular
E. Initiate a video EEG study

Correct Answer is: D

A recent randomized controlled trial indicated that IM midazolam is equal to

intravenous lorazepam for the treatment of status epilepticus. Phenytoin should not be given intramuscularly because the risk of purple glove syndrome. The other choices are important considerations in the management of this patient, but treatment with a benzodiazepine should not be delayed.

Suggested Reading

Silbergleit R, Durkalski V, Lowenstein D, Conwit R, Pancioli A, Palesch Y, Barsan W. NETT Investigators. Intramuscular versus intravenous therapy for prehospital status epilepticus. N Engl J Med. 2012;366(7):591–600.

144. You are evaluating a 16-month-old girl in the ER after her first seizure. The mother describes this event with the girl is stiffening up and then rhythmically shaking for 4 min. On arrival she has a temperature of 39 °C (102.2 °F). After treatment with antipyretics, the patient is now awake and alert and routine laboratory results are normal.
What is your next best step in management?
    A. Discharge patient with pediatric neurology follow up
    B. Lumbar puncture and empiric antibiotics
    C. Video EEG monitoring for 24 h
    D. MRI brain with and without gadolinium
    E. Admit for observation for 23 h

Correct Answer is: A
This is a classic presentation of a child with a simple febrile seizure. Febrile seizures occur in 2–5% of the population. Work up is typically only be initiated in febrile seizures with focal seizure or in the setting of febrile status epilepticus.

Suggested Reading

Gupta A. Febrile Seizures. Continuum (Minneap Minn). 2016;22(1 Epilepsy):51–9.

145. You are seeing a 7-month-old baby in the ED with new onset of seizures. You ordered an EEG which showed hypsarrhythmia.
What is your next best step in management?
    A. Routine pediatric neurology consultation
    B. Treat with adrenocorticotropic hormone (ACTH)
    C. Lumbar puncture
    D. Referral for corpus callosotomy
    E. Levetiracetam 10 mg/Kg/dose

Correct Answer is: B
Hypsarrhythmia on the EEG is part of the diagnosis for infantile spasms. Prompt treatment with ACTH is recommended.

Suggested Reading

Wilmshurst JM, Gaillard WD, Vinayan KP, Tsuchida TN, Plouin P, et al. Summary of recommendations for the management of infantile seizures: Task Force Report for ILAE Commission of Pediatrics. Epilepsia. 2015;56(8):1185–97.

146. You are seeing a 16-month-old boy for his an unprovoked generalized tonic clonic seizure (GTC). Previously, he had 2 complex febrile seizures. They were prolonged alternating unilateral convulsions. His mother reported recent some jerking movements of his arms. This jerking occurred as increased clusters prior to onset of the GTC. Recently he has also increased falls. While he is in the hospital, he underwent an EEG and MRI of the brain, both of which are normal. One day later, he is awake, but has some mild truncal ataxia on exam.
Which gene is responsible for his condition?
    A. CACNA1A
    B. DMPK gene
    C. KCNQ2
    D. SCN1A
    E. TSC1

Correct Answer is: D

The child has Dravet syndrome which is one of the genetic epileptic encephalopathies. Usually, unprovoked seizures start in the first or second year of life in an otherwise healthy infant. However, recurrent spells of hemiconvulsive febrile status epilepticus in the first year of life may delay the diagnosis. The term "severe myoclonic epilepsy of infancy (SMEI)", has been not used any more because there are too many cases are being identified without obvious myoclonic events. Classical, the child has normal development at the onset of seizures, though most patients will have very obvious delays in motor, language and cognitive development by 3–4 years of age. Progressive ataxia has is a common finding in this syndrome. Up to 80–90% of cases meeting clinical criteria of Dravet syndrome will have a mutation identified in the SCN1A gene region.

Mutations in the CACNA1A region lead to multiple phenotypes including sporadic and familial hemiplegic migraine, episodic ataxia and spinocerebellar ataxia, type 6. KCNQ2 mutations typically lead to benign familial neonatal convulsions, though a more aggressive phenotype with a severe epileptic encephalopathy has been described (though without myoclonic seizures or prolonged hemiconvlusive febrile status). TSC1 mutations lead to tuberous sclerosis, unlikely given the normal MRI scan in this patient and DMPK mutations are seen in myotonic dystrophy.

Suggested Reading

- Dravet C. The core Dravet syndrome phenotype. Epilepsia. 2011;52(s2):3–9.

147. You are seeing a 6-month-old baby boy for his intractable seizures and encephalopathy. He started to have seizure at 2 months of age and have been unresponsive to therapy with phenobarbital, levetiracetam and oxcarbazepine. He has microcephaly and developmental delay. CSF reveals a cell count of 3, protein of 25 ug/dL and glucose of 20 mg/dL. An extensive metabolic work-up was done immediately prior to the procedure was normal including a glucose level of 85 mg/dL. His brain MRI is normal.

What would be the most appropriate treatment for his intractable seizures?

A. Corpus callosotomy
B. High dose nightly benzodiazepine usage
C. Ketogenic diet
D. Topiramate
E. Vagal nerve stimulation

Correct Answer is: C

The most likely diagnosis of this child is glucose transporter type 1 (GLUT-1) deficiency. The diagnosis is based on the combination of intractable seizures and developmental delays in infancy or childhood with hypoglycorrhachia (low glucose in the CSF) in the absence of any other abnormality. Almost all patients have a CSF glucose of less than 40 mg/dL, and a ratio of glucose in the CSF/blood ratio less than 0.33 (normal range is 0.5–0.67). The above phenotypic presentation is the most common, though milder cases may present with complex movement disorders and other paroxysmal symptoms triggered by fasting or exercise. A majority of the patients have a de-novo mutation in the SLC2A1 gene, leading to impaired active transport of glucose into the CSF through the glucose transporter. A variety of seizure types are seen and although EEG is frequently abnormal, no specific pattern is diagnostic. Similarly, brain imaging is either normal or non-specific. The ketogenic diet is highly effective in both control of seizures and prevention of progressive mental decline, and early

9

institution of the diet is recommended as soon as the diagnosis is established. Commercial testing of the SLC2A1 gene is available for confirmation.

Suggested Reading

- DeGiorgis, V, Veggiotti, P. GLUT1 deficiency syndrome 2013: Current state of the art. Seizure. 2013;(22):803.
- Klepper, J. GLUT1 deficiency syndrome in clinical practice. Epilepsy Research. 2012;(100):272.

148. You are seeing a 5-month-old boy with history of spasms. His mother reports that he is very sensitive to any noise and reacts with an exaggerated startle response with muscle spasms involving the whole body. The symptoms will recur if the stimulation has been repeated. It was becoming increasingly difficult for her to take care of him as he would become very stiff every time she picks him up for change of clothes or to feed him. His muscle tone appears normal when lying in bed by himself. **What is the correct answer?**
    - A. Serum anti-glutamic acid decarboxylase (GAD) antibodies will be positive.
    - B. EEG will show generalized 3 Hz spike and wave activity.
    - C. CSF will be positive for 14-3-3 protein.
    - D. Autosomal recessive inheritance is most common.
    - E. It involves mutation in the gene for alpha-1 subunit of the glycine receptor.

Correct Answer is: E
This is the clinical presentation of exaggerated startle disease or hyperekplexia. The main feature to differentiate from a normal infantile startle response is that the event with hyperekplexia is markedly exaggerated and does not habituate with repetition of the stimulus. Symptoms include massive flexion of the neck (severe enough to at times compromise the airway of the infant) and trunk with abduction and flexion of the arms. It can also result in tonic muscle spasms. They may resemble tonic seizures, but the consistent ability to be provoked by a stimulus is atypical for seizures. An EEG would be expected to show only movement artifact during the spells. The disorder most commonly is due to mutations in the glycine receptor alpha1-subunit (GLRA1) gene and inherited as an autosomal dominant trait (though autosomal recessive and x-linked inheritance has been reported.) Mutations typically result in deficient production and activity of glycine (a major inhibitory neurotransmitter) in the central nervous system. Anti-GAD antibodies are not seen in this disorder, rather being best known for their presence in "stiff-person syndrome." CSF exam is typically normal in these patients. The condition can improve over time, but benzodiazepines, such as clonazepam, provide effective symptomatic treatment for this condition.

Suggested Reading

- Espay A, Chen R. Myoclonus. Continuum Lifelong Learn Neurol. 2013;19(5):1264.
- Bode A, Lynch J. The impact of human hyperekplexia mutations on glycine receptor structure and function. Molecular Brain. 2014;7:2.

149. You are evaluating a 15-year-old boy for his epilepsy. His seizures stared 5 months ago and he is on carbamazepine. He has a total of 8 seizures. His seizure occurs about 1–2 h after waking from sleep, either early in the morning and or after awakening from a midday nap. He has no loss of consciousness and no jerky movements of the hands have

been reported. No family history of epilepsy. His exam and brain MRI are normal. EEG shows 3–4 Hz generalized spike wave discharges and photosensitivity.

What is the most accurate diagnosis?

A. Autosomal dominant nocturnal frontal lobe epilepsy (ADNFLE)
B. Epilepsy with grand mal seizures on awakening
C. Left frontal lobe epilepsy
D. Juvenile myoclonic epilepsy
E. Progressive myoclonic epilepsy

Correct Answer is: B

Epilepsy with grand mal seizures upon awakening is an idiopathic generalized epilepsy (IGE) syndrome characterized by generalized tonic clonic seizures occurring predominantly on awakening (independent of the time of day.) The typical EEG findings of an IGE including predominantly generalized spike and slow waves (though focal abnormalities can also be noted) and photosensitivity. The syndrome shares too many manifestations with the more common juvenile myoclonic epilepsy, including similar provoking features (sleep deprivation, alcohol use and bright flickering lights), but the diagnosis of JME would typically require either clinical absence or myoclonic events in addition to generalized tonic-clonic seizures. Treatment for both conditions would involve broad spectrum agents such as lamotrigine, levetiracetam, sodium valproate, topiramate or zonisamide. Carbamazepine (narrow spectrum sodium channel blocking agent) is relatively contraindicated.

Though frontal lobe seizures can occur during sleep-wake transitions, they most commonly occur out of sleep, and not 1–2 h after awakening. Additionally, although very rapidly generalizing discharges can be present on EEG, photosensitivity is rare. Without a suggestive family history, a diagnosis of ADNFLE would be hard to confidently make. The patient has not been identified to have myoclonic seizures, and has not have the typical progressive cognitive decline seen with the disorders leading to a progressive myoclonic epilepsy.

Suggested Reading

- Janz D. Epilepsy with grand mal on awakening and sleep-waking cycle. Clin Neurophysiol. 2000;111(S2):S103–10.
- Rudzinski LA, Shih JJ. The classification of Seizures and epilepsy syndromes. Continuum 2010;16(3):15–35.

150. You are seeing a 6-month-old baby in the ED for his left arm shaking seizure which became generalized and lasted for 15 min. Birth and delivery were normal. He has reached all developmental milestones on time. There is a family history of febrile seizures in his father. On examination, he smiles and coos, but does not reach with his left hand. On examination, he has a right otitis media and is febrile.

Which **of the following is consistent with a simple febrile seizure in this patient?**

A. Age of the patient
B. Family history
C. Length of seizure
D. Neurologic examination
E. Seizure semiology

Correct Answer is: A

Febrile seizure is very common in the young child, with an age onset of onset 6 months to 5 years of age (other author's reported onset as young as 3 months and as late as 6 years). Simple febrile seizures are characterized by

seizures accompanied by fever that are generalized in onset, last less than 15 min, and do not occur more than once in 24 h. Febrile seizures are complex due to either longer duration, focal signs at onset, or recurrence within 24 h. Achievement of normal neurodevelopmental milestones and a normal neurologic exam are required to classify the episode as a febrile seizure. Prominent encephalopathy prior to or after the seizure should raise suspicion of a secondary cause such as a central nervous system infection and focal onset seizures with post-ictal hemiparesis may suggest a structural cause such as tumor, stroke or abscess. Although the genetics of febrile seizures is still not well known (other than for syndromes such as generalized epilepsy febrile seizures plus- GEFS+), a family history of such events is very common, though not effective in differentiating between simple and complex febrile seizures.

Suggested Reading

- Waruiru C, Appleton R. Febrile seizures: a consensus of their significance, evaluation, and treatment. Consensus development conference of febrile seizures. 1980. National Institute of Health. Pediatrics.1980;66:1009–12.
- Shinnar S, Glauser TA. Febrile Seizures. J Child Neuro. 2002:17(1):s44–52.

151. You are seeing a 10-year-old girl for her loss of consciousness and convulsions. She was exercising and had sudden loss of consciousness with witnessed convulsions and urinary incontinence. Few minutes later, she regaines her consciousness and reports no recall of any warning symptoms. Her developmental history is normal. Her family history is remarkable of her father had a seizure in his 20s after diving into cold water. A paternal uncle had childhood seizures and died while swimming as a teenager. She has a normal general and neurological examinations.

What is the most urgent diagnostic test?

A. 12-lead electrocardiogram
B. Transthoracic echocardiogram
C. Routine EEG
D. MRI brain
E. Tilt table test

Correct Answer is: A

The patient has a spell of exercise-induced syncope with convulsions. Her family history is suggestive of autosomal dominant pattern of convulsions possibly induced by cold water immersion. This is most concerning for a congenital long QT syndrome and a 12-lead electrocardiogram (EKG) is necessary for diagnosis. If normal, the patient should have exercise testing or be referred to pediatric cardiology, as occasionally the initial resting EKG can be normal. Majority of congenital long QT syndrome patients have a normal structural heart exam on echocardiography so this is not a high priority test in this population. A routine EEG may be warranted if the EKG is normal or the patient has recurrent episodes outside the setting of exercise. Typically, however, convulsions associated with long QT syndrome are due to anoxic seizures, and would not be likely to reveal any interictal abnormalities on EEG. Likewise, brain MRI is not indicated for this condition but may be indicated if the patient is felt to have epilepsy rather than anoxic seizures. A tilt table test may be helpful is cases neurocardiogenic syncope due to orthostatic hypotension. Patients with this etiology for syncope do not typically have syncope during active phases of exercise.

Suggested Reading

- McLeod KA. Syncope in childhood. Arch Dis Child. 2003; 88(4):350–3.

152. You are following an 18-year-old woman with juvenile myoclonic epilepsy for preconception planning. When she has her menarche, she had her first seizure. She has not had a seizure in 3 years. She is on valproic acid 500 mg twice a day and folate 1 mg daily. She is using a barrier method of contraception. She has no side effects. Her neurologic examination, EEG, and MRI are normal.

Based on evidence-based medicine, what is appropriate advice to give her at this point regarding pregnancy planning?

A. increase dose of valproic acid as her seizure control will worsen during pregnancy
B. increase folate dose to 5 mg daily and proceed with plans for pregnancy
C. she should not have children due to risk of teratogenicity
D. substitute extended release valproic acid, which will decrease risk of teratogenicity
E. transition to another broad-spectrum antiepileptic drug prior to pregnancy

9

Correct Answer is: E

Valproate (VPA) exposure in the first trimester has a higher risk of major congenital malformations and likely reduced cognitive outcomes. In addition, monotherapy exposure to phenytoin or phenobarbital possibly reduces cognitive outcomes. The AAN Practice Guideline recommends, if possible, avoidance of valproate during the first trimester of pregnancy to decrease the risk of major congenital malformations (Level B) and throughout pregnancy to prevent reduced cognitive outcomes (Level B). If possible, avoidance of phenytoin and phenobarbital during pregnancy may be considered to prevent reduced cognitive outcomes (Level C). There is also evidence of potentially less risk with other broad-spectrum AEDs, lamotrigine and levetiracetam, making one of these agents a better choice for this patient. There is no evidence that seizure control is likely to worsen during pregnancy although it may for a minority of women. Although increased folate is recommended during pregnancy, there is a paucity of evidence-based medicine to recommend a specific dose although 4 mg a day is commonly used.

Suggested Reading

- Harden CL, Meador KJ, Pennell PB, et al. Practice parameter update: Management issues for women with epilepsy–focus on pregnancy (an evidence-based review): Teratogenesis and perinatal outcomes: report of the Quality Standards Subcommittee and Therapeutics and Technology Assessment Subcommittee of the American Academy of Neurology and American Epilepsy Society. Neurology. 2009;73:133–41.
- Hernández-Díaz S, Smith CR, Shen A, et al. Comparative safety of antiepileptic drugs during pregnancy. Neurology. 2012;78(21):1692–9.

Ethics and Professionalism

Y. M. Awaad, *Absolute Pediatric Neurology*, https://doi.org/10.1007/978-3-319-78801-2_10

1. A 7-year-old boy is admitted to the ICU after an out-of-hospital cardiac arrest. He was being treated for vomiting and headache that became daily after initially being intermittent, paroxysmal and focal on the right side. There was a family history of migraine and he reported visual blurring at the onset of vomiting and headache in the left visual field. He had a non-contrast CT scan that was unremarkable and no sign of intercurrent illness. He was initially treated with sumatriptan but as this produced no real relief he was hospitalized and given ondansetron with analgesia. After 2 days in the hospital he was discharged slightly improved on scheduled ondansetron and acetaminophen. The following morning he was discovered pulseless in his bed. His father began CPR and emergency medical technicians arrived within 5 min. He was intubated and ECG showed ventricular fibrillation. By the time he was transported to the ER at 30 min he had a sinus rhythm and blood pressure. His exam in the ER showed no pupillary light reflex and absent corneal reflex, extraocular movements, and gag. CT scan was normal except for indistinct gray-white differentiation. An EEG at 10 h post-arrest showed electrocerebral silence. Evaluation for cause of his arrest was negative except for the presence of a prolonged QT interval of 0.48 suggesting he may have acquired long QT syndrome secondary to ondansetron. A repeat EEG shows electrocerebral silence and his exam is unchanged.
What is your approach with the family?
   A. "If only I had seen this child…" You explain that you never use ondansetron for nausea and vomiting in the setting of migraine and your approach to migraine would have likely resulted in resolution of his symptoms prior to discharge making only rescue medications necessary. You suggest they withdraw support since he is brain dead on your exam.
   B. "Your child is dead according to my tests…" You explain that after cardiac arrest loss of pupillary light response is associated with death or vegetative state 95% of the time and he has not improved so he cannot recover. The EEG confirms your opinion.
   C. "Let me summarize what I know about your son…" You describe the history as you know it and then your exam and test results describing how you arrive at the conclusion the child is brain dead. After asking for questions you give your opinion that support should be withdrawn.
   D. To be sure we understand each other, could you tell me what you understand is going on with your son…" You listen to the family's ideas and answer any questions that arise from your opening statement and then explain your exam and the EEG results. After allowing questions and discussions with the family you state your recommendation that support be withdrawn.
   E. "The studies and my exam show there is no hope…" You present the data from the CT scan, EEG and your exam and state that the child is brain dead. You wait for questions and when there are none excuse yourself.

Correct Answer is: D
The approach in "d" addresses many of the issues that have been identified in the literature on end-of-life care. In

the case of children the parents' views of their and their child's rights to act autonomously is the foremost principle of contemporary medical ethics, but the importance of autonomous choice to individual parents varies greatly, with some preferring to delegate or share decision making with family members or physicians. Physicians need to determine each family's preferences in this regard. This is one of many areas where communication with the family is important. The list shows the areas identified in reports (see reference) that are crucial to good ICU communication.

Identify a private place for communication with family members

Increase proportion of time spent listening to family rather than talking

Identify commonly missed opportunities

- Listen and respond to family members
- Acknowledge and address family emotions
- Explore and focus on patient values and treatment preferences
- Explain the principle of surrogate decision making to the family
- Affirm no abandonment of patient and family

Assure family that the patient will not suffer

Provide explicit support for decisions made by the family

Use of the VALUE mnemonic during family conferences:

- V = value statements made by family members
- A = acknowledge emotions
- L = listen to family members
- U = understand who the patient is as a person
- E = elicit questions from family members

Provide consistent communication from different team members

Suggested Reading

- Schwani H, Wenrich MD, Tonelli MR, Curtis JR. Meeting physician's responsibilities in providing end-of-life care. Chest. 2008;133:775–86.

2. A 16-year-old girl whose parents are friends of yours is evaluated for possible seizure activity. She was observed to have episodes of staring, morning jerks, and had one convulsion. A diagnosis of juvenile myoclonic epilepsy (JME) was made and confirmed on EEG. Additional testing revealed that she tested positive for marijuana and cocaine. She was also found to have genital herpes. The patient asks that her parents not be told of her drug or sexual activities.

Which of the following is the most appropriate management?

A. Begin treatment for JME with valproate and inform her parents of the social problems described.
B. Begin treatment for JME with valproate and consult your state law on disclosing information to parents.
C. Begin treatment for JME with lamotrigine and inform her parents of the social problems described.
D. Begin treatment for JME with lamotrigine and consult your state law on disclosing information to parents.
E. Refrain from treatment of her JME until social problems described are adequately resolved.

Correct Answer is: D

Juvenile myoclonic epilepsy and patient confidentiality Discussion: The patient presents with a relatively obvious epileptic syndrome. Given her sexual proclivities, the use of valproate should be avoided because of its potential teratogenic effect. The main issue has to do

with what to tell the parents. Child neurologists might disagree as to whether we think the patient's welfare is best served by discussing the problems with the parents or abiding by the secrecy requested by the patient. However, we need to be aware laws vary from state to state and need to be carefully addressed before decisions are applied.

Suggested Reading

- Weddle M, Kokotailo P. Adolescent substance abuse: confidentiality and consent. Pediatr Clin North Am. 2002;49(2).

10

3. A 7 year old presents to your office with headaches. The symptoms are consistent with migraines. Family history is negative for migraines but mom states that the child's father was recently diagnosed with Huntington's disease. Although the child is asymptomatic, mom would like genetic testing.

   The best response should be:

   A. The child is not at risk for Huntington's disease
   B. If testing is done, the child should not be informed of the results until he/she reaches adulthood
   C. Since there is no cure for Huntington's disease, the testing should never be done until a child reaches adulthood
   D. The testing should not be done until the child becomes symptomatic
   E. The recommendations are that predictive genetic testing for adult onset conditions generally should be deferred unless an intervention initiated in childhood may reduce morbidity or mortality

Correct Answer is: E

The American Academy of Pediatrics published a policy statement in 2013 on the Ethical and Policy Issues in Genetic testing and screening of children. A summary of the statement:

1. **Decisions about whether to offer genetic testing and screening should be driven by the best interest of the child.**
2. **Genetic testing is best offered in the context of genetic counseling.**
3. **In a child with symptoms of a genetic condition, the rational for genetic testing is similar to that of other medical diagnostic evaluations.**
4. **When performed for therapeutic purposes, pharmacogenetics testing of children is acceptable, with permission of parents or guardians and, when appropriate, the child's assent.**
5. **The AAP and ACMG support the mandatory offering of newborn screen for all children.**
6. **The AAP and ACMG do not support the routine carrier testing in minors when such testing does not provide health benefits in childhood.**
7. **For pregnant adolescents or for adolescents considering reproductive, genetic testing and screening should be offered as clinically indicated.**
8. **Parents or guardians may authorize predictive genetic testing for asymptomatic children at risk for childhood-onset conditions.**
9. **Predictive genetic testing for adult-onset conditions generally should be deferred unless an intervention initiated in childhood may reduce morbidity and mortality. An exception might be made if diagnostic uncertainty poses a significant psychosocial burden, particularly when an adolescent and his or her parents concur in their interest in predictive testing.**
10. **For ethical and legal reasons, health care providers should be cautious about providing predictive genetic testing to minors without the involvement of their parents or guardians, even if a minor is mature.**

11. **Tissue compatibility testing of minors of all ages is permissible to benefit immediate family members but should be conducted only after a thorough exploration of the psychosocial, emotional and physical implications.**
12. **The rationale for genetic testing of children in biological families should apply for adopted children awaiting placement for adoption.**
13. **At the time of genetic testing, parents and guardians should be encouraged to inform their child of the test results at an appropriate age. Under most circumstances, a request by a mature adolescent for test results should be honored.**
14. **Results from genetic testing of a child may have implications for the parents and other family members.**
15. **The risk of misattributed paternity, use of donor games, adoption, or other questions about family relationships may be uncovered "incidentally" whenever genetic testing is performed.**

Suggested Reading

- Ethical and policy issues in genetic testing and screening of children. 2013. AAP.

4. A 6-month-old male infant is brought to the emergency room by his father after suffering a seizure. The father states he has been more irritable than usual since waking from his nap, then suddenly became unresponsive and stiffened all over, followed by 2 min of generalized clonic jerking. He has not been awake since the event. While in the emergency room, he has 2 more short seizures, and is given 20 mg/kg of phenobarbital. Per the father, he has had no prior seizures and only a history of reflux, for which he takes ranitidine. On examination, he is somnolent, with little responsiveness, has a full and tense anterior fontanelle. Pupils are small and reactive; corneal and gag reflexes are present. Tone is decreased, with little spontaneous movement, but withdrawal to pain. Reflexes are brisk throughout with 4–6 beats of clonus at both ankles. CT of the head reveals acute on chronic subdural hemorrhages bilaterally, with patchy areas of intraparenchymal edema. Chest x-ray shows multiple rib fractures in various stages of healing. The child is admitted to the pediatric intensive care unit. After receiving a brief update on the child's condition, the father asks to be alone with his son.

Which of the following would be the most appropriate response to his request?

A. advise the father to retain legal counsel
B. further testing, including MRI of the brain, need to be performed to exclude non-accidental head trauma (i.e., child abuse) prior to allowing his visitation
C. given the nature of the injuries noted, specialists in child protection will need to further assess the situation to determine who is eligible to be left alone with the child
D. inform the father he is suspected of child abuse and will not be allowed to see his son
E. inform the father that his son can have no visitors until his seizures have been controlled for at least 24 h

Correct Answer is: C

When treating young children with injuries suspected to be secondary to nonaccidental trauma (i.e., child abuse), the main goal of the treating physician is to stabilize the patient and focus on treatment of the affected organ systems.

It is not the job of the clinician to assign blame to caregivers, or make primary determinations over safety of caregiver contact, either during the ongoing hospitalization or regarding discharge planning. It is also imperative to remember that there are rare cases of metabolic or genetic disorders that can mimic injury produced by nonaccidental injury. Physicians with expertise in the field of child abuse are often employed to assist with reviewing the history, physical exam findings and response to treatment to determine if one of these rare masquerading conditions exists. Although a history needs to be obtained by the treating physicians, detailed questioning of the caregiver(s) should be left to law enforcement and child protective agents.

Suggested Reading

- Swaiman K, Ashwal S, Ferriero DM, Schor N. Swaiman's pediatric neurology. 5th ed. Philadelphia: Elsevier; 2012. p. 1126–48.

5. A 16-year-old boy presents with weakness in his left arm, following a motorcycle accident 6 weeks ago. He is referred for an EMG due to concern that he may have a brachial plexopathy. He is with his mother, who is anxious to see what findings the EMG will reveal. After explaining the procedure to the boy, he refuses to undergo the test. **Which of the following choices is ethically advisable?**
   A. cancel the EMG, explaining that the boy's wishes should be honored
   B. cancel the EMG, explaining that diagnostic testing cannot be provided when family members disagree
   C. proceed with the EMG, explaining that what is most important is ascertaining the diagnosis
   D. proceed with the EMG, explaining the boy is not of age to give informed consent
   E. proceed with the EMG, explaining that the risks of the test are minimal

Correct Answer is: A
Electromyography, which is a painful test, should be performed only when the patient consents to the procedure. At issue is not whether family members disagree, but who has the capacity and the right to make a medical decision. The need for a diagnosis does not take precedence over informed consent, and competent patients have a moral and a legal right to refuse diagnostic (or therapeutic) interventions. Although the boy is not of legal age (usually 18, except for emancipated minors) to give informed consent, at 16 he is likely developmentally mature enough to have the capacity to participate in medical decision making and is capable of giving, or refusing, assent. Assent is the capacity to agree to a medical procedure. A minor's refusal to assent should be weighed against how essential the test result is to the minor's welfare. Honoring the boys wish, in this case, is likely to foster trust and a better partnership with his physicians.

Suggested Reading

- Evans P. Assent and refusal by children and adolescents. In: Williams MA, McGuire D, Rizzo M, editors. Practical ethics in clinical neurology: a case-based learning approach. Philadelphia: Lippincott Williams & Wilkins; 2012. p. 149–50.

6. A 12-year-old girl is evaluated in the ED and diagnosed with bacterial meningitis. Her parents are divorced; her mother, who has sole custody, refuses treatment.

Which of the following is the best course of action in this case?

A. A court order should be sought for treatment
B. The mother's wishes should be respected, but the child should be admitted for observation and placed in isolation
C. Treat the patient without regard for the mother's wishes
D. The health care provider cannot treat the patient in this case unless consent is obtained from the father
E. An ethics consult should be obtained before treating the patient

Correct Answer is: C
If there is a clear and imminent danger to the life of a child, with a risk of death as a result of a delay in treatment, the health care provider can proceed with treatment without judicial review against the wishes of the custodial parent. In divorce, only parents with custody of the child are able to consent to treatment. If both parents have custody, only one parent must give consent. The health care provider's decision should be based upon the best interest of the patient, so if treatment is required urgently, the health care provider can proceed.

Suggested Reading

- ▶ http://www.educus.com/Journals/12612264.
- ▶ http://pediatrics.aappublications.org/content/111/3n03.long ▶ http://pediatrics.aappublications.org/content/92/2/290.Abstract key=66ab600cb23cd0b00b7b35050f371bcfff895a50&keytype2=tf _ipsecsha (▶ http://pediatrics.aappublications.org/content/92/2/290. abstract? ij key=66ab600cb23cd0b00b7b35050f371bcfff895aSO&keytype2=tf ipsecsha) ▶ https://www.acponline.org/running_practice/ethics/manual/manual6th.htm (▶ http://www.acponline.org/runni ng_practice/ethics/manua l/manual6th.htm) ▶ http://pediatrics.aappublications.org/content/128/Supplement_4/5167.full (▶ http://pediatrics.aappublications.org/content/128/Supplement_4/S167.full).

7. A 17-year-old male patient arrives at the ED in police custody, suspected of ingesting illicit medications to avoid arrest. The patient was arrested in a raid on an apartment where he has lived for several months with 2 friends. The police request a nasogastric aspirate for evidence, but the patient refuses.
Which of the following is correct?

A. The health care provider should comply with the request because ingestion could result in death for the patient
B. The health care provider is legally obligated to comply with the evidentiary request in a criminal investigation
C. The health care provider should honor the patient's wishes
D. The health care provider should seek a court order to pass a nasogastric tube
E. Parental permission should be obtained to treat the patient, but evidence should not be supplied to the police against the patient's wishes

Correct Answer is: C
Minors who live apart from their parents who are older than age 13 are considered emancipated minors and are authorized to consent to medical care. This includes refusal of care. The health care provider should inform the patient of the risks of refusal of care and should also tell the patient that evidence will be collected for the police if the patient consents to care.

A health care provider cannot perform a medical procedure at the direction of the police without a patient's consent.

Suggested Reading

- ▶ https://www.acponline.org/running_practice/ethics/manual/manua16th.htm
- ▶ http://pediatrics.aappublications.org/content/128/Supplement_4/5167.full.
- Fischer C, Oneto C. USMLE medical ethics: The 100 cases you are most likely to see on the exam. New York: Kaplan; 2009.

Headache

Y. M. Awaad, *Absolute Pediatric Neurology*, https://doi.org/10.1007/978-3-319-78801-2_11

1. Cyclic vomiting in children is a syndrome in which of the following groups?
   A. Migraine with aura
   B. Classic Migraine
   C. Migraine without aura
   D. Migraine equivalent

Correct Answer is: D
Children can have three types of migraine; migraine with aura (classic migraine) migraine without aura (common migraine) and migraine equivalent syndromes. Migraine equivalent syndromes is characterized by the transitory disturbance in neurological function. Abdominal migraine, benign paroxysmal vertigo, cyclic vomiting syndrome, benign paroxysmal torticollis, alternating hemiplegia of childhood, and vestibular migraine are different presentations of migraine equivalents. The child has normal neurological examination between attacks, there typically a family history of migraine and a clinical evolution over the years to the more classic types of migraine.

Suggested Reading

- Lagman-Bartolome A, Lay C. Pediatric migraine variants: a review of epidemiology, diagnosis, treatment, and outcome.

2. You are evaluating an 18-year-old female for her episodic vertigo, which not associated with headache and lasting hours to days for the last 6 months. She always complains of occasional bi-frontal, pulsatile headaches without photo- or phonophobia or vertigo. Those headaches got relived by ibuprofen. No family history of migraine, but the mother gets sinus headaches not associated with fever or nasal drainage, but she gets relieve when she lies down in a quiet, dark room. Her younger brother gets motion sickness if he reads in the car back seat. On examination, she has two 0.5-cm café au lait spots, one on the left leg and one on the right back. Her MRI scan showed a 4 mm Chiari I malformation without abnormalities of the ventricles, brain parenchyma, or extra-axial spaces.
   What is your explanation to the girl and her family?
   A. The anatomic abnormality of her brain seen on MRI scan.
   B. Her mother's chronic sinusitis.
   C. The family's predisposition to migraine and its equivalents.
   D. Her café au lait spots and likely neurofibromatosis.
   E. A brain tumor too small to be seen on the MRI scan.

Correct Answer is: C
Benign paroxysmal vertigo is a "migraine equivalent" which could happen with migraine in families. The mother's headaches are a migraine headache and it is not a sinus headache, and her brother's motion sickness is also a migraine equivalent. Her café au lait spots are neither large nor numerous enough to be of consequence. Her Chiari I malformation is also likely a variant of no medical significance.

3. A PCP referred a 14 years old female to you because she missed 3 months of school because of her headaches. She has been getting "homebound schooling" and has not been doing well; the school wants her to repeat the year. She has a daily headache and it is all day but not pulsatile. The headaches do not have a specific location and it gets worse by the end of each day. She has mild asthma for which she takes a prn inhaler. Family history is remarkable for depression in his mother, sleepwalking in his younger brother, and a maternal

grandmother had menstrual headaches that required her to sleep when they occurred. The parents are divorced and there is a restraining order against the father because he physically abused the mother. She is always having a normal general and neurological on multiple occasions. She is on amitriptyline at night and sumatriptan twice a week for the worst of the headaches, but still she has no relief.

What is your recommendations?

A. Obtain a CT scan of the child's head.
B. Switch from amitriptyline to nortriptylline.
C. Tell the mother to have the restraining order against the father lifted.
D. Get toxic screens on the child's blood and urine in case the father poisoned him.
E. Arrange for psychiatric evaluation and counseling for the mother and children.

Correct Answer is: E

The family needs psychiatric evaluation and counseling. She has chronic daily headache with many psychosocial stressors causing it. There is a family history of migraine and also migraine-equivalent (sleepwalking), but her headaches do not have the character or temporal features of common migraine. Her school absence requires urgent action and return to school may be therapeutic for her but will likely require considerable psychological and scholastic support.

Suggested Reading

- Waldie KE, Thompson JM, Mia Y, Murphy R, Wall C, Mitchell EA. Risk factors for migraine and tension-type headache in 11-year-old children. J Headache Pain. 2014;15(1):60.

4. The EMS brought an 8-year-old girl accompanied with her teacher after she was seen wandering around the playground, and then vomited at school. The teacher reported that she is clumsy, which was unusual for her. You examined her and found that, she is pale. She complains of nausea, headache in the back of her head, which started after arrival in the ED. When the mother arrives, she reports that the girl had a similar episode twice before in the last few months, and she will go back to baseline after an extended nap.

What is your most likely diagnosis?

A. Abdominal migraine
B. Acute confusional migraine
C. Acute post-traumatic migraine, after unwitnessed fall on the playground
D. Basilar migraine
E. Cyclic vomiting syndrome

Correct Answer is: D

This is a case of basilar migraine, which is one of the most common complicated migraine variants, represents 3–19% of all migraine. The onset is usually by 7–8 years. You have to have two or more clear signs and symptoms of posterior fossa involvement to diagnose it. The signs and symptoms include: vertigo, nausea or vomiting, ataxia, visual field deficits, diplopia, tinnitus, hearing loss, confusion, dysarthria, weakness, syncope, with the first 4 being the most common. The typical child will begin with the posterior fossa symptoms such as intense dizziness, vertigo, ataxia and diplopia, which can last for minutes to an hour, and then are followed by the headache phase. The headache is often occipital in location.

5. A 16-year-old female with known history of intermittent migraines treated with sumatriptan nasal spray who has a 4-year history for the last

5 years, she is complaining of a new type of pain. It is a burning pain with numbness on the left side of her face. She has no fever or other sickness. She recently had four wisdom teeth extracted. She has unremarkable past medical history, but she has a family history of migraines in her mother and grandmother. She has subjective decreased sensation to touch over the right cheek on examination.

What is the most likely diagnosis?

A. Glossopharyngeal neuralgia
B. Nervus intermedius neuralgia
C. Periodic migrainous neuralgia
D. Trigeminal dysesthesia
E. Trigeminal neuralgia

Correct Answer is: D

Trigeminal dysesthesia is a continuous pain following complete or partial damage to a peripheral nerve. Wisdom tooth extraction or root canal is a frequent cause. The pain can be self-limiting, depending on nerve regeneration. It can be treated with local anesthetic blockade, topical application of capsaicin, or oral tricyclic antidepressants.

Periodic migrainous neuralgia is a type of cluster headache that presents as orofacial pain, usually in the maxilla, and is not precipitated by oral surgery, but is a primary headache disorder.

Trigeminal neuralgia is a painful, unilateral occurrence of brief, electric, shock-like pain limited to one or more divisions of the trigeminal nerve. The pain is often evoked by minor stimuli, such as washing the face or brushing the teeth. It is unrelated to oral surgery, and is usually due to a tumor, such as acoustic neuroma, or a demyelinating lesion.

Glossopharyngeal neuralgia similar in quality to that of trigeminal neuralgia, but occurs in the distribution of the glossopharyngeal nerve, often triggered by chewing, swallowing, or rotating the head. It is due to an elongated stylohyoid process that irritates or compresses the nerve, and radiograph shows a calcified stylohyoid ligament; treatment is resection of this ligament with microvascular decompression of the nerve.

Nervus intermedius neuralgia is localized to the middle ear, otherwise described similarly to trigeminal neuralgia.

11

Suggested Reading

- David Dodick, et al, editor. Wolff's headache and other head pain. 8th ed. Oxford University Press; 2008. p. 431–2.

6. Which of the following can be seen in patients with idiopathic increased intracranial pressure?

A. Constant continuous headache
B. 6th nerve palsy
C. Neck pain
D. All of the above

Correct Answer is: D

The idiopathic increased intracranial pressure can present with different clinical symptoms in different patients. Usually, patient will complain of a severe headache, most commonly in the morning, and usually in the occipital region. Diplopia, transient visual obscurations, and blurred vision may be also present. Some patients report pulsatile tinnitus, and many can describe severe neck pain. This can at times be the presenting symptom and can be mistaken for signs of meningitis.

Suggested Reading

- Tibussek D, Distelmaier F, von Kries R, Mayatepek E. Pseudotumor cerebri in childhood and adolescence – results of a Germany-wide ESPED-survey. Klin Padiatr. 2013;225(2):81–5.

- Per H, Canpolat M. Clinical spectrum of the pseudotumor cerebri in children: etiological, clinical features, treatment and prognosis. Brain Dev. 2013;35(6): 561–8.

7. Familial Hemiplegic Migraine (FHM) includes all of the following except:
   A. 50% of those with FHM type 1 develop a progressive cerebellar ataxia
   B. Autosomal recessive inheritance
   C. Although sensory auras and aphasia can be present, the diagnosis requires the presence of a motor aura
   D. Some attacks can be associated with a CSF pleocytosis

Correct Answer is: B
Familial hemiplegic migraine is an autosomal dominant inheritance. Patients typically have hemiparesis along with other focal neurological signs or symptoms. The focal neurological deficit can be prolonged, at times lasting days. It is typically occurring in the first or second decade with attacks decreasing in frequency over time. Patients can have cerebellar signs or deficits with time. Mutations in the *CACNA1A*, *ATP1A2*, *SCN1A*, and *PRRT2* genes have been found to be associated with FHM.

- Suggested Reading

- Russel M, Ducros A. Sporadic and familial hemiplegic migraine: pathophysiological mechanisms, clinical characteristics, diagnosis, and management. Lancet Neurol. 2011;10(5):457–70.

8. Medication overuse headache is defined by which of the following?
   A. Overuse of particular medications used to treat an acute headache for greater than 3 months
   B. Headache present for >15 days a month
   C. Headache has markedly worsened during the time of medication overuse
   D. All of the above

Correct Answer is: D
Medication overuse is a reason for chronic daily headache. To diagnose medication overuse headache, medications have to be used more than 3 months, and for > 15 days a month. Treatment includes starting the patient on a preventative medication, significantly decreasing the use of the acute medications, and possibly an admission to the hospital to break the headache cycle.

- Suggested Reading

- Cuvellier JC, Nasser H, Vallée medication headache. 2013;53(2):387–8.
- Pakalnis A, Kring D. Chronic daily headache, medication overuse, and obesity in children and adolescents. J Child Neurol. 2012; 27(5):577–80.
- ICHD II Revision of criteria for 8.2 Medication overuse headache. Silberstein, et al. Cephalalgia. 2005;25:460–5.

9. Which of the following are considered contraindications to triptan use?
   A. Hemiplegic migraine
   B. Migraine with aura
   C. Hypothyroidism
   D. Previous history of benign paroxysmal torticollis

Correct Answer is: A
You cannot use the triptans in patients with a hemiplegic migraine because their vasoconstrictive action.

- Suggested Reading

- Gelfand AA. A neurologist's guide to acute migraine therapy in the emergency room. Neurohospitalist. 2012; 2(2):51–9.

- Hershey A. Current approaches to the diagnosis and management of paediatric migraine. Lancet Neurol;2010;9.

10. Headaches attributed to Chiari I malformations include all of the following except:
    A. Typically, occipital in location
    B. Exacerbated by valsalva maneuvers
    C. Signify that the Chiari is symptomatic and needs decompression
    D. May be associated with bilateral sensory symptoms if a syrinx is present

Correct Answer is: C
To diagnose Chiari I malformation, the cerebellar tonsils has to be extended downward into the foramen magnum, at least 5 mm. Headaches associated with Chiari I malformations are typically occipital in location, associated with neck pain, and are exacerbated by Valsalva maneuvers. Usually, Chiari I malformations are discovered accidently when the patient is undergoing neuroimaging for an unrelated problem. The presence of headache does not always signify the Chiari is symptomatic. A trial of medication for headaches should be done first to see if the headache is unrelated to the Chiari malformation. Chiari malformations can be associated with spinal cord syrinx. If this is the case, then they are considered "symptomatic" and typically require decompression.

11

Suggested Reading

- Aitken LA, *Lindan CE, et al. Chiari type I malformation in a pediatric population. Pediatr Neurol. 2009;40(6):449–54.
- Benglis D Jr., Covington D, et al. Outcomes in pediatric patients with Chiari malformation type I followed up without surgery. J Neurosurg Pediatr. 2011;7(4):375–9.

11. In the pediatric headache patient, neuroimaging is recommended in the following circumstances:
    A. Adolescent patients with chronic daily headache
    B. Patients with headaches that are predominantly occipital in location
    C. Patients with chronic recurrent headaches
    D. Patients with >10 missed school days a month

Correct Answer is: B
Routine neuroimaging is not recommended for headaches that do not have any atypical features. Morning headache or headache waking up patient out of sleep requires imaging. If patient has any focal neurological signs or symptoms associated with the headache, neuroimaging is indicated. Studies have shown that headaches that are predominantly occipital in location may have a higher association with structural abnormalities and imaging should be considered.

Suggested Reading

- Sheridan DC, Meckler GD, Spiro DM, Koch TK, Hansen ML. Diagnostic testing and treatment of pediatric headache in the emergency department. J Pediatr. 2013;► https://doi.org/10.1016/j.jpeds.2013.07.006.
- Lewis DW, Ashwal S, Dahl G, Dorbad D, Hirtz D, Prensky A, Jarjour I. Practice parameter: evaluation of children and adolescents with recurrent headaches: Report of the Quality Standards Subcommittee of the American Academy of Neurology and the Practice Committee of the Child Neurology Society. Neurology. 2002;59:490–8.
- Hershey A. Current approaches to the diagnosis and management of pediatric migraine. Lancet Neurol. 2010;9:190–204.

12. Which medication is typically used to treat hemicrania continua?
    A. Amitriptyline
    B. Topiramate
    C. Propranolol
    D. Indomethacin

Correct Answer is: D

Hemicrania continua is included in the trigeminal autonomic cephalgias along with chronic paroxysmal hemicrania. This syndrome is associated with a moderate to severe unilateral headache that can be associated with ptosis, tearing and swelling of the eyelid. These disorders are felt to part of the indomethacin responsive headache syndromes. Although there are some reports of response to the migraine prophylactic agents such as topiramate and amitriptyline, indomethacin is still the drug of choice for this headache syndrome.

Suggested Reading

- Rozen TD. Indomethacin-responsive TACs (proxysmal hemicrania, hemicrania continua, and LASH): further proof of a distinct spectrum of headache disorders. Headache. 2012.
- Moorjani BI, Rothner AD. Indomethacin-responsive headaches in children and adolescents. Semin Pediatr Neurol. 2001;8(1):40–5.

13. The cyclic vomiting syndrome includes which of the following:
    A. At least 5 attacks of vomiting, which occurs at least 4 times per hour for at least 1 h
    B. Often associated with a diagnosis of delayed gastric emptying
    C. Frequent single episodes of vomiting are noted in-between attacks
    D. Nystagmus is a frequent accompanying sign

Correct Answer is: A

Pediatric cyclic vomiting syndrome (CVS) is a periodic syndrome associated with attacks of vomiting occurring at least 4 times per hour for at least 1 h. The vomiting cannot be caused by any other gastrointestinal disorder. Patients are typically symptom free between attacks so should not have frequent single episodes of vomiting. Nystagmus is not a frequent accompanying sign. Reports of prevalence of CVS are approximately 2% of children in the US. Attacks are strikingly similar in a patient, beginning around the same time of day and lasting typically a certain number of days. CVS is considered a childhood "migraine variant" syndrome. Various reports suggest 40–60% of children will go on to develop typical migraine in adolescence.

Suggested Reading

- Cuvellier JC. Childhood periodic syndromes. Pediatr Neurol. 2010;42(1):1–11.
- Stickler GB. Relationship between cyclic vomiting syndrome and migraine. Clin Pediatr (Phila). 2005; 44(6):505–8.

14. Considering basilar migraine: All of the following are true except
    A. Motor weakness is a frequent finding
    B. Ataxia is common
    C. The aura commonly involves diplopia
    D. Dysarthria is common

Correct Answer is: A

Basilar migraine is a migraine syndrome that typically includes ataxia, slurred speech, diplopia, vertigo, and bilateral visual symptoms. Weakness is uncommon.

Suggested Reading

- The international classification of headache disorders. 2nd ed. Cephalalgia. 2004;24 suppl 1:1–160.

15. Which of the following medications used to treat pediatric headache might not be the best choice for obese patients?
   A. Topiramate
   B. Verapamil
   C. Cyproheptadine
   D. Gabapentin

Correct Answer is: C
Cyproheptadine is a medication frequently used as a migraine prophylactic agent. Its side effects include sedation and a significant stimulation of appetite that limit its use.

Suggested Reading

- Lewis DW, Yonker M, Winner P, Sowell M. The treatment of pediatric migraine. Pediatr Ann. 2005;34(6):448–60.
- Termine C, Ozge A, Antonaci F, Natriashvili S, Guidetti V, Wöber-Bingöl C. Overview of diagnosis and management of paediatric headache. Part II: therapeutic management. J Headache Pain. 2011;12(1):25–34.

16. You are seeing a 7-year-old boy who told his family that he has a cool "superpower". He said, "I can sit in my seat in class and make the teacher get bigger and smaller and bigger and smaller just by really concentrating hard." His mother is concerned and she took him to an optometrist to have his eyes checked. By taking the history, you find that there is a family history of migraine in the boy's maternal grandmother and aunt. The boy's father was a sleepwalker as a child and his mother has to sit in the front seat of the car when she is a passenger, otherwise she will vomit. You should:
   A. Order an MRI scan for the child.
   B. Tell the child to stop scaring his parents.
   C. Reassure the family by telling them what the episodes likely are.
   D. Have the mother bring her other children in for neurological evaluation.
   E. Refer the child to a psychiatrist or psychologist.

Correct Answer is: C
Alice in Wonderland syndrome is a migraine variant that is unaccompanied by pain, nausea, or photo-/phonophobia and that serves as a marker for the migraine-susceptible genotype. It generally occurs in children who have a family history of migraine and associated phenomena and who are otherwise neurologically normal.

Suggested Reading

- Ilik F, Ilik K. Alice in Wonderland syndrome as aura of migraine. Neurocase. 2014;20:474–5.

17. You are seeing a 16-year-old female with daily headache after she has a mild head trauma a week ago. She had no loss of consciousness and the pain of the impact was gone within a minute. She described the headache as bilateral, pulsatile, and diffuse with a frontal predominance. She has no headache when she wakes up in the morning, but she will have a moderate headache by lunch time. She had difficulty concentrating at school. When she comes home from school every day, she is irritable, which was very unusual for her. She will take a nap for couple of hours before doing her homework. Taking short naps make the headache tolerable enough to finish her work. She has a past medical history of headache before her period every month. Her family history is remarkable for a younger brother gets motion sickness and a "sinus headaches" that are preceded by zigzag lines in front of her mother eyes and associated with nausea. She

has a normal general and neurological examinations.

What is your next step?

A. Order an MRI scan of the head
B. Begin a therapeutic trial of amitriptyline
C. Have a school psychologist evaluate the girl for school phobia
D. Do a lumbar puncture
E. Refer the girl to an otolaryngologist for sinus evaluation

Correct Answer is: B
Migraine like headache that occurs within days-to-weeks of a minor head injury in a child with the genetic susceptibility to migraine is called post-traumatic migraine. The mother's headaches are not sinus headaches, as they are preceded by a scotoma, accompanied by nausea, related to motion sickness, and unrelated to fever, cough, or nasal discharge. The girl herself has had menstrual headache, also a migraine-associated syndrome. Amitriptylline is among the most commonly used and efficacious agents for post-traumatic migraine.

Suggested Reading

- Kuczynski A, Crawford S, Bodell L, Dewey D, Barlow KM. Characteristics of post-traumatic headaches in children following mild traumatic brain injury and their response to treatment: a prospective cohort. Dev Med Child Neurol. 2013;55:636–41.

18. A mother of 10-year-old boy brought him to the ED after he awakened this morning with a bad frontal headache and blurry vision. His past medical history is remarkable of chronic ear infections for years requiring bilateral PE tube insertion. The tubes fell out 1 year ago, and never been replaced. He had ear pain and fever 1 week ago and it was treated by amoxicillin, but it has not helped. He developed a bony swelling behind his left ear, but he did not tell his mother about it. Finally, he told his mother this morning. On examination in the ED, he was sick looking with 38.5 °C fever, tenderness over the left mastoid, and bilateral papilledema. The rest of his general and neurological examination is normal. A CT scan has been ordered and showed, lack of aeration of the left mastoid air cells and a white area inside of the left lateral venous sinus posteriorly.

You decide to obtain:

A. An EEG with sphenoidal leads now and a CT angiogram later
B. A lumbar puncture with opening pressure now and an MRI/MRV later
C. An MRI of the orbits now and an MRI of the spine late
D. A Humphrey's visual field test now and a serum vitamin A level later
E. A CBC and ESR now and a blood culture later

Correct Answer is: B
Mastoiditis and lateral cerebral venous sinus thrombosis became much less common after the antibiotic era. They do occur, however, and are often associated with an acute, antibiotic-resistant exacerbation of chronic otitis media. Occlusion of the dural venous flow can cause pseudotumor cerebri and a lumbar puncture is both diagnostic and therapeutic. His CT scan demonstrates left dural venous sinuses thrombosis, and neither the CT scan nor his examination demonstrates evidence of focal differential intracranial pressure, so there is no need to obtain an MRI/MRV urgently. Visual fields should be obtained, but are not of emergent importance. Neither an EEG nor an MRI of the spine would be likely to be useful in this child. In a febrile child with systemic spread of a presumed bacterial infection,

a blood culture should be obtained expediently. While vitaminosis A can cause pseudotumor cerebri, that is unlikely to be the cause of this youngster's difficulties.

Suggested Reading

- Kuczkowski J, Dubaniewicz-Wybieralska M, Przewoźny T, Narozny W, Mikaszewski B. Otitic hydrocephalus associated with lateral sinus thrombosis and acute Mastoiditis in children. Int J Pediatr Otorhinolaryngol. 2006;70:1817–23.

19. You are seeing a 14-year-old boy in the PICU after he lost his consciousness while he was playing a game at school. His father told you that the boy was fine before the game although he had headed the ball once or twice during the game, nothing unusual seemed to have happened until he suddenly lost his consciousness. The boy was running down the field and he did not make contact with the ball, suddenly stopped, grimaced, held his head with both hands crying out, and fell to the ground. He had generalized jerky movement for couple of minutes and then lay unconscious, intermittently extending both arms and arching his back. He has been unconscious ever since. His father also reports that 3 weeks ago, he woke up with headache and neck stiffness in 3 different occasions, but the symptoms went away shortly after he got out of bed. His family history is remarkable of a maternal grandmother who died from glioblastoma. His father and paternal grandfather have polycystic kidney disease
The boy is most likely had an intracranial hemorrhage because of:
   - A. A brain tumor
   - B. Head trauma
   - C. An arteriovenous malformation
   - D. An infection
   - E. An aneurysm

11

Correct Answer is: E
This boy sustained an intracranial hemorrhage with a subarachnoid component after several episodes during the prior month of sentinel bleeding. His family history is remarkable for one elderly individual with a glioblastoma, generally not a hereditary condition, and two relatives with polycystic kidney disease, a disorder which is genetically linked to the occurrence of cerebral aneurysms.

Suggested Reading

- Ruggieri PM, Poulos N, Masaryk TJ, Ross JS, Obuchowski NA, Awad IA, Braun WE, Nally J, Lewin JS, Modic MT. Occult intracranial aneurysms in polycystic kidney disease: screening with MR angiography. Radiology. 1994;191:33–9.
- Fehlings MG, Gentili F. The association between polycystic kidney disease and cerebral aneurysms. Can J Neurol Sci. 1991;18:505–9.

20. A 17-year-old female with a long history of childhood migraine which occurs once or twice per month and well controlled by ibuprofen. Recently, she increases in her headache frequency, headaches come most days of each week, and she has to take ibuprofen 2 or 3 times a day almost every day. In the last 2 weeks, her headaches became more severe and less responsive to ibuprofen. There is no change in her headache character. She told you that her mother is taking a medicine every night at bedtime to prevent the mother's headache from coming. She has a normal general exam except her BMI is 30. You instructed her to stop the ibuprofen all of a sudden and prescript her a triptan to use no more than twice a week.
You might best decide to also give her daily preventive treatment with:
   - A. Naproxen sodium
   - B. Valproic acid
   - C. Botulinum toxin
   - D. Verapamil
   - E. Topiramate

Correct Answer is: E

The girl has an increase of her headaches after a long history of migraine for years during adolescence. This is a very common phenomenon in young women. This led her to take more ibuprofen daily most of the days. She has therefore developed medication overuse headaches. Interestingly, NSAIDs is very effective and even protective in patients with infrequent headaches, but likely to trigger medication overuse headaches in those with frequent or chronic headaches as in her case. Treatment involves discontinuation of NSAID, symptomatic use of triptans no more than twice a day for no more than 2 days in any week, and starting the patient on a daily preventive medication for migraine. Of those listed, verapamil is not particularly efficacious and valproic acid is likely to cause weight gain and, possibly, ovarian cysts in this already overweight youngster. On the other hand, topiramate is both efficacious and likely to cause weight loss, so it is a good first-line preventive drug for this adolescent.

Suggested Reading

- Starling AJ, Hoffman-Snyder C, Halker RB, Wellik KE, Vargas BB, Dodick DW, Demaerschalk BM, Wingerchuk DM. Risk of development of medication overuse headache with nonsteroidal anti-inflammatory drug therapy for migraine: a critically appraised topic. Neurologist. 2011;17:297–9.
- Carod-Artal FJ. Tackling chronic migraine: current perspectives. J Pain Res. 2014;7:185–94.

21. A 13-year-old girl stared to have daily episodic lancinating pains in the back of her head for the last 3 months after she hit her left occiput on the floor. She is not complaining of photophobia, nausea, tearing, and conjunctival injection with the headaches. On examination, she has tenderness over her right greater occipital nerve. Treatment with acetaminophen, ibuprofen, naproxen, and indomethicin have been ineffective.

What is your likely diagnosis?

A. Chronic daily headache
B. Chronic paroxysmal hemicrania
C. Cluster headache
D. New daily persistent headache
E. Occipital neuralgia

Correct Answer is: E

International Headache Society criteria for ICHD-II criteria for occipital neuralgia includes paroxysmal stabbing pain, with or without persistent aching between paroxysms, in the distribution(s) of the greater, lesser and/or third occipital nerves; tenderness over the affected nerve; and pain is eased temporarily by local anesthetic block of the nerve. It is very important to differentiate between, Chronic daily headache occurs when a patient has > 15 headaches days per month, for more than 4 h per day for more than 3 months, and a new daily persistent headache occurs in a patient without a previous significant headache history, and the features of the headache are similar to a chronic tension-type headache.

Cluster headaches are severe headaches that are typically located behind the eye or over the eye, with autonomic features such as tearing, conjunctival injection, nasal congestion or ptosis. The patient often appears agitated during a cluster headache, in contrast to the typical migraine headache patient who wants to go to sleep in a quiet, dark room. Cluster headaches are also unilateral side-locked headaches, and never switch between sides.

Chronic paroxysmal hemicrania (CPH), like cluster, belongs to a group of headaches referred to as the trigeminal autonomic cephalgias. However, in CPH the headaches occur multiple (1–40) times a day and lasts for a shorter duration (minutes. CPH is, by definition, responsive to indomethicin.

Suggested Reading

- International classification of headache disorders (ICHD-II). Cephalalgia. 2004;24 (s1):23–136.

22. A 10-year-old girl who practice gymnastic is complaining of pain in her right foot. She describes the pain as constant and aching, but sometimes, there is a burning sensation that makes her stop practicing. When her mother tries to rub her foot, the girl cries and pulls her foot away. She has unremarkable past medical history. You examined her and you found that, the skin appears slightly cooler on the right foot than on the left, and somewhat mottled. She guards the foot on examination, wincing even with light touch. She has a normal DTRs. She is able to walk independently, and currently describes the pain as a 3 on a scale of 10. She states that she can practice when it is this level, but when it increases, she has to stop.
What are you going to order to establish her diagnosis?
    A. MRA of ankle for blood flow aberration
    B. Radiograph of ankle to evaluate for subtle fracture
    C. Somatosensory evoked potential to assess for spinal plexus injury
    D. Venous doppler to assess for deep venous thrombosis
    E. Sudomotor function test to assess for greater sweat output

Correct Answer is: E
Sudomotor axon reflex test (QSART), which is a quantitative teat can be used to show sympathetic hyperactivity which is associated with altered sweat output. It helps to confirm clinical impressions of a complex regional pain disorder. It usually occurs after an initiating noxious event. A specific fracture on x-ray might be seen, but would not make the diagnosis in this child. The inciting event can be mild or significant, and in a gymnast, can be a combination of minor injuries. The diagnosis is primarily clinical, and usually requires at least 2 of the following symptoms: sensory (hyperesthesia), vasomotor (temperature or skin color abnormalities), sudomotor/fluid balance (edema, sweating abnormalities), or motor (decreased range of movement, weakness, tremor, or neglect), and at least 2 of the following signs: sensory (allodynia or hyperalgesia), vasomotor (objective temperature or skin color abnormalities), sudomotor/fluid balance (objective edema or sweating abnormalities), or motor (objective decreased range of motion, weakness, tremor, or neglect).

Suggested Reading

- Johnson RT, et al., editors. Current therapy in neurologic disease. 6th ed. St. Louis: Mosby Press;2002. p. 71–4.

11

23. A 16-year-old girl with a long history of migraines came to the ED after 2 day history of unrelenting head pain associated with severe photophobia and phonophobia, anorexia, nausea and vomiting. Her Previous headaches occurred 3–4 times per month, lasting 3–5 h. She is on amitriptyline 30 mg daily at night, and has been taking sumatriptan intranasal twice a day for the last 2 days. Her past medical history is remarkable for asthma, treated with Singulair, and acne treated with doxycycline. She is pale, tired appearing and in moderate distress. Neurological examination is normal. ED physician gave her 20 mg of metaclopromide orally and 15 mg of ketorolac intramuscularly. Her headache has not resolved after 30 min, and she is given 0.2 mg of dihydroergotamine intravenously. 15 min later, she develops repeated forced head turning episodes with

eye deviation to either side. She is very anxious during the episodes and cries repeatedly.

What do you have to do?

A. Administer fosphenytoin 1000 mg intravenously
B. Administer diphenhydramine 50 mg intravenously
C. Administer repeat doses of dihydroergotamine, metaclopramide, and ketoralac
D. Start baclofen 10 mg every 8 h
E. Start gabapentin 300 mg every 6 h

Correct Answer is: B

Acute dystonic reaction can occur in some patients immediately after the administration of the offending medication, such as metaclopromide, or slightly delayed. Recognition of the disorder is the key to appropriate treatment and prevention of further episodes in the future. Diphenhydramine is the treatment of choice.

Suggested Reading

- Johnson RT, et al., editors. Current therapy in neurologic disease. 6th ed. St. Louis: Mosby Press; 2002. p. 339–40.

24. You are seeing a 16-year-old male with a long history of once a week migraine headache, who has an increase in his headache frequency for the last year. He was on acetominophen with codeine, and a combination medication with butalbital (Acetominophen/butalbital/caffeine; Fioricet) for abortive therapy. These medications had initially helped with the headache pain, but no longer seem to be effective, and his severe headaches have continued to increase in frequency. He uses one of these medications at least four times a week. He currently has severe migraine headaches four times a week, as well as a lower grade "all the time" headache. He has normal exam and has no papilledema. His MRI is normal.

What is the most appropriate next step in management?

A. Continue current treatment and add corticosteroid
B. Discontinue current medications and observe
C. Perform lumbar puncture
D. Replace acetaminophen/codeine with oxycodone
E. Taper opiate and barbiturate and start topiramate

Correct Answer is: E

This presentation is for a chronic daily headache syndrome, which meets the International Headache Society Criteria for Chronic Migraine, with the exception of his overuse of both opiate and barbiturate compounds. These compounds should be withdrawn in the patient. Care should be taken, depending on the patient's dose and duration of use, not to trigger an abrupt withdrawal syndrome. Recent evidence suggests that starting a preventative medication during this withdrawal phase is helpful.

Suggested Reading

- Revised International Headache Society criteria for chronic migraine. Appendix 1.5.1 chronic migraine
  - Headache (tension-type and/or migraine) on ≥15 days per month for at least 3 months*
  - Occurring in a patient who has had at least 5 attacks fulfilling criteria for 1.1 Migraine without aura

25. A 16-year-old girl came to your office with a complaint of sharp pain which varies in location headaches. Each headache lasts less than 1 min, but it is quite severe. When the headache is over, she feels tired, but the pain is gone. The headache has been

increased in frequency lately, occurring multiple times each day. She is worried and she is looking for an answer to her worries. She does not have any other type of headaches, and she has a normal neurological exam.

What is the most appropriate treatment?

A. Indomethacin 50 mg three times a day for 2 weeks
B. Naproxen sodium 500 mg twice a day for 10 days
C. Propranolol twice a day for 2–4 months
D. Sumatriptan nasal spray at onset of headache
E. Topiramate 25 mg at night for 1 week, increasing weekly to 100 mg at night

Correct Answer is: A

The clinical presentation of an icepick headache, which is a type of primary stabbing headache and is responsive to indomethacin. The age of onset ranges from 12 to 70 years, and it is more common in females. The pain is experienced as a sharp stab, exclusively or predominantly felt in the distribution of the first division of the trigeminal nerve, lasting seconds to a minute, recurring irregularly. A response to indomethacin is often supportive of the diagnosis, and doses of 25–150 mg are usually effective. Primary stabbing headaches can also co-occur with migraine. Other diagnostic considerations include trigeminal autonomic cephalgias, such as hemicrania cicrania or chronic paroxysmal hemicrania. These conditions are also responsive to Indomethicin, but are side locked to one side of the head.

Suggested Reading

- Dodick D, et al., editors. Wolff's headache and other head pain. 8th ed. Oxford University Press; 2008:p. 431–2.

11

26. You are seeing a 14-year-old girl with a history of intermittent once a month headache for the last 3 years. She describes the headaches as a visual aura of flashing lights, followed by severe throbbing headache (9 out of 10 on a visual analog scale) 10 min later. The headache is associated with phonophobia and photophobia, and she has to go to sleep in order to relieve the headaches. The headaches last for several hours. She has tried acetaminophen and ibuprofen without success.

What is the best medication for her pain control at the onset of a headache?

A. Almotriptan
B. Aspirin/butalbital/caffeine
C. Oxycodone
D. Prochlorperazine
E. Valproic acid

Correct Answer is: A

Migraine is a moderate to severe headache of pulsating quality and is made worse with activity according to the International Headache Society. Headache usually is associated with either nausea and vomiting or photophobia and phonophobia. Children tend to have shorter duration headaches than adults, usually between 1–72 h in duration, and (in contrast to adults) may have bilateral pain.

Acetominophen and ibuprofen have been shown to be effective in patients with migraine. These are good first choices for children and adolescents to use in the treatment of episodic migraine. On June 2009, the FDA extended the indication for almotriptan to include treatment of migraines in adolescents between 12 and 17 years of age, making it the first triptan to be approved for pediatric patients. Published data also support a role for the other triptans in the treatment of headaches in children under the age of

18, although many of these compounds have not yet approved by the FDA for children under the age of 18. Opiates, such as oxycodone, and barbituate containing compounds such as Aspirin/ butalbital/caffeine (Fiorinal), can make a headache patient prone to rebound, or medication overuse, headaches and should be avoided in this situation. Prochlorperazine alone or in combination with ketorolac can be useful in an emergency room setting for the treatment of childhood migraine. Oral valproic acid is not used for the acute treatment of migraine, although some suggestive evidence exists that intravenous valproic acid may be helpful.

Suggested Reading

- Bigal ME, Lipton RB. Excessive acute migraine medication uses and migraine progression. Neurology. 2008;71(22):1821–8; Brousseau DC, Duffy SJ, Anderson AC, Linakis JG. Treatment of pediatric migraine headaches: a randomized, double-blind trial of prochlorperazine versus ketorolac. Ann Emerg Med. 2004;43(2):256–62.
- Damen L, Bruijn JK, Verhagen AP, Berger MY, Passchier J, Koes BW. Symptomatic treatment of migraine in children: a systematic review of medication trials. In Pediatrics. 2005;116(2):e295–302.
- International classification of headache disorders (ICHD-II). Cephalalgia. 2004;24:(s1):23–136; Lewis D, Ashwal S, Hershey A, Hirtz D, Yonker M, Silberstein S; American Academy of Neurology Quality Standards Subcommittee; Practice Committee of the Child Neurology Society. Practice parameter: pharmacological treatment of migraine headache in children and adolescents: report of the American Academy of Neurology Quality Standards Subcommittee and the Practice Committee of the Child Neurology Society. Neurology. 2004;63(12):2215–24.
- Linder SL, Mathew NT, Cady RK, Finlayson G, Ishkanian G, Lewis DW. Efficacy and tolerability of almotriptan in adolescents: a randomized, double-blind, placebo-controlled trial. Headache. 2008;48(9):1326–36.

27. A 15-year-old right handed girl presented to the ED with a sudden onset of a right sided paresis, lasting for 15 min, followed by an intense throbbing left sided headache. Previously she has migraine with visual auras. There is a family history of her mother and aunt have had similar episodes of weakness and headaches as teenagers. On exam, she is uncomfortable with headache pain, is photophobic, but her weakness has resolved.
    What diagnostic tests are you going to order to reveal the etiology of her condition?
    A. Carotid ultrasound
    B. Diffusion weighted imaging on a Head MRI
    C. EEG
    D. Genetic testing for the Calcium channel gene CACNA1A
    E. Thematic Apperception Test

Correct Answer is: D
A sudden onset of hemiplegia in an adolescent is of great concern. MRI study with diffusion weighted imaging should be strongly considered. However, in this particular scenario, this young woman most likely has familial hemiplegic migraine. This can be associated with three different genes (CACNA1A, ATP1A2 and SCNA1), with calcium channel mutations (CACNA1A) being commonly detected, particularly if the symptoms first appear before 16 years of age. The hemiplegia may occur before the headache, as is typical for most migraines auras. A Todd's paralysis, acute stroke, or functional disorder could also be

considered in this scenario. Given the strong family and personal history of migraine, this is most likely familial hemiplegic migraine.

Suggested Reading

- Lewis DW. Pediatric migraine. Neurol Clin. 2009;27(2):481–501.
- International classification of headache disorders (ICHD-II). Cephalalgia. 2004;24(s1):23–136.
- Roach ES, Golomb MR, Adams R, Biller J, Daniels S, Deveber G, Ferriero D, Jones BV, Kirkham FJ, Scott RM, Smith ER. Management of stroke in infants and children: a scientific statement from a Special Writing Group of the American Heart Association Stroke Council and the Council on Cardiovascular Disease in the Young. Stroke. 2008;39(9):2644–91.

28. A 16-year-old girl came with a 1-year history of daily headaches. She reports that her daily continuous headache does not prevent her from attending her school, but it does not improve with sleep. She has a consistently right-side head headache. She has no family history of headache. She has unremarkable examination and a normal brain MRI.
What medication should be used initially?
A. Ibuprofen
B. Prednisone
C. Sumatriptan
D. Valproic acid
E. Indomethacin

11

Correct Answer is: E
Classification of headaches is essential to their optimal treatment. Unilateral headaches can represent ominous conditions, such as arteriovenous malformations, or can represent hemicranias continua which is a primary headache disorder which is partly defined by its response to indomethacin. Not all patients with hemicrania continua with resolve with indomethacin, but all patients with unilateral headache should be given a trial of indomethacin.

Suggested Reading

- Marmura MJ, Silberstein SD, Gupta M. Hemicrania continua: who responds to indomethacin? Cephalalgia. 2009;29(3):300–7.
- Ji T, Mack KJ. Unilateral chronic daily headache in children. Headache. 2009;49(7):1062–5. Epub 2009 Jun 1.

29. A 14-year-old girl is complaining of headaches. She has 2–3 headache per week of pounding pain in her forehead which occasionally cause her to miss school. They are 8/10 in severity on a scale of 0/10. They occur more often in the afternoons, and never awaken her at night. She has light and sound sensitivity with her headache. When she takes Ibuprofen, the headache goes away within 30 min but occasionally she has to sleep to get relief. She takes accutane for acne. She has a family history of sinus headaches in her mother and grandmother. She has a normal exam. Venous pulsations are present on ophthalmoscopic exam.
Which of the following is the most likely diagnosis?
A. Tension headache
B. Cluster headache
C. Migraine
D. Sinus headache
E. Pseudo tumor cerebri

Correct Answer is: C
Classification of headaches is important in assisting with treatment and prognosis issues. Migraine diagnosis requires specific criteria to be met, including photophobia, nausea, and relief by

sleep, and exacerbation with exercise. Family history is important during this assessment, and further delineation of the specific nature of headache in her family members would be advised, as "sinus" headaches are occasionally actually misdiagnosed migraines Rebound headaches or transformed migraines can be misdiagnosed if the medication history is not adequately assessed. Age of onset of headaches is not relevant in diagnosis of migraines, though there is a typical age of onset around puberty.

Suggested Reading

- Winner P. Classification of pediatric headache. Curr Pain Headache Rep. 2008;12(5):357–60. Review.

30. You are seeing a 16-year-old female in the ED because off her headache for 2 months. Her headache was intermittent, but now it became worse, daily for the last 2 weeks, and it is 5/10. She describes it as being generalized. She has tried over the counter medications, but never been on any prescribed medications. Her body mass index is 30, she is in moderate distress but the rest of her general and neurological exams are normal. She does not have any signs and symptoms meningitis. You ordered a LP, which demonstrates an opening pressure of 29 cm. but the rest of the CSF parameters are normal. She has relief of her headache shortly after the LP but the headache came back after 24 h and she came back to the ED because her headache worsens. She is lying flat on bed and every time she gets up her headache will worse. You admitted her to the hospital and put her on strict bedrest, but her headache fails to improve over the next 24 h.

What is your next step in her management?

A. Repeat the lumbar puncture and remove a larger volume of CSF
B. Increase fluids, administer IV caffeine, and consider an epidural blood patch
C. Administer intravenous antibiotics and antiviral medications
D. Administer intranasal sumatriptan followed by intravenous dihydroergotamine
E. Administer intravenous corticosteroids

Correct Answer is: B
She has worsening chronic recurrent headaches, but her headache does not have any migraines features described. Most properly she has a rebound or chronic daily headache due to daily over-the-counter analgesic use. The lumbar puncture was performed to rule out pseudo tumor cerebri, and did show elevated opening pressure. This case is dealing with a low-pressure headache which is the sequelae of the LP. Headache after a lumbar puncture is common, but is usually resolved within a day or two. If there is no relief after 48 h, strong consideration should be made to diagnosing and treating the low-pressure headache with bedrest, hydration, and caffeine and, if needed, an epidural blood patch.

Suggested Reading

- Candido KD, Stevens RA. Post-dural puncture headache: pathophysiology, prevention and treatment.

31. You are seeing a 17-year-old female in the ED because off her sudden, acute, and severe (10/10) headache. It is bi-temporal in location, pulsatile, and associated with photophobia and phonophobia. She has vomited once

in the emergency room. She had three similar episodes in the last 6 months, all requiring emergency room visits due to dehydration from repeated vomiting. **What is the most appropriate treatment recommendation?**

A. Acute treatment with intravenous fluids, non-steroidal anti-inflammatory agent and anti-emetic, followed by rescue medication only
B. Acute treatment with narcotic, followed by 6-month course of prophylactic medication
C. Acute treatment with non-steroidal oral anti-inflammatory, followed by daily use of non-steroidal anti-inflammatory agent for 2 weeks
D. Acute treatment with intravenous valproic acid followed by preventative treatment with sodium valproate for 1 year
E. Acute treatment with intravenous steroids, followed by daily use of indomethacin for 6 weeks

Correct Answer is: A
Acute treatment of migraines in a child is dictated by the severity of the headache and the concomitant symptoms. Migraine pain needs to be treated with pain medication and the severe nausea needs to be treated with anti-emetics and intravenous rehydration. Specific migraine medications such as triptans can often treat the pain as well as the associated symptoms, though most are not FDA-approved in adolescents. The use of daily medications should be reserved for those patients who have headaches unresponsive to rescue medications or whose headaches are so frequent as to cause disability, such as missed school days.

Suggested Reading

- Lewis DW. Pediatric migraine. Neurol Clin. 2009;27(2):481–501.

32. You are evaluating an 8-year-old boy for his headaches which started 1 year ago, but they became more frequent and severe over time. They occur 2–3 times/ week, are 8/10 in severity, and last for an hour after he takes acetaminophen. On one occasion, the pain was so severe that he passed out for a few minutes. The headache is located in the mid-forehead and he cannot characterize its nature. He has normal exam. A midsagittal MRI is shown here.

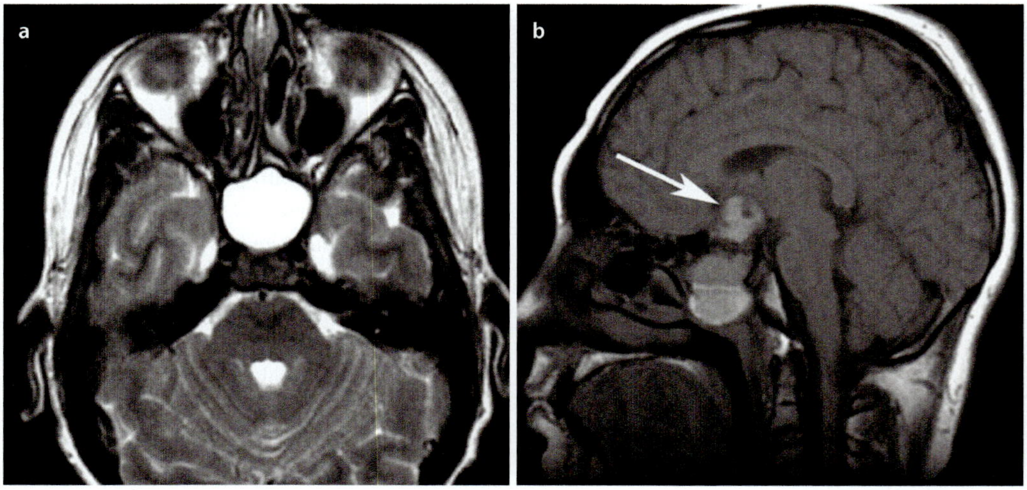

Fig. 11.1 **a** Coronal MRI. **b** Midsagittal MRI showing Sephenoid mucocele. Sphenoid mucocele. Permission by Lui YW, Dasari SB, Young RJ. Am J Neuroradiol. 2011;32(4):617–26. ▶ https://doi.org/10.3174/ajnr.A2144

What is the most likely diagnosis regarding the area identified by the arrow?

A. Hypothalamic hamartoma
B. Pituitary tumor
C. Sphenoid mucocele
D. Cribriform plate lipoma
E. Chondrosarcoma of the skull base

Correct Answer is: C
Child neurologist has to be fully aware with neuroanatomy as seen on MRI imaging and all films should be viewed personally, without relying on the neuro-radiologist report. This image shows a sphenoid mucocele of fairly significant size. These are rare in children, but can cause significant headache that is often medically refractory. Treatment is with surgical resection of the mucocele, usually with complete resolution of the headaches.

Suggested Reading

- Uren BA, Berkowitz RG. Isolated inflammatory sphenoid sinus disease in children. Ann Otol Rhinol Laryngol. 2003;112(4):370–2.

33. A 12-year-old boy is complaining of headache every time he is doing a valsalva maneuver which have been increased in frequency and severity in the last 2 months, now rated 8/10. They are occipital in location, and non-radiating. He denies any photophobia or phonophobia. Sleep does not improve the pain. He has a blurred optic disc margins on funduscopic examination. His brain MRI is shown.

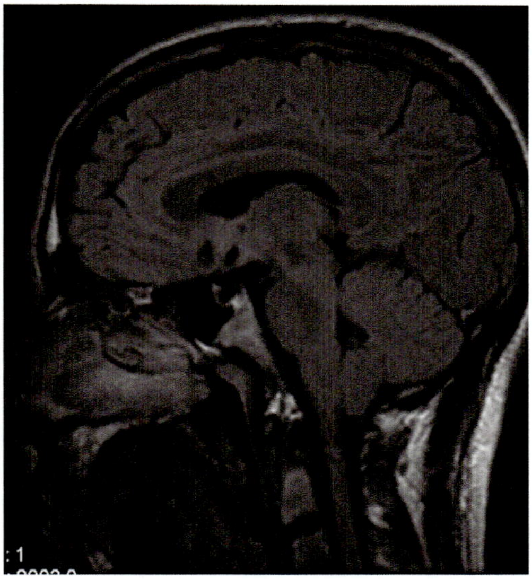

Fig. 11.2 Image of a Type 1 Arnold-Chiari Malformation. The cerebellum has descended 7 mm and there are herniated cerebellar tonsils into the foramen magnum. (Basket of Puppies)

What is on the image could explain his headache?

A. Thrombosis of the torcula
B. Cerebellar tonsillar ectopia
C. Sphenoid mucocele
D. Empty sella
E. Frontal sinus air-fluid levels

Correct Answer is: B
Many structural lesions can cause headaches in children, including sinus disease, pituitary lesions, pineal lesions, venous sinus thrombosis, and AVM. Chiari I malformation with ectopia or excessive descent of the cerebellar tonsils can cause increased intracranial pressure leading to headaches that can be refractory to medication. Cine flow studies at the level of the foramen magnum can help in determining the extent of obstruction of the Chiari.

34. A 16-year-old female has had several spells of severe (rated 8/10) unilateral headache associated with contralateral weakness and numbness, each lasting for several hours. She is normal in between the attacks. Her family history is remarkable of her mother had similar spells as a teenager.
What is the most likely underlying pathophysiology regarding these episodes?
A. Mitochondrial oxidative phosphorylation disorder
B. Glutamate neurotoxicity
C. Ion channelopathy
D. Vasoconstriction
E. Acetylcholine receptor blockade

Correct Answer is: C
Hemiplegic migraine is a relatively rare form of migraine with aura, and has both familial and non-familial (sporadic) forms. Genetic tests are available, and the known genes encode ion-transporters. The pathophysiologic mechanisms are complex, but are best explained by abnormalities in the trigeminal-vascular system.

Suggested Reading

- Cady R, Biondi DM. An update on migraine pathophysiology and mechanism-based pharmacotherapeutics for migraine. Postgrad Med. 2006; Spec No: 5–13. Review.

35. You are evaluating a 15-year-old boy for his worsening in frequency and duration headache which stared 3 weeks ago. They are as 6/10 rate. They are diffuse in nature, no nausea or vomiting, and no change in appetite. He complains of photophobia, but no phonophobia. He has seasonal allergies, exercise-induced asthma, and moderately severe inflammatory acne. His is taking loratadine, albuterol, fluticasone, minocycline, and salicylic acid. His examination is remarkable for absence of venous pulsations and mild papilledema.
Which of the following medications is the most likely cause of his headaches?
A. loratadine
B. Albuterol
C. Minocycline
D. Fluticasone
E. Salicylic acid

Correct Answer is: C
You have to be fully aware of medication triggers of pseudo-tumor cerebri to be able to treat it rapidly. Minocycline and other antibiotics such as tetracycline are known to promote increased intracranial pressure in some patients, precipitating pseudo- tumor cerebri. Other agents can include lithium and retinoids.

Suggested Reading

- Friedman DI. Medication-induced intracranial hypertension in dermatology. Am J Clin Dermatol. 2005;6(1):29–37. Review.

36. A 10-year-old girl is complaining of frequent headaches which have caused her to miss many school days this year. The lights and noise of the classroom are increasing her headache. She goes to the office 4–5 times a week to get ibuprofen 200 mg orally. She reports that she also has headache at home as well. Acetaminophen or ibuprofen does help to relieve her headache, and estimates she goes through a bottle per month of each medication. Patient and mother state the medication is helpful in relieving the pain, and deny any associated side effects.
Treatment of which of the following conditions would most likely lead to improvement in her headache frequency?
A. Migraine
B. Cluster
C. Tension-type
D. Analgesia overuse
E. Hemicranias continua

Correct Answer is: D
Chronic daily headaches in children and adolescents can cause significant disability,

but they are not as common as intermittent headaches. The diagnosis of analgesic overuse syndrome, and/or transformed migraine, is necessary for effective treatment. The use of a prophylactic agent combined with removal of the overused rescue medication, and educating the patient and family as to the cause of the change in frequency of the headaches, can be dramatic in returning the child to a functional state in terms of school attendance.

Suggested Reading

- Moore AJ, Shevell M. Chronic daily headaches in pediatric neurology practice. J Child Neurol. 2004;19(12):925–9.

37. A 14-year-old girl is brought to the ED after a syncope spell at school. She has a history of chronic, recurring headaches and mild attention-deficit disorder for which she takes methylphenidate. Her MRI is shown.

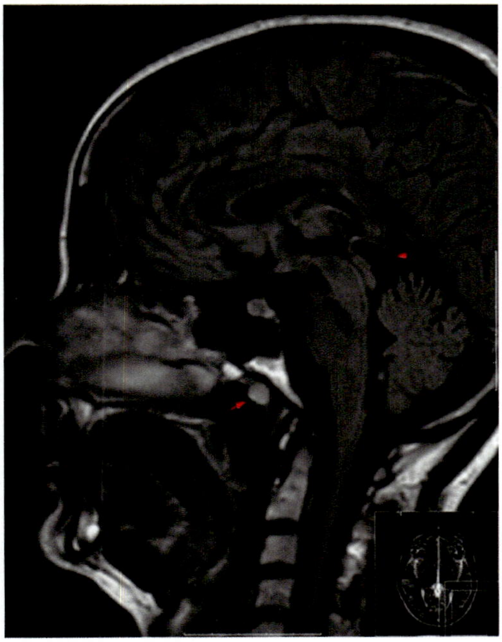

Fig. 11.3 Tornwaldt's cyst in sagittal MRI (FLAIR). The cyst appears hyperintense in the midline of the nasopharynx. In this case there is also a cyst of the pinealis gland showing a signal intensity slightly higher than the CSF. (Hellerhoff Wikipedia)

What is the most likely explanation for the abnormality demonstrated?

A. Hypothalamic hamartoma
B. Simple pineal cyst
C. Pineal teratoma
D. Choroid plexus cyst
E. Optic nerve schwannoma

Correct Answer is: B
Glial cysts of the pineal are often found incidentally on neuroimaging or at autopsy, and are usually benign. The finding can be seen in 20–25% of healthy individuals on MRI so are usually incidental and do not usually need repeat imaging, unless they have worrisome characteristics such as large size or multi-locuated cyst. They very rarely become symptomatic, causing headache, syncope, insomnia, or sudden death.

Suggested Reading

- Pu Y, Mahankali S, Hou J, Li J, Lancaster JL, Gao JH, Appelbaum DE, Fox PT High prevalence of pineal cysts in healthy adults demonstrated by high-resolution, noncontrast brain MR imaging. AJNR Am J Neuroradiol. 2007;28(9):1706–9. Epub 2007 Sep 20.

38. A 14-year-old female fell in the school yard. She did not have any skin abrasion anywhere, but she twisted her left ankle so that it was mildly painful all day. At home that night, her ankle was mildly swollen and she held an ice compress against it on and off all evening. Her symptoms disappeared over the next couple of days. A week later, she noticed the onset of episodes of redness, heat, and intense burning pain over the whole lower 1/3 of her left leg and foot that last for a few minutes to a few hours, and then remit completely until the next episode.

What is your explanation?

A. Cellulitis caused by MRSA
B. Erythema multiforme

C. Pellagra
D. Complex regional pain syndrome
E. Erythromelalgia

Correct Answer is: D
This is a case of a complex regional pain syndrome because the predated history of minor trauma and episodic nature of the color and temperature change and pain. Erythromelalgia usually occurs in older individuals and is not preceded by injury. Pellagra involves desquamation and usually there is an identified risk factor for vitamin deficiency. Erythema multiforme has a characteristic pattern on the skin and is usually not this focal or lateralized. Finally, cellulitis does not produce episodic symptoms.

Suggested Reading

- Fukushima FB, Bezerra DM, Villas Boas PJ, Valle AP, Vidal EI. Complex regional pain syndrome. Brit Med J. 2014;348:g3683.

11

39. An 8-year-old girl fell off her Bick on the sidewalk. The child's right leg hit the sidewalk, scraping the skin and bruising it, and the Bick toppled on top of her, but did not cause serious injury. She cried briefly but walked back to her house. Two weeks later, she began refusing to walk on that leg. Her parents noticed that the leg would become bright red, hot, and swollen from the knee down and stay that way for hours at a time.
The child might benefit from:
A. Bed rest and pampering.
B. Antibiotics and topical vasoconstrictors.
C. Physical therapy
D. Oxycodone and prednisone.
E. Casting and avoidance of weight bearing.

Correct Answer is: C
Complex regional pain syndrome (formerly known as reflex sympathetic dystrophy) is well-described in children but poorly understood in any age group. Multifactorial etiology and predisposition are suspected and therapy is almost always multidisciplinary, involving graded physical therapy, individual and family psychotherapy, agents aimed at decreasing neurogenic pain, and agents that affect the autonomic nervous system.

Suggested Reading

- Katholi B, Daghstani SS, Banez GA, Brady KK. Non-invasive treatments for pediatric complex regional pain syndrome – a focused review. PM R. 2014. pii: S1934-1482(14)00175-0. ► https://doi.org/10.1016/j.pmrj.2014.04.007. [Epub ahead of print] PMID 24780851.
- Goldschneider KR. Complex regional pain syndrome in children: asking the right questions. Pain Res Manag. 2012;17:386–90.

40. A 9-year-old boy who was involved in a car accident presents to the ED, is complaining of worsened progressively for the last 2 weeks. There is no history of loos of consciousness and was not seen immediately after the accident. He has a history of intermittent headaches, typically in the back of his head and neck for 1 year. Now, he has daily headache, and over the counter medication does not of any help. He cannot characterize the headache quality, but denies any has photophobia or phonophobia. Yesterday, his headache has intensified after having a bout of coughing secondary to a flare up of his asthma. His past medical history is unremarkable beside his asthma. Family history is remarkable of

migraine in his father (mainly occipital headaches) and the paternal side of the family. He has a normal neurologic exam, including funduscopic exam.
What is your next step in the evaluation and management of this case?

A. amitriptyline 10 mg nightly
B. indomethacin every 8 h as needed
C. MRI of the brain
D. reassurance, no intervention needed unless headache frequency persists for another month
E. spinal tap for opening pressure and cerebrospinal fluid analysis

Correct Answer is: C
Occipitally located migraine in adults is common, but in children, occipital headache always increase concern to find a potential secondary etiology. Headache increases with cough (Valsalva-like maneuver) can indicate either an increased intracranial pressure, or headaches associated with a Chiari I malformation. Posterior fossa tumors (the most common location for primary brain tumors in children) often present with pain in the occipital region as well. Cough headache in adults can be treated with daily indomethacin, though this primary headache disorder is also unusual, and up to 25% of adults with headache induced with coughing have been found to have a Chiari malformation on imaging. Neither acute treatment with sumatriptan, nor chronic treatment with amitryptline would be indicated without a more clear history of migraine and exclusion of a more obvious cause of headache in this patient.

41. You are evaluating a 14-year-old boy with 1-year history of headache. The headache has been increased in frequency and intensity in the last 3 months. The school has to call his mother to pick him up and he missed a lot of school days. When he has the headaches, he prefers to lie in a dark, quite room. Also, vomiting relieves the headache. He used to use the over-the-counter medications such as acetaminophen or ibuprofen, but they are not helping any more. Because his frequent absences, his school grades have been dropped. There is a family history of migraines in his mother. He has a normal neurologic exam.
What is your next step in his evaluation?

A. CT scan of the sinuses
B. EEG
C. MRI of the brain with and without gadolinium
D. perform lumbar puncture
E. reassure mother and child and begin treatment with a triptan

Correct Answer is: E
This is a case of migraine headaches without aura. He has intermittent headaches that meet the IHS criteria for migraine. He prefers to lie in a quiet dark room, because movement can trigger the headache. Also, he has vomiting associated with the headaches.

According to the AAN Guidelines for the evaluation of episodic headaches in adolescents an imaging procedure would only be indicated in patients with a recent change in the type of headache; associated features of neurological dysfunction; or if there are neurologic abnormalities noted on examination.

In addition, the Guidelines did not recommend an EEG as part of the evaluation of any child with episodic headaches.

According to the AAN Guidelines of the Pharmacological Treatment of

Migraines in Children and Adolescents, sumatriptan nasal spray was found to be effective in the treatment of migraines in adolescents and children. A recent study also found that almotriptan was effective in treating migraines in children. His history is not suggestive of sinus disease nor CNS infection.

Suggested Reading

- Linder SL, Mathew NT, Cady RK, et al. Efficacy and tolerability of almotriptan in adolescents: a randomized, double-blind, placebo-controlled trial. Headache. 2008;48:1326–36.
- Lewis, DW, Ashwal S, Dahl G, et al. Practice parameter: evaluation of children and adolescents with recurrent headache. Neurology. 2002;59(4):490–8.

42. An 8-year-old girl is brought to the ED 2 days after having an acute onset of headache that has not relived by over-the-counter medications use. Her PCP suspected migraine because of the nausea and vomiting near the onset. This morning, it was difficult to arouse her from a nap so her family brought her for evaluation. Her medical history is remarkable for small stature. Family history is remarkable for acquired hearing loss, type II diabetes and early onset heart disease on her maternal side. Her general examination is significant for weight and height in the 5rd percentile, with head size at the 20th percentile. Blood pressure and pulse are normal. On your exam, she was drowsy, though with stimulation she awakens, has fluent speech and can follow limited directions. Cranial nerve examination show evidence of a left homonymous hemianopsia on confrontation testing, but is otherwise normal. The rest of her exam was normal. Laboratory studies show a normal CBC; a comprehensive metabolic profile with serum bicarbonate of 14; and an increased anion gap. Serum lactate returns at 4.5 mmol/L (normal less than 2.3). Her CT and MRI are shown.

11

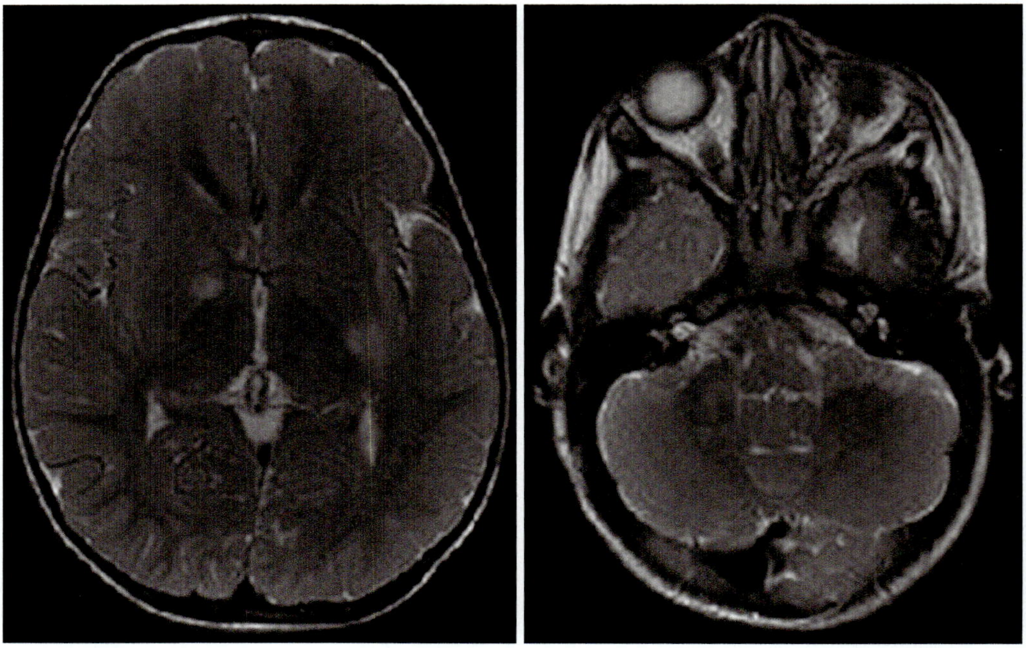

Fig. 11.4 Imaging revealed an apparent stroke in the right posterior cerebral artery distribution. American Academy of Neurology Institute, produced by permission

Which of the following results are most likely given her presentation and imaging findings?

A. cerebral angiography showing diffuse irregular narrowing and beading
B. hemoglobin electrophoresis showing 90% hemoglobin S
C. magnetic resonance angiography showing abrupt tapering of the right carotid artery in the neck
D. muscle biopsy showing ragged-red fibers
E. skin biopsy showing electron-dense granules in the media of arterioles on electron microscopy

Correct Answer is: D

This patient, though initially thought to have primary headache, has focal neurologic findings several days into the headache prompting imaging. Imaging revealed an apparent stroke in the right posterior cerebral artery distribution. Her CT scan also shows subtle hyperdense lesions of the basal ganglia, likely calcifications. Given the lactic acidosis noted on presentation, short stature of the patient and family history of cardiomyopathy, hearing loss and type II diabetes in maternal relatives, a mitochondrial disorder would be the most likely diagnosis, in particular mitochondrial encephalopathy, lactic acidosis and stroke (MELAS). This multisystem disorder typically has onset between 2 and 10 years of age, with normal early developmental milestones. Initially seizures, recurrent headaches, intermittent ataxia and focal neurologic deficits arising from stroke-like episodes predominate. Eventually there is progressive loss of function due to the aftereffects of the metabolic disturbance of the brain. The initial attacks often involve the occipital lobe, with infarctions not always conforming to definitive vascular territories (though this patient did have what was felt to be a PCA distribution infarction.) Recovery from the "stroke" is often quite good. Diagnosis relies initially on elevated lactate and pyruvate in the blood or cerebrospinal fluid. Muscle biopsy commonly reveals ragged-red fibers (even if there is not clear evidence of a myopathy on exam), and specific mutations can be searched for in plasma or muscle in multiple mitochondrial genes. There is no specific treatment for this mitochondrial disorder, though supplementation with vitamins (to include coenzyme Q10, thiamine and carnitine) and l-arginine may be somewhat protective in decreasing the severity of the stroke-like events. There is some evidence that intravenous infusion of L-argining early in the "stroke" can reverse the process and result in complete recovery. Ischemic stroke is very rare in children outside of the immediate perinatal time frame. The placenta is a wonderful clot former and due to the patent foramen ovale in normal prenatal cardiac physiology, there is a natural right to left shunt for clots to enter the arterial circulation. It is very uncommon (less than 2–5% likely) that an additional stroke risk factor will be identified in such perinatal infarctions. Conversely, stroke occurring outside the neonatal time frame is often secondary to another disorder including coagulopathies and hemoglobinopathies (sickle cell disease in particular), congenital or acquired heart disease, neck or head trauma, vasculitis (primary CNS or secondary) and multiple vasculopathies to include Fabry disease, homocystinuria, MELAS and moyamoya disease or syndrome. The workup needs to be extensive, unless particular clues from the personal or family history suggest a specific diagnosis.

Suggested Reading

Tarnopolsky MA. Mitochondrial cytopathies in children and adults. Continuum Lifelong Learning Neurol. 2009;5(6): 98–125.

- Fenichel GM. Clinical pediatric neurology. 6th ed. Philadelphia: Saunders Elsevier; 2009;256–63.

43. A 10-year-old girl is referred to you because of several spells of altered perception. She has three spells which she experienced nausea and headache and perceived people in her immediate environment as being very near, but she had no loos of consciousness. She is doing excellent at school. She denies the use of recreational drug. Her general, neurologic examinations are normal, as well as her brain MRI and EEG.

What is the most likely diagnosis?

A. Alice in wonderland syndrome
B. Conversion disorder
C. Delusional disorder
D. Focal seizures with dyscognitive features
E. Schizophrenia

11

Correct Answer is: A

Alice in Wonderland syndrome, is a benign syndrome usually related to migraine and typically affecting young children. During spells, patients may perceive objects or other people as being larger, smaller, broader, thinner, nearer or farther away than they really are. Altered perception of body image may also occur. Migraine headaches may occur before, during, or after the perceptual alteration. Evaluation for hallucinogenic drugs, even if denied, is very important. The patient is quite young to be presenting with schizophrenia or delusional disorder, which would also require indications of a thought disorder, which is not specified in this case. Focal epilepsy, while important to exclude, is less likely based on the normal EEG and absence of altered consciousness. Conversion disorder would be a diagnosis of exclusion.

Suggested Reading

- Liu AM, Liu JG, Liu GW, Liu GT. Alice in wonderland syndrome: presenting and follow-up characteristics. Pediatr Neurol. 2014;51(3):317–20.
- Illik F, Illik K. Alice in Wonderland syndrome as aura of migraine. Neurocase. 2014;20(4):474–5.
- Hamed SA. A migraine variant with abdominal colic and Alice and Wonderland syndrome: a case report and review. BMC Neurol. 2010;10:2. ▸ https://doi.org/10.1186/1471-2377-10-2.

44. Which of the following can be caused by defects in a calcium channel gene?

A. Familial hemiplegic migraine
B. Myotonia congenital
C. Hyperkalemia periodic paralysis
D. Paramyotonia congenital

Correct Answer is: A

Mutations in calcium channel can cause familial hemiplegic migraine. It is a voltage dependent, P/Q type, alpha 1A subunit (CACNA1A) which codes for a calcium channel. Mutations in the same gene can cause alternating hemiplegia of childhood, episodic ataxia type 2, and spinocerebellar ataxia type 6. Familial hemiplegic migraine can also be caused by mutations in Sodium Channel, Voltage Gated, Type I Alpha Subunit) (SCN1A1) or ATPase, Na+/K+ Transporting, Alpha 2 Polypeptide (ATP1A2).

Mutations in the gene CLCN1 which codes for a chloride channel can cause mytonia congenita. A condition which is characterized by a "warm up phenomenon" where repeated motions improves symptoms. This can be inherited in an autosomal dominant or in an autosomal recessive manner; in each case, the same gene is implicated.

Hyperkalemic periodic paralysis is caused by mutations in Sodium channel, Voltage Gated, Type IV Alpha Subunit

(SCN4A) are implicated in up to 70% of cases of. This is characterized by episodes of weakness exacerbated by high potassium food, cold exposure, and moderate exercise followed by rest.

Mutations in (Calcium Channel, Voltage Dependent, L Type, Alpha 1S Subunit) CACNA 1S may underlie up to 70% of cases of hypokalemic periodic paralysis. Weakness can be triggered by carbohydrate rich meals or by exercise after a period of rest.

Paramyotonia congenita is similar to myotonia congenita; however, the warm up phenomenon is not present and symptoms may actually be exacerbated by repeated movement. Mutations in Sodium Channel, Voltage Gated, and Type IV Alpha Subunit (SCN4A) are implicated.

Suggested Reading

- Knupp K, Parsons JA, Brooks-Kayal AR. Channelopathies. In: Swaiman K, Ashwal S, Ferriero OM, Ferriero D, editors. 5th ed. Edinburgh: Elsevier Saunders; 2012: 544–53.

45. An 8-year-old girl complains of dizziness and frequently vomiting while riding in back seat of her mother car. She has normal development, general and neurological exams.
    What is your recommendation to the parents?
    A. She should wear an eye mask while the car is moving
    B. Make sure she can see forward out the window
    C. She should read in the car
    D. Provide DVD video player for her to watch

Correct Answer is: B

Motion sickness can be induced by motion in the visual filed opposed to the actual forward movement of the body in the car. Looking out the window while driving in the car can minimize this affect. Younger children in the back seat typically have visual input only of the car interior. A higher set seat with greater window exposure, such as in a minivan, would reduce the incidence of motion sickness as the child can watch the environment pass in the direction opposite of their body.

An eye mask would eliminate the visual input of the motion in the direction opposed to the body movement and increases motion sickness symptoms.

Focusing on a book is providing stationary input compared to the movement of the body and will increase motion sickness symptoms.

Focusing on a video player again is providing stationary input compared to the movement of the body and will increase motion sickness symptoms.

Suggested Reading

- Golding JF, Gresty MA. Pathophysiology and treatment of motion sickness. Curr Opin Neurol. 2015; 28(1):83–8.

46. What is the recommendation of the American Academy of Neurology and The Child Neurology Society recommendations in the evaluation of a 12-year-old girl with a 15-month history of frontal headaches and a non-focal neurological exam?
    A. Non-contrast CT
    B. MRI with venogram
    C. EEG
    D. No study required

Correct Answer is: D

Brain imaging in children with a history of chronic headaches is not cost effective because there is minimal chance of identifying a treatable intracranial pathology if a thorough history, general physical and neurological examinations are normal and non-focal.

Non-contract CT is rarely helpful in the evaluation of chronic headaches, with the exception of headaches secondary to chronic sinusitis. In this case the general physical examination and history would be suggestive of sinusitis-associated symptoms. In addition, non-contrast CT is also preferred in cases of acute onset headache when intracranial bleeding is suspected.

MRI with MRV is utilized in suspected venous sinus thrombosis when increased intracranial pressure is present.

EEG changes are not common, are non-specific and play no role in the diagnosis or management of headaches.

Suggested Reading

- Hershey AD. Pediatric headache: update on recent research. Headache: J Head Face Pain. 2012;52(2):327–32.

47. Which of the following would be the earliest step in the proposed development of migraine?
    A. Release of vasoactive neuropeptides from trigeminal sensory nerves
    B. Meningeal blood vessel dilation
    C. Activation of trigeminal sensory afferents in the meningeal vessels
    D. Cortical spreading depression
    E. Meningeal blood vessel constriction

Correct Answer is: D
Cortical spreading depression is felt to occur first. However, it is uncertain whether the trigger for cortical spreading depression occurs in the brain stem or within the cortex.

The pathophysiology of migraine is as follows:

1. **Activation of hypersensitive "central generator" (it is debated whether the initiating trigger for migraine occurs in the cortex or in the brain stem).**
2. **Disrupted ion homeostasis, release of neurochemicals, and transient dysfunction of neuronal function.**
3. **Meningeal blood vessel dilation and activation of trigeminovascular system.**
4. **Release of vasoactive neuropeptides (calcitonin gene-related peptide (CGRP), neurokinins, prostaglandins, substance P, etc.) from activated trigeminal sensory nerves leads to sterile neurogenic inflammation.**
5. **Worsening vasodilation, increasing firing of trigeminal afferents causing pain intensification.**
6. **Trigeminal nociceptive afferents carry pain signals to trigeminal nucleus caudalids (TNC) for processing and ascent through thalamus to cortex**
7. **Continuous ascending pain signals activate more neurons leading to associated symptoms such as photo/phonophobia, nausea, and vomiting.**
8. **Continuous TNC firing, leads to central sensitization if activated pathways are not stopped.**

Suggested Reading

- Silberstein SD, Lipton RB, Dodick O, et al. Wolffs headache and other head pain. 8th ed. New York: Oxford University Press; 2008.

48. An 18-year-old girl complains of headaches, blurred vision, nausea, and vomiting. She has no previous history of migraines, and had no known thrombotic disorders. Fundus examination showed papilledema. MRI was normal, and she has elevated cerebrospinal fluid pressure.
    This disorder may be associated with:
    A. Oral contraceptive use
    B. Hypervitaminosis A
    C. Hypoparathyroidism
    D. Obesity
    E. All of the above

Correct Answer is: E

The patient has pseudo tumor cerebri, also called idiopathic intracranial hypertension or benign intracranial hypertension. It is a disorder of chronically elevated intracranial pressure, resulting in papilledema, which may progress to sub-retinal hemorrhages, optic atrophy, and blindness. Symptoms include headache, diplopia, visual loss and distortion (typically peripheral), nausea, and vomiting. The disorder is often idiopathic and commonly occurs in women of childbearing age with obesity. Pseudo tumor cerebri is also associated with a number of conditions, including endocrine dysfunction (e.g. hypoparathyroidism, Addison's disease, and Cushing's disease), pregnancy, oral contraceptive use, steroid withdrawal, hypervitaminosis A, and tetracycline therapy. The goal of treatment is to preserve vision and decrease intracranial pressure.

Medical management may include acetazolamide and steroids. Surgical approaches include optic nerve sheath fenestration and ventricular shunting. Historically, patients were treated with repeated lumbar punctures.

Suggested Reading

- Gans MS. Idiopathic intracranial hypertension. ► http://emedicine.medscape.com/article/1214410-overview. Updated 5/2/14 accessed 5/29/14.
- Simon RP, et al. Clinical neurology. 4th ed. Stamford, CT: Appleton & Lange. p. 91, 152.

49. An 18-year-old 34 weeks pregnant female is complaining of daily headaches that are unilateral, throbbing, associated with nausea, vomiting, photophobia and phonophobia, lasting for about 4–5 h every day. These headaches are not different from the headaches that she used to have before her pregnancy. Her neurologic exam is normal. M RI and MRV of the brain are normal as well. You suggest initiating this patient on a preventive medication.

What is the safest medication to be used?

A. Amitryptiline
B. Topiramate
C. Valproic acid
D. Atenolol
E. Lithium

Correct Answer is: A

Amitryptiline is a pregnancy category C. It has a very low level in the breast milk. There is a conflicting data regarding limb deformities on high doses of amitryptline, but there is no association reported with doses of 10–50 mg a day, which is what is used as preventive dosing. It is recommended that the dose be tapered 3–4 weeks prior to the delivery. Otherwise, babies should be monitored for drowsiness, hyper excitability, and suckling problems.

Topiramate is associated with cleft palates and cleft lips and also hypospadias.

Valproic acid is associated with neural tube defects as well as lower IQ in children exposed in utero.

Atenolol is a pregnancy category D. It is associated with babies with low weight for gestational age.

Lithium is teratogenic and is a category D in pregnancy.

Suggested Reading

- MacGregor, A. Headache in pregnancy. Continuum. Am Acad Neurol. Review Article. 2014;20(1):128–47.

50. Psychosocial factors that differ in adolescents with migraine headaches compared to age matched controls, include which of the following?

A. A More often have divorced parents
B. Have social skill deficient
C. Experience more school problems
D. Families are more likely to be in the lower socioeconomic class
E. There are no significant psychosocial differences

Correct Answer is: E
Headaches are common in children and up to 80% of adolescent's report experiencing a headache before the age of 14. Psychosocial factors in children with migraine do not differ significantly from headache-free controls, but are absent more days from school on average. In contrast, children with tension-type are more likely to have problems with family (primarily divorce) and housing conditions, school and relations in peer groups.

Suggested Reading

- Karwautz A. Psychosocial factors in children and adolescents with migraine and tension-type headache: a controlled study and review of the literature. Cephalalgia; 1999;(19)1:32–43.

11

51. Headache from cerebral vasculitis is uncommon in children, but occurs in children with which disease?
 A. Type I diabetes
 B. Asthma
 C. Cerebellar astrocytoma
 D. Systemic lupus erythematosus
 E. Osteogenesis imperfecta

Correct Answer is: D
Headaches are frequently seen in the course of a child with a connective tissue disease, such as systemic lupus erythematosus (SLE).

Connective tissue disease related vasculitis occurs as a result of hypersensitivity of cerebra l vessels to an autoimmune process.

Approximately 10% of children with SLE and mixed connective tissue disease will experience severe headaches and may be the presenting feature.

Treatment includes corticosteroids.

Asthma, type I diabetes and osteogenesis imperfecta are seen in children but are not associated with vasculitis.

Cerebellar astrocytoma represents approximately 20% of all brain tumors in children, much less common in adults, are typically low grade with a good prognosis and rarely associated with vasculitis.

Suggested Reading

- Malattia C, Martini A. Pediatric-onset systemic lupus erythematosus. Best Pract Res Clin Rheumatol. 2013;27(3):351–62.

52. Which of the following medications is specifically FDA-approved for the treatment of acute migraine attacks in pediatric patients?
 A. Codeine
 B. Frovatriptan
 C. Frovatriptan with acetaminophen
 D. Diazepam
 E. Sumatriptan and naproxen in a single oral formulation

Correct Answer is: E
Treximet is a combination of sumatriptan and naproxen and was approved for pediatric use in 2015, 7 years after approval for adults. The recommend dose for children 12 years and older is one tablet with1 0 mg of Sumatriptan and 60 mg of naproxen sodium (10/60 mg) and the maximum dose is 85/500 mg.

Zolmitripan (Zomig) and almotriptan (Axert) are triptans also FDA-approved for children 12 and older.

Frovatriptan is used in adults and off-label in children. Narcotics are commonly used in emergency department settings for the treatment of severe

childhood migraines, but are not specifically FDA-approved for this indication.

Benzodiazepines are not effective in migraine headaches.

Suggested Reading

- Freitag FG, Shumate D. Current and investigational drugs for the prevention of migraine in adults and children. CNS Drugs. 2014;28(10):921–7.

53. An 18-year-old obese female came with a 5-month history of intermittent headaches. The pain is characterized as pressure-like and throbbing, but without photophobia. Headaches are not associated with nausea or vomiting. She reports that she is able to "hear my pulse in my head" and occasionally has blurred vision, especially in the morning when she awakens. Her past medical history is significant only for severe menstrual cramping, for which she was recently started on an oral contraceptive. She has no papilledema on fundus exam. Rest of the neurological exam is normal.

    What is most likely the diagnosis?
    - A. Classic migraine
    - B. Migraine without aura
    - C. Benign intracranial hypertension
    - D. Subarachnoid hemorrhage
    - E. Tension headache

Correct Answer is: C

The transient visual loss is most commonly seen in patients with benign intracranial hypertension than migraines, and results from changes in intracranial pressure that can relate to position. Retinoids, vitamin A toxicity, tetracycline, lithium, and oral contraceptives use is associated with pseudo tumor cerebri. Obesity is also a strong risk factor for benign intracranial hypertension.

Suggested Reading

- Mowzoon N, Flemming KD. Neurology board review: an illustrated study guide. Rochester: Mayo Clinic Scientific; 2007. Print.

54. Which of the following symptoms is a "red flag" in the diagnosis of childhood migraine that may suggest more serious intracranial pathology?
    - A. Head ache in a child less than 4 year of age
    - B. A consistent headache pattern over a one-year period
    - C. Headaches associated with vomiting
    - D. Headache associated with distorted vision
    - E. Pain correlates with episode of vertigo

Correct Answer is: A

Headaches, head pain and migraine are rare in children under the age of 4 and warrant neuroimaging to rule-out causes of increased intracranial pressure. Headaches occurring at an increasing frequency or increasing severity over several weeks in a child under the age of 12 are not characteristic of a migraine pattern. Headaches with vomiting upon awakening suggest increased intracranial pressure. Transient visual auras occur in classic migraines and benign paroxysmal vertigo is a migraine variant in young children and is associated with nausea, vomiting and nystagmus.

Suggested Reading

- Raieli V, et al. Migraine in a pediatric population: a clinical study in children younger than 7 years of age. Dev Med Child Neurol. 2015;57(6):585–8.

55. Which of the following statements regarding migraine headaches in children is true

A. The prevalence of migraine in children 7 and younger is 2.5%
B. It is a hereditary disorder transmitted by autosomal recessive inheritance
C. A history of migraine in at least one parent is 50%
D. Boys and girls are affected equally in all pediatric age groups
E. About one-quarter will continue to have migraines into adulthood

Correct Answer is: A
In pediatric neurology practice 75% of headaches in young children referred for neurological consultation are Migraines headaches. Muscle tension and psychogenic headaches are less likely to be experience in children. Under the age of 7 is the only age category in children that both sexes are affected equally. The incidence of migraines in ages 7 to puberty is 5%, with a female predominance of 3:2. In post-pubertal boys the incidence is 5% and in girls it is 10%. There is a strong autosomal dominant hereditary pattern and there is a history of migraines in at least 90% of parents. Approximately three quarters will continue to experience migraines by the age of 25 and half will continue until the age of 50.

11

Suggested Reading

Lewis DW. Pediatric migraine. Neurol Clin. 2009;27(2):481–501.

56. An 18-year-old female with a 5-year history of severe migraine headaches. She has a visual aura, she has a unilateral temporal headache occurring either on her left or right side, nausea and photophobia are associated with her headache, falling asleep is relieving the headache. Her headaches occurred once a month, but in the last year they have occurred twice a week. The headaches are severe enough to prevent her from attending school, and engaging in social activities. Her past medical history was significant for an allergy to sulfa, and she has a family history of kidney stones. Her neurologic examination is normal, and she has no papilledema.
What is the appropriate next step in management?
A. lumbar puncture
B. Start amitriptyline
C. Head MRI and MRA
D. Start Topiramate
E. Start Valproic acid

Correct Answer is: B
This is a female with frequent migraine headaches, without recent change, and a normal examination. An MRI scan is unlikely to reveal a treatable cause in patients with chronic (>6 months) headaches, with no focal neurologic deficits, papilledema or a history of seizures. Similarly, the MRA or CSF studies would unlikely be of value.

Preventative or prophylactic therapy are daily medications to be taken by the patient to decrease the headache frequency. More than 20 medications have been used for migraine prevention, but we have no studies to clearly indicate which would be the optimal to use in children or teenager.

However, in this patient one would want to avoid the use of Valproic acid because of potential teratogenic side effects. Topiramate is chemically related to sulfa compounds, and occasional patients will show an allergic cross-reactivity. Topiramate also predisposes to renal stones. Amitriptyline is frequently used in children and teens. With amitriptyline, EKG has to be done to detect a prolonged QT interval.

Suggested Reading

- Hershey AD, Powers SW, Bentti AL, Degrauw TJ. Effectiveness of amitriptyline in the prophylactic management of childhood headaches. Headache. 2000;40:539–49.
- Lewis DW, Ashwal S, Dahl G, Dorbad D, Hirtz D, Prensky A, Jarjour I; Quality Standards Subcommittee of the American Academy of Neurology; Practice Committee of the Child Neurology Society. Practice parameter: evaluation of children and adolescents with recurrent headaches: report of the Quality Standards Subcommittee of the American Academy of Neurology and the Practice Committee of the Child Neurology Society. Neurology. 2002;59(4):490–8.
- Lewis D, Ashwal S, Hershey A, et al. Practice parameter: pharmacological treatment of migraine headache in children and adolescents: report of the American Academy of Neurology Quality Standards Subcommittee and the Practice Committee of the Child Neurology Society. Neurology. 2004;63:2215–24.
- Lewis D, Winner P, Saper J, Ness S, Polverejan E, Wang S, Kurland CL, Nye J, Yuen E, Eerdekens M, Ford L. Randomized, double-blind, placebo-controlled study to evaluate the efficacy and safety of topiramate for migraine prevention in pediatric subjects 12 to 17 years of age. Pediatrics. 2009;123(3):924–34.

57. What drug can be used as substitute for sumatriptan in a patient with medication-overuse headache who requires bridge therapy?
    - A. butorphanol 2 mg intranasally every 4 h
    - B. hydromorphone 4 mg four times daily
    - C. naproxen 750 mg extended release once daily
    - D. oxycodone 30 mg twice daily
    - E. rizatriptan 10 mg twice daily

Correct Answer is: C

Naproxen 750 mg extended release once daily can be used in mediation-overuse headache require bridge therapy to decrease the transient increase in headaches that occurs during discontinuation of the overused agent. The choice of bridge therapy is based on the specific overused treatment and the tolerability of the acute treatment alternative. For patients who overuse sumatriptan, long-acting NSAIDs are recommended as bridge therapy. Opioids are not recommended for this purpose because of the potential for dependence. Rizatriptan would not be an appropriate substitute since it, like sumatriptan, is a short-acting triptan, although long-acting triptans such as naratriptan or frovatriptan may be appropriate as rescue therapy.

Suggested Reading

- Giamberardino, Mitsikostas, Martelletti. Update on medication overuse headache and its treatment. Curr Treat Options Neurol. 2014;17(8):368.
- Lipton. Risk factors for and management of medication overuse headache. Continuum Lifelong Learning in Neurology. 2015;21(4):1118–31.

58. You are evaluating a 17-year-old obese girl with worsening headache. She has borderline hypertension. Her headaches bifrontal and bioccipital band-like pressure and pain. Occasionally, she experiences brief visual loss or graying, especially with straining, which lasts only seconds, but no photophobia or phonophobia. When

the pain is severe, she feels her vision is becoming increasingly blurred and she will have nausea and vomiting. **Which of the following is not a proposed mechanism in the pathogenesis of this condition?**

A. Decreased CSF absorption
B. Increased venous pressure
C. Increased CSF formation
D. Congenital stenosis of venous sinuses
E. Aqueduct stenosis

Correct Answer is: E

This is a case of Idiopathic intracranial hypertension (IIH), also known as benign intracranial hypertension or pseudotumour cerebri, which is a syndrome with signs and symptoms of increased intracranial pressure but where a causative mass or hydrocephalus is not identified. The typical demographic are middle-aged obese females. Presentation is usually with headaches, visual problems and papilledema. Papilledema may not always be present, or may be unilateral, making the clinical diagnosis less than straightforward. Neurological examination is usually normal, with a sixth cranial nerve palsy sometimes encountered. Additional clinical findings include normal CSF composition with elevated opening pressure (opening pressure varies however, with a mean pressure of less than 35 mmHg, with pressure waves as high as 80 mmHg which last 5–20 min).

Treatment options include CSF letting, acetazolamide and lumboperitoneal shunts. In patients with progressive visual deterioration, optic nerve fenestration may be required to preserve vision. Topiramate can be used if there is a contraindication to Acetazolamide (such as a sulfa allergy) because of its carbonic anhydrase inhibitor effect. IIH is a poorly understood condition. Various mechanisms have been proposed to explain its pathogenesis, including decreased CSF absorption, increased CSF production, increased intravascular volume, and increased intracranial venous pressure. Of the possible etiologies listed, aqueductal stenosis is not a cause of idiopathic intracranial hypertension (IIH), although it would be a secondary cause of hydrocephalus.

11

Suggested Reading

- Acheson JF, Green WT, Sanders MD. Optic nerve sheath decompression for the treatment of visual failure in chronic raised intracranial pressure. J Neurol Neurosurg Psychiatry.1994; 57:1426–29.
- Burgett RA, Purvin VA, Kawasaki A. Lumboperitoneal shunting for pseudotumor cerebri. Neurology. 1997;49:734–9.
- Headache Classification Subcommittee of the International Headache Society. The international classification of headache disorders: 2nd ed. Cephalalgia. 2004;24 (Suppl 1):9–160.

59. You are asked to see a 9-year-old female because she has several spells of altered perception. In three of her episodes, she had nausea and headache and perceived people in her immediate environment as being larger than they are. She is doing very good at school and denies any loss of consciousness or recreational drug use. Her neurologic examination, MRI of the brain and EEG are normal. **What is the most likely diagnosis?**

A. Alice in wonderland syndrome
B. Conversion disorder
C. Delusional disorder
D. Focal seizures with dyscognitive features
E. Schizophrenia

Correct Answer is: A

Alice in Wonderland syndrome is a benign syndrome often related to migraine and typically affecting young children. During spells patients may perceive objects or other people as being larger, smaller, broader, thinner, nearer or farther away than they really are. Altered perception of body image may also occur. Migraine headaches may occur at any time during or after the perceptual alteration. It is important in the evaluation of perceptual alterations to consider the use of hallucinogenic drugs even if denied. The patient is quite young to be presenting with schizophrenia or delusional disorder, which would also require indications of a thought disorder, which is not mentioned in the vignette. Focal epilepsy, while important to exclude, is less likely based on the normal EEG and absence of altered consciousness. Conversion disorder would be a diagnosis of exclusion.

Suggested Reading

- Liu AM, Liu JG, Liu GW, Liu GT. Alice in wonderland syndrome: presenting and follow-up characteristics. Pediatr Neurol. 2014;51(3):317–20.
- Illik F, Illik K. Alice in Wonderland syndrome as aura of migraine. Neurocase. 2014;20(4):474–5.
- Hamed SA. A migraine variant with abdominal colic and Alice and Wonderland syndrome: a case report and review. BMC Neurol. 2010;10:2. ▶ https://doi.org/10.1186/1471-2377-10-2.

60. You are evaluating an 18-year-old girl in the ED with severe headache for the last 5 days. She has a history of migraine since she was 9 years of age. Her headaches usually respond to a combination of Ibuprofen with oral Sumatriptan. Sometimes she needs to use injectable Sumatriptan if she has no response to the oral combination. The current headache started 5 days ago and there was no response to the oral combination. She ran out of her injectable Sumatriptan, so she kept using oral Sumatriptan and Ibuprofen for the last 5 days, but the headache did not improve, so she decide to go to emergency department.
She has a stable vital sign and her neurological exam is normal.
After initiating IV fluids, what treatment is the most appropriate first line therapy in this patient?
A. IV prochlorperazine
B. IV magnesium sulfate
C. IV sodium valproate
D. IV methylprednisolone
E. IV hydromorphone

Correct Answer is: A

This is a clinical presentation of status migrainosus. The proper treatment of status migrainosus is IV therapy. Dihydroergotamine (DHE) is the gold standard therapy. Between the choices given here, IV prochlorperazine would be the most appropriate next step. Anti-emetics parentally are considered first-line pharmacologic treatment for status migrainosus in the ED with high-quality evidence supporting their use. Between antiemetics, the strongest data exists for prochlorperazine and metoclopramide.

Steroids, including methylprednisone, can be used in status migrainosus, but data does not support its use in the reduction of headaches.

Hydromorphone and other opioids should not be used in almost all cases, as they may lead to dependence and increase the headache relapse rate.

Magnesium sulfate can be used in status but not as a first line treatment. Studies have shown mixed evidence of effectiveness for acute migraine in ED.

No placebo-controlled studies have evaluated the efficacy of valproate sodium in patients with status migrainosus. So it cannot be used as a first line agent. Although it can be tried if other first line agents (DHE, *NSAIDs, antiemetics*) have failed.

Suggested Reading

- Continuum. Headache. 2015;21(4):1004–1010.

61. You are seeing an 18-year-old male with history of recurrent, severe migraine headaches and some progressive mild cognitive impairment brings. He brought a recent brain MRI which shows multiple white matter lesions. His mother recently died at 59 from dementia but the autopsy suggested cerebral autosomal dominant arteriopathy with subcortical infarcts and leukoencephalopathy (CADASIL). He would like to know if his MRI shows that he has the disease. **Affection of what brain area is most supportive of the diagnosis of (CADASIL)"?**
    - A. Corona radiata
    - B. Posterior limb of internal capsule
    - C. External capsule
    - D. Anterior limb of internal capsule
    - E. Centrum semiovale

11

Correct Answer is: C
Cerebral autosomal dominant arteriopathy with subcortical infarcts and leukoencephalopathy (CADASIL) is an inherited, autosomal dominant condition caused by mutations of the Notch3 gene. Affected individuals usually have migraine, mood disturbance, and recurrent strokes, often progressing to subcortical dementia. T2-weighted hyper-intensity of the temporal white matter and external capsule are characteristic findings that may help to distinguish the disease.

Suggested Reading

- O'Sullivan M, Jarosz JM, Martin RJ, et al. Neurology. 2001;56:628–34.

62. What is the most reasonable substitute for sumatriptan in an 18 years-old-female patient with medication-overuse headache who requires bridge therapy?
    - A. butorphanol 2 mg intranasally every 4 h
    - B. hydromorphone 4 mg four times daily
    - C. naproxen 750 mg extended release once daily
    - D. oxycodone 30 mg twice daily
    - E. rizatriptan 10 mg twice daily

Correct Answer is: C
Some patients with mediation-overuse headache require bridge therapy to ease the transient increase in headaches that occurs during discontinuation of the overused agent. The choice of bridge therapy is based on the specific overused treatment and the tolerability of the acute treatment alternative. For patients who overuse sumatriptan, long-acting NSAIDs are recommended as bridge therapy. Opioids are not recommended for this purpose because of the potential for dependence. Rizatriptan would not be an appropriate substitute since it, like sumatriptan, is a short-acting triptan, although long-acting triptans such as naratriptan or frovatriptan may be appropriate as rescue therapy.

Suggested Reading

- Giamberardino, Mitsikostas, Martelletti. Update on medication overuse headache and its treatment. Curr Treat Options Neurol. 2014;17(8):368.
- Lipton. Risk factors for and management of medication overuse headache. Continuum Lifelong Learning in Neurology. 2015;21(4):1118–31.

Infections

Y. M. Awaad, *Absolute Pediatric Neurology*, https://doi.org/10.1007/978-3-319-78801-2_12

1. A 14-year-old female is brought to the ED because she has altered consciousness, headache and fever of (102 F.) for 2 days. You examined her and you found no meningeal signs, but she requires repeated tactile stimulation to maintain arousal, she is not oriented except to person, makes frequent paraphasic errors, and can recall just one of three objects after a distracting task. The rest of the neurologic examination is unremarkable. Lumbar puncture was done and CSF analysis shows a red blood cell count of 25 cells/hpf; white blood cell count of 120 cells/hpf with a lymphocytic predominance; glucose of 70 mg/dL; and protein of 95 mg/dL.
What is the best treatment to be initiated at this time?
A. Iduroxidine
B. Ceftriaxone
C. Vidarabine
D. Solumedrol
E. Acyclovir

12

Correct Answer is: E
the clinical presentation is indicative of herpes simplex encephalitis (HSE), which affects 1 in 250,000 to 1 in 500,000 individuals per year in the United States, with approximately one-third of cases occurring in patients between the ages of 6 months and 20 years. HSE can occur as a primary infection or a reactivation of the herpes simplex virus (HSV). Patients present with a variety of non-specific findings, including fever, headache, altered consciousness, dysphasia, seizures, and/or focal neurologic deficits. CSF analysis could be normal in 5–10%. In majority of cases, CSF analysis shows an elevated white blood cell count with a lymphocytic predominance and an elevated protein. Red blood cells are often present but are non-diagnostic. PCR form the CSF has a sensitivity of 94% and specificity of 98% in confirming the diagnosis. EEG, CT, and MRI are supportive studies in the diagnosis. Treatment consists of intravenous acyclovir 10 mg/kg every 8 h (30 mg/kg/d) for 14–21 days. Idoxuridine was the first antiviral drug used to treat HSE; however, it proved to be both ineffective and toxic. Acyclovir was demonstrated to be superior to vidarabine in a head-to-head trial. Neither ceftriaxone, nor solumedrol would be appropriate treatments, as both the clinical presentation and CSF studies suggest viral encephalitis.

Suggested Reading

- Whitley RJ, Kimberlin DW. Herpes simplex: encephalitis children and adolescents. Semin Pediatr Infect Dis. 2005;16:17–23.

2. A 2 days old full-term infant has been evaluated for irritability and microcephaly. He is a product of uncomplicated pregnancy, labor and delivery for a healthy mother. Head ultrasonography and CT scan showed enlarged posterior horns of the lateral ventricles and punctuate calcifications which are both periventricular and diffuse. On neurological examination, he has increased tone and hyperreflexia. A dilated funduscopic exam shows a large area of absent retina with hyperpigmented margins.
What is the most likely diagnosis?
A. Congenital cytomegalovirus infection
B. Congenital toxoplasmosis
C. Congenital herpes simplex type 1
D. Congenital rubella
E. Congenital syphilis

Correct Answer is: B
Congenital toxoplasmosis (CT) is a rare disorder despite the ubiquitous presence of the parasite in the environment and high incidence of sero-positivity in the population. Domestic cats are the

reservoir and human transmission occurs from oral ingestion of ova in fecal contaminated dirt or litter boxes. Infected mothers during pregnancy will transmit the congenital infection to their babies in 50–80%, via hemaotgenous spread of the parasite to the placenta and fetus. Only 5% of children will have neurological sequelae, approximately 35% develop chorioretinitis by age 12 with many lesions being subclinical. In the US, Massachusetts routinely screens newborns for the condition with a yearly incidence of new cases of 0.8 per 10,000. Treatment is not known to prevent chorioretinitis or neurologic injury but this is debated. The case presented represents the minority of CT cases with only 1 of 22 cases reported in a 2-year period in the UK having this constellation of signs and symptoms.

The calcifications in CT is diffuse involving the cortex and may also be periventricular with hydrocephalus, but calcification in congenital CMV involve the periventricular region only. Maternal prenatal screening has been suggested and is carried out in France for example, however, opponents point out that it is expensive, raises anxiety in positives and there is no evidence that maternal treatment prevents CT. The prognosis for a child affected as above is poor.

Suggested Reading

- Gilbert R, Tan H, Cliffe S, Guy E, and Stanford M. Symptomatic toxoplasma infection due to congenital and postnatally acquired infection. Arch Dis Child 2006;91:495–8.

3. You have been consulted on a 4-year-old boy for his headache, progressive vomiting and fever for 10 days. His mother reports that he has no current respiratory symptoms, but she has been sick with intermittent respiratory symptoms for the last few months. Today, he starts to have double vision and he becomes dysarthric. His brain CT shows enlarged ventricles without any obvious mass lesion. On examination, he has bilateral papilledema, an incomplete bilateral 6th CN paresis and mild right facial weakness. He has trouble swallowing liquids. You performed a LP and shows 250 WBC's (lymphocyte predominant), protein of 350 mg/dL and glucose of 30. Opening pressure was 300 mm. Routine gram stain and bacterial culture of the cerebrospinal fluid are negative at 48 h. His brain MRI shows enhancement of the basilar meninges and two nodular enhancing lesions in the temporal lobes.

What are you going to order on the remaining spinal fluid?

A. Enterovirus PCR
B. Herpes simplex virus PCR
C. Human herpesvirus PCR
D. Lymphocytic choriomeningitis virus PCR
E. Mycobacterium tuberculosis PCR

Correct Answer is: E

this is a case of basilar meningitis confirmed by the neurologic and radiographic findings. The cranial nerve palsies typically develop from a thickened exudate at the base of the brain that either entraps the cranial nerve itself or leads to a vasculitis and ischemia of the nerve. This exudative process suggests a more localized inflammatory process, seen more commonly with tubercular, Lyme, fungal and parasitic meningitis. This process is also seen in cases of sarcoidosis, neoplastic meningitis and some forms of CNS vasculitis. Basilar meningitis is extremely rare with viral meningitis. Lymphocytic choriomeningitis virus can cause the intrauterine infection with

clinical and radiologic features that can be confused with the congenital CMV infection, but would not present in the above fashion. Central nervous system tuberculosis follows the dissemination of tuberculosis after primary infection (most commonly the lung). This process can occur at the same time as the primary disease or several years later. Basilar meningitis and at times parenchymal infections called tuberculomas (noted on this patient's MRI scan) can be caused by multiplying organisms in the subarachnoid space. Hydrocephalus is also seen frequently. Tuberculosis can also involve the spinal cord, either from a vertebral body abscess or an arachnoiditis. Diagnosis of central nervous system tuberculosis can be quite challenging. Only 5–25% of patients have a positive acid-fast stain. Only in 20–40% of patients, bacteria by routine single lumbar puncture (AFB culture) can be isolated. Increasing the volume collected to 10 mL (20 mL or more in adult patients) and performing repeated sampling of the spinal fluid yield a positive result in up to 50–80%. PCR assay has a sensitivity on a single sample of 50–75%. Treatment of CNS tuberculosis is quite challenging. Initial therapy involves four drugs (combination of isoniazid, rifampin, pyrazinamide and ethambutol or streptomycin) for 2 months. As sensitivity tests allow, two agents can be used as a treatment. Response to treatment is usually seen within 2 weeks, though therapy should continue for 9–12 months. Treatment of the primary TB infection reduces the incidence of CNS infection. A shunting procedure of the CSF is occasionally required and corticosteroids may reduce the mortality and morbidity of the disease, especially in children with altered level of consciousness, papilledema, focal deficits or elevated intracranial pressure.

4. You are evaluating a 5-year-old boy for his behavior changes. He has a history of mild developmental, but recently he became more subdued and less interested to play with his brother. He used to talk in full sentences, now he is speaking in 2-word phrases. He has no other focal neurological abnormality except bilateral mild spastic Para paresis. His past medical history is unremarkable. Recently, his mother was tested positive for HIV. You ordered ELISA and Western blot studies on the child which came back positive for HIV. His CSF studies shows 10 WBCs/hpf, protein 40 mg/dL, glucose 65 mg/dL. India ink and AFB stains are negative. PCR and serology for CMV is negative. Toxoplasmosis serology (IgM and IgG) are negative. Serum and CSF cryptococcal antigen testing is normal. PCR of the spinal fluid for JC virus DNA is sent and pending. Brain MRI shows global cerebral atrophy and bilaterally symmetric hyperintense signal in the white matter on T2-weighted sequences; these same regions appear isointense on T1-weighted images.

   What treatment is most likely to improve him clinically?

   A. Amphotericin
   B. Gangcyclovir
   C. Anti-retroviral therapy
   D. Isoniazid and rifampin
   E. Pyrimethamine and sulfadiazine

Correct Answer is: C

this is a HIV positive child patient who develop signs and symptoms of progressive encephalopathy and spastic diparesis. This is acquired prenatally form his mother. The differential diagnosis includes many different infectious agents, as well as primary CNS lymphoma. Toxoplasmosis is ruled out because of the negative serology and

lack of mass lesions on MRI. Tuberculous infection usually produces a striking basilar meningitis. Although a negative acid-fast stain of the CSF does not exclude this possibility, the child's clinical and radiology presentation is not consistent with CNS tuberculosis. The laboratory markers for both cryptococcal and CMV meningitis were negative.

In this case 2 entities have to be consider, progressive multifocal leukoencephalopathy (PML) and HIV encephalopathy. Both can cause a subacute encephalopthy, but PML is unlikely to produce isolated cognitive decline, without other focal neurologic deficits (especially visual field loss). Neuroimaging of PML also shows more focal abnormalities, extending into the subcortical white matter, and tend to be hypointense on T1-weighted images.

The incidence of congenital HIV encephalopathy has decreased greatly in developed countries since the use of highly active anti-retroviral therapy (HAART) in affected women. There are multiple presentations for this disorder, including a progressive, static or indolent course. Pre-existing global developmental delay is not unusual in the progressive course. After a varied period of time, the child usually develops a combination of behavioral deterioration, cognitive regression and motor impairment (with both pyramidal and extra-pyramidal findings). Diagnosis is one of exclusion, with neuroimaging and spinal fluid examination necessary to rule out the many other infectious and neoplastic processes contributing to encephalopathy in children with HIV infection. The CSF in HIV encephalopathy is often normal, though can have a mildly increased cell count and protein level. The most common radiographic findings include cortical atrophy, nonspecific white matter changes and basal ganglia calcifications (best seen on computed tomography.) Aggressive use of anti-retroviral therapy has been shown to either slow or reverse the features of progressive HIV encephalopathy in both pediatric and adult patients.

Suggested Reading

- Barton, et al. The neurologic manifestations of pediatric infectious diseases and immunodeficiency syndromes. 2008:157–72 AAN Continuum, April 2006, 111–32.

5. You are seeing an 8-year-old boy in the PICU for his new onset status epilepticus. He has a history of a large, tender lymph node in the right neck for 3 days, and he was on a 14-day course of Augmentin as a treatment. His mother had difficulty getting him to arouse this morning and called the EMS. While he was in his way to the ER, he developed right face and arm clonic activity, and was given 3 doses of lorazepam and a loading dose of fosphenytoin which stopped the seizure. You ordered an EEG showed intermittent non-convulsive electrographic seizures from the left hemisphere. His brain CT was normal. His CSF showed a white blood count of 18 cells/mm^3, with normal glucose and protein levels. You started him on vancomycin, ceftriaxone and acyclovir. Herpes simplex PCR testing was negative.

   Which of the following laboratory tests is most likely to be abnormal?

   A. Acid fast bacilli culture of the cerebrospinal fluid
   B. Cerebrospinal fluid for cryptococcal antigen
   C. Repeat cerebrospinal fluid PCR for HSV I/II
   D. Serum Bartonella henselae titers

Correct Answer is: D

Skin abrasion or scratch from a young kitten can cause Bartonella infections.

The most striking manifestations the prominent lymphadenopathy in the cervical, axillary or inguinal region. Other systemic symptoms such as fever, anorexia, fatigue and headache may also be present. Atypical cases with neurologic features can occur. Encephalopathy (presenting with mental status changes or new-onset seizures, often status epilepticus) is the most common neurologic presentation, representing about 2% of cases of cat scratch disease in the largest case series reviewed. Less likely neurologic presentations include acute or subacute monocular blindness due to retinitis, a peripheral neuritis resembling Guillain-Barre syndrome, meningitis and a transverse myelitis. Fever is not necessarily present during the encephalopathy and CSF may not show pleocytosis. Imaging studies are typically normal but hyperintense lesions on T2-weighted and FLAIR MRI in the deep grey structures and rarely the cortex can be seen. A consideration of the disease should be maintained in anyone with acute or subacute encephalopathy and either lymphadenopathy and/or recent kitten exposure. The benefits of multiple antibiotic in patients with focal brain lesions or encephalitis from bartonella infections are uncertain. Spontaneous resolution is the rule for this disease, though rarely chronic epilepsy may develop. Seizures and status epilepticus are not common in Lyme disease. Subacute or chronic meningitis and unilateral or bilateral facial nerve palsies are the most common neurologic presentations in Lyme disease. Rarely, initial PCR testing for herpes simplex encephalitis can have a false negative result. In cases with a high index of suspicion, especially with focal seizures and hemorrhagic infarctions in the temporal or orbital frontal cortices, repeat PCR testing should be considered. Both cryptococcal and M. tuberculosis infections of the central nervous system would typically present in an immune compromised host. Although atypical mycobacterial infections can lead to prominent cervical lymphadenopathy, this feature is not present in M. tuberculosis infection.

12

Suggested Reading

- Barton, et al. The neurological manifestations of pediatric infectious diseases and immunodeficiency syndrome. 2008:243–50.

6. You are seeing a 10-year-old boy in the ED with new-onset seizure activity and 1 month of headaches. He is not febrile. He moved with his family recently form South America. His neurologic examination is unremarkable. EEG is characterized by continuous, polymorphic delta slowing in the left frontal region. His brain MRI is shown.

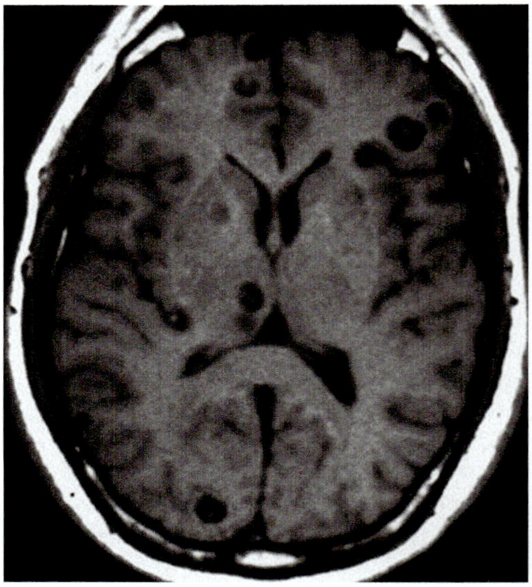

Fig. 12.1 Neuro-cysticercosis (NCC). American Academy of Neurology Institute, produced by permission

Which test are you going to order to confirm his diagnosis?

A. Blood culture
B. HIV test

C. ELISA for serum IgG antibodies to T. solium
D. Sedimentation rate
E. Stool analysis

Correct Answer is: C
Neuro-cysticercosis (NCC) is a parasitic disease caused by the larval form of the pork tapeworm, Taenia solium. It is the most common parasitic disease of the nervous system and the main cause of acquired epilepsy in developing countries. There are four subtypes of NCC based on where the larvae lodge—parenchymal, subarachnoid/cisternal, intraventricular, and spinal. You have to consider the following in your differential diagnosis, tuberculoma, pyogenic brain abscesses, fungal abscess, toxoplasmosis, a primary or metastatic brain tumor and infectious vasculitis. When there is a clinical suspicion for NCC, the next step is to obtain an enzyme-linked immunosorbent assay (ELISA) for serum IgG antibodies to T. solium. Since there is cross-reactivity between cysticercosis and echinococcus antibodies (approximately 23%) a positive result by ELISA should be confirmed by Western blot. Calcified lesions in the chronic stage can be seen by the CT scan. Albendazole and praziquantel have both been shown to be cysticidal; however, a recent meta-analysis suggests that albendazole is superior to praziquantel in terms of its ability to control seizures in affected patients and to completely eradicate cysts.
Treatment is not required in patients without significant symptomatology. Hydrocephalus is a common complication, often necessitating placement of an intraventricular shunt.

Suggested Reading

- Nash TE, et al. Treatment of neuro-cysticercosis: current status and future research needs. Neurology. 2006;67:1120–27.
- Matthaiou DK, Panos G, Adamidi ES, Falagas ME. Albendazole versus Praziquantel in the treatment of neurocysticercosis: a meta-analysis of comparative trials. PLOS N`egl Trop Dis. 2008;2(3):e194.

7. You have been asked to see a 5-day-old baby girl in the NICU for possible seizures. She was small for gestational age and born at 32 weeks gestation. On day 2 of life, she has had feeding difficulties and has received phototherapy for jaundice. On your exam, she is micro cephalic, has hepatosplenomegaly, and a purpuric rash. You ordered head ultrasound which shows ventriculomegaly. Her blood labs elevated aminotransferases, direct and indirect hyperbilirubinemia, thrombocytopenia, and hemolytic anemia.
Which test is most likely to confirm this patient's diagnosis?
A. Bone marrow biopsy
B. Head CT scan
C. Ophthalmologic examination
D. Rapid plasma reagin (RPR) test
E. Urine CMV culture

Correct Answer is: E
Cytomegalovirus is one of the herpesviridae family. Infected immunocompetent adults are asymptomatic; on the other hand, congenital infection is the most prevalent infection-related cause of congenital neurologic impairment. Vertical transmission—during pregnancy through the placenta, during delivery through cervical secretions or blood, or postnatally through breast milk—occurs in 30% of cases; however, not all infected fetuses are affected. Symptomatic Infants at birth (10%) are typically small for gestational age with feeding problems, ocular problems (chorioretinitis, retinal scars, optic atrophy, and central vision loss), sensorineural hearing loss,

organomegaly, thrombocytopenia, jaundice, microcephaly, seizures, and abnormal neurologic examinations. Neuroimaging may reveal periventricular cysts and calcifications, ventriculomegaly, vasculitis, hydranencephaly, and/or neuronal migration abnormalities. Perinatal mortality for symptomatic newborns ranges from 2–30%, with survivors having poor neurodevelopmental prognoses. Infected infants who are asymptomatic at birth are still at risk for neurodevelopmental issues, such as learning disabilities and attention deficit hyperactivity disorder. In addition, 5–15% of these infants will develop sensorineural hearing loss, which is typically bilateral and progressive. If CMV infection is suspected in utero, an amniocentesis should be performed to confirm vertical transmission. Fetal ultrasound or MRI can help to predict the risk that the fetus will be affected at birth. Urine culture or CMV-DNA testing by PCR can help in confirming congenital infection within 3 weeks of birth. Infected newborns should be further evaluated with a complete blood count, platelet count, transaminase level, and bilirubin levels (direct and indirect) and should have both an ophthalmologic examination and auditory brainstem evoked responses. Symptomatic newborns should be treated with gancyclovir 6 mg/kg/dose twicw a day for 6 weeks, as this improves hearing outcomes. Treatment of asymptomatic newborns is not currently recommended.

12

Suggested Reading

- Coll O, et al. Guidelines on CMV congenital infection. J Perinat Med. 2009;37:433–45.

8. You are seen a one-week-old baby in the ED for her focal seizure which consisted of shaking of the left side of her body, with apparent apnea and cyanosis of the lips. The seizure stopped spontaneously after few minutes, but on exam, she is lethargic and has a rectal temperature of 40.6 °C. She has a full and open anterior fontanelle. She has an uncomplicated pregnancy, labor, and delivery at full term.

Which of the following is the most likely cause of her condition?

A. Coccidiomycosis systemic infection
B. Congenital CMV
C. Congenital toxoplasmosis
D. Focal cortical dysplasia
E. Neonatal herpes simplex encephalitis

Correct Answer is: E

Vertical transmission (from infected mother to neonate at the time of birth) is common in neonatal HSV, though congenital infection can occur, and postpartum virus exposure similar to that found in older children can occur in the young infants depending on their exposure to the appropriate source. Patient age, level of consciousness at presentation, and duration of symptoms before the initiation of therapy are the most three important outcome measures are. The last one of the three is the only one that can be controlled, so treatment for HSV encephalitis with intravenous acyclovir must be initiated immediately for there to be optimal chance at neurological recovery. The therapy should not be delayed too long for evaluation purposes, because diagnostic information can still be obtained 24–48 h after the initiation of treatment.

Suggested Reading

- Current therapy in neurologic disease. In: Johnson RT, et al., editors 6th ed. St. Louis: Mosby Press: 2002 123–24.

9. The following scenario is part of a two-question series, Discussion & References included at the end of series.

A 16-year-old female came to the office with 2 days history of right facial weakness and she is unable to close her right eye. She has trouble sucking from a straw and also, she has drooling from her right side of the mouth. She denies paresthesias, ear pain or hyperacusis. On skin examination you note the following:

The most likely infectious agent causing the above symptoms is:

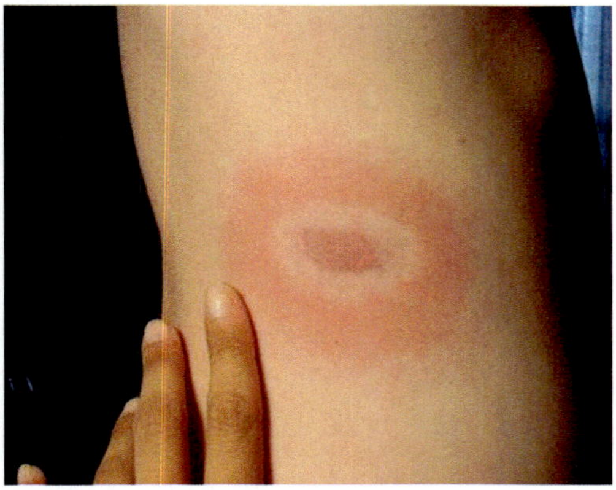

Fig. 12.2 Erythematous rash in the pattern of a "bull's-eye" from Lyme disease. ► en:User:Jongarrison. Hannah Garrison

A. Herpes Simplex Virus Type 1
B. Borrelia burgdorferi
C. Rickettsia rickettsii
D. Mycoplasma pneumonia

Correct Answer is: B

10. The following scenario is part 2 of a 2-question series, Discussion & References included at the end of series.

The best treatment option for this patient is:

A. Acyclovir
B. Forscarnet
C. Doxycycline
D. Azithromycin
E. Fluconazole

Correct Answer is: C

The skin manifestation is the target sign of the Lyme disease which is caused by the tick-transmitted spirochete, *B. burgdorferi*. Clinical manifestations may include erythema migrans, lymphocytic meningitis, cranial neuritis, and polyradiculitis. Diagnosis includes an ELISA on serum for anti-*B. burgdorferi* antibodies. If serum is positive, then Western blot is completed. Treatment options include oral doxycycline, ampicillin, and cefuroxime axetil.

Suggested Reading

- Halperin JJ. Lyme disease: a multisystem infection that affects the nervous system. Continuum. 2012; 18(6)

11. You are evaluating a 7-year-old girl for her new-onset headache and nausea. She had a slight headache last night and was given children Motrin. Early morning, she woke up complaining of a "really bad headache," as well as nausea. She felt warm by her mother. Her past medical history is unremarkable. All of her vaccinations are up to date. On examination, temperature is 39 °C. She is uncomfortable and prefers the lights to be dimmed. She refuses to flex her neck and resists passive flexion of the neck. She has a positive Kernig sign. She is alert and oriented in all three spheres. Although in significant pain, she is cooperative in the rest of the neurological exam which is normal. There is no papilledema. She has a vesiculopapular rash on her palms and soles; and small ulcerations on her lips. CSF examination reveals normal opening pressure; 2 RBC/mm^3; 156 WBC/mm^3

(80% lymphocytes, 20% PMN); protein 51 mg/dL; and glucose 70 mg/dL.

What is your likely diagnosis?

A. acute disseminated encephalomyelitis
B. cerebral toxoplasmosis
C. encephalitis due to herpes simplex virus-1
D. meningitis due to enterovirus
E. neuro-cysticercosis

Correct Answer is: D

This is a clinical presentation of meningitis. She has fever, headache, and nuchal rigidity. The CSF profile (lymphocytic pleocytosis, normal glucose) is typical of a viral process. The rash on the palms, soles, and mouth are characteristic for enterovirus. Enteroviruses cause about 80% of all cases of viral meningitis and are more likely to cause infection in the autumn. Acute disseminated encephalolmyelitis (ADEM) is unlikely to be associated with a rash, and children usually appear more ill with focal neurologic deficits and seizures. Cerebral toxoplasmosis and neuro-cysticercosis would be unlikely to present with meningitis symptoms. HSV encephalitis may have a similar CSF profile, but the clinical picture would not be compatible as there are no behavioral or cognitive symptoms.

12

Suggested Reading

- DeBiasi RL, Tyler K. Viral meningitis and encephalitis. Continuum Lifelong Learing Neurol. 2006;12(2):58–94.

12. A 5-week-old baby infant is brought to the ED with lethargy, irritable and refusal to eat. He is a full-term infant who was born via uncomplicated vaginal delivery and had been doing very well until 1 day before admission. He has a low-grade fever this morning. On examination, he has a 39.5 °C fever. Anterior fontanelle is full. He is lethargic, but does become more alert when his neck is moved and moves all four extremities symmetrically. His reflexes are symmetric, 2+ and the plantar responses are extensor. CSF examination reveals cell count 290 WBC/mm^3 with 98% polymorphonuclear cells; 4 RBC/mm^3; protein 45 mg/dL; glucose 10 mg/dL. MRI with gadolinium is obtained with imaging as shown.

What is your likely diagnosis?

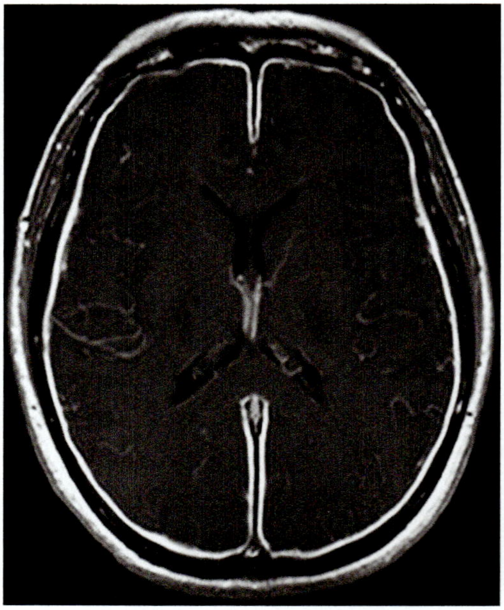

Fig. 12.3 MRI, bacterial meningitis; T1. Own work (Original text: *selbst erstellt.* MBq Disk 12:01, 26. Okt. 2010 (CEST). Wikipedia

A. acute disseminated encephalomyelitis
B. bacterial meningitis
C. cerebral toxoplasmosis
D. fungal meningitis
E. viral encephalitis

Correct Answer is: B

He has fever and lethargy and has meningeal, signs on examination. CNS infec-

tion has to be number one on your list. The CSF showed, polymorphonuclear pleocytosis and depressed glucose, so bacterial meningitis is the most likely diagnosis. The MRI adds further information by demonstrating gadolinium enhancement in the walls of the lateral ventricles, suggesting that this child also has ventriculitis as a complication of meningitis. The MRI is not consistent with acute disseminated encephalomyelitis (ADEM), which would demonstrate T2 lesions in the white matter. Cerebral toxoplasmosis would demonstrate ring-enhancing lesions. Fungal meningitis is possible, but less likely than bacterial meningitis and the CSF profile would usually demonstrate a lymphocytic, or mixed pleocytosis. Viral encephalitis is also unlikely due to the depressed CSF glucose and polymorphonuclear cells.

Suggested Reading

- Bartt R. Acute bacterial and viral meningitis. Continuum Lifelong Learning Neurol. 2012;18(6):1255–89.

13. A 16-year-old healthy female came back from a summer camping trip, is complaining of headache and facial weakness which started upon awakening this morning. She had been sick with generalized headaches for the past 2 weeks. She does not recall having a rash. She is afebrile, but has a mild nuchal rigidity. She has bilateral lower motor neuron facial weakness otherwise the rest of her neurological exam is unremarkable. CSF shows 110 white blood cells (90% lymphocytes), protein of 95 mg/dL, and glucose of 60 mg/dL.
    What is your diagnosis?
    A. Acute HIV infection
    B. Carcinomatous meningitis
    C. Lyme disease
    D. Miller Fisher syndrome
    E. Neurosarcoidosis

Correct Answer is: C
The correct answer is Lyme disease. The clinical scenario is consistent with Lyme disease because of the subacute to chronic meningitis and bifacial weakness, especially she has a recent camping trip with possible recent tick exposure. Not all patients recall having the typical rash, as it is generally painless and may be in a region of the body the patient cannot easily see. Acute HIV infection, neuro-sarcoidosis, and carcinomatous meningitis can cause a similar presentation, but is less likely given the travel history. Miller Fisher syndrome can cause bilateral facial weakness but the CSF profile would not demonstrate a pleocytosis.

Suggested Reading

- Halperin J. Lyme disease: a multisystem infection that affects the nervous system. Continuum Lifelong Learning Neurol. 2012;18(6):1338–50.

14. The mother of a 3-year-old girl brought her for her ongoing poorly controlled seizures despite the use of multiple anti-epileptic medications. Her mother brought a recent CT performed 1 week ago, but the rest of her medical records is not available. On examination, her head circumference is below 5th percentile, she has no visual fixation, and spasticity bilaterally in the lower extremities more than the upper. Reflexes are brisk with sustained clonus at both ankles. No family history of similar condition, and she has two older siblings who are both healthy. She is taken levetiracetam and phenobarbital.
    What abnormal results would you be looking for as a neonate?

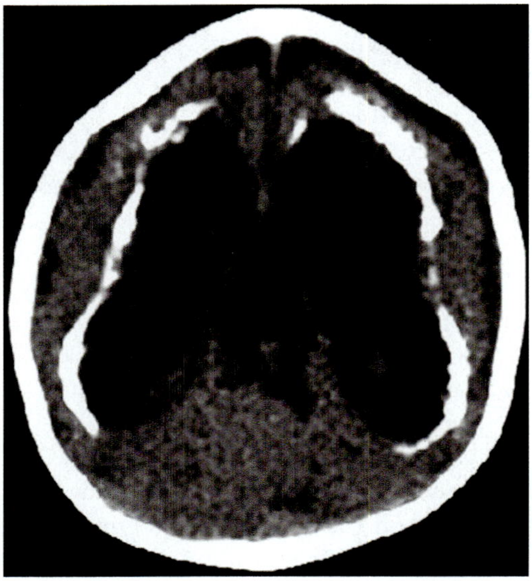

Fig. 12.4 CT, congenital cytomegalovirus (CMV) infection. American Academy of Neurology Institute, produced by permission

A. CT scan revealing a Dandy-Walker malformation
B. genetic testing revealing a mutation in the TSC1 gene region
C. karyotype showing three copies of the 21st chromosome
D. MRI showing aqueductal stenosis
E. urine from the infant positive for cytomegalovirus

Correct Answer is: E

This girl has uncontrolled epilepsy, spasticity, and prominent microcephaly. Her head CT shows very large ventricles with hyperdense signal in the immediate periventricular region, and a very simple appearing cerebral cortex, without any apparent sulcation consistent with lissencephaly. This is a presentation of congenital cytomegalovirus (CMV) infection. Children with Down syndrome (trisomy 21) do not develop a prominent microcephaly and are usually hypotonic on examination, and intracranial calcifications would not be expected. Children with either Dandy-Walker malformation or aqueductal stenosis are at risk for macrocephaly due to non-communicating hydrocephalus. Tuberous sclerosis can lead to calcified sub-ependymal nodules and rarely regions of pachygyria or polymicrogyria, though not lissencephaly. Tuberous sclerosis (TS) does not have such extreme microcephaly. CMV is the most common congenital viral infection, occurring in 1–2% of live births. Fortunately, less than 10% of infants are symptomatic. Severe migrational defects are a consequence of infection early (in the first trimester). Clinical manifestations include intrauterine growth retardation, jaundice, petechiae and purpura (the so-called blueberry muffin spots), severe microcephaly, cerebral calcifications (peri-ventricularly), glaucoma and chorioretinitis. Due to the ubiquitous nature of this virus it is essential that the virus be isolated from one of many different locations in the newborn (most commonly urine and saliva) within the first 2–3 weeks of life to confirm that infection was acquired congenitally. Antiviral therapy may modify the degree of retinal involvement but does not modify the CNS features of the infection. Symptomatic treatment of associated seizures and spasticity is needed for most patients. The outcome can be predicted by the severity of the associated migrational defect. Children with lissencephaly (reported in severe cases of CMV which can impair neuronal migration) have profound delays in development, whereas those with only mild microcephaly and intracranial calcifications may have a milder degree of developmental delay.

15. You are seeing a previously healthy 16-year-old female with 1 day of left facial droop 14 days after camping trip up north. She was seen by her PCP, who prescribed oral prednisone.

3 days later she has right face weakness. On examination, she has moderate to severe bilateral facial weakness but the rest of her general and neurologic examination are unremarkable, and she has no rash.

What test are you going to order to find out the cause of her facial weakness?

A. Serum angiotensin converting enzyme level
B. Serum HIV antibody and antigen testing
C. Serum Lyme antibody
D. CSF cell count and protein
E. CSF varicella zoster virus PCR

Correct Answer is: C

A patient has bilateral facial nerve palsies and coming back from an area of endemic Lyme disease, most likely the cause of her presentation either idiopathic (Bell's) palsy or Lyme disease. Lyme disease is the more likely diagnosis because the simultaneous facial nerves involvement. Bilateral facial nerves involvement can happen in Bell's palsy but less common. As this neurological complication typically occurs within weeks of initial infection of the borrelia burgdorferi organism, serum Lyme antibodies are usually positive (if not, they should be rechecked within 1–2 weeks and the patient treated empirically for Lyme disease). In cases of facial palsy without meningitis, CSF testing is not required to make the diagnosis, though should be performed if there are any signs of meningitis (nuchal rigidity or persistent headache.) Cranial neuropathy is the most common neurological manifestation of sarcoidosis, and the facial nerve is the most frequently involved. Multiple cranial nerve involvement is not rare. The serum ACE level may be elevated in neuro-sarcoidosis but is not sensitive or specific. Sarcoidosis is a less likely diagnosis in this case especially in the absence of other systemic clues and the clear risk factors for Lyme disease. Acute HIV seroconversion has rarely been associated with unilateral or bilateral facial palsy. Because this is an early manifestation, both serum HIV antibody and antigen testing should be obtained as the patient may not have seroconverted. While unlikely to be causative in this case due to the demographics, HIV testing should still be considered based on multiple guidelines recommending routine screening in patients aged 13–65 years of age. Another relatively common cause of simultaneous bilateral facial palsy is the Miller-Fisher variant of Guillain-Barré syndrome. In these cases CSF cell count and total protein showing cytoalbuminologic dissociation is supportive. With the lack of areflexia or ataxia, however, this is an unlikely diagnosis. There are cases reported with preserved reflexes, however, and a spinal fluid exam might be considered if Lyme testing is unrevealing. Varicella zoster reactivation in the geniculate ganglion may lead to vesicular eruption in the ear canal and ipsilateral facial palsy (Ramsay Hunt syndrome). It may rarely occur in the absence of shingles. This is a clinical diagnosis and it may occur without CSF spread of virus, as detected in CSF VZV PCR. Given the young age of the patient, absence of shingles, and the more common occurrence of Lyme disease in this setting, VZV is unlikely.

Suggested Reading

- Halperin JJ, Shapiro ED, Logigian E, Belman AL, Dotevall L, Wormser GP, et al. Practice parameter: treatment of nervous system Lyme disease (an evidence-based review): report of the Quality Standards Subcommittee of the American Academy of Neurology. Neurology. 2007;69(1):91–102. 125.

16. A 16-year-old boy is complaining of a rapid onset lower extremity weakness and facial paralysis, more on the right side than the left. Two days after a He was on a camping trip and 2 days later he started to have congestion, cough and muscle aches. Over the course of the next 48 h he began having trouble walking. He has no rash and but he has remarkable weakness in right leg extensors and flexors, accompanied by flaccid muscle tone, right facial drooping with symmetrical forehead wrinkling. He has normal mental status. EMG indicates severe denervation in affected muscle regions.

What is your diagnosis?

A. Lyme disease
B. West Nile virus infection
C. Acute demyelinating encephalomyelitis
D. Enterovirus infection

Correct answer is: B

Since 1999, West Nile virus has become the most important cause of arboviral meningitis, encephalitis and acute flaccid paralysis in the U.S. The virus is transmitted by an infected mosquito. A flu-like illness develops 3–14 days after the mosquito bite. Sensory symptoms are minimal and encephalopathy does not occur. MRI of the brain can be normal or show white matter demyelination. In this case, the facial weakness is lower motor neuron and there is sparing of the forehead muscle. In West Nile infections, MRI of the spine and electro diagnostic studies are consistent with lower motor neuron and ventral horn pathology.

Lyme meningitis is presented initially by intermittent attacks of severe headache and mild meningismus. Some will develop signs of mild encephalitis and cranial neuritis, most commonly lower motor neuron facial palsy. Peripheral nerve disease is characterized with symmetrical, distal paresthesias with sensory loss on examination.

The presenting features of acute disseminated encephalomyelitis include a rapid onset encephalopathy with multifocal neurologic signs and deficits. Peripheral nerve deficient are not characteristic of this condition.

Poliovirus is the most devastating enterovirus infection and causes severe paralysis. Coxackie virus and echovirus are enterovirus, but more likely to cause aseptic meningitis. Initial symptoms are fever, sore throat, and malaise and gastrointestinal illness.

Suggested Reading

- Solomon T, Ooi MH, Beasley DW, Mallewa M. West Nile encephalitis. BMJ: Br Med J. 2003;326(7394):865.

17. A 14-year-old female symptoms were not improved after been on amoxicillin for 2 days for her otitis media and low-grade fever and she developed episodes of severe vertigo.

What is the cause of her vertigo?

A. Hypervolemia secondary to illness
B. Meningitis
C. Amoxicillin toxicity
D. Acute serous labyrinthitis

Correct answer is: D

Viral or bacterial ear infection can be followed by rapid onset of vertigo. Labyrinth mechanisms can be irritated and stimulate vestibular actions can occur secondary to direct extension of the infection to the inner ear, as well as local effects of bacterial toxins.

Hypervolemia, orthostatic hypotension and syncope can occur with illnesses due to reduced intake and fever but the symptom is mainly light-headedness.

Meningitis is a major cause of vestibular and auditory dysfunction in chil-

12

dren, but meningismus must be present. Amoxicillin toxicity is not associated with vertigo, but aminoglycosides, anticonvulsants, streptomyci n and minocycline toxicity can cause vestibular symptoms.

Suggested Reading

Kishore A. Assessment and management of pediatric vestibular disorders. ECAB Dizziness and Vertigo across Age Groups, 2014.

18. A 16-year-old female was admitted to the hospital with a two-day history of fever, headache, nausea and vomiting. This morning her mother found her confused and lethargic. On your examination, you found that she had a moderate left hemiparesis. Her CSF showed: 250 white blood cells/mm^3 (79% leukocytes), 350 red blood cells/mm^3, protein of 95 mg/dl and normal glucose levels.
   What test findings will provide sufficient presumptive evidence to make a diagnosis?
   A. Periodic lateralizing epileptiform discharges
   B. Right cerebral slowing on EEG
   C. Non-contrast CT
   D. Right temporal increased signal intensity on T2 MRI

Correct answer is: D
Temporal regions are significantly have been affected more than other brain regions in herpes encephalitis. T2 weighted imaging identifies the earliest stage of herpes encephalitis that most commonly involves the cortex and white matter in the temporal and inferior frontal lobes. On subsequent imaging, independent foci enlarge then coalesce and in severe cases result in encephalomalacia of the temporal lobe. The confirmatory test is spinal fluid PCR for the herpes virus.

Before the MRI era, periodic lateralizing epileptiform discharges (PLEDS) was the most the predictive study.

Although background slowing is seen with encephalitis, slowing itself is not specific to herpes encephalitis. Focal slowing is seen commonly in areas of cortical strokes or large tumors. Noncontrast CT is most useful in acute trauma or suspected arterial hemorrhage, as it can rapidly be utilized to identify intracranial blood.

Suggested Reading

Songmen S, Panta OB, Maharjan S, Paudel S, Ansari MA, Ghimire RK. A Retrospective Study of Magnetic Resonance Imaging Findings in Acute Encephalitis Syndrome. J Inst Med. 2015;38(2).

19. You are evaluating a 17-year-old male in the ER for his headache, nausea, vomiting, photophobia, neck pain, and fever of 39C. On examination, he has right VI CN palsy and right upper and lower facial droop. Funduscopic examination revealed no papilledema and spontaneous venous pulsations are present. The boy cries out in pain and lifts his knees on passive neck flexion during his exam. He has no other focal neurological signs.
   What is your next step in management?
   A. Head CT followed by administration of vancomycin and ceftriaxone IV followed by a lumbar puncture
   B. Lumbar puncture followed by head CT followed by administration of vancomycin and ceftriaxone IV
   C. Lumbar puncture followed by immediate administration of vancomycin and ceftriaxone IV
   D. Immediate administration of vancomycin and ceftriaxone IV with no further action because lumbar puncture is contraindicated

Correct answer is: C

Head CT is recommended prior to lumbar puncture based on the recommendations of the Infectious Diseases Society of America if the patient has papilledema, focal neurological deficits, recent neurosurgery or trauma, hydrocephalus, or a CSF shunt, or immunocompromised. In this case, the patient does have focal neurological deficits on exam. However, cranial nerve VI and VII palsies are specifically excluded and thus, this patient does not need a head CT prior to lumbar puncture. When the lumbar puncture can be done immediately, this should be performed followed by empiric therapy which in this case includes vancomycin and a third-generation cephalosporin.

If the patient needs a CT scan before the LP based on the criteria described above, treatment should not wait until head CT is done. Poorer outcomes are associated with delays in therapy. Typically, the head CT would precede the lumbar puncture if it is even necessary. Again, empiric treatment should not be delayed.

12

Empiric treatment with antibiotics in this age group vancomycin and a third-generation cephalosporin like ceftriaxone, should be started prior to gram stain and culture results. The major pathogens are Neisseria meningitidis and Streptococcus pneumoniae in patients between the ages of 24 months and 50 years old.

Suggested Reading

- Tunkel AR, Hartman BJ, Kaplan SL, et al. Practice guidelines for the management of bacterial meningitis. Clin Infect Dis. 2004;39:1267.
- Kaplan SL. Bacterial meningitis in children older than one month: clinical features and diagnosis. In: Up-to-date, Edwards MS, Nordli DR, Armsby C, editors. Up-to-date. Waltham. Accessed on 20 Dec 2015.
- Kaplan SL. Bacterial meningitis in children older than one month: treatment and prognosis. In: Up-to-date, Edwards MS, Nordli DR, Armsby C, editors Up-to-date. Waltham. Accessed on 20 Dec 2015.

20. You are seeing a 12-year-old male in the ED for his fever, headache, nausea, vomiting, lethargy, and a seizure just after he arrived to the ED. You have done a lumbar puncture and you will send CSF for analysis.

What set of orders will you send for?

A. Opening pressure, protein, glucose cell count and differential, PCR for Herpes Simplex 1 and 2, PCR for enterovirus, PCR for varicella zoster virus, and bacterial culture
B. Opening pressure, protein, glucose, cell count and differential, and bacterial culture
C. Opening pressure, protein, glucose, cell count and differential, bacterial culture, and herpes simplex 1 and 2 viral culture.
D. Opening pressure, protein, glucose, cell count and differential, and west
E. Nile virus PCR

Correct answer is: A

If you are ordering CSF analysis as part of the work up for suspected viral encephalitis, the minimum you have to order includes, opening pressure, protein, glucose, cell count and differential, and PCR for herpes virus 1 and 2, varicella zoster, and enterovirus. Other viral testing can be performed as well based on clinical presentation or geographic area, but HSV1, HSV2, VZV, and enterovirus are the highest yield.

Viral culture is not recommended. PCR for HSV 1 and 2 should be performed, not culture.

HSV, VZV, and enterovirus PCR are recommended in the initial examination of cerebrospinal fluid. While in some cases, it is appropriate to order testing for West Nile virus, this is not the best answer as HSV and enterovirus testing are not included in this order set. And actually, in those with West Nile Virus which is causing central nervous system disease, viral PCR of the cerebrospinal fluid is only 55% sensitive. A diagnosis can be made based on IgM antibodies specific to west Nile virus in the cerebrospinal fluid. Thus, even if west Nile virus is suspected, PCR may be negative and thus insufficient for diagnosis.

Suggested Reading

- Di Pentima C. Viral meningitis: clinical features and diagnosis in children. In: Up-to-date, Edwards MS, Nardi DR, Armsby C, editors. Up-to-date. Waltham. Accessed on 20 Dec 2015.
- Tunkel AR, Glaser CA, Bloch KC, Sejvarl J, Marra CM, Roos KL, Hartman BJ, Kaplan SL, Scheid WM, Whitley RJ. The management of encephalitis: clinical practice guidelines by the infectious diseases society of America. Clin Infect Dis. 2008;47:303–27.
- Hardarson HS. Acute viral encephalitis in children and adolescents: clinical manifestations and diagnosis. In: Up-to-date, Kaplan SL, Fleisher GR, Nordli DR, Armsby C, editors. Up-to-date. Waltham. Accessed on 20 Dec 2015.
- Hardarson HS. Acute viral encephalitis in children and adolescents: pathogenesis and etiology. In: Up-to-date, Edwards MS, Armsby C, editors. Up-to-date. Waltham. Accessed on 20 Dec 2015.
- Keen R, Michael BO, Menson E, Mehta B, Easton A, Hemingway C, Klapper PE, Vincent A, Lim M, Carrol E, Solomon T. Management of suspected viral encephalitis in children e Association of British Neurologists and British Paediatric Allergy Immunology and Infection Group National Guidelines. J Infect. 2012;64:449–77.
- Solomon T, Hart IJ, Beeching NJ. Viral encephalitis: a clinician's guide. Pract Neural. 2007;7(5):288–305.
- Petersen LR. Clinical manifestations and diagnosis of West Nile virus infection. In: Up-to-date, Hirsch MS, Mitty J, editors. Up-to-date. Waltham. Accessed on 20 Dec 2015.

21. A 6-month-old baby boy is brought to the ED with severe hypotonia and respiratory distress. His mother started him on different solid foods in the last 2 weeks. 3 days ago, he had constipation and "seemed weak". One day ago, the infant had a poor suck, droopy eyelids and was unable to feed normally. On neurological exam, he has severe hypotonia, absent tendon reflexes, limited facial movement, and ptosis and dilated pupils.
What test will you order to make the diagnosis?
A. CT of the brain
B. MRI of the cervical spinal cord
C. Edrophonium test
D. Stool culture

Correct answer is: D
Clostridium botulinum infects the infants from contaminated formula, ingestion of contaminated honey or inhaled from dust from nearby construction. The solid foods in this vignette may have included honey.

The growth of clostridium botulinum can be tested by Stool culture. The typical prodromal symptoms are constipation and poor feeding. The pathophysiology is a cholinergic blockade of skeletal muscle and autonomic nerves caused by the exotoxin. Progressive facial, pharyngeal weakness, ptosis, dilated pupils, absent reflexes and constipation differentiate infantile botulism from other inflammatory demyelinating and neuromuscular junction disorders.

Brain MRI is of no value in the diagnosis, because it is a neuromuscular junction disease.

The spinal cord is not affected in infantile botulism.

Familial infantile myasthenia is a rare form of myasthenia. Administration of edrophonium will rapidly reverse the symptoms in myasthenia related conditions. The condition occurs: in the absence of myasthenia in the mother, with respiratory depression at birth, episodic weakness and apnea during the first 2 years of life. Familial infantile myasthenia typically improves with age. Since the condition responds to anticholinesterase medication, early diagnosis is important. Infantile myasthenia syndromes does not present with dilated pupils, absent reflexes or constipation.

Suggested Reading

- Mitchell WG, Tseng-Ong L. Catastrophic presentation of infant botulism may obscure or delay diagnosis. Pediatrics. 2005;116(3):e436–8.

12

22. A 13-year-old male came to the ED with headache, nuchal rigidity, and fever. On examination, he has no focal neurological signs. A lumbar puncture was performed, and showed that the patient has viral meningitis.
Which CSF results from below are most consistent with viral meningitis?
    A. WBC < 5 cells/mm^3, no neutrophils, protein of 20 mg/dl, glucose of 60 mg/dl
    B. WBC 100 cells/mm^3, 30% neutrophils, protein of 50 mg/dl, glucose of 60 mg/dl
    C. WBC 200 cells/mm^3, 70% neutrophils, protein of 110 mg/dl, glucose of 30 mg/dl
    D. WBC 200 cells/mm^3, 40% neutrophils, protein of 209 mg/dl, glucose of 30 mg/dl

Correct answer is: B

B is most consistent with viral meningitis. Neutrophils may be present, typically early in the infection, but typically do not account for more than 50% of the white blood cells present. White blood cells range from 100 to 500 cells per mm^3. Protein may be elevated but is typically under 100 mg/dl. Glucose is usually normal although may be decreased in patients with mumps or herpes simplex.

In normal adults, up to 5 cells per mm^3 leukocyte is acceptable with no neutrophils. Normal leukocyte count may be higher in preterm infants; in this case normal cerebrospinal fluid has less than 20 cells per mm^3. In term infants, up to 2 months of age, cerebrospinal fluid may contain up to 15 cells per mm^3, and still be considered normal Protein should be between 15 and 50 mg/dl.

In acute bacterial meningitis, WBC cells are more than 100 to 500 cells per mm^3, mostly neutrophils, and protein is 100–500 mg/dl. Glucose is often low, under 40 mg/dl; if the patient is hyperglycemic, glucose may be corrected to under 60% of the total serum value.

In tuberculous meningitis, WBC may range from 10 to 500 cells per mm^3, glucose is often decreased, and protein may range from 100 to 500 mg/dl. Neutrophils may be present in greater numbers earlier in the infection. In 3% of children and 6% of adults with tuberculous meningitis, cell count is normal. 16% of children, and 6% of adults may have normal protein and 77% of children and 72% of adults have glucose of under 45 mg/dL in the cerebrospinal fluid.

Suggested Reading

- Pomar V, Domingo P. Acute viral meningitis. In: Garda-Monc JC, editors. CNS infections: a clinical approach. London: Springer;2014:45–55.

- Garcfa-Monc JC, Rodriguez-Sainz A. CNS tuberculosis and other mycobacterial infections. In Garda-Monc, JC, editors. CNS Infections: a clinical approach. London: Springer;2014:139–61.
- Gomez-Beldarrain M, Garcfa-Monc MDJC. Lumbar puncture and CSF analysis and interpretation. In Garcfa-Monc, JC, editors. CNS infections: a clinical approach. London: Springer;2014:1–16.

23. A 16-year-old boy from Cuba came to the ED after having a focal right arm shaking seizure for 5 min and resolved spontaneously. Head CT was ordered and shows a round 10 mm hypodense cystic lesion in the left frontal lobe. You ordered MRI which showed a small, hyperintense spot within the cystic lesion. The radiology attending reads as a scolex.
Which of the following is most likely true?
    A. The patient has definitive neuro-cysticercosis
    B. A diagnosis of definitive neuro-cysticercosis can be made in this case in the absence of brain biopsy.
    C. Again, the patient has definitive neuro-cysticercosis based on imaging findings and does not need serological testing
    D. The patient does not need cerebrospinal fluid testing in order to confirm this diagnosis.

Correct answer is: A
Absolute criteria include (1) demonstration of parasite histologically on brain biopsy, (2) the presence of a cystic lesion with scolex on neuro imaging, and (3) the presence of sub-retinal parasites, seen on funduscopic exam.

Major criteria include (1) Lesions that are highly suggestive of the diagnosis on imaging, (2) anticysticercal antibodies in serum determined by enzyme-linked immunoelectrotransfer blot assay (EITB), (3) intracranial lesion resolution with appropriate treatment (albendazole or praziquantel), and (4) the presence of one enhancing lesion that resolves spontaneously.

Minor criteria include (1) lesions that are compatible with the diagnosis, (2) clinical findings that are suggestive of this diagnosis, (3) anticysticercal antibodies or antigens within cerebrospinal fluid determined by ELISA, and (4) cysticercosis documented outside the central nervous system.

Epidemiologic criteria include (1) known household member who has Taenia solium infection, (2) frequent travel to areas where the disease is endemic, and (3) history of living in an area where the disease is endemic.

The presence of one absolute criterion- in this case the presence of a scolex on neuro imaging- allows for a definitive diagnosis of neuro-cysticercosis. A definitive diagnosis can be made in the presence of 1 epidemiologic criterion, 1 minor criterion, and 2 major criteria. If a patient has 1 major criterion and 2 minor criteria, a diagnosis of probable neuro-cysticercosis can be made. If a patient has 1 major criterion, 1 minor criterion, and 1 epidemiologic criterion OR if a patient has 3 minor criteria and 1 epidemiologic criterion, a diagnosis of probable neuro-cysticercosis can be made.

A diagnosis of definitive neuro-cysticercosis can be made in this case in the absence of brain biopsy.

Again, the patient has definitive neuro-cysticercosis based on imaging findings and does not need serological testing.

The patient does not need cerebrospinal fluid testing in order to confirm this diagnosis.

Suggested Reading

- White AC. Epidemiology, transmission, and prevention of cysticercosis. In: Up-to-date, Weller PF, Baron EL, editors. Up-to-date. Waltham. Accessed on 20 Dec 2015.
- White AC. Clinical manifestations and diagnosis of cysticercosis. In: Up-to-date, Weller PF, Baron EL, editors. Up-to-date. Waltham. Accessed on 20 Dec 2015.
- White AC. Treatment of cysticercosis. In: Up-to-date, Weller PF, Baron EL, editors. Up-to-date. Waltham. Accessed on 20 Dec 2015.
- Dhawan VK. Pediatric neuro-cysticercosis. In: Kumar A, Barton LL, Kossoff EH, editors. Medscape Reference. ▶ http://emedicine.medscape.com/article/999053-overview (▶ http://emedicine.medscape.com/article/999053-overview). Updated March 3 2015, Accessed 21 Dec 2015.
- Rodriguez S, Wilkins P, Dorny P. Immunological and molecular diagnosis of cysticercosis. Path Glob Health. 2012;106:286–98.
- Baird RA, Wiebe S, ZuntJR, HalperinJJ, Gronseth G, Roos KL. Evidence-based guidelines: Treatment of parenchymal neuro-cysticercosis: Report of the guideline development subcommittee of the American Academy of Neurology. Neurology. 2013;80:1424–29.
- Garcia Prof HH, Nash TE, Del Brutto OH. Lancet Neurol. 2014;13(1):1202–15.
- Lucato LT, Guedes MS, Sato JR, Bacheschi LA, Machado LR, Leite CC. The role of conventional MR imaging sequences in the evaluation of neuro-cysticercosis: impact on characterization of the scolex and lesion burden. Am J Neuroradiol. 2007;36(12):1501–04.

12

24. A 2-day old baby was treated empirically with gentamicin and ampicillin for suspected meningitis. His CSF results showed an infection with group B streptococcus.

What is your next best step in management?

A. Gentamicin should be discontinued immediately
B. Repeat lumbar puncture should be performed in a week; if cells, protein, and glucose are normal, all antibiotics can be discontinued.
C. Repeat lumbar puncture should be performed in 24–48 h; if cells protein, and glucose are normal, gentamicin and ampicillin can be discontinued, although penicillin G should be started for a total treatment period of 14–21 days
D. Repeat lumbar puncture should be performed in 24–48 h; if cells protein, and glucose are normal, ampicillin can be discontinued, although treatment with gentamicin should continue for 14 to 21 days.

Correct answer is: C
Premature rupture of membranes, chorioamnionitis, and GBS bacteriuria during pregnancy, prior delivery of an infected infant, the presence of fever during labor and delivery, or delivery at under 37 weeks are the risks factors for early onset group B streptococcal disease (GBS). Gentamicin and ampicillin is recommended as an empiric treatment for infants with suspected meningitis at 2 days of age. Penicillin G is the treatment of choice if GBS meningitis has been confirmed. However, it is recommended that CSF to be obtained 24–48 h after the onset of therapy. If sterilization is confirmed, then gentamicin and ampicillin can be discontinued; penicillin G should be started and antibiotics should continue for 14–21 days.

Suggested Reading

- Tunkel AR, Hartman BJ, Kaplan SL, et al. Practice guidelines for the management of bacterial meningitis. Clin Infect Dis. 2004;39:1267.

- Edwards MS, Baker CJ. Bacterial meningitis in the neonate: clinical features and diagnosis. In: Up-to-date, Kaplan SL, Weisman LE, Armsby C, editors. Up-to-date. Waltham. Accessed on 20 Dec 2015.
- Edwards MS, Baker CJ. Bacterial meningitis in the neonate: treatment and outcome. In: Up-to-date, Kaplan SL, Weisman LE, Armsby C, editors. Up-to-date. Waltham. Accessed on 20 Dec 2015.

25. A 14-year-old boy has been admitted to hospital with headache and altered mental status after he had a generalized seizure. A lumbar puncture is performed, opening pressure is normal, and there is a white cell count of 50 mainly neutrophil, protein is slightly elevated at 55 and glucose is normal. He was treated with acyclovir empirically for suspected herpes simplex encephalitis. Finally, the diagnosis is confirmed by HSV1 and 2 PCR. After a few days of acyclovir treatment, the drug becomes unavailable nationwide and becomes expensive to the patients and the hospital. The patient has confirmed herpes simplex encephalitis.

    What should the worried you do?

    A. You should do nothing- if there is no acyclovir, he cannot treat herpes simplex encephalitis
    B. You should start ganciclovir immediately at a dose of 5 mg/kg every 12 h.
    C. You should start foscarnet IV immediately at a dose of 60
    D. Mg/kg every 12 h
    E. You should wait for acyclovir to become available- surely the person responsible will end up in jail for securities fraud soon

Correct answer is: B

A dose of 10 mg/kg has to be used to treat HSV encephalitis in a child of at least 12 years of age for 3 weeks. Although if the CSF is still positive for infection on repeat testing, the treatment may need to be prolonged. IV ganciclovir is recommended as a substitution if acyclovir becomes unavailable, given every 12 h at a dose of 5 mg/kg.

You have to monitor the patient for thrombocytopenia, leukopenia, or anemia.

If ganciclovir is not available, foscarnet can be used. Although foscarnet can also be used in place of acyclovir during drug shortages, ganciclovir is recommended as a first choice. Foscarnet can cause renal insufficiency and electrolytes should be monitored.

The patient needs to be treated. He cannot wait for acyclovir to become available.

Suggested Reading

- Hardarson HS. Acute viral encephalitis in children and adolescents: Treatment and prevention. In: Up-to-date, Edwards MS, Fleisher GR, Nordli DR, Armsby C, editors. Up-To- Date. Waltham. Accessed on 20 Dec 2015.
- Zachary KC. Acyclovir: an overview. In: Up-to-date, Hirsch MS. Mitty J, editors. Up-to-date. Waltham. Accessed on 20 Dec 2015.

26. A 22-month-old boy was seen with his family in your office for a second opinion. 2 weeks ago, he was admitted to the PICU with a 101.5 F temperature, irritability, and lethargy and neck pain because of the suspicion of meningitis. You reviewed the lab results provided to his family upon discharge. The CSF showed 25 leukocytes/mm^3, 95% lymphocytes, protein concentration of 65 mg/dl and glucose concentration of 70. He was treated with antibiotics and his blood and spinal fluid cultures were negative at discharge 5 days later.

    What is the likely diagnosis?

    A. Migraine headache
    B. Asceptic meningitis
    C. Self-limiting mild encephalitis
    D. Lyme disease

Correct answer is: B
Aseptic meningitis and bacterial meningitis can have the same clinical presentation. But, bacterial meningitis can cause more aggressive and severe symptoms and sequela. The relatively low spinal fluid protein level, normal glucose and the moderately elevated cell count with lymphocytic predominance are highly suggestive of viral or aseptic meningitis.

In older children and adults, migraine headaches can present with stiff neck and focal neurological disturbances. Migraine headaches are uncommon in children under 2, and typically do not present with a fever.

By definition, persons with encephalitis present with an altered mental status and most progress to seizures with a prolonged recovery phase. The spinal fluid analysis may be similar to those described in this case.

Although Lyme disease can cause meningitis, it is rarely a presenting manifestation and is rarely occurs in children this age.

Suggested Reading

- Cohn KA, Thompson AO, Shah SS, Hines EM,Lyons TW, Welsh EJ, Nigrovic LE. Validation of a clinical prediction rule to distinguish Lyme meningitis from aseptic meningitis. Pediatrics. 2012;129(1):e46–53.

27. You are examining a 16-month-old boy comes with vomiting, irritability, and appetite loss. His immunizations are not up to date because his mother has a concern over the side effects. On exam, he is febrile with temperature of 39C and appears lethargic. When you attempted to check his pupils, he cried, and closed his eyes. He resisted attempts to bend his head forward. There are no focal deficits on neurological exam.

What is your next step in management?

A. Obtain blood and cerebrospinal fluid samples, send for cultures, and treat based on the results
B. Obtain blood and cerebrospinal fluid samples but immediately start ampicillin and meropenem while waiting for results
C. Obtain blood and cerebrospinal fluid samples but immediately start dexamethasone, vancomycin and, cefotaxime while waiting for results
D. Obtain blood and cerebrospinal fluid samples but immediately start vancomycin; dexamethasone can be given an hour after the antibiotics are started.

Correct answer is: C
If you suspected bacterial meningitis in children over 1 year of age, and in adults up to 50 years of age, vancomycin and a third-generation cephalosporin should be started for empiric coverage.

Potential pathogens include Streptococcus pneumonia, Neisseria meningitidis, Streptococcus agalactiae, Haemophilus influenza, and Escherichia coli. In patients between 1 and 3 months of age, Streptococcus agalactiae is most common followed by Streptococcus pneumonia and then Neisseria meningitidis. In those at least 3 months of age but under 3 years of age, Streptococcus pneumonia is most common, followed by Neisseria meningitidis, Streptococcus agalactiae and then gram-negative bacilli.

Patients at least 3 years of age but under 10 years of age tend to have Streptococcus pneumonia and Neisseria meningitidis. Overall, the most common pathogens in fully vaccinated children are Streptococcus pneumonia and Neisseria meningitidis although in this

case, the child is not fully vaccinated. Regardless, vancomycin and a third-generation cephalosporin are used empirically to cover the most common pathogens, accounting for antibiotic resistance. Dexamethasone is recommended in those with meningitis due to Haemophilus influenza type b to mitigate hearing loss. Use in other cases is controversial; clinicians can consider giving this drug in those older than 6 weeks who have meningitis due to Pneumococcal bacteria. This is the best answer only because there are no obvious contraindications to dexamethasone use, and also, it is the only answer that includes immediate use of the correct empiric therapy. If antibiotic therapy is given immediately, dexamethasone is not recommended if over an hour has passed.

Anti-microbial therapy should be started at once in an individual with suspected bacterial meningitis. It is not prudent to wait for cultures, gram stain, cell count, protein level, or glucose within the spinal fluid prior to treating. Ideally, cerebrospinal fluid is obtained prior to the start of antibiotics; however, one should not wait for any results. Treatment should start at once. If cerebrospinal fluid cannot be obtained immediately, treatment should start regardless and cerebrospinal fluid obtained later if possible.

Meropenem coverage includes Listeria monocytogenes, Staphylococcus aureus, Escherichia coli, Streptococcus pneumoniae, Haemophilus influenza, and Pseudomonas aeruginosa.4 Ampicillin coverage includes, among other pathogens, Listeria monocytogenes and Streptococcus agalactiae. In a child under 1 month old, empiric treatment includes ampicillin and cefotaxime or ampicillin and an aminoglycoside like gentamicin, to cover for Streptococcus agalactiae, Escherichia coli, Listeria monocytogenes, and Klebsiella. In those over age 50, ampicillin is added empirically to vancomycin and a third-generation cephalosporin to cover Listeria monocytogenes. Meropenem may be used empirically with vancomycin in suspected cases of meningitis occurring post neurosurgery. In this case, coverage should include Pseudomonas aeruginosa and other aerobic gram-negative bacilli, Staphylococcus aureus, and Staphylococcus epidermidis. Similarly, vancomycin and meropenem may be used in patients with suspected meningitis occurring after penetrating head trauma. The same regimen may be used empirically in a patient with a CSF shunt in place, when bacterial meningitis is suspected. In this case, coverage needs to include Staphylococcus epidermidis, Staphylococcus aureus, Pseudomonas aeruginosa, and Propionibacterium acnes.

If dexamethasone is given, it should be given within 20 min of the first dose of antibiotics, if it is not given just prior to the first dose. Dexamethasone may actually interfere with the ability of anti-microbials to cross the blood brain barrier. Dexamethasone is not recommended an hour after antibiotics have been given.

Suggested Reading

- Kaplan SL. Bacterial meningitis in children: dexamethasone and other measures to prevent neurological complications. In: up-to-date, Edwards MS, Nordi DR, Armsby C, editors. Up-To –Date. Waltham. Accessed on 20 Dec 2015.
- Kaplan SL. Bacterial meningitis in children older than one month: clinical features and diagnosis. In: up-to-date, Edwards MS, Nordli DR, Armsby C, editors. Up-to-date. Waltham. Accessed on 20 Dec 2015.

- Kaplan SL. Bacterial meningitis in children older than one month: treatment and prognosis. In: up-to-date, Edwards MS, Nordli DR, Armsby c, editors. Update. Waltham. Accessed on 20 Dec 2015.
- Tunkel AR, Hartman BJ, Kaplan SL, et al. Practice guidelines for the management of bacterial meningitis. Clin Infect Dis. 2004;39:1267.

28. A 7-year-old female is seen in the ED with suspected bacterial meningitis. After you done with her history and physical and reviewed her lab tests, you determined that she has a very low risk of bacterial meningitis, despite having 15 white blood cells per microliter in her cerebrospinal fluid.

Which of the following is most likely correct?

A. She has a positive CSF gram stain and presented with a seizure
B. She has a peripheral blood absolute neutrophil count of 15,000 cells per microliter
C. Her CSF protein is 40 mg/dl
D. She has an absolute neutrophil count of 1500 cells per microliter in the cerebrospinal fluid

12

Correct answer is: C

The Bacterial Meningitis Score can be used to determine whether a child has a lower risk of bacterial meningitis in the setting of cerebrospinal fluid with at least 10 cells per microliter. Those who do NOT have (1) a positive cerebrospinal fluid gram stain (2) history of seizure (3) peripheral blood absolute neutrophil count (ANC) of at least 10,000 cells per microliter (4) cerebrospinal fluid absolute neutrophil count (ANC) of at least 1000 cells per microliter, or (5) a cerebrospinal fluid protein of at least 80 mg/dl are at low risk of having bacterial meningitis. The patient in this case has a protein of under 80 mg/dL.

Patients who do NOT have CSF gram stain positivity and who did NOT present with seizure are at lower risk of bacterial meningitis.

Patients who do NOT have an absolute neutrophil count of at least 10,000 cells per microliter in the peripheral blood are at lower risk of having bacterial meningitis. Patients who do NOT have an absolute neutrophil count in the cerebrospinal fluid of at least 1000 cells per microliter are at lower risk of having bacterial meningitis.

Suggested Reading

- Nigrovic LE, Kuppermann N, Macias CG, et al. Clinical prediction rule for identifying children with cerebrospinal fluid pleocytosis at *very* low risk of bacterial meningitis. JAMA. 2007;297:52.

29. Which of the following is most true about pediatric neuro-cysticercosis?

A. Most pediatric cases involve multiple cysts.
B. Enzyme linked immunoelectrotransfer blot assay (EITB) can be used to confirm a diagnosis in a child with a single intracranial lesion given specificity of 100% and sensitivity of 90%
C. The most common initial clinical manifestation in children is a seizure
D. This condition is most often diagnosed in children in the first 24 months of life

Correct answer is: C

Seizures are the most common presentations in children up to 65–80% of cases. Majority have a single lesion at diagnosis as well. Focal sensory or motor deficits, headache, vomiting, or mental status changes are less common presentations.

¾ of children will have single intracranial lesion at diagnosis. About 50% may have a scolex visible as a small focus of hyperdensity within the lesion.

ELISA (enzyme linked immunoelectrotransfer) can be used in order to determine whether antibodies to Taenia solium are present in the CSF or blood. The sensitivity and specificity of this test may vary, however. In those with at least 2 known viable central nervous system cysts, sensitivity is as high as 98%. However, in those with 1 cyst, sensitivity may be between 50 and 60%. In children with 3 or more lesions, sensitivity is 90% while specificity is up to 100%.

In children below 24 months of age, the diagnosis cannot be made because the life cycle and incubation period of the parasite. Taenia solium is ingested by pigs; following this, oncospheres, which have passed through the intestinal wall during digestion, travel to the muscles where cysticerci form. Humans, upon ingestion of the cysticerci through improper cooking and/ or handling of pork, are not immediately infected with cysticercosis. Adult worms grow in the small intestine until eggs (via the fecal oral route) are ingested. After this, oncospheres travel through the body, reaching the liver, central nervous system, musculature, and other tissues. Thus, infection is not instantaneous and tends not to manifest in babies or children under 24 months of age.

Suggested Reading

- White AC. Epidemiology, transmission, and prevention of cysticercosis. In: up-to-date, Weller PF, Baron EL, editors. Up-to-date. Waltham. Accessed on 20 Dec 2015.
- Dhawan VK. Pediatric neuro-cysticercosis. In: Kumar A. Barton LL, Kossoff EH, editors. Medscape Reference. ▶ http://emedicine.medscape.Com/article/999053-overview (▶ http://emedicine.medscape.com/article/999053-overview). Updated March 3 2015, Accessed 21 Dec 2015.
- Rodriguez S, Wilkins P, Dorny P. Immunological and molecular diagnosis of cysticercosis. Path Glob Health. 2012;106:286–98.
- White AC. Clinical manifestations and diagnosis of cysticercosis. In: Up-to-date, Weller PF, Baron EL, editors. Up-to-date. Waltham. Accessed on 20 Dec 2015.

30. A 16-year-old female was admitted to the ICU after she has a sudden onset of altered mental status and seizures. Her mother reported that the girl had a temperature of 102 F 2 days ago accompanied with, vomiting, diarrhea, headache, myalgia, hypotension and desquamating rash. She started to be agitated and confused in the last 24 ours. She experienced a generalized seizure 2 h before. She has a negative toxicology screens. A lumbar puncture showed normal opening pressure and protein level with no cells. Brain MRI was normal. She has a normal past medical history and developmental history is normal. **What is the likely etiology of this condition?**
    A. Staphylococcus aureus
    B. Measles virus
    C. Rhabdovirus
    D. Ecstacy (MOMA) overdose

Correct answer is: A

The presentation is most likely of toxic shock syndrome, which can be a fatal illness that is caused by infection or colonization of staphylococcus. This can result from tampon use in menstruating females, but has also been reported to occur in children requiring occlusive surgical dressings. The onset is sudden, rapid and presents as described above. Signs of lethargy, obtundation, encephalopathy and generalized seizures can have happened rapidly. Complications can include cardiac arrhythmias, pulmonary edema and renal failure. Clinical course and cultures of the infected areas are diagnostic.

Measles presents with a morbilform rash and the clinical presentation does not progress to the described severity.

Rabies occurs from a bite or scratch from an infected animal and presents with fever, myalgia and paresthesias. Neurological symptoms include hyper-excitability, autonomic dysfunction. The paralytic manifestations include flaccid paralysis in the bitten limb that progressively ascends to involve the remainder of the body.

Ecstacy overdose presents in a similar fashion to other stimulant class drugs. High does have been reported to cause hyperpyrexia, rhabdomyolysis, intravascular coagulopathy, hepatic necrosis, cardiac arrhythmia and stroke. These symptoms can occur in reported doses associated with "recreational" doses.

Suggested Reading

- Chan BC, Maurice P. Staphylococcal toxic shock syndrome. New Eng J Med. 2013;369(9):852.

12

31. A 16-year-old male presents with headache and severe pain radiating down his low back to the right leg 4 weeks after he came back from a camping trip. He complains also from paresthesias in his left hand and right foot. He reports having a rash that started 2 weeks ago, which seems to be migrating and looks round and erythematous with a paler center. **Which of the following is incorrect regarding this condition?**
    - A. Ceftriaxone is used for the treatment of this condition
    - B. Doxycycline can be used for the treatment in the setting of normal CSF
    - C. Bacterial meningitis with predominance of neutrophils is a common manifestation
    - D. There are early and late neurologic manifestations of the disease
    - E. Approximately 10% of asymptomatic people in endemic areas may be seropositive for this organism

Correct answer is: C

The clinical presentation is of Lyme disease. Lyme disease has a wide variety of neurologic presentations; but bacterial meningitis with neutrophilic predominance is unlikely to occur. Subdural empyema is not seen in Lyme disease. It is caused by Borrelia burgdorferi. It is more commonly acquired in the Northeastern United States and is transmitted by a tick bite, more specifically the Ixodes tick. Neurologic complications can occur in both early phase and a late phase of the disease. A rash called erythema migrans, which is characteristic and has a "bull's eye" appearance occurs in the early phase. Other non- neurologic manifestations include carditis, arthralgias, lymphadenopathy, and fever.

Neurologic manifestations in the early phase include the following: - Aseptic meningitis: these patients have a mononuclear pleocytosis and mild elevation of protein levels in the CSF, as well as intrathecal production of antibodies against Borreliaburgdorferi. - Encephalitis. - Cranial neuropathy: commonly cranial nerve VII, and this can be uni- or bilateral. - Peripheral nervous system: including mononeuritis multiplex, peripheral neuropathy, polyradiculopathy, or even a Guillain-Barre type presentation (which is not common). Neurologic presentations in the late phase are encephalopathy, encephalomyelitis, and peripheral neuropathy. CNS Lyme disease diagnosis is based on clinical and epidemiological suspicion, supported by the presence of positive serology, CSF abnormalities, and intrathecal production of antibodies.

Serology is positive in 10% of people living in endemic areas, and this should be taken into account. Intravenous ceftriaxone, up to 2 g daily for 2–4 weeks is the treatment of choice. For late presentations, a longer course may be required. Oral antibiotic therapy with doxycycline can be used in patients without CSF abnormalities.

Suggested Reading

- Comprehensive Review in Clinical Neurology: A Multiple-Choice Question Book for the Wards and Boards ©2011 Wolters Kluwer Health Lippincott Williams & Wilkins. All rights reserved.

32. The classic triad of symptoms in congenital toxoplasmosis includes:
    A. Seizures, psychomotor retardation, hydrocephalus
    B. Seizures, rash, intracranial calcifications
    C. Hydrocephalus, chorioretinitis, intracranial calcifications
    D. Chorioretinitis, rash, spastic paraparesis
    E. Psychomotor retardation, hypotonia, chorioretinitis

Correct answer is: C
Congenital toxoplasmosis is secondary to placental transmission of the protozoan toxoplasmosis gondii, most often in the third trimester. Hydrocephalus, chorioretinitis, and intracranial calcifications are the classic triad of symptoms in congenital toxoplasmosis. Other manifestations may include fever, rash, hepatosplenomegaly, jaundice, thrombocytopenia, seizures, and psychomotor retardation. Approximately 25% of affected children will have systemic symptoms at birth. Premature infants are typically more severely affected than babies born at full term. Develop learning disabilities or ocular manifestations may occur later in life in normal newborns. The treatment of choice in newborn includes pyrimethamine, sulfadiazine, and leukovorin for 1 year. Prednisone may be added in the setting of elevated cerebrospinal fluid protein levels or chorioretinitis.

Suggested Reading

- Fenichel GM. Clinical pediatric neurology. 5th ed. Philadelphia: Elsevier Saunders. p. 122.
- Jones J, et al. Congenital toxoplasmosis. Am Fam Physician. 2003;67(10):2131–8.

33. A 3-day old full term with no prenatal care. You suspected meningitis and ordered cerebrospinal fluid analysis. Pending the CSF results.
    what should be started empirically?
    A. Vancomycin n and ceftriaxone should be started
    B. Ampicillin and vancomycin should be started
    C. Ampicillin and gentamicin should be started
    D. Vancomycin should be started

Correct answer is: C
Ampicillin and gentamicin can be started empirically; the most common pathogens in infant under 3 days of age will be Streptococcus agalactiae, Escherichia coli, Listeria monocytogenes and other enteric bacilli.

On the other hand, the most common pathogens after 4 days of life are, Serratia marcescens, Pseudomonas aeruginosa, and Citrobacter koseri.

In infants under the age of 1-month, common pathogens include Streptococcus agalactiae, Escherichia coli, Listeria monocytogenes, and Klebsiella. Ampicillin and cefotaxime may also be used in patients under 1 month of age, but this is not listed as an answer choice.

In children over 1 month of age, and in adults up to the age of 50, Vancomycin and a third-generation cephalosporin such as ceftriaxone can be started empirically because the coverage for Listeria monocytogenes is required.

Streptococcus pneumoniae, Streptococcus agalactiae, Haemophilus influenza, Neisseria meningitidis, and Escherichia coli are common between 1 month and 23 months of age. Vancomycin and third generation cephalosporin are usually sufficient.

Streptococcus pneumoniae and Neisseria meningitidis are common between 2 and 50 years of age.

Ampicillin and vancomycin are not recommended for empiric coverage in neonates with suspected bacterial meningitis.

Vancomycin n is not recommended for empiric treatment of suspected bacterial meningitis in infants under 1 month of age.

Suggested Reading

- Edwards MS, Baker CJ. Bacterial meningitis in the neonate: clinical features and diagnosis is. In: Up-to-date, Kaplan SL, Weisman LE, Armsby C, editors. Up-to-date. Waltham. Accessed on 20 Dec 2015.
- Kaplan SL. Bacterial meningitis in children older than one month: Clinical features and diagnosis. In: Up-to-date, Edwards MS, Nordli DR, Armsby C, editors. Up-to-date. Waltham. Accessed on 20 Dec 2015.
- Tunkel AR, Hartman BJ,Kaplan SL, et al. Practice guidelines for the management of bacterial meningitis. Clin Infect Dis. 2004;39:1267.

34. A 16-year-old boy has fever and progressive right leg weakness. His neurological evaluation including EMG/NCS indicates a motor neuron disease.

What is the most likely cause of his symptoms?

A. Poliomyelitis
B. Subacute sclerosing panencephalitis (SSPE)
C. Progressive multifocal leukoencephalopathy (PML)
D. Subacute HIV encephalomyelitis
E. Kuru

Correct answer is: A

Poliomyelitis is the only choice that can cause a pure motor neuron disease. Only1% of cases, the virus enters the central nervous system, preferentially infecting and destroying motor neurons, leading to muscle weakness and acute flaccid paralysis but the majority of cases, infection cause no symptoms at all. Different types of paralysis may occur, depending on the nerves involved. Spinal polio is the most common form, characterized by asymmetric paralysis that most often involves the legs. Between 25% and 50% of patients who have recovered from paralytic polio in childhood can develop additional symptoms decades after recovering from the acute infection, notably new muscle weakness and extreme fatigue. This condition is known as post-polio syndrome (PPS). The symptoms are thought to involve a failure of the over-sized motor units created during the recovery phase of the paralytic disease. PPS is a slow, progressive disease, and there is no specific treatment for it. Post-polio syndrome is not an infectious process, and patients experiencing the syndrome do not shed poliovirus.

Suggested Reading

Bradley WG, Daroff RB, Fenichel GM, Jankovic J. Neurology in clinical practice. 5th ed. Philadelphia: Elsevier; 2008.

35. Which of the following statements regarding congenital AIDS is correct?
    - A. 80% of infants born to mothers with AIDS will show evidence of infection at birth
    - B. Macrocephaly is a common complication of the disorder
    - C. Basal ganglia calcifications are more common in children than adults with AIDS
    - D. HIV encephalopathy results in hypotonia
    - E. None of the above

Correct answer is: C

Infants of HIV mothers can be infected via placental transmission, perinatal exposure, or breastfeeding. The incidence of HIV transmission to newborns is approximately 30% with the use of retroviral therapies. Children disease progression is the reflection of the disease severity in the mother. 20% will have a rapidly progressive course with death in infancy if the HIV is positive. Hepatosplenomegaly, bone marrow failure, lymphocytic interstitial pneumonia, chronic diarrhea, failure to thrive, microcephaly, and basal ganglia calcifications, are more common symptoms in children than adult. HIV encephalopathy may be evident 2 months to 5 years post-exposure, with developmental regression, microcephaly, dementia, spasticity, ataxia, pseudobulbar palsy, movement disorders, myoclonus, and seizures. Death typically occurs within a few months of onset. Treatment of HIV in children includes zidovudine, didanosine, and nevirapine.

Suggested Reading

Fenichel GM. Clinical pediatric neurology. 5th ed. Philadelphia: Elsevier Saunders; 2005. p. 124–5.

36. An 8-year-old boy became unsteady and unable to walk all of a sudden, this afternoon. Despite of being scared, he is very cooperative and well-spoken. On examination, he has mild bilateral lateral gaze nystagmus, past-pointing on finger-nose-finger test, and normal reflexes. He has a normal strength, but he cannot balance while standing, and he has a lurching gait. He had chicken pox 14 days ago, but he is otherwise healthy. Developmental milestones are normal.
    What is your most likely diagnosis?
    - A. Acute postinfectious cerebellitis
    - B. Friedreich ataxia (FRDA)
    - C. Medulloblastoma
    - D. Miller Fisher syndrome
    - E. Multiple sclerosis

Correct answer is: A

Acute post-infectious cerebellitis can present as acute onset of cerebellar symptoms (maximal within a few hours) following any viral infection by 10–14 days. Usually, the sensorium should remain clear. MRI of the brain may show increased T2 intensities in the cerebellum. Improvement should begin within a few days of onset, and gait should normalize within 1–5 months.

Suggested Reading

Fenichel GM. Clinical pediatric neurology: a signs and symptoms approach. Philadelphia: WB Saunders; 1997.

Montenegro MA, Santos SL, Li LM, Cendes F. Neuroimaging of acute cerebellitis. J Neuroimaging 2002;12:72–4.

37. An 8-year-old female is admitted with continued shaking of her left arm. Her brain CT scan is shown.

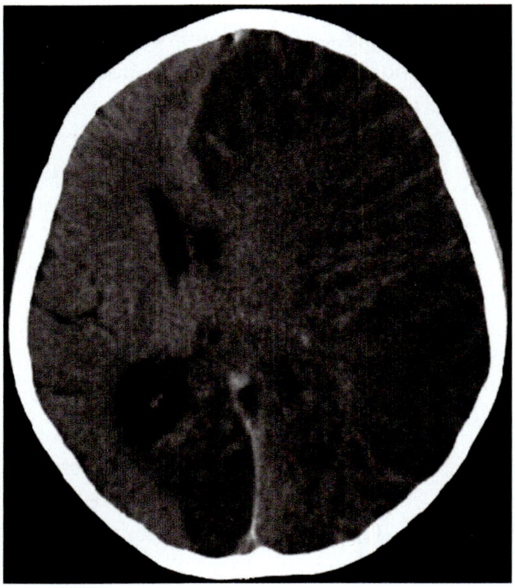

Fig. 12.5 Brain CT scan without contrast enhancement of a patient, female, 8 years old, with Rasmusen's encephalitis. (Own work. Mikhail Kalinin. Wikipedia)

12

Which of the following is true regarding treatment?

A. Immunotherapy represents the best chance for seizure remission
B. Anti-epileptic drug polytherapy represents the best chance for seizure remission
C. Hemispherotomy represents the highest chance for seizure remission
D. Vagus nerve stimulator represents the highest chance for seizure remission
E. No treatment offers any sizable chance for seizure remission.

Correct Answer is: C

This patient has Rasmussen's encephalitis. A recent case series of 13 patients some patients do have transient benefit from immunotherapy. However, surgery was associated with seizure freedom in 63% of patients treated with surgery. Despite the aggressive nature of Rasmussen's encephalitis, hemispherectomy does offer a chance of seizure freedom in this population.

Suggested Reading

- Hoffman CE, Ochi A, Snead OC 3rd, Widjaja E, Hawkins C, Tisdal M, Rutka JT. Rasumussen's encephalitis: advances in management and patient outcomes. Childs Nerv Syst. 2016;32(4):629–40.

38. You are evaluating an 18-year-old female for her diplopia and right facial and retro-orbital pain. Her symptoms were preceded by a severe ear infection for the last few weeks. Examination reveals a right sixth (abducens) nerve palsy and diminished sensations on the right face. Motor strength is normal in all extremities. A CT scan reveals opacity of the right mastoid air cells and petrous part of temporal bone.
What is your diagnosis?

A. Bell palsy
B. cavernous sinus thrombosis
C. Gradenigo syndrome
D. Millard-Gubler syndrome
E. Ramsay-Hunt syndrome

Correct Answer is: C

The clinical presentation is suggestive of Gradenigo syndrome. It is characterized by the triad of suppurative otitis media, pain in the distribution of the trigeminal nerve, and abducens nerve palsy. Cranial nerve (CN) VII can also be involved. The cranial nerves involvement occurs when otitis media infection spreads to involve the petrous apex. Diabetics or immunosuppressed patients are at higher risk. Awareness of the symptom complex is important for early diagnosis and intervention with high dose antibiotics or surgery as indicated to avoid the morbidity and poten-

tially life-threatening complications associated with this condition.

Ramsay-Hunt syndrome is secondary to herpes zoster infection which can involve cranial nerves V (ophthalmic branch), VI and VII palsy with vesicular eruption in the auditory canal.

Bell palsy involves cranial nerve VII causing ipsilateral lower motor type weakness of the facial muscles.

Cavernous sinus thrombosis can present with chemosis, proptosis and painful ophthalmoplegia and multiple cranial nerve deficits. Depending upon the extent of the involvement this can include CN III, IV, V (divisions I and II), and VI and post-ganglionic sympathetic axons to the eye.

Millard-Gubler syndrome is caused by a pontine lesion affecting cranial nerves VI and VII and corticospinal tract with ipsilateral facial and abducens palsy and contralateral hemiplegia.

Suggested Reading

- Motamed M, Kalan A. Gradenigo syndrome. Postgrad Med J. 2000;7(899):559–60.
- Bradley's neurology in clinical practice. Daroff R, Fenichel G, Jankovic J, Mazziotta J, editors. 6th ed. Philadelphia: Elsevier, 2012; 1754.

39. A 16-year-old boy complains of sudden onset vertigo and nausea which is continuous and severe for 3 days. He had an upper respiratory symptom 1 week ago which resolved. He has no history of hearing loss, tinnitus or aural fullness. On examination, he has horizontal nystagmus with fast component towards the right as well as decreased caloric response in the left ear.
What is your diagnoses?
A. acute labyrinthitis
B. benign paroxysmal positional vertigo
C. bilateral vestibular neuritis
D. Ménière disease
E. unilateral vestibular neuritis

Correct Answer is: E

This is a presentation of a vestibular neuritis which results from viral inflammation of the vestibular nerve. The main features of unilateral vestibular neuritis include severe and prolonged vertigo, nausea, vomiting, and nystagmus with fast component away from the affected side, normal hearing and otherwise normal neurologic exam. Incidence is highest in middle age and there is frequently a recent history of viral illness. Patients with bilateral vestibulopathy typically present with imbalance and oscillopsia and do not have vertigo or spontaneous nystagmus. Acute labyrinthitis can also result from similar viral etiology but the involvement of the labyrinth causes hearing loss in addition to the vestibular symptoms.

Benign paroxysmal positional vertigo is characterized by recurrent episodes of vertigo brought on by a sudden change in head position which is thought to be caused by abnormal stimulation of the ampulla of one of the semicircular canals, by gravity induced movement of free floating otoliths during changes in head position. Typically, there are no hearing abnormalities and other neurologic deficits. Ménière disease is characterized by attacks of vertigo lasting from minutes to hours associated with nausea and vomiting, sensation of fullness or pressure in the ears, fluctuating hearing loss and tinnitus. Symptoms can be unilateral or bilateral.

Suggested Reading

- Ropper A, Samuels M. Adams and Victor's principles of neurology. 8th ed. New York:Mcgraw Hill, 2005; 261.
- Baloh R. Acute unilateral and bilateral peripheral vestibular loss. Continuum Lifelong Learning Neurol 2006;12(4):46–64.
- Zee DS. Pathophysiology of vestibular symptoms and signs: the clinical examination. Continuum Lifelong Learning Neurol 2006;12(4):13–32.

Mental Retardation/ Cognitive Disorders

Y. M. Awaad, *Absolute Pediatric Neurology*, https://doi.org/10.1007/978-3-319-78801-2_13

1. A 5-year-old boy with a history of speech delay. He still does not know his colors or shapes. He has no significant past medical history. He is not any treatment. During your exam, he is friendly and loquacious. You heard a systolic murmur that radiates to the neck. He has several dysmorphic features, including a long philtrum and prominent lips with an open mouth.
What is the most likely diagnosis?
   A. Fragile X syndrome
   B. William's syndrome
   C. Velocardiofacial defect
   D. Mitochondrial disorder
   E. Down's syndrome

Correct Answer is: B
William's syndrome is associated with a deletion at 7q11.23. It is associated with mental delay, unusual elfin facies, and cardiovascular anomalies, including supra-valvular aortic stenosis, mild prenatal growth deficiency and occasionally, hypercalcemia. They are very friendly and have an outgoing and loquacious personality. However, they may also have mood lability. Although they have good verbal skills, they may have delayed adaptive skills.

Other cardiac anomalies include peripheral pulmonic stenosis and mitral valve prolapse (13%).

13

Suggested Reading

- Jones KL. Smith recognizable patterns of human malformation. 6th ed. Philadelphia: Elsevier; 2006. p. 122–4.
- Menon Deepa. Williams syndrome. In: Accardo PJ, editor. Developmental disabilities in infancy and childhood. vol. 2. 3rd ed. Baltimore: Brooke's Publishing; 2008. p. 353–61.

2. A 9-year-old boy has been evaluated for deterioration of his behavior and school performance. His psychological testing reveals IQ of 65. On examination, he has significant dysmorphic features with prominent ears. He has a sister with learning disabilities and a maternal uncle with Parkinsonism.
What is the most appropriate test to obtain at this time?
   A. MRI of the Head
   B. FMR1 trinucleotide repeat
   C. Serum ceruloplasmin
   D. EEG
   E. High resolution chromosomes

Correct Answer is: B
The boy has mild mental retardation, behavioral difficulties, a family history of learning difficulties in a sister and movement disorder in his maternal uncle. In boys, Fragile X is the most common inherited cause of mental retardation. Usually, they have large protruding ears, macro-orchidism, moderate to severe mental retardation, hyperextensible finger joints, hypotonia and autism or autistic like behavior. Also it might be associated with ADHD and social anxiety. It is secondary to an unstable triplet repeat amplification of the CGG within the FMR1 gene on chromosome Xq27.3. More than 200 triplet repeats are needed to have the full phenotypic expression. A triplet repeats above 55–200 is considered a pre-mutation state. The maternal uncle is the pre-mutation carrier manifesting with the Fragile X tremor/ataxia syndrome (FXTAS). It is a late onset, neurodegenerative condition that is characterized by an intention tremor, cerebellar ataxia and executive dysfunction. This is usually seen in pre-mutation carriers. Patients may have weakness, fatigue, anxiety and irritability.

Suggested Reading

- Bodensteiner J, Ellis C, Schaeffer GB. Mental retardation. In: Maria B, editor. Current management in child neurology. 4th ed. Helton: BC Decker; 2009. 346–57, 285–95.

3. A 7-year-old girl was referred by her school teacher because school difficulties. Her teacher mentioned in her referral that the child does not seem to understand spoken instructions. She witnessed a violent crime in her neighborhood 3 months ago. Her mother also reported that for the last 3 months she has had difficulty following directions and seems irritable because the family does not understand her. She had one seizure 2 weeks ago. Her sleep EEG is shown.

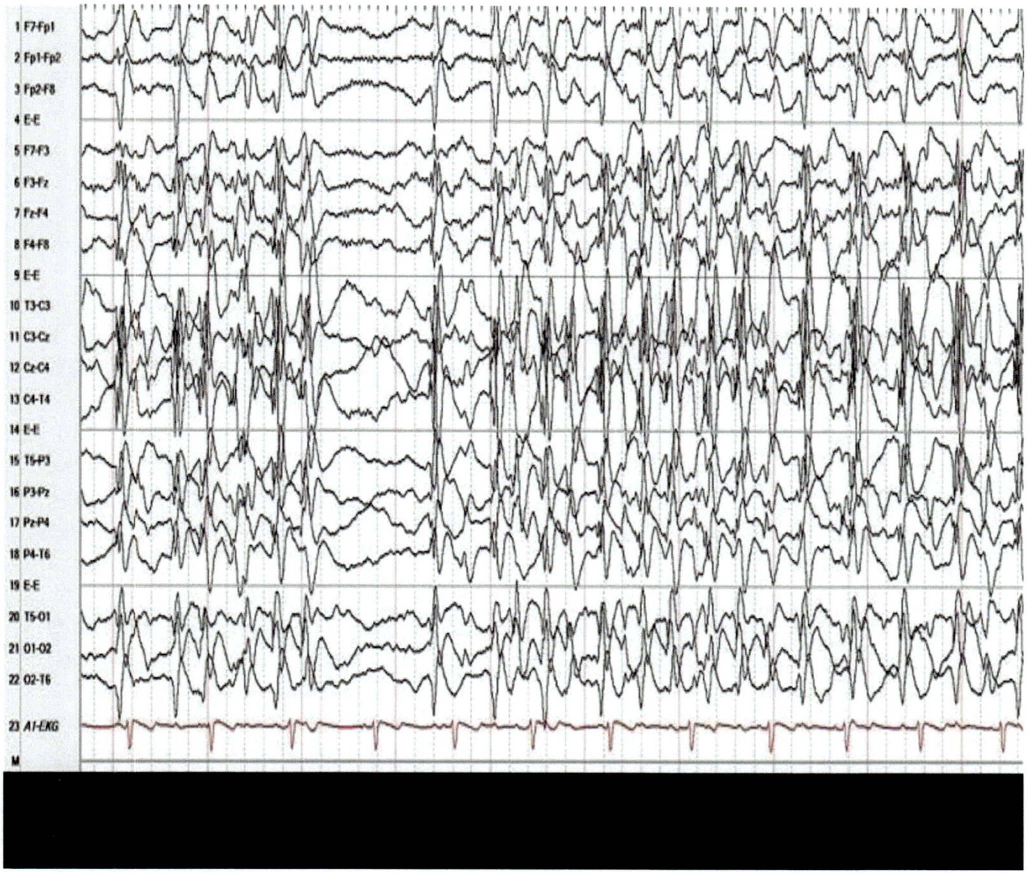

Fig. 13.1 EEG findings of Landau-Kleffner syndrome. American Academy of Neurology Institute, produced by permission

What is your diagnosis?

A. Rett syndrome
B. Landau-Kleffner syndrome
C. Angelman syndrome
D. Lennox-Gastaut syndrome
E. Benign Rolandic Epilepsy

Correct Answer is: B
Landau-Kleffner syndrome is one of the epileptic encephalopathies. It is characterized by verbal auditory agnosia (loss of understanding of spoken words). The patient has normal psychomotor development initially followed by loss of language milestones. Seventy to eighty percent of patients have epilepsy. Behavioral abnormalities characterized by hyperactivity, inattention, aggressiveness and social withdrawal are very common. EEG findings are continuous

generalized slow spike and wave in sleep or bilateral independent temporal spike and wave discharge.

Suggested Reading

- Nickel K, Wirrell E. Electrical status epilepticus in sleep. Semin Pediatr Neurol. 15:50–60.

4. A 12-year-old girl with Down's syndrome came to the office with her family. Her family is complaining of her self-help skills regression and she became very irritable lately. She is attending special education classes but her school grades have been dropping. She has dysmorphic features consisting of a flat facial profile with almond shaped palpebral fissures.
   Which of the following is the most appropriate next step in her evaluation?
   A. CT of the brain
   B. Thyroid function tests
   C. Cervical spine films
   D. Electroencephalogram
   E. Spinal fluid for neurotransmitters

13

Correct Answer is: B
Down's syndrome is one of the most common chromosomal disorder that results from complete trisomy of the chromosome 21 due to non-disjunctions during gamete formation. There are a complex medical issues that may vary from birth to adulthood in children with Down's syndrome.

There are certain considerations have to be addressed in children with Down's syndrome between the ages of 1 to puberty. There may be delayed eruption of the first tooth. Hypo-thyrodism is on the rise in children with Down's syndrome and the signs and symptoms maybe subtle.

Autoimmune thyroiditis may present at any age. Refractive errors which increases with age have to be monitored and a substantial number of children have high myopia. Astigmatism and hyperopia are also seen but are less common.

Cervical spine X - Rays are routinely recommended in children with Down's syndrome because of atlantoaxial subluxation. The boy is presenting with cognitive decline rather than the typical gait changes, loss of bladder or bowel control or quadriparesis that is seen in patients with cord disorders.

Suggested Reading

- Roger P, Roizen N, Capone GT. Down syndrome. In: Accardo PJ, editor. Developmental disabilities in infancy and childhood. vol 1. 3rd ed. Baltimore: Brookes Publishing; 2008. p. 285–303.

5. A 12-month-old female brought to the office by her family because they have a concern about her development. She has a normal development in her first sixth month of life. Few months ago she stopped playing with her toys, and wrings her hands together constantly. On exam, her head circumference at 10th percentile, which had been at the 25th percentile at her 6-month checkup. She is hypotonic and unable to walk independently. She does not babble, point, nor gesture.
   What test is most likely to identify the correct diagnosis?
   A. Brain magnetic resonance imaging
   B. Electrocencephalogram
   C. MecP2 sequencing
   D. Muscle biopsy
   E. Serum lactate

Correct Answer is: C
Rett syndrome is one of a neurodevelopmental disorders characterized by loss of communication skills. Usually,

children have a normal prenatal and perinatal period. It affects mainly females because it is X-linked dominant disorder. It is a genetic disorder on chromosome Xq28. Genetic testing with sequencing abnormalities of the MeCP2 gene can be used to confirm the diagnosis. The mecp2 gene is a DNA binding protein that acts as a global transcriptional repressor. Nonsense mutations patients present with a sever phenotypes, while patients with missense mutations present with mild phenotypes. Clinical manifestations include acquired microcephaly, seizures, respiratory abnormalities, and psychomotor retardation with loss of manual praxis and stereotypic hand wringing movements.

Suggested Reading

- Menkes JH. Heredodegenerative disease. In: Menkes JH, Sarnat H, Maria B, editors. Child neurology. 7th ed. Philadelphia: Lippincott Williams and Wilkins; 2000. p. 210–11.
- Bibat G, Naidu S. Rett syndrome. In: Accardo PJ, ed. Developmental disabilities in infancy and childhood. vol. 2. 3rd ed. Baltimore: Paul Brookes Publishing; 2008. p. 545–50.

6. A 4-year-old foster boy presented for a developmental delay evaluation. He has been with his foster parents for three, but they do not know his previous medical history. He eats toys, paper, wood and clay.

   What test are you going to order?

   A. Electroencdephalogram
   B. Lead level
   C. Liver function tests
   D. Cranial MRI
   E. Thyroid function tests

Correct Answer is: B

Lead is the most common environmental toxin. High serum lead levels has a strong correlation with the clinical symptoms, and cognitive deficits. Although blood levels have dramatically dropped in the past decades (from 15 ug/dl to 2.7 in 1991 to 1994), there are still a significant number of children who may have blood levels equal or greater than 10ug/dl. The consensus guidelines indicated targeted screening of all children with identifiable risk factors including children living in housing before 1950, children of ethnic or racial minority groups who may be exposed to lead containing food remedies, children who have emigrated (or adopted) from countries where lead poisoning is prevalent, children with iron deficiency, children exposed to contaminated dust or soil, children with developmental delay whose oral behavior places them at risk for lead exposure, children whose parents are expose to lead (vocationally, avocationally, and during home renovation), children of low income families and victims of abuse and neglect.

Suggested Reading

- Shevell M, Ashwal S. Practice parameter: evaluation of the child with global developmental delay: report of the Quality Standards subcommittee of the American Academy of Neurology and the practice committee of the Child Neurology Society. Neurology. 2003;60:367–80.
- Davioli CT and Chisolm J.J. Childhood lead poisoning. In: Capute AJ, Accardo PJ, editors. Developmental disabilities in infancy and childhood. vol 1. 2nd ed. Baltimore: Brooke's Publishing.1996. p. 232–3.

7. A 4-year-old female with developmental delay has seen by you. Her family describes her as a very slow feeder, who often choked while taking her bottle. She started to stand at 18 months of age and started walking at 24 months. At 4-years of age,

she started to combine two words together. She has moderate hypotonia and has a voracious appetite.
What test would most likely confirm the diagnosis?
A. High resolution chromosome studies
B. Muscle biopsy
C. Fish testing of 15q11.2-13
D. MECP2 sequencing
E. Brain magnetic resonance imaging

Correct Answer is: C
Clinical manifestations of Prader Willi syndrome are hypotonia (usually during infancy), failure to thrive, obesity (childhood onset), hypogonadism, small hands and feet, short stature, hypopigmentation and almond shaped eyes. Methylation analysis is the test of choice to diagnose the syndrome. 75% of affected individuals have a deletion of the long arm of chromosome 15 at q 11-q13. The paternally derived chromosome has been deleted. Maternal uniparental disomy accounts for 20% of cases.

Suggested Reading

- Jones KL. Smith recognizable patterns of human malformation. 6th ed. Philadelphia: Elsevier; 2006. p 223–7.

8. A couple is in the process of adopting a 4-year-old boy who has a history of hyperactivity and behavioral problems. On examination, he has a remarkable short stature, microcephaly, short palpebral fissures, a long, smooth nasal philtrum, and thin upper lip.
Exposure to which agent during the pregnancy is most likely to account for his clinical presentation?
A. Methamphetamine
B. Cocaine
C. Valproic acid
D. Alcohol
E. Phenytoin

Correct Answer is: D
Prenatal exposure to alcohol is well recognized as a teratogen to the developing fetus. The condition is known as Fetal alcohol spectrum (FAS) disorder. The clinical features include dysmorphic facial characteristics (microcephaly, facial anomalies: short palpebral fissures, long smooth nasal philtrum and thin upper vermillion border). The behavioral profile in children with FAS is consistent with Attention deficit hyperactivity disorder.

Suggested Reading

- Lipkin P. Attention-deficit hyperactivity disorders mimic disorder. In: Accardo PJ, editors. Developmental disabilities in infancy and childhood. Vol. 2. 3rd ed. Baltimore: Paul Brookes Publishing; 2008. p. 684.

9. A 52-year-old woman with the history of progressive tremor for the last 1–2 years. She has both resting and action tremors on exam. Her action tremors are worst at end point. She has a past medical history of primary ovarian failure. Her grandson has a severe developmental delay, but no other family history of neurologic disease. Brain MRI shows hyper intense signal changes in the middle cerebellar peduncles and periventricular white matter on T2-weighted images.
What is the diagnosis?
A. Spinocerebellar ataxia type 1
B. Pantothenate kinase-associated neurodegeneration (PKAN)
C. Huntington disease
D. LRRK2 mutation
E. Fragile X tremor ataxia syndrome

Correct Answer is: E
Fragile X syndrome is one of the most common identifiable causes of intellectual disability in children (mainly male). It is a result of an abnormal

trinucleotide triplet repeat in the FMR1 gene region on the X chromosome. Female patients have a highly variable phenotype, with a different neuropsychiatric presentation, but typically the IQ scores are not in the intellectual disabled range. Patients who have only a per-mutation (and not the full mutation in the FMR-1 gene region) develop two other clinical phenotypes. Fragile X tremor ataxia syndrome (FXTAS) occurs in men and women, but the neurologic manifestations typically developing after the age of 50. The tremor can be variable, having essential, cerebellar or mixed features. Mild cognitive changes in executive function are also common. The cause of The well described MRI findings listed above in this syndrome have no well-known cause. Females with these permutations may also develop primary ovarian failure.

SCA-1, Huntington disease and PKAN all lead to progressive neurologic decline, though with different clinical phenotypes, and not simply progressive tremor. All of them do not have the MRI findings described. LRRK2 mutations result in a classic Parkinson's phenotype.

Suggested Reading

- Pandolfo M, Manto M. Cerebellar and afferent ataxias. Continuum. 2013; 19(5 Movement Disorders):1312–43.

Metabolic

Y. M. Awaad, *Absolute Pediatric Neurology*, https://doi.org/10.1007/978-3-319-78801-2_14

1. You are evaluating a 5-year-old boy for his development and speech delay. He was born full term. He rolled on time, but he sat very late and has never walked. Excessive movements of his hands started at 13 months of age and he never was able to feed himself and had no hand coordination. He has very limited speech. His family history is unremarkable of developmental or speech delay. On examination, he has significant areas of injury to his lips and cheeks and healing wounds on his tongue, but skin exam is normal. His mother reported that he has orange crystals in the urine sediment in his diaper. Prominent choreoathetoid movements are noted. He has decrease truncal tone, with mild spasticity in his lower extremities.
Which of the following is most likely to be abnormal?
   A. glycine
   B. ammonia
   C. lactate
   D. uric acid
   E. very long-chain fatty acids

Correct Answer is: D
This is a classic clinical presentation of Lesch-Nyhan disease, which is an X-linked disorder of purine metabolism leads to an overproduction of uric acid, affecting multiple organ systems. The underlying neurological pathophysiology is unclear, but it could be secondary to abnormality in neurotransmitter metabolism, including dopamine, rather than direct toxicity of uric acid itself. Affected children have normal development initially, followed by motor development delay at 3–6 months of age. Involuntary movements of the limbs and face appear in the second year of life, and also progressive changes in tone (axial hypotonia and limb spasticity). Oral auto-mutilation, a very classic feature of the disorder, develops between 2 and 4 years of age, though is not uniformly noted. Motor skills like sitting and walking are lost (if they were ever acquired) and 50% of patients develop seizures. Speech is much delayed, and mental retardation is common.

Elevated levels of uric acid are noted in both urine and serum and are very helpful in screening for the disease. Confirmatory enzyme activity of hypoxanthine-guanine-phosphoribosyltransferase (HGPRT), in erythrocytes or culture fibroblasts, provides a definitive diagnosis. Treatment with allopurinol may prevent the renal complications of the disorder; including kidney stones, obstructive uropathy, and eventual renal failure, but is not effective in treating the neurologic manifestations. Typically, drastic methods—such as tooth extraction, or continuous restraint of limbs— are needed to prevent self-mutilation.

Suggested Reading

Pagon RA, Adam MP, Bird TD, et al., editors. Gene reviews [Internet]. Seattle: University of Washington, Seattle; 1193–2013.

2. You are evaluating a 5-year-old boy for his development delay. He achieved his milestones as follows: sat late at 11 months, began pulling to stand at 17 months, but has never walked independently. He starts losing his ability to stand and is not supporting his weight in a seated position over the last year. He has sever speech delay, only some grunts and no babbling. He cannot reach or grasp for objects. Head circumference is in the 50th percentile. On examination, he has a very large tongue with prominent supraorbital ridges and thick eyebrows. The liver edge is palpated 5 cm below the costal margin. On neurologic exam, he has poor visual attention with limited tracking; axial tone is decreased with normal

extremity tone and normal reflexes. His brain MRI shows prominent perivascular spaces, without other obvious abnormality.

What is most likely diagnosis?

A. adrenoleukodystrophy
B. fragile X syndrome
C. metachromatic leukodystrophy
D. mucopolysaccharidosis
E. Rett disease

Correct Answer is: D

This boy has sever global developmental delay. Majority of those children will never have a definitive etiology for their delays. The AAN guidelines have found brain MRI and chromosome microarray testing to be of the highest yield in patients with non-specific and non-syndromic global delay. In other cases, a full medical history and physical exam can often assist the child neurologist in reaching the appropriate diagnosis. This is especially true if there is progressive loss of previously acquired developmental skills (neuro-regression.) Certain exam findings are very helpful; evaluation of growth parameters including head circumference, assessment for dysmorphic features or neuro-cutaneous stigmata and other signs of storage which include macro-glossia and hepatosplenomegaly can be of great importance to recognize. The neurologic exam should document whether there is presence or absence of concomitant white matter (spasticity, brisk reflexes, optic atrophy), deep grey nuclear (abnormal movements or rigidity) or cerebellar (truncal or limb ataxia) involvement. When particular clues do arise from the history or exam more focused laboratory testing can often improve the diagnostic yield. This patient has evidence of enlarged non-neuronal tissue, including bone (supraorbital ridging), tongue and liver. Sometimes referred to as the Hurler phenotype presence of such enlargement is highly indicative of lysosomal storage disorder (and more specifically one of the mucopolysaccharidoses). The specific form of MPS can be suggested by the abnormal excretion of urinary glycosaminoglycans, and confirmatory testing involves assessing and quantifying the specific enzyme deficiency. A spectrum of severity is present with patients with some residual activity, having in general a milder and less rapidly progressive form of the disease.

On the other hand, the oligosaccharidoses, present in a similar fashion with global developmental delay (and/or regression) with evidence of extra neuronal storage and must be screened for separately by assessing for abnormal urinary oligosaccharide excretion.

Another way to divide global delay children with or without regression, is by signs indicating a white matter (leukodystrophy) versus grey matter (poliodystrophy) disorder. Both metachromatic and adrenoleukodystrophy are disorders affecting the white matter primarily leading mostly to motor regression early in the course, with evidence of spasticity, brisk reflexes and optic atrophy. Neither of these disorders would be expected to have prominent early cognitive delays nor signs of storage on exam.

Fragile X syndrome presents with global developmental delay and in particular, prominent intellectual disability, though would not be expected to lead to regression in skills nor signs of progressive storage with time (though mild dysmorphic features are present).

Rett syndrome, (identified by MECP2 mutational analysis) is X-linked dominant and thus typically affects females (most often lethal before birth in males). Surviving males with this disorder have duplications of the genetic region, rather than deletion, and have prominent difficulties early on in life with feeding due to low muscle tone; and although they may have dysmorphic features, they do not develop progressive coarsening with time.

Suggested Reading

- Fenichel GM. Clinical pediatric neurology. 6th ed. Philadelphia: Saunders Elsevier; 2009. p. 119–51.
- Michelson DJ, Shevell MI, Sherr Eh, et al. Evidence report: genetic and metabolic testing on children with global developmental delay: Report of the Quality Standards Subcommittee of the American Academy of Neurology and the Practice Committee of the Child Neurology Society. Neurology. 2011;77:1629–35.
- Muenzer J. Overview of the mucopolysaccharidoses. Rheumatology (Oxford). 2011;50 Suppl 5:v4–12.

3. You are seeing a 9-year-old female with a history of progressively worsening dystonia, choreoathetosis, dysarthria and intellectual deterioration for the last 3 years. On your examination for noted, pigmentary retinopathy and extensor plantar responses. MRI is shown.

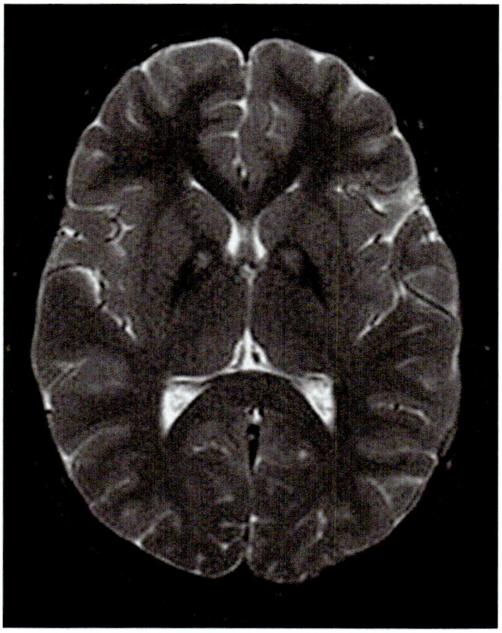

Fig. 14.1 MRI image shows iron deposits in the basal ganglia, the so-called eye-of-the-tiger sign (T2w GRASE sequence). (Enro2002. Wikipedia)

What is the most likely diagnoses?

A. Wilson disease
B. acute disseminated encephalomyelitis
C. hereditary spastic paraplegia
D. metachromatic leukodystrophy
E. pantothenate kinase-associated neurodegeneration

Correct Answer is: E
The clinical and radiological findings are classic of Pantothenate kinase-associated neurodegeneration (PKAN), formerly Hallervorden-Spatz syndrome. It is one of brain iron accumulation (NBIA) neurodegenerative disorders. Infantile neuroaxonal dystrophy, neuroferritinopathy and aceruloplasminemia are other types of NBIA. It is an autosomal recessive disorder and associated with mutations in the PANK2 gene. MRI shows the "eye of the tiger" sign, with hyper-intensity in the medial globus pallidus surrounded by hypo-intensity.

Suggested Reading

- Gregory A, Hayflick SJ. Pantothenate kinase-associated neurodegeneration. In: Gene Reviews at Gene Tests: Medical Genetics Resource (online resource). Copyright University of Washington, Seattle. 1997–2012. Available at ▶ www.ncbi.nlm.nih.gov/books/NBK1490/. 2002. Accessed 9-4-12.

4. You are evaluating a 6-year-old boy for his gait. He was born prematurely at 33 weeks gestation, stayed in the regular nursery for 1 week because he had feeding and temperature control problems, he was discharged home without other complication. His early milestones were on target, including walking at 13 months of age. Over the last few months, he has had difficulty with his walking and running, start to trip and fall more often. Simultaneously, he started to have some

behavioral regression with increased outbursts and difficulty understanding his speech. You examined him and noticed that, he has poor eye contact, some dysfluent speech, and is not interested in following most directions. He has mild spasticity in both legs, with brisk reflexes. Gait is spastic in nature, with a mild crouch and some scissoring. His brain MRI is shown.

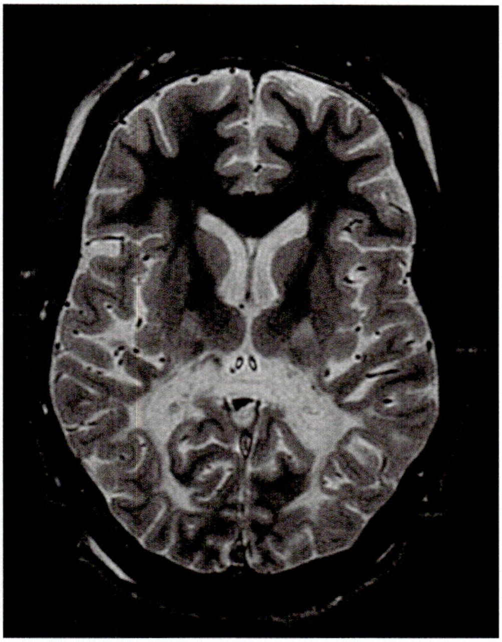

Fig. 14.2 Adrenoleukodystrophy and MRI showing T2 weighted axial scan at the level of the caudate heads demonstrates marked loss of posterior white matter, with reduced volume and increased signal intensity. The anterior white matter is spared. Features are consistent with X-linked adrenoleukodystrophy. (Sources: Radiopediacase. ► http://radiopaedia.org/images/318699 and ► http://radiopaedia.org/uploads/radio/0031/8699/T2.jpg. Frank Gaillard)

What is the most likely diagnosis for this boy?

A. adrenoleukodystrophy
B. cerebral palsy
C. dopa-responsive dystonia
D. Lesch-Nyhan syndrome
E. Menkes disease

Correct Answer is: A

The boy has clinical and radiographic manifestations of a white matter function disorder. With the A diagnosis of cerebral palsy (a static disorder of motor control by definition) is incorrect because of the progressive nature of the disease.

Lesch-Nyhan syndrome and Menkes disease are primarily grey matter disorders with progressive dementia and seizures. Additional deep grey matter dysfunction is seen with the former as well.

Dopa-responsive dystonia can have misdiagnosed as a cerebral palsy, though a careful history will have demonstrated its diurnal nature (with patients often unaffected in the morning upon awakening) and the exam will disclose dystonia rather than spasticity.

Adrenoleukodystrophy (ALD) is an X-linked disorder of oxidation of very long-chain fatty acids (by peroxisomes) leading to accumulation in tissues and plasma. The classic presentation occurs in young boys aged 4–8 years, with concomitant change in behavioral regulation, cognition and gait. Corticotropin stimulation test can detect early subclinical adrenal dysfunction. The disease is relentless, leading to death within 3 years of presentation in most children. Different treatments modalities have been tried in the form of vitamin or enzyme therapy without much success. Bone marrow transplantation is useful if initiated early in the disease. Unfortunately, by the time the diagnosis is made it is often too late to affect the disease process. Diagnosis is often suggested by the pattern of white matter hyper-intensity on MRI. Posterior predominant changes, sometimes also involving the splenium of the corpus callosum and not uncommonly contrast-enhancing along the leading edge of the actively demyelinating areas, which

should suggest the diagnosis and differentiate ALD from other primary leukodystrophies. Elevated levels of very long-chain fatty acids (24 and 26 carbon length molecules) are found in the plasma, as is found in most peroxisomal disorders.

Suggested Reading

- Fenichel GM. Clinical pediatric neurology. 6th ed. Philadelphia: Saunders Elsevier; 2009. p. 150–51.

5. You are evaluating a 14-year-old male who was referred by his coach because the boy has had difficulties during training. His father reports that the coach has noticed that the boy's endurance is poor and that he complains frequently of cramps and muscle pain. The boy told you that he is able to continue his training as long as he is able to rest briefly as this allows the muscle pain to lessen. Even resuming exercise after rest, he must resume at a slightly reduced level to prevent recurrence of muscle pain and cramping. Also, he told you that his urine becomes very dark colored after football practices. You suspect a common disorder of carbohydrate metabolism resulting in a metabolic myopathy.
Which statement is true regarding myophosphorylase deficiency?
A. Needle EMG typically demonstrates myotonic discharges.
B. It is inherited in an autosomal dominant fashion.
C. It is characterized by progressive proximal weakness in a limb-girdle pattern.
D. It occurs as a result of deficiency of debranching enzyme.
E. CK remains persistently elevated even in between episodes of myoglobinuria.

14

Correct Answer is: E
Myophosphorylase deficiency (McArdle disease) is a common disorder of carbohydrate metabolism caused by mutations in the PYGM gene encoding myophosphorylase. It is inherited as an autosomal recessive disorder, and presents with episodes of myoglobinuria occurring as a result of brief intense or prolonged low-level exercise. The classic manifestations in childhood are exercise intolerance, fatigue, myalgias, poor endurance and cramping. "Second-wind phenomenon" in which brief rest allows for dissipation of muscle pain is an associated finding. Although fixed weakness can occur later in the course of the disease, its early presentation is with episodic muscle pain and exercise intolerance.

Unlike patients with adult-onset carnitine palmitoyltransferase II deficiency, CK remains elevated even between episodes of myoglobinuria. Needle EMG is usually normal, although occasional myotonic discharges, muscle irritability and myopathic potentials with rapid recruitment may be seen.

Cori or Forbes disease (glycogen storage disease, type III) is secondary of debranching enzyme deficiency. Muscle weakness may present late in life, with a distal predominant weakness. Systemic symptoms are much more common in childhood and include hepatomegaly, short stature, intermittent hypoglycemia and rarely seizures.

Suggested Reading

- Tobon, Alejandro. Metabolic myopathies. CONTINUUM: Lifelong Learn Neurol. 2013;19(6):1571–97.

6. Mutations of the FBN1 gene encoding fibrillin are associated with which of the following disorders?
A. Ehlers-Danlos syndrome

B. Hereditary hemorrhagic telangiectasia (Rendu-Osler-Weber syndrome)
C. Marfan syndrome
D. Sturge-Weber syndrome
E. Susac syndrome

Correct Answer is: C
Marfan syndrome is a connective-tissue disorder inherited in an autosomal dominant manner and caused mainly by mutations in the gene FBN1. This gene encodes fibrillin-1, a glycoprotein that is the main constituent of the micro-fibrils of the extracellular matrix. Most mutations are unique and affect a single amino acid of the protein. Reduced or abnormal fibrillin-1 leads to tissue weakness, increased transforming growth factor beta signaling, loss of cell-matrix interactions, and finally, to the different phenotypic manifestations of Marfan syndrome. Since the description of FBN1 as the gene affected in patients with this disorder, great advances have been made in the understanding of its pathogenesis.

The development of several mouse models has helped our understanding of this disease, and it would change the treatment and the prognosis of patients in the coming years. Cardiovascular involvement which is one of many different clinical manifestations of Marfan syndrome, deserves special consideration, due to its impact on prognosis. Ghent criteria which requires a comprehensive clinical assessment of multiple organ systems helps in the diagnosis of Marfan syndrome. Genetic testing can be useful in the diagnosis of selected cases.

Suggested Reading

- Cunha L. Marfan's syndrome. In: Uncommon cause of stroke. Caplan L, editor. 2nd ed. New York: Cambridge University Press; 2008. p. 131–8.
- Cañadas V, Vilacosta I, Bruna I, Fuster V. Marfan syndrome. Part 1: pathophysiology and diagnosis. Nat Rev Cardiol. 2010;7(5):256–65. Epub 2010 Mar 30.

7. Which of the following is X linked?
   A. Ornithine transcarbamylase (OTC) deficiency (OTC)
   B. Carbamoyl phosphate synthetase deficiency (CPS1)
   C. Argininosuccinate acid lyase deficiency (ASL)
   D. Argininosuccinate acid synthetase deficiency (ASS)

Correct answer is: A
Ornithine transcarbamylase deficiency is the only urea cycle disorders is inherited as an X linked disorder; the rest are autosomal recessive. Elevated ammonia, respiratory alkalosis, vomiting, and encephalopathy are the characteristic findings in urea cycle disorders. If there is a suspicion for a urea cycle disorder if ammonia is elevated, suggested testing includes arterial blood gas, serum glucose, electrolytes, lactate, and amino acids in addition to urine orotic acid and amino acids. OTC deficiency is marked by low or absent serum citrulline, and high urine orotidine/ orotic acid.

Carbamoyl phosphate synthetase deficiency, is inherited in an autosomal recessive fashion like most other urea cycle disorders. In OTC deficiency, there is elevated plasma ammonia and low or absent citrulline. In this case, urine orotidine/ orotic acid is low or normal.

Lethargy, encephalopathy, and eye movement abnormalities may be present at birth.

Argininosuccinic aciduria is secondary to argininosuccinate lyase deficiency, and inherited as an autosomal recessive manner. Laboratory tests are significant for elevated ammonia and citrulline. Urine, plasma, and cerebrospinal fluid may have increased levels of

argininosuccinic acid. Urine orotic acid is also elevated.

Citrullinemia type I is caused by defects in argininosuccinate synthetase. It affect neonates who will have hypotonia and seizures. Ammonia and citrulline levels are usually increased.

Suggested Reading

- Haberle J, Boddaert M, Burlina A, Chakrapani A, Dixon M, Huemer M, Karail D, Martinelli D, Sanjurjo Crespo P, Santer R, Servais A, Valayannopoulos V, Lindner M, Rubio V, Dionisi-Vici C. Suggested guidelines for the diagnosis and management of urea cycle disorders. Orphanet J Rare Dis. 2012;7(32):1–30.
- Lee B. Urea cycle disorders; clinical features and diagnosis. In: Hahn S, TePas E, editors. Up-to-date. Waltham. Accessed on 12 Dec 2015.
- Menkes JH, Wilcox WR. Inherited metabolic diseases of the nervous system. In: Menkes JH, Sarnat HB, Maria BL, editors. Child neurology. 7th ed. Philadelphia: Lippincott Williams and Wilkins; 2006L. p. 29–142.

8. Which of the following protein is defective in phenylketonuria?
   A. Dihydropteridine reductase
   B. Sepiapterin reductase
   C. Phenylalanine hydroxylase
   D. GTP cyclohydrolase
   E. 6-pyruvoyl tetrahydrobiopterin synthase

14

Correct answer is: C

Phenylketonuria is caused by mutations in the phenylalanine hydroxylase (PAH) gene. Seizures, developmental delay, and mental retardation will occur because of the inability to process phenylalanine. Rough dry skin, musty odor, microcephalus, and tremor are other clinical features. Much of this can be avoided if a phenylalanine restricted diet is followed.

Mutations in the quinoid dihydropteridine reductase (QDPR) gene lead to dysfunction of quinoid dihydropteridine reductase which is involved in the creation of tetrahydrobiopterin (BH4) from quinoid dihydropterin. The resultant deficiency of BH4, which is necessary for hydroxylation of phenylalanine and processing of tyrosine and tryptophan, leads to defects in serotonin, epinephrine, and norepinephrine and dopamine synthesis. This is associated with hypotonia, oculogyric crisis, seizures, and involuntary movements.

Mutations in sepiapterin reductase (7, 8-dihydrobiopterin: NADP+ oxidoreductase) (SPR) lead to altered function of sepiapterin reductase, another molecule involved in the production of tetrahydrobiopterin. Dystonia, spasticity, and mental retardation are common with Sepiapterin reductase deficiency. Phenylalanine levels in the blood may be normal, although elevated levels sepiapterin, biopterin, and dihydropterin may be present in the cerebrospinal fluid.

Mutations in GTP cyclohydrolase 1 (GCH1) lead to alterations in in the protein cyclohydrolase. This is also required for tetrahydrobiopterin synthesis and dysfunction of this protein results in hypotonia, hyperthermia, and seizures. Mutations in this gene also cause dopa responsive dystonia. Mutations in 6-pyruvoyltetrahydropteri n synthase (PTS) lead to dysfunction in the processing of tetrahydrobiopterin. In this case, phenylalanine hydroxylase activity is normal although phenylalanine levels are high. Patients may have hypotonia, seizures, and involuntary movements.

Suggested Reading

- Menkes JH, Wilcox WR. Inherited metabolic diseases of the neNous system. In: Menkes JH, Sarnat HB, Maria BL, editors. Child neurology. 7th ed.

Philadelphia: Lippincott Williams and Wilkins; 2006L. p. 29–142.
- National Library of Medicine (US). Genetics Home Reference [Internet]. Bethesda: The Library; 2015 Dec 7. Tetrahydrobiopterin deficiency; [reviewed 2011 July; cited 2015 Dec 13]; Available from: ► http://ghr.nlm.nih.gov/condition/tetrahydrobiopterin-deficiency.
- National Library of Medicine (US). Genetics Home Reference [Internet]. Bethesda: The Library; 2015 Dec 7. SPR; [reviewed 2012 May; cited 2015 Dec 13]; Available from: ► http://ghr.nlm.nih.gov/gene/SPR.
- National Library of Medicine (US). Genetics Home Reference [Internet]. Bethesda: The Library; 2015 Dec 7. GCH1; [reviewed 2012 May; cited 2015 Dec 13]; Available from: ► http://ghr.nlm.nih.gov/gene/GCH1

9. Which of the following is associated with deficiency of alpha L Iduronidase?
   A. Hurler syndrome
   B. Hunter syndrome
   C. Sanfilippo syndrome type A
   D. Sanfilippo syndrome type B
   E. Morquio syndrome type A

Correct answer is: A

Mucopolysaccharidoses type1 is a lysosomal storage disease caused by mutations in the Iduronidase, alpha-L (IDUA) gene which codes for alpha L Iduronidase. Mucopolysaccharidoses type1 encompasses Hurler syndrome, Hurler Scheie syndrome, and Scheie syndrome. Hurler is the most severe with hepatosplenomegaly, breathing difficulties, dystosis multiplex, valvular heart disease, hearing loss, hydrocephalus, myelopathy, and coarse facial features. Death usually occurs in the first decade. Hurler Scheie is less severe with death occurring by age 20. Micrognathia, toe walking, and coarse facies may be present. Intelligence may be normal.

Scheie syndrome is the least severe-with life expectancy in the decades.

Hunter disease refers to mucopolysaccharidoses type 2, a deficiency of iduorate sulfatase. Presentation is similar to that of Hurler syndrome although corneal clouding is not present. Mucopolysaccharidoses type 3, which encompasses Sanfilippo A, B, C, and D, is another subtype. Type A is associated with sulfamidase deficiency, type B is associated with alpha N acetylglucosami nidase deficiency, type C is associated with acetyl-CoA: alpha glucosaminide n-acetyl transferase deficiency, and type D is associated with N acetylglucosami ne 6 sulfatase deficiency. All lead to build up of heparan sulfate. Presentation includes behavioral problems, developmental delay, and sleep disorders. Sanfilippo syndrome type B is associated with alpha-N-acetylglucosaminidase deficiency with buildup of heparan sulfate, aggressive behavior, and neurological decline.

Mucopolysaccharidoses type 4 encompasses Morquio syndrome type A and Morquio syndrome type B. Morquio type A is caused by defects in galactosamine-6-sulfatase, while Morquio type B is caused by dysfunction of beta galactosidase. Mucopolysaccharidoses type 4 is characterized by short stature, lax ligaments, genu valgum, C1-2 subluxation, hearing loss, coarse facial features, and valvular heart disease.

Suggested Reading

- Wynn R. Mucopolysaccharidoses: clinical features and diagnosis. In: Hahn, Patterson MC, TePas E, editors. Up-to-date, Waltham. Accessed on 12 Dec 2015.
- Murali HR, Renaud DL. Inborn errors of metabolism. In: Mowzoon N, Flemming KO, editors. Neurology board review: an illustrated study guide. Rochester: Mayo Clinic Scientific Press; 2007. p. 933–80.

10. Which of the following is caused by defects in mitochondrial DNA?
    A. Carnitine palmitoyltransferase I deficiency
    B. Carnitine palmitoyltransferase II deficiency
    C. Carnitine-acylcarnitine translocase deficiency
    D. Cytochrome b deficiency

Correct answer is: D
Defects in the mitochondrial gene MT-CYB (mitochondrial encoded cytochrome b) can cause the cytochrome b deficiency. This leads to dysfunction of mitochondrial complex III. include Fatigue, myopathy, exercise intolerance, encephalopathy, cardiomyopathy, and renal dysfunction are the classic manifestations.

Defects in the gene carnitine palmitoyltransferase 1A (liver) (CPT1A) can cause the carnitine palmitoyltransferase I deficiency. This is nuclear DNA, not mitochondrial DNA. Hepatic encephalopathy, myopathy of adult onset, or acute fatty liver of pregnancy are the clinical findings.

Carnitine palmitoyltransferase II deficiency is caused by mutations in nuclear DNA; CPT2 (carnitine palmitoyltransferase 2) is the specific gene implicated. This has a wide variation in phenotypes. In its more severe form, patients die in the neonatal period after presenting with liver failure, seizures, encephalopathy, cardiomyopathy, and hypoglycemia.

Defects in nuclear, not mitochondrial, DNA can cause the carnitine-acylcarnitine translocase deficiency. The gene implicated is solute carrier family 25 (carnitine/acylcarnitine translocase), member 20 (SLC25A20). It appears in the neonatal period with elevated ammonia, hypoglycemia, and encephalopathy. Dilated cardiomyopathy may also be present.

14

Suggested Reading

- National Library of Medicine (US). Genetics Home Reference [Internet]. Bethesda: The Library; 2015 Dec 7. Complex III deficiency; [reviewed 2014 Apr; cited 2015 Dec 13]; Available from: ▸ http://ghr.nlm.nih.gov/condition/mitochondrial-complex-iii-deficiency.
- O'Farrell E. Mitochondrial myopathies caused by disorders of lipid and purine metabolism. In: Patterson MC, Dashe JF, editors. Up-to-date. Waltham. Accessed on 12 Dec 2015.
- Darras BT. Mitochondrial myopathies: clinical features and diagnosis. In: Shefner JM, Dashe JF, editors. Up-to-date. Waltham. Accessed on 12 Dec 2015.

11. You are evaluating a suspected cerebral palsy 3-year-old male with a history of psychomotor delay, retinitis pigmentosa, failure to thrive with persistent large volume loose stools. His past laboratory results include a hemoglobin level of 6.8 g/dl, plasma cholesterol level of 85 mg/dl and triglyceride level of 22 mg/dl.
    What blood tests are going to order to reach the diagnosis?
    A. Apolipoprotein B
    B. Carnitine
    C. Creatine kinase
    D. Plasma phenylalanine

Correct answer is: A
This is a clinical presentation of Abetalipoproteinemia. It results in fat malabsorption from birth and is characterized by low density lipoprotein deficiency. This results in insufficient cholesterol, triglyceride and vitamin absorption for normal development. Chronic vitamin E deficiency is the reason for the neurological complications. Retinitis pigmentosa is present in almost all cases.

Carnitine is a cofactor that aids in the transfer of long chain fatty acids across the inner mitochondrial

membrane. Carnitine deficiency presents with progressive proximal muscle weakness.

Creatine kinase levels are elevated in myopathies and muscular dystrophies that typically present with muscle weakness in children and gait disturbance in older children.

Phenylketonuria presents with similar developmental delays but is not associated with anemia and abnormal lipid profile.

Suggested Reading

- Burnett JR, Hooper AJ. Vitamin E and oxidative stress in abetalipoproteinemia and familial hypobetalipoproteinemia. Free Radical Biol Med. 2015;88:59–62.

12. What is the most likely diagnosis is a 16-year-old boy with a 6-month history of progressive dysarthria, dystonia and Kayser-Fleischer rings on examination?
    - A. Mercury poisoning
    - B. Hepatolenticular degeneration
    - C. Lead encephalopathy
    - D. Gauchers Type III disease

Correct answer is: B

Hepatolenticular degeneration (Wilson disease), is a disorder of copper metabolism and can present with hepatic, neurological or psychiatric symptoms. Excess copper accumulation in the liver, brain and cornea damage tissue. The most common neurological symptoms in children are dysarthria and dystonia. Children under the 10 year of age present with liver failure. The Kayser-Fleischer ring is a prominent predictor of the disease and is evident when copper deposits along the limbus of the cornea as a yellow-brown pigment.

Exposed to mercury is common in general population from food with fish being the major source of methyl mercury exposure. Neurological manifestations like peripheral neuropathy, tremor, ataxia, blindness and seizures are common with high blood levels.

Lead intoxication in children at low levels causes slowed developmental progress with greatest effect on language development. However, acute lead encephalopathy can be rapidly fatal.

Gauchers type III presents with hepatosplenomegaly, impaired bone marrow production of red blood cells and platelets and progressive neurological symptoms due to an accumulation of glycolipids in reticuloendothelial cells.

Suggested Reading

- Lorincz MT. Recognition and treatment of neurologic Wilson's disease. Semin Neurol. 2012; 32(5):538.

13. You are seeing a 4 days old newborn who developed ketoacidosis, hypoglycemia, hypotonia, and lethargy. His urine has a characteristic sweet odor. **Which statement regarding this disorder is true?**
    - A. It is a disorder of lysosoma l storage
    - B. It results in an accumulation of alanine
    - C. A variant is responsive to vitamin B6 (pyridoxine
    - D. There is a deficiency of branched-chain ketoacid dehydrogenase
    - E. MRI demonstrates basal ganglia calcifications

Correct Answer is: D

The clinical scenario is indicative of maple syrup urine disease. It is a result of a deficiency of branched-chain ketoacid dehydrogenase. The enzyme decarboxylates branched chain amino acids, and its deficiency results in the accumulation of isoleucine, leucine, and valine. Dysmyelination, heterotopias, diffuse spongy degeneration, and a failure

of cortical lamination are the main manifestations. Severe deficiency has a neonatal onset, and occurs in babies who are normal at birth, but develop ketoacidosis, hypoglycemia, hypotonia, lethargy, seizures, and cerebra l edema after beginning feedings containing protein. If untreated, coma and respiratory failure will result in death. A milder form has later onset, with a moderate deficiency of the enzyme. Ketoacidosis, ataxia, and intellectual disability are the main symptoms. The characteristic feature is a sweet smell of the urine. Subcortical white matter changes and cerebral edema, particularly after a protein-containing meal are seen on MRI. Hemodialysis and diets low in branched-chain amino acids are the treatment of choice. A thiamine responsive variant exists; hence a trial of thiamine is warranted.

Suggested Reading

- Fenichel GM. The disorder has autosomal recessive inheritance. Clin Pediatr Neurol. 5th edition. Philadelphia: Elsevier Saunders; 2005. p. 4–5.

14. You are evaluating a 15-year-old female in the ED with a history of severe abdominal pain, nausea, and vomiting for 2 days. All her labs including liver enzymes are normal. She received intravenous fluids in the ED. Today, she has a generalized tonic-clonic seizure followed by hallucinations and delusions. Brain MRI with contrast and CSF analysis are normal. On day 4 of her admission to the hospital, she is noted to have mild weakness of wrist extension; 1 week later, examination shows bilateral wrist drop.
What is your diagnosis in this patient?
A. Wilson's disease
B. Systemic lupus erythematosuis
C. Acute inflammatory demyelinating polyneuropathy
D. Acute disseminated encephalomyelitis
E. Acute intermittent porphyria

Correct Answer is: E
This is a case of an acute hepatic porphyria. It is an autosomal dominant and involve multiple areas of the nervous system. They are secondary to enzymatic dysfunction in porphyrin metabolism with subsequent abnormalities in heme synthesis and metabolism. These disorders include acute intermittent porphyria (AIP), which results from various mutations that lead to reduced activity of the enzyme porphobilinogen deaminase, variegate porphyria, which results from reduced activity of the enzyme protoporphinogen IX oxidase, hereditary coproporphyria which results from reduced activity in the enzyme coprophorphinogen oxidase, and plumboporphyria, which results from reduced enzymatic activity of Li-aminolevulinic acid (ALA) dehydratase.

Symptoms often do not appear until adolescence or later because the dysfunctional enzymes have some residual enzyme activity, with some symptoms occurring in episodes with exposure to certain triggers. Medications, menstruation, and alcohol exposure are common triggers. With exposure to these triggers, activity of the hepatic enzyme ALA synthase increases, leading to overproduction of heme precursors that cannot be sufficiently metabolized by the involved downstream enzymes.

In spite the different porphyries differ in several biochemical aspects, their neurologic manifestations are similar. Symptoms typically manifest in early adulthood, with females being more commonly and more severely affected as compared to males. The early symptoms

typically is abdominal pain and other gastrointestinal symptoms, followed by neurologic symptoms, including most prominently manifestations of autonomic instability (tachycardia, labile hypertension, orthostasis, and urinary retention). Neuropsychiatric symptoms including psychosis occur, and seizures may be present as well. In some patients, a subacute predominantly motor neuropathy occurs; the arms may be affected prior to the legs, and proximal muscles are involved more than distal muscles.

Involvement of the radial nerve in isolation may occur. The neuropathy is both axonal and demyelinating. Cranial nerve involvement, and even respiratory muscle involvement leading to respiratory failure, may occur.

In AIP, photosensitivity is not present, whereas with variegate porphyria and hereditary coproporphyria, photosensitivity with skin blistering and hyperpigmentation occur. During an attack, elevated levels of porphobilinogen and aminolevulinic acid are detectable in the urine and serum. Elevated protoporphyrinogen and coproporphyrinogen in the stool distinguish variegate porphyria and hereditary coproporphyria from AIP.

Treatment of the porphyrias involves prevention of attacks by avoidance of drugs that may precipitate the attack (including anti-epileptics, particularly barbiturates) and other triggers. Treatment of attacks includes supportive care, a high-carbohydrate diet, and in some cases hematin, which suppresses delta ALA synthase activity.

Although Wilson's disease is on the differential diagnosis of patients with neuropsychiatric symptoms, it does not typically lead to peripheral motor mono-neuropathies or abdominal pain, except in the setting of hepatic impairment, and there is no evidence of liver disease in the case presented.

The history in this vignette is not consistent with acute disseminated encephalomyelitis, in which the MRI would be abnormal, or acute inflammatory demyelinating polyneuropathy. Although systemic lupus erythematosuis can lead to a similar clinical picture, normal MRI of the brain and CSF analysis make this less likely.

Suggested Reading

- Bradley WG, Daroff RB, Fenichel GM, et al. Neurology in clinical practice, 5th ed. Philadelphia: Elsevier; 2008.
- Ropper AH, Samuels MA. Adams and Victor's principles of neurology, 9th ed. New York: McGraw-Hill; 2009.
- Comprehensive review in clinical neurology: a multiple-choice question book for the wards and boards ©2011 Wolters Kluwer Health Lippincott Williams & Wilkins. All rights reserved.

15. You were asked to see a newborn, who is lethargic with poor feeding and rapidly becomes encephalopathic and develops seizures. His lab tests form the nursery shows hyperammonemia with respiratory alkalosis and normal anion gap. The NICU team has to intubate him and start mechanical ventilation. You suspected a urea cycle disorder.

Which of the following is correct regarding this group of disorders?

A. This is a group of disorders that are all inherited in an X-linked fashion
B. Ornithine transcarbamylase deficiency is the most common cause
C. Hyperammonemia and organic acidemias are commonly found in patients with these disorders
D. Arginase deficiency commonly presents in the newborn period
E. High protein diet is indicated for their treatment

Correct Answer is: B
Urea cycle disorders are a group of conditions caused by deficiency of enzymes responsible for urea synthesis and more importantly ammonia and ammonia-containing compound removal. The most common disorder is Ornithine transcarbamylase (OTC) deficiency which is X-linked. Carbamyl phosphate synthetase deficiency, argininosucci nic acid synthetase deficiency, argininosuccinic acid lyase deficiency, and arginase deficiency are an autosomal recessive disorder. These enzyme defects will lead to hyper-ammonemia, which is the main cause of the clinical manifestations. Ammonia induces glutamine accumulation, which leads to astrocyte swelling and brain edema. Hyper-ammonemia, encephalopathy, and respiratory alkalosis is the triad suggesting of those disorders. This infant has very high concentrations of ammonia, no evidence of organic acidemias, normal anion gaps, and normal serum glucose level.

Liver biopsy specimens can help in the amino acid analyses and enzyme activity for specific urea cycle disorders.

The clinical presentation often begins in the newborn period with progressive lethargy, vomiting, hypotonia, and seizures. Higher levels of ammonia may be associated with coma and eventually death.

Females with OTC deficiency, and some patients with partial deficiencies, may have late-onset presentations and become symptomatic after large amounts of protein ingestion or intercurrent sickness.

Arginase deficiency does not cause symptoms in the newborn, whereas newborn presentation is common in the rest of urea cycle disorders.

Treatment includes limitation of nitrogen intake in the diet and administration of essential amino acids. Calories can be supplied with carbohydrates and fat. During acute episodes, sodium benzoate and sodium phenylacetic acid are used, and sometimes dialysis may be required. Mannitol has been used for brain edema and increased intracranial pressure. Long-term treatment with low-protein diet and essential amino acids, as well as arginine supplementation (except in arginase deficiency), may stabilize the neurologic deterioration.

16. You are seeing a newborn baby who developed encephalopathy secondary to metabolic acidosis and hyper-ammonemia. There is also keto-acidosis and elevated methylmalonic acid levels. You suspect methylmalonic acidemia.
Which of the following is incorrect regarding this condition?
A. The deficient enzyme is D-methylmalonyl-CoA mutase
B. Propionyl-CoA levels are not altered in this enzymatic disorder
C. Adenosylcobalamin acts as cofactor in the involved enzymatic step
D. Protein restriction in the diet is part of the treatment plan
E. The enzyme affected participates in the conversion of L-methylmalonyl CoA to succinyl-CoA

14

Correct Answer is: B
In methylmalonic acidemia, the level of propionyl-CoA increases because its accumulation. It is an autosomal recessive condition caused by the deficiency of D-methylmalonyl-CoA mutase. This enzyme normally catalyzes the isomerization of L-methylmalonyl-CoA to succinyl CoA, which then enters the Krebs cycle. Adenosylcobalamin is a required cofactor. A defect in this metabolic pathway leads to accumulation of propionyl- CoA, propionic acid, and methylmalonic acid, causing metabolic acidosis, hyperglycinemia, and hyper-ammonemia. At birth those children are

normal, becoming symptomatic within the first week of life, manifesting with lethargy, failure to thrive, vomiting, dehydration, hypotonia, and respiratory distress. Hematologic abnormalities, including bleeding disorders leading to intracranial hemorrhage, may also occur. Survivors are left with intellectual disability, developmental delay, and recurrent acidosis.

The diagnosis should be suspected in newborn patients with metabolic acidosis, ketosis, hyperglycinemia, and hyper-ammonemia. Methylmalonic acid is elevated in plasma and urine, and the enzyme activity can be analyzed in fibroblasts.

The treatment is a protein restricted diet and supplementation of hydroxycobalamin and carnitine. Antibiotics are also helpful to reduce the production of propionic acid. In the acute setting, these patients need hydration and glucose administration with discontinuation of protein intake. This condition is screened for by extended newborn screening, thus allowing for pre-symptomatic treatment in most patients with the classic or severe form of the disease.

17. You are evaluating a 1-year old boy for his axial hypotonia, limb hypertonia, myoclonus, intellectual disability, and episodic hypoglycemia. His symptoms are worse throughout the day, and improve after sleep.
The most likely diagnosis is:
A. Phenylketonuria
B. Hartnup disease
C. Canavan disease
D. DOPA decarboxylase deficiency
E. Homocysteinuria

Correct Answer is: D
Phenylketonuria is secondary to a deficiency of phenylalanine hydroxylase, which causes dysmyelination, heterotopias, diffuse spongy degeneration, and a failure of lamination. It begins between 2–3 months of age with a musty odor of the skin and urine, intellectual disability, hyperactivity, irritability, tremor, spasticity, dry and hypo-pigmented skin, microcephaly, and infantile spasms that later evolve to a generalized tonic-clonic seizure disorder.

Hartnup disease results from an abnormality of the neutral amino acid transport protein, such that it impairs intestinal and renal absorption of neutral amino acids (i.e. tryptophan). Symptoms are unrelated to diet, and include photosensitive pellagra-like dermatitis (due to nicotinamide deficiency), developmental delays, headaches, psychiatric changes, hypotonia, and ataxia. Clinical presentations may be due in part to intestinal absorption of toxins resulting from amino acid breakdown. Stress or infection can trigger symptomatic episodes, and take up to 1 month for resolution. The disorder is of autosomal recessive inheritance, with a mutation on chromosome 5.

Canavan disease is an autosomal recessive deficiency of aspartoacylase, which results in accumulation of N-acetylaspartate (NAA). NAA serves as an osmolyte, causing edema and spongiform changes of white matter. Symptoms include developmental regression, hypotonia that evolves to spasticity, macrocephaly, dysphagia, optic nerve atrophy, seizures, and posturing with stimulation (extension of the lower extremities and head, with arm flexion).

DOPA decarboxylase deficiency prevents conversion of L-dopa to dopamine, and 5-hydroxytryptophan to serotonin. Its symptoms begin within the first two years of life, and consist of axial hypotonia, limb hypertonia, dystonia, startle myoclonus, intellectual disability, and autonomic dysfunction (e.g. sweats, temperature instability, ptosis, miosis, and episodic hypoglycemia). A main

feature is the worsening of symptoms throughout the day, with improvement after sleep.

In homocysteinuria, heterozygous mutations lead to accelerated atherosclerosis, while homozygous mutations lead to increased platelet aggregation. Homocysteinuria consists of three subtypes: (1) Cystathionine 13-synthase deficiency. Homozygous mutations may result in strokes, myocardial infarctions, intellectual disability, glaucoma, lens dislocations, a marfanoid body type, and osteoporosis. Symptom onset occurs prior to age five. (2) Methylenetetrahydrofolate reductase (MTHFR) deficiency. This form leads to a more severe phenotype. (3) Deficiency of B12 coenzyme synthesis and transport.

Suggested Reading

- Fenichel GM. Clinical pediatric neurology. 5th ed. Philadelphia: Elsevier Saunders; 2005. p. 125–8,138, 222.

18. You are evaluating a newborn baby for encephalopathy in association of metabolic acidosis and hyper-ammonemia. There is also ketoacidosis, and elevated blood propionic acid and glycine levels with normal methylmalonic acid levels. You suspect propionic acidemia.

    Which of the following is correct regarding this condition?

    A. It is caused by deficiency of D-methylmalonyl-CoA mutase
    B. It is X-linked
    C. High protein diet is recommended for these patients
    D. Hematologic disorders occur in this condition
    E. Propionyl-CoA carboxylase activity is increased

Correct Answer is: D

This is a clinical presentation of propionic acidemia, in which hematologic manifestations such as pancytopenia and bleeding disorders may occur. It is an autosomal recessive disorder caused by a deficiency of propionyl-CoA carboxylase. This enzyme normally participates in the carboxylation of propionyl-CoA to D-methylmalonyl-CoA, a step that requires the coenzyme biotin.

Children with propionic acidemia are normal at birth but develop symptoms either in the early neonatal period, in infancy, or later in childhood. The classic presentation is feeding difficulty, lethargy, hypotonia, dehydration, and attacks of metabolic acidosis and hyperammonemia. They may progress to have seizures and coma. Hepatomegaly, pancytopenia, and bleeding disorders including intracranial hemorrhage are also other findings. Survivors have intellectual disability and basal ganglia abnormalities.

Newborn babies with ketoacidosis, with an anion gap, and elevated propionic acid levels in the blood and sometimes in the urine, diagnosis should be suspected. Elevation of glycine levels in plasma and urine and of methylcitrate and B-hydroxypropionate in urine are also observed. Enzyme activity in leukocytes or fibroblasts is reduced.

Treatment is restricted protein diet, IV fluids for hydration, as well as carnitine and biotin supplementation. Dialysis may be required in some patients. Antibiotics such as metronidazole may decrease the production of propionate by enteric bacteria. D-methylmalonyl-CoA mutase deficiency causes methylmalonic academia. Propionic acidemia is screened for by extended newborn screening, thus allowing for presymptomatic treatment in most patients with the classic or severe form of the disease.

19. You are evaluating a 12- month-old boy for his hypotonia, alopecia, and seizures. His Lab shows ketoacidosis,

14

hyperammonemia, and elevated urine organic acid levels. You suspect Biotinidase deficiency.

Which statement below is incorrect?

A. Biotin levels are elevated in biotinidase deficiency and should not be supplemented
B. Hearing and vision loss can occur
C. Biotinidase cleaves biocytin and participates in biotin recycling
D. Biotinidase participates in processing of dietary protein-bound biotin
E. Patients have ketoacidosis, hyperammonemia, and organic aciduria

Correct Answer is: A
Biotin is a water-soluble B-complex vitamin that is necessary in multiple metabolic reactions including gluconeogenesis, fatty acid synthesis, catabolism of amino acids, and gene expression. Biotinidase deficiency can cause biotin deficiency. This enzyme normally cleaves biocytin, thereby recycling biotin, and also participates in processing of dietary protein-bound biotin, making it available to the free biotin pool. Biotinidase deficiency has previously been known as late-onset multiple carboxylase deficiency, and it is inherited in an autosomal recessive fashion. Children with this enzymatic defect manifest with seizures, hypotonia, ataxia, developmental delay, hearing and visual loss, spastic para-paresis, and cutaneous abnormalities, including alopecia. Laboratory studies demonstrate ketoacidosis, hyper-ammonemia, and organic aciduria. The enzyme activity can be analyzed in serum. Treatment is biotin supplementation, which prevents intellectual disability and reverses most of the symptoms. This condition is screened for by extended newborn screening, thus allowing for pre-symptomatic treatment in most patients with the classic or severe form of the disease.

Suggested Reading

- Comprehensive review in clinical neurology: a multiple-choice question book for the wards and boards © 2011 Wolters Kluwer Health Lippincott Williams & Wilkins. All rights reserved.

20. You saw a 2 days old newborn for his seizures. The nurse told you that the baby refused feeding and seemed irritable in the first few hours of life. The infant subsequently developed respiratory failure and required intubation. You have ordered an extensive workup including a brain MRI (shown below). His CSF showed a high glycine level.
Which of the following is incorrect regarding this condition?

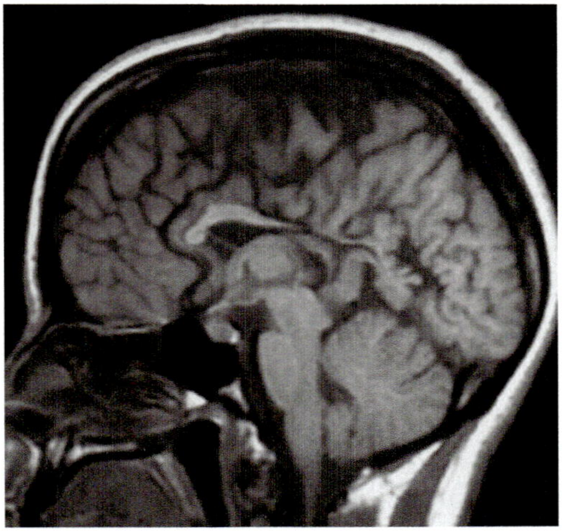

Fig. 14.3 Corpus callosum, agenesis. Sagittal T1-weighted MRI of the brain shows partial agenesis of the corpus callosum. The genu and anterior body of the corpus callosum are visualized, whereas the posterior body, splenium, and rostrum are absent. Wikipedia

A. This patient has a disturbance of glycine degradation
B. Patients who survive the acute phase are left with intellectual disability, spasticity, and epilepsy
C. Treatment with sodium benzoate is effective and prevents progression of the disease

D. It is autosomal recessive
E. EEG may show burst suppression

Correct Answer is: C
There is a partial agenesis of the corpus callosum on the MRI. A diagnosis of glycine encephalopathy (non-ketotic hyperglycinemia) is based on the MRI finding, the clinical picture and the high CSF glycine levels. Available treatment options are limited and not effective. Glycine encephalopathy is an autosomal recessive. The onset is in newborns who, within a few hours after birth, become irritable with poor feeding and hiccups. Subsequently, they develop a progressive encephalopathy with hypotonia, myoclonic seizures, and respiratory failure requiring mechanical ventilation. Survivors will have intellectual disability, spasticity, and epilepsy. Brain MRI may reveal a hypoplastic or absent corpus callosum and gyral malformations and cerebellar hypoplasia. In the acute phase, the EEG shows burst suppression and hypsarrhythmia. Non-ketotic hyperglycinemia or glycine encephalopathy is caused by a defect in the P-protein (glycine decarboxylase) gene, which encodes a component of the mitochondrial glycine cleavage system, therefore affecting the degradation of glycine, with accumulation of this substance. Serum and CSF glycine levels are elevated, and the ratio of CSF to plasma glycine concentration is more than 0.6, whereas normally, it is less than 0.4. No effective treatments are available; sodium benzoate decreases plasma glycine concentrations, but the CSF level does not normalize with this therapy, and neurologic dysfunction is not reversible. Benzodiazepines can be used for seizures. Dextromethorphan and ketamine can be used to inhibit NMDA receptor excitation by glycine.

14

21. What is the treatment of a 12-month-old boy that presents with a history of acute episodes of ataxia, irritability and lethargy accompanied by the appearance of dark blood in the urine?
A. Maintenance anti-convulsive medication
B. Carnitine and Coenzyme Q supplementation
C. A phenylalanine free diet
D. Protein restricted diet

Correct Answer is: D
Maple syrup urine disease is a metabolic disorder caused by defect in the enzyme branched-chain keto acid dehydrogenase. It is a recessively inherited disorder. Trigger factors are minor infections, surgery or a protein rich diet. During an episode, the urine has a maple syrup smell and is made dark by blood and urine containing high levels of branched-chained amino acids and ketoacids.

Carnitine and coenzyme Q10 are commonly administered to maximize function in mitochondrial disorders.

Phenylketonuria is an autosomal recessive disorder caused by a deficiency of the hepatic enzyme phenylalanine hydroxylase and presents at birth. The treatment is a phenylalanine free diet.

Suggested Reading

- Strauss KA, Puffenberger EG, Morton DH. 2013. Maple syrup urine disease.

22. You are seeing a 17-year-old male in the PICU with left-sided weakness and aphasia. His head CT showed an acute ischemic infarct in the territory of the right middle cerebral artery. On examination, he is tall, thin, has long fingers, and high arched feet. Past medical history is remarkable of lens dislocation, pigeon chest and osteoporosis.

What single blood test is likely to be of diagnostic use in this patient?

A. Peripheral blood smear
B. Thyroid-stimulating hormone
C. Homocysteine
D. Branched chain amino acids
E. Lactic acid

Correct Answer is: C

This is a classic manifestation of homocystinuria. It is an AR disorder; caused by Cystathion ine-13-synthase deficiency --> elevation of blood and urine levels of homocysteine and methionine. Usually, patients are normal at birth; but they will have developmental delay and intellectual disability later. They may have seizures and psychiatric manifestations.

They have a collagen metabolism abnormality --> eye, bones, and the vascular system --> Ectopia lentis and lens dislocation. Other clinical manifestations include, marfanoid habitus with tall and thin stature, pectus carinatum, pes cavus, genu valgum, and osteoporosis. Intimal thickening of the blood vessel walls and high incidence of thromboembolism, including strokes.

Elevation of plasma and urine homocysteine, methionine in the plasma and CSF can confirm the diagnosis.

Majority of patient respond to pyridoxine, so give this first. Betaine, folate and vitamin 812 supplements. Low-protein diet, specifically low in methionine with cysteine supplementation.

Suggested Reading

- Mowzoon N, Flemming KD. Neurology board review: an illustrated study guide. Rochester: Mayo Clinic Scientific; 2007. Print.

23. A mother of a newborn reported that the baby is lethargic with poor feeding. At the hospital he rapidly becomes encephalopathic and develops seizures. He has hyperammonemia with respiratory alkalosis and normal anion gap. Eventually, the baby requires intubation and mechanical ventilation. A urea cycle disorder is suspected.

Which statement below is correct?

A. This is a group of disorders that are all inherited in an X-linked fashion
B. Ornithine transcarbamylase deficiency is the most common cause
C. Hyperammonemia and organic acidemias are commonly found in patients with these disorders
D. Arginase deficiency commonly presents in the newborn period
E. High protein diet is indicated for their treatment

Correct Answer is: B

Urea cycle disorders are a group of conditions caused by deficiency of enzymes responsible for urea synthesis and more importantly ammonia and ammonia-containing compound removal.

Ornithine transcarbamylase (OTC) deficiency is the most common and is X-linked. All others are inherited in an autosomal recessive fashion and include carbamyl phosphate synthetase deficiency, argininosuccinic acid synthetase deficiency, argininosuccinic acid lyase deficiency, and arginase deficiency. These enzyme defects will lead to hyperammonemia, which is the main cause of the clinical manifestations. Ammonia induces glutamine accumulation, which leads to astrocyte swelling and brain edema. Hyperammonemia, encephalopathy, and respiratory alkalosis are the triad suggestive of this group of disorders. These patients have very high concentrations of ammonia, no evidence of organic acidemias, normal anion gaps, and normal serum glucose level. Amino acid analyses help to

distinguish specific urea cycle disorders, and enzyme activity can be evaluated in liver biopsy specimens. Clinical manifestations often begin in the newborn period with progressive lethargy, vomiting, hypotonia, and seizures. Higher levels of ammonia may be associated with coma and eventually death. Females with OTC deficiency, and some patients with partial deficiencies, may have late-onset presentations and become symptomatic after large amounts of protein ingestion or inter-current illnesses.

Arginase deficiency does not cause symptoms in the newborn, whereas newborn presentation is common in the rest of urea cycle disorders.

Treatment includes limitation of nitrogen intake in the diet and administration of essential amino acids. Calories can be supplied with carbohydrates and fat. During acute episodes, sodium benzoate and sodium phenylacetic acid are used, and sometimes dialysis may be required.

Mannitol has been used for brain edema and increased intracranial pressure. Long-term treatment with low-protein diet and essential amino acids, as well as arginine supplementation (except in arginase deficiency), may stabilize the neurologic deterioration.

14

Suggested Reading

- Comprehensive review in clinical neurology: a multiple-choice question book for the wards and boards ©2011 Wolters Kluwer Health Lippincott Williams & Wilkins.

24. You are asked to see a 5 -day-old baby boy at the hospital because of persistent vomiting and diarrhea, predominantly after being fed. He has jaundice, hypotonia and hepatosplenomegaly on examination. Reducing substances are detected in the urine. A presumptive diagnosis of galactosemia is made.

Which of the following is not true regarding this disorder?

A. Galactose-1-phosphate uridyltransferase deficiency is the only defect associated with galactosemia
B. Galactitol accumulation produces cataracts that are reversible
C. It is autosomal recessive
D. The treatment is removal of lactose and ga lactose from the diet
E. Patients with this disorder may develop ataxia and tremor despite treatment

Correct Answer is: A

Galactosemia occurs in newborns and it is an autosomal recessive disorder. There are three enzymatic defects that account for galactosemia: galactose-1-phosphate uridyltransferase deficiency, galactokinase deficiency, and uridine diphosphate galactose 4_ epimerase deficiency.

Galactose-1-phosphate uridyltransferase deficiency causes classic galactosemia and is the only type associated with intellectual disability. Patients present in the first days of life with feeding difficulties, vomiting, diarrhea, and jaundice.

Hepatomegaly, failure to thrive, lethargy, and hypotonia are also a clinical manifestation. Cataracts also occur and are caused by an accumulation of galactitol. Developmental delay, cognitive impairment, ataxia, and tremor are late neurologic sequelae. B rain MRI shows white matter changes and cortical and cerebellar atrophy. Prenatal diagnosis of galactosemia is available, and newborn screening is available for this condition, thus allowing for treatment prior to the onset of symptoms. The diagnosis can be presumed in patients presenting with the clinical manifestations described, and the detection of reducing substances in the urine, especially

after feeding. The enzymatic defect can be detected in plasma and/or erythrocytes. Lactose and galactose should be immediately restricted from the diet. This intervention may reverse cataracts and hepatomegaly and may prevent progression of neurologic disease. However, despite this intervention, these patients may develop long-term neurologic sequelae, including learning disability, cognitive impairment, ataxia, and tremor.

25. Which of the following is not true regarding mucopolysaccharidoses (MPS)?
    A. There is accumulation of glucosaminog lycans, which are detected in urine
    B. Hurler syndrome is caused by A-L-iduronidase deficiency
    C. Sanfilippo syndrome is a group of MPS with accumulation of heparan but not dermatan sulfate
    D. Morquio syndrome manifests with prominent intellectual disability
    E. Zebra bodies can be seen on electron microscopy

Correct Answer is: D

There is no intellectual disability in patients with Morquio syndrome. Mucopolysaccharidoses (MPS) are caused by impaired lysosomal degradation of glucosaminoglycans, which are long unbranched molecules of repeating disaccharides. Various enzymatic defects lead to the accumulation of glucosaminoglycans in lysosomes and the extracellular matrix. All MPS are autosomal recessive except Hunter disease, which is X-linked. In general, MPS are a group of progressive multisystem disorders that affect the cornea, cartilage, bone, connective tissue, reticuloendothelial system, and nervous system.

Hurler syndrome is type I MPS and is caused by A-L-iduronidase deficiency. The gene is localized to chromosome 4, and there is accumulation of both dermatan and heparan sulfate. These patients are normal at birth, but within the first 2 years of life, they will develop coarsening of facial features, with progressive skeletal dysplasia with dysostosis multiplex and growth impairment (dwarfism). There is a restricted range of motion of the joints, hearing loss, corneal clouding, macroglossia, hernias, visceromegaly, valvular heart disease, and prominent intellectual disability.

Scheie syndrome is a mild MPS type I, and the intermediate form is known as Hurler-Scheie syndrome.

Most recently, MPS type I has been classified as severe MPS type I and attenuated MPS type I. The diagnosis of MPS type I is based on elevated urinary excretion of dermatan and heparan sulfate and confirmed with enzyme analysis in leukocytes and fibroblasts. Pathologically, there are cells with vacuolated appearance, expansion of perivascular spaces in the CNS, and neuronal lipidosis. Electron microscopy demonstrates reticulogranular material in epithelial and mesenchymal cells, and lamellar material in neurons, some of which adopt a layered appearance and are called zebra bodies. Enzyme replacement therapy can be used to treat non-central nervous system manifestations of the disease. Stem cell transplantation can be potentially helpful.

Hunter syndrome or MPS type II is caused by a defect in iduronate sulfatase, with accumulation of dermatan sulfate and heparan sulfate. These patients have the Hurler phenotype but lack the corneal clouding and have characteristic nodular ivory-colored lesions on the back, shoulders, and upper arms. These children have short stature, macrocephaly, macroglossia, hoarse voice, hearing loss, visceromegaly, dysostosis multiplex, joint contractures,

entrapment neuropathies such as carpal tunnel syndrome, and intellectual disability. The diagnosis is based on mucopolysacchari duria and confirmed with analysis of the enzyme activity. Treatment is symptomatic.

Other MPS include types III, IV, VI, VII, and IX as follows: - MPS type III or Sanfilippo syndrome has several subtypes (A, B, C, and D) and is associated with accumulation of heparan sulfate only. The main manifestation is intellectual disability. - MPS type IV or Morquio syndrome has two subtypes (A and B), and they manifest with corneal clouding, dysostosis multiplex, and heart disease, with normal intelligence. - MPS type VI is also known as Maroteaux-Lamy syndrome and manifests with normal intelligence, dysostosis multiplex, corneal clouding, heart disease, and other features similar to Hurler syndrome. - MPS type VII is also known as Sly syndrome, and these patients have hydrops fetalis, intellectual disability, dysostosis multiplex, corneal clouding, and other features of Hurler syndrome.

26. Which of the following conditions has mutation in gene ATP7B?
    - A. Wilson's disease
    - B. Hemochromatosis
    - C. Parkinson's disease
    - D. Huntington's disease
    - E. All of the above

Correct Answer is: A
Wilson's disease has a common gene defect in ATP7B. Hemochromatosis has mutations in HFE gene. Parkinsonism and Huntington's disease are neurodegenerative disorders. Huntington's disease is autosomal dominant and is a trinucleotide repeat disease whose severity and onset is determined by the number of CAG repeats. The disease has variable penetrance depending on the number of repeats. The number of repeats is unstable and increases with each subsequent generation a phenomenon known as a dynamic mutation. Encephalitis is an infectious disorder.

Suggested Reading

Sadock BJ, Sadock VA, Kaplan HI. Kaplan & Sadock's synopsis of psychiatry: behavioral sciences/clinical psychiatry. Philadelphia: Lippincott Williams & Wilkins; 2013.

27. You are evaluating a 14- year-old boy with a history of severe generalized myoclonus, ataxia, and loss of color vision. On examination, he has a cherry red spots. His EEG showed slow background, and photosensitive bilateral fast spike and wave activity. **What finding would establish the diagnosis?**
    - A. An alpha-N-acetylgalactosaminidase deficiency
    - B. A decrease in cultured skin fibroblast alpha-neuraminidase
    - C. A response to oral biotin
    - D. A hexoaminidase A deficiency
    - E. A muscle biopsy with ragged red fibers

Correct Answer is: B
Schindler disease is caused by an alpha-N-acetylgalactosaminidase deficiency. It is a rare autosomal recessive disorder with acute infant and chronic adult-onset forms. The main manifestations in infants are severe psychomotor deterioration with spasticity, cortical blindness, and myoclonic epilepsy with an exaggerated startle response. The adult form is characterized by mild cognitive deficits.

Sialidosis type 1A occurs in adolescent and is characterized by severe generalized myoclonus, night blindness, and loss of color vision, ataxia, cherry-red spots, and generalized convulsions.

The EEG usually shows progressive slowing and bilateral, photosensitive fast spike-wave discharges. A decrease in cultured skin fibroblast alpha-neuraminidase is diagnostic.

Biotinidase deficiency responses to oral biotin. Its clinical manifestations include hypotonia, generalized tonic-clonic and myoclonic seizures, rash, and alopecia, and occurs in infancy. The EEG demonstrates multifocal spikes and slow waves.

Tay-Sachs disease is secondary to a hexoaminidase A deficiency, with the onset of development delay, cherry-red spots, and "startle seizures" in infancy.

A muscle biopsy with ragged red fibers is indicative of myoclonic epilepsy with ragged red fibers (MERRF), which is a mitochondrial disorder. The clinical features include myoclonus, epilepsy, myopathy, intellectual disability, and cerebellar dysfunction. Patients may also have short stature, deafness, optic atrophy, cutaneous lipomas, and neuropathy. The onset is typically in childhood or early adulthood.

Suggested Reading

- Varma A, Moraes CT. Mitochondrial disorders. In: Bradley WG, Daroff RB, Fenichel GM, Jankovic J, editors. Neurology in clinical practice, 4th ed. Elsevier, Inc.; 2004. p. 781–808.
- Pastores GM, Kolodny EH. Inborn errors of metabolism of the neNous system. In: Bradley WG, Daroff RB, Fenichel GM, Jankovic J, editors. Neurology in clinical practice. 4th ed. Elsevier, Inc.; 2004. p. 1811–32.

28. Which of the following is correct regarding sialidosis?
    - A. Sialidosis type I has infantile onset
    - B. Sialidosis type II has adult onset
    - C. A cherry-red spot is rarely seen in this condition
    - D. Coarse facial features are almost never seen in sialidosis type II
    - E. These patients have myoclonic epilepsy

Correct Answer is: E

Sialidosis is one of the glycoproteinoses. Myoclonic epilepsy is one of its features. Glycoproteinoses are a lysosomal storage disorders, and they are inheritance as autosomal recessive disorders, in which the enzymatic defect leads to accumulation of oligosaccharides, glycopeptides, and glycolipids. Vacuolization of multiple cell types occur secondary to accumulation in the brain and viscera. There are multiple phenotypes depending on the enzyme affected.

Usually, patients have coarse facial features, skeletal abnormalities, and psychomotor retardation.

Sialidosis is caused by deficiency of lysosomal A-neuraminidase (sialidase), leading to increased urinary excretion of sialic acid-containing oligosaccharides. Type I sialidosis (cherry red spot myoclonus syndrome) occurs in adolescence to adulthood and manifests with myoclonic epilepsy, visual deterioration, and cherry-red spots without dysmorphism.

Type II occurs in childhood, and these patients have not only myoclonic epilepsy and cherry-red spots in the retina but also severe neurologic abnormalities, coarse facial features, severe dysostosis, and psychomotor retardation.

The neonatal form is characterized by hydrops fetalis, nephrotic syndrome, and early death. Other glycoproteinoses include A-mannosidosis caused by A-mannosidosidase deficiency, B-mannosidosis caused by B-mannosidosidase deficiency, fucosidosis caused by fucosidase deficiency, aspartylglucosami nuria caused by aspartylglucosaminidase deficiency, and Schindler disease caused by A-N acetylgalactosaminidase deficiency.

Abnormal urinary excretion of oligosaccharides and glycopeptides, as well as vacuolated lymphocytes with membrane-bound vacuoles, are present. Analysis of enzyme activity can give you the definitive diagnosis.

29. You are evaluating an 11-year-old boy for his developmental delay and psychomotor retardation. You examined him and noticed, there is limited horizontal gaze, ataxia, and generalized spasticity. On general examination, he has hepatosplenomegaly. Enzymatic activity of glucocerebrosidase in leukocytes is depressed.
What is correct regarding this disorder?
    A. There is accumulation of lysosomal glucocerebrosides
    B. Patients with type 1 of this disease have severe neurologic impairment by age 2
    C. Type 3 has its onset before age 2 and progresses rapidly to death between age 2 and 4
    D. Enzyme replacement therapy is not available for this condition
    E. It is more prevalent in Asian populations than in Ashkenazi Jews

14

Correct Answer is: A
This is a clinical presentation of Gaucher disease. It is an autosomal recessive disorder, and is caused by deficiency of the enzyme glucocerebrosidase (acid 8-glucosylceramidase) leading to lysosomal accumulation of glucocerebrosides (glucosylceramide). It is caused by mutations in the gene GBA on chromosome 1q21 and is more common in Ashkenazi Jews.

There are three phenotypes:

- **Type 1 is the most common and does not involve the CNS. It is characterized by hepatosplenomegaly with anemia and thrombocytopenia, skeletal involvement, and pulmonary infiltrates.**
- **Type 2 has its onset before the age of 2 years, with psychomotor involvement, spasticity, choreoathetosis, oculomotor abnormalities, and progresses to death by 2–4 years of age. These patients may also have hepatosplenomegaly, hydrops fetalis, and cutaneous changes.**
- **Type 3 begins after the age of 2 years and progresses slowly, with hepatosplenomegaly, psychomotor deterioration, spasticity, ataxia, and oculomotor involvement.**

The diagnosis can be made with an analysis of the enzyme B-glucosylceramidase or glucocerebrosidase in leukocytes. This enzyme can also be tested for in amniocytes and through chorionic villous sampling, allowing for prenatal diagnosis.

Gaucher cells are caused by the lysosomal storage of glucocerebroside in macrophages. These cells are found in the liver, spleen, lymph nodes, and bone marrow, and have large a cytoplasm with striated appearance, what has been likened to "wrinkled tissue paper."

In the CNS, the brain stem and deep nuclei are most severely affected, and neuronal degeneration is seen, likely from neurotoxic action of glucosylsphingosine.

Enzyme replacement with imiglucerase can be effective for liver and spleen involvement and for the hematologic abnormalities.

Type 3 may benefit from bone marrow transplantation.

30. You were asked to see a 15-year-old girl in the ED who came in with severe headache and vomiting that was consistent with migraine. She was treated with IV fluids, ketorolac and diphenhydramine with no relief. She was admitted to the hospital and was given intravenous valproic acid

and her headache completely has been subsided. Later that evening she felt better and drank two protein shakes. The following morning, the nurse could not arouse her. All tests including a toxicology screen and MRI which were negative. An ammonia level was elevated at 250 mmol/l. The valproic acid was stopped. She was treated with intravenous fluids and the ammonia level fell to 50 mmol/l. She was discharged home. One month later, she came back with severe headache, vomiting and confusion. Her mother mentioned that she could not eat for a couple of days due to headaches so she substituted meals with several protein shakes. The mother reported that she often drank protein shakes and had subsequent irritability but she thought that was due to the headaches. On examination she was lethargic and had myoclonic jerks. An ammonia concentration was ordered and was 400 mmol/l. Repeat ammonia was 450 mmol/l.

What is the most likely diagnosis is?

A. Hyperammonemia due to Valproic acid
B. Ornithine transcarbamylase deficiency
C. Lafora disease
D. Status epilepticus
E. Viral Encephalitis

Correct Answer is: B

The patient is heterozygous for Ornithine Transcarbamylase (OTC) Deficiency. Female heterozygotes can present as early as the first week of life or as late as 30 years of age. Symptoms before diagnosis can be nonspecific: episodic extreme irritability, headaches, episodic vomiting and lethargy, ataxia, stage II coma, delayed growth, developmental delay, and seizure. There have been cases of valproic acid sensitivity. In males with OTC deficiency, sodium valproate may precipitate acute liver failure (Tripp et al. 1981). Hjelm et al. (1986) concluded that the vulnerability of toxic effects of valproate extends to heterozygotes as well. They described a family in which 2 daughters and a son died in childhood, all with clinical features suggesting a metabolic disorder; in one, valproate seemed to have accelerated death. They concluded that the mother was a heterozygote for OTC deficiency. Honeycutt et al. (1992) reported a previously undiagnosed heterozygous woman who had symptomatic hyperammonemia during initiation of valproate therapy.

Suggested Reading

- Ornithine Transcarbamylase Deficiency. OMIM Entry # 31125.

31. A 16-year-old boy presents to your office with facial dystonia and dysarthria. On ophthalmologic exam, you have seen picture show below.

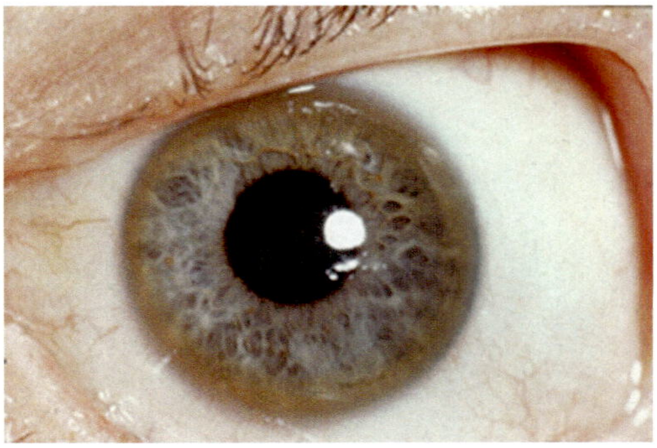

Fig. 14.4 Kayser-Fleischer ring: copper deposition in Descemet's membrane of the cornea. These rings can be either dark brown, golden, or reddish-green, are 1–3 mm wide, and appear at the corneal limbus. With rare exceptions, they are diagnostic of inherited hepatolenticular degeneration—Wilson's disease. This 32-year-old patient complained of longstanding difficulty speaking. He also had a tremor. (▶ http://cnx.org/content/m15007/latest/. Herbert L. Fred, MD, Hendrik A. van Dijk. Wikipedia)

What is your first choice for treatment of this condition?

A. Deferoxamine
B. Hemodialysis
C. Lactulose
D. D-penicillamine
E. Disodium edetate

Correct Answer is: D
The picture shows the Kayser-Fleischer rings which are classic presenting symptoms of Wilson disease, a disorder of copper metabolism. D-penicillamine, a chelation therapy is first choice therapy in this condition, though several other agents, such as dimercaprol, may be used. Deferoxamine chelates iron. Edetate salts chelate heavy metals, but is not used for copper chelation. Lactulose helps with clearance of ammonia. Hemodialysis is not used for this condition.

Suggested Reading

- White H. Neurologic manifestations of acute and chronic liver disease. Continuum. 2014;20(3 Neurology of Systemic Disease):670–80.

Movement Disorders

Y. M. Awaad, *Absolute Pediatric Neurology*, https://doi.org/10.1007/978-3-319-78801-2_15

1. A 12-year-old female came for an evaluation for her complex motor tics including excessive eye blinking, facial movements and neck stretching. She has daily tics which are annoying to her, but no social embarrassment for her and her family. She is an excellent student, socially well-adjusted, and has no obsessive-compulsive, anxiety or ADHD symptoms. **What is your first-line treatment options?**
   A. Atomoxetine 40 mg daily
   B. Risperdone 1 mg daily
   C. Comprehensive Behavioral Intervention for Tics (CBIT)
   D. Clonidine 0.1 mg tid
   E. Neurofeedback

Correct Answer is: C
Treatment should be individualized in tics and Tourette syndrome patients. CBIT or other behavioral interventions and treatments should be considered before pharmacological treatments especially in cooperative children. CBIT is a "package" of approaches with "habit reversal" techniques as a major component. If unsuccessful, and if tics are causing loss of self-esteem, social dysfunction, provoking anxiety, limiting participation in activities, physical discomfort, school issues or other functional difficulties, adjunctive pharmacological therapies can be considered. Medications used for tic-suppression include alpha-2 adrenergic agonists as first-line consideration, and typical and atypical neuroleptics as second-tier medications. Co-morbid ADHD, obsessive-compulsive disorder, anxiety or depression should be treated with specific pharmacological therapies.

15

Suggested Reading

- Roessner V, Schoenefeld K, Buse J, et al. Pharmacological treatment of tic disorders and Tourette syndrome. Neuropharmacology. 2013;68:143–9. Epub 20 Jun 2012.
- Singer HS. Treatment of tics and Tourette syndrome. Curr Treat Options Neurol. 2010;12:539–61.

2. The diagnosis of benign paroxysmal torticollis of childhood includes all of the following except:
   A. Typical age of onset is 5–7 years of age.
   B. Episodic attacks of head tilting lasting minutes to days
   C. Attacks remit spontaneously and tend to reoccur monthly
   D. Associated signs and symptoms may include ataxia, pallor, irritability and vomiting

Correct Answer is: A
Benign paroxysmal torticollis is an episodic torticollis syndrome, classically starts before age 12 months and resolving by age 3–5 years of age. Family history of migraine is very common. Episodes can last hours to days, typically associated with pallor and occasionally vomiting.

Suggested Reading

- Rosman NP, Douglass LM, Sharif UM, Paolini J. The neurology of benign paroxysmal torticollis of infancy: report of 10 new cases and review of the literature. J Child Neurol. 2009;24(2):155–60.

3. A 6-year-old boy came with his family with complain of in-toeing of his left foot with walking. His dystonic posturing generalizes to involve his left arm, and the right side of his body as well over the following year. He has no cognitive problems, and he has had no seizures. There is no change in his dystonia during the day. When you examined him, he has a generalized dytsonia involving all extremities. Brain MRI is normal.

Which gene is involved in this patient genetic disease?

A. Epsilon-sarcoglycan (SCGE)
B. GTP cyclohydrolase 1 (GTPCH 1)
C. Pantothenate kinase (PANK2)
D. Thyroid transcription factor 1 (TITF1)
E. Torsion A (DYT1)

Correct Answer is: E
Torsion dystonia (DYT1 dystonia) or also referred as dystonia musulorum deformans, usually presents with dystonic posturing of a foot, leg, or arm. It appears first with specific actions; e.g., writing or walking. Finally, the contractions frequently become evident with less specific actions and spread to other body regions.

Myoclonus-dystonia (M-D) is a movement disorder characterized by a combination of myoclonus and dystonia. Depression, anxiety, and obsessive-compulsive disorder (OCD) are common co-morbid features. It is secondary to mutations in the epsilon-sarcoglycan gene.

GTP cyclohydrolase 1-deficient dopa-responsive dystonia (GTPCH1) is usually respond to low doses of levodopa. The typical presentation is a gait disturbance caused by foot dystonia, later development of Parkinsonism, and diurnal fluctuation of symptoms.

Pantothenate kinase-associated neurodegeneration (PKAN) is a neurodegenerative disease characterized by brain iron accumulation and was formerly called Hallervorden-Spatz syndrome. PKAN is characterized by progressive dystonia and basal ganglia iron deposition that results in an "eye of the tiger" sign on MRI.

Benign hereditary chorea is an autosomal dominant disorder with nonprogressive chorea. It is a result of mutations in the thyroid transcription factor (TITF-1) gene.

Suggested Reading

- Please see ► http://www.ncbi.nlm.nih.gov/sites/GeneTests/?db=GeneTests for up to date reviews on these topics.

4. A 10-year-old boy with the history of frequent eye blinking for the last 6 months. The eye blinking is bothering him, his teachers and family. He has a normal physical examination with the exception of frequent eye blinking and facial grimacing.
What is your the most likely diagnosis?

A. Chronic Vocal Tic Disorder
B. Chronic Motor Tic Disorder
C. Tourette's Disorder
D. PANDAS
E. Transient Tic Disorder

Correct Answer is: E
Tic disorders occur in nearly 1% of children. Tics usually start between 7–12 years of age. Motor tics typically appear first, followed by the onset of vocal tics in some individuals. "Transient Tic Disorder" should be considered if tics are longer than 4 weeks, but less than a year. On the other hand, Tourette's will have multiple motor and at least one vocal tic for more than 1 year in duration. Chronic motor or Chronic Vocal tic disorder may be used to define other children. (DSM-IV TR for the tic disorders DSM-IV-TR Criteria 307.23 (Tourette's Disorder). Both multiple motor and one or more vocal tics have been present at some time during the illness, although not necessarily concurrently. (A tic is a sudden, rapid, recurrent, non-rhythmic, stereotyped motor movement or vocalization). The tics occur multiple times a day, (usually in bouts,) nearly every day or intermittently throughout a period of more than 1 year, and during this period there was never a tic-free period of more than 3 consecutive months. The onset is

before age 18 years. The disturbance is not due to the direct physiological effects of a substance (e.g. stimulants) or a general medical condition (e.g. Huntington's disease or post viral encephalitis) DSM-IV-TR Criteria 307.22 (Chronic Motor or Vocal Tic Disorder). Single or multiple motor or vocal tics (i.e. sudden, rapid, recurrent, non-rhythmic, stereotyped motor movements or vocalizations), but not both, have been present at some time during the illness. Criteria have never been met for Tourette's disorder DSM-IV-TR Criteria 307.21 (Transient Tic Disorder). Single or multiple motor and/or vocal tics (i.e. sudden, rapid, recurrent, non- rhythmic, stereotyped motor movements or vocalizations). Criteria have never been met for Tourette's disorder or chronic motor or vocal tic disorder Diagnostic and Statistical Manual of Mental Disorders. 4th ed., Text Revision DSM-IV-TR. Washington, DC: American Psychiatric Association; 2000. Walkup JT, Ferrão Y, Leckman JF, Stein DJ, Singer H. Tic disorders: some key issues for DSM-V. Depress Anxiety. 2010 Jun; 27(6):600–10.

5. A 12-year-old girl came to your office for an evaluation for her repetitive jerky movements of her hands and arms that have appeared over the last 2 weeks. She cannot control them and they are interrupting her handwriting. Her school teacher complained of her behavioral outbursts in class which is not in character. On examination, she is thin, and no dysmorphic features. She has a soft systolic murmur noted anteriorly, and has no hepatosplenomegaly noted. She has moderate facial acne, and an elevated body mass index of 35. She was diagnosed with attention deficit disorder, but she is not taking any medications.

15

What tests are you going to order at this time?

A. Erythrocyte sedimentation rate
B. Anti-streptolysin antibody
C. Cholesterol and triglyceride panels
D. Anti-phospholipid antibody
E. Liver function tests

Correct Answer is: B
Sydenham chorea is one of the complications of acute rheumatic fever which has to be considered in any child presenting with a movement disorder, especially due to the long-term treatment requirements. It is a complication of untreated streptococcal infections. The onset can be insidious, and therefore the diagnosis can be delayed. The cardinal features are chorea, emotional lability, and hypotonia; trouble at school may be the reason for seeking medical attention. In addition to treating the chorea, these patients should have treatment of the active streptococcal infection for 10 days and then prophylactic penicillin therapy until age 21.

Suggested Reading

- Fenichel GM (ed.). A Signs and Symptoms Approach. In: Clinical Pediatric Neurology. 2nd ed. Philiadelphia: W.B. Saunders Company; 1993.

6. At 6 years of age, a boy was diagnosed with ADHD, but no medication was prescribed. He started having frequent twitching of his face and eye blinking behavior at 7 years of age. By 8 years of age, he was disruptive in class by making frequent whistling noises.
Which of the following is the most likely additional symptom that this patient may experience?

A. Myoclonus
B. Dystonia
C. Learning disorder
D. Coprolalia
E. Wing beating tremor

Correct Answer is: C
This is a classic presentation for Tourette's Disorder, which is defined as having frequent multiple motor tics and at least one verbal tic for 1 year in duration. The initial presentation can include ADD or ADHD, which often is present before the onset of the tics. Anxiety, depression, obsessions, compulsions, and learning disabilities are common. Coprolalia or copropraxia are uncommon, but may occur. The presence of additional movement disorders, such as dystonia, a wing-beating tremor, or myoclonus should alert the clinician to additional potential diagnoses including myoclonus dystonia, Wilson's disease, or neuroacanthocythosis.

Suggested Reading

- Jankovic J. Tourette's syndrome. N Engl J Med. 2001;345(16):1184–92.

7. A 14-year-old female has one-month history of rapidly worsening involuntary movements causing her to be unable to write and walk. She had slurred speech 1 week before presentation. In spite of she is doing well at school, teachers reported that she is crying more easily than usual. She has unremarkable past medical and birth histories. She is not taking any medications. She has a normal general exam. Neurologic examination shows, severe dysarthria and motor impersistence with tongue protrusion. She has mild, diffuse hypotonia and marked generalized chorea, which causes her to bump into things while ambulating. DTRs are 2+ but are hung-up at the knees. Her routine blood work, including a basic metabolic panel, complete blood count, sedimentation rate, and pregnancy test, all of which were normal/negative.

   An abnormal/positive result on which of the following tests would alter the patient's treatment?

   A. Anti-DNase B
   B. C-reactive protein
   C. Toxicology screen
   D. Echocardiogram
   E. ASO titer

Correct Answer is: D
10% to 20% of patients with acute rheumatic fever (ARF) will have Sydenham's chorea, usually weeks to months after a group A β-hemolytic streptococcal (GABHS) infection. The classical presentations include chorea, hypotonia, and emotional lability. The mechanism of the disease is not fully understood, the pathological explanation is that molecular mimicry between streptococcal and basal ganglia peptides leads to immune-modulated damage of the basal ganglia. The diagnosis is based on elevated anti-streptolysin O and/or anti-DNase B titers may corroborate the diagnosis. Negative titers do not exclude the diagnosis. Throat culture to determine whether the patient has an active GABHS infection should be done; if positive, the patient should be treated with antibiotics. Other laboratory and imaging studies may be necessary to exclude other causes of chorea, such as drug reactions, systemic lupus erythematosus, and Wilson's disease. Echocardiogram has to be done on all patients to assess for carditis and should be started on long-term antibiotic prophylaxis to prevent rheumatic recurrences. If chorea is disabling, treatment options include valproate, carbamazepine, and/or dopamine receptor antagonists.

8. An 8-year-old female with one-year history of eye rolling, facial grimacing, and head jerking that occur multiple times per day. She has a tingling sensation in her neck that is temporarily

relieved by jerking her head. She reported that she can stop the movements if she wants for several seconds at a time. She has been on loratadine 10 mg/day for the last 2 years for her repetitive sniffing and throat clearing, and ibuprofen 400 mg as needed for neck pain related to her head jerking movements. Sniffing has stopped over the past year but she has started audibly inhaling. She has no school troubles. Her family and teachers have no concerns about her mood or behavior. She has a family history of anxiety in her mother and ADHD in her brother. Her general and neurologic examinations are normal, with the exception of the aforementioned adventitious movements.
What is your choice as a first-line treatment for her abnormal movement?
A. Guanfacine
B. Sertraline
C. Pimozide
D. Risperidone
E. Haloperidol

Correct Answer is: A
Tourette syndrome (TS) affects an estimated 0.1 to 3% of the population. Diagnosis of Tourette syndrome is based on, patient will have multiple motor and one or more vocal tics, which occur many times a day nearly every day for more than 1 year, though not necessarily concurrently. Onset must be prior to age 18 years, and the tics cannot be due to the effects of a substance or general medical condition. Obsessive-compulsive disorder (OCD), attention deficit hyperactivity disorder (ADHD), anxiety, depression, learning disorders, and/or oppositional behavior/conduct disorder are very common co-morbidity. You do not have to treat it unless the tics are causing morbidity. In this case, pharmacotherapy should be initiated with low doses of α-adrenergic drugs (clonidine, guanfacine). Although, haloperidol, pimozide, and risperidone can be used for patients who have failed an α-adrenergic agent, they have significant side effects, including extrapyramidal symptoms, weight gain, and electrocardiographic changes.

15

Suggested Reading

- Swain JE, Scahill L, Lombroso PJ, King RA, Leckman JF. Tourette syndrome and tic disorders: a decade of progress. J Am Acad Child Adolesc Psychiatry. 2007;46(8):947–68.

9. An 8-year-old boy is presented to your office with a gradual worsening of his gait for the past 2 years. His family reports a tendency for his right foot to turn down and in. He has no problem in the morning, but his foot begins to turn by late afternoon each day, even if he has not been physically active. He has no significant past medical history, and he is doing fine at school. No medications were prescribed. His family history is remarkable of a father has similar but less severe symptoms which began in his early 20's. He has a normal general and neurological examination except his tone and tendon reflexes are increased in the distal right lower extremity. He has a flexor plantar response. Sensation is intact.
What test are you going to order to reach the diagnosis?
A. MRI brain
B. Genetic study for DYT1
C. CSF neurotransmitters
D. Ceruloplasmin
E. Genetic study for hereditary spastic paraplegia

Correct Answer is: C
Segawa disease (Autosomal dominant GTP cyclohydrolase deficiency) is a dopa-responsive dystonia caused by a heterozygous mutation of the GCH1

gene on chromosome 14q22.1–2. The term "hereditary progressive dystonia with marked diurnal fluctuation" is not in use any more. Onset is usually around 6 years of age and starts with postural dystonia of a lower extremity, mostly with talipes equinovarus. Action dystonia (especially retrocollis or oculogyric crisis) can occur in some patients. Postural high-frequency (8–10 Hz) tremor develops in an upper extremity at around 10 years of age. Usually, it starts asymmetric with marked diurnal fluctuation (aggravation towards the evening and near complete if not complete recovery after overnight sleep). Growth decelerates such that patients are 2 standard deviations below age norms for height by the late teens. Eventually, the dystonia becomes more generalized and tremor becomes more pronounced and constant rather than fluctuating. Anticipation occurs in some families with a wide variation in age of onset. Neuroimaging is usually normal. Low levels of homovanillic acid, biopterin, and neopterin can be detected on CSF examination. It is recommended to start patients on levodopa/carbidopa 4–5 mg/kg/day to alleviate the symptoms.

Suggested Reading

- Segawa M. Chang Gung Med J. 2009; 32:1–11.

10. A 10-month-old boy, 3 months ago he was acutely sick then he developed severe dystonia and rigidity which worsen over time. He was admitted to the PICU after he had a fever and vomiting accompanied by hypoglycemia and metabolic acidosis and he was treated with IV fluids. During his PICU admission he became acutely hypotonic and lost head control and had seizures. An EEG was normal. Brain MRI showed atrophy of the frontoparietal areas with widening of the Sylvian fissures and increased signal of the bilateral putamen and caudate nuclei on T2 weighted images. He has a large head size since early infancy. Family history is unremarkable. On examination, he has severe diffuse rigidity, dystonia, and tongue thrusting.

Which of the following is the most likely diagnosis?

A. Glutaric acidemia type 1
B. MELAS
C. Wilson's disease
D. Carbon monoxide poisoning
E. Methylmalonic aciduria

Correct Answer is: A

Glutaric acidemia type 1 is an autosomal recessive inborn error of lysine, hydroxylisine, and tryptophan metabolism caused by deficiency of glutaryl-CoA dehydrogenase. This enzyme is located in the mitochondrial matrix. More than 60 mutations of the gene encoding this enzyme have been identified, including missense, nonsense, and intronic variants. There is a correlation between residual enzyme activity and biochemical phenotype, but not between phenotype and severity of the genetic lesion, as siblings within the same family and with the same mutation have discordant phenotypes. Fever, infections, and fasting play can precipitate neuronal damage. It is rare (worldwide incidence 1:100,000) except in certain populations such as the Old-Order Amish community of Pennsylvania and North American Ojibway-Cree in Canada.

Patients have macrocephaly at birth or shortly thereafter, with atrophy of the frontoparietal cortical areas creating a "bat-wing" appearance (widening of the Sylvian fissures), creating a "micrencephalic macrocephaly". Subdural hemorrhages due to stretching of veins from large CSF extra-axial collections can occur in those patients. Bouts of acute decompensation usually occur between 6 and 18 months and if not present by 5 years of age are unlikely to occur. These bouts are

associated with edema of the putamen and caudate nuclei and present clinically with hypotonia and loss of head control. Seizure-like episodes are common, but EEG does not show epileptiform features. Hypotonia disappear after few weeks and is replaced by rigidity and dystonia. Patients will end up with severe motor disability but they have normal cognition. Usually, urine organic acid analysis shows elevated levels of 3-OH-glutaric acid which is diagnostic. Urine glutarylcarnitine is also typically elevated (acylcarnitine urine testing). Early detection by newborn screen helps to prevent the acute decompensation episodes by use of a special diet with protein restriction, supplemented with lysine-free special formula and carnitine.

Suggested Reading

- Hedlund GL, Longo N, Pasquali M. Glutaric acidemia type 1. Am J Med Genet Part C Semin Med Genet. 2006;142C:86–94.

11. A 10-year-old male came to the office with his foster mother for evaluation of random, rapid, involuntary flowing movements after sudden stopping his medication he was on after he was removed from his biological parents due to concerns of neglect.
Which of the following types of medication has most likely been discontinued?
    - A. Antibiotic agent
    - B. Antiepiletpic agent
    - C. Bronchodilator agent
    - D. Neuroleptic agent
    - E. Nonsteroidal anti-inflammatory agent

Correct Answer is: D

Sudden discontinuation of neuroleptics can cause chorea in children and adolescents. This is known as withdrawal-emergent syndrome and is generally self-limited. Chronic treatment with neuroleptics can also cause tardive chorea. Anticonvulsants (particularly phenytoin), oral contraceptives, and stimulants can induce chorea.

Suggested Reading

- Shannon KM. Treatment of chorea. Continuum Lifelong Learning Neurol. 2007;13(1):72–93.

12. A 10-year-old girl with the diagnosis of cerebral palsy came for an abnormal gait, her symptoms are significantly worse at the end of the day compared to the morning. She has hyperreflexia and equinovarus posturing of the feet on her examination.
What is your first step in management?
    - A. Implantation of an intrathecal baclofen pump
    - B. Injections of botulinum toxin into calf muscles
    - C. Oral carbidopa/levodopa
    - D. Oral tetrabenazine
    - E. Referral to a pediatric orthopedic surgeon

Correct Answer is: C

This is a clinical presentation of hereditary dopa-responsive dystonia; the diurnal variation is characteristic of this disorder. Low-dose levodopa provides a dramatic benefit that usually is sustained for years. Recently, this syndrome has been renamed as autosomal dominant GTP cyclohydrolase 1 deficiency or Segawa disease. The reason is a mutation of the GCH-1 gene located on 14q22.1 to q22.2. Because of heterozygous mutation, partial deficiency of tetrahydrobiopterin affects tyrosine hydroxylase (TH) rather selectively and causes decrease of TH in the terminals of the nigrostriatal dopamine (NS DA) neurons, projecting to the D1 receptors on the striosome, the striatal direct pathways and the sub-thalamic

15

nucleus (STN) and the D4 receptors of the tuberoinfundibular tract.

The activities of TH in the terminal are high in early childhood decrease exponentially to the stational level around early 20s, and show circadian oscillatron. TH in HPD follows these variations with around 20% of normal levels and with development of the downstream structures show appears characteristic clinical symptoms age dependently. In late fetus period to early infancy, through the striosome-substantia nigra pars compacta pathway failure in morphogenesis of the DA neurons in substantia nigra, in childhood around 6 years postural dystonia through the D1 direct pathways and the descending output of the basal ganglia. Diurnal fluctuation is apparent in childhood but decrease its grade with age. TH deficiency at the terminal on the STN causes action dystonia from around 8 years and postural tremor from around 10 years, focal dystonia in adulthood.

Adult onset cases in the family with action dystonia start with writer's cramp, torticollis or generalized rigid hypertonus with tremor but do not show postural dystonia. TH deficiency on the D4 receptors causes stagnation of the body length in childhood. With or without action dystonia depends on the locus of mutation. Postural dystonia is inhibitory disorder, while action dystonia is excitatory disorder. The TH deficiency at the terminal does not cause morphological changes or degenerative process. Thus, levodopa shows favorable effects without any relation to the duration of illness.

Suggested Reading

- Geyer HL, Bressman, SB. Treatment of dystonia. Continuum Lifelong Learning Neurol. 2007;13(1):94–121.
- Segawa M. Hereditary progressive dystonia with marked diurnal fluctuation. Brain Dev. 2011;33(3):195–2.

13. A 10-year-old boy came with his family to your office because his family suspecting him to have Tourette syndrome because off his occasional blinking, sniffing, or grunting. The movements do not bother him; even him and his teachers do not notice them. He does not have any hyperactivity, attentional difficulty, or psychiatric dysfunction, and the neurologic examination is normal.

What is the most reasonable treatment at this time?

A. Botulinum toxin injections
B. Clonidine patch
C. Oral methylphenidate
D. Oral pimozide
E. Reassurance and education of the parents

Correct Answer is: E

The child has tics, but they are mild and you do not have to use any pharmacotherapy. Because the prognosis is good the family should be reassured. Clondine, or neuroleptics like pimozide, can be used if the tics were more severe. The role of botulinum toxin in treating tics is promising, but certainly would not be first-line therapy in a mildly affected patient of this age. If the child has attention deficit hyperactivity disorder as a comorbid with the tic disorder Stimulants like methylphenidate can be useful; despite a longstanding concern that stimulants can exacerbate tic, the evidence for this association is not very strong.

Suggested Reading

- Sanger TD. Tic disorders and Tourette syndrome in children. Continuum Lifelong Learning Neurol. 2007;13(1):139–53.

14. Four months after a 9-year-old boy has frequent blinking, grimacing, and grunting, these completely stopped completely without any intervention.

What is your diagnosis?

A. Sydenham's chorea
B. Tourette syndrome
C. Meige syndrome
D. Chronic motor tic disorder
E. Transient tic disorder

Correct Answer is: E

Tics are stereotyped and repetitive movements or vocalizations that are quite common in childhood with age of onset typically between 6 and 12, and peak intensity often between 10 and 14 years of age. If symptoms persisted for more than 1 month, but less than 1 year, a transient tic disorders could be considered in the majority of children. If tics are present for more than 1 year, it is a chronic tic disorders by definition, and may involve motor or vocal (phonic) tics. On the other hand, Tourette syndrome has at least 1 year of multiple motor tics and at least one phonic tic. Additional neuropsychiatric disorders are commonly seen with Tourette syndrome, with up to 50% of patients meeting criteria for an attentional disorder (ADD or ADHD) and 15–20% an anxiety or obsessive-compulsive disorder. Sydenham's chorea is the movement disorder associated with rheumatic fever, secondary to an immune reaction to a streptococcal infection. Meige syndrome is a form of oro-facial or cervical idiopathic dystonia, commonly affecting patients in their 50–70 years of life. Both disorders have no tics as part of their symptomatology.

15

Suggested Reading

- Martino D, Mink J. Tic disorders. Continuum (Minneap Minn). 2013;19(5):1287–311. ▶ pediatrics.aappublications.org/content/121/6/1281.full.pdf.

15. A 10-year-old girl with 2 weeks history of involuntary movements in her limbs. 5 weeks earlier she had streptococcal pharyngitis and she was treated with antibiotics. On examination, she has rapid muscle contractions flowing randomly from one body part to another, as well as mild dysarthria, hyperactivity, and inattentiveness. Her Antistreptolysin O titer is elevated.
What is the most important next investigation?

A. MRI of the brain
B. Genetic testing
C. Lumbar puncture
D. Echocardiogram
E. Slit lamp examination

Correct Answer is: D

The patient has Sydenham chorea, which is one of the major Jones criteria for rheumatic heart disease. Carditis, another of the major Jones criteria, is present in up to 80% of patients with Sydenham chorea.

Suggested Reading

- Cardoso F, Silva CE, Mota CC. Sydenham's chorea in 50 consecutive patients with rheumatic fever. Mov Disord. 1997;12:701–3.

16. A 9-year-old girl has gait disturbance in the morning but it is worse later in the day. You decided to exam her in the afternoon. On exam, she has reduced facial expression, increased tone in the limbs, and hyperreflexia. When you asked her to walk, there is plantar flexion and inversion of the ankles.
What medication is likely to dramatically improve her symptoms?

A. Acetazolamide
B. Carbidopa/levodopa
C. Mexiletine
D. Tetrabenazine
E. Zinc

Correct Answer is: B

Dopa-responsive dystonia is characterized by diurnal fluctuation of Parkinsonism and dystonia in a child. Treatment with

low-dose levodopa is both diagnostic and therapeutic, as it is expected to confer dramatic and sustained improvement.

Suggested Reading

Geyer HL, Bressman SB. Treatment of dystonia. Continuum Lifelong Learning Neurol. 2007;13(1):94–121.

17. 15-year-old boy has Tourette syndrome for the last 4 years, asking you for a pharmacologic treatment for his bothered tics.
What medications from below list can cause tardive dyskinesia?
    A. guanfacine
    B. clonidine
    C. pimozide
    D. methylphenidate
    E. tetrabenazine

Correct Answer is: C
Pimozide blocks dopamine receptors in the striatum like other neuroleptic medications and its use can cause tardive syndromes. Stimulants like methylphenidate traditionally can worsen tics, although more recent controlled trials have not supported this association. Guanfacine and clonidine are used to treat tics and attention deficit hyperactivity disorders but do not cause tardive syndromes. Tetrabenazine is a dopamine depletor rather than a dopamine receptor-blocking agent and does not cause tardive dyskinesias.

Suggested Reading

Kenney C, Hunter C, Mejia N, Jankovic J. Tetrabenazine in the treatment of Tourette syndrome. J Pediatr Neurol. 2007;5:11–6.

18. An 8-year-old girl with a history of restlessness, irritability and inattentiveness in school for the last 3 weeks. 5 weeks ago, she had a sore throat for few days. Now she has facial grimacing and rapid, jerky movements in both arms and legs that she cannot suppress.
Which of the following findings is most likely to be found on further evaluation?
    A. positive urine toxicology screen
    B. Koplik spots
    C. expanded CAG repeats in the gene coding for the huntingtin protein
    D. low serum ceruloplasmin
    E. carditis

Correct Answer is: E
Sydenham chorea is a complication of infection with group A beta Hemolytic.

Streptococci that cause pharyngitis few weeks before onset of the neurologic.

Symptoms. Patients usually have emotional or behavioral disturbances.

Chorea is one of the major Jones criteria for rheumatic fever. Carditis is another major criteria and can affect as many as 80% of patients with Sydenhams chorea. Cardiac Work-up is should be done in children with Sydenham chorea. This patient's presentation is not typical of Wilson disease (low ceruloplasmin), Huntington disease (expanded CAG repeats), measles (Koplik spots) or acute intoxication.

Suggested Reading

Leffler J. Sydenham chorea. Movement Disorder Virtual University. Accessed 27 June 2012.

19. A 7-year-old girl is complaining of difficulty walking secondary to right leg stiffness and involuntary inversion of her ankle. Her symptoms begin by late morning and worsen as the day progresses, although she is normal upon waking up in the morning or after a nap. She has generalized hyperreflexia.

Which of the following medications is most likely to be effective?

A. acetazolamide
B. baclofen
C. carbamazepine
D. haloperidol
E. levodopa

Correct Answer is: E

The patient presented with a dopa-responsive dystonia (DRD) which is successfully treated with low-dose levodopa. Trihexyphenidyl and benztropine (Anticholinergic medications) can also be effective but are associated with more side effects. Carbamazepine has been effective in a few patients, but this benefit is mild and inconsistent. Hereditary progressive dystonia with marked diurnal fluctuation (HPD) is a dopa-responsive dystonia described by Segawa et al. in 1976. After discovery of the causative gene, the gene of GTP cyclohydrolase 1 (GCH-1) located on 14q22.1 to q22.2, this is called autosomal dominant GCH-1 deficiency or Segawa disease. Clinically there are two types: postural dystonia and action dystonia type. In most cases the symptoms at onset is dystonic posture, with rigidity in one lower extremity, pes equinovarus, around 6 years. Postural dystonia expands to other limbs, and all limbs and trunk muscles are affected by late teens, the rigidity aggravates progressively until around 20 years of age, but the progression subsides in the 20s and becomes stationary in the 30s. Postural tremor with high cycles of 8 Hz to 10 Hz appears after 10 years in an upper extremity and expands to all limbs by thirties. However, locomotion is preserved throughout the course. In action dystonia type, besides postural dystonia, dystonic movements of an upper extremity or action retrocollis appear around 8 years. The latter may associate oculogyric crises. In families with action dystonia type, there are adult onset cases who start with writer's cramp, torticollis or generalized rigid hypertonus with postural tremor, but do not show dystonic posture or apparent progression. Symptoms show marked diurnal fluctuation in childhood, which becomes progressively less apparent over time. In adult onset cases it is not observed. Childhood onset cases show stagnation of body length with onset of dystonia. This is not observed in cases with onset after adolescence.

Suggested Reading

- Nygaard TG, Marsden CD, Fahn S. Dopa-responsive dystonia: long-term treatment response and prognosis. Neurology. 1991;41:174–81.
- Segawa M. Hereditary progressive dystonia with marked diurnal fluctuation. Brain Dev. 2011;33(3):195–201.

20. A 9-year-old boy has been evaluated for being off balance. His parents reported that his symptoms come on in attacks and in between attacks he appears completely normal. In the office, he had his symptoms for a few hours. On examination, he has dysarthria, ataxia and nystagmus. His symptoms gradually resolved and he complained of a throbbing headache.

What statement below is correct?

A. This condition is associated with mutation in the voltage-gated potassium channel gene KCNA1.
B. This condition can be associated with progressive cerebellar atrophy.
C. This condition is associated with mutation in the glial glutamate transporter gene SLC1A3.
D. It is caused by a triple repeat mutation in the calcium channel gene CACNA1A.
E. It has autosomal recessive mode of inheritance.

15

Correct Answer is: B

The clinical presentation is consistent with episodic ataxia type 2 (EA2). There are 8 different of this ataxia. It is caused by mutations of ion channel genes and present as attacks of ataxia with or without additional neurologic symptoms. They are autosomal dominant.

Episodes of ataxia in type 1 (EA1) can be associated with brief facial myokymia or neuromyotonia, lasting seconds to minutes. EA2 has longer lasting episodes of ataxia and can be associated with nystagmus and dysarthria. Progressive cerebellar atrophy on neuroimaging can present over time in these patients.

The causative gene is known in four of the episodic ataxias; types 1, 2, 5, and 6. EA1 is due to a mutation in the voltage-gated potassium channel gene KCNA1 on chromosome 12. EA2 results from a non-sense mutation and not a triple repeat mutation in the calcium channel CACNA1A. This is the same gene mutation causing familial hemiplegic migraine and hence patients can have positive history of migraines. EA6 is associated with mutation in the glial glutamate transporter gene SLC1A3.

Stress, exertion, caffeine, alcohol and heat can trigger EA2 attacks, which can be treated by acetazolamide. Over time, ataxia and nystagmus may become more pervasive symptoms. The pathophysiology for the progressive nature of symptoms and atrophy on imaging is unknown at this time.

Suggested Reading

- Pandolfo M, Manto M. Cerebellar and afferent ataxias. Continuum Lifelong Learning Neurol. 2013;19(5):1312.
- Ropper A, Samuels M, Klien J. Adams and Victor's principles of neurology. 10th ed. New York: Mcgraw Hill; 2014. p. 946.

21. A 14-year-old boy develops episodes of left-sided writhing movements, especially when getting up quickly from his desk at school. They last 10 s or fewer, without any accompanying alteration in consciousness. He may have up to 20 episodes per day. He is started on carbamazepine by his pediatrician for possible epilepsy which leads to a significant reduction in the frequency of episodes. His parents bring him to your office for a second opinion. On further history, his father and paternal uncle had similar but milder symptoms as children, which eventually subsided in middle age. His examination is normal.
Which of the following is the most likely explanation for his symptoms?
    A. Paroxysmal kinesogenic dyskinesia
    B. Paroxysmal nonkinesogenic dyskinesia
    C. Paroxysmal exertional dyskinesia
    D. Paroxysmal hypnogenic dyskinesia
    E. Episodic ataxia type 1

Correct Answer is: A

The patient has episodes of chorea (form of dyskinesia) triggered by sudden movement and lasting only seconds, with an autosomal dominant pattern of inheritance. There is brisk response to carbamazepine. This is most consistent with paroxysmal kinesogenic dyskinesia, which is more common in males than females with median age of onset of 12 years. For unknown reasons, it responds well to carbamazepine and other anticonvulsants although EEG reveals no seizures. Paroxysmal nonkinesogenic dyskinesia also manifests with intermittent dyskinesias, but the episodes last minutes to hours rather than seconds to minutes. They are not triggered by movement (although alcohol or caffeine may precipitate) and do not respond to anticonvulsants. Paroxysmal exertional dyskinesia is triggered by prolonged exertion and may last 5–30 min. Episodes of paroxysmal hypnogenic dyskinesia are short in duration and may respond to anticonvulsants, but are often due to

frontal lobe (supplementary motor) seizures and by definition occur out of sleep rather than occurring with movements while awake. Patients with episodic ataxia type 1 have brief episodes lasting seconds and that may be triggered by movement and relieved with anticonvulsants. However, the episodes are characterized by ataxia and myokimia is present during and between episodes.

Suggested Reading

- Fahn S. The paroxysmal dyskinesias. In: Principles and practice of movement disorders. Elsevier; 2011. p. 476–95.

22. A 17-year-old male presents with facial dystonia and dysarthria. On ophthalmologic exam, he has brown discoloration around the periphery of his iris.
What is the treatment of choice in his case?
A. Lactulose
B. Deferoxamine
C. D-penicillamine
D. Hemodialysis
E. Disodium edetate

Correct Answer is: D
This is the classic presentation of Wilson disease, a disorder of copper metabolism. The Kayser-Fleischer rings are a cardinal symptom of the disease. Chelation therapy is the treatment of choice. D-penicillamine is first choice, though several other agents, such as dimercaprol, may be used. Deferoxamine chelates iron. Edetate salts chelate heavy metals, but is not used for copper chelation. Lactulose helps with clearance of ammonia. Hemodialysis is not used for this condition.

Suggested Reading

- White H. Neurologic manifestations of acute and chronic liver disease. Continuum. 2014;20(3 Neurology of Systemic Disease):670–80.

15

23. What is the safest treatment for a 7-month-old boy with a 12-days history of binocular dysconjugate, rotary nystagmus that was preceded by torticollis?
A. Focused radiation treatments
B. Vascular embolization
C. Monitor with no intervention
D. ACTH treatment

Correct answer is: C
Spasmus nutans happens between 6–12 months of age. First symptom is either a head tilt or torticollis, sometimes accompanied with titubation. It lasts for 1–2 years and spontaneously resolves.

Rarely these symptoms can occur in children with anterior visual pathway glioma. Glioma should be considered if nystagmus is monocular, and the optic nerve is pale and the onset after 1 year of age.

There is no vascular location that would present with these symptoms as a result of an aneurysm.

Infantile spasms can be treated with ACTH, but spams are episodes of repetitive whole body flexion.

Suggested Reading

- Halachmi-Eyal O, Kowal L. Assessing abnormal head posture: a new paradigm. Curr Opin Ophthalmol. 2013;24(5):432–37.

24. A 16-year-old girl with a history of persistent abnormal mouth and facial movements for the last 4 months. She has severe mental retardation and has been on different medications for severe behavioral outbursts. Currently she is taking valproate and clonazepam for her behavior, but past medications history is not available. The movements are seen all day, but they disappear in sleep.
You observed several periods of masticatory movements with lip smacking and episodic tongue protrusion.

What is the most likely etiology of these movements?

A. Seizures
B. Behavioral disorder
C. Lesch-Nyhan syndrome
D. Neuroleptic medication

Correct answer is: D
Tardive dyskinesia can be caused by Dopamine receptor targeting drugs such as neuroleptics and antimimetics. In all children with abnormal facial or limb movements with a current or recently history of taking neuroleptics drug-induced dyskinesia should be suspected. Neuroleptic medications are administered to the pediatric population for mania and severe behavioral disorders with increasing frequency. Tardive dyskinesia symptoms can manifest long after the medication has been discontinued. Neuroleptics are also an effective treatment for refractory, problematic motor tic and phonic tics. Focal motor seizures would rarely manifest as isolated oral-buccal movements. Subtle movements can be seemed in in partial seizures and associated with absence seizures. These oral-buccal movements are not consistent with a behavioral disorder or an intentional habitual behavior.

Lesch-Nyhan occurs almost exclusively in males and is characterized by severe neurological and behavioral abnormalities. Abnormal movements include dystonia, chorea and Ballismus but not symptoms similar to tardive dyskinesia.

Suggested Reading

- Correll CU, Leucht S, Kane JM. Lower risk for tardive dyskinesia associated with second generation antipsychotics: a systematic review of 1-year studies. Am J Psychiatry. 2014.

25. What is your treatment for a 9-month-old boy that presents with increasing binocular nystagmus, persistent head tilt with titubation and normal optic discs on examination?

A. ACTH or high dose steroids for 2 weeks
B. Specific amino acid diet restriction
C. Chemotherapy
D. Observation only

Correct answer is: D
Spasmus nutans appears between ages 6–12 months and lasts up to 2 years. It consists of high frequency, low amplitude nystagmus (bi- or unilateral) that can be horizontal, vertical or rotary and is often dysconjugate. The reason of the syndrome is unclear, but it is benign and transitory. Therefore, no medical or surgical intervention is required.

Glioma of the anterior visual pathway can present similarly in some children, but characteristically the nystagmus is monocular with a pale optic nerve.

Progressive cognitive and motor impairment occur gradually in Phenylketonuria if a diet containing the amino acid, phenylalanine was continued in the child diet. Infantile spams consist of generalized episodes of body flexion and the first line treatment is ACTH or steroids until the spasms resolve.

Suggested Reading

- Sanger TD, Delgado MR, Gaebler-Spira D, Hallett M, Mink, JW. Classification and definition of disorders causing hypertonia in childhood. Pediatrics. 2003;111(1):e89–97.

26. What is your diagnosis of a developmentally appropriate 10-year-old boy with a one-year history of chorea, dysarthria, emotional liability and a recent finding of mitral valve insufficiency?

A. Glutaric acidemia type 1
B. Fahr disease
C. Neuroacathocytosis
D. Sydenham chorea

Correct answer is: D

Sydenham chorea is the most common cause of chorea in childhood. The etiology is an underlying untreated streptococcal infection and chorea is a cardinal feature. The onset is approximately 4 months after the streptococcal infection is contracted. Anti-streptococcal anti-bodies cross react with basal ganglia cells to activate the abnormal movements and obsessive-compulsive symptoms. The chorea typically begins unilaterally by will generalize in most cases.

Glutaric academia type 1 occurs in infancy and include cognitive regression, excessive sweating and irritability followed by progressive choreoathetosis and dystonia.

Fahr disease (idiopathic basal ganglia calcification), occurs secondary to infection, metabolic disturbance or genetic disorders. Age of onset is in 3-4th decade, but may occur in children and comprises of neuropsychiatric symptoms and a variety of abnormal movements.

The features of neuroacanthocytosis, or choreoacanthocytosis, include motor tics, oromandibular dyskinesia, and dystonia and occasionally self-mut ilation of the lips. Onset may occur in the teens, but most commonly presents in adulthood.

Suggested Reading

- Swedo SE. Sydenham's chorea: a model for childhood autoimmune neuropsychiatric disorders. Jama. 1994;272(22):1788–91.

15

27. A 10-year-old boy was evaluated for a history of paroxysmal right arm and shoulder movements in the last 4 months. The movements consist of sudden flexion of his arm with extension of his shoulder of 1–2 s duration. There is no change in his mental status. The patient cannot anticipate when the movements will occur. The movements happened more often in the evening or when he is tired. At age 4, he had 3 generalized seizures, Carbamazepine was prescribed and after one-year seizure free, the medication was discontinued. His EEG at the time showed "seizure" activity. **Which of the below questions would help distinguish between seizures and movement disorder?**
    A. Can you suppress the movements if you try?
    B. Have the movements ever occurred during sleep?
    C. Are the movements identical each time?
    D. Did the current movements occur during the time the child was monitored for seizures?

Correct answer is: B

Involuntary movements, such as chorea, characteristically abate or completely disappear during sleep, spinal myoclonus is an exception. Periodic movements of sleep are one movement disorder that occurs during sleep, but it not problematic during waking hours. Seizures do occur during sleep and some forms occur more often.

Most movement disorder cannot be suppressed, with the exception of temporary suppression of vocal and motor tics of childhood. Seizures cannot be willfully suppressed.

Focal motor seizures will manifest in similar motor patterns with each seizure. Most movement disorders motor component vary and will not provide diagnostic benefit to differentiate between seizure and movement disorders.

Frontal lobe or temporal lobe focal motor seizures may manifest with movements described in this case. Nocturnal paroxysmal dystonia was once believed to be a movement disorder, but subsequent research has proven this condition to be frontal lobe epilepsy. In addition, children can have both epilepsy and a movement disorder.

Suggested Reading

Silveira-Moriyama L, Lin JP. A field guide to current advances in pediatric movement disorders. Curr Opin Neurol. 2015;28(4):437–46.

28. A 7-year-old boy with normal behavior and he has a good academic performance. He has a three-month history of rapid facial contractions with forced eye blinking that occur more frequently under stress and are not present in sleep.
    What is your diagnosis?
    A. Tourette syndrome
    B. Chronic motor tics of childhood
    C. Transit motor tics of childhood
    D. Nervous child

Correct answer is: C

Transient motor tics of childhood is an isolated motor tic of childhood with a duration of less than 6 months. Motor tics are abrupt, uncontrollable movements that most commonly involve head, neck and facial muscles. 10% of all children can have tics at some time during the school years. Transient tics may also include phonic or vocal tics.

A Tourette's syndrome diagnosis requires the presence of both motor and phonic tis, Attention Deficit Disorder and Obsessive Compulsive Disorder. Chronic motor tics require at least a 6-month duration of tics. Individuals with chronic motor tics are at risk for maintaining longer-term tic presence and for developing Tourette's syndrome. Tics could occur in a nervous child is an outdated and incorrect statement. This originates from the fact that stress and anxiety include the presence of tics in a child predisposed to the condition or activates tics in a child with a tic disorder.

Suggested Reading

Swedo SE, Leonard HL. Childhood movement disorders and obsessive compulsive disorder. J Clin Psychiatry. 1994.

29. A 10-year-old boy with a history of renal failure who was on dialysis and he had encephalopathy, developed rapid muscle jerks of his arms and shoulders. The movements are symmetrical of about 3 cycles of rapid contraction and relaxation. Sometimes, the movements in the arms are asymmetric and even just unilateral. He has no change in mental status and he cannot suppress the movements.
    What is the classification of those movement?
    A. Motor tics
    B. Myoclonus
    C. Chorea
    D. Tremor

Correct answer is: B

Myoclonus is classified as several involuntary movements manifested as rapid muscle jerks that can be rhythmic or non-rhythmic, focal, multifocal or generalized, spontaneous or activated.

Myoclonus occurs during sleep tend to have greater amplitude. There are many causes of myoclonus, including metabolic disturbances associated with renal failure.

Motor tics are typically including motor complex, stereotyped movements that can be at least temporarily suppressed.

Choreaform movements are usually more random, single larger movements that are often incorporated into a voluntary action.

Rhythmic myoclonus can look very similar to a tremor, but a tremor is a continuous to and fro movement where rhythmic myoclonus has a characteristic pause between contraction and relaxation of the muscle groups involved.

Suggested Reading

Silveira-Moriyama L, Lin JP. A field guide to current advances in pediatric movement disorders. Curr Opin Neurol. 2015;28(4):437–46.

30. A 7-year-old girl is diagnosed at 5 years of age with moderate quadriplegic cerebral palsy because of significant variability of her spasticity and restriction of movement. The symptoms are much better when she awakens in the morning, then her muscle tone gradually increases as the day progresses. The gait disturbance was noticed by her family at 4 years of age, with her right lower leg being most affected. The abnormal tone spread to her arms, and then became generalized. On examination, she has no cerebellar, sensory or autonomic disturbances and her intelligence is age appropriate.
What treatment is most likely to benefit this child the most?
A. Baclofen
B. Rhizotomy
C. Levodopa
D. Dantrolene sodium

Correct answer is: C
Her symptoms with diurnal variation indicates Dopa-responsive dystonia. Usually, it starts at 4–8 years of age and the initial features can be foot dystonia or abnormal hand posturing. The increased tone and posturing progress to include arms and legs and is commonly diagnosed as cerebral palsy. A trial of carbadopa-levodopa is recommended if generalized dystonia is suspected in children. Baclofen is prescribed for the treatment of spasticity associated with cerebral palsy and spinal cord injury. The clinical course symptoms onset at age 4 years with continued progression is not characteristic of cerebral palsy. Rhizotomy is a neurosurgical procedure for the treatment of medically refractory spasticity mainly in diplegic amulatory patients.

Dantrolene sodium reduces the excitation contraction in spasticity associated with cerebral palsy and spinal cord injury.

15

Suggested Reading

- Sanger D, Delgado MR, Gaebler-Spira D, Hallett M, Mink W. Classification and definition of disorders causing hypertonia in childhood. Pediatrics. 2003;111(1): e89–97.

31. A parents of a 10-year-old boy have a concern regarding their sons "unusual behavior"? He has a rapid, random involuntary movements of his arms that he appears to end in a voluntary action. His arms move simultaneously down to his sides, and then he slips them into his pockets. He will also jerk his leg up, and then act as if he is re-tying his shoe.
What is your classification of this movement?
A. Ballismus
B. Athetosis
C. Chorea
D. Motor tics

Correct answer is: C
Chorea is a rapid, involuntary movement that can affect any body that culminates with the patient attempting to integrate the end of the movement into a purposeful action. The rate of movements can be sporadic or almost continuous.

Ballismus is a high-amplitude rapid violent movement of a limb, shoulder or pelvis. In children is occurs with cerebral palsy, kernicterus, Sydenham chorea and lupus.

Athetosis are low-amplitude writing movements that occur alone or associated with chorea in choreoathetosis. The most common cause of independent Athetosis is perinatal brain injury and is seen in children with cerebral palsy.

Motor tics usually involve head, neck and facial movements in transient or chronic motor tic of childhood or Tourette's syndrome.

Suggested Reading

Boyd KN, Mailman RB. Dopamine receptor signaling and current and future antipsychotic drugs. In Current Antipsychotics. Springer Berlin: Heidelberg; 2012. pp. 53–86.

32. An 18-year-old boy presents for evaluation of recurrent episodes of weakness and headaches. He states that he typically sees bright flickering lines, accompanied by difficulty speaking and right-sided weakness. Shortly afterwards he gets a unilateral pounding debilitating headache, associated with nausea, photo- and phonophobia. He has been hospitalized 3 times for these episodes, and has been treated twice for stroke with a "clot-buster". All episodes resolve spontaneously within 24 h. His mother who passed away in a car accident last year had similar symptoms. His current neurological examination is unremarkable. MRI brain is normal. Subsequent work-up reveals a gene defect involving a calcium channel. **The gene defect responsible for this patient's condition is also the cause for which of the following?**
   A. Episodic Ataxia 1
   B. Episodic Ataxia 2
   C. Benign familial neonatal convulsions
   D. Myotonia congenital
   E. Generalized epilepsy with febrile seizures (GEF+)

Correct answer is: B
This patient has familial hemiplegic migraine (FHM). FMH is an autosomal dominant chanellopathy resulting in migraines with auras associated with unilateral hemiparesis that can last up to several hours. Occasionally cerebellar sign and symptoms are present. Patients frequently get treated for ischemic stroke, however, MRI is always normal. Symptoms resolve spontaneously within several hours. FHM comes in several genetic variants, the most common being FHM1, which is due to defect in the CACNA 1A gene on Chromosome 19, encoding a P/Q-type calcium channel. B: Mutations in the CACNA1A gene also cause Episodic Ataxia 2, and spinocerebellar ataxia type 6. All other choices are channellopathies as well, however, none of them involve calcium channels. A and C: Episodic Ataxia 1 and benign familial neonatal convulsions are both potassium chanellopathies. D and E: Myotonia congenital is a chloride chanellopathy, and generalized epilepsy with febrile seizures (GEF+) is a sodium chanellopathy. It should be noted that these characteristics may be seen in several other neurological disorders. Specifically, Generalized epilepsy with febrile seizures plus (GEFS+) is related to familial hemiplegic migraine type 3 (FHM3), yet also comes up in relation to severe myoclonic epilepsy of infancy (SMEI), temporal lobe epilepsy (TLE),and benign familial neonatal- infantile seizures (BFNIS). In addition, CACNA1A is involved in FHM1, SCA6, childhood absence epilepsy (CAE), and episodic ataxia type 2 (EA2).

Suggested Reading

Barrett CF, van den Maagdenberg AM, Frants RR, Ferrari MD. Advances in Genetics. 2008;63:57–83.

33. A 14-year-old boy complaining of multiple attacks of dystonic posturing of his arm and leg per day. These attacks usually occur when he is playing with his friends, but can occur at any time. He is an excellent baseball player, but has not been participating as much in baseball lately because the attacks occur frequently during

such activities, and he has fallen or dropped the ball several times during these attacks. They last about 15–30 s, and can occur multiple times a day, depending on his level of activity. They also occur if he is startled. In between episodes. His exam is entirely normal.

Which of the following statements is correct regarding this patient's condition?

A. This disorder results from a mutation in the nicotinic acetylcholine receptor
B. This patient has paroxysmal non-kinesigenic dyskinesia
C. A good response to anticonvulsants is seen in this disorder
D. A good response to acetazolamide is seen in this disorder
E. This is an epileptic disorder

Correct answer is: C

The clinical presentation is consistent with paroxysmal kinesigenic dyskinesias (PKOs). There are several categories of paroxysmal dyskinesias, all sharing in common episodes of hyperkinetic abnormal movements with intervening normalcy. The abnormal movements may include dystonia, chorea or choreoathetosis, ballism, or dysarthria. These disorders differ in the length of the paroxysm, triggers for the episodes, pharmacologic therapy, and genetics. PKO is characterized by episodes that last seconds to at most 5 min, triggered by sudden movement as well as by startle and hyperventilation. PKO may be either familial or sporadic, and secondary forms occur in multiple sclerosis, following trauma, in patients with a history of perinatal hypoxic encephalopathy, and in the setting of other underlying neurologic disorders. The primary form responds well to anticonvulsant such as carbamazepine. In paroxysmal non-kinesigenic dyskinesia (PNKD), attacks last 2 min to several hours, and there are sometimes no clear triggers, although episodes can be aggravated by alcohol, caffeine, and fatigue. Episodes are less frequent than in PKD. PNKD does not typically respond to anticonvulsants. A third form of paroxysmal dyskinesias is referred to as paroxysmal exertional dyskinesias, in which episodes are triggered by prolonged exercise and last typically 5–30 min but sometimes up to 2 h. Paroxysmal hypnogenic dyskinesias were previously thought to be non-epileptic dyskinesias but are now known to be frontal lobe seizures as part of the syndrome autosomal dominant nocturnal frontal lobe epilepsy, which results from mutations in the nicotinic acetylcholine receptor, among other genetic mutations. The paroxysmal dyskinesias are not epileptic, but there is an association between PKO or PNKD and epilepsy; families have been reported that have both PNKD and infantile convulsions with choreoathetosis, and a mutation in the gene encoding a sodium/glucose transporter on chromosome 16 has been identified.

15

Suggested Reading

- Fahn S, Jankovic J. Principles and practice of movement disorders. Philadelphia: Elsevier; 2007.

34. Which of the following statements is incorrect regarding acquired causes of cerebellar ataxia?
    A. Hypothyroidism can lead to gait ataxia, and thyroid-stimulating hormone should be checked in patients with gait ataxia
    B. Celiac autoantibodies should be checked in patients with gait ataxia only if there are gastrointestinal symptoms to suggest gluten intolerance
    C. The chemotherapeutic agent cytarabine can lead to irreversible cerebellar ataxia

D. Mercury and bismuth both can lead to cerebellar ataxia in toxic amounts
E. Chronic phenytoin can lead to cerebellar atrophy due to Purkinje cell loss

Correct answer is: B
Celiac disease can cause isolated cerebellar dysfunction without gastrointestinal symptoms. In a patient with ataxia of unclear etiology, celiac antibodies should be checked as gluten free diet can improve the ataxia. There are several causes of acquired cerebellar ataxia. Hypothyroidism can cause gait ataxia, and checking serum thyroid stimulating hormone is indicated in an adult presenting with ataxia. Supplementation with thyroid hormone can lead to improvement of the gait disorder. Chemotherapeutic agents including 5-fluorouracil and cytarabine can cause significant cerebellar toxicity. In cytarabine toxicity, Purkinje cell loss and gliosis occur, and there is loss of dentate neurons as well; the cerebellar dysfunction is typically irreversible. Metals such as mercury can cause cerebellar toxicity as well as visual cortex toxicity, leading to a syndrome of ataxia, visual field deficits, and paresthesias. Bismuth salicylate can cause cerebellar toxicity if ingested in high amounts. Other cerebellar toxins include the solvent toluene. Chronic intake of phenytoin can cause cerebellar atrophy due to damage to Purkinje cells. Acute phenytoin toxicity can cause a reversible cerebellar ataxia. Other causes of acquired cerebellar ataxia include infection (as in HIV infection, Creutzfeldt Jakob disease, and Whipple's disease) or post infection (such as is seen after varicella zoster infection in children). The Miller-Fisher variant of Guillain Barre leads to ataxia in addition to areflexia, ophthalmoplegia, and involvement of other cranial nerves.

Suggested Reading

- Bradley WG, Oaroff RB, Fenichel GM, et al. Neurology in clinical practice, 5th ed. Philadelphia: Elsevier; 2008.
- Ropper AH, Samuels MA. Adams and Victor's principles of neurology, 9th ed. New York: McGraw-Hill; 2009.

35. A 6-year-old boy came to the office with his parents for concern of seizures. His family reported that he has episodes of flapping his arms repeatedly against his sides and then against his head, sometimes for several minutes. He ignores everyone around him during those episodes. Episodes happens when he is upset, but also in the evening around the time his father gets back home from work, particularly when his father brings home ice cream or other treats. He has a motor and language delay, and has been in special education classes at school. He does not have many friends and spends most of his free time playing with the same train set, assembling and disassembling it repeatedly.
What is your impression?
A. He likely has seizures and he should undergo video-EEG monitoring
B. He likely has a complex motor tic disorder
C. This patient's history is consistent with Tourette's syndrome
D. He has paroxysmal dyskinesias
E. This patient likely has stereotypies

Correct answer is: E
From the history, the episodes of arm flapping are likely stereotypies. Stereotypies are patterned, repetitive, stereotyped movements, or vocalizations that occur in response to an external or internal stimulus. Common stereotypies are head nodding, arm flapping, body rocking, head banging, grunting, humming, or moaning.

They may occur in otherwise normal children during times of excitement or boredom, but more often occur in children with developmental delay and autism. When associated with the latter, self-injurious stereotypies may be present. In Rett's syndrome, several stereotypies are often seen, including hand wringing, body rocking, and others. Stereotypies have no urge with relief after executing the movement or vocalization like complex motor tics. This patient's history is not consistent with Tourette's syndrome or paroxysmal dyskinesias.

Suggested Reading

- Fahn S, Jankovic J. Principles and practice of movement disorders. Philadelphia: Elsevier; 2007.

36. An 18-year-old girl presents for evaluation of new abnormal movements of the right arm. The movements began shortly after she got into an argument with her mother. The movements have persisted since then. The movement disappears during sleep. On examination, she has continued tremor of the right hand that is equal at rest and with posture. The frequency of the tremor varies during your exam, and it increases when talking about the argument that triggered her symptoms. The frequency also entrains to a different examiner-provided frequency, and disappears during a motor examination of the left arm. You suspect she has a psychogenic movement disorder.

    What is the most important initial intervention for this condition?

    A. Diagnostic debriefing
    B. Cognitive behavioral therapy
    C. Dynamic psychotherapy
    D. Physical therapy
    E. Start an SSRI for depression

15

Correct answer is: A

Treatment of psychogenic movement disorders is a process that often requires multiple steps and interventions. The most important first step is the diagnostic debriefing, in which the diagnosis is disclosed in an empathetic and nonjudgmental way. The most important predictor of favorable outcome after treatment for these patients is acceptance of their diagnosis. The 3 important points of emphasis should be that the movements are real and disabling, that they are not deliberate, and that they are not necessarily indicative of psychiatric disease. It is crucial to emphasize the certainty of the diagnosis, and further neurological tests are not necessary or recommended. Ultimately, psychological intervention may be appropriate for many of these patients, and multidisciplinary approaches with physical therapy and rehab medicine may be also useful.

Suggested Reading

- Morgante F, Edwards M, Espay A. Psychogenic movement disorders. CONTINUUM: Lifelong Learning in Neurol. 2013;19(5):1383–96.

37. You are evaluating a 9-year-old boy with symptoms of being off balance. The symptoms come on in attacks and he is completely normal in between attacks. In the office, he had been having symptoms for a few hours. On examination, he has dysarthria, ataxia and nystagmus. While still in the clinic, his symptoms gradually resolved and he complained of a margin like headache.

    What is the correct statement regarding his condition?

    A. This condition is associated with mutation in the voltage-gated potassium channel gene KCNA1.

B. This condition can be associated with progressive cerebellar atrophy.
C. This condition is associated with mutation in the glial glutamate transporter gene SLC1A3.
D. It is caused by a triple repeat mutation in the calcium channel gene CACNA1A.
E. It has autosomal recessive mode of inheritance.

Correct answer is: B
This is a clinical presentation of episodic ataxia type 2 (EA2). There are 8 subtypes of these ataxias group, caused by mutations of ion channel genes and present as attacks of ataxia with or without additional neurologic symptoms. They have autosomal dominant mode of inheritance.

Episodes of ataxia in type 1 (EA1) can be associated with brief facial myokymia or neuromyotonia, lasting seconds to minutes. EA2, as in this case, has longer lasting episodes of ataxia and can be associated with nystagmus and dysarthria. Additionally, progressive cerebellar atrophy can be seen over time in these patients.

There are 4 known causative genes for the episodic ataxias; types 1, 2, 5, and 6. EA1 is due to a mutation in the voltage-gated potassium channel gene KCNA1 on chromosome 12. EA2 results from a non-sense mutation and not a triple repeat mutation in the calcium channel CACNA1A. This is the same gene mutation causing familial hemiplegic migraine and hence patients can have positive history of migraines. EA6 is associated with mutation in the glial glutamate transporter gene SLC1A3.

Stress, exertion, caffeine, alcohol and heat can trigger the attacks of EA2, and can be ameliorated by use of acetazolamide. Over time, ataxia and nystagmus may become more pervasive symptoms. The pathophysiology for the progressive nature of symptoms and atrophy on imaging is unknown at this time.

Suggested Reading

- Pandolfo M, Manto M. Cerebellar and afferent ataxias. Continuum Lifelong Learning Neurol. 2013;19(5):1312.
- Ropper A, Samuels M, Klien J. Adams and Victor's principles of neurology. 10th ed. New York: Mcgraw Hill; 2014. p. 946.

Neuro-cutaneous Syndromes

Y. M. Awaad, *Absolute Pediatric Neurology*, https://doi.org/10.1007/978-3-319-78801-2_16

1. Which of the following statements is incorrect regarding epidermal nevus syndrome (ENS)?
   A. This syndrome is a manifestation of a heterogeneous group of disorders that share in common the presence of epidermal nevi
   B. Hemimegalencephaly may occur ipsilateral to a facial nevus
   C. The epidermal nevi in this disorder may undergo malignant transformation
   D. There is increased risk of astrocytoma and other tumors in patients with ENS
   E. Lisch nodules are a feature of ENS

Correct Answer is: E
E. Lisch nodules are a feature of neurofibromatosis, not epidermal nevus syndrome (ENS). Iris colobomas are the most frequent ocular abnormality in patients with ENS. ENS includes several disorders that are characterized by the presence of epidermal nevi and neurologic manifestations. These disorders include Proteus syndrome, which is characterized by asymmetric and often marked hypertrophy of soft tissues and bones, and other rare disorders such as sebaceous nevus syndrome and Becker nevus syndrome. Epidermal nevi are slightly raised patches of hyperpigmentation that are present at birth or appear in childhood. They enlarge over time. Not all patients have neurologic manifestations; occurrence of nevi over the face and scalp predict neurologic involvement. Neurologic manifestations may include intellectual disability, seizures, and cranial neuropathies. In patients with hemimegalencephaly (which often occurs ipsilateral to a facial nevus), contralateral hemiparesis may be seen. Other brain malformations seen in patients with ENS include focal pachygyria, agenesis of the corpus callosum, Dandy-Walker syndrome, and neural tube defects. Cerebral vascular abnormalities including leptomeningeal hemangiomas and arteriovenous malformations may also occur. Patients with ENS are at increased risk of malignancy; the nevus itself may undergo malignant transformation into basal cell carcinoma or other skin malignancies, and there is an increased risk of astrocytoma and other, systemic, malignancies. Various skeletal abnormalities may occur in ENS, including kyphoscoliosis. Ocular abnormalities include iris colobomas (most common), retinal lesions, and strabismus. Cardiac and genitourinary abnormalities also occur.

16

2. Regarding the finding in a patient with neurofibromatosis type 1 shown in the Figure, which of the following statements is incorrect?

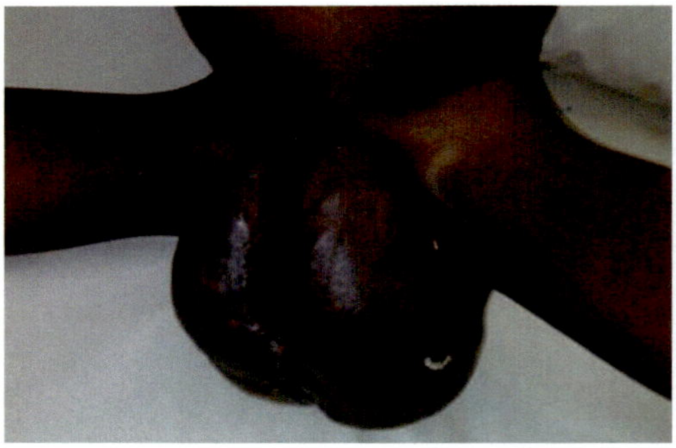

Fig. 16.1 Genitourinary Plexiform Neurofibroma Mimicking Sacrococcygeal Teratoma. (▶ http://openi.nlm.nih.gov/imgs/512/348/3461780/3461780_JSTCR-4-50-g001.png. Nasir AA, Abdur-Rahman LO, Ibrahim KO, Adegoke MA, Afolabi JK, Adeniran JO – *J Surg Tech Case Rep* (2012) Wikipedia)

   A. It is a plexiform neurofibroma
   B. These types of neurofibromas can invade the skin, causing thickening and skin hypertrophy
   C. Plexiform neurofibromas consist of mainly Schwann cells and fibroblasts

D. In a minority of cases, plexiform neurofibromas undergo malignant degeneration into malignant peripheral nerve tumors
E. Plexiform neurofibromas typically regress with age, particularly when they first form at younger age.

Correct Answer is: E
Figure shows a plexiform neurofibroma. Plexiform neurofibromas enlarge in approximately half of patients, particularly when they are present prior to the age of 10 years. Neurofibromas, seen in neurofibromatosis type 1, occur in two types: cutaneous neurofibromas, which originate in the dermis or adjacent layers, and plexiform neurofibromas, which originate in peripheral nerves. They consist predominantly of Schwann cells and fibroblasts but also contain mast cells. Plexiform neurofibromas may occur in the face and can be disfiguring; invasion into the overlying skin causes hypertrophy, hyperpigmentation, and thickening of the skin. Neurofibromas that arise from dorsal root ganglia can grow in a dumbbell shape, invading the spinal canal and leading to nerve root and even spinal cord compression. Neurofibromas can arise also in the GI tract, leading to intestinal obstruction or gastrointestinal bleeding. As mentioned, in almost 50%, plexiform neurofibromas enlarge and can become disfiguring when superficial, particularly when present from an early age (before the age of 10 years). These lesions should be monitored closely, since in minority they can undergo malignant.

Suggested Reading

- Degeneration into a malignant peripheral nerve sheath tumor. ©2011 Wolters Kluwer Health Lippincott Williams & Wilkins N2013E.All rights reserved.

3. You are seeing a 9-year-old boy with a history of headache. His headaches increase when he lie down and accompanied with nausea and vomiting. You ordered an MRI which showed a 1 centimeter enhancing mass close to the foramen of Monro. As a baby he had a cardiac rhabdomyoma.
What gene is responsible for his condition?
A. The patient has a mutation in the NF1 gene
B. The patient has a mutation in the TSC1 gene
C. The patient has a mutation in the PTCH1 gene
D. The patient has a mutation in the PTEN gene
E. The patient has a mutation in the NF2 gene

Correct Answer is: B
This is a clinical presentation of tuberous sclerosis complex. TS is caused by mutations in the TSC1 or TSC2 genes, coding for hamartin and tuberin, respectively. Major criteria include facial angiofibromas, forehead plaques, ungula or peri-ungual fibroma, 3 hypomelanotic macules, shagreen patch, retinal nodular hamartomas, cortical tubers, sub-ependymal nodules, sub-ependymal giant cell astrocytoma, cardiac rhabdomyoma and lymphangiomyomatosis/ renal angiomyolipoma. Minor criteria include hamartomatous rectal polyps, multiple pits in dental enamel that are randomly distributed, bone cysts, cerebral white matter radial migration lines, gingival fibromas, nonrenal hamartomas, retinal achromatic patch, confetti skin lesions, and renal cysts. The diagnosis of definite tuberous sclerosis complex can be made in the presence of either 2 major features or 1 major feature and 2 minor features. The

presence of 1 major feature and 1 minor feature is sufficient for a diagnosis of probable tuberous sclerosis complex. The presence of 1 major feature in isolation, or the presence of at least 2 minor features is suggestive of possible tuberous sclerosis complex. The patient's enhancing brain mass, located near the foramen of Monro, is consistent with sub-ependymal giant cell astrocytoma (SEGA). This, and the patient's cardiac rhabdomyoma, allow for a diagnosis of definite tuberous sclerosis complex.

Mutations in the NF1 gene, encoding for the protein neurofibromin, cause neurofibromatosis type I. This is diagnosed in the presence of 2 or more of the following:(1) the presence of > 6 cafe au lait macules (5 mm in diameter pre-pubertal, 15 mm in diameter post pubertal) (2); 2 neurofibroma or 1 plexiform neurofibroma (3) freckling of the inguinal or axillary region (4) an optic glioma, (5) iris hamartomas (6) osseous lesion (thinning of long bone cortex, sphenoid wing dysplasia) or (7) first degree relative with NF.

Mutations in the PTCH1 gene encoding for Patched 1 are associated with nevoid basal cell carcinoma, or Gorlin syndrome. Major features include > 2 basal cell carcinomas (12: is sufficient for people under 20 years of age), odontogenic keratosis of the jaw, 3 > palmar or plantar pits, bilamellar calcification of falx cerebri, rib abnormalities (bifid, fused, or markedly splayed), and a first degree relative with the condition. Minor features include (1) frontal bossing/ hypertelorism/ cleft lip or palate (2) sprengel deformity/ pectus/ syndactyly of digits, (3) bridging of sella turcica/ hemivertebrae flame shaped radiolucensies (4) ovarian fibroma and (5) medulloblastoma. A diagnosis of Nevoid basal cell carcinoma can be made in the presence of either 2 major criteria or 1 major and 2 minor criteria.

16

Suggested Reading

- Jozwiak S, Migone N, Ruggieri M. The tuberous sclerosis complexes. In: Ruggieri M, PascualCastroviejo I, Di Rocco C, eds. Neurocutaneous Disorders Phakomatoses and Hamartoneoplastic Syndromes. Morlenbach: Springer-Verlag/Wien; 2008:181–227.
- Tabori U, Laberge A-M, Ellezam B, Carret A-S. Cancer predisposition in children with brain tumors. In: Scheinemann K, Bouffet E, editors. Pediatric Neuro-Oncology. New York: Springer; 2015. p. 69–89.
- Gorlin RJ. Nevoid basal cell carcinoma. In: Ruggieri M, Pascual-Castroviejo I, Di Rocco C, editors. Neurocutaneous Disorders Phakomatoses and Hamartoneoplastic Syndromes. Morlenbach: Springer/Wien; 2008. p. 669–94.
- Chan TSY, Wang X, Spence T, Taylor MD, Huang A. Embryonal brain cell tumors. In: Scheinemann K, Bouffet E, editors. Pediatric Neuro-Oncology. New York: Springer; 2015. p. 127–13.

4. Which of the following is not correct regarding neurofibromatosis type 1 (NF1)?
   A. Renal artery stenosis and pheochromocytoma are on the differential diagnosis of hypertension occurring in NF1 patients
   B. There is an association between NF1 and Moyamoya disease
   C. The majority of patients with NF1 have severe developmental delay
   D. Macrocephaly is the most common head size abnormality seen in NF1 Patients and is independent of the extent of hydrocephalus
   E. NF1 patients have an increased risk of intracranial aneurysms

Correct Answer is: C

The majority of patients with neurofibromatosis type 1 (NF1) have normal cognition or mild developmental delay. Other neuropsychiatric manifestations in NF1

include behavioral problems and learning disabilities, which may be present in approximately half of NF1 patients.

Renal artery stenosis due to renal artery dysplasia occurs in some patients with NF1 and can lead to hypertension.

Pheochromocytoma has also been associated with NF1 and the latter two causes of hypertension should be considered in an NF1 patient with hypertension.

Moyamoya disease and other cerebral artery abnormalities including intracranial aneurysms may occur in NF1 patients.

Macrocephaly is the most common head size abnormality seen in NF1 patients and occurs independent of hydrocephalus, although aqueductal stenosis may occur in NF1.

Thinning of the cortex of long bones and other long bone dysplasias may lead to pathologic fractures and pseudoarthrosis. Other skeletal abnormalities in NF1 include scoliosis and sphenoid wing dysplasia.

5. You are evaluating a 5-month-old child with developmental delay, infantile spasms, a renal tumor and sub ependymal nodules on MRI most likely has the presence of which of the following genes?
   A. TSC1
   B. TSC2
   C. SMN1
   D. SMN2
   E. PMP2

Correct Answer is: A

The tuberous sclerosis complex (TSC) is an autosomal dominant disorder with variable phenotypic transmission. Two genes responsible for are TSC1 on chromosome 9 and TSC2 on chromosome 16. Children with TSC1 are more likely to have more severe symptoms than those with TSC2.

SMN1 is responsible for approximately 95% of the cases of spinal muscular atrophy. SMN2 produces a protein product that appears to improve the phenotype in patients with SMN1. The larger the copy of SMN2, the milder the disease.

PMP2 is peripheral myelin protein gene that is duplicated on chromosome 17 in persons with Charcot-Marie-Tooth type 1.

Suggested Reading

Northrup H, Koenig MK, Au KS. Tuberous sclerosis complex. 2011.

6. You diagnosed a 12-year-old boy recently with tuberous sclerosis complex. You ordered an MRI of the brain as part of his work-up. His MRI is shown below. **Which of the following statements is incorrect regarding the findings on this MRI**
   A. These are known as cortical tubers
   B. These lesions are hamartomas
   C. The burden of such lesions correlates with cognitive function
   D. The burden of such lesions correlates with the occurrence and severity of seizures
   E. These lesions are premalignant

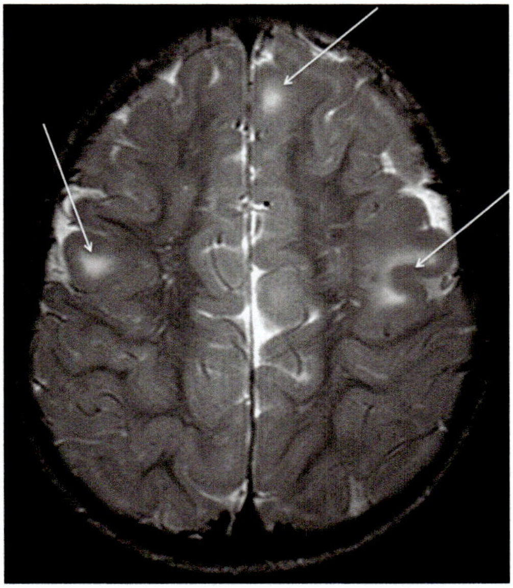

Fig. 16.2 ILAE.org. EpilepsyDiagnosis.org, Diagnostic Manual

Correct Answer is: E
There are multiple hyper-intense lesions in the cortex and gray white junction. These are cortical tubers, also known as cortical hamartomas, findings seen in tuberous sclerosis complex (TSC). Cortical tubers contain large bizarre neurons, abnormal glia, predominantly astrocytes, and hypomyelinated axons. These lesions are not premalignant. CNS manifestations of TSC include intellectual disability, although up 50% of the patients with TSC have normal intelligence. Seizures occur in the majority of TSC patients; the majority of patients with TSC and intellectual disability will have seizures, but not all TSC patients with seizures will have intellectual disability. A variety of seizure types may occur in patients with TSC; TSC is the most common cause of infantile spasms and, in such cases, treatment with vigabatrin is very effective. Other common neuropsychiatric manifestations of TSC include behavioral problems including attention deficit/hyperactivity disorder and learning disabilities.

The burden of cortical tubers correlates to some extent with cognitive function and presence, frequency, and severity of seizures.

7. You are evaluating a 3-month-old baby for developmental delay. His brain MRI shows atrophy with bilateral subdural hematomas. He is hypotonic. He has a coarse, brittle hair, hyperelastic skin, and absent eyebrows.
   What is the most likely diagnosis?
   A. Menkes disease
   B. Wilson disease
   C. Ehlers-Danlos syndrome
   D. No accidental injury (child abuse)
   E. Hypomelanosis of Ito

16

Correct Answer is: A
Menkes disease, also known as kinky hair syndrome, is a neuro-cutaneous disorder characterized by the presence of brittle hair (pili torti), hyper-elastic skin, and thin or absent eyebrows. Abnormal fullness of the cheeks, high arched palate, micro-gnathia, osteoporosis, and metaphyseal dysplasia are also seen. Neurologic manifestations include cerebral vasculopathy and progressive cerebral atrophy leading to subdural hematomas and/or hygromas. Seizures and severe developmental delay occur. Other organ systems are involved, including the skeletal, gastrointestinal, and genitourinary tract. Menkes disease is an X-linked recessive disorder resulting from a mutation in ATP7A, a copper transporter, resulting in defective copper transport across the intestines and widespread copper deficiency in the brain and other organs. Various enzymes require copper as a cofactor, including cytochrome c oxidase, dopamine 8-hydroxylase, and lysyl oxidase among others. Histopathologically, the cortex, thalamus, and subcortical nuclei demonstrate loss of neurons and gliosis. The cerebellum shows loss of granular neurons and Purkinje cells. Laboratory studies demonstrate low serum levels of ceruloplasmin and copper. The presence of subdural hematomas in an infant may raise question of non-accidental injury, although the cutaneous findings and other manifestations allow the distinction to be made. Menkes disease is a disorder of copper, deficiency, unlike Wilson disease, a disorder of copper toxicity, which is due to a mutation in the ATP7B enzyme.

8. What medications would be helpful in the treatment of this patient?

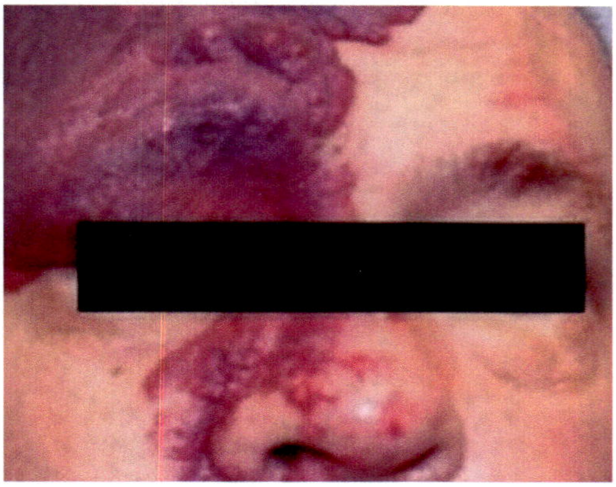

Fig. 16.3 Courtesy of Dr. David Rothner. Shown also in color plates. Comprehensive Review in Clinical Neurology: A Multiple-Choice Question Book for the Wards and Boards ©2011 Wolters Kluwer Health Lippincott Williams & Wilkins. All rights reserve

A. Famotidine 25 mg PO BID
B. High-dose vitamin D daily
C. Dorzolamide 2% (Trusopt) drops to affected eye q8h
D. Amitriptylene 10 mg qHS
E. Minocycline 50 mg BID

Correct Answer is: C

This is a case of Sturge-Weber Syndrome (also called also called encephalotrigeminal angiomatosis) and his likely medications include AED such as phenytoin and glaucoma drops such as Dorzolamide or Brinzolamide. Sturge-Weber (SWS) is caused by residual embryonal blood vessels. These vessels develop around the cephalic portion of the neural tube part of which is in the ectoderm destined to become facial skin. Normally, these vessels regress around the ninth week of gestation but failure of regression results in residual vascular tissue, which forms the abnormal vascular collections which can be in the leptomeninges, face, and eye. Besides the Port-Wine stain usually seen on the face, SWS patients often have developmental delay, ADHD, seizures, and glaucoma. Neurologic damage can progress from small focal seizures to frequent generalized seizures, and even worsening cognitive function and hemiparesis.

9. You got a call from the radiologist regarding a 9-year-old female, who you referred her for an MRI as part of her seizure work-up. Her neurological examination was non-focal and on her skin exam, there was a unilateral cutaneous angioma over the left maxillary region of her face.
What is the brain abnormality and where is it is most likely located?

A. Right temporal grey matter-lined cleft extending from the ependyma to the pia mater
B. Left hemispheric cyst
C. Venous angioma of the pia matter
D. Cortical tubers and sub-ependymal nodules

Correct Answer is: C

Sturge-Weber syndrome is a sporadic neuro-cutaneous disorder consisting of a port-wine stain (cutaneous angioma) of the face and ipsilateral venous angioma of the pia matter. The clinical presentation might include cognitive impairments, contralateral hemiparesis with hemiatrophy and homonymous hemianopia. A 15–50% of newborn with a facial port-wine birthmark in the upper face region has a risk of developing Sturge-Weber syndrome with the accompanied brain and ocular involvement, and up to 80% will have seizures.

Grey matter-lined cleft extending from the ependyma to the pia mater is characteristic of a schizencephalic cleft and is not associated with a neuro-cutaneous manifestation.

A porencephalic cyst is a broad categorization of the presence of a cerebral cyst and most are formed as a result of cell loss. The most common etiologies include prenatal or antenatal infarction or trauma. There is no associated neuro-cutaneous findings.

Cerebral cortical tubers and sub-ependymal nodules are seen in individuals

with Tuberous Sclerosis. Associated dermatologic features include hypomelanotic macules and raised plaques of thickened skin, referred to as Shagreen patches.

Suggested Reading

- Comi AM. Sturge-Weber syndrome. Handbook of clinical neurology. 2014;132:157–68.

10. Neuro-cutaneous syndromes (phakomatoses) represent a group of central nervous system disorders that can be associated with lesions in the skin, eye, brain and other visceral organs. **The neuro-cutaneous syndrome least likely to have comorbid epilepsy is:**
    - A. Sturge Weber
    - B. Tuberous Sclerosis
    - C. Neurofibromatosis Type 1
    - D. Hypomelanosis of Ito
    - E. Incontinentia Pigmenti

Correct Answer is: C
Epilepsy can be seen as a feature in many of the Neuro-cutaneous syndromes. The occurrence rate of seizures varies. Seizures occur in approximately 80% of patients with Sturge Weber, 80% of patients with Tuberous Sclerosis, 50% of children with Hypomelanosis of Ito, 13% of patients with Incontinentia Pigementi and 1% of patients with NF 1.

Suggested Reading

- Cross JH. Neuro-cutaneous Syndromes and Epilepsy –Issues in Diagnosis and Management. Epilepsia. 2005;46(Supp 10);17–23.

16

11. An 18-year-old female has been evaluated for left ear hearing loss with vertigo. You ordered a MRI, which shows bilateral vestibular schwannomas. Her family history is remarkable of bilateral vestibular schwannomas and multiple meningioma in her mother. **What is incorrect regarding the disorder depicted?**
    - A. It is autosomal dominant in inheritance
    - B. It results from a mutation in the merlin gene on chromosome 22
    - C. Various CNS tumors including schwannomas, meningiomas, astrocytomas, and ependymomas can occur in this disorder
    - D. Cutaneous findings such as neurofibromas and axillary freckling are common in this disorder
    - E. Sub-capsular cataracts are a feature of this disorder

Correct Answer is: D
Neurofibromatosis type 2(NF2) has less cutaneous findings than (NF1). NF2 is less common than NF1 and has distinct diagnostic criteria, clinical manifestations, and pathophysiology. Diagnostic criteria for NF2 include one of the following:

- **Bilateral schwannomas of cranial nerve (CN) VIII (although other CNs can be affected, most commonly CN V).**
- **A unilateral CN VIII schwannoma with a first-degree relative with NF2.**
- **A family history of a first-degree relative with NF2 combined with any two of the following lesions: neurofibroma, meningioma, glioma, subcapsular (pre-senile) cataracts.**

In contrast to NF1, cutaneous lesions such as cafe au lait spots and neurofibromas are uncommon in NF2, but they may occur. The main cutaneous findings seen in NF2 are cafe au lait spots and plexiform cutaneous schwannomas. On the other hand, various CNS tumors occur more commonly in NF2, often in the same patient, including schwannomas, meningiomas, ependymomas, and astrocytomas of the brain and spine. Lisch nodules do not occur in NF2, but sub-capsular cataracts and epi-retinal folds may occur. NF2 is one of the neuro-cutaneous

syndromes that is often not diagnosed until adulthood. NF2 is autosomal dominant, with variable expression and complete penetrance. It results from a mutation in the merlin (also known as schwannomin) gene on chromosome 22.

Merlin is a tumor suppressor gene, and mutations in this gene account for the various neoplasms seen in NF2. A variety of mutations in the NF2 gene have been identified, and the type of mutation correlates with clinical severity, with missense mutations leading to some functional protein production and milder clinical phenotype, and frame shift mutations leading to more severe disease.

Gorlin syndrome and Rubinstein-Taybi syndrome are rare syndromes associated with multiple meningiomas, but this patient's history of bilateral schwannomas combined with the family history is suggestive of NF2.

Tuberous sclerosis complex has distinct cutaneous and CNS findings.

Schwannomatosis is a distinct disorder characterized by the occurrence of multiple schwannomas affecting various CNs but not CN VIII. It may be segmental, and a pure spinal form also exists. It may be familial and has in some cases been associated with a mutation on chromosome 22 in a gene near, but different from, the gene mutated in NF2; less than 15% of cases of schwannomatosis are hereditary.

Suggested Reading

- Comprehensive Review in Clinical Neurology: A Multiple-Choice Question Book for the Wards and Boards © 2011 Wolters Kluwer Health Lippincott Williams & Wilkins. All rights reserved.

12. You ordered a brain CT scan for a patient with tuberous sclerosis complex (TSC), and it shows hyperdensities, as shown in the figure.

Which of the following statements is correct regarding these lesions?

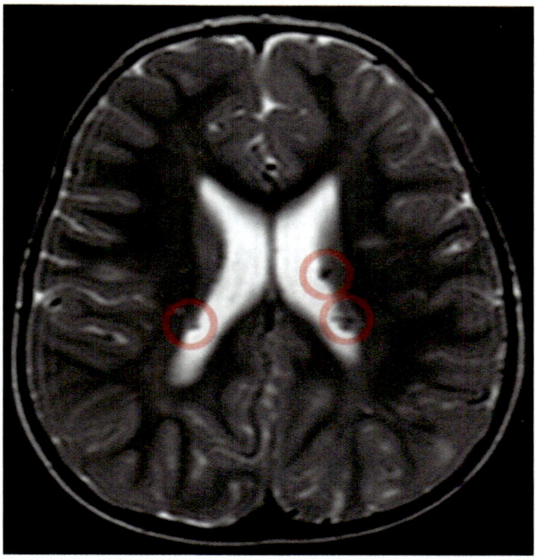

Fig. 16.4 Tuberous sclerosis in MRI: Sub-ependymal nodules; T2 axial. Hellerhoff. Wikipedia

A. These are all malignant and should be resected
B. This patient likely has, in addition to TSC, benign hereditary calcification of the basal ganglia (Fahr disease)
C. The burden of these lesions correlates with the severity of mental retardation in TSC patients
D. These are calcified sub-ependymal nodules and are one of the major diagnostic criteria for TSC
E. These are malignant sub-ependymal giant cell astrocytomas

Correct Answer is: D

There are multiple periventricular hyperdense lesions. Those are sub-ependymal nodules, and their presence is one of the major diagnostic criteria of tuberous sclerosis complex. Sub-ependymal nodules mainly occur in the periventricular region, often at the caudo-thalamic groove. They are thought to arise from remnants of the germinal matrix. They have the potential to grow over time and, in a minority, transform

into sub-ependymal giant cell astrocytoma. Unlike cortical tubers, the presence and number of sub-ependymal nodules are not thought to correlate with cognitive function or seizures. Benign hereditary calcification of the basal ganglia is on the differential diagnosis of subcortical calcifications, but the distribution of these calcifications is typically within the striatum or thalamus and they are not as nodular as these sub-ependymal nodules are. There is no association between TSC and Fahr disease.

13. The shown skin lesion is characteristic in a neuro-cutaneous disorder associated with seizures and hamartomas in multiple body parts.
What is this lesion?

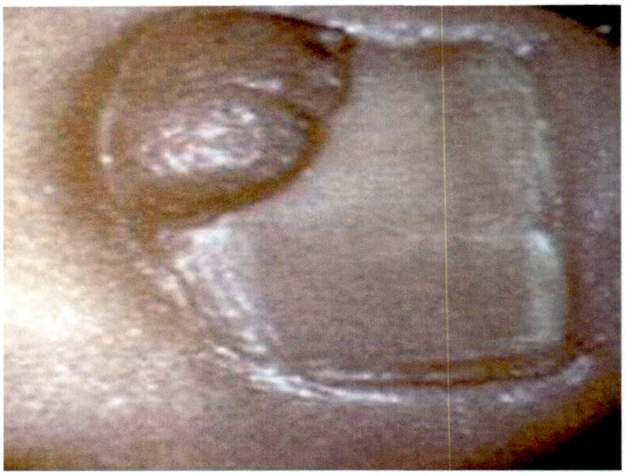

Fig. 16.5 Is Courtesy of Dr. David Rothner. Shown also in color plates. Comprehensive Review in Clinical Neurology: A Multiple-Choice Question Book for the Wards and Boards

16

A. Periungual hematoma
B. Cutaneous neuro-fibromas
C. Subungual fibroma
D. Periungual fibroma
E. Angiokeratoma

Correct Answer is: D
Periungual fibroma is one of the major criteria the cutaneous findings of tuberous sclerosis complex (TSC). On the other hand, traumatic periungual hematomas are typically darker in color and resolve with time.

Subungual fibromas occur under the nail and are also one of the major criteria for TSC.

Angiokeratomas are purplish lesions seen in intertriginous regions in patients with Fabry disease.

14. You are evaluating a 12-year-old boy for his seizures. On examination, he has multiple hypo-pigmented lesions on his trunk, and also lesions on his face as shown in the figure.
What term best describes the face lesions?

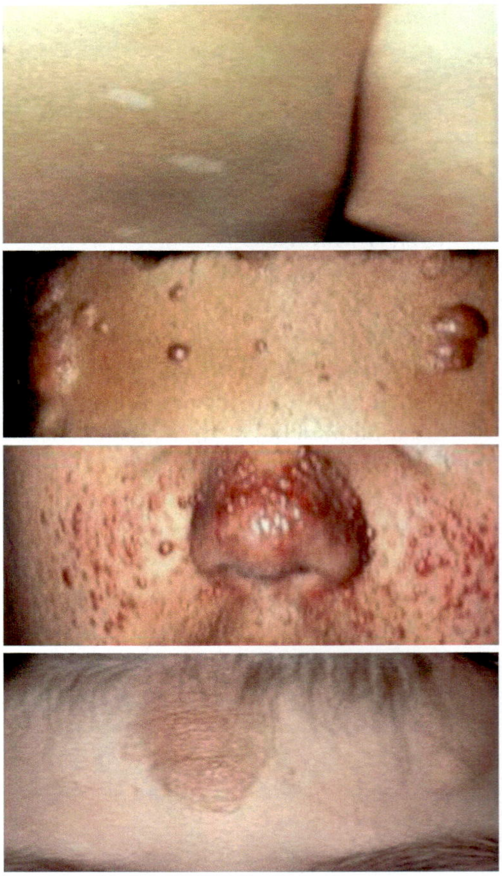

Figs. 16.6, 16.7 and 16.8 Is Courtesy of Dr. David Rothner. Shown also in color plates. Comprehensive Review in Clinical Neurology: A Multiple-Choice Question Book for the Wards and Boards

A. Ashleaf spots
B. Cutaneous neurofibromas
C. Angiofibromas
D. Shagreen patche
E. Severe acne

Correct Answer is: C
This boy has tuberous sclerosis complex (TSC), because of the combination of the ash leaf spots and the facial angiofibromas. TSC is a neuro-cutaneous disorder that affects multiple organ systems including the skin, brain, heart, lungs, and kidneys and others. The diagnosis of TSC can be made when two of the following major criteria or one major and two minor criteria are present.

Major criteria: facial angiofibroma or forehead plaque, periungual, ungual, or subungual fibroma; shagreen patch; more than three hypomelanotic macules (including ash leaf spots); retinal hamartomas; cortical tubers; sub-ependymal nodules; sub-ependymal giant cell astrocytoma, cardiac rhabdomyoma, lymphangiomyomatosis, or renal angiomyolipoma.

Minor criteria: dental pits, rectal hamartomatous polyps, bone cysts, radial migration lines in the cerebral white matter, gingival fibromas, nonrenal hamartomas, retinal achromic patches, confetti skin lesions (hypo-pigmented, stippled lesions on the extremities), and multiple renal cysts. Ash leaf spots are not specific for TSC but occur in the majority of patients with TSC and are often present at birth but become more obvious with age; in newborns, examination under ultraviolet light makes them more apparent. Tinea corporis, a fungal infection, also leads to circular lesions on the trunk, but tinea has a different appearance.

Facial angiofibromas, also known as adenoma sebaceum, which are hamartomatous lesions consisting of vascular and connective tissue. They often become apparent in early childhood as papules in the malar region and become more apparent and numerous with time: they characteristically progress to involve the nasolabial folds and sometimes the chin. Facial angiofibromas may resemble acne if not examined closely and if other historical and clinical features are not taken into consideration.

Shagreen patches are cutaneous hamartomas that have irregular borders and are raised. Shagreen patches most often occur on the trunk (back or flank). These lesions may not be present in childhood but may appear later in life.

Hamartomas can occur in a variety of body parts in TSC including the retina and gastrointestinal tract.

15. You are seeing an infant in the ED with a history of seizures manifest by flexor and extensor spasms. On examination, there is a hypo-melanotic macule on his back.
Which of the following syndromes should be considered?
A. Hypomelanosis of Ito
B. NF1
C. NF2
D. Tuberous sclerosis

Correct Answer is: D
This child has Tuberous Sclerosis (TSC). TSC is associated with seizures that typically begin in infancy. The flexor/extensor myoclonus may indicate infantile spasms, which are associated with hypsarrhythmia on EEG. The hypo-melanotic macule may be shaped like a leaf and thus has been deemed an "ash leaf spot"; this is the most common lesion associated with this disease.

Suggested Reading

- Fenichel GM. Clinical pediatric neurology: a signs and symptoms approach. Philadelphia: WB Saunders; 1997.

16. Regarding the phakomatoses, which of the following finding is not associated with the specified disorder?
   A. Hyper-pigmented cutaneous lesions and leptomeningeal melanoma neuro-cutaneous melanosis
   B. Hemi-facial atrophy-Parry-Romberg syndrome
   C. Multiple endochondromas and secondary hemangiomas-Maffucci syndrome
   D. Hypo-pigmented streaks or patches that follow skin lines-incontinentia pigmenti
   E. Retinal, cerebellar, and spinal hemangioblastomas-von Hippel-Lindau disease

Correct Answer is: D

Hypo-pigmented streaks or patches that follow skin lines occur in Hypomelanosis of Ito, not in incontinentia pigmenti. The phakomatoses are a group of disorders that share in common the occurrence of dysplastic lesions and the tendency for tumor formation. They include neurofibromatosis, tuberous sclerosis, Sturge-Weber syndrome, epidermal nevus syndrome, in addition to a variety of other rare disorders. In incontinentia pigmenti, skin involvement occurs in stages including vesiculobullous lesions present at birth, verrucous lesions that appear at approximately 6 weeks of age, then hyper pigmented lesions that appear "splashed-on." Some patients have normal cognition and no evidence of neurologic dysfunction; neurologic manifestations include intellectual disability, pyramidal tract findings, and ocular abnormalities. It is X-linked dominant in inheritance and affects only females; it is thought to be lethal in males. It results from a mutation in the NEMO gene, which encodes a protein involved in the nuclear factor K-B pathway. Neuro-cutaneous melanosis is characterized by the presence of various types of congenital cutaneous lesions that are abnormally pigmented (such as giant hair pigmented nevi and congenital melanocytic nevi) in association with leptomeningeal melanoma. The leptomeningeal areas most often affected include those around the base of the brain, brain stem, and cerebellum. The pathophysiology of this disorder is not well defined; the cells of origin of the leptomeningeal melanomas are thought to be melanoblasts, pigmented cells normally found in the pia mater.

Parry-Romberg syndrome is marked by the occurrence of facial atrophy, which involves atrophy of facial bone, cartilage, and soft tissue, often with ipsilateral loss of eyelashes, eyebrows, and scalp hair. This begins typically after birth or in early childhood and the atrophy ceases by the third decade of life. Neurologic manifestations include headaches, Horner syndrome, seizures, and hemiparesis. Patients with Parry-Romberg syndrome are at increased risk for a variety of benign tumors.

In Maffucci syndrome, multiple endochondromas (tumors of cartilage) occur, in association with secondary hemangioma formation, and various skin findings including vitiligo and cafe au lait spots. These endochondromas grow over time, leading to disfigurement and skeletal abnormalities. Neurologic manifestations result from the association of this syndrome with various CNS tumors, including CNS teratomas and pituitary adenomas, as well as compression of nervous system structures by the endochondromas, such as cerebral compression by calvarial endochondromas.

In von Hippel-Lindau disease, multiple retinal, cerebellar, and spinal hemangioblastomas occur. Benign hemangiomas and cysts in various body parts can also occur. Cutaneous manifestations are not a feature of this disorder. This disorder is autosomal dominant and results from a mutation in a gene on chromosome 3 that encodes for a tumor suppressor protein.

Suggested Reading

- Comprehensive Review in Clinical Neurology: A Multiple-Choice Question Book for the Wards and Boards © 2011 Wolters Kluwer Health Lippincott Williams & Wilkins. All rights reserved.

17. A 14-year-old female is brought to the ED because a sudden onset of weakness of the right face and arm. She has a history of a focal motor seizures and intellectual disability. On exam, she has a port wine stain in the left V1 distribution, and she has weakness of the right face and arm. CT was ordered.

    This disorder may be associated with which finding(s)?

    A. Meningeal angiomas
    B. Hydrocephalus
    C. Tram tracking calcifications
    D. Intracerebral parenchymal angiomas
    E. All of the above

Correct Answer is: E

This is a presentation of Sturge-Weber syndrome. Findings are variable, and may include angiomas of the face, meninges and brain (typically ipsilateral to the facial lesion, often involving the occipital region), with contralateral weakness and atrophy, and homonymous hemianopia. The cutaneous angiomas are termed "port wine stains," and typically occur in a V1 distribution. Glaucoma is a possible complication when angiomas involve the choroid. Intellectual disability is evident in 70% of patients, and seizures are noted in the majority of cases. Seizures are most often focal motor or generalized tonic-clonic initially, although other types may develop. In addition to angiomas, imaging may reveal cerebral atrophy, hydrocephalus, and tram tracking gyral calcifications. Sturge-Weber syndrome was believed to occur sporadically, although a responsible gene mutation has recently been identified on chromosome 9 (GNAQ). The sudden onset of weakness may reflect hemorrhage of an angioma (a rare occurrence) or a post-ictal Todd's paralysis. Weakness often develops in the setting of the initial flurry of seizures, although unlike a typical Todd's paralysis, it may be long-lasting or even permanent. Other patients have TIA or stroke-like episodes unrelated to seizure activity. Although initially progressive, the condition typically stabilizes over time.

Suggested Reading

- Santos CC, et al. Neuro-cutaneous syndromes. In: Bradley WG, Daroff RB, Fenichel GM, Jankovic J, editors. Neurology in Clinical Practice. 4th ed. Elsevier Inc.; 2004. p. 1867–900.

18. A 10-year-old boy with a history of seizures and headache came to your office for an evaluation. You ordered a brain MRI, which is shown. The lesion shown in the MRI is resected and pathologic analysis is consistent with sub-ependymal giant cell astrocytoma.

    What is the most likely diagnosis?

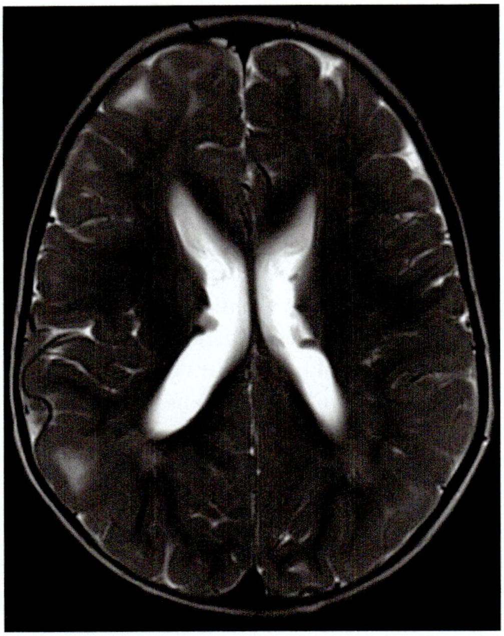

Fig. 16.9 ILAE.org. EpilepsyDiagnosis.org, Diagnostic Manual

A. Tuberous sclerosis complex
B. Neurofibromatosis type 1 (NF1)
C. Neurofibromatosis type 2 (NF2)
D. Sturge-Weber syndrome
E. He probably does not have a neuro-cutaneous disorder; this tumor is most often seen sporadically

Correct Answer is: A
MRI shows a sub-ependymal giant cell astrocytoma (SEGA), which is an uncommon tumor, but it is seen almost exclusively in patients with tuberous sclerosis complex (TSC) and is a major diagnostic criterion for TSC. It is a benign, low-grade astrocytoma but leads to symptoms due to mass effect and ventricular obstruction. Surgery is usually curative. Rapamycin may be of benefit in the treatment of SEGA. SEGA does not typically occur in the other neuro-cutaneous disorders described.

16

19. Which of the following statements is incorrect regarding the genetics of tuberous sclerosis complex (TSC)?
A. It is autosomal recessive with complete penetrance
B. It is autosomal dominant with variable penetrance
C. It can be caused by a mutation in the TSC1 gene that encodes for the protein hamartin
D. It can be caused by a mutation in the TSC2 gene that encodes for the protein tuberin
E. The presence of specific clinical features does not reliably distinguish between the different genetic mutations that can cause this condition

Correct Answer is: A
Tuberous sclerosis complex (TSC) is an autosomal dominant disorder with variable penetrance. TSC may be either inherited or more commonly sporadic. TSC is caused either by a mutation in the TSC1 gene on chromosome 9 that encodes for the protein hamartin or by a mutation in the TSC2 gene on chromosome 16 that encodes for the protein tuberin.

Tuberin and hamartin interact with each other and normally function as tumor suppressor genes, and abnormalities in these proteins lead to unregulated cell growth and proliferation. Although there are some genotype phenotype correlations, the clinical manifestations of each mutation overlap significantly, so the two mutations cannot be distinguished between reliably on the basis of clinical features alone.

Suggested Reading

Comprehensive Review in Clinical Neurology: A Multiple-Choice Question Book for the Wards and Boards ©2011 Wolters Kluwer Health Lippincott Williams & Wilkins. All rights reserved.

20. The findings shown in the figures are consistent with which neuro-cutaneous syndrome? Fig. (A) Courtesy of Dr. David Rothner; (B) Coronal T1-weighted pre-contrast MRI.
What is your diagnosis?

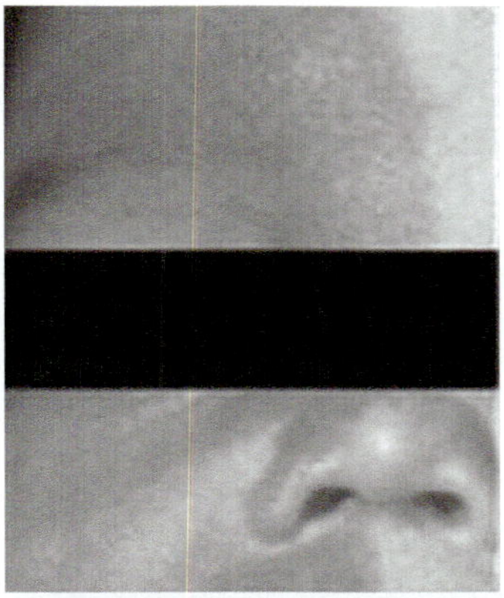

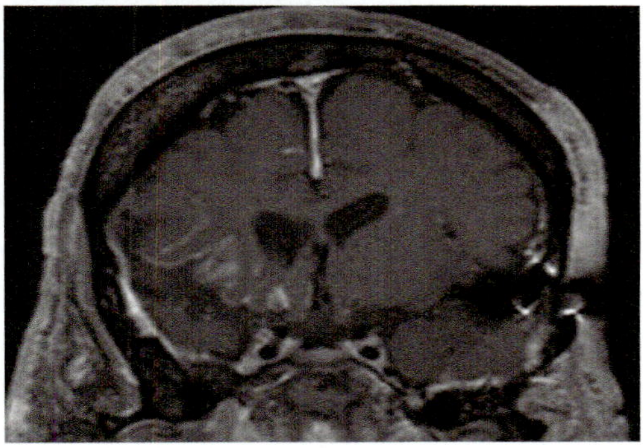

Figs. 16.10 and 16.11 Coronal T1-weighted pre-contrast MRI. (Courtesy of Dr. David Rothner)

A. Neuro cutaneous melanosis
B. Incontinentia pigmenti
C. Hypomelanosis of Ito
D. Sturge-Weber syndrome
E. Epidermal nevus syndrome

Correct Answer is: D
The findings shown are indicative of Sturge-Weber syndrome, in which gyral calcifications result from angiomatosis of the leptomeninges and the brain. The manifestation of Sturge-Weber syndrome includes cutaneous angioma of the face (port-wine nevus), which often occurs in a trigeminal distribution, but may involve any part of the body. Associated features in some cases include angiomatosis of the ipsilateral and less commonly bilateral leptomeninges and the cortex. Some patients have only cutaneous findings without CNS involvement; this is most often the case if cutaneous angiomas are present only in the limbs (without facial involvement). Neurologic manifestations are variable; some patients may have no neurologic signs or symptoms, whereas others may have seizures, contralateral hemiparesis, and/or developmental delay. CNS involvement is most common in those with cutaneous angiomas involving the face. Cobb syndrome, or cutaneomeningospinal angiomatosis, is a variant of Sturge Weber syndrome (SWS) in which cutaneous angiomas occur in a dermatome corresponding to spinal dural angioma. Glaucoma may be a complication of Sturge-Weber syndrome but pre-senile cataracts are not. The pathophysiology of SWS is thought to relate to persistence of embryonal blood vessels that normally regress during gestation; it is considered a congenital malformation rather than a genetic disorder and is not hereditary. The classic radiographic finding is one of gyral calcifications giving a tram-track appearance that may be initially best seen on a CT scan. Cerebral hemiatrophy, rather than hemimegalencephaly, is also seen. MRA is useful in assessing the extent of intracranial involvement. Cerebral venous thrombosis may occur uncommonly.

21. You are examining a 7-year-old boy, you found out that he has more than six hyper pigmented lesions.
What term best describes these lesions?

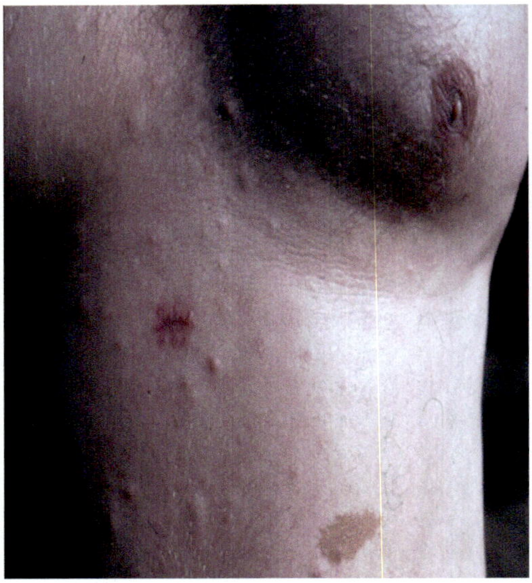

Fig. 16.12 Patient with multiple small cutaneous neurofibromas and a "café au lait spot" (bottom of photo, to the right of centre). A biopsy has been taken of one of the neurofibromas. Haymanj. Wikipedia

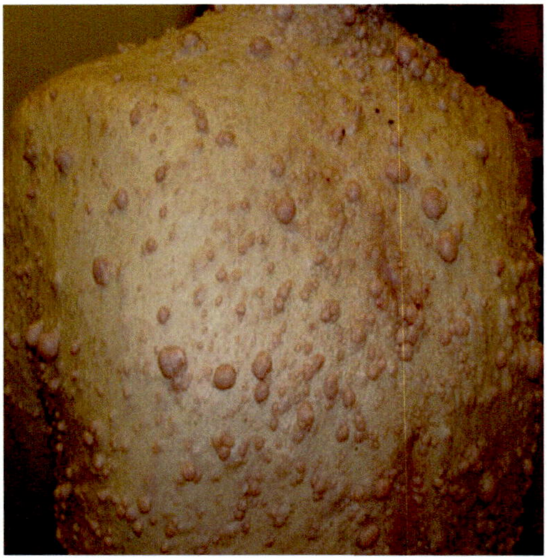

Fig. 16.13 Neurofibromi cutanei sulla schiena di un individuo affetto da neurofibromatosi di tipo 1. Article of MedMedicine.it. Unknown. Wikipedia

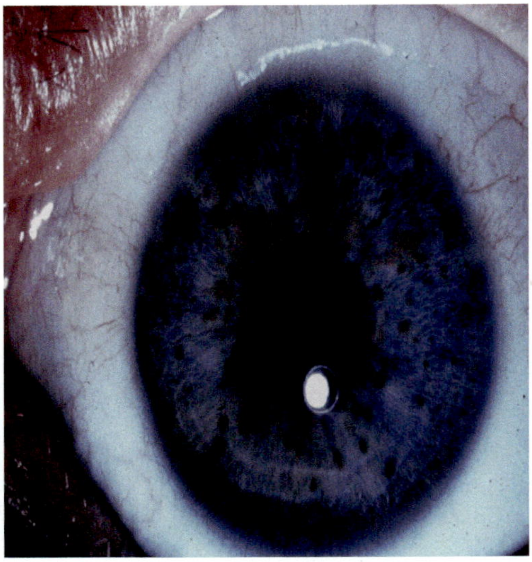

Fig. 16.14 The patient was a 14-year-old male with pulsating exophthalmos of the left eye and poor vision of this highly myopic left eye. There was also some ptosis of the left eye with mild puffiness. Upward gaze of the left eye was limited. Slit lamp examination showed multiple, slightly raised nodules of the right iris. National Eye Institute. National Eye Institute. Wikipedia

A. Ash leaf spots
B. Cutaneous neuro-fibroma
C. Plexiform neuro- fibroma
D. Shagreen patches
E. Cafe au lait spots

Correct Answer is: E
The cutaneous findings shown in Figures are seen in neurofibromatosis type 1 (NF1), or von Recklinghausen disease. NF1 is a neuro-cutaneous disorder that involves multiple organs including the skin, brain, eyes, and bones. The hyperpigmented macules seen are known as cafe au lait spots. Axillary freckling is seen in Fig. 1, and cutaneous neuro-fibromas are seen in Fig. 2. To make a diagnosis of NF1, two or more of the following must be present:

- **Six or more cafe au lait macules measuring more than 5 mm in diameter in pre-pubertal children or more than 15 mm in diameter post-puberty.**
- **Two or more cutaneous neuro-fibromas or one plexiform neuro-fibroma.**

16

- Inguinal or axillary freckling
- Optic nerve gliomas.
- Two or more Lisch nodules.
- NF1 diagnosed in a first-degree relative.
- Sphenoid wing dysplasia, pseudoarthrosis, or cortical thinning of long bones.

Cafe au lait spots may be seen in localized, segmental form in isolation in the setting of post-somatic mutations in the NF1 gene. In contrast to cafe au lait spots, ash leaf spots are hypo-pigmented and are seen in tuberous sclerosis complex. Shagreen patches are connective tissue hamartomas also seen in tuberous sclerosis. The other disorders listed are also neuro-cutaneous disorders, collectively known as the phakomatoses.

Unlike NF1, neurofibromatosis type 2 (NF2) is not diagnosed by the presence of specific cutaneous findings but rather by other criteria.

Sturge-Weber syndrome is marked by the presence of hemangiomas.

TSC and epidermal nevus syndrome have specific cutaneous findings that differ from NF1.

22. A 5-month-old boy is referred to you for an evaluation of his hypo-pigmented streaks on his skin that occurred in a V-shape on his back, and in a linear pattern on his legs, following the skin lines since birth. He has history of seizures. On ophthalmologic exam, he has cataracts. Head circumference was 2 standard deviations above the mean.
What is your most likely diagnosis?
A. Neuro-cutaneous melanosis
B. Incontinentia pigmenti
C. Hypomelanosis of Ito
D. Sturge-Weber syndrome
E. Epidermal nevus syndrome

Correct Answer is: C
Hypo-melanosis of Ito (HI) is a neuro-cutaneous disorder that involves multiple organ systems including the skin, eyes, brain, and skeleton. The cutaneous features of HI include multiple hypo-pigmented streaks or patches that are present at birth and in some follow Blaschke lines (skin lines that form specific patterns over the trunk and extremities, such as a V shape over the back and linear lines over the limbs). Skin lesions are present at birth or appear in infancy and are best detected by ultraviolet light in light-skinned children. The severity of the skin lesions does not correlate strongly with neurologic involvement. Intellectual disability as neurological finding is seen in some but not all patients, and may be severe in some cases. Seizures are another major neurologic manifestation. Macrocephaly or microcephaly may be seen, with the former being more common. Cerebral and cerebellar hypoplasia are also often seen, although various malformations of cortical development may occur in patients with HI, including hemimegalencephaly, lissencephaly, and polymicrogyria. Eye involvement (microphthalmia, cataracts, optic atrophy, and retinal detachment) are common findings. Other manifestations include, skeletal hemi-hypertrophy, cleft lip and palate, and congenital heart disease such as tetralogy of Fallot. Various karyotype abnormalities have been found in patients with HI, including autosomal mosaicism for aneuploidy or unbalanced translocations, mosaic trisomy 18, ring chromosome 22, and translocations involving the X chromosome. There is not a clear genotypic-phenotypic correlation.

23. A brain MRI of a 17-year-old male with neurofibromatosis type complaining of diplopia, shows abnormalities in the left optic nerve and in the pons. **Which of the following statements is incorrect regarding these abnormalities?**

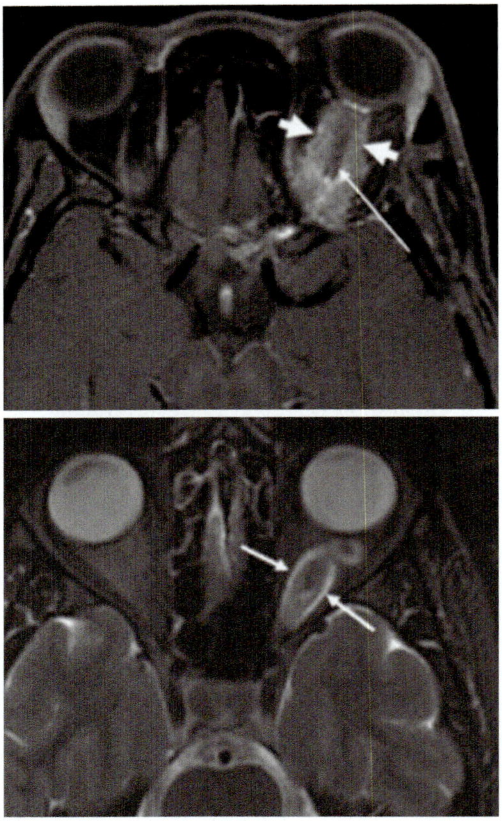

Figs. 16.15 and 16.16 Optic nerve sheath meningioma (*thick arrows*) and optic nerve (*thin arrow*). Glioma of optic nerve. ► https://openi.nlm.nih.gov/detailedresult.php?img=2765171_IJRI-19-135-g010&query=optic+nerve+glioma&it=xg&lic=by&req=4&npos=1. Chavhan G. B., Shroff M. M.W.

16

A. He likely has an optic nerve glioma
B. Optic nerve gliomas are common in NF1
C. Schwannomas and ependymomas are the most common tumors occurring in NF1 patients
D. Optic nerve gliomas in patients with NF1 typically are low grade and often can be monitored for years without intervention

Correct Answer is: C
Schwannomas and ependymomas are rare in neurofibromatosis type 1 (NF1); they more commonly occur in neurofibromatosis type 2 (NF2). Thickening of the left optic nerve represents an optic nerve glioma. Optic nerve gliomas are the most common tumor of the CNS seen in NF1 patients and may be unilateral or bilateral. These are often low-grade lesions but may cause symptoms due to mass effect, including diplopia, pain, and proptosis. Optic pathway gliomas can occur anywhere along the optic pathways, from the optic nerve to the optic radiations. Optic chiasm gliomas may present with precocious puberty when they lead to pressure on diencephalic structures. Because these lesions are often benign, serial imaging over time is often used to monitor these tumors, with chemotherapy, radiation, or surgery instituted as necessary.

Nonspecific subcortical hyper-intensities (in the basal ganglia, thalamus, and other regions) are common in NF1 patients and are of unclear etiology and significance. Figure shows enlargement of the pons, which likely represents a low-grade glioma. NF1 patients are at an increased risk of cerebral, cerebellar, and brain stem astrocytomas. NF1 patients are also at an increased risk for leukemia.

24. Which of the following statements is incorrect regarding the genetics and molecular biology of neurofibromatosis type 1 (NF1, van Recklinghausen disease)?
A. NF1 results from a mutation in the neurofibromin gene on chromosome 17
B. Neurofibromin activates a GTPase that inhibits the ras proto-oncogene, a protein involved in cell proliferation.
C. Several mutations in the NF1 gene have been identified, but in general, strong phenotype genotype correlations do not occur

D. NF1 is an autosomal recessive disorder
E. NF1 has complete penetrance but variable expressivity

Correct Answer is: D
Neurofibromatosis type 1 (NF1) is an autosomal dominant disorder with markedly variable expression but complete penetrance. It results from a mutation in the neurofibromin gene on chromosome 17. Approximately half of cases are sporadic. Neurofibromin is a tumor suppressor protein that normally activates a GTPase that inhibits ras, a proto-oncogene involved in cell proliferation. More than 100 mutations in the NF1 gene have been identified, but no specific genotype-phenotype correlations occur.

25. Which is not a common cutaneous presentation of tuberous sclerosis (TS)?
A. Ash-leaf hypo-pigmented macules
B. 1-3 mm stippled hypo-pigmented areas on the extremities
C. iris hamartomas
D. sub-epidermal fibrous patches
E. ungual fibromas

Correct Answer is: C
Up to 90% of patients with TS have Ash-leaf hypo-pigmented macules. They are typically present at birth, but difficult to visualize, requiring the use of ultraviolet light. Confetti macules are evident in patients with TS, and consist of 1-3 mm stippled hypo-pigmented areas on the extremities. Lisch nodules are iris hamartomas, common in neuro-fibromatosis type 1. Shagreen patches are sub-epidermal fibrous patches, which have an "orange-peel" appearance. They are typically 1–10 cm, irregularly shaped, flat or slightly raised, flesh colored plaques, most often located on the back or flank in patients with TS. They are present in 20–30% of patients with TS, although may not be evident in childhood. Koenen tumors are ungual fibromas, which are nodular or fleshy lesions under or next to the nails. They commonly appear in patients with TS during puberty, and are seen in 15–20% of patients.

Suggested Reading

Santos CC, et al. Neurocutaneous syndromes. In: Bradley WG, Daroff RB, Fenichel GM, Jankovic J, editors. Neurology in Clinical Practice. 4th ed. Elsevier Inc.; 2004. p. 1867–900.

26. You are seeing a 16-year-old male with a history of moderate intellectual disability and new-onset generalized tonic-clonic seizures. You ordered an MRI, which is shown.
What are you expecting to see on his physical examination?
A. adenoma sebaceum
B. bilateral hearing loss
C. café au lait spots
D. facial port wine stain
E. Lisch nodules

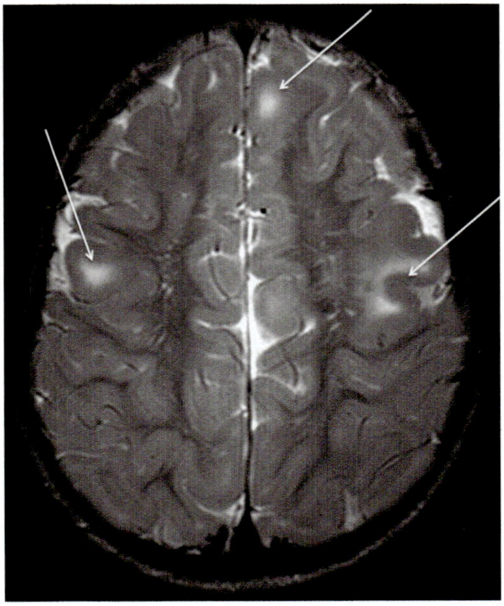

Fig. 16.17 ILAE.org. EpilepsyDiagnosis.org, Diagnostic Manual

Correct Answer is: A
There are multiple areas of T2 signal abnormality that are most consistent with cortical tubers. Also, there is a sub-ependymal giant cell astrocytoma (SEGA) on the right side periventricular. The MRI findings suggest a diagnosis of tuberous sclerosis. Adenoma sebaceum is a common cutaneous feature associated with tuberous sclerosis. Other physical exam features of tuberous sclerosis include periungual fibromas, hypomelanotic macules, gingival fibromas, shagreen patches, randomly distributed pits in dental enamel, achromatic retinal patches, and "confetti" skin lesions.

Café au lait spots and Lisch nodules are features of neurofibromatosis type I.

Facial port wine stains are a feature of Sturge-Weber syndrome.

Bilateral hearing loss may be seen in many conditions, but is often a feature of neurofibromatosis type II.

Suggested Reading

- Roach ES, Sparagana SP. Diagnosis of tuberous sclerosis complex. J Child Neurol 2004; 19(9):643–49.

27. Which of the following are not included in the required features of neurofibromatosis type 1 (NF1) as established by the NIH, of which two are needed to make a clinical diagnosis:
    A. Optic pathway glioma
    B. Distinctive osseous lesion such as sphenoid wing dysplasia or cortical thinning of the cortex of long bones
    C. First degree relative with NF1
    D. Increased T2 signal intensity on MRI of the brain

Correct Answer is: D
"NF1 is a multisystem disorder in which some features may be present at birth and others are age-related manifestations. A National Institutes of Health (NIH) Consensus Development Conference (2) regarding NF1 demarcated the following 7 features, of which 2 or more are required to establish the diagnosis of NF1:

1. **Six or more cafe-au-lait spots (CLSs) equal to or greater than 5 mm in longest diameter in pre-pubertal patients and 15 mm in longest diameter in post- pubertal patients.**
2. **Two or more neurofibromas of any type or 1 plexiform neurofibroma.**
3. **Freckling in the axillary or inguinal regions.**
4. **Optic glioma (optic pathway glioma).**
5. **Two or more Lisch nodules (iris hamartomas).**
6. **A distinctive osseous lesion, such as sphenoid wing dysplasia or cortical thinning of the cortex of long bones, with or without pseudoarthrosis; and**
7. **A first-degree relative (parent, sibling, or child) with NF1 according to the aforementioned criteria.**

In addition, although areas of increased T2 signal intensity are commonly identified on MRI of the brain, they do not represent an obligatory feature of NF. Therefore, the NIH Consensus Development Conference did not recommend routine neuroimaging of the brain as a means of establishing a diagnosis of NF1."

Suggested Reading

- Joseph H. Hersh and Committee on Genetics. Health Supervision for Children with Neurofibromatosis. Pediatrics. 2008;121:633. ▸ https://doi.org/10.1542/peds.2007-3364.

28. What would be the most other abnormal finding in the 16-year-old male whose brain MRI is shown?

16

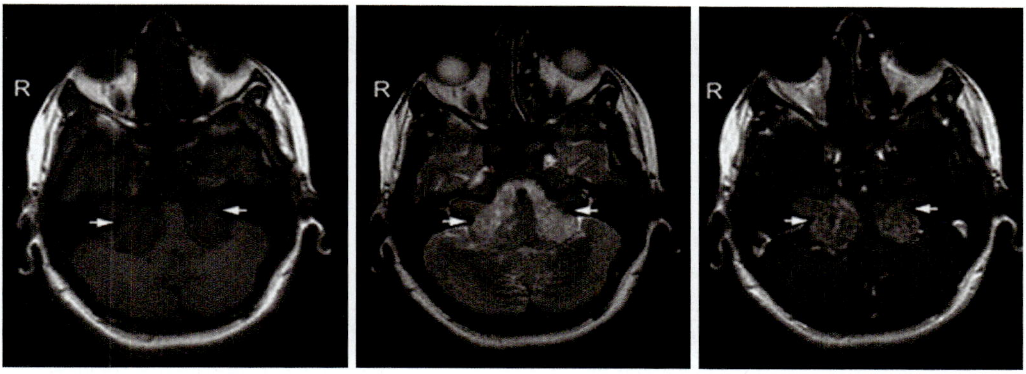

Fig. 16.18 American Academy of Neurology Institute, produced by permission

A. Axillary freckling
B. Café-au-lait spots
C. Cataracts
D. Iris hamartomas
E. Scoliosis

Correct Answer is: C
The brain MRI shows vestibular schwannomas, which are the hallmark of neurofibromatosis type 2. Another common feature of neurofibromatosis type 2 are juvenile cataracts. The other options are typical of neurofibromatosis type 1 but are rarely present in neurofibromatosis type 2.

Suggested Reading

- Hilton DA, Hanemann CO. Schwannomas and their pathogenesis. Brain Pathol 2014;24(3):205–20.
- Lloyd SK, Evans DG. Neurofibromatosis type 2 (NF2): diagnosis and management. Handb Clin Neurol 2013;115:957–67.
- Evans DG. Neurofibromatosis type 2 (NF2): a clinical and molecular review. Orphanet J Rare Dis. 2009;4:16. ► https://doi.org/10.1186/1750-1172-4-16.

29. An 8-year-old boy came with his family to your office for evaluation. The family brought a previous MRI to the visit, shown below.

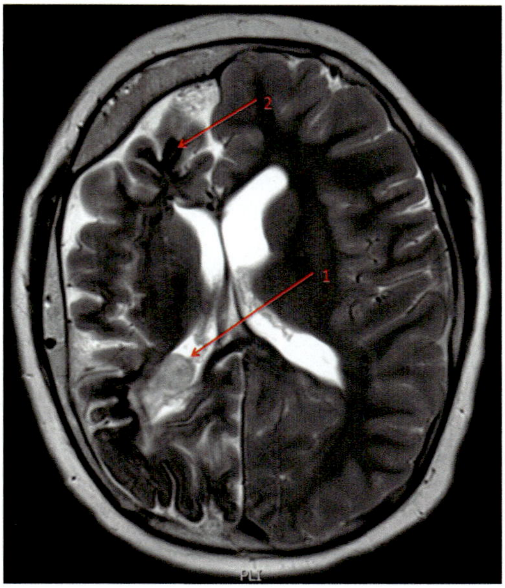

Fig. 16.19 STURGE WEBER SYNDROME. ILAE.org. EpilepsyDiagnosis.org, Diagnostic Manual

What feature, if present, would be most specific in making a definitive diagnosis?

A. Autosomal recessive inheritance pattern
B. Facial capillary malformation
C. Failure to meet developmental milestones in the first few months of life
D. Retinal astrocytoma on dilated eye exam
E. Seizures in the first year of life

Correct Answer is: B

The MRI shows right parieto-occipital pial enhancement, gyral calcifications, and atrophy consistent with leptomeningeal capillary-venous malformation. The presence of facial capillary malformation (a port wine stain) in the 1st or 2nd division of the trigeminal nerve in this setting would be diagnostic of Sturge-Weber syndrome (SWS). This neuro-cutaneous finding is typically ipsilateral to the cerebral vascular malformation. An autosomal dominant inheritance pattern would be atypical. SWS, although congenital, is a sporadic disease and so unlikely to occur in siblings or offspring of affected individuals.

Glaucoma is a common but inconsistent feature of SWS, occurring in 30–70% of patients with SWS. Glaucoma may be congenital or develop later in life. In the rare patient without facial capillary malformation, the presence of glaucoma and typical MRI pattern is highly suggestive of SWS. Retinal astrocytoma is seen in patients with tuberous sclerosis, not SWS.

Though seizures and developmental delay occur commonly in patients with SWS, (with 95% having developed seizures by age five), neither are specific to SWS and may occur in a multitude of congenital and developmental diseases.

Suggested Reading

- Thomas-Sohl KA, Vaslow DF, Maria BL. Sturge-Weber syndrome: a review. Pediatr Neurol. 2004;30(5):303–10.

Neurologic Complications of Systemic Disease

Y. M. Awaad, *Absolute Pediatric Neurology*, https://doi.org/10.1007/978-3-319-78801-2_17

1. **The following scenario is part of a two-question series, Discussion & References included at the end of series.** You are evaluating a 16-year-old female with a history of increasing headache for the last 2 months. The headache is episodic pounding but has become daily. She reported increasing of her weight by 5 lb., and she is abnormally sweaty. On exam she has mild proximal muscle weakness, hyperreflexia and a new intention tremor. **What lab test are you going to order to reach the diagnosis?**
   A. Creatine Kinase
   B. Electrolytes
   C. Tissue Transglutaminase IgA
   D. Thyroid Hormone
   E. Bun/Cr

Correct Answer is: D

2. **The following scenario is question two of the two question series, Discussion & References included at the end of this series.** **What other finding on your exam can be associated with this diagnosis?**
   A. Urinary Incontinence
   B. Papilledema
   C. Hemiplegia
   D. Distal Sensory Loss
   E. Facial Weakness

Correct Answer is: B
Increasing headache without other manifestations may be associated with hyperthyroidism, but may also be associated with intracranial hypertension or rarely sinus venous thrombosis. Hyperthyroidism or Grave's Disease patients can compline of acceleration of linear growth, weight loss or poor weight gain, tachycardia, feeling warm, and increased sweating. Neurological symptoms can include headache, tremor, behavior or mood changes and rarely ataxia. Hyperthyroidism is not associated with focal neurological changes, facial weakness, incontinence and focal sensory changes, but if present should trigger further evaluation. It is very important to consider the possibility of elevated increased intracranial pressure in patients with abnormal thyroid status, although the ICP typically returns to normal after treatment of the hyperthyroidism.

Suggested Reading

- Author, Stephen La Franchi, MD, Section Editor, Mitchell Geffner, MD. Deputy Editor, Alison G. Hoppin, MD.Up-To-Date Clinical manifestations and diagnosis of hyperthyroidism in children and adolescents Accessed 12/8/2014.

3. You are seeing a 16-year-old female in the ICU because of her unresponsiveness for 5 h after having a seizure. One week ago, she had her first generalized tonic-clonic seizure, she was seen in the ER, had a normal CT scan of the brain, and was discharged home. Her family reported that she has increasing unsteadiness in her gait for 2 days before admission. Her medical history is unremarkable and she is not taken any medications. Family history is remarkable for type I diabetes in her mother and hypothyroidism in a maternal aunt. On examination, she is minimally responsive to sternal rub. Vital signs were temperature 98.8 F, pulse 88/min., BP 110/70, respiratory rate 12/min. and oxygen saturation 99% on 2 L nasal cannula. Pupils were 4 mm and reactive, no gaze preference was noted. Corneal and gag reflexes were present. DTRs are hyperactive throughout. Basic laboratory studies, including a CBC, comprehensive metabolic profile, serum lactate and ammonia were normal. An EEG showed diffuse background slowing with no epileptiform discharges. Brain MRI was normal.

17

Lumbar puncture showed 6 WBC/ mm^3, normal glucose and protein 60 mg/dL. Thyroid function tests were normal. Anti-microsomal antibodies were markedly elevated.

What is the best treatment interventions being most likely to produce improvement in her case?

A. IV acyclovir
B. IV fosphenytoin
C. IV solumedrol
D. IV thiamine
E. Oral thyroid replacement

Correct Answer is: C

The patient has subacute encephalopathy. The list of differential diagnosis is long and has many disorders. Toxic or traumatic etiologies have to be considered from her history. Treatable or modifiable conditions should be considered, including hypoglycemia, hyponatremia, uremia and hyper-ammonia, which respond quickly to treatment. Structural lesions of the brain, such as tumors or vascular insults should be considered, though would be more likely to present with focal neurologic findings in addition to the encephalopathy. Infectious causes should always be considered, though would be unlikely without fever and CSF pleocytosis. Acute disseminated encephalomyelitis is a fairly common cause of subacute encephalopathy in childhood, but it usually has radiological findings in the cerebral white and/or deep gray matter. Non-convulsive status epilepticus should be considered in a patient with a history of seizure, though there was no evidence in this case based on the EEG findings. Nutritional deficiencies would be a rare cause in a previously healthy child, though thiamine deficiency should be considered with a history of ophthalmoparesis, ataxia and alteration in mental status. Rarer diagnostic possibilities should be considered if the etiology remains undefined despite an in-depth search for the above conditions. One such cause is Hashimoto's encephalopathy. In spite it is an adult disorder, many cases of Hashimoto's encephalopathy have been reported in children, usually in females over the age of 10 years. Although many neurologic symptoms may be present, alterations in consciousness, seizures and status epilepticus have been the most commonly reported in pediatric patients. Patients themselves are usually euthyroid or mildly hypothyroid but have markedly elevated titers of anti-microsomal (and less commonly anti-thyroglobulin) antibodies. The exact pathophysiologic role of these antibodies has not been clearly understood, most likely they represent an immunologic marker for an as yet unidentified autoimmune mechanism. Although replacement of thyroid hormones is indicated for long term treatment of clinically hypothyroid individuals, this thyroid replacement has no impact on the neurologic features of the disorder. Immune suppressive therapy, most commonly with oral or intravenous steroids has resulted in rapid clinical improvement. The duration of immune suppressive therapy is variable, although most patients are able to taper off medication within months. The diagnosis requires a high index of suspicion. Ancillary tests other than the antibodies mentioned above are nonspecific. EEG typically reveals only slowing of the background, a majority of patients have normal neuroimaging studies and cerebrospinal fluid shows a normal cell count with a modestly elevated protein in most patients.

Suggested Reading

- Watemberg, et al. Encephalopathy Associated with Hashimoto Thyroiditis: a pediatric perspective In J. Child Neurol. 2006;21(1):1–5.

4. You were asked to see a 16-month-old girl with a history of 4 weeks of fussiness and repeated falling. Her

past medical history is remarkable of a viral illness 2 weeks ago and her PCP diagnosed her with acute cerebellar ataxia. Her exam at that time was significant for mild ataxia but she was able to walk on discharge. Her brain MRI was normal. Today, she has had worsening of her symptoms; she is not able to stand and cannot sit without support. Her family noted a tremor when she reaches for objects and jerky eye movements.

What test from below list would change her management?

A. Serum VMA/HVA
B. Scan of her torso
C. EMG/Nerve Conduction study
D. Testing for autoantibodies
E. CSF Neurotransmitters

Correct Answer is: B

This is the clinical presentation of opsoclonus myoclonus syndrome (OMS) and search for underlying neuroblastoma is essential. Neither serum VMA/HVA nor urine VMA/HVA are sensitive enough to rule out or detect an underlying neuroblastoma in patients with OMS. Finding an underlying neuroblastoma is critical as 48% of children with OMS. If there is no neuroblastoma on CT or MRI of the torso, one could consider MIBG scan, and/or follow up scan several months after the initial normal scan. If neuroblastoma is detected it should be removed and treated appropriately but treatment of the OMS with immunomodulatory therapy (ACTH, IVIG etc.) is also critical.

17

Suggested Reading

- Gorman MP. Update on diagnosis, treatment, and prognosis in opsoclonus-myoclonus-ataxia syndrome. Curr Opin Pediatr. 2010;22(6):745–50.

5. A 6-year-old boy came to the ED after having 2 clonic seizures involving his left arm and leg, 15 min each. His past medical history is unremarkable. Many of his family members were ill with a gastrointestinal illness few weeks ago. On examination, his blood pressure is 140/94, he is afebrile and pulse is 140/min. He has weakness and decreased tone of his left arm greater than leg and an extensor plantar response on the left side. His labs are, hemoglobin of 7.6, hematocrit of 25 and platelet count of 25,000. The peripheral smear shows multiple Schistocytes. Serum sodium is 134, bicarbonate 20, glucose 165, BUN 40, creatinine 3.9. A non-contrast head CT scan is unremarkable.

What is the most likely diagnosis for this patient?

A. Hemolytic-uremic syndrome
B. Hypertensive encephalopathy
C. Hyponatremia
D. Kawasaki syndrome
E. Sickle cell vasculopathy

Correct Answer is: A

This patient has symptomatic focal seizures secondary to a recent ischemic stroke. Hyponatremia is a cause of symptomatic seizures, though not secondary to stroke. Typically, serum sodium level need to be less than 120–125 meq/L to produce seizures. The remainder of the choices listed above are potential causes of seizures and ischemic stroke, though hypertensive encephalopathy usually produces bilaterally symmetric abnormalities on imaging, especially in the more posterior brain regions. Focal infarctions respecting vascular distributions are not commonly seen. The constellation of

hemolytic anemia, acute renal failure and thrombocytopenia is most suggestive of hemolytic-uremic syndrome. Although sickle cell disease can cause anemia with seizures secondary to ischemic stroke, sickle cells and not schistocytes (red blood cells that have been fragmented by passage through damaged small blood vessels) would be noted on the peripheral smear. Hemolytic-uremic syndrome is most commonly triggered by a diarrheal associated illness, often shiga-toxin producing strains of E. coli. The toxins have a direct effect on the kidney, causing injury to the sub-endothelial capillary spaces, leading to acute renal failure. Several other infectious, immunologic, familial and endocrine causes have been reported. Neurologic manifestations are seen in 30–40% of cases, and are most commonly a combination of behavioral changes, motor seizures, stroke and varying degrees of encephalopathy. Treatment is mainly supportive, with renal dialysis required in 30–50% of cases. Plasmapheresis has been utilized in some cases.

Suggested Reading

- Ariceta G, Besbas N, Johnson S, Karpman D, Landau D, Licht C, Loirat C, Pecoraro C, Taylor CM, Van de Kar N, Vandewalle J, Zimmerhackl LB; European Paediatric Study Group for HUS. Guideline for the investigation and initial therapy of diarrhea-negative hemolytic uremic syndrome. Pediatr Nephrol. 2009;24(4):687–96. Epub 2008 Sep 18.

6. You are asked to see a 9-year-old female at the hospital because she is significantly obtunded. She was admitted 2 days ago by a pediatric gastroenterologist for vomiting and anorexia, and was diagnosed with acute hepatitis secondary to non-A, non-B hepatitis. She has not responded well to supportive care, and has developed a significant coagulopathy, requiring treatment with cryoprecipitate and recombinant Factor VII (rFVII). You examined her and she is able to open her eyes to voice, but cries in response to questions, and will not respond verbally. Her neck is supple and her optic disc margins are blurred. There is no tremor or asterixis. Her parents stated that she has been confused for the last 2 days. **What is the most likely neurological complication from her systemic disease?**
   - A. Obstructive hydrocephalus
   - B. Large-vessel ischemic stroke
   - C. Cerebral edema with compromised cerebral perfusion
   - D. Coma secondary to elevated serum carnitine levels
   - E. Hyperglycemia

Correct Answer is: C
Acute hepatic failure in children is uncommon. In infants, it is more likely to be associated with an inborn error of metabolism (such as tyrosinemia), whereas in older children and adolescents it is more often due to viral hepatitis or drug exposure (such as acetaminophen). Wilson's disease should also be considered in older children. Children with encephalopathy associated with acute hepatic failure may not have asterixis or tremor. The presence of severe coagulopathy or coma is associated with an increased risk of death. Liver transplantation is required for those children who do not recover spontaneously with supportive care.

Suggested Reading

- Cochran JB, Losek JD. Acute liver failure in children. Pediatr Emerg Care 2007;23:129–135.

7. You are evaluating a 14-year-old female after her tonic-clonic seizure, preceded by unresponsiveness with head and gaze deviation to the right side. She has a change in her behavior for the last 2 days, mainly agitation and possible visual hallucinations. She has a similar event 6 months ago which has been resolved over 1 week, but no diagnosis has been made. She is afebrile, awake, but agitated, unable to settle in bed. Her gait is ataxic. Brain CT and MR imaging are normal. You ordered a LP, shows normal opening pressure and CSF profile. Her EEG shows generalized slowing with multifocal epileptiform discharges. Her complete blood count and serum chemistries are normal, including serum thyroid levels. However, she has markedly elevated anti-thyroglobulin serum antibodies.

What is the most likely diagnosis?

A. Herpes simplex encephalitis
B. Schizophrenia
C. Idiopathic frontal lobe epilepsy
D. Hashimoto encephalopathy
E. Rasmussen chronic encephalitis

Correct Answer is: D

The pathogenesis of Hashimoto encephalopathy (HE) is unknown, but likely relates to the activity of autoantibodies against CNS antigens. Serum levels of thyroid hormone may be either normal or low for patients with this disorder. It is an important diagnosis to consider in children and adolescents with unexplained seizures, ataxia, myoclonus, encephalopathy, or atypical psychosis, since it can be successfully treated with corticosteroid administration. It is likely under-diagnosed in children and adolescents due to the failure to consider HE on the differential diagnosis. The diagnosis is usually made by identifying the presence of high serum levels of anti-thyroglobulin and anti-microsomal antibodies. A relapsing-remitting course may be observed.

Suggested Reading

- Watemberg N, Greenstein D, Levine A. Encephalopathy associated with Hashimoto thyroiditis: pediatric perspective. J Child Neurol. 2006;21:1–5.
- Alink J, de Vries TW. Unexplained seizures, confusion or hallucinations: think Hashimoto encephalopathy. Acta Paediatr. 2008;97:451–453.
- Castillo P, Woodruff B, Caselli R, Vernino S, Lucchinetti C, Swanson J, Noseworthy J, Aksamit A, Carter J, Sirven J, Hunder G, Fatourechi V, Mokri B, Drubach D, Pittock S, Lennon V, Boeve B. Steroid-responsive encephalopathy associated with autoimmune thyroiditis. Arch Neurol. 2006;63(2):197–202.

8. You are evaluating a 6 -year-old boy presents for his uncontrollable seizures despite he was treated with several different anticonvulsant medications. He is currently on oxcarbazepine and topiramate, but continues to have complex partial seizures monthly. His medical history is remarkable for poor weight gain, abdominal cramping and intermittent diarrhea. His development is on target. He has a normal examination. He has no neuro-cutaneous stigmata. Brian CT scan is shown:

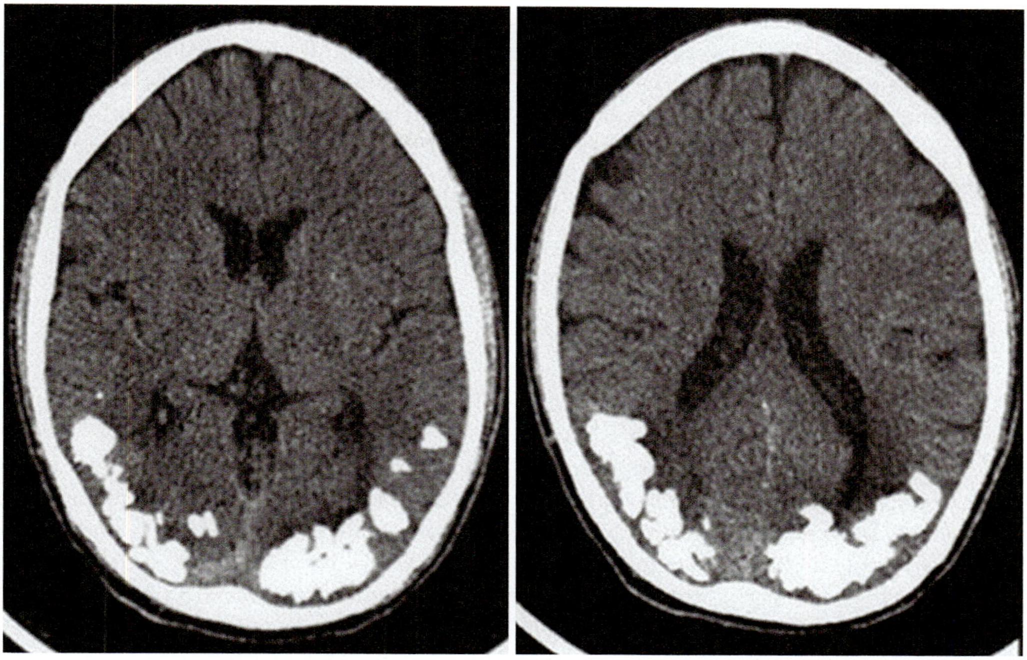

Figs. 17.1 and 17.2 A CT scan of the patient revealed calcification (*white*) in the back of his brain, caused by celiac disease. (Permission: The New England Journal of Medicine ©2014)

What test are you going to order to reach the diagnosis of his epilepsy?

A. Cerebrospinal lactate and pyruvate levels
B. Genetic testing for TSC1 and TSC 2
C. Serum parathyroid hormone
D. Serum toxoplasmosis titers
E. Anti-endomysial antibodies followed by a small bowel biopsy

Correct Answer is: E

Many assumptions have been made to link celiac disease to many neurologic disorders. Celiac disease results secondary to a permanent sensitivity in genetically susceptible patients to gluten products in wheat, barley and rye, and presents with features of an immune mediated enteropathy. The most common neurologic symptoms include chronic progressive ataxia and/or neuropathy in adults. Recent studies have shown an increased rate of celiac disease in children with epilepsy. A specific syndrome of epilepsy and occipital calcifications has been reported. Complex partial seizures, which is refractory to traditional anticonvulsant agents are common in those children. Gluten free diet improve the seizures control. It is felt chronic folic acid deficiency may lead to the development of the calcifications. A majority of affected children will have some form of gastrointestinal involvement, such as chronic diarrhea, constipation or failure to thrive, though neurologic dysfunction can be the sole presenting feature of the disorder.

Once celiac disease is suspected, a practical approach to diagnosis starts with screening serum laboratory testing. Traditionally this was done via anti-gliadin antibodies (IgA mediated), though these antibodies are not specific for celiac disease and have been replaced with anti-endomysial antibodies and/or assay of tissue transglutaminase. Although a positive antibody test is indicative of celiac disease, a formal diagnosis can be confirmed by small bowel biopsy before starting a gluten-free diet. A false-negative biopsy can happened if the biopsy has been done after initiation of the diet.

Calcifications seen in tuberous sclerosis complex typical are located sub-ependymal. The calcified lesions resulting from leptomeningeal angiomatosis in Sturge-Weber syndrome often have a similar appearance to those described above. However, the lack of an associated facial port-wine nevus or severe developmental delay would make this diagnosis highly unlikely in this patient. Those seen in mitochondrial disorders traditionally affect the deep gray structures. Hyper- or hypoparathyroidism has been associated with bilateral basal ganglia calcifications in adults (often cases of Fahr's disease). Neuroimaging of patients with congenital toxoplasmosis often reveals subtle punctate calcifications in the parenchyma, but either microcephaly or significant developmental delay is usually noted as well.

Suggested Reading

- Journal of Clinical Neuromuscular Disease. 2004;5:129–37.
- Journal of Child Neurology. 2002;17(11):800–6.

9. The floor nurse has noted that her 3-year-old boy patient is not using his right arm. The boy was admitted for induction chemotherapy for his precursor B cell acute lymphoblastic leukemia. He has received intrathecal cytarabine; systemic methylprednisolone, doxorubicin, vincristine, and asparaginase; and intrathecal triple therapy with cytarabine, methotrexate, and hydrocortisone. His last intrathecal treatment was 10 days ago, and he had no complication at that time. You examined him and you found that, he has slurred speech, right lower facial droop, and right arm paralysis. DW- MR imaging shows bilateral areas of restricted diffusion in the cerebral white matter, most prominently within the left temporal lobe. He recovered gradually over the following week, and repeat MR imaging 1 month later shows complete resolution of the diffusion abnormalities.

   Which of the following medications is most likely to have caused this patient's symptoms?

   A. Doxorubicin
   B. Intrathecal hydrocortisone
   C. Intrathecal methotrexate
   D. Methylprednisolone
   E. Vincristine

Correct Answer is: C

Several central nervous system complications are associated with childhood leukemia, some secondary to the disease itself and others secondary to its treatment. Leukemia can cause neurologic dysfunction through direct invasion of the nervous system, which generally occurs through leptomeningeal metastasis with dissemination of leukemic cells throughout the subarachnoid space. It can also cause dysfunction indirectly, often through disturbances of coagulation and blood flow (e.g. disseminated intravascular coagulation, hyper-viscosity/leukostasis, venous sinus thrombosis). Finally, the CNS is a common site of relapse, as seen in 3–8% of children with either ALL or AML.

The treatments for childhood leukemia—systemic/intrathecal chemotherapy, cranial irradiation, and bone marrow transplantation—can also cause neurologic dysfunction. The side effects of chemotherapy vary based on the specific agents used. Intrathecal and high-dose intravenous methotrexate have been shown to cause immediate, acute to subacute, and chronic neurologic syndromes. The acute to subacute syndrome usually occurs within days to several weeks of treatment and is characterized by a variety of neurologic signs, including seizures, mental status changes, and focal neurologic deficits (e.g. aphasia, anesthe-

sia, paresis, ataxia, tremor, blurred vision). Brain imaging reveals leukoencephalopathy, but the lesions are usually reversible. Intrathecal chemotherapy—whether with methotrexate or other agents—can also be associated with complications such as Post-Dural puncture headache, CNS hemorrhage, spinal cord dysfunction, chemical meningitis, and neuropsychological dysfunction. Cranial irradiation is a very effective form of CNS-directed treatment, but attempts have been made to eliminate or reduce its use given its substantial rates of secondary neoplasms, endocrine diseases, growth impairment, neurocognitive dysfunction, and other neurotoxic effects. Patients who undergo bone marrow transplantation are at risk for seizures, which occur in about 5% of patients treated with cyclosporine; CNS infections; and graft-versus host disease.

Suggested Reading

- Pui, C-H, Howard SC. Current management and challenges of malignant disease in the CNS in paediatric leukemia. In Lancet Oncolo. 2008;9:257–68.
- Shuper A, et al. Methotrexate treatment protocols and the central nervous system: significant cure with significant neurotoxicity. In J Child Neurol. 2000;15:573–80.
- Demopoulous A, DeAngelis LM. Neurologic complications of leukemia. In Curr Opin Neurol. 2002;15:691–99.

10. You are seeing a 4-year-old boy in the ED who has his first generalized convulsive seizure for 5 min. He has watery diarrhea for 3 days, which became bloody today. On examination, he has a low-grade fever (38 degrees Celsius) and a mildly full abdomen, but no rash or neurocutaneous stigmata. He is minimally arousable, only moaning with examination. Laboratory studies show a low hematocrit of 32%, a white blood cell count of 13.5/mm^3, and a platelet count of 52,000/uL. His basic metabolic panel shows a BUN of 110, a creatinine of 2.1 mg/dL and glucose of 136 mg/dL. His urine shows moderate blood and protein, and hyaline casts. **What is the most likely diagnosis?**
    A. Celiac disease
    B. Febrile seizure
    C. Hemolytic uremic syndrome
    D. Idiopathic thrombocytopenic purpura
    E. Shigellosis

Correct Answer is: C
Hemolytic uremia is a triad of: microangiopathic hemolytic anemia, thrombocytopenia, and acute renal failure. More than 75% of all cases occur in children younger than 3 years, with few cases after 5 years of age. In older adults it can occur, usually with an identifiable provocation. Thirty-three percent of patients can have neurological manifestations. Most of these tend to be mild and transient, but convulsions and ischemic cerebral infarctions, especially in the basal ganglia, can be severe.

Suggested Reading

- Rust R Hemolytic Uremic Syndrome. On ▶ http://emedicine.medscape.com/article/1183555-overview, updated April 3, 2009.

11. You are seeing an 8-year-old boy in the PICU because of progressive confusion and drowsiness for 2 days. His past medical history is unremarkable and takes no medications. He has been vomiting several times a day for 4 days, and this has continued. He has normal vital signs. Scleral icterus and right upper quadrant abdominal tenderness are present. He is drowsy and unable repeat his name, and he does not know his age or his siblings' names. His speech is mildly dysarthric. Cranial nerves are intact. He has low truncal tone but normal extremity

tone and strength. Reflexes are brisk in the upper and lower extremities, with 3–4 beats of clonus at the ankles. He is not able to sit unsupported. His laboratory studies show a mild normocytic anemia, with an ALT of 450 U/L and AST of 680 U/L. Bilirubin is elevated at 6.5 mg/dL. Serum ammonia is elevated at 120 ug/dL. EEG is ordered because of intermittent arms twitching movements, and showed diffuse background slowing with tri-phasic waves. Brain CT scan is normal.

What is most appropriate initial intervention management of this patient?

A. Lactulose
B. Liver transplantation
C. Lorazepam
D. Manganese chelation
E. Mannitol

Correct Answer is: A

The boy has an encephalopathy associated with a hepatic disease. The causes of hepatic encephalopathy in children differ greatly from those in adults (where chronic liver disease and cirrhosis are most common. Children with hepatic encephalopathy most often have acute fulminant liver failure, either from viral hepatitis, toxic ingestion or inborn errors of metabolism. Although encephalopathy is the most constant clinical finding, also noted are variations in muscle tone, hyperreflexia, parkinsonian features, ataxia, and dysarthria and action tremor. Asterixis, a hallmark of adult metabolic encephalopathies, including those of hepatic origin, can be absent in pediatric cases.

The pathophysiology behind hepatic encephalopathy appears to arise from harmful effects of compounds toxic to the brain that would typically be filtered by the portal circulation. Although ammonia has been the chief toxin identified, other compounds including short chain fatty acids, false neurotransmitters and gamma aminobutyric acid have been implicated as well, helping to explain the few patients with hepatic encephalopathy without hyper-ammonemia. Cerebral edema is a frequent complication in the later stages of hepatic encephalopathy, and is often the cause of death.

Reducing the ammonia concentration and treating various complications including infections, renal and cardiovascular dysfunction, and bleeding secondary to ruptured varices, hypersplenism or clotting factor deficiencies are the most effective treatments for hepatic encephalopathy. Ammonia production can be reduced by lowering dietary protein intake and increasing osmotic removal from the gut by non-absorbable disaccharides such as lactulose.

Lorazepam would be indicated in the setting of seizures, which are associated in only 10–30% of cases of hepatic encephalopathy. In fact, the benzodiazepine receptor antagonist flumazenil has shown some evidence in adult studies improving clinical features of the encephalopathy.

Mannitol or hypertonic saline administration is effective when cerebral edema is present, though not present in the current case.

Liver transplantation should be considered for any severe and progressive cases of hepatic encephalopathy, not responding to more conservative measures.

Manganese deposition in the basal ganglia has been postulated to lead to extrapyramidal features of hepatic encephalopathy in adults with chronic liver cirrhosis. Trials of manganese chelation are underway in adults, since chronic cirrhotic liver disease is rare in children, the utility in this age patient is quite unclear.

Suggested Reading

- Swaiman, et al. Pediatric neurology, principles and practice, 4th ed. pp. 2294–7.

12. A 16-year-old male with history of sickle cell disease and previous strokes (the most recent occurring 4 months prior) came to the ED for his left-sided weakness which happened 20 min ago. His NIH stroke scale is 8 because the combination of dysarthria, facial weakness and left-sided weakness. His brain MRI showed a right frontal-parietal infarct. His previous 2 transcranial Doppler (TCDs) revealed velocities >250 cm/s, though he was lost to follow up and never started receiving regular monthly transfusions.
    What is the most appropriate acute intervention for this patient?
    A. Exchange transfusion to reduce the concentration of sickle hemoglobin to less than 30%
    B. Hypotonic saline boluses
    C. Permissive hyperglycemia
    D. Tissue plasminogen activator
    E. Urgent extracranial-intracranial bypass procedure

Correct Answer is: A
The use of tissue plasminogen activator in pediatric patients with stroke secondary to sickle cell disease has no data to support it, which is a treatment option for adult patients. Supportive care measures including correction of hypoxemia and hypotension and maintenance of normoglycemia are standard procedures, as in any patient with stroke. Hypotonic saline should be avoided in patients with cerebral edema after large infarctions as this could aggravation this condition. The current standard of care is exchange transfusion to keep sickle hemoglobin <30% is, and shows a lower recurrent stroke risk than simple transfusion alone. The combination of vigorous hydration and exchange transfusion decrease viscosity and allow improved perfusion to the penumbra. Primary prevention of stroke risk in children with sickle cell disease remains a very important part of ongoing medical surveillance of patients with this disorder. Screen transcranial Doppler studies are recommended starting at age two. Individuals with elevated flow velocities over 200 cm/sec are recommended to begin month transfusions, with the goal of keeping the hemoglobin S concentration under 30%. Data from the major trial (the STOP trial) showed a 90% reduction in stroke risk using this treatment plan. Over time, patients with sickle cell disease are at risk for development of moyamoya syndrome, with progressive narrowing of the proximal intracranial carotid artery and development of multiple small collateral vessels. Consideration of EC-IC bypass procedures may be necessary for such patients, but this therapy would not be used in the therapy of acute stroke.

Suggested Reading

- Holmstedt C, Adams RJ. Neurologic complications of hemoglobinopathies. Continuum (Minneap Minn). 2011;17(1):56–72.

13. You are evaluating an 18-year-old man for his hearing loss. After few hours after he got his first dose of chemotherapy for testicular cancer, he developed bilateral tinnitus and muffled hearing that progressed over the next 48 h. He denies vertigo. He has a normal neurological examination except reduced hearing to finger rub bilaterally. Weber test does not lateralize and air conduction is greater than bone conduction bilaterally. Audiometry demonstrates significant high- and middle-frequency hearing loss bilaterally.
    Which chemotherapeutic agent likely caused this syndrome?
    A. Bleomycin
    B. Cisplatin

C. Etoposide
D. Ifosfamide
E. Vinblastine

Correct Answer is: C
Ototoxicity is a well-known complication of cisplatin chemotherapy. Tinnitus is common and hearing loss is often bilateral, symmetric and permanent. High-frequency hearing loss is most common, but medium frequencies may also be affected. Other drugs that lead to ototoxicity include aminoglycosides, quinine and salicylates. Ifosfamide can cause acute encephalopathy.

Suggested Reading

- Mattox DE. Assessment and management of tinnitus and hearing loss. Continuum Lifelong Learning Neurol. 2006:12(4); 135–50.

14. You are evaluating a 13-year-old boy with chronic renal disease on monthly cyclophosphamide pulse therapy regimen. He is complaining of headaches that are not responsive to acetaminophen. He is brought to the ED after having focal seizure in his left hand and arm which became generalized. On your exam, he is still quite sleepy, but is waking up. His left hand is clumsy and his left arm is weak. You could not understand his speech he is frustrated by this. His blood pressure is 180/100 and his temperature is 38 °C. He is complaining of a diffuse headache. His MRI scan is shown below:
Three days later, he is feeling better. He has normal speech but his hand and arm are weak and clumsy. His blood pressure is 150/85 and his temperature is 37.5 °C.
He is discharged from the hospital and you see him 7 months later. His examination is completely normal. His MRI scan is below.

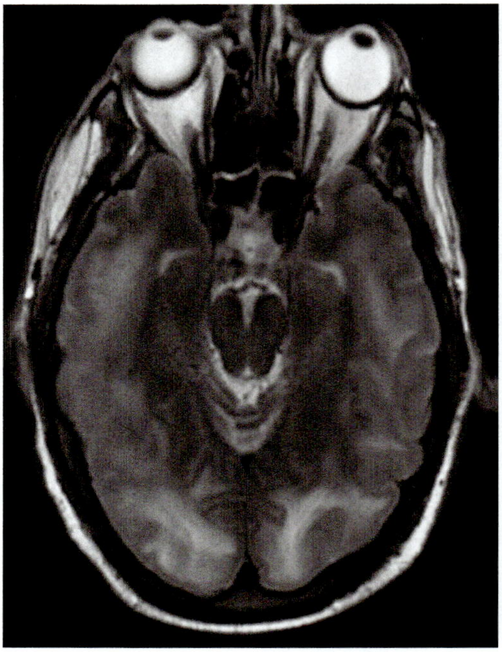

Fig. 17.3 Magnetic resonance image showing multiple cortico-subcortical areas of hyperintense signal involving the occipital and parietal lobes bilaterally and pons in a patient with posterior reversible encephalopathy syndrome. Near fatal posterior reversible encephalopathy syndrome complicating chronic liver failure and treated by induced hypothermia and dialysis: a case report. (J Medical Case Reports 2009, 3:6623. doi: https://doi.org/10.1186/1752-1947-3-6623. Rashmi Chawla, Daniel Smith and Paul E Marik. Wikipedia)

The clinical and MRI findings confirm your suspicion of:
A. ADEM
B. A brain abscesses
C. PRES
D. A hypertensive hemorrhage
E. MELAS

Correct Answer is: C
Posterior reversible encephalopathy syndrome (PRES) most often occurs in the setting of renal failure, hypertension, and/or immunosuppression and is characterized by headache, confusion, and visual loss. It often reverses completely over weeks with effective treatment for the underlying disease. The rapidity with which this

17

patient improves back to baseline and the reversal of his MRI findings in a patient with renal disease requiring immunosuppressive treatment marks this as PRES.

Suggested Reading

- Gera DN, Patil SB, Iyer A, Kute VB, Gandhi S, Kumar D, Trivedi HL. Posterior reversible encephalopathy syndrome in children with kidney disease. Indian J Nephrol. 2014;24(1):28–34.
- Akın F, Kılıçaslan C, Solak ES, Uzun M, Aygün S, Arslan Ş. Posterior reversible encephalopathy syndrome in children: report of three cases. Childs Nerv Syst. 2014;30(3):535–40.
- Raj S, Overby P, Erdfarb A, Ushay HM. Posterior reversible encephalopathy syndrome: incidence and associated factors in a pediatric critical care population. Pediatr Neurol. 2013;49(5):335–9.

15. An 18-years old healthy male has a change in his mental status right after he finished running a full marathon. His coach brought him to the first aid tent at the finish line, as he was unable to walk. He was delirious when the physician was examining him and did not have orientation to time and place. He had generalized weakness without focal findings on neurological exam. Few minutes later, he developed a generalized tonic-colonic seizure.

    What is the most likely cause for his symptoms?

    A. Hypoglycemia
    B. Hypokalemia
    C. Hyponatremia
    D. Hypocalcemia
    E. Hypomagnesemia

Correct Answer is: C

Patient's symptoms of delirium with mental status change and weakness followed by seizure is highly suggestive of hyponatremia. Hyponatremia can occur in about 13% of marathon runners and this patient developed both systemic and neurological manifestations of hyponatremia.

Hypoglycemia and sometime hypocalcemia can cause mental status change, but not the delirious type; also, seizures are less likely to occur.

Hypokalemia and hypomagnesemia very unlikely to cause mental status change.

Suggested Reading

- Continuum. Acute symptomatic seizure and systemic illness. 2014;20(3):601–23.

16. You are evaluating an 18-year-old female for her double vision. This is started 4 months ago mostly in the morning upon waking, and then it subsides. She reports double vision as side-by-side double vision (horizontal diplopia). She has no associated headache.

    Her exam is remarkable for proptosis and weak abduction of the left eye. Pupils are symmetric and reactive to light equally. MRI of orbit shows enlargement and increased enhancement of the muscles and soft tissue of the left orbit.

    What is your likely etiology for her diplopia?

    A. Tumor of the orbit
    B. Idiopathic intracranial hypertension
    C. Lambert-Eaton myasthenic syndrome
    D. Ocular myasthenia gravis
    E. Thyroid ophthalmopathy

Correct Answer is: E

Worsening in the morning for her diplopia is a key feature for her condition. Thyroid ophthalmopathy (which is sometimes referred to as thyroid-associated orbitopathy) is associated with diplopia that is worse upon awakening due to orbital congestion when in the supine position. A lymphocytic inflammatory infiltration of

the orbital tissues occurs in approximately 50% of patients with graves disease and can be detected in a MRI of the orbit.

Horizontal diplopia also could be the first symptom of Idiopathic intracranial hypertension, but she denies headache or any other feature in the history to support this diagnosis. Lack of the any other symptoms rules out the Lambert-Eaton myasthenic syndrome. Diplopia could be an initial symptom of ocular myasthenia gravis, but in myasthenia, diplopia is conversely better in the morning and worsens at the end of the day.

Suggested Reading

- Continuum. Neuro-ophthalmology. 2014;20(4):952–3.

Neuromuscular

Y. M. Awaad, *Absolute Pediatric Neurology*, https://doi.org/10.1007/978-3-319-78801-2_18

1. A family of a 2-month-old baby boy brought him for evaluation because he is floppy compared to its first child. On examination, he does not lift his head or roll over, he perspires profusely on his head and face when feeding, and hypotonic and weak. He is alert and smiles appropriately but has scant limb movements and a weak cry. He is areflexic and the muscles are difficult to palpate. **What study are going to order to establish the diagnosis?**
   - A. Serum CK
   - B. Blood spot for alpha 1–4 glucosidase deficiency.
   - C. Determination of CTG repeat number in the PK gene.
   - D. Survival motor neuron gene mutation analysis
   - E. Electromyography

Correct Answer is: D
Perspiration when feeding is an indication of the work the infant is doing to breathe and eat at the same time. The expressive face would be expected in SMA at this stage but not in myotonic dystrophy (type 1 associated with PK gene abnormality). Although Pompe's disease would not affect the facial expression at this age, the fact that the muscles are not firm and easily palpated would be unexpected. Though the serum CK, EMG, MRI and muscle biopsy are reasonable tests to consider, the most common cause of hypotonia and weakness in this age group, particularly given the alert and expressive face and flabby muscles would SMA-1.

Suggested Readings

- Bodensteiner JB. The evaluation of the hypotonic child. Semin Pediatr Neurol. 2008;15:10–20.

18

2. A pediatrician referred a 5-month-old infant to you because his eyelids look droopy and his muscle tone is floppier than usual. He saw the infant few days ago for constipation and puts him on Karo syrup, and also the infant is not feeding well. Three days later, her mother brings her back to the pediatrician's office because she. You asked the mother if anything new or different is being fed to the baby or is present in the baby's environment. The mother says she has not fed the baby anything other than breast milk, but she and her husband are having an extension put on their home for which they just broke ground 3 weeks ago. There is no family history of neuromuscular disease and no one else has been sick at home.

   On examination, the infant is hypotonic, areflexic, and has ptosis and dysconjugate gaze although he seems to be awake and alert. An EMG demonstrates an incremental response to rapid repetitive nerve stimulation.

   The baby's condition is likely the result of:
   - A. The Karo syrup being given before 2 years of age
   - B. The recent digging up of soil outside of the home
   - C. An occult viral infection
   - D. A genetic disorder of muscle
   - E. A congenital disorder of the neuromuscular junction

Correct Answer is: B
Infant botulism often starts with constipation and rapidly progresses to include areflexic hypotonia and paresis of eye movement. It can be the result of ingestion of Clostridium botulinum spores in honey; more often, it is the result of spores in soil that is unearthed during construction. EMG findings include an incremental response to rapid repetitive nerve stimulation.

Suggested Readings

- Domingo RM, Haller JS, Gruenthal M. Infant botulism: two recent cases and literature review. J Child Neurol. 2008;23(11):1336–46.

3. You are following a 14-year-old morbidly obese boy for metabolic syndrome. His fasting glucose was 150 and his fasting cholesterol was 250, so he was started on a sulfonylurea and a statin. Two weeks later, he awaked unable to lift either arm sufficiently to comb his hair. His proximal arm muscles ached as if he had done chin-ups in gym class.
He is likely to have:
A. Statin-induced myopathy
B. Deconditioning syndrome
C. FSH muscular dystrophy
D. Endogenous steroid myopathy
E. Hypothyroidism

Correct Answer is: A
An uncommon side effect of statins exists along a spectrum that includes myolysis, myopathy, and myalgias in various patients. It generally involves proximal musculature and is painful and reversible with early withdrawal of the statin.

Suggested Readings

- Scripko PD, Amato AA, Puig A. Mystery case: a 63-year-old man with progressive proximal pain and weakness. Neurology. 2014;82(4): e26–9.

4. You are evaluating a 3-year-old girl with congenital hypotonia, severe intellectual disability, and dysphagia, neonatal diagnosis of hydrocephalus and recent onset of seizures. She cannot sit independently but does smile and respond to her environment. She has not had any neurological regression. Fundus exam revealed optic nerve hypoplasia and retinal dysplasia. Her MRI at 2-days of life is shown.

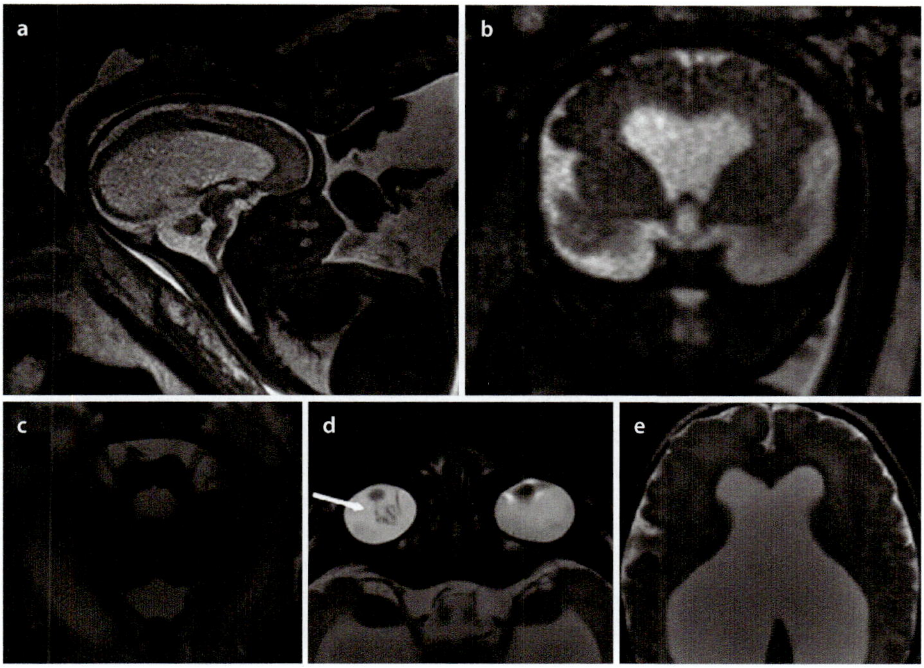

Fig. 18.1 Fetal (**a**, **b**) and 2-day-old (**c**–**e**) brain MRI showing malformations consistent with muscle-eye-brain disease. **a** Sagittal-T2: brainstem hypoplasia and "kinked" pontomesencephalic contour. **b** Coronal-T2: absent septum pellucidum and severe ventricular dilation. **c** Axial-T2: hypoplastic pons with an abnormal posterior indentation; dysplastic cerebellum with small cysts. **d** Axial-T2: retinal detachment (arrow); microphthalmia. **e** Axial-T2: abnormal gyral sulcal pattern with a nodular cobblestone-appearing cortex. (Teaching NeuroImages: Prenatal MRI of muscle-eye-brain disease. Resident and Fellow Section. Neurology **June 1, 2010** vol. 74 no. 22 **e101**)

What is your most likely cause of her syndrome?

A. LMNA-related congenital muscular dystrophy
B. Muscle Eye Brain Disease
C. Merosin Positive Muscular Dystrophy
D. SEPN1-related congenital muscular dystrophy
E. Fukuyama Congenital muscular dystrophy

Correct Answer is: B

MRIs show poly-microgyria, pontine hypoplasia, patchy T2/FLAIR subcortical and periventricular white matter signal abnormality, partial posterior commisural dysgenesis, and absent septum pellucidum. Those findings are suggestive of a congenital muscular dystrophy/cobblestone complex malformation. MRI findings together with her clinical symptoms suggested that she was mostly likely to have a more severe form of a dystroglycanopathy, in particular, Muscle Eye Brain (MEB) disease. Her genetic testing confirmed this with 2 mutations of the *POMGNT1* gene, which is the most common cause of MEB.

LMNA-related CMD (L-CMD) can present with a severe picture in the first 6 months of life (absence of head or trunk support) or with progressive loss of head support after acquisition of sitting or walking ability (dropped head syndrome). Often hypotonia and weakness of the axial-cervical muscles is rapidly progressive, followed by more slowly progressive weakness of the proximal upper limbs and distal lower limbs. However, facial muscles are spared. With time, the characteristic findings are head lag, thoracic and lumbar spinal hyperextension (rigidity), lower limb contractures, and talipes equinovarus but no significant upper limb contractures. MRI is typically normal.

Fukuyama Congenital muscular dystrophy is another dystroglycanopathy, but the neurological and eye findings are typically less severe. In addition, the brainstem is typically normal.

Merosin positive congenital muscular dystrophy and *SEPN1*-related congenital muscular dystrophy are other forms of congenital muscular dystrophy, but typically brain MRI is normal and intelligence is normal in merosin positive CMD.

Suggested Readings

- Bertini E, D'Amico A, Gualandi F, Petrini S. Congenital muscular dystrophies: a brief review. Semin Pediatr Neurol. 2011;18(4):277–88.
- Congenital Muscular Dystrophy Overview, Gene Reviews, Susan Sparks, MD, PhD, Susana Quijano-Roy, MD, PhD, Amy Harper, MD, Anne Rutkowski, MD, Erynn Gordon, MS, CGC, Eric P Hoffman, PhD, and Elena Pegoraro, MD, PhD. January 22, 2001; Last Revision: August 23, 2012 accessed 12/8/2014.

5. You are seeing a newborn infant with hypotonia and respiratory failure. The mother had polyhydramnios but her delivery was normal. Mother had a long narrow face and release of a hand grip is delayed.
In the first year of life this infant is most likely to have which of the following?

A. Cognitive delay, cardiac rhythm disturbances and hepatitis
B. Myotonia, cognitive delay and dysphagia
C. Cardiac rhythm disturbance, dysphagia and myotonia
D. Cognitive delay, facial weakness and pneumonia
E. Facial weakness, myotonia and pneumonia

Correct Answer is: D

This is clinical presentation is most likely congenital myotonic dystrophy 1. DM1 results from an expansion of a CTG trinucleotide repeat in the 3′-untranslated

18

region of the dystrophia myotonica protein kinase gene (DMPK gene) on chromosome 19q 13.3. Usually the mother has only mild symptoms and is diagnosed after she has an infant with the severe congenital form as there may be significant expansion of the trinucleotide repeat when passed from mother to child. In general, longer CTG repeat expansions correlate with an earlier age of onset and more severe disease. Small but abnormal repeats (50–99) are often associated with a mild or asymptomatic phenotype. Maternal anticipation of the DM1 gene is more common than paternal anticipation. Infants with congenital DM1 have hypotonia, and often subsequent respiratory failure. They are also at significant risk for intellectual disability (50–60%). However, the myotonia is not typically present in the first year of life and cardiac conduction abnormalities, while significant, do not typically present until the 2nd decade. Hepatitis is not typically associated with DM1.

Suggested Readings

- Myotonic Dystrophy Type 1 in Gene Reviews, Thomas D Bird, MD, Initial Posting: September 17, 1999. Last Update: May 16, 2013.

6. ***The following scenario is part of a two-question series, Discussion & References included at the end of series.***

   You are seeing an 11old boy who has been toe walking since he was toddler and has difficulty straightening his arms. On exam he has mild weakness and atrophy of biceps and triceps muscles, slight facial weakness and cannot fully extend his arms at the elbow. However, his hand strength is normal. CK is mildly elevated. Family history is remarkable for maternal uncle has similar symptoms as a child. **What is the most likely cause of his symptoms?**

   A. Limb-Girdle Muscular Dystrophy
   B. Becker's Muscular Dystrophy
   C. Fascioscapulohumeral Dystrophy
   D. Emery-Dreifuss Muscular Dystrophy
   E. Merosin-Deficient Congenital Muscular Dystrophy

Correct Answer is: D

The following scenario is part of a two-question series. Please proceed to the next question. Discussion & References included at the end of series.

7. At 16 years of age, this boy developed recurrent dizzy spells and fainted once. **What is the most likely cause of his dizziness?**

   A. Dilated Ventricular Cardiomyopathy
   B. Vagal Nerve Dysfunction
   C. Aortic Stenosis
   D. Cardiac Conduction Deficits
   E. Vertebrobasilar Arterial Disease

Correct Answer is: D

Emery-Dreifuss muscular dystrophy presents in childhood or early adolescence with relatively mild weakness and contractures at the elbows and ankles. It is characterized by the triad of early contractures of the Achilles tendons, elbows, and posterior cervical muscles; slowly progressive muscle weakness and wasting with humeroperoneal distribution in the early stages; and later cardiomyopathy with conduction deficits. The disease is most commonly x-linked (mutations in X-EMD at Xq28), less commonly autosomal recessive (lamin A/C gene on chromosome 1q21) and rarely autosomal dominant. The neuromuscular symptoms may be relatively mild.

The cardiac conduction deficits usually occur later, in the 3rd decade, but may present as early as 5 years of

age. While the weakness may be mild and missed in childhood, the cardiac conduction deficits, which can initially include first degree AV-Block, sinus bradycardia and supraventricular tachycardia and may progress to atrial flutter, atrial fibrillation, and atrial stand-still, can be lethal and increase the risk of ischemic stroke.

Suggested Readings

- Deymeer F. Emery-Dreiffus muscular dystrophy In: Jones H, De Vivo D, Darras B, editors. Neuromuscular disorders of infancy, childhood and adolescence, A clinician's approach. Philadelphia: Butterworth Heinmann; 2003. p. 753–63.

8. You are evaluating a 6-year-old boy with difficulty walking and trouble going up stairs. For the last year his family noticed that he was falling more often and was not able to jump well or keep up with his friends on the playground. On examination, he has proximal muscle weakness, calf hypertrophy and he use Gowers' maneuver to stand. CK is 23,000.
   What is the most appropriate treatment advice for this family?
   A. Prednisone treatment should be offered as it has been demonstrated to have a beneficial effect on muscle strength and function
   B. Prednisone can be considered but reliable data to support its use in this disorder is lacking
   C. Prednisone may be used but should be stopped if their son is unable to tolerate the recommended dose as lower doses of prednisone are not effective
   D. IVIG may be used to treat crises in this disorder with or without prednisone use
   E. Prednisone use in this disorder can hasten deterioration and should be avoided

Correct Answer is: A
As stated in the AAN and CNS Practice Parameter on Corticosteroid treatment of Duchenne Dystrophy (DMD), boys with DMD should be offered treatment with 0.75 mg/kg/d of prednisone or Deflazacort (0.9 mg/kg/day) as these treatments have been shown to have a beneficial effect on muscle strength and function for boys with DMD. Even lower doses of steroid can have benefit and so if side effects require a decrease in prednisone, tapering to dosages as low as 0.3 mg/kg/day have been shown to provide a less robust but significant improvement. IVIG does not typically have a role in the management of DMD.

Suggested Readings

- AAN Practice Parameter: Corticosteroid treatment of Duchenne dystrophy, Report of the Quality Standards Subcommittee of the American Academy of Neurology and the Practice Committee of the Child Neurology Society, R. T. Moxley III, MD, S. Ashwal, MD, S. Pandya, MS, PT, A. Connolly, MD, J. Florence, MHS, PT, K. Mathews, MD, L. Baumbach, MD, C. McDonald, MD, M. Sussman, MD and C. Wade, PhD, PT, RN, Neurology January 11, 2005 vol. 64 no. 1 13–20.

9. You were asked to see a 3-month-old girl in the hospital with a 5-day history of constipation followed over the next 3 days by poor feeding with a weak suck, decreased urinary output and irritability. No systemic manifestations or fever. Her pregnancy and delivery were unremarkable. On examination, her heart rate is 140/min, systolic blood pressure 60, respirations 40/min, temperature 36.7 degrees. She is listless, with a weak cry, weak suck, and poor head control and decreased DTRs. Eye movements are decreased and pupillary reactions sluggish.

What study is most likely to establish the etiology?

A. Acetylcholine receptor antibodies
B. Cerebrospinal fluid examination
C. CPK level
D. Stool sample for botulinum toxin
E. Thyroid function studies

Correct Answer is: D

This is a classic presentation of infantile botulism. There are 4 types of human disease which may result from botulinum toxin, including food-borne or "classical" botulism, wound botulism, adult intestinal toxemia, and infant botulism.

Food-borne botulism occurs via the ingestion of foods contaminated with preformed toxin, whereas the remaining forms of human disease occur through the infection with and growth of clostridial organisms that germinate in situ in wounds or in the gastrointestinal tracts of those afflicted, thereafter producing toxins which are absorbed and exert systemic effects.

Iatrogenic botulism has been reported to rarely result from the injection of toxin for medical and cosmetic purposes. Inhalational botulism could result from aerosolization of botulinum toxin, and has been of interest in recent years as a potential weapon of bioterrorism. Since it was first described as a recognizable and discrete entity in 1976, infant botulism has become the most frequently reported syndrome related to botulinum toxin, accounting for roughly 75% of all annual cases in the United States. In approximately 85% of cases, a source of ingestion is never found. The clinical syndrome of infant botulism usually occurs between 2 weeks and 1 year of age, with a median age of about 10 weeks. The symptoms described in infant botulism are related to peripheral cholinergic blockade due to botulinum toxin. These include constipation or a change in stool pattern with decreased frequency of bowel movements related to autonomic dysfunction, bulbar weakness manifesting as hypophonia and a weak cry, poor suck, and diminished gag, leading to difficulty swallowing, drooling, and often dehydration, cranial nerve palsies such as ptosis, sluggish papillary light reflexes and ophthalmoplegia, facial weakness, and diminished head control with neck and shoulder-girdle weakness, then progressing to generalized hypotonia and a descending, symmetric flaccid paralysis of the skeletal muscles with reduced spontaneous movement, delayed motor developmental milestones, and diminished or absent muscle stretch reflexes. Other findings of autonomic dysfunction may result, including anhydrosis, dry mouth and throat, often leading to mucosal irritation and an incorrect initial clinical suspicion for pharyngitis, hypertension alternating with postural hypotension, brady- and tachydysrhythmias, flushing, decreased anal sphincter tone, and bladder atony. Respiratory compromise, hypoventilation, hypoxia, and the need for mechanical ventilation in a majority of cases ensue as the diaphragmatic and accessory respiratory musculature becomes affected. Treatment is supportive and administration of Botulism immune globulin. This compound has been found to have a half-life of 28 days in vivo, and a single infusion has been shown to neutralize botulinum toxin for at least 6 months. It immediately neutralizes all circulating botulinum toxin and remains present in neutralizing amounts in the circulation for several months, allowing for the regeneration of nerve endings to take place. It consists of immune globulin prepared from the plasma of donors immunized with pentavalent (AB-CDE) botulinum toxoid.

Suggested Readings

- Domingo RM, Haller JS, Gruenthal M. Infant Botulism: two recent cases and literature review. J Child Neurol. 2008;23(11):1336–46.

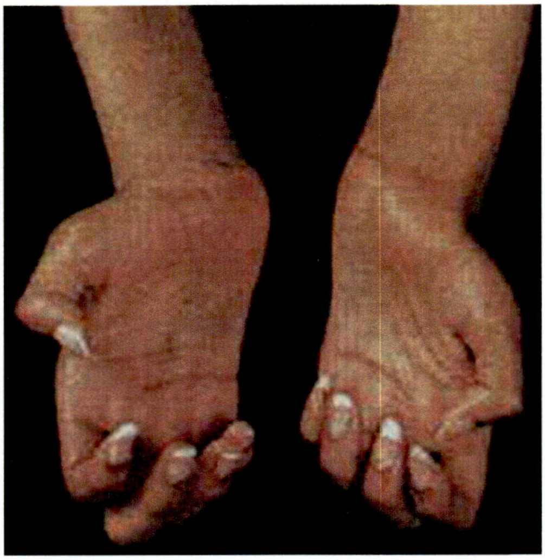

Fig. 18.2 Own work (Original text: *Own work, originally from en.wikipedia; description page is/ was here.*). Benefros at English Wikipedia

10. You are evaluating a 12-year-old girl with progressive weakness of the distal extremities. She has no family history of weakness. She wears AFOs to prevent a foot drop and aid his walking. Her hands are nearly non-functional due to weakness and atrophy of the intrinsic muscles and she cannot oppose the thumb and little finger. Her reflexes are absent and she has normal strength in the proximal muscles and face.
What is your next step in her evaluation?
A. Genetic CMT evaluation.
B. Genetic study of CTG repeats in the PK gene.
C. Muscle biopsy with immunohistochemical stains.
D. Nerve conduction velocity.
E. Serum CK

18

Correct Answer is: D.
Although the clinical picture is indicative of a peripheral neuropathy, the lack of family history means it is impossible to determine the exact type of disease or the inheritance pattern.

The approach to this condition in the absence of family history or inheritance pattern should be to first determine if the disease is demyelinating or axonal or mixed. If the MNCV is normal or near normal the condition is axonal and the causes of axonal hereditary motor sensory neuropathy should be sought. The full CMT battery is expensive and wasteful. In considering the axonal forms of disease, mitofuscin-2 mutations are the most common but only make up about 20% of the cases. If the mitofuscin-2 gene is normal the MPZ protein gene and the gap junction binding protein (GJB1, Connexin 32) should be tested.

Suggested Readings

- Bird TD Charcot Marie Tooth Hereditary Neuropathy Overview. In Genetests.com last revised 1/25/11.

11. You are evaluating a 3-year-old boy for developmental delay. He was a product of full term pregnancy with no complications and acquired normal early milestones, however did not stand until 12 months and walk until 15 months. Also, he has speech delay. There is negative family history of developmental delay, mental retardation or other neurological problems. On examination, he is mildly hypotonic with low amplitude tendon reflexes in all limbs. He is not dysmorphic and has average weight and height. His urine organic acid and serum amino acid screen, a metabolic panel including lactate, and acyl-carnitine profile were normal. AST and ALT both are 2–3 times the upper limit of normal. There is no history of jaundice or hepatitis.
What is the next test being you going to order?
A. Complete genomic microarray analysis.
B. Gene testing for fragile X syndrome.
C. Liver biopsy.

D. MRI of brain, with and without contrast.
E. Serum creatine kinase determination.

Correct Answer is: E
The MDA currently recommends CK screening in male children with developmental delay if there are no other features which would suggest a direction for diagnostic evaluation. Children with dystrophinopathies (Duchenne muscular dystrophy) on average have a 15-point decrease in IQ and may not show weakness, calf hypertrophy, absent reflexes or other signs of the muscle disease until later in childhood. The so called "liver enzymes" AST and ALT are also produced in muscle whereas creatine kinase (CK) is produced only in muscle (skeletal and cardiac) and brain. In patients with high "liver enzymes" and apparently normal liver function, you should always check the CK before proceeding to a liver biopsy.

Suggested Readings

Srour M, Bejjani BA, Rorem EA, et al. An instructive case of an 8-year-old boy with intellectual disability. Sem Ped Neurol. 2008;15:154–7.

12. You are evaluating a 7-month-old infant with delayed acquisition of motor developmental milestones. She seems to be cognitively intact but cannot roll, sit, support her weight or crawl. She can sit if placed in the sitting position. Her reflexes are absent and her muscles are flabby on palpation. Her mother reports that she has been affected since birth and does not appear to be getting worse. Her MRI is shown.

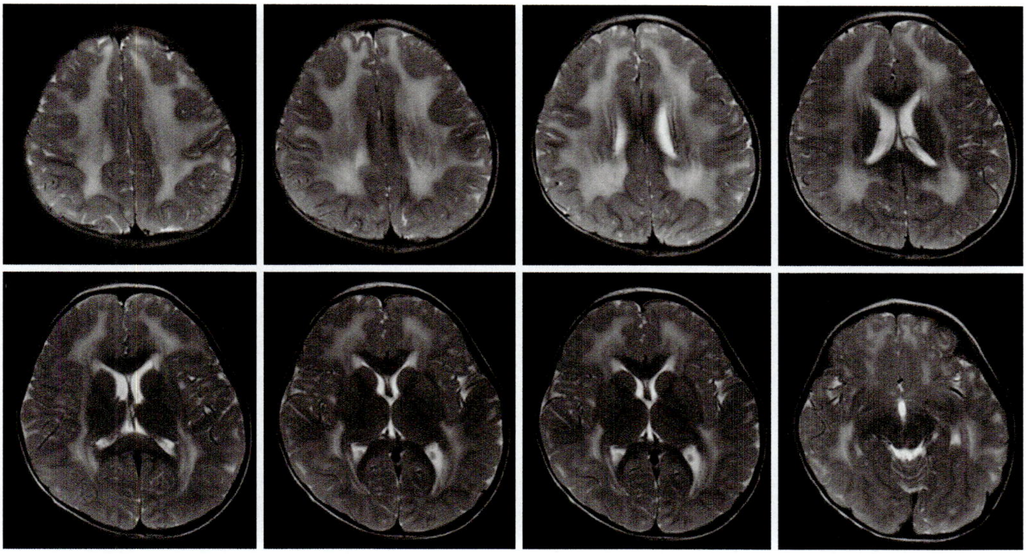

Fig. 18.3 A 3-year-old girl suffered from merosin-deficient congenital muscular dystrophy (MDCMD). Magnetic Resonance Imaging (MRI) brain shows diffuse and symmetrical increase in T2W signal in white matter of cerebral hemispheres. Signal characteristic of corpus callosum, internal capsule, basal ganglia and thalami are normal. Brain stem and cerebellum are structurally normal (not shown). Ventricles are not dilated. The major abnormality is abnormal T2 prolongation in cerebral white matter, without involvement of corpus callosum, internal capsule, brain stem and cerebellum or other structural abnormalities. (Protocol: Magnet strength 1.5 Tesla, TR 4500, TE 1086/Ef, without contrast, 5 mm slice thickness). (J Radiol Case Rep. 2012 Aug;6(8):1–7. doi: ► https://doi.org/10.3941/jrcr. v6i8.997. Epub 2012 Aug 1. PubMed.gov)

What is the most likely diagnosis?

A. Adrenal leukodystrophy
B. Globoid cell leukodystrophy
C. Multiple sclerosis
D. Periventricular leukomalacia
E. Merosin deficient muscular dystrophy

Correct Answer is: E
The absence of encephalopathy makes Krabbe and ALD unlikely. The absence of reflexes argues against all of the above but E although some cases of ALD will have depressed reflexes for a time during the development of the disease. The extensive white matter changes in the brain without cognitive impairment, particularly in the context of a non-progressive congenital muscle disease is so characteristic of Merosin deficient congenital muscular dystrophy that some feel muscle biopsy is not necessary in the diagnostic evaluation of these patients.

Suggested Readings

Bodensteiner JB. The evaluation of the hypotonic child. Semin Pediatr Neurol. 2008;15:10–20.

13. You are evaluating a full-term male infant in the NICU who has developed difficulty feeding, generalized hypotonia, and a weak cry in his first day of life. The mother had "extreme fatigue" during her pregnancy to the point that she had difficulty keeping her eyes open and chewing her food at dinnertime. She was not taking any medications or illicit substances. Birthweight was 3475 g. APGAR scores were 9 at 1 and 5 min, and a physical examination performed in the delivery room was unremarkable. On repeat next day examination, the infant has a weak cry and intercostal retractions. He is awake and alert, but his face appears expressionless. He has generalized hypotonia, resulting in a frog-legged posture, and a paucity of spontaneous movements. DTRs are 2+ throughout, but he has a weak suck. **What is the most appropriate next step in determining this patient's diagnosis?**

A. SMN gene dosage analysis
B. Acetylcholine receptor antibody assay
C. Head MRI
D. Methylation analysis of chromosome 15q
E. Botulinum toxin assay

Correct Answer is: B
Transient neonatal myasthenia gravis (TNMG) is a disorder of postsynaptic neuromuscular transmission that occurs in 21% of infants born to mothers with acquired myasthenia gravis, particularly mothers with active, acetylcholine receptor (AChR) antibody-positive disease. Although the putative mechanism involves passive transfer of anti-AChR or anti-MUSK antibodies across the placenta, the actual mechanism may be more complicated. The majority of patients develop symptoms within a few hours of birth; onset after 72 h has never been reported. Typical findings include generalized hypotonia and difficulty sucking/swallowing, as well as weak cry, facial diplegia, and respiratory distress. Atypical cases may present with arthrogryposis. Gavage feeding and mechanical ventilatory support may be necessary in severe cases. If the mother is known to have anti-AChR or anti-MUSK antibodies, the diagnosis of TNMG may be fairly obvious. On the other hand, if the mother is undiagnosed or has seronegative MG, it may be necessary to confirm the diagnosis by administering an acetylcholinesterase agent (e.g. neostigmine, edrophonium, pyridostigmine) and observing for clinical improvement. False-negative pharmacologic tests can occur, in which case repetitive nerve stimulation before and after the administration of an acetylcholinesterase

agent improves the accuracy of the diagnosis. There is conflicting data about whether maternal serum AChR antibody titers are helpful in predicting which newborns will develop symptoms. Neonatal AChR antibody titers are not helpful in predicting the disease course, but their decline correlates with clinical improvement. Treatment consists of supportive care and, when necessary, acetylcholinesterase agents. Recovery generally occurs within 4 months.

Suggested Readings

- Niks EH, Verrips A, et al. A transient neonatal myasthenic syndrome with anti-MUSKantibodies. Neurology 2008;70:1215–16.

14. You are seeing a 5-month-old baby girl with difficulty feeding and inability to handle secretions. She has been progressively less active for the last 5 days and has been constipated for the last 7 days. On examination she has bilateral ptosis, is drooling, and is unable to hold her head up. single fiber EMG (S-SFEMG) shows incremental response with high-rate repetitive nerve stimulation.

What is the most likely diagnosis?

A. Myasthenia Gravis
B. Congenital Myasthenic Syndrome
C. Infantile botulism
D. Hypokalemic periodic paralysis
E. Myotonia Congenita

Correct Answer is: C

The incremental response at high rates of repetitive stimulation is one of the major criteria for botulism. Other features would include decreased amplitude of the CMAPs, post tetanic facilitation which is prolonged. Infant botulism is a more insidious disease than the adult form as the disease results from the colonization of the upper GI tract with the absorption of tiny amounts of the toxin at a time rather than the ingestion of a larger quantity of preformed toxin as in the adult form. Thus the onset may be subacute and difficult to recognize at first. These children are almost all constipated for several days before the clinical presentation. They clearly suffer from an acquired motor deficit rather than one present at birth and they have prominent involvement of the cranial musculature. The diagnosis can be made by inoculation of mice with serum from the affected individual but electro diagnosis can be done more quickly and is quite reliable. Since these patients can be treated with antiserum it's important to make the diagnosis and initiate therapy as early as possible to limit the duration and severity of the disease. The source of the botulism organisms is frequently not ascertained but classically includes honey and inadequately sterilized bottles and nipples.

Suggested Readings

- Bale JF, Infant Botulism in Gilman S, Goldstein GW, Waxman SG (eds.), Medlink, San Diego, Arbor Publishing, Medlink 2007. 12th ed. Gutierrez AR. Electro diagnosis of infant botulism. J Child Neurol. 1994;9:362–6.

15. You are seeing a 4-year-old boy because he has trouble keeping up with his peers when running or jumping. He is a little slower cognitively than his sister who is 14 months younger. No family history of neurologic and neuromuscular diseases. On examination his tendon reflexes are present but uniformly depressed and his muscles are firm on palpation. He has a serum CK 10,200 IU.

The laboratory examination most likely to yield the definitive diagnosis is which of the following?

A. Deletion analysis of the SMN gene
B. Deletion analysis of the dystrophin gene
C. Analysis of the CTG repeat number in the PK gene

D. Electromyogram and nerve conduction velocity studies
E. Alpha 1–4 glucosidase enzyme activity determination

Correct Answer is: B
Few diseases are associated with high CK. In the face of muscle weakness, cognitive delay and depressed reflexes and this very elevated CK the dystrophinopathies are the most obvious concern and would be the first test to do. SMN gene testing for SMA, CTG repeats for myotonic dystrophy and alpha 1–4 glucosidase activity for Pompe's disease would be considerations if the CK were only slightly elevated. EMG and MNCV testing will help to distinguish myopathy from neuropathic disease but will not yield a specific diagnosis.

Suggested Readings

- Engel AG, Yamamoto M, Fishback KH. Dystrophinopathies. In: Engel AG, Frenzine-Armstrong C, editors. Myology. 2nd ed. 1994. p. 1133–1187.

16. You are evaluating an 18-year-old female who had episodes of generalized stiffening of her muscles that last for several hours since she was 9 years of age. Exposure to cold temperature or exercise can provoke those episodes. On examination, she has delayed muscle relaxation after voluntary contraction and this becomes more marked with continued attempts. Her upper arm muscles are hypertrophied and the CPK is 850. **A mutation affecting the function of which of the following is likely to be present?**
    A. Calcium channel
    B. Chloride channel
    C. Potassium channel
    D. Sodium channel
    E. Sodium/potassium pump

18

Correct Answer is: C
This is a case of paramyotonia congenita, caused by mutations in the SCN4A gene which encodes the alpha subunit of the muscle sodium channel. In paramyotonia congenita, the myotonia typically becomes more pronounced with repeated muscle contractions. This "paradoxical myotonia" contrasts with that of myotonia congenita (due to mutations in CLCN1, which encodes a chloride channel), associated with a warm-up phenomenon of improvement in stiffness with repeated use. Other disorders due to SCN4A mutations include hyperkalemic periodic paralysis and hypokalemic periodic paralysis.

Suggested Readings

- Statland, JM, Barohn, RJ. Muscle Channelopathies: the Nondystrophic Myotonias and Periodic Paralyses. CONTINUUM: Lifelong Learn Neurol. 2013;19(6):1598–614.

17. You are seeing a 6-year-old boy with a history of delay in attaining his motor milestones, prolonged toe walking, frequent falls, and difficulties performing basic motor tasks, such as running and jumping. On examination he has symmetric calf hypertrophy, a mildly lordotic posture, waddling of gait, and poor hip excursion during running. He has a head lag when you pulled him forward from a supine position. He performs a Gower's maneuver when rising from a seated position on the floor to a standing position. Serologic testing reveals a CK of 31,400 U/L. **What treatment options should be offered?**
    A. Achilles tendon lengthening
    B. Coenzyme Q supplementation
    C. Mexiletine 150 mg orally 3 times per day
    D. Prednisone 0.75 mg/kg/d
    E. Pyridostigmine 30 mg every 6 h

Correct Answer is: E

The diagnosis of Duchenne muscular dystrophy (DMD) should be your first thought in a 3–5-year-old boy with difficulty running/jumping, toe walking, large calves, neck weakness, a partial Gower's sign, and a CK level greater than3000 U/L. Corticosteroids should be offered to all boys with DMD. Corticosteroids prolong walking; transiently increase, and then slow the decline in, muscle strength; reduce falls; improve pulmonary measures; decrease scoliosis; and may improve cardiac and cognitive function. The timing for initiation of steroids, and the specific dosage to be used remain undefined. Alternate regimens of weekend-only dosing have shown similar benefits with fewer long term side effects of steroid use (growth and adrenal suppression, bone health, hypertension). Achilles tendon lengthening is contraindicated in this disorder, with likely worsening of pre-existent weakness. Early institution of stretching and orthotic use is standard of care to prevent worsening ankle contractures in this disorder. Coenzyme Q supplementation has shown no benefit for patients with DMD, though might provide benefit (in addition to other nutritional supplements) in mitochondrial myopathies. Mexilietine would be helpful for patients with myotonic disorders and pyridostigmine for disorders of the neuromuscular junction (classic autoimmune myasthenia gravis or for many of the congenital myasthenic syndromes.) Neither of these disorders should present with such classic features of DMD, including such a markedly elevated creatine kinase level.

Suggested Readings

- The Muscular Dsytrophies. Wicklund, Matthew P. CONTINUUM: Lifelong Learn Neurol. 2013;19(6):1535–70.

18. You are evaluating a 15-year-old boy with progressive running difficulties and occasional falls. These tended to occur when he was at sports practice; although he was still active, his athletic performance was deteriorating and he was having increasing difficulty arising from a chair, climbing stairs or riding a bicycle. His past medical history is unremarkable expect for tremor beginning at age 9 years. On examination, he has a normal cranial nerves exam but mildly reduced muscle tone throughout. DTRs were reduced. Proximal strength was reduced with some resistance preserved (4/5). He has Trendelenburg gait and he could walk on his toes, but not on his heels. He has Gower's sign. Electro diagnostic studies performed soon thereafter showed normal motor nerve conduction velocities with a reduced compound muscle action potential in multiple muscles. Sensory nerve conductions are also normal. EMG shows evidence of acute denervation and re-innervation in several muscles of the proximal and distal extremities. CK is elevated at 550. A muscle biopsy was performed showing grouped atrophy, consistent with denervation.
The clinical, electro diagnostic and pathologic manifestations of the case suggest which of the choices as the most likely diagnosis?
A. Becker muscular dystrophy
B. Early-onset amyotrophic lateral sclerosis
C. Limb-girdle muscular dystrophy
D. Paraneoplastic Lambert-Eaton mysasthenia
E. Spinal muscular atrophy

Correct Answer is: E

The clinical presentation demonstrates progressive, primarily proximal muscle

weakness, which would typically be seen primarily with disorders of skeletal muscle or neuromuscular junction. However, the electro diagnostic testing and biopsy are more consistent with disease of the anterior horn cells. There are no concomitant upper motor neuron findings on exam, making any type of ALS unlikely. The most likely diagnosis would be late-onset spinal muscular atrophy (SMA) type 3 or 4 (also known as Kugelberg-Welander syndrome). Late childhood/early adolescence is the typical time of presentation with proximal neurogenic muscular atrophy that may be confused clinically with LGMD. An elevated CK level can be seen with later-onset SMA, though is more likely to be elevated with early-onset forms. It is distinguished from early onset ALS but the absence of UMN signs. Grouped atrophy on muscle biopsy is a hallmark of the disease. Genetic testing is available, showing abnormalities in the survival motor neuron (SMN) region on chromosome 5. The SMN1 gene protein product is important in the formation of spliceosomes, which are important agents in the processing of pre-mRNA into mRNA. Homozygous recessive gene deletions are lethal to motor neurons but the phenotype is predicated by the presence of a second gene, SMN2; more copies of SMN2 modify the clinical presentation of SMA. Patients with 0 or 1 copy of SMN2 typically present in infancy at the more common SMA, type I (Werdnig-Hoffman disease), never achieving ability to sit, with death from respiratory compromise by age 2, if not supported with mechanical ventilation. At the other end of the spectrum, with 4 or more copies of the SMN2 protein product, types III and IV can have a normal lifespan, though usually undergo some degree of progressive muscular weakness at varying ages.

Suggested Readings

- Tiryaki E, Horak HA. ALS and other motor neuron diseases. CONTINUUM Lifelong Learn Neurol. 2014;20(5):1185–207.
- Barohn RJ. Clinical spectrum of motor neuron disorders. CONTINUUM Lifelong Learn Neurology. 2009;15(1, Myasthenic Disorders and ALS):111–131.

19. You are following a 9-year-old boy in the DMD clinic. When he was a toddler, he was diagnosed based on a workup for elevated liver function tests. At that time, his CPK was found to be elevated at 5880 U and muscle biopsy confirmed his diagnosis. His examination is significant for lumbar lordosis and thick calves. When walking, he toe walks, has a Trendelenburg gait and demonstrates a Gower sign on arising from the floor.
What is correct regarding therapeutic interventions for this patient?
A. as an alternative to chronic corticosteroid therapy, immunosuppression with azathioprine should be considered for long-term treatment
B. chronic corticosteroid treatment should be offered now, using either prednisone or deflazacort
C. exposure to sunshine and a balanced diet rich in vitamin D and calcium has no role in the management of these patients
D. physical therapy should not include passive stretching exercise, which is associated with increased pain
E. prednisone treatment should be deferred until he becomes wheelchair confined

Correct Answer is: B
This is a case of Duchenne muscular dystrophy (DMD). This is an X-linked degenerative muscle disorder which affects males in early childhood. Patients have thickened calves and toe walk. Progression occurs over years, becoming wheelchair-bound by 12 years of age. The AAN and the CNS have published national

practice parameters for the use of corticosteroid therapy` in DMD/BMD.

Recommendations include offering boys older than 5 years of age treatment with prednisone at a dose of 0.5 mg per kilogram per day. Recommendations also include the use of deflazacort at 0.9 mg per kilogram per day. Management should include also include physical therapy, especially for passive stretching exercises to prevent contractures of the iliotibial band, Achilles tendons and flexors of the hip.

To prevent secondary complications patients should receive exposure to sunshine as well as a balanced diet rich in vitamin D and calcium to improve bone density and reduce the risk of fractures. Immunosuppression with azathioprine has not been demonstrated to be beneficial and is not recommended as therapy.

Suggested Readings

- Darras BT. Muscle diseases. Continuum Lifelong Learn Neurol. 2006;12(3):33–75.

20. You are seeing a 6-year-old boy who refused to walk. 3 weeks ago, he had an upper respiratory tract infection which resolved with supportive measures. Six days prior to presentation he complained of back pain and difficulty walking. This rapidly progressed to complete refusal to walk over the next few days. On examination, he has severe leg weakness and milder arm weakness. He had reduced withdrawal to pin to the neck. Muscle stretch reflexes are absent. He has normal CSF studies. Motor and sensory nerve conduction studies show low compound muscle action potentials (CMAPs) and sensory responses are unobtainable. There is no conduction block or temporal dispersion. Lower limb F wave responses are unobtainable. There are fibrillation potentials and reduced recruitment of normal appearing motor unit potentials on needle examination of weak muscles.

What prognoses is most likely for this child?

A. good due to the normal appearing motor unit potentials
B. good in the pediatric population overall
C. poor due to the absent sensory responses
D. poor due to the low CMAPs
E. poor in the pediatric population overall

Correct Answer is: B

This is a case of pediatric acute inflammatory demyelinating polyneuropathy (AIDP), presenting with Guillain-Barre syndrome (GBS). In children, the spinal fluid examination is normal more commonly than in adults, and can be normal early in either population. Sensory responses are frequently absent or abnormal, but not universally so. F wave responses are frequently abnormal as an early finding. Indicators of a potentially poor prognosis in adults (low CMAP amplitudes and fibrillation potentials) are not necessarily predictors of a poor prognosis in the pediatric population where series have demonstrated a favorable outcome overall.

Suggested Readings

- Bradshaw DY, Jones HR Jr. Guillain-Barré syndrome in children: clinical course, electrodiagnosis, and prognosis. Muscle Nerve. 1992;15:500–506.

21. You are seeing a 9-year-old girl in the ED for muscle stiffness and an inability to walk after receiving a shot of epinephrine for a presumed allergic reaction. Her family history is remarkable for her father has "muscle stiffness" on awakening in the morning that improves when he does "warm up exercises." Her older son was

evaluated for frequent falls and "clumsiness" by his pediatrician but no diagnosis was rendered. The patient's neurologic examination is remarkable for well-developed musculature in both lower extremities. Needle EMG of these affected muscles demonstrates ongoing waxing and waning discharges.

Which of the following abnormal ion channels is most likely responsible for her condition?

A. calcium
B. chloride
C. magnesium
D. potassium
E. sodium

Correct Answer is: B
This is a clinical presentation of myotonia congenita. This is an autosomal inherited condition that affects the function of chloride channels. The autosomal dominant form, known as Thomsen disease, appears earlier in childhood, but tends to have less severe symptoms than the autosomal recessive form known as Becker disease. People with Becker disease present later in childhood and have a more severe form of the disease, characterized by temporary attacks of muscle weakness, usually in the upper extremities, often brought on by activity after periods of rest. The Becker form is far more common than the autosomal dominant Thomsen form. The myotonia is often precipitated by release of adrenaline during periods of excitement or with the use of epinephrine. Symptomatic treatment is available with anticonvulsants and mexiletine for severe cases.

18

Suggested Readings

- Bertorini TE, editor. Neuromuscular disorders: treatment and management. Woburn:Butterworth-Heinemann; 2010.
- Ropper AH, Samuels MA. Adams and Victor's principles of neurology. 9th ed. New York: McGraw Hill; 2009.

22. You are seeing a 9-year-old girl, with a 7-month history of onset of proximal weakness, presents for further evaluation of muscle weakness. Her mother mentioned that she fell on her left arm 2 months ago, and a plain film shows no fracture, but the PCP mentioned something about "extra calcium". On examination she has erythema over her cheeks and elbows and proximal limb weakness. Serum creatine kinase (CK) level is normal. EMG demonstrates fibrillation potentials and short duration, low amplitude motor unit potentials in proximal muscles, without myotonic discharges. She is admitted to the hospital with severe abdominal pain and bloody stools.

What is your likely diagnosis?

A. childhood acid maltase deficiency
B. congenital myotonic dystrophy type 1
C. early onset myotonia congenita
D. juvenile dermatomyositis
E. pediatric mitochondrial myopathy

Correct Answer is: D
The subacute onset of proximal muscle weakness and EMG with fibrillation potentials and myopathic motor unit potentials are relatively nonspecific. The associated abnormalities assist with the diagnosis in this case. Plain films likely revealed subcutaneous calcification, and she ultimately likely developed gastrointestinal vasculitis leading to intestinal hemorrhage or perforation. This is all compatible with juvenile dermatomyositis. Serum CK values are not uncommonly normal and do not exclude the diagnosis. EMG typically shows fibrillation potentials and myopathic motor unit potentials in the affected muscles. Muscle biopsy shows peri-fascicular atrophy and muscle fiber structural changes with a perimysial and perivascular predominance of the inflammatory infiltrate.Mitochondrial myopathy can be associated with pseudo-

obstruction in some cases or gastrointestinal dysmotility or cachexia. Myotonic congenita is rarely diagnosed in childhood, and myotonic discharges are typical on EMG in the pediatric population. Childhood acid maltase deficiency frequently causes delayed motor development, proximal weakness, and respiratory insufficiency and failure. Myotonic discharges are frequently seen. Congenital myotonic dystrophy presents at birth rather than in childhood.

Suggested Readings

- Shah DU, Darras BT, Markowitz JA, et al. The spectrum of myotonic and myopathic disorders in a pediatric electromyography laboratory over 12 years. Pediatr Neurol. 2012;47:97–100.
- Mastaglia FL, Garlepp MJ, Phillips BA, Zilko PJ. Inflammatory myopathies: clinical, diagnostic and therapeutic aspects. Muscle Nerve. 2003;27:407–25.

23. You are evaluating a 7-year-old boy for gait disturbance. He has normal birth history; he started crawling at 10 months and walked at 18 months. Around the age of 3, he was noted to fall. He has not been able to climb stairs, and he has difficulty running. His general examination is remarkable for a protuberant abdomen, enlarged gastrocnemius muscles, and a waddling gait. The rest of his family is normal including his two sisters. Family history is remarkable for a maternal uncle who was wheelchair bound and died of "heart problems." His CK is markedly elevated (10,000). An EMG shows increased insertional activity, with fibrillation potentials and small polyphasic motor unit potentials diffusely, but most prominent in proximal muscles. A muscle biopsy is performed and the results are shown.

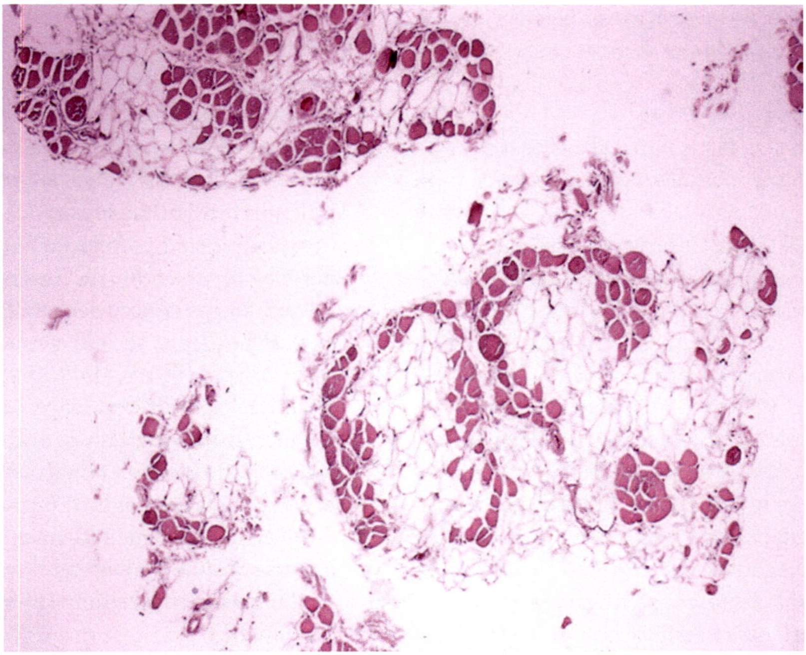

Fig. 18.4 Histopathology of gastrocnemius muscle from patient who died of pseudohypertrophic muscular dystrophy, Duchenne type. Cross section of muscle shows extensive replacement of muscle fibers by adipose cells. (► http://phil.cdc.gov/phil/home.asp ID#: 70 US Department of Health and Human Services. Dr. Edwin P. Ewing, Jr. Permission: None - This image is in the public domain and thus free of any copyright restrictions. As a matter of courtesy. we request that the content provider be credited and notified in any public or private usage of this image. Wikipedia)

What is your diagnosis?

A. Duchenne muscular dystrophy
B. Nemaline rod
C. Normal muscle
D. Polymyositis
E. Spinal muscular atrophy

Correct Answer is: A
The pathological slide shows the characteristic changes of Duchenne muscular dystrophy. Duchenne muscular dystrophy is caused by a defect at the Xp21 site. The abnormal gene produces a reduced muscle content of dystrophin, a structural muscle protein. The dystrophin content is less than 3% of normal. The incidence of Duchenne dystrophy is 1/3500 male births. The initial features of this disease are delayed motor milestones and gait disturbance. Motor function declines throughout childhood. The immediate cause of death may be caused by arrhythmia, aspiration, and inter-current infection. Respiratory insufficiency is a contributing factor in most cases.

Suggested Readings

- Heffner RR. Neuromuscular diseases. From Neuropathology review. AFIP course 2002.
- Fenichel GML. Clinical pediatric neurology: a signs and symptoms approach. 4th ed. Philadelphia: WB Saunders, 2001;176–8.

24. You are evaluating 2 siblings, ages 8 and 10 in the DMD clinic for weakness. Both had a weak cry as neonates and ptosis by age 1. Ocular ductions were noted to be reduced by age 3. Both children fatigue easily and were never able to run. An EMG shows decremental response which repairs with exercise and edrophonium.

In this genetic condition, where would the highest frequency of mutations be found?

A. acetylcholine receptor
B. acetylcholinesterase
C. agrin
D. choline acetyltransferase
E. rapsyn

Correct Answer is: A
This is a typical presentation of congenital myasthenic syndrome (CMS). It was initially described in 1977 with the identification of a case due to acetylcholinesterase deficiency. Since that time, many families have been identified, and through analysis it has been determined that mutations in the acetylcholine receptor account for the majority of cases, well over 50%. Of these mutations, the majority are found in the epsilon subunit of the acetylcholine receptor, leading to a marked decrease in the amount of receptor available in the postsynaptic cleft. However, mutations which also alter the kinetics of the channel have also been defined, so called slow and fast channel mutations. These mutations lead to failure of postsynaptic depolarization.Mutations in choline acetyl transferase lead to failure to produce sufficient acetylcholine. Whereas, mutations in agrin and rapsyn lead to failure of post-synaptic aggregation of receptors at the synapse. The absence of the acetylcholinesterase prolongs the lifetime of acetylcholine in the synaptic space, which increases the duration of the end-plate current so that it outlasts the refractory period of the muscle fiber and excites a second compound muscle action potential (CMAP). The prolonged end-plate currents lead to overload of the synaptic space with cations and end-plate myopathy, loss of junctional folds, and loss of acetylcholine receptors. Transmission of the CMS is autosomal recessive, except in the case of slow channel syndrome, which is inherited as an autosomal dominant trait.

Suggested Readings

- Engel AG, Ohno K, Sine SM. Sleuthing molecular targets for neurological diseases at the neuromuscular junction. Nat Rev. Neurosci. 2003;4(5):339–52.

25. You were asked to see a previously healthy 6-month-old infant presents to the emergency room with a 2-day history of irritability and constipation; then hypotonia, weakness, weak cry, and respiratory distress. On examination she is hypotonic diffusely, with diffuse limb weakness, ptosis, ophthalmoplegia, poor cry and suck, and reduced reflexes. Routine nerve conduction studies show very low compound muscle action potential (CMAPs) amplitudes, less than 20% of normal, in the median and peroneal motor nerves. Motor nerve conduction velocities and sensory nerve responses are normal. 2 Hz repetitive nerve stimulation of the peroneal motor nerve reveals no decrement. On 50 Hz repetitive nerve stimulation for 20 s.

Which of the following diagnostic findings would be expected?

A. decrement greater than 10%
B. decrement greater than 100%
C. facilitation greater than 10%
D. facilitation greater than 100%
E. no decrement or facilitation is diagnostic

Correct Answer is: C

This is a classic case of infantile botulism. The diagnosis is ultimately made via bacteriological testing on stool samples, but electro diagnostic findings are quite specific. Typical findings include very low CMAP amplitudes at rest. The remainder of routine nerve conduction studies is normal. Repetitive nerve stimulation at slow rates may produce decrement, but decrement may be absent when CMAP amplitudes are very low, such as in this case.At higher rates of repetitive stimulation (20 Hz or 50 Hz), facilitation is typical, but often does not reach the degree that is expected in Lambert-Eaton myasthenia syndrome. An increment of 30–200% in the CMAP amplitude can be expected. This also, however, may be absent in particularly severe cases. Needle examination usually demonstrates fibrillation potentials and short duration, low amplitude motor unit potentials, with or without polyphasia.

Suggested Readings

- Cornblath DR, Sladky JT, Sumner AJ. Clinical electrophysiology of infantile botulism. Muscle Nerve. 1983;6:448–52.

26. You are evaluating an 18-year-old male for episodes of hand numbness. He has noticed hand numbness after playing video games for long periods of time for several years. He reports that the tingling and diminished sensation would persist for several days then resolve. He also had similar sensations after sleeping with his arm back behind his head. On one occasion he had arm weakness after driving a long distance with his arm resting out the car window. This persisted for 10 days before resolving.

On examination he has mildly reduced pinprick on the finger pads of the index fingers bilaterally and very mild left finger abduction weakness. Muscle stretch reflexes are diffusely diminished. Electro diagnostic studies of both arms show prolonged median sensory nerve peak latencies bilaterally, and focal slowing of left ulnar motor nerve conduction on short segment incremental stimulation ("inching") studies localizing to the medial epicondyle. Median and ulnar sensory nerve conduction velocities are mildly slow.

What is the most appropriate next step?

A. alpha-galactosidase enzyme assay
B. genetic testing
C. lower limb nerve conduction studies
D. mRI of the cervical spine
E. left upper limb needle examination

Correct Answer is: C
Hereditary neuropathy with liability to pressure palsies (HNPP) must be considered in a young patient with multiple mono-neuropathies at common sites of compression and diffusely reduced reflexes. Classic findings on EMG include multiple entrapment neuropathies superimposed on a mild polyneuropathy, often characterized by sensory nerve conduction slowing and distal motor latency prolongation. This is often most helpful when found in the lower limbs where fewer nerves are typically compressed. Therefore, lower limb nerve conduction studies would be the most appropriate next step to evaluate for findings typical for HNPP.Needle examination would be appropriate to perform following that, and genetic testing for a deletion in the peripheral myelin protein-22 gene (PMP22) would be confirmatory. Alpha-galactosidase enzyme assay would be utilized to evaluate for Fabry disease, also presenting in young men but with painful neuropathy, angiokeratomas, and renal insufficiency. MRI of the cervical spine would be appropriate if the history or examination were compatible with radiculopathy or myelopathy.

Suggested Readings

- Anderson PB, Yuen E, Parko K, So YT. Electro diagnostic features of hereditary neuropathy with liability to pressure palsies. Neurol. 2000;54:40–4.

27. The most reliable predictor of non-awakening (death or vegetative state) in post- anoxic coma is provided by which of the following neurophysiology tests?
    - A. alpha coma on electroencephalography
    - B. bilateral absence of the N20 somatosensory response to median nerve stimulation
    - C. burst suppression on electroencephalography
    - D. frontal intermittent rhythmic delta on electroencephalography
    - E. low-voltage delta activity on electroencephalography

Correct Answer is: B
Bilateral absence of the N20 somatosensory response to median nerve stimulation constitutes the most reliable predictor of non-awakening in post-anoxic coma. The other indices listed also predict a poor prognosis, but with less specificity. Bilateral absence of the N20 somatosensory response to median nerve stimulation is not, however, diagnostic of brain death and can also occur in severe bilateral supra-tentorial lesions, drug intoxication, or severe cerebral edema.

Suggested Readings

- Guérit JM. Neurophysiological testing in neurocritical care. Curr Opin Crit Care. 2010;16:98–104.
- Carter JL, Stevens JC. Somatosensory evoked potentials. In: Daube JR, Rubin DI, editors. Clinical neurophysiology. 3rd ed. New York: Oxford University Press; 2009. p. 276.

28. You are seeing a 16-year-old boy who is referred to you by his school soccer coach after he noticed slowing in his speed with running and loss of power when kicking the ball. His mother also noticed that there have been changes in the appearance of his running and walking over the past year. In particular, she relates his "steps are shorter" when he runs and that he has a slight "waddle" to his walking. On examination he has a mild, limb-girdle pattern of weakness with associated mild calf hypertrophy. His facial and extraocular muscles are spared. Serum CK was elevated at 1850 U/L. Needle EMG

18

of a proximal muscle revealed trace fibrillation potentials and positive sharp waves, most of the motor units however were myopathic in appearance and recruitment was notably increased. A muscle biopsy is deferred for genetic analysis.

Which of the following genetic defects is most likely to be found in this boy?

A. A PMP22 duplication of chromosome 17
B. Out-of-frame mutation in the DMD gene
C. CCTG repeat expansion in the ZNF9 gene on chromosome 19q13.3
D. D4Z4 repeat contraction on chromosome 4q35
E. In-frame mutation in the DMD gene

Correct Answer is: E

A male patient with a limb-girdle pattern of weakness should be evaluated for a dystrophinopathy even in the absence of family history. The elevated CK supports a myopathic etiology as do the needle EMG findings. Mildly increased abnormal spontaneous activity with notably myopathic recruitment suggests a dystrophic myopathic process. An out-of-frame mutation in the DMD gene disrupts the reading frame, creating a truncated RNA transcript that is degraded (nonsense-mediated decay). Because the transcript is degraded, there is absence of dystrophin protein, resulting in a more classic Duchenne phenotype, which this patient certainly does not have, given the preserved independent ambulation at age 16. A Becker phenotype (which this patient does resemble) typically results from in-frame mutations with retained amino- and carboxy-terminus domains and therefore retained function, leading to some dystrophin protein production.

CCTG repeat expansion in the zinc finger protein 9 gene results in proximal myotonic myopathy (DM2). Calf hypertrophy is not expected, and myotonic discharges should be noted on needle EMG. A D4Z4 repeat contraction on chromosome 4q35 results in facioscapulohumeral muscular dystrophy. Duplications in the PMP22 region are the most common genetic cause of Charcot-Marie-Tooth neuropathy, type 1A, which would produce neuropathic rather than myopathic electro diagnostic abnormalities.

Suggested Readings

Wicklund, Matthew P. The Muscular Dystrophies. CONTINUUM Lifelong Learn Neurol. 2013:19(6):1535–70.

29. You were asked to see an infant with hypotonia. The child is in respiratory distress and has a very weak suck. He demonstrates no contractures or dysmorphic features. You noticed that his mother has bilateral ptosis with mild perioral weakness. His grandmother has some mild loss of temporalis bulk does not have the features his mother demonstrates. His mother has difficulty letting go when she shakes your hand. His grandmother does not but comments that she notices this at times when she is in the cold.

You suspect a trinucleotide expansion in which gene?

A. ZNF9
B. D4Z4
C. FXN
D. DMPK
E. EMD

Correct Answer is: D

The infant's presentation suggests congenital myotonic dystrophy based on the characteristic features in his undiagnosed mother, and suggestive features in his grandmother. This is consistent with

anticipation as occurs in the setting of a trinucleotide expansion. Myotonic dystrophy type 1 is caused by a CTG repeat expansion in the *DMPK* gene. The phenotype in infants (due to a markedly expanded repeat number most classically inherited through the maternal copy of the gene) is typically marked peripheral hypotonia. Infants do not have clinically myotonia, so it is critical to briefly examine the mothers of such infants for features of more classic myotonic dystrophy.

ZNF9 mutations results in myotonic dystrophy type 2, which does not have infantile presentation. D4Z4 mutations result in facioscapulohumeral muscular dystrophy; and EMD mutations cause Emery-Dreifuss muscular dystrophy. Although infantile onset is rarely reported with either, mom nor grandmother possess features of these disorders. Repeat expansion in the FXN (Frataxin) gene results in Friedreich's ataxia, which is autosomal recessively inherited and presents in the second decade of life with progressive ataxia amongst other systemic features.

Suggested Readings

- Wicklund MP. The muscular Dystrophies. CONTINUUM Lifelong Learn Neurol. 2013;19(6):1535–70.

30. Regarding the various manifestations of the different subtypes of Charcot-Marie-Tooth (CMT).
Which of the following statements is not true?
    A. Hammertoes and spine deformities are more prominent in CMT1 than CMT2
    B. CMT2 typically has a later age of onset as compared to CMT1
    C. CMT3, or Dejerine-Sottas syndrome, presents in infancy and typically leads to disabling weakness
    D. Respiratory muscle involvement is common in the most common type of CMT
    E. In some subtypes of CMT4, one of the axonal CMTs, vision or hearing loss occurs

Correct Answer is: D
The clinical presentation suggests the diagnosis of Charcot-Marie-Tooth (CMT) 1. Respiratory compromise is not usually seen in the most common forms of CMT, but occurs in some cases of CMT2C. The CMTs, also known as hereditary sensorimotor neuropathies or peroneal muscular atrophy, are a large, heterogeneous group of inherited peripheral neuropathies. The CMTs can be divided into demyelinating, axonal, and combined demyelinating and axonal forms. They are genetically heterogeneous. The demyelinating CMTs include CMT1 and CMTX.CMT4, involves both demyelination and axon loss. In the demyelinating CMTs, NCS generally show diffuse, uniformly slow conduction velocities without conduction blocks or temporal dispersion, indicating a hereditary as opposed to acquired demyelinating process. There may be evidence of axon loss in the demyelinating forms as well, particularly in patients with long standing disease; this is secondary axon loss, and conduction velocities as well as CMAP and SNAP amplitudes will be reduced. In contrast, with the axonal forms, motor and sensory potential amplitudes will be reduced, but conduction velocities will be normal or minimally reduced. At the time of this publication, there were seven subtypes of CMT1; they are all inherited in an autosomal dominant fashion. CMT1A is the most common inherited demyelinating neuropathy. Clinical manifestations typically begin in the first two decades of life and include slowly progressive weakness, muscle atrophy, kyphosis, and mild (often

asymptomatic) sensory loss. Other signs include hammertoes, high-arched feet, palpably enlarged nerves due to peripheral nerve hypertrophy (which more commonly occurs in the CMT1 group compared to the other CMTs), and pes cavus. Involvement of the upper extremities typically occurs later in life. There is often a family history of neuropathy, though due to variable expression, some affected family members may only have mild features such as hammertoes and may remain undiagnosed for a large part of their life; sporadic cases without a clear family history also exist. Other forms of CMT may be congenital and severe. In the CMT1 group, many of the genes involved are related to myelin synthesis. CMT1A is due to a duplication in the peripheral myelin protein 22 (PMP22) gene on chromosome 17, whereas CMT1 B is due to a mutation in the myelin protein 0 gene. CMT1 B is more severe in terms of clinical manifestations as compared to CMT1A.In patients with CMT1, CSF shows elevated protein levels in some cases. Roussy-Levy syndrome is phenotypically similar to CMT1A but is associated with the presence of a static tremor and gait ataxia. It has been associated with mutations in both the PMP22 and myelin protein O genes. On nerve biopsy, pathologic features of the demyelinating inherited polyneuropathies include demyelination and an onion-bulb appearance due to Schwann cell proliferation. Onion bulbs are not specific for CMT, and also occur with chronic inflammatory demyelinating polyneuropathy. CMTX is the second most common type of CMT. It is demyelinating and is clinically similar to CMT1, but it is X-linked in inheritance; males therefore tend to be more severely affected compared to females. It is due to a mutation in the connexin 32 gene. CMT2 accounts for approximately one-third of the autosomal dominant inherited neuropathies. The CMT2 group are axonal neuropathies; NCS show normal conduction velocities, and nerve biopsy shows axon loss without evidence of significant demyelination. Compared to CMT1, in CMT2, symptoms and signs typically appear later and foot and spine deformities are less severe. Clinical manifestations do not always help distinguish the different CMTs, but some clinical features occur more frequently in the different subtypes. Optic atrophy occurs more in CMT2A2, foot ulcerations in CMT2B, and vocal cord paralysis, intercostal, and diaphragmatic weakness in CMT2C. In CMT2D, unlike in the other CMTs, the hands are involved more than the feet. Peripheral nerve hypertrophy does not occur. They are all autosomal dominant in inheritance, except for a subtype of CMT2A. The genes implicated in the CMT2 group are involved in axonal transport and membrane trafficking. CMT2A2 is one of the most common of this group and is due to mutations in mitofusin 2. CMT3, also known as Dejerine-Sottas syndrome or hypertrophic neuropathy of infancy, is one of the more severe forms of the demyelinating CMTs. It presents in infancy with proximal weakness, absent deep tendon reflexes, and hypertrophy of the peripheral nerves. Prominent sensory symptoms including pain and dysesthesias occur. Patients typically have extensive disability early in life. Both autosomal recessive and dominant forms exist. CSF protein is usually elevated. Congenital hypomyelination is seen along the spectrum of this disorder. CMT3 is genetically heterogeneous; mutations in several genes including PMP22, protein myelin 0, and other genes implicated in defective demyelination are associated with CMT3.The CMTs can be misdiagnosed as muscular dystrophy; NCS findings, as well as the presence of hammertoes and high-arched foot, distinguish between the two.

Suggested Readings

- Bradley WG, Daroff RB, Fenichel GM, et al. Neurology in clinical practice, 5th ed. Philadelphia: Elsevier; 2008.
- Rapper AH, Samuels MA. Adams and Victor's principles of neurology, 9th ed. New York: McGraw-Hill; 2009.
- Comprehensive Review in Clinical Neurology: A Multiple-Choice Question Book for the Wards and Boards ©2011 Wolters Kluwer Health Lippincott Williams & Wilkins. All rights reserved.

31. You are seeing a 13-year-old boy for "trouble walking". The child has problems walking up stairs and standing on his toes when has to reach for something. In addition, his mother has noted he has developed a "very high arch in his feet". On neurological examination, he has weakness in peroneal and anterior tibial muscles. The ankle tendon reflex is diminished compared to the patellar and brachial reflexes. The boys gait is slow and he lifts his leg up high in order to lift his foot of the ground as he steps forward.

What protein is affected in this condition?

A. Dystrophin
B. Survival motor neuron protein
C. Myelin basic protein
D. Peripheral myelin protein 22

Correct Answer is: D

Charcot-Marie-Tooth 1 (CMT1), also referred to as hereditary motor and sensory neuropathy type1 (HMSN1), is a demyelinating neuropathy that typically begins in the second decade of life and progresses gradually throughout the patient's life. The distal nerves in legs are affected first causing weakness and foot drop. Pes cavus is described as a high instep/arch, or that develops in several neurological conditions of hereditary peripheral neuropathies. As the CMT1 progresses, the proximal leg and hands become affected. The peripheral myelin protein 22 is a critical component of the myelin sheath. In CMT1 this protein production is limited and results in improper myelination and decay of peripheral nerve function.

Dystrophin is structural muscle protein that is absent or present at very low amounts in patients with Duchenne muscular dystrophy. Proximal muscles are predominately affected.

The survival motor neuron (SMN) protein is deficient in spinal muscular atrophy type I. This protein is found in the spinal cord at high levels, but is present throughout the body. This condition presents in the first 2 years of life.

Myelin basic protein is a major constituent in the sheath of oligodendrocytes and Schwann cells. This protein is found in elevated levels in the spinal fluid of patients with central nervous system demyelinating conditions, such as multiple sclerosis, as well as in central nervous system infections.

Suggested Readings

- Suter U. "MOTOR AND SENSORY NEUROPATHI ES." Cell biology and pathology of Myelin: evolving biological concepts and therapeutic approaches. 4 (2012):51.

32. You are evaluating a 6-year-old boy with a history of proximal muscle weakness, pain and stiffness for the last 2 months. 2 weeks before this he had fever, generalized fatigue and anorexia. On examination he has erythema and mild edema of the upper eyelids.

Electromyography (EMG) results will show which of the following findings?

A. Normal
B. Fasciculation at rest with increased mean amplitude of motor unit potentials

C. Increased insertional activity, fibrillations and positive sharp waves
D. Short-duration, low amplitude motor unit potential

Correct Answer is: C
Dermatomyositis is a systemic inflammatory angiopathy resulting from vascular occlusion and infarction of muscle, skin, connective tissue, gastrointestinal tract and small diameter peripheral nerves. Peak incidence is between 5–10 years. The initial proximal weakness will eventually generalize and flexion contractures may develop. The muscle biopsy diagnostic feature is peri-fasicular atrophy. The inflammatory process may remain active for 2 years and corticosteroids are used to suppress the inflammatory response and reduce muscle damage.

The EMG study would not be normal. EMG aids in distinguishing between myopathic and neuropathic disease processes, and provides supportive evidence of pathophysiology peripheral neuropathy and motor neuron disease.

These EMG findings are most consistent with a denervation process, such as in spinal muscular atrophy type I.

These findings would more likely be found in conditions associated with cholinergic blockade at the neuromuscular junction, as seen in infantile botulism.

Suggested Readings

- Mills KR. The basics of electromyography. J Neurol Neurosurg Psychiatry. 2005;76(suppl. 2): ii32–ii35.
- Dalakas MC. editors. Polymyositis and dermatomyositis. Butterworth Heinemann; 2013.

33. You are evaluating a 4-year-old boy with a history of normal motor development until he began to have frequent falls at the age of 2. On neurological exam at 2 years of age, he had distal leg weakness with absent tendon reflexes, and appropriate cognitive development?
What is the most likely diagnosis?
A. Late infantile neuronal ceroid lipofuscinosis
B. Gauchers type III disease
C. Spinal muscular atrophy type II
D. Spinal muscular atrophy type III

Correct Answer is: D
The age of onset of spinal muscular atrophy type III is after 18 months, compared to type 1 at 0–6 months and type II, 6–18 months. Type III clinical course is less severe and initial symptoms include gait instability, fine action tremor, and weakness of distal leg muscles or proximal arm muscles. Facial muscle may be weak, extraocular muscles are not affected and hand strength is the last muscle groups to be involved.

Symptoms of late infantile neuronal ceroid lipofuscinosis begin between 2 and 4 years of age and include progressive cognitive impairment and abnormal movements. Visual impairment begins by 4–6 years of age and progresses to blindness.

Gauchers type III presents between the ages of 2 and 12 with hepatosplenomegaly, impaired bone marrow involvement and progressive motor and cognitive impairment.

The age of onset on of spinal muscular atrophy type II is 6–18 months and the initial feature are delayed motor milestones with limited achievement. The children will attain the ability to sit with balance, but will be unable to stand or ambulate.

Suggested Readings

- Kaufmann P, McDermott MP, Darras BT, Finkel R, Kang P, Oskoui M, Constantinescu A et al. Observational study of spinal muscular atrophy type 2 and 3: functional outcomes over 1 year. Arch Neurol. 68(6): 779–86.

34. You are evaluating a 17-year-old male for episodic weakness and fatigue. He states that he tends to wake up with weakness when he eats Chinese food or pizza for dinner in large quantities. Family history is remarkable of his father also has episodic weakness and at one point was brought to the emergency room when he awoke with weakness after eating a large pasta meal the night prior. The mother recalls that the father's potassium was low on arrival.

What is the most likely diagnosis?

A. Hypokalemic periodic paralysis
B. Hyperkalemic periodic paralysis
C. Myotonia congenital
D. Paramyotonia congenital

Correct Answer is: A

This a case of hypokalemic periodic paralysis. Hypokalemic periodic paralysis type I is caused by a mutation in calcium channel, voltage-dependent, L type, alpha 1S subunit (CACNA 1S) while type II is caused by sodium channel, voltage gated, type IV alpha subunit (SCN4A) mutations. Typically, weakness follows emotional stress, ingestion of carbohydrates or alcohol, rest after exercise, or cold. In particular, weakness may occur in the morning following a large carbohydrate meal the night prior. Attacks can be hours to days and the onset of the disease is usually in adolescence. Weakness may progress to flaccid quadriplegia and deep tendon reflexes may be lost. Respiratory muscles may be affected. Preventive treatments include potassium sparing diuretics such as spironolactone or daily acetazolamide or dichlorphenamide acutely, patients may receive potassium supplementation.

Hyperkalemic periodic paralysis tends to present earlier than hypokalemic periodic paralysis. This is also autosomal dominant and typically caused by mutations in sodium channel, voltage gated, type IV alpha subunit (SCN4A). Generalized myotonia may be present. Attacks tend to be shorter than those associated with hypokalemic periodic paralysis, lasting minutes to hours. Rarely, attacks may last days. Weakness tends not to include the face. Triggers include rest after exercise, cold, fasting, and potassium ingestion; symptoms are alleviated by inhaled beta adrenergic agents and carbohydrate ingestion. Patients are managed by avoiding high potassium meals and by avoiding rest following strenuous activity. Intravenous calcium, inhaled beta agonists, or thiazide diuretics may be used in acute attacks. Prophylaxis involves avoiding potassium rich foods and avoiding strenuous exercise. Additionally, dichlorphenamide, acetazolamide, hydrochlorothiazide, and metaproterenol may be effective in preventing attacks.

Myotonia congenita may be autosomal dominant or recessive; in each case, mutations in chloride channel, voltage sensitive 1 (CLCN1) may be causative. Thomsen disease is the autosomal dominant form; in this case, patients may present in early childhood or in infancy. A "warm up" phenomenon is present where stiffness improves with repeated movement. Becker type myotonia is the autosomal recessive form. This tends to present later in life although the "warm up" phenomenon is present in this form too. Weakness may occur following myotonia in the recessive form. In both forms, stiffness is more prominent in the cold. Para-myotonia congenita is caused by mutations in sodium channel, voltage gated, type IV alpha subunit (SCN4A), as in hypokalemic periodic paralysis type II and hyperkalemic periodic paralysis in individuals with para-myotonia congenita, the "warm up" phenomenon is not present and repeated movements may worsen myotonia and weakness; cold is also a potential trigger. Pharyngeal muscles and muscles of the hand and face are all

affected. Avoidance of cold, the use of mexiletine (a lidocaine derivative), and hydrochlorothiazide are all preventive. In particular, mexiletine is used to prevent cold induced weakness.

35. You are seeing an 18-year-old female for generalized weakness. On electro diagnostic testing the initial compound muscle action potentials (CMAP) were normal. After a train of 6 stimuli at a rate of 3 per second, the amplitude of the CMAP's decreased by 35%.
What is the likely diagnosis?
A. Dermatomyositis
B. Guillain-Barre syndrome
C. Myasthenia gravis
D. Hypothyroidism

Correct Answer is: C
The test of the neuromuscular junction is based on the Jolly principle that first described the electro diagnostic findings in patients with myasthenia gravis in which the strength of muscle contractions is progressively diminished during a train of electrical stimuli. This progressive failure of neurotransmission is similar to the ones found with administration of curare (or other non-depolarizing neuromuscular blockers) and can be partially corrected by neostigmine.

Electro diagnostic findings in dermatomyositis include myopathic features of increased insertional activity, fibrillations and positive sharp waves.

Electro diagnostic findings in Guillain-Barre syndrome include a reduction in amplitudes of muscle action potentials slowed conduction velocity, or complete conduction block in motor nerves. The initial symptoms in this condition are most commonly paresthesias and numbness.

Neuropathy associated with hypothyroidism is not common and is characterized by a significant reduction in nerve conduction velocities.

Suggested Readings

- Chiou-Tan FY, Gilchrist JM. Repetitive nerve stimulation and single-fiber electromyography in the evaluation of patients with suspected myasthenia gravis or Lambert-Eaton myasthenic syndrome: review of recent literature. Muscle Nerve. 2015;52(3):455–62.

36. You are seeing an8 month-old girl who developed mild to moderate generalized hypotonia over the last 3 months and the electromyography study revealed fibrillations, fasciculation, sharp waves on needle insertion at rest with large, prolonged and polyphasic motor unit potentials.
What disease classification do these findings support?
A. Neuropathic process
B. Myopathic process
C. Mitochondrial disorder
D. Inconclusive

Correct Answer is: A
The needle electrode examination is accomplished by recording the firing response during the muscle insertion of spontaneous and then voluntary muscle activity. Denervation disease results in fibrillations, fasciculation, sharp waves on needle insertion at rest with large, prolonged and polyphasic motor unit potentials. Myopathic disease is characterized by brief, small amplitude, polyphasic potentials.

Mitochondrial myopathies will have myopathic features on electromyography studies.

Fibrillations, fasciculation and sharp waves are pathological findings.

Suggested Readings

- Brown WF. The physiological and technical basis of electromyography. Butterworth Heinemann; 2013.

37. Charcot-Marie-Tooth (CMT) type 1 differs from CMT type 2 in that:
   A. Type 1 is an axonal neuropathy
   B. Type 1 is associated with upper extremity nerve conduction velocities >40 mis
   C. Type 2 has autosomal recessive inheritance
   D. Type 1 is a severe infantile form of CMT
   E. None of the above

Correct Answer is: E
CMT is currently classified as type 1, type 2, and type 4. The term "type 3" (Dejerine-Sottas syndrome) is no longer used, with Dejerine-Sottas syndrome now referring to severely affected infants with any type of CMT. The letter designations (e.g. CMT1A, CMT2B, etc.) indicate the different causative mutations.

Type 1 includes hypertrophic demyelinating neuropathies with nerve conduction velocities (NCVs) slowed to less than 38 *mis* in the upper extremities. The disorder is of autosomal dominant inheritance, with mutations including duplications of the peripheral myelin protein gene, PMP22 (in CMT1A) and mutations of the myelin protein zero gene, MPZ (in CMT1 B). CMT1X, although X-linked, is categorized as a CMT type 1 disorder as it is a demyelinating process. CMT1X is caused by mutations of the GJB1 gene, which encodes the protein connexin-32.

Type 2 includes axonal neuropathies with relatively normal nerve conduction velocities. They are also of autosomal dominant inheritance, with mutations in the mitofusin 2 gene, MFN2 (in CMT2A) and the RAB7A gene of the RAS oncogene family (in CMT2B).

Type 4 includes the CMT subtypes of autosomal recessive inheritance.

18

Suggested Readings

Patzko A, Shy ME. Charcot-Marie-Tooth disease and related genetic neuropathies. Continuum. 2012;18(1):39–59.

38. You are evaluating a 15-year-old male with intermittent muscle pain and weakness when he exercises, with normal motor status between events and age appropriate cognitive abilities? **What test result will support your diagnosis?**
   A. Serum CK levels
   B. Impaired lactate response to ischemic exercise test
   C. Fasciculation and fibrillations on EMG
   D. Low ammonia response to forearm ischemia test

Correct Answer is: D
Myoadenylate deaminase deficiency presents with several different phenotypes; infants with hypotonia, children with progressive myopathies and recurrent rhabdomyolysis and in children and adults with exercise intolerance. The forearm ischemia test helps in the differential diagnosis of muscle pain and weakness associated with exercise. Patients with myoadenylate deaminase deficiency do not generate ammonia but have appropriately elevated lactate levels in ischemic conditions. The pain associated with the exercised induced phenotype, is described as diffuse aching to more severe localized cramping, along with muscle swelling and tenderness.

Duchene muscular dystrophy presents before the age of 5 with a gait disturbance with proximal leg weakness.

McArdle disease is a myophosphorylase deficiency that limits the first step of glycogenolysis in muscle and therefore results in low glucose availability in muscle cells. Serum CK levels, mutational analysis

and muscle biopsy are used for diagnosis. This condition may present with exercise intolerance and weakness but usually is not diagnosed until the person is in their 20's.

Denervation neuropathies are progress live disorders and will not have intermittent symptoms with complete resolution.

Suggested Readings

- Devanshi J, Kaminski HJ. Rhabdomyolysis and Myoglobinuria. In: Neuromuscular disorders in clinical practice. Springer: New York; 2014. p. 1545–59

39. Myophosphorylase deficiency (McArdle's disease) is characterized by:
   A. Autosomal dominant inheritance
   B. Prominent distal weakness
   C. Lack of a second wind phenomenon
   D. Elevations of ammonia and lactic acid in the exercise forearm test
   E. None of the above

Correct Answer is: E

McArdle's disease results from a disruption of the carbohydrate metabolism chain due to a deficiency of myophosphorylase. It is caused by mutations of chromosome 11, of autosomal recessive inheritance. Onset is during childhood. Initially, children tire easily, then progress to the classic symptoms of pain and contractures with exercise. An EMG performed during a contracture, however, would not demonstrate any muscle activity, differentiating this phenomenon from a true muscle cramp. Patients experience a second wind phenomenon, in which exercise intolerance may be overcome by brief rests. Most patients have no weakness. When present, weakness is typically mild and affects proximal muscles and upper extremities. An exercise forearm test (also called an ischemic exercise test or ischemic forearm test) may aid in diagnosis. In this test, the arm muscles are contracted in the setting of restricted blood flow, with an inflated blood pressure cuff on the upper arm. Patients will develop pain and contractures. Following the exercise, bloodwork demonstrates that ammonia levels are elevated, while lactic acid levels do not rise. This contrasts with myoadenylate deaminase deficiency, in which patients will have elevated lactic acid levels, but fail to increase ammonia.

Suggested Readings

- Amato AA and Brooke MH. Disorders of skeletal muscle. In: Bradley WG, Daroff RB, Fenichel GM, jankovic j, editors. Neurology in Clinical Practice (4th edition). Elsevier, Inc.; 2004. p. 2463–2510.

40. You are evaluating a 2-year-old girl is because of she would never sweat no matter what fluctuations occurred in her body temperature. She had suffered from recurrent fevers since childhood, but an infectious etiology to her fevers could not be identified. Her family noticed that she did not cry when she received her vaccinations, and since she had started walking, if she bumped into an object or fell, she did not seem to feel pain, even when she sustained a significant abrasion or bruise. She has also been seen by a psychiatrist for self-mutilating behaviors (severe lip biting) and intellectual delay.
   What is your most likely diagnosis in this patient?
   A. Hereditary sensory and autonomic neuropathy (HSAN) type 1
   B. Charcot-Marie-Tooth 1
   C. HSAN type
   D. HSAN type
   E. HSAN type 4

Correct Answer is: E
The HSANs are a relatively rare, genetically and phenotypically heterogeneous group of hereditary neuropathies. As a group, they share in common prominent sensory signs and symptoms, including pain, sensory loss, and autonomic features with little motor involvement. Because of the sensory loss, patients with HSANs are prone to painful calluses, stress fractures, neuropathic (Charcot) joints, skin ulcerations that heal poorly, and infections with deep tissue involvement, such as osteomyelitis, leading to disfiguring acral mutilations. Hereditary sensory and autonomic neuropathy type I (HSAN I) is the most frequent type of hereditary neuropathy that primarily affects sensory neurons. Hereditary sensory and autonomic neuropathy type II (HSAN2) is characterized by progressively reduced sensation to pain, temperature, and touch.

Hereditary sensory and autonomic neuropathy type III features marked ataxic gait that progressively worsens over time. HSAN 4 is characterized by insensitivity to pain, anhidrosis, and intellectual disability as well as self- mutilation. Sense of touch, vibration, and position are normal. Congenital insensitivity to pain with anhidrosis is extremely rare entity, in which patients are subjected to repeated injuries which are often neglected. There is no specific treatment but patient training and family education are key to avoid further neglect and damage.

41. You are seeing an 18-year-old boy with episodes of weakness and inability to move his arms and legs. Extraocular movements and bulbar and respiratory muscles are spared. The patient says that he gets these episodes with emotional stressors, after exercise, or after eating heavy desserts. His family history is remarkable of his father has similar episodes. **What is the most likely diagnosis?**
    - A. Hyperkalemic periodic paralysis
    - B. Hypokalemic periodic paralysis
    - C. Andersen-Tawil syndrome
    - D. Paramyotonia congenital
    - E. Myotonia congenital

Correct Answer is: B
This is a clinical presentation of hypokalemic periodic paralysis, which is inherited in an autosomal dominant fashion; however, sporadic cases have been reported. There are two types: type 1 caused by a mutation in the calcium channel gene CACNA 1S on chromosome 1q31, and type 2 caused by a mutation in the sodium channel gene SCN4A. These patients present with episodes of weakness without myotonia that could be focal or generalized and ranges from mild to severe, associated with hyporeflexia during the attacks, each of which can last for hours, with some persistent mild weakness for a few days. During attacks, the creatine kinase level may be elevated and the serum potassium is usually reduced. These episodes are triggered by exercise, meals rich in carbohydrates, ethanol, cold exposure, and emotional stressors. Provocative testing can be done with glucose administration. The main treatment focus is to avoid triggers; carbonic anhydrase inhibitors such as acetazolamide and potassium-sparing diuretics are useful in treating this condition. Hyperkalemic periodic paralysis, on the other hand, presents with episodes of weakness triggered by resting after exercise and fasting. This condition is autosomal dominant and is caused by a mutation in the sodium channel gene SCN4A. Provocative testing is done with administration of potassium. The treatment is focused on avoiding triggers. During attacks, glucose can be provided, and as prophylactic therapy, thiazide diuretics can be used. Andersen-Tawi l syndrome is also a channelopathy characterized by periodic paralysis,

ventricular arrhythmias, and dysmorphic features. It is associated with a mutation in the potassium channel gene KCN J2.

Suggested Readings

Comprehensive review in clinical neurology: a multiple-choice question book for the Wards and Boards © 2011 Wolters Kluwer Health Lippincott Williams & Wilkins. All rights reserved.

42. You are evaluating a 4-year boy with a history of normal motor development until he was first noted to begin to have frequent falls at the age of 2, he had distal leg weakness with absent tendon reflexes, and appropriate cognitive development on his exam at this time.

What is the most likely diagnosis?

A. Late infantile neuronal ceroid lipofuscinosis
B. Gauchers type III diseas
C. Spinal muscular atrophy type II
D. Spinal muscular atrophy type III

Correct Answer is: D

The age of onset of spinal muscular atrophy type III is after 18 months, compared to type I at 0–6 months and type II, 6–18 months. Type III clinical course is less severe and initial symptoms include gait instability, fine action tremor, and weakness of distal leg muscles or proximal arm muscles.

Facial muscle may be weak, extraocular muscles are not affected and hand strength is the last muscle groups to be involved.

Symptoms of late infantile neuronal ceroid lipofuscinosis begin between 2 and 4 years of age and include progressive cognitive impairment and abnormal movements. Visual impairment begins by 4–6 years of age and progresses to blindness.

Gauchers type III presents between the ages of 2 and 12 with hepatosplenomegaly, impaired bone marrow involvement and progressive motor and cognitive impairment.

The age of onset on of spinal muscular atrophy type II is 6–18 months and the initial feature are delayed motor milestones with limited achievement. The children will attain the ability to sit with balance, but will be unable to stand or ambulate.

Suggested Readings

Kaufmann P, McDermott MP, Darras BT, Finkel R, Kang P, Oskoui M, Constantinescu A et al. Observational study of spinal muscular atrophy type 2 and 3: functional outcomes over 1 year. Arch Neurol. 2011;68:(6):779–86.

43. You are seeing a 7-year-old boy with a muscular dystrophy was normal at birth, but at 4 years of age, was unable to jump or run properly. He developed calf pseudo-hypertrophy, and difficulty standing when seated on the floor. He now reports difficulty climbing, with frequent falls due to weakness.

What do you expect to see on your evaluation?

A. An absence of dystrophin staining on muscle biopsy
B. An EMG with myopathic changes
C. A frameshift mutation at the locus Xp21
D. An electrocardiogram with tachycardia
E. All of the above

Correct Answer is: E

Duchenne's muscular dystrophy (DMD) is the most common form of muscular dystrophy, affecting 1 in 3500–5000 newborn males. DMD is less common in girls, as it is an X-linked recessive disorder. The mutation is at the Xp21 locus, and in DMD (in contrast to Becker's muscular dystrophy), is most often a frame shift mutation. The

mutation results in absence of dystrophin, which forms part of the support structure that anchors the contractile proteins to the outside of the muscle cell. Affected patients are normal at birth, and like most toddlers, are clumsy when learning to walk. The clumsiness, however, may persist, and children do not learn to jump or run properly. Patients have difficulty when rising from the floor, and may need to use their hands to push up against their knees to assist (Gower's maneuver). Calf pseudo-hypertrophy develops. Patients begin to have difficulty climbing and have frequent falls, eventually requiring the use of a wheelchair. Contractures develop at the hips, knees, and ankles. Cardiac musculature is involved, with a dilated cardiomyopathy, degeneration and fibrosis of the posterolateral wall of the lateral ventricle, and/or valvular and wall motion abnormalities. An abnormal EKG is common, often with tachycardia, even in young children. Evaluation reveals an elevated creatine kinase (CK) level, and an EMG with myopathic changes. The diagnosis may be established by DNA testing or muscle biopsy. Biopsy often demonstrates muscle necrosis, phagocytosis, fiber size variation, fibrosis, basophilia, and hyaline fibers, with the absence of staining for dystrophin. Patients may experience some benefits to strength and function from administration of prednisone. Death, usually in early adulthood, is typically due to respiratory failure or cardiomyopathy.

Suggested Readings

- Amato AA, Brooke MH. Disorders of skeletal muscle. In: Bradley WG, Daroff RB, Fenichel GM, Jankovic J, editors. Neurology in Clinical Practice. 4th ed. Elsevier, Inc.; 2004. p. 2463–510.

18

44. You are seeing a 4-month-old boy was hypotonic at birth, with microphthalmia and cataracts. MRI reveals hydrocephalus with cobblestone lissencephaly.

What is the most likely diagnosis?

A. Walker-Warburg syndrome
B. Muscle-Eye-Brain disease
C. Phosphoglycerate mutase deficiency
D. Welander myopathy
E. Phophofructokinase deficiency

Correct Answer is: A

Walker-Warburg syndrome consists of muscular dystrophy, with cerebral and eye malformations. Retinal and eye malformations are severe, and may include microphthalmia, cataracts, retinal dysplasia, and optic atrophy. Cerebral malformations include aqueductal stenosis, pontine hypoplasia, Dandy-Walker malformations, and agyric or pachygyric cortices. A "cobblestone" lissencephaly is common, with nodular, disorganized cortex of variable thickness. MRI may also demonstrate white matter changes. Death typically occurs in 2 years. The disorder is caused by a mutation of chromosome 9 and is of autosomal recessive inheritance. Muscle-eye-brain disease also presents with muscular dystrophy, but the associated cerebral and eye findings are of a much less severe phenotype than evident with Walker-Warburg syndrome. Patients may have myopia and a preretinal membrane or gliosis, but there are no major malformations. The cortical changes are also less severe, with focal white matter changes. Muscle-eye-brain disease is due to a mutation in the gene for 0-mannose-1, 2 N-acetylglucosaminyl transferase, located on chromosome 1, and is of autosomal recessive inheritance. Phosphoglycerate mutase deficiency is a rare autosomal recessive disorder, due to mutations on chromosome 7. It presents with attacks of muscle pain and myoglobinuria, of onset in childhood or adolescence. Welander myopathy is a disorder of adult onset (40–60 years of age), with weakness of the hands followed by foot drop. It may also be associated with a

distal small fiber neuropathy. The disorder is of autosomal dominant inheritance.

Phophofructokinase deficiency affects the conversion of fructose-6- phosphate to fructose-1, 6-diphosphate in the glycolytic chain. It results in nausea, vomiting, and muscle pain elicited by exercise. An infantile-onset type is associated with blindness and psychomotor retardation, while a late onset type is associated with cardiac dysfunction. The disorder is due to a mutation on chromosome 1, of autosomal recessive inheritance.

Suggested Readings

Amato AA, Brooke MH. Disorders of skeletal muscle. In: Bradley WG, Daroff RB, Fenichel GM, Jankovic J, editors. Neurology in clinical practice. 4th ed. Elsevier, Inc.; 2004. p. 2463–510.

45. You are evaluating a 7-year-old boy with motor development delay and difficulty walking. His weakness is predominantly in the proximal muscles, with severe weakness of hip flexors, quadriceps, gluteal, and pretibial muscles. He also has pectoral and shoulder weakness and winging of both scapula. His calves are enlarged, with a "rubbery" texture. His intelligence quotient (IQ) is low. His serum CPK is 11,560 IU/L (normal 220 IU/L).

What is the most likely diagnosis?

A. Becker muscular dystrophy
B. Duchenne muscular dystrophy
C. Emery-Dreifuss muscular dystrophy
D. Fascioscapulohumeral muscular dystrophy
E. Limb-girdle muscular dystrophy

Correct Answer is: B

This is a case of Duchenne muscular dystrophy. This condition is a dystrophinopathy, inherited in an X-linked recessive fashion, and is the most common genetic muscle disease, affecting 1 in 3500 live male births. About a third of the cases are caused by spontaneous mutations in the dystrophin gene, so there may not be a positive family history. This condition presents early in life and manifests with weakness and delayed development of motor milestones. These children have frequent falls, and difficulty walking, running, and rising from supine and sitting positions. Weakness is significant in the proximal muscles, predominantly in the iliopsoas, quadriceps, and gluteal muscles, as well as the shoulder girdle and upper limbs. It also tends to affect the pretibial muscles. These patients have pseudohypertrophy of the calves due to fibrosis. They also have scapular winging and contractures.

Ocular, facial, and bulbar muscles are usually spared. Cardiac involvement includes arrhythmias, cardiomyopathy, and heart failure. Mild intellectual disability with a subnormal intelligence quotient (IQ) may be seen. These children become wheelchair- or bed-bound, and may eventually die of respiratory failure and pulmonary infections. CPK values range from 10 to 100 times higher than normal. Needle EMG shows fibrillations, positive waves, and myopathic motor unit potentials. In general, myofiber necrosis, degeneration, regeneration, increased fiber size variation, endomysial inflammation, and fibrosis are collectively called dystrophic changes, which are characteristic for Duchenne muscular dystrophy, but not specific, and can be seen in other dystrophies. Dystrophin is the affected gene product and is absent in patients with Duchenne. Dystrophin is a cytoplasmic protein that binds and interacts with other intracytoplasmic proteins such as F- actin, and is linked to the trans-sarcolemmal dystroglycan protein complex, providing a structural link between the sub-sarcolemmal cytoskeleton and the extracellular matrix. If dystrophin is lost or

altered, this sarcolemmal structure is affected, making it susceptible to rupture. The diagnosis of Duchenne muscular dystrophy is made by genetic testing of the dystrophin gene or by absent dystrophin immunostaining on muscle biopsy.

Suggested Readings

- Comprehensive review in clinical neurology: a multiple-choice question Book for the Wards and Boards ©2011 Wolters Kluwer Health Lippincott Williams & Wilkins. All rights reserved.

46. You are seeing a 7-year-old boy for stiffness. His legs are stiff, and he has difficulty relaxing muscles after contracting them. He cannot release objects easily once grasped with his hands, and when he closes his eyes, it takes a few seconds before he is able to open them completely. If he performs the same motor task multiple times, it becomes easier. When his thenar eminence is percussed, there is prolonged contraction and delayed relaxation. Family history is remarkable of his father and grandfather have similar clinical features that started around the same age.

    What is the most likely diagnosis?

    A. Paramyotonia congenital
    B. Myotonia congentia, Becker' disease
    C. Myotonia congenita, Thomsen's disease
    D. Hyperkalemic periodic paralysis
    E. Hypokalemic periodic paralysis

Correct Answer is: C

This boy has myotonia congenita, more specifically Thomsen's disease. There are two types of myotonia congenita: Thomsen's disease, which is autosomal dominant, and Becker's disease, which is autosomal recessive. This group of disorders is caused by a channelopathy secondary to a mutation in the chloride channel gene CLCN1 on chromosome 7q. The main manifestation is myotonia, which is an impaired muscle relaxation as seen when the patients cannot relax their handgrip after grasping an object, and also manifested on percussion, leading to contraction and delayed relaxation. Myotonic potentials can be detected on EMG. In myotonia congenita, as opposed to para-myotonia, there is a "warm-up" phenomenon, in which the myotonia improves after repetitive muscle activation.

Thomsen's disease is autosomal dominant and begins in the first decade of life manifesting with painless myotonia, but not weakness, and is milder than the recessive form. Becker's disease is the recessive form that presents later, usually in the second decade of life, is more severe than the dominant form, and may manifest with weakness after severe episodes of myotonia. Propofol and depolarizing neuromuscular blocking agents may aggravate the myotonia, and patients may have prolonged recovery. Mexiletine is the treatment of choice.

47. You are evaluating a 16-year-old boy for acute onset of ataxia and dysarthria after he recovered from a streptococcal pharyngitis, associated with fever, and was successfully treated with penicillin. He had difficulty running with several sprained ankles since early childhood, but is otherwise healthy. He has a family history of Charcot-Marie-Tooth (CMT) neuropathy. His MRI showed acute white matter changes, particularly within the posterior fossa.

    The acute neurological changes are most likely related to an underlying:

    A. CMT1A
    B. CMT2A
    C. CMT1X
    D. CMT2A
    E. CMT4C

18

Correct Answer is: C
CMT1X neuropathy is associated with acute episodes of ataxia, dysarthria, and in some cases, asymmetric weakness. White matter changes are evident, particularly within the posterior fossa, during these episodes. The symptoms resolve in weeks to months, and typically do not recur. They are often triggered by metabolic stressors such as travel to high altitudes, febrile illnesses, hyperventilation, and concussion. These CNS changes have been reported in patients with CMT1X due to TSSI, R75W, E102del, R142W, R164W and C168Y mutations of the GJB1 gene, which encodes the protein connexin-32.

The presence of CNS symptoms does not correlate with the duration or severity of neuropathy. The neuropathy typically presents as distal lower extremity weakness, with slowed running and frequent sprained ankles, typically beginning by 10 years of age in affected males. Hands, particularly the thenar muscles, may be affected later in the course. Distal sensory loss with painful sensory paresthesia may also occur. Heterozygous females may be asymptomatic, but often have mild manifestations.

Suggested Readings

- Kleopa KA. The role of gap junctions in Charcot-Marie-Tooth disease. J Neurosci. 2011;31(49): 17753–60.
- Patzko A, Shy ME. Charcot-Marie-Tooth disease and related genetic neuropathies. Continuum. 2012;18(1):39–59.

48. You are seeing a 9-year-old female who experiences 2–4 episodes of proximal muscle weakness per day. The attacks are precipitated by rest following exercise and last 1 to 2 h. Serum potassium concentration during the attack of weakness is normal.

What is most likely to cause the muscle weakness in periodic hyperkalemic paralysis?

A. Decreased potassium conductance in muscle cells
B. Hyperpolarization of muscle cells
C. Inactivation of sodium channels in muscle cells
D. Increased duration of action potentials produced by a-motoneurons
E. Increased release of neurotransmitters from a-motoneurons

Correct Answer is: C
Periodic hyperkalemic paralysis is a disorder of muscle membrane excitability resulting from a sodium channel disorder. Inactivation of the sodium channels on the skeletal muscle membrane prevents action potentials from being produced, and therefore leads to muscle weakness or paralysis. Although the exact mechanism of periodic hyperkalemic paralysis is not known, it appears to be due to a mutation in the gene coding for the sodium inactivation gate. Attacks are usually frequent, focal, short duration (usually 15 min to 1–2 h, up to 4–5 h); may occur several times daily. May be precipitated by exposure to cold, rest after exercise or oral intake of potassium, emotional stress, and pregnancy. Episodes more frequent when poor oral intake and high potassium diet. Myotonia may or may not be present, serum potassium measured during an attack is often normal but may be high or even low. Myotonic discharges may be present on EMG. Treatment - ingestion of carbohydrates and sugars may prevent or abort attack; prophylaxis with hydrochlorothiazide and carbonic anhydrase inhibitors (acetazolamide).

Suggested Readings

- Mowzoon N, Flemming KD. Neurology Board Review: an illustrated study guide. Rochester: Mayo Clinic Scientific; 2007. Print.

49. You are seeing an infant with generalized hypotonia and weakness, you ordered a muscle biopsy, with a Gomori trichrome stained, which is shown.

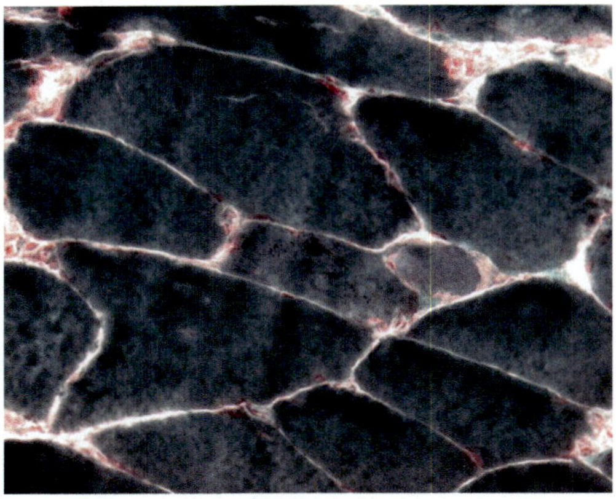

Fig. 18.5 Muscle biopsy showing rod-like inclusions in a myofiber as seen in Nemaline myopathy (Gomori trichrome stain). (Own work. Jensflorian. Wikipedia)

What is the most likely diagnosis?

A. Central core disease
B. Nemaline myopathy
C. Centronuclear myopathy
D. Myofibrillar myopathy
E. Congenital fiber type disproportion

Correct Answer is: B

Gomori trichrome staining of the muscle biopsy shows red punctuate inclusions within the skeletal muscle cytoplasm, representing nemaline rods. Rods may be visible with electron microscopy, as well. They are composed of alpha-actin, desmin, and nebulin. Biopsies in nemaline myopathy also reveal type 1 fiber predominance, type 1 atrophy, and type 28 deficiencies. Both autosomal dominant and recessive forms of nemaline myopathy have been documented, with various mutations affecting alpha-tropomyosin, beta tropomyosin, nebulin, troponin T, and alpha-actin. Clinical manifestations include early onset of hypotonia, followed by diffuse limb weakness, with mild weakness of the face and other bulbar muscles. The face is typically long and narrow, with an abnormally long or short jaw. Other malformations include high arches of the feet and palate and kyphoscoliosis. An associated cardiomyopathy may occur. A fatal infantile form consists of hypotonia and respiratory failure.

Suggested Readings

- Image adapted from: Lawlor MW, et al. Novel mutations in NEB cause abnormal nebulin expression and markedly impaired muscle force generation in severe nemaline myopathy. Skelet Muscle. 2011;1(1):23.
- Amato AA, Brooke MH. Disorders of skeletal muscle. In: Bradley WG, Daroff RB, Fenichel GM, Jankovic J, editors. Neurology in Clinical Practice. 4th ed. Elsevier, Inc.; 2004. p. 2463–510.

50. Which of the following is correct regarding Lambert-Eaton Myasthenic Syndrome (LEMS)?

A. Presynaptic stores of acetylcholine are decreased
B. Antibodies are typically present against post-synaptic motor nerves
C. Antibodies are most commonly directed against voltage-gated potassium channels
D. All of the above
E. None of the above

Correct Answer is: E

In LEMS, the quantal release of acetylcholine is impaired, although the presynaptic stores of the neurotransmitter and the postsynaptic response remain normal. The result is a syndrome including proximal weakness, hyporeflexia, and dysautonomia (i.e. dry mouth), with particular involvement of the lower extremities. Ocular findings such as ptosis and opthalmoparesis are

less common, and milder, than in myasthenia gravis. Symptoms may worsen in heat or with febrile illnesses. A characteristic feature of LEMS is that rapid repetitive stimulation or voluntary activity aids in the release of quanta to allow generation of muscle action potentials. Clinically, this may be evident as an increased response of previously hypoactive reflexes after contraction of the associated muscle, for example. The phenomenon may also be evident with facilitation of compound muscle action potential (CMAP) amplitudes with repetitive nerve stimulation on EMG/NCS. In the majority of patients, LEMS results from antibodies against voltage-gated calcium channels (VGCCs) on the presynaptic motor nerve terminal. The VGCC antibodies are often presumed to result from cross-reactivity with antigens of an underlying tumor. An associated cancer is found in approximately 40% *of* patients, most often small cell lung cancer (SCLC). LEMS may also be seen in the setting of autoimmune disorders, non-SCLC, lymphosarcomas, malignant thymomas, and cancers of the breast, stomach, colon, prostate, bladder, kidney, and gallbladder. LEMS often precedes the diagnosis of cancer. If no cancer is detected within 2 years of LEMS onset, an autoimmune disorder should be suspected. Prednisone, plasma exchange, 4-diaminopyridine, and intravenous immunoglobulin are available treatment options.

Suggested Readings

- Stickler DE. Lambert-Eaton Myasthenic Syndrome (LEMS). ▶ http://emedicine.medscape.com/article/1170810-overview. Updated 5/3/13. Accessed 5/16/14.

51. Regarding the pathophysiology of myasthenia gravis, which of the following is correct?
    A. In its most common form, it is autoimmune due to antibodies against presynaptic voltage-gated calcium channels
    B. It is due to inhibition of exocytosis of presynaptic vesicles containing acetylcholine
    C. In its most common form, it is autoimmune due to antibodies against the acetylcholine receptor
    D. It results from increased degradation of acetylcholine at the neuromuscular junction
    E. In its most common form, it is due to mutations in the acetylcholine receptor gene

Correct Answer is: A
The pathophysiology of autoimmune myasthenia gravis relates to the presence of circulating anti-acetylcholine receptor antibodies, which bind to the acetylcholine receptor causing immune-mediated destruction of the junctional folds that contain dense concentrations of this receptor, and a higher rate of internalization and destruction of acetylcholine receptor. In some cases, the antibodies might block binding of acetylcholine to its receptor at the neuromuscular junction. Antibodies against presynaptic voltage-gated calcium channels occur in Lambert-Eaton myasthenia syndrome. Botulinum toxin inhibits exocytosis of presynaptic vesicles containing acetylcholine. Rarely, myasthenia results from mutations in the acetylcholine receptor gene.

Suggested Readings

- Comprehensive Review in Clinical Neurology: a multiple-choice question Book for the Wards and Boards ©2011 Wolters Kluwer Health Lippincott Williams & Wilkins. All rights reserved.

52. You were evaluating an infant has severe diffuse weakness and hypotonia and ordered a muscle biopsy with an H&E stained, which is shown below.

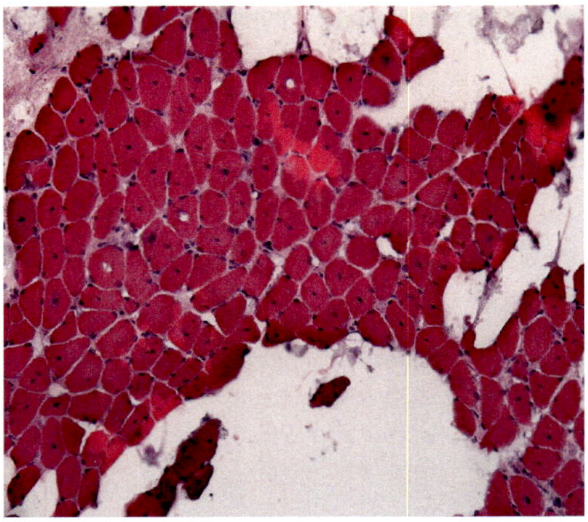

Fig. 18.6 Muscle biopsy of a 70-year old female showing histological picture of centrunuclear myopathy, am adult-onset congenital myopathy. (Own work. Jensflorian. Wikipedia)

What is the most likely diagnosis?

A. Central core disease
B. Nemaline myopathy
C. Centro-nuclear myopathy
D. Myofibrillar myopathy
E. Congenital fiber type disproportion

Correct Answer is: C

Centro-nuclear or myotubular myopathy is characterized by muscle fibers with central nuclei, as evident in the above image. The nuclei are surrounded by a halo devoid of myofilaments, containing mitochondrial and glycogen aggregates. Up to 90% of fibers may be affected. Biopsy may also show fiber size variation, type 1 predominance, and type 1 atrophy. The severe, often fatal, infant phenotype consists of extra-ocular, facial, and limb weakness, hypotonia, and respiratory failure. It is caused by an X-linked recessive mutation of the MTM1 gene, which codes for myotubularin. The infantile form is most common. Less severe forms may be evident in adolescents and adults, caused by other mutations (e.g. MTMR2, MTMR3), both autosomal dominant and recessive. EMG demonstrates fibrillation potentials, positive sharp waves, complex repetitive discharges, and occasionally, myotonic discharges.

Suggested Readings

- Image from: Jungbluth H, et al. Centronuclear (myotubular) myopathy. Orphanet J Rare Dis. 2008;25;3:26.
- Amato AA, Brooke MH. Disorders of skeletal muscle. In: Bradley WG, Daroff RB, Fenichel GM, Jankovic J, editors. Neurology in Clinical Practice. 4th ed. Elsevier, Inc.; 2004. p. 2463–510.

53. Other physical symptoms of Duchenne muscular weakness include:

A. Awkward manner of walking, stepping, or running
B. Increased lumbar lordosis
C. Higher risk of neurobehavioral disorders such ADHD
D. Skeletal deformities such as scoliosis
E. All of the above

Correct Answer is: E

Patients tend to walk on their forefeet, because of an increased calf tonus. Also, toe walking is a compensatory adaptation to knee extensor weakness. Increased Lumbar lordosis leads to shortening of the hip-flexor muscles.

There is a higher risk of neurobehavioral disorders (e.g., ADHD) and learning disorders (dyslexia).

54. You are seeing a 19-month-old girl who has had weakness since birth, and has been unable to learn to walk. She is developing contractures at the knees, but with hypermobility at the wrists and ankles.

What is the most likely diagnosis?

A. Ullrich's congenital muscular dystrophy
B. Laminin a2 deficiency
C. Emery-Dreifuss dystrophy
D. Dysferlin deficiency
E. Sarcoglycan deficiency

18

Correct Answer is: A

Hypermobility is evident in disorders of collagen, as seen in the muscular dystrophies due to collagen type VI mutations (i.e. Ullrich's congenital muscular dystrophy). It is not a feature of the other disorders listed. Ullrich's congenital muscular dystrophy is due to a mutation of collagen type VI. It presents with neonatal weakness and multiple contractures. The characteristic feature is distal hypermobility with protrusion of the calcanei.

Laminin a2 (merosin) deficiency results from a mutation of chromosome 6, of autosomal recessive inheritance. Laminin is a protein in the basement membrane, which attaches to dystroglycan. Absence of the protein results in hypotonia at birth, severe weakness of the trunk and limbs, and contractures of the feet and hips. Seizures occur in up to 20% of patients. White matter abnormalities may be evident on imaging. A partial deficiency causes a milder phenotype.

Emery-Dreifuss muscular dystrophy is caused by a deficiency of emerin, a structural protein of the inner nuclear membrane coded by the STA gene. It is of X-linked inheritance. Slowly progressive weakness affects the anterior legs, upper arms, and shoulders. Early contractures are evident. The disorder is associated with cardiomyopathies.

Dysferlin deficiency (limb girdle muscular dystrophy type 28) is caused by a mutation on chromosome 2, of autosomal l recessive inheritance. Although the function of the protein is unknown, its deficiency leads to limb-girdle weakness. Onset is typically in the teenage or early adult years.

Sarcoglycan deficiency causes limb girdle muscular dystrophies of types 2C, 20, 2E, and 2F. The disorders are of autosomal recessive inheritance, and lead to trunk and limb weakness with calf hypertrophy.

Suggested Readings

- Amato AA, Brooke MH. Disorders of skeletal muscle. In: Bradley WG, Daroff RB, Fenichel GM, Jankovic J, editors. Neurology in clinical practice. 4th ed. Elsevier, Inc.; 2004. p. 2463–510.

55. You were asked to see a 6-year-old boy because of weakness and a possible muscle problem. You ordered a muscle biopsy, is shown below. **Which of the following is not true regarding this condition?**
    - A. It is autosomal dominant, and the gene involved is RYR1
    - B. These patients are at risk for malignant hyperthermia
    - C. There is prominent proximal weakness, especially in the pelvic girdle
    - D. Pathologically, there are small cores that lack mitochondria, occurring only in some segments of the muscle fiber
    - E. Facial, bulbar, and ocular muscles are usually spared

Correct Answer is: D

The muscle biopsy shown is for a central core myopathy. This nicotinamide adenine dinucleotide-stained specimen demonstrates loss of oxidative activity within the center of muscle fibers, seen as paler areas where there is absence of mitochondria. These central cores run along the length of the muscle fiber, as opposed to multicore or mini-core disease in which the cores are small, extending through only segments of the fiber length. Central core myopathy is an autosomal dominant disease, caused by a mutation in the ryanodine receptor gene RYR1 on chromosome 19q13.1. These patients are at risk for the development of malignant hyperthermia and this should be considered when general anesthesia is needed. The clinical presentation is that of weakness and hypotonia soon after birth, and

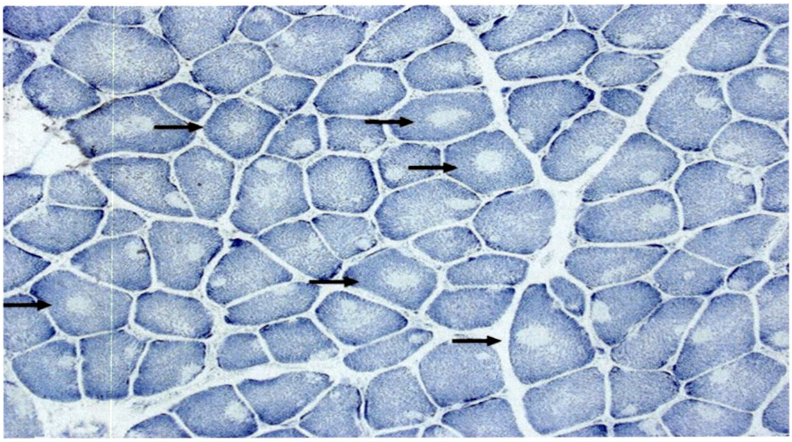

Fig. 18.7 Heinz Jungbluth W Histopathologie der Central-Core-Myopathie. (Orphanet J Rare Dis. 2007;2:25 ► https://doi.org/10.1186/1750-1172-2-25)

subsequent delay in motor development. The weakness is proximal, and the pelvic girdle is usually more affected than the shoulder girdle. Facial, bulbar, and ocular muscles are usually spared. CK levels are slightly elevated.

56. Both myotonic dystrophy type I and myotonic muscular dystrophy type II are inherited as:
    - A. Autosomal recessives
    - B. X-linked recessives
    - C. Autosomal dominants
    - D. Mutations in the DMPK genes
    - E. None of the above

Correct Answer is: C
Both types of myotonic dystrophy are inherited in an autosomal dominant pattern, which means one copy of the altered gene in each cell is sufficient to cause the disorder. In most cases, an affected person has one parent with the condition.

57. You are evaluating an 18-year-old male because of weakness. The patient has frontal balding, atrophy of the temporalis and masseter muscles, and weakness of the sternocleidomastoids and bilateral ptosis. He has also upper extremity weakness especially in forearm extensors, as well as atrophy in the anterior tibial muscles, with weakness of dorsiflexion of the feet. After percussion of his thenar eminence, there is prolonged contraction and slow relaxation. In addition, you observed a significant decline in compound motor action potential (CMAP) amplitude in DM1 with both short exercise test (SET) and short exercise test with cooling (SETC) immediately after effort.
    What is the most likely diagnosis?
    - A. Becker muscular dystrophy
    - B. Dystrophic myotonia type 1 (DM1) myotonic dystrophy
    - C. Emery-Dreifuss muscular dystrophy
    - D. Fascioscapulohumeral muscular dystrophy,
    - E. DM2 myotonic dystrophy

Correct Answer is: B
This is a case of dystrophic myotonia type 1 (DM1) myotonic dystrophy, which is an autosomal dominant condition with high penetrance, caused by a CTG expansion in the myotonic dystrophy protein kinase gene on chromosome 19q. These patients present in early adult life with ptosis and facial weakness, and characteristic features such as frontal balding, atrophy of the masseters and temporalis, and weakness and atrophy of small muscles of the hands and extensors of the forearms and peroneal muscles. Pharyngeal and

laryngeal weakness may be present, but this finding is rare. Patients have myotonia, which is a phenomenon of prolonged contraction and slow relaxation. Patients may also have diaphragmatic weakness, leading to respiratory failure, and cardiac abnormalities, especially conduction defects. Various other tissues are also involved, and patients may exhibit esophageal dilatation, megacolon, lenticular opacities and cataracts, intellectual disability, testicular atrophy with infertility, and androgen deficiency. CK levels may be slightly elevated. EMG demonstrates myotonic discharges and short, rapidly recruiting motor unit potentials with fibrillations. Histo-pathologically, muscle biopsy demonstrates marked central nucleation, type 1 fiber atrophy, peripherally placed sarcoplasmic masses, ring fibers, and pyknotic nuclear clumps. In addition, a significant decline in CMAP amplitude in DM1 with both SET and SETC immediately after effort is consistent with DM1. In DM2, there is no marked change in CMAP amplitude with either SET or SETC.

Suggested Readings

- Comprehensive Review in Clinical Neurology: a multiple-choice question Book for the Wards and Boards ©2011 Wolters Kluwer Health Lippincott Williams & Wilkins. All rights reserved.
- Value of short exercise and short exercise with cooling tests in the diagnosis of myotonic dystrophies {DM1 and DM2).
- Gawel M, Szmidt-Salkowska E, Lusakowska A, Nojszewska M, Sulek A, Krysa W, Rajkiewicz M, Seroka A, Kaminska AM. Muscle Nerve. 2014;49(2);277–83.

58. Early signs of Duchenne muscular dystrophy may include:
    - A. Truncal hypotonia
    - B. Difficulty in sitting
    - C. Atrophy of the deltoid and calf muscles
    - D. Pseudo-hypertrophy of the deltoid and calf muscles
    - E. Speech impairment

Correct Answer is: D
Early signs of Duchenne muscular dystrophy may include pseudo-hypertrophy (enlargement of calf muscles), low endurance, and difficulties in standing unaided or inability to ascend staircases.

59. Which of the following are associated with myotonic dystrophy type 1?
    - A. Christmas tree cataracts
    - B. Cardiac conduction defects
    - C. Distal weakness
    - D. Endocrine abnormalities
    - E. All of the above

Correct Answer is: E
Myotonic dystrophy type 1 is a muscular dystrophy caused by a mutation in the gene coding for myotonic dystrophy protein kinase (DMPK) on chromosome 19. The disorder results from CTG repeats, with anticipation and the size of expansion correlating with severity. The clinical manifestations include weakness with muscle wasting and myotonia (involuntary sustained contractions elicited by percussion or strong voluntary contraction, particularly when cold). The weakness is most pronounced distally, and the disease often presents with hand weakness and foot drop. The face appears long and mournful with ptosis and an open, slack mouth, due to weakness. A curious feature is the denial of illness. Myotonic dystrophy type 1 is associated with a number of systemic manifestations, including: Cardiac abnormalities, e.g. conduction defects, tachy-arrhythmias, fibrosis of the conduction system. It should be noted that the cardiac effects are not cardiomyopathies, in contrast to many other muscle diseases. Disturbed sleep with excessive daytime sleepiness, due to depression of the respiratory drive. Christmas tree cata-

racts. Testicular atrophy, impaired glucose tolerance, and other endocrine abnormalities. Gallbladder disease.

Suggested Readings

Amato AA, Brooke MH. Disorders of skeletal muscle. In: Bradley WG, Daroff RB, Fenichel GM, Jankovic J, editors. Neurology in clinical practice. 4th ed. Elsevier, Inc.; 2004. p. 2463–510.

60. Spinal muscular atrophy (SMA) is a hereditary disease affecting the lower motor neurons.
Which of the following statements about SMA are correct?
   A. It is an autosomal dominant disorder
   B. SMA in children is classified into three types, based on ages of onset, severity, and progression of symptoms. All three types are caused by defects in the SMN1 gene
   C. SMA type I, also called Werdnig-Hoffmann disease, is evident by the time a child is 6 months old.
   D. (b) and (c)
   E. None of the above.

Correct Answer is: D
SMA is an autosomal l recessive disorder.

61. You are seeing a 2-month-old baby because he is unable to breastfeed due to poor latching and sucking. His mother switched him to formula but he is still a "lazy eater" and doesn't suck much, preferring to let it drop into his mouth. He is smiling and cooing. His mother is concerned, however, because he does not move as much as the other children in his daycare. On examination, he is in the 15 percentiles for height and 10 percentiles for weight and 10 percentiles for head circumference. There are no dysmorphic features, his pupils are equal, round, and reactive to light and accommodation, extraocular eye movements are intact without nystagmus, mucous membranes are moist with tongue fasciculation present. Lungs are clear to auscultation bilaterally, heart has a regular rate and rhythm without murmurs, and abdomen is soft, non-tender and non-distended with no hepatosplenomegaly. Patellar reflexes are 0/4, Achilles reflexes are 0/4, and brachioradialis reflexes are 0/4. He is floppy, unable to support his head when pulled to a seated position, and does not kick or bat at objects although he does move his fingers and toes. In horizontal suspension he lays limp on the physician's hand and in vertical suspension he starts to slip through the physician's hands.
Which of the following is true regarding his likely diagnosis?
   A. This is an autosomal dominant trait
   B. His lower extremities will be weaker than his upper extremities
   C. His mother has myasthenia gravis
   D. There is a vaccine that can prevent infection of this illness
   E. This child will have impaired intellect

Correct Answer is: B
This is a clinical presentation of spinal muscular atrophy (SMA) type 1, also known as Werdnig-Hoffmann disease. The main features in this case that differentiate SMA from other conditions that cause hypotonia or developmental delay are the areflexia and tongue fasciculation exhibited by this baby. SMA is one of the most frequent autosomal recessive disorders and does not exhibit an ethnic preference. Although the phenotype is variable, 95% of children with SMA can be diagnosed with gene-mutation testing of the SMN1 gene on chromosome 5q. There are 3 types of SMA.

SMA presents with symmetric muscle weakness however the proximal muscle groups are weaker than the distal muscle groups and lower extremities are weaker than the upper extremities. Thus, over time, the legs will stop moving but the child can continue to play with toys that are placed in their hands.

Neonates born to mothers with myasthenia gravis can develop a transitory myasthenic syndrome as a result of anti-acetylcholine receptor antibody. Symptoms include ptosis, ophthalmoplegia, weak facial movements, poor sucking and feeding, hypotonia, and variable extremity weakness. Symptoms will persist from 1–10 weeks. Diagnosis is confirmed by the demonstration of clinical improvement lasting approximately 45 min after intramuscular administration of neostigmine. The infant described in this case does not show evidence of ptosis, ophthalmoplegia, or weak facial movements, making neonatal transitory myasthenia gravis unlikely.

Poliomyelitis is an acute enterovirus illness that presents with a prodromal of vomiting, diarrhea and aseptic meningitis followed by evolution of asymmetric flaccid weakness. This weakness is the result of infection of groups of anterior horn cells. This is similar to SMA, which also presents with flaccid weakness due to anterior horn cell degeneration. The difference between SMA and poliomyelitis is the prodromal illness and acute onset in poliomyelitis in contrast to progressive symmetric weakness.

Infants with SMA have normal mental, social, and language skills and sensation. For this reason, it is very important that social, language, and intellectual skills be maximized while providing symptomatic therapy.

Suggested Readings

- Schroth M. Special considerations in the respiratory management of spinal muscular atrophy. Pediatrics. 2009;123(4):245–9.
- Chung B, et al. Spinal muscular atrophy: survival pattern and functional status. Pediatrics. 2004;114(5):e548–53.
- Kliegman RM, et al. Nelson essentials of pediatrics.5th ed. Philadelphia: Elsevier Saunders; 2006.

62. You are evaluating an 18-year-old male with weakness of his hands bilaterally, which he first noticed several months prior to the office visit. On examination, he has atrophy of the thenar muscles, as well as impaired vibratory sensation in his feet.

Which of the following subtype of Charcot-Marie-Tooth (CMT) disease is the most likely diagnosis?

A. CMT1 B
B. CMT2D
C. CMT1X
D. CMT2A
E. CMT4C

Correct Answer is: B

In many forms of CMT, the patient presents with symmetrical distal limb weakness and sensory loss, pes cavus, and a family history of neuropathy. CMT2D is unique amongst the CMT disorders, in that the hands are affected early in the course. The disorder typically presents in adolescence or early-adulthood with bilateral weakness and atrophy of thenar and first dorsal interosseus muscles, initially sparing the hypothenar eminence. Patients may also report transient cramping and pain in the hands when cold and cramping in calf muscles with exercise. Sensory deficits may follow, with impaired pinprick, temperature, touch, and vibration sense in the feet, and less often, the hands, in a stocking-glove distribution. CMT2D is due to a mutation of the GARS gene, which encodes glycyl-tRNA synthetase. A mutation of the same gene also causes distal hereditary motor neuropathy (dHMN) type V. When sensory deficits are present, the disorder is classified as CMT2D. When sensory deficits are absent, the disorder is classified as dHMN type V.

Suggested Readings

- Goldfarb LG, Sivakumar K. GARS-associated axonal neuropathy. ▶ http://www.ncbi.nlm.nih.gov/books/NBK1242/. Updated 8/25/11. Accessed 5/16/14.
- Patzke A, Shy ME. Charcot-Marie-Tooth disease and related genetic neuropathies. Continuum. 2012;18(1):39–59.

63. You are evaluating a 14-year-old female with bilateral foot drop. She has been clumsy and seemed to trip on her own feet, and could not participate in ballet classes as a young child. In the recent years, her feet became noticeably weak. On examination, she had bilateral symmetric weakness of foot dorsiflexion and plantarflexion. She had hammertoes and high-arched feet. Ankle and knee-deep tendon reflexes were absent. Examination of the mother also revealed hammertoes and high-arched feet. Conduction velocities of approximately 30 cm/second were revealed in all NCS of the legs, with no identifiable conduction block.
What is the most likely diagnosis in this patient?
A. Charcot-Marie-Tooth (CMT) 1
B. CMT2
C. A muscular dystrophy
D. CMT3
E. CMT4

Correct Answer is: A
This clinical presentation is consistent with Charcot-Marie-Tooth (CMT) 1. The clinical manifestations are discussed further below, but respiratory compromise is not usually seen in the most common forms of CMT, but occurs in some cases of CMT2C. The CMTs, also known as hereditary sensorimotor neuropathies or peroneal muscular atrophy, are a large, heterogeneous group of inherited peripheral neuropathies. The CMTs can be divided into demyelinating, axonal, and combined demyelinating and axonal forms. They are genetically heterogeneous. The demyelinating CMTs include CMT1 and CMTX. CMT4, involves both demyelination and axon loss. In the demyelinating CMTs, NCS generally show diffuse, uniformly slow conduction velocities without conduction blocks or temporal dispersion, indicating a hereditary as opposed to acquired demyelinating process. There may be evidence of axon loss in the demyelinating forms as well, particularly in patients with long standing disease; this is secondary axon loss, and conduction velocities as well as CMAP and SNAP amplitudes will be reduced. In contrast, with the axonal forms, motor and sensory potential amplitudes will be reduced, but conduction velocities will be normal or minimally reduced. At the time of this publication, there were seven subtypes of CMT1; they are all inherited in an autosomal dominant fashion. CMT1A is the most common inherited demyelinating neuropathy. Clinical manifestations typically begin in the first two decades of life and include slowly progressive weakness, muscle atrophy, kyphosis, and mild (often asymptomatic) sensory loss. Other signs include hammertoes, high-arched feet, palpably enlarged nerves due to peripheral nerve hypertrophy (which more commonly occurs in the CMT1 group compared to the other CMTs), and pes cavus. Involvement of the upper extremities typically occurs later in life. There is often a family history of neuropathy, though due to variable expression, some affected family members may only have mild features such as hammertoes and may remain undiagnosed for a large part of their life; sporadic cases without a clear family history also exist. Other forms of CMT may be congenital and severe. In the CMT1 group, many of the genes involved are related to myelin syn-

thesis. CMT1A is due to a duplication in the peripheral myelin protein 22 (PMP22) gene on chromosome 17, whereas CMT1 B is due to a mutation in the myelin protein O gene. CMT1 B is more severe in terms of clinical manifestations as compared to CMT1A. In patients with CMT1, CSF shows elevated protein levels in some cases. Roussy-Levy syndrome is phenotypically similar to CMT1A but is associated with the presence of a static tremor and gait ataxia. It has been associated with mutations in both the PMP22 and myelin protein 0 genes. On nerve biopsy, pathologic features of the demyelinating inherited polyneuropathies include demyelination and an onion-bulb appearance due to Schwann cell proliferation. Onion bulbs are not specific for CMT, and also occur with chronic inflammatory demyelinating polyneuropathy. CMTX is the second most common type of CMT. It is demyelinating and is clinically similar to CMT1, but it is X-linked in inheritance; males therefore tend to be more severely affected compared to females. It is due to a mutation in the connexin 32 gene. CMT2 accounts for approximately one-third of the autosomal dominant inherited neuropathies. The CMT2 group are axonal neuropathies; NCS show normal conduction velocities, and nerve biopsy shows axon loss without evidence of significant demyelination. Compared to CMT1, in CMT2, symptoms and signs typically appear later and foot and spine deformities are less severe. Clinical manifestations do not always help distinguish the different CMTs, but some clinical features occur more frequently in the different subtypes. Optic atrophy occurs more in CMT2A2, foot ulcerations in CMT28, and vocal cord paralysis, intercostal, and diaphragmatic weakness in CMT2C. In CMT2D, unlike in the other CMTs, the hands are involved more than the feet.

Peripheral nerve hypertrophy does not occur. They are all autosomal dominant in inheritance, except for a subtype of CMT2A. The genes implicated in the CMT2 group are involved in axonal transport and membrane trafficking. CMT2A2 is one of the most common of this group and is due to mutations in mitofusin 2. CMT3, also known as Dejerine-Sottas syndrome or hypertrophic neuropathy of infancy, is one of the more severe forms of the demyelinating CMTs. It presents in infancy with proximal weakness, absent deep tendon reflexes, and hypertrophy of the peripheral nerves. Prominent sensory symptoms including pain and dysesthesias occur. Patients typically have extensive disability early in life. Both autosomal recessive and dominant forms exist. CSF protein is usually elevated. Congenital hypomyelination is seen along the spectrum of this disorder. CMT3 is genetically heterogeneous; mutations in several genes including PMP22, protein myelin 0, and other genes implicated in defective demyelination are associated with CMT3. The CMTs can be misdiagnosed as muscular dystrophy; NCS findings, as well as the presence of hammertoes and high-arched foot, distinguish between the two.

Suggested Readings

- Bradley WG, Daroff RB, Fenichel GM, et al. Neurology in Clinical Practice, 5th ed. Philadelphia: Elsevier; 2008.
- Ropper AH, Samuels MA. Adams and Victor's Principles of Neurology, 9th ed. New York: McGraw-Hill; 2009.
- Comprehensive Review in Clinical Neurology: a multiple-choice question Book for the Wards and Boards

64. You are seeing a 20-week-old infant girl with a one-week onset of diffuse hypotonia, ptosis, dysphagia, weak cry and dilated, sluggish pupils. The infant has been constipated and has a poor suck when feeding. EMG

showed, after 20–50 Hz stimulation, a reversal of a presynaptic block, then a gradual increase in the size of the motor unit potentials.

What is the likely diagnosis?

A. Infantile myasthenia
B. Infantile botulism
C. Infantile spinal atrophy
D. Infantile myotubular myopathy

Correct Answer is: B

Clostridium botulinum infects the infants from contaminated formula, ingestion of contaminated honey or inhaled from dust from nearby construction. The exotoxin produced causes a cholinergic blockade of skeletal muscle and autonomic nerves. Progressive facial, pharyngeal weakness, ptosis, dilated pupils, absent reflexes and constipation differentiate infantile botulism from other inflammatory demyelinating and neuromuscular junction disorders. The peak incidence is between March and October with prodromal symptoms of constipation and poor feeding.

Infantile myasthenia syndromes do not present with dilated pupils, absent reflexes or constipation.

Infantile spinal muscular atrophy symptoms do not include bulbar manifestations (facial and pharyngeal weakness, ptosis, dilated pupils).

Infantile myotubular myopathy (mild/moderate form) typically manifests with low tone at birth, subsequent motor delay and may include ophthalmoplegia and cognitive impairment.

Suggested Readings

- Brown N, Desai S. Infantile Botulism: a case report and review. J Emerg Med. 2013;45(6):842–5.

18

65. You are evaluating a floppy baby. You diagnosed him with Centro nuclear myopathy based on a muscle biopsy. **Which of the following characteristics are not true regarding this condition?**

A. Respiratory failure occurs in severe forms
B. The muscle fibers occur show central nucleation
C. Pharyngeal and laryngeal muscles may be affected
D. Extraocular movements are rarely affected
E. Could be autosomal dominant, autosomal recessive, or X-linked

Correct Answer is: D

Centro-nuclear myopathy (also known as myotubular myopathy) is a congenital myopathy, manifesting characteristically with ptosis and ocular palsies, as well as weakness of facial, pharyngeal, laryngeal, and neck muscles. It typically presents with hypotonia and weakness at birth, or in early childhood. Proximal and distal weakness and hypo-reflexia can be seen. Severe forms may be fatal due to respiratory failure in the first few months of life. CK levels are mildly elevated. Needle EMG shows a myopathic pattern with positive waves and fibrillations. Pathologically, there are small muscle fibers and central nucleation, as well as predominance of type I fibers, which are small and hypotrophic. This condition is inherited in an X-linked or autosomal dominant or recessive fashion. The X-linked form is severe and presents in the neonatal period, the autosomal dominant form is an adult-onset milder form, and the autosomal recessive form is intermediate in severity.

66. Which of the following statements is not true regarding the disorder depicted in the figure?

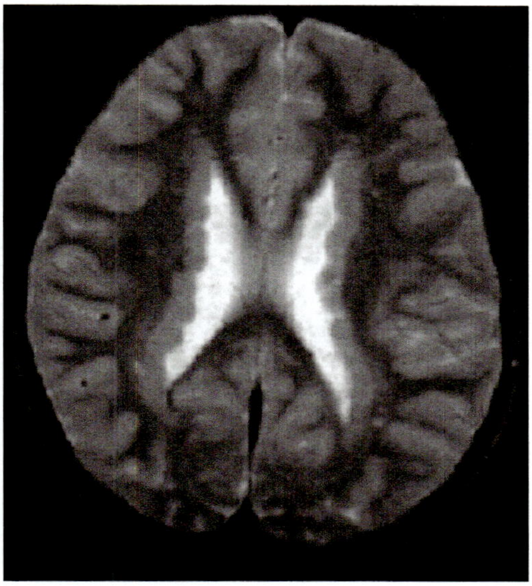

Fig. 18.8 Subcortical band heterotopia, or double cortex. ILAE.org. EpilepsyDiagnosis.org, Diagnostic Manual

A. It is a disorder of neuronal migration
B. It results from abnormalities in a protein involved in microtubule organization and stabilization
C. It is an X-linked disorder
D. Mutations in the DCX gene lead to this disorder in females and lissencephaly in males
E. This disorder is classically associated with muscular dystrophy

Correct Answer is: E
The MRI shows subcortical band heterotopia. The neuronal migration disorder associated with muscular dystrophy is cobblestone lissencephaly. The lissencephaly syndromes result from neuronal migration abnormalities and include subcortical band heterotopia, or double cortex, in which there is relatively normal cortex with an underlying band of white matter, underneath which is a band of gray matter. This disorder results from a mutation in the DCX gene on chromosome X, which encodes for the protein doublecortin, which is involved in microtubule organization and stabilization. The same mutation can lead to classic lissencephaly (smooth brain, agyria, or pachygyria) when occurring in males. This difference in manifestations in females as compared with males is thought to result from lyonization (random X inactivation) in females, such that in neurons in which the mutated gene is inactivated, normal migration occurs. Clinical features include intractable seizures, microcephaly, hypotonia, spastic quadriparesis, recurrent aspirations necessitating feeding tube, and shortened life expectancy. Lissencephaly type I characterized by agyria or pachygyria rather than the presence of two bands of gray matter separated by a band of white matter. Cobblestone lissencephaly (rather than subcortical band heterotopia), or lissencephaly type II, is seen in several disorders, including Walker-Warburg syndrome, Fukuyama muscular dystrophy, and muscle-eye-brain disease of Santavuori. In polymicrogyria, there are excess, abnormal gyri.

67. Symptoms of Duchenne muscular dystrophy usually occur in:
A. Female children before age 6
B. Male children before age 6
C. Male children between ages 6 and 12
D. Adolescent males
E. Adolescent females

Correct Answer is: B
Symptoms usually appear in male children before age 6 and may be visible in early infancy. Progressive proximal muscle weakness of the legs and pelvis associated with a loss of muscle mass is observed first. Eventually this weakness spreads to the arms, neck, and other areas.

68. You are seeing a baby who is diagnosed with a congenital muscular dystrophy. Clinically, he is weak and has multiple contractures with distal hyperlaxity. There are protrusions of the calcanei in the feet.
What is the most likely diagnosis?
    - A. Fukuyama-type congenital muscular dystrophy
    - B. Laminin alpha 2 deficiency
    - C. Walker-Marburg syndrome Muscle-eye-brain disease
    - D. Muscle-eye-brain disease
    - E. Ullrich's congenital muscular dystrophy

Correct Answer is: E
This patient has Ullrich's congenital muscular dystrophy, which presents with neonatal weakness, contractures and distal hyperlaxity, as well as protrusion of the calcanei. It is associated with mutations of collagen type VI and is thought to be related to Bethlem myopathy. Walker-Marburg syndrome is an autosomal recessive condition characterized by muscular dystrophy and brain and ocular abnormalities. Patients are hypotonic at birth with elevated CK levels. The ocular malformations include microphthalmia, colobomas, cataracts, glaucoma, corneal opacity, retinal dysplasia, and optic atrophy. There are multiple brain CNS malformations including hydrocephalus, aqueductal stenosis, cerebellar hypoplasia, and cortical abnormalities. Muscle-eye-brain disease is an autosomal recessive condition in which there is also muscular dystrophy and brain and ocular abnormalities; however, the cortical changes are milder and the white matter changes are more focal. The eyes are also affected to a lesser degree than Walker-Marburg syndrome.

69. What is the most common sign or symptom at presentation of McArdle's Disease {Type V Glycogen Storage Disease)?
    - A. Hypoglycemia
    - B. Leg cramps
    - C. Hepatomegaly
    - D. Cardiomegaly
    - E. Feeding difficulties

Correct Answer is: B
McArdle's disease is caused by Myophosphorylase deficiency and occurs in 1/100,000 live births. It was the first metabolic myopathies to be recognized. Though its onset is at birth, it often goes undiagnosed until adulthood well into the 3rd and 4th decades. Signs and symptoms include exercise-induced muscle cramps, myalgias, and myoglobinuria. A classic finding is the "second wind phenomenon", where the muscular symptoms abate somewhat around 10 min into activity. Patients eventually present to the ED or physician with severe pain, muscle contractures, or rhabdomyolysis.

There are more than a dozen types of GSDs, but the four that cause the most clinically significant neurologic and muscle problems are: (1) Pompe disease (Type II, acid maltase deficiency) --> cardiomegaly, cardiomyopathy, (2) Cori disease (Type III, debranching enzyme deficiency) --> Hypoglycemia, hepatomegaly, (3) McArdle disease (Type V, myophosphorylase deficiency), (4) Tarui disease (Type VII, phosphofructokinase deficiency).

70. You are evaluating a 4-year-old boy for delayed gross motor development. He is a very engaging child who is a great eater but always appears

18

to be fatigued and has difficulty with standing. When he tries to walk he falls frequently and has difficulty getting back up. Past medical history is remarkable for two liver biopsies for elevated liver enzymes.

What is the most appropriate next step in evaluation?

A. EMG with nerve conduction
B. Plasma lactate
C. Ammonia
D. Creatine kinase
E. MRI of the brain

Correct Answer is: D

This is a case of Duchenne muscular dystrophy. Clinical manifestations of muscle weakness and calf pseudohypertrophy are typically not recognized until 3 years of age or later. Walking often begins later than in normal children and affected boys experience more falling than is expected for age. Gait abnormalities often become apparent at 3–4 years of age.

Muscle fiber necrosis can cause elevation in purported liver enzymes. Serum alanine transaminase (ALT) and aspartate transaminase (AST) levels are commonly used as biochemical indicators of hepatocellular injury but can also detect occult muscle disease. High concomitant serum CK levels can point to muscle as the source of high transaminase levels.

Suggested Readings

- McMillan et al. Serum transaminase levels in boys with Duchenne and Becker muscular dystrophy. Pediatrics. 2011;127(1).
- Swaiman. Pediatric Neurology Principals& Practice.

Neuro-Oncology

Y. M. Awaad, *Absolute Pediatric Neurology*, https://doi.org/10.1007/978-3-319-78801-2_19

1. You are evaluating a 6-year-old boy who fell down in his school playground and he has a head trauma. EMS has been called because he vomited several times. In the ER, the attending physician ordered a head CT scan which showed large mass filling the fourth ventricle, and hydrocephalus. His parents reported that he was clumsy in his walking and he had mild headaches for 1 week. His past medical history is unremarkable. On exam, he has bilateral papilledema, mild truncal instability while seated, a broad-based gait, and no skin stigmata. His brain MRI sample is shown. Contrast administration showed patchy enhancement of the lesion. Tissue biopsy reveals small round undifferentiated blue cells with hyperchromatic nuclei. No rosettes or pseudo rosettes are identified.

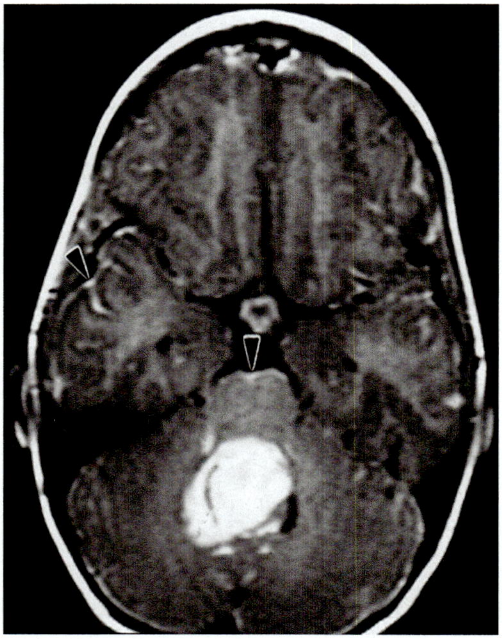

Fig. 19.1 MEDULLOBLASTOMA. As seen in this MRI study of a vermian lesion, medulloblastomas are contrast-enhancing masses. Diffuse enhancement in the cerebral subarachnoid space (*arrows*) indicates leptomeningeal dissemination. (▶ http://peir2.path.uab.edu/scripts/acdis.dll?cmd=see&fp=/dbih/AFIP/00405851.tif&fmt=jpg&q=100&h=512. The Armed Forces Institute of Pathology. Wikipedia)

Which of the following tumors is most likely?

A. Ependymal
B. Juvenile pilocytic astrocytoma
C. Medulloblastoma
D. Oligodendroglia
E. Sub ependymal giant cell astrocytoma

Correct Answer is: C

In the first decade of life, posterior fossa region are the most common brain tumors in children. Clinical manifestations include: a progressive subacute ataxia, truncal if located in the vermis and appendicular if located primarily in one cerebellar hemisphere. Signs of increased intracranial pressure, such as vomiting, headache and occasionally a sixth nerve palsy are due to the compressive effects these tumors have on the outflow of cerebrospinal fluid through the cerebral aqueduct or fourth ventricle itself. The most common posterior fossa tumors in childhood include medulloblastoma, juvenile pilocytic astrocytoma and ependymoma. Oligodendroglioma is a rare tumor in children, accounting for 1% of childhood brain tumors, and is chiefly supratentorial in location. Sub-ependymal giant cell astrocytomas are juxtaventricular tumors, usually located at the region of the foramen of Monro, and seen exclusively in patients with tuberous sclerosis.

Medulloblastoma among the above mentioned posterior fossa tumors is notable for its midline location, fairly diffuse contrast enhancement on MRI and histologic presence of small round blue cells with hyperchromatic nuclei. Medulloblastomas are currently felt to be histologically similar to primitive neuro-ectodermal tumors, differentiating along several cell lines, not dissimilar to tumors of stem cell origin. Subarachnoid seeding of the tumor can occur, with "drop metastases" present

along the spinal axis. With the advent of radiation treatment and more aggressive neurosurgical resection, the survival rate has increased markedly over the past 30 years. The overall best survival rate is for children older than age 3, with less than 1.5 cm^3 residual tumor after resection, and no evidence of subarachnoid seeding, with 5-year survival rates greater than 80%. Adjuvant chemotherapeutic regimens are added for higher risk groups and those with recurrent disease.

Pilocytic astrocytoma can occur anywhere in the cerebellum. About 80% are cystic with a large mural nodule that contrast enhances on MRI. Pathology reveals compact, strongly fibrillated cells alternating with loose, spongy areas composed of micro cysts. Leptomeningeal spread is quite rare. Treatment for well demarcated astrocytomas is total surgical resection, with survival rates approaching 90% at 10 years.

Ependymomas arise in relation to any part of the ventricular system, with infratentorial location being most common in children younger than three. Older patients more commonly have a supra-tentorial location. MRI appearance can mimic that seen with medulloblastoma, and metastatic spread through the spinal neuro-axis can occur as well. Histologically, they appear quite different, with ependymal rosettes or pseudo-rosettes lining a small central lumen. Treatment regimens utilize a combination of surgical resection, radiation and chemotherapy.

Suggested Reading

- Swaiman et al. Pediatric neurology, principles and practice. 4th ed. p. 1707–16.

2. You were asked to see an 18-month-old girl with one-week history of "twitching" that started in her legs but eventually affected all four extremities. Now, she is not able to ambulate. Two days ago, her mother noted that her eyes were moving abnormally. No history any recent viral infections or immunizations. On examination, she has significant involuntary, chaotic, multi-directional saccadic eye movements, action myoclonus, and both appendicular and truncal ataxia. Her head MRI is normal, but CSF analysis shows a mild pleocytosis and a mildly elevated protein. Urine catechol amines, shows a homovanillic acid of 61.5 mg/g (normal 0–32.6) and vanillyl mandelic acid of 20 mg/g (normal 0–16.7).
What is your next step in management?
A. CT scan of the chest and abdomen
B. Anti-Hu antibody titers
C. Ceruloplasmin level
D. CSF measles antibody titers
E. ENT consultation

Correct Answer is: A
This is a clinical presentation of an opsoclonus-myoclonus-ataxia (OMA) syndrome, also referred to as "dancing eye and dancing feet syndrome." The term opsoclonus refers to involuntary, chaotic, multidirectional saccades, which are present during fixation and smooth pursuit and persist during eyelid closure and sleep. Opsoclonus often occurs in association of appendicular myoclonus and cerebellar ataxia. Behavioral disturbances, postural tremor, and/or encephalopathy can be exhibited. Opsoclonus has different etiologies: paraneoplastic, para-infectious, toxic-metabolic, or idiopathic phenomenon. In children, more than half of paraneoplastic opsoclonus is secondary to neuroblastoma. Although a variety of anti-neuronal antibodies have been identified in this disorder, the majority of patients are seronegative. All children presenting with OMA should be evaluated for occult neuroblastoma with

urine catechol amines, including homovanillic acid and vanillyl mandelic acid, imaging of the chest and abdomen, and, if negative, 123I-metaiodobenzylguanidine (MIBG) scan. When negative, the evaluation should be repeated after several months. The prognosis for survival of neuroblastoma patients with opsoclonus is better than for those without opsoclonus. Management involves treatment of the underlying process, as well as symptomatic treatment with corticosteroids, intravenous immunoglobulin (IVIG), or adrenocorticotrophic hormone (ACTH). Low-dose cyclophosphamide may be beneficial in refractory cases. With or without treatment, children with opsoclonus and neuroblastoma usually experience resolution of the opsoclonus, though most experience relapses.

Suggested Reading

- Wong A. An update on opsoclonus. Curr Opin Neurol. 2007;20:25–31.

3. You are seeing a 9-month-old boy in the hospital, who has been vomiting (non-bloody, non-bilious) for 4 weeks and progressive off balance for 2 weeks. He achieved his milestones on target like sitting independently at 7 months but he cannot do so for the last week. You examined him, he is alert but irritable, with impaired up gaze and significant truncal ataxia. You ordered head CT, shows a high density, enhancing posterior fossa mass with significant hydrocephalus. Because the finding on the CT, you ordered an MRI, shows a round, slightly lobulated mass within the cerebellar vermis and fourth ventricle, which is isointense to gray matter on T1- and T2-weighted images and is homogenously enhancing.

What is your most likely diagnosis?

A. Hemangioblastoma
B. Medullary glioma
C. Teratoma
D. Medulloblastoma
E. Juvenile pilocytic astrocytoma

Correct Answer is: D

Different posterior fossa tumors can be presented with the same symptoms, but both neuroimaging suggest a medulloblastoma. Astrocytomas are more common than medulloblastomas but are predominantly cystic. Medullary gliomas, teratomas, and hemangioblastomas have different radiological characteristics and are less common. Several different radiological techniques are used in the medulloblastoms diagnosis, but the defined diagnosis is based on WHO-defined histological criteria. Classic medulloblastoma is characterized by sheet-like areas of small, round, blue cells with scant cytoplasm and dense hyperchromatic nuclei. Homer-Wright rosettes, which are circular groupings of tumor cells, are present in less than half of cases. Other subtypes of medulloblastoma include desmoplastic, large cell anaplastic, medullomyoblastic, and melanotic variants. Staging requires a gadolinium-enhanced MRI of the brain and entire spine and a lumbar puncture to assess for disseminated disease, which is present in 30% of children at presentation; however, drop metastases are readily apparent on imaging may obviate the need for a lumbar puncture. CSF should be obtained 2 weeks post-operatively to avoid false positive results.

Suggested Reading

- Crawford JR, MacDonald TJ, Packer RJ. Medulloblastoma in childhood: new biological advances. Lancet Neurol. 2007;6:1073–85.

4. An 18-year-old girl came for evaluation, she is complaining of blurry

19

vision, headache and difficulty ambulating for 4 months. On examination, she has bilateral papilledema, multiple retinal angiomas, dysmetria, ataxia, brisk deep tendon reflexes, extensor plantar responses, and ankle clonus. You ordered a brain MRI, shows a large enhancing midline cerebellar lesion compressing the fourth ventricle and brainstem. A follow -up cervical MRI shows multiple nodular enhancing lesions.

What is the most likely diagnosis?

A. Medulloblastoma
B. Cerebellar astrocytoma
C. Arteriovenous malformation
D. Von Hippel Lindau disease
E. Ependymoma

Correct Answer is: D

In von Hippel Lindau disease patients, diagnosis can be made by the presence of a single retinal angioma or cerebellar hemangioblastoma, renal cell carcinoma, or pheochromocytoma. If there is no family history, patients have to have 2 or more retinal angiomas, hemangioblastomas within the central nervous system, or one such lesion and a characteristic visceral tumor. Hemangioblastomas can affect not only the retina and cerebellum, but the brainstem and spinal cord as well, thus resulting in heterogeneous neurological findings. Von Hippel Lindau disease patient's prognosis is based on the brain and spinal cord localization, the underlying biology of the central nervous system tumors, and comorbid entities such as carcinomas. Management of von Hippel Lindau patients is best by a multidisciplinary approach because of the potential for multi-organ involvement.

Suggested Reading

- Clark PE, Cookson MS. The von Hippel-Lindau gene: turning discovery into therapy. Cancer. 2008 Oct 1;113(7 Suppl):1768–78. Kaelin WG. Von Hippel-Lindau disease. Annu Rev. Pathol. 2007;2:145–73.
- Maher ER. Von Hippel-Lindau disease. Curr Mol Med. 2004;4(8):833–42.
- Lonser RR, Glenn GM, Walther M, Chew EY, Libutti SK, Linehan WM, Oldfield EH. Von Hippel-Lindau disease. Lancet. 2003; 361(9374):2059–67.

5. You are seeing a 19-month-old girl in the hospital who has normal walking and understandable two-word phrases for the last few months, suddenly she became unsteady walking and wobble irregularly when sitting. One day ago, she starts to have irregular, jerky, conjugate movements of her eyes and is unable to bring a spoon smoothly to her mouth while eating.

What is your expectations?

A. Good prognosis medulloblastoma
B. Bad prognosis medulloblastoma
C. Good prognosis neuroblastoma
D. Bad prognosis neuroblastoma
E. Bad prognosis glioblastoma

Correct Answer is: A

Opsoclonus-myoclonus-ataxia (OMA) syndrome is a paraneoplastic syndrome most often associated with neuroblastoma. The neuroblastomas with which it occurs tend to be the more differentiated, less malignant tumors, and often, the neuroblastoma can be cured, but the progressive course of OMA syndrome and its cognitive sequelae are the cause of long-term disability. Both anti-T-cell and anti-B-cell therapies are useful in this disorder.

Suggested Reading

- Stefanowicz J, Izycka-Swieszewska E, Drozyńska E, Pienczk J, Połczyńska K, Czauderna P, Sierota D, Bień E, Stachowicz-Stencel T, Kosiak W, Balcerska A. Neuroblastoma and opsoclonus-myoclonus-ataxia syndrome–clinical and pathological characteristics. Folia Neuropathol. 2008;46(3):176–85.

- Aydin GB, Kutluk MT, Buyukpamukcu M, Akyuz C, Yalcin B, Varan A. Neurological complications of neuroblastic tumors: experience of a single center. Childs Nerv Syst. 2010;26(3):359–65.

6. You are evaluating a previously 6-years old boy who has been having nausea, vomiting and double-vision for the last month. On exam, he has weakness in right eye abduction, mild right facial weakness, and a decreased gag. He also has dysmetria more in the right upper extremity than left. His DTRs are increased on the left more than the right. His brain MRI is shown.

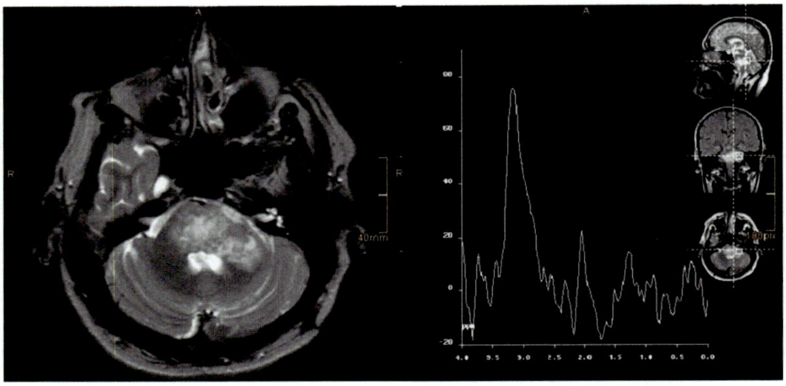

Fig. 19.2 The single voxel spectrum is derived from a glioma within the brain stem. The T2-weighted image on the left side shows the extension of the tumor. The spectrum exhibits a large peak of choline compounds at about 3.2 ppm. (Own work. Mschocke. W)

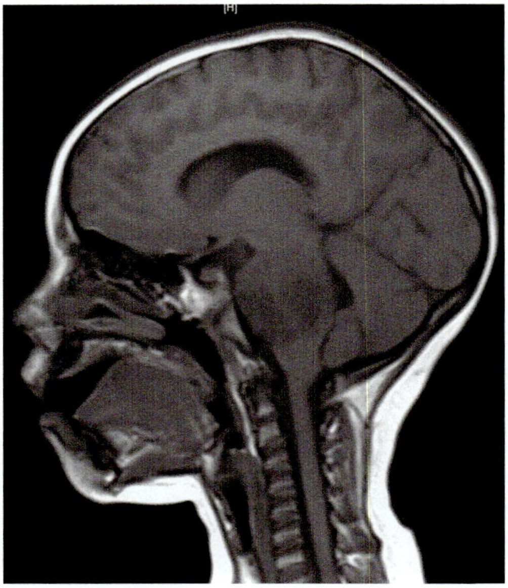

Fig. 19.3 Brainstem Glioma in 4-year-old. MRI sagittal, without contrast. (Own work. Tdvorak. W)

What is the most likely prognosis?

A. Good long-term survival following surgical resection
B. Full recovery following IV antibiotic treatment
C. Good long-term survival following radiation therapy
D. Good long-term survival following chemotherapy
E. Poor prognosis despite any therapy

Correct Answer is: E

Diffuse intrinsic brainstem gliomas typically has the triad of cranial neuropathies, ataxia, and long tract signs. The pontine gliomas have the worst prognosis of all brainstem gliomas. Less than 10% of patients are alive and free of progressive disease 18 months following diagnosis, even after treatment with radiotherapy.

Suggested Reading

- Recinos PF, Sciubba DM, Jallo GI. Brainstem tumors: where are we today?. Pediatr Neurosurg. 2007;43(3):192–201.
- Korones DN. Treatment of newly diagnosed diffuse brain stem gliomas in children: in search of the Holy Grail. Expert Rev. Anticancer Ther. 2007;7(5):663–74.

7. A 10-year-old female is complaining of early morning headaches with vomiting for 1 month. She has a history of mild ASD, seizures and multiple hypo-pigmented spots. A T2 weighted axial MRI image is shown below. Microscopic pathology showed numerous pleomorphic giant cells. **What is your diagnosis?**
   - A. Segmental neurofibromatosis
   - B. Sturge Weber syndrome
   - C. Linear nevus sebaceous syndrome
   - D. Tuberous sclerosis complex
   - E. None of the above

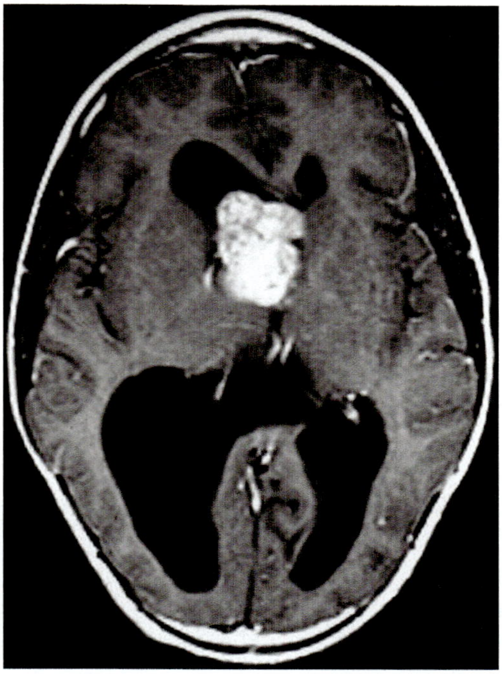

Fig. 19.4 Subependymal Giant Cell Astrocytoma (Tuberous Sclerosis) s of the type associated with en:tuberous sclerosis are typically bulky, contrast-enhancing masses in the region of the en:foramen of Monro. Most overlie the head of the en:caudate nucleus. Foramen obstruction has produced en:hydrocephalus. Image and description are from the AFIP Atlas of Tumor Pathology, according to entry #405677 in Pathology Education Instructional Resource. The Armed Forces Institute of Pathology Electronic Fascicles (CD-ROM Version of the Atlas of Tumor Pathology) contains U.S. Government work which may be used without restriction [1]. (The Armed Forces Institute of Pathology. W)

Correct Answer is: D
The MRI showed a large intraventricular mass in a child with epilepsy, mild ASD and hypo-pigmented macules. The pathology of the mass revealed numerous pleomorphic giant cells consistent with a sub-ependymal giant cell astrocytoma or SEGA. This consolation is consistent with a tuberous sclerosis complex diagnosis. SEGAs can occur in 10–15% of patients with tuberous sclerosis. It is thought that they develop from the sub ependymal nodules near the foramen of Monro.

Suggested Reading

- Jóźwiak S1, Nabbout R, Curatolo P. Participants of the TSC Consensus Meeting for SEGA and Epilepsy Management. Management of subependymal giant cell astrocytoma (SEGA) associated with tuberous sclerosis complex (TSC): clinical recommendations. Eur J Paediatr Neurol. 2013;17(4):348–52.
- Roth J, Roach ES, Bartels U, Jóźwiak S, Koenig MK, Weiner HL, Franz DN, Wang HZ Sub-ependymal giant cell astrocytoma: diagnosis, screening, and treatment. Recommendations from the International Tuberous Sclerosis Complex Consensus Conference 2012. Pediatr Neurol. 2013;49(6):439–44.

8. You are seeing a 6-year-old girl in the ED, who complains of dizziness and ataxia for the last 3 weeks. She is very scary to walk by herself and she has to hold on her parents. Her PCP diagnosed her with acute labrynthitis because she had an upper respiratory infection at the time of onset. On examination she has a left 7th nerve palsy affecting her eye and face. In addition, she has inability to abduct her right eye. She has a wide based gait and hyperreflexia with clonus. Her sagittal T1 imaging is shown below.

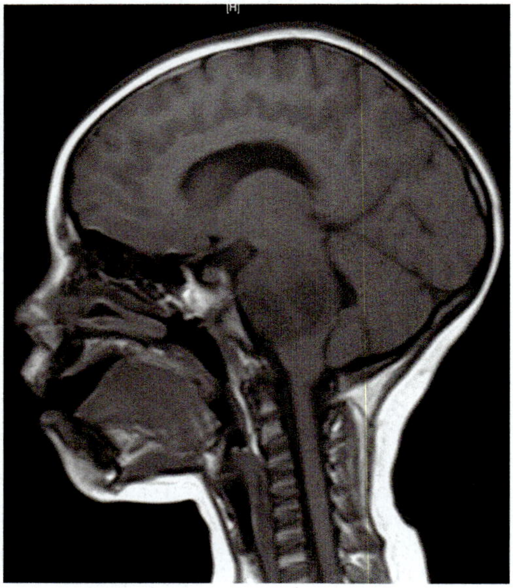

Fig. 19.5 Brainstem Glioma in 4-year-old. MRI sagittal, without contrast. (Own work. Tdvorak. W)

Which of the following statements are true?

A. Surgery followed by radiation is the conventional approach to treatment of this lesion
B. This lesion is highly radiosensitive and carries a 55% 5-year survival
C. This lesion has a high rate of metastatic spread
D. Despite treatment the median survival for this lesion less than 1 year from the time of diagnosis
E. None of the above

Correct Answer is: D

The sagittal image provided The MRI shows large and abnormal signal of the pons as well as compression of the cerebellum and obstructive hydrocephalus. This is consistent with a diagnosis of diffuse intrinsic pontine glioma. They are typically high-grade tumors with a very poor prognosis. The typical age at diagnosis is between 5 and 9 years of age. Patients typically present with ataxia, cranial nerve abnormalities or signs of increased intracranial pressure. These lesions are very hard to be surgical resected. Their response to radiation and chemotherapy is variable and short lived. The median survival is less than 1 year from diagnosis.

Suggested Reading

- Warren K. Diffuse intrinsic pontine glioma: poised for progress. Front Oncol. 2012;2:205.

9. A 12-year-old girl is brought by her family because her teacher reported to them that the girl is not listen, does not pay attention, is very distractible presented, and has a slow decline in her school performance. She has decreased hearing on examination. Her axial MRI imaging is shown below.
What is your most likely diagnosis?

A. Inflammatory pseudo tumor
B. Sarcoidosis
C. Neurofibromatosis type 2
D. Tuberous sclerosis
E. None of the above

Correct Answer is: C

The MRI shows 2 enhancing vestibular schwannomas and an extra axial mass in the right cerebellar hemisphere, most

19

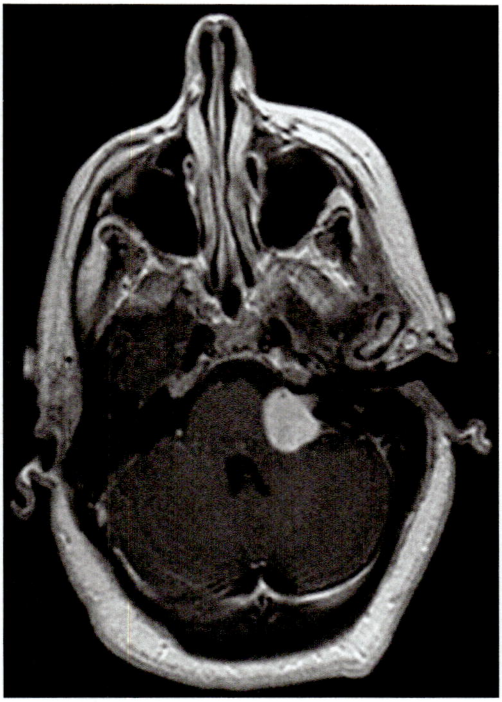

Fig. 19.6 Vestibular schwannoma. (RadsWiki. RadsWiki. W)

likely a meningioma. This is consistent with a probable diagnosis of neurofibromatosis type 2. Although NF2 is mainly an adult disorder, it can occur in the pediatric age group. The average age of onset is from 18 to 24 years. In addition to the vestibular schwannomas, patients also develop meningioma and ependymomas. This is an autosomal dominant disorder, with 50% of cases a result of a de novo mutation. Treatment has been mainly symptomatic. Bevacuzumab (Avast in) has been used to treat progressive vestibular schwannoma. Studies have shown improved hearing and tumor shrinkage.

Suggested Reading

- Evans, Gareth, D, Neurofibromatosis 2, Gene Reviews: August 18, 2011 (update).
- D Gareth R Evans Neurofibromatosis type 2 (NF2): a clinical and molecular review. Orphanet J Rare Dis. 2009;4:16.
- Plotkin SR1, Merker VL, Halpin C, Jennings D, McKenna MJ, Harris GJ, Barker FG 2nd. Bevacizumab for progressive vestibular schwannoma in neurofibromatosis type 2: a retrospective review of 31 patients. Otol Neurotol. 2012;33(6):1046–52.

10. A 7-year-old girl has a history of progressive ataxia for the last 2 months. She has been having morning vomiting for the past 2 weeks. Her MRI is shown. Treatment consisted of surgical resection. The child remains well 8 years post-operative.

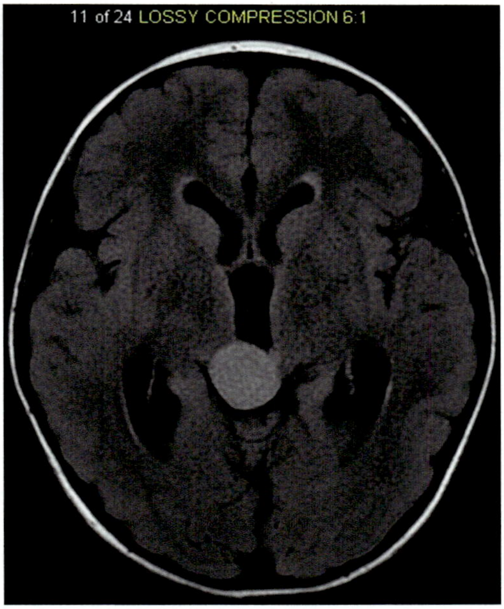

Fig. 19.7 Axial CSF suppressed FLAIR image showing a circumscribe hyperintense mass in the tectum of the brainstem presumed to be a pilocytic astrocytoma. In the course of my work as a radiologist. (Jto410. W)

What is the most likely diagnosis?

A. Choroid plexus papilloma
B. Juvenile pilocytic astrocytoma
C. Glioblastoma multiform
D. Oligodendroglia
E. None of the above

Correct Answer is: B

There is a multi-cystic enhancing lesion involving the cerebellar hemisphere on

the MRI. This is the radiological presentation of a juvenile pilocytic astrocytoma. This is the most common cerebellar tumor in children. Typical age of presentation is between 5 and 13 years old. Surgical resection is typically the only treatment that is necessary. The other choices listed may require chemotherapy and/or radiation.

Suggested Reading

- Chourmouzi D, Papadopoulou E, Konstantinidis M, Syrris V, Kouskouras K, Haritanti A, Karkavelas G, Drevelegas A. Manifestations of pilocytic astrocytoma: a pictorial review. Insights Imaging. 2014;5:387–402.

11. You are evaluating a 16-month-old girl in the ED for her 2-week history of left head tilt and decreased left facial movement. By history, she has been very irritable and clingy for the last month. In addition, her right leg has been "stiff", and she is not able to take steps or pulling to stand as before. She has normal language and fine motor skills. Her birth and past medical histories are unremarkable. On examination, she is alert but irritable. She has limited abduction, decreased blinking, and incomplete closure of her right eye; left lower facial droop; limited elevation of the left palate; leftward tongue deviation; and right lower extremity spasticity. Knee jerks are asymmetric, with a crossed adductor response on the right only. She is unable to pull to stand. Her brain MRI is shown.
    What is your most likely diagnosis?
    A. Ependymal
    B. Hemangioblastoma
    C. Medulloblastoma
    D. Pontine glioma
    E. Schwannoma

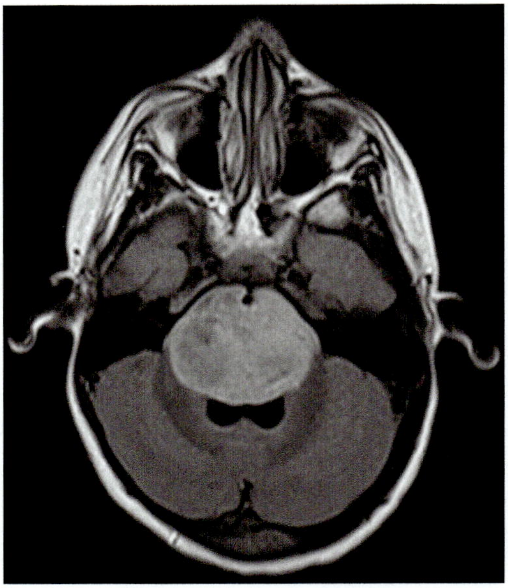

Fig. 19.8 Brain stem glioma. MRI axial, with contrast. (Own work. Tdvorak. W)

Correct Answer is: D
Diffuse intrinsic pontine gliomas account for 60–75% of all pediatric brainstem tumors, with approximately 200–300 cases diagnosed in the USA each year. The most clinical presentations of those tumors are signs of cranial nerve, long tract, and cerebellar dysfunction. The mean age at diagnosis is 7–9 years, and there is no sex predilection. Diagnosis is generally based on MR imaging with and without gadolinium. Classically, pontine gliomas are associated with diffuse infiltration and hypertrophy of the pons. They are typically >2 cm at the time of presentation. On T1-weighted sequences, they appear hypo-intense with indistinct margins; on T2-weight images, they appear hyper-intense. Administration of gadolinium results in little to no contrast enhancement. In some cases, newer imaging techniques, such as FDG-PET and diffusion tensor imaging, may aid in diagnosis and/or treatment planning. The role of stereotactic biopsy remains controversial, though it may be of benefit in cases with atypical imaging characteristics. Standard treatment remains conventional radiotherapy to a total

dose of 54–59.4 Gy, as studies conducted to assess the efficacy of hyperfractionated radiotherapy and various chemotherapeutic regimens have failed to demonstrate improved outcomes. The prognosis for pontine gliomas is dismal, with a median onset of disease progression following irradiation of <6 months, median survival of ~10 months, and prolonged survival (>/=24 months) in <10% of all patients.

Suggested Reading

- Frazier JL, Lee J, Thomale UW, Noggle JC, Cohen KJ, Jallo GI. Treatment of diffuse intrinsic brainstem gliomas: failed approaches and future strategies. A review. In J Neurosurg. 2009;3:259–69.

12. You are evaluating a 4-year-old boy with a history of strabismus for 3 weeks ago. The strabismus is just on the right eye, and occurs mainly when he is tired. There is a family history of brain tumors in 2 of his mother aunts. His brain and orbits MRI, which was ordered by an ophthalmology 1 week ago, showed enlargement and mild contrast enhancement of the right optic nerve consistent with a glioma. No involvement of the chiasm or hypothalamus is noted.

What is your next step in management?

A. Detailed skin examination
B. Lumbar puncture
C. MRI of the spinal cord
D. Surgical debulking of the left optic glioma
E. Radiation therapy

Correct Answer is: A

Optic pathway gliomas are about 3–5% of all childhood tumors. There is an extremely high incidence with neurofibromatosis, type 1. Up to 5–15% of children with NF-1 will show evidence of an optic pathway glioma by the age of 6. Conversely, of all children with optic gliomas, 50% will meet criteria for the diagnosis of NF-1. In fact, optic pathway glioma is one of the diagnostic criteria for the disorder. As part of the initial evaluation of a child with a unilateral or bilateral optic pathway glioma, a skin examination looking for other cutaneous manifestations of neurofibromatosis (café-au-lait macules, axillary freckling and neuro-fibromas) should be done. In the setting of neurofibromatosis, most optic nerve gliomas are identified on routing surveillance screening, many will not even manifest visual symptoms. Slowly progressive visual loss is the most common presenting sign in children without NF-1. Additional findings may include proptosis, nystagmus or an acquired strabismus. Examination might reveal any combination of afferent papillary defect, visual field loss and either optic atrophy or papilledema (especially in cases of extension to the hypothalamus which can lead to obstructive hydrocephalus.) In general, optic chiasm lesions and those with extension to the hypothalamus have the highest morbidity and mortality. Lesions confined to the optic nerve tend to be stable over time, with even a small percentage undergoing spontaneous resolution amongst the patients with neurofibromatosis. Treatment is therefore reserved for patients with progression of disease, which can either be clinical (progressive visual field loss) or radiologic. Radiotherapy with chemotherapy is indicated for children over the age of 5. In younger children, or in those with neurofibromatosis, chemotherapy alone may be utilized. Patients with NF have a much higher incidence of secondary malignancies after cranial irradiation due to the defective tumor suppression inherent with the disorder. There is no metastasis through the neuroaxis with optic nerve glioma, therefore imaging of the spine is not indicated. Lumbar puncture has no place in the evaluation or management of optic pathway gliomas.

Suggested Reading

- Willhelm H. Primary optic nerve tumors In Curr Opin Neurol. 2009;22(1):11–8.
- Swaiman et al. Pediatric neurology, principles and practice. 4th ed. p. 1702–3.

13. You are evaluating a 14-year-old girl for her chronic headaches for 3 years. Her headaches are bi-frontal, squeezing in nature. She has been taken ibuprofen and lay down to relief the headaches. She has no aura, phono-phobia but sometimes have photophobia. Sometimes she will have nausea. When she has the headaches, she will be a little more irritable. She has normal social interaction and cognitive performance. Her family history is remarkable for migraine, her mother and several other females on the maternal side of the family. On examination, she is at the 3rd percentile for height and the 75th percentile for weight. Neurologic examination, shows bilateral papilledema, and her visual fields show inconsistent finger counting in the left temporal field. Basic laboratory studies, sodium is 158 mEq/L, potassium 4.2 mEq/L. Urine is dilute, with a specific gravity of 1.003. Her head CT shows a 5×4 cm partially calcified mass in the sellar region.

What is the most likely diagnosis?

A. Craniopharyngioma
B. Dysembryoplastic neuroepithelial tumor (DNET)
C. Medulloblastoma
D. Oligodendroglioma
E. Pleomorphic Xanthroastrocytoma (PXA)

Correct Answer is: A

The typical location for craniopharyngioma is the sellar region.

Medulloblastoma occurs in the posterior fossa, and DNET, oligodendroglioma and PXA occur in the cerebral cortex.

The most common manifestations of the sellar and supra-sellar region are, headache, visual field defects (classically bitemporal hemianopia) and endocrine abnormalities. Craniopharygioma, pituitary adenoma, optic pathway glioma, meningioma, epidermoid/dermoid, teratoma and hypothalamic hamartoma are the most common sellar and suprasellar region. Aneurysms/ arteriovenous malformation, granulomatous lesions associated with sarcoidosis or tuberculosis and congenital arachnoid cysts should be included in the differential diagnosis. Imaging, sometimes including magnetic resonance arteriography, should help distinguish tumor from other lesions.

Craniopharyngiomas account for 5% of all childhood brain tumors. These very slow-growing tumors are believed to originate from embryonic rest cells near Rathke's pouch. Due to the indolent nature, symptoms are often present for 1–2 years prior to the identification of the tumor. Headache can result from direct effects of the tumor itself or as a result of increased intracranial pressure due to obstruction of either the third ventricle or foramen of Monro. Visual disturbance are quite common, frank visual field abnormalities depend on whether the tumor affects pre-chiamal, chiasmal or post chiasmal pathways. In the past, endocrine abnormalities contributed to a majority of the morbidity and mortality of the tumor. Thyroid and growth hormone deficiencies, as well as diabetes insipidus, tend to be more consistent concomitant disorders, though any aspect of the hypothalamic/pituitary axis may be affected. Post-operatively, morbid obesity due to hyperphagia, is a striking complication. Radiologic appearance is varied though classically reveals a sellar/supra-sellar mass that is partially solid, with cystic components. Calcification is observed in up to 80% of the patients.

Treatment is depending on the degree of infiltration of the hypothalamus, optic nerve/chiasm and carotid arteries. If gross total resection is possible, this provides the least chance of tumor recurrence. On the other hand, partial resection with adjunctive radiation therapy (currently using stereotactic or gamma knife technology) is the treatment of choice if total resection is not possible. In younger children, radiation therapy may be delayed until recurrence or progression is noted. Systemic chemotherapy has no role in management of craniopharyngioma, though for tumors of primarily cystic nature, intra-cystic Bleomycin has been utilized. Overall, the tumor itself tends to be fairly benign, with only rare reports of metastasis, but the endocrinologic, visual and cognitive effects of both the tumor and the late effects of treatment can cause significant quality of life issues.

Suggested Reading

- Garnett et al. Craniopharyngioma. In Orphaned J Rare Dis. 2007;2:18.

14. You are evaluating a 3-year-old girl for her progressive loss of balance control for 1 week. Two days ago, she developed jerking movements in the arms and legs. She started walking independently at 12 months of age, but last week she became too unsteady to walk and even struggled to sit up independently. You ordered a brain MRI with contrast and a lumbar puncture, both were normal. On examination, she has some multidirectional rapid eye oscillation movements, spontaneously and at times gaze-evoked. You strongly suspect a paraneoplastic syndrome.

    What is the most likely neoplasm to be found in this girl?

    A. Acute myeloid leukemia
    B. Angiomyolipoma
    C. Craniopharyngioma
    D. Neuroblastoma
    E. Ovarian teratoma

Correct Answer is: D

This is a classic presentation of opsoclonus-myoclonus syndrome (OMS). Most cases occur in preschool age children, but it can occur throughout the life span. The usual presentation is either acute or subacute and progressive ataxia, raising the suspicious of acute cerebellar disease due to toxins, post-infectious inflammation, infection or tumor. The characteristic finding of opsoclonus (involuntary multidirectional saccades without inter-saccadic intervals) may not be identified for days or even weeks into the course of the disease. Truncal and extremity myoclonus typically presents early on, though can be subtle, and often confused for seizures. Behavioral changes, sleep dysfunction, and psychomotor retardation are common in affected children. About 50% of cases to be paraneoplastic in nature, secondary to a neuroblastoma, with the remainder of patients felt to have a post-infectious etiology. A well-defined antibody has not been identified in pediatric cases. In adults, the most commonly associated cancers are small-cell lung cancer and gynecologic and breast cancers. Rarely, acute infectious encephalitis can produce opsoclonus, though not typically the entire spectrum of neurologic disease seen in OMS. Treatment of this syndrome can be very challenging. In paraneoplastic cases, removal of the tumor (and at times adjuvant chemotherapy) is indicated, but unlikely to produce neurologic remission. A combined immunomodulatory regimen, including high-dose corticosteroids (or ACTH), intravenous immune globulin, and rituximab is often applied, with varying degrees of success. Though the motor manifestations will

improve with time with effective treatment, a chronic static encephalopathy often results. Ovarian teratoma has been associated with anti-NMDA receptor encephalitis in children, there has not been a well-established para-neoplastic syndrome associated with leukemia, craniopharyngioma or angiomyolipoma.

Suggested Reading

- Rosenfeld MR, Dalmau JO. Paraneoplastic Disorders of the CNS and Autoimmune Synaptic Encephalitis. Continuum Lifelong.

15. A 14-year-old boy has been evaluated for gait ataxia. On neurologic examination, he has truncal and extremity ataxia, oculomotor apraxia, intermittent extremity dystonia and chorea, and multiple scleral telangiectasias. His mother stated that his eyes have seemed progressively more "bloodshot" over the past year. His past medical history is remarkable for frequent pulmonary infections. Family history is remarkable of a 10-year-old brother is similarly affected.

    What serum screening tests is most likely to be abnormal in this case?

    A. alpha-fetoprotein
    B. ammonia
    C. creatine kinase
    D. lactate
    E. uric acid

Correct Answer is: A

Patients in this case have ataxia-telangiectasia, an autosomal recessive condition with childhood onset causing ataxia, oculomotor apraxia, choreoathetosis and dystonia, and telangiectasias on skin and conjunctivae. Immunodeficiency and susceptibility to cancer (especially lymphoma and leukemia) are significant causes of morbidity and mortality. An elevated alpha-fetoprotein level (over 90%) can help in diagnosis, and genetic testing of the ATM gene is available for confirmatory diagnosis.

19

Suggested Reading

- Pandolfo M, Mando M. Cerebellar and Afferent Ataxias. Continuum (Minneap Minn) 2013;19(5):1312–134. Arning Neurol 2012;18(2):366–83.

16. The gadolinium-enhanced T-1 weighted sagittal brain MRIs for a patient complaining of headache and ataxia. It has a posterior fossa mass. Surgical resections have been done.

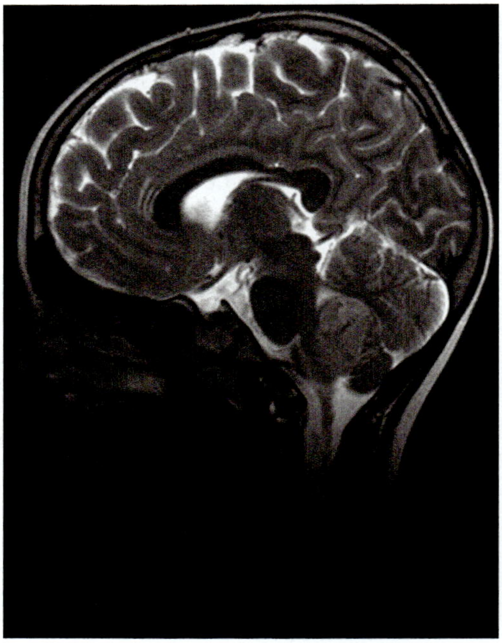

Fig. 19.9 Anaplastisches Ependymom. MRT in verschiedenen Wichtungen und Ebenen. (Own work. Hellerhoff. W)

What is your most likely diagnosis?

A. Choroid plexus neoplasm
B. Ependymoma
C. Meningioma
D. Metastatic neoplasm
E. Sub-ependymoma

Correct Answer is: B

Ependymomas account for 3–5% of intracranial neoplasms. They arise from the ventricular wall, and 60% occur in the posterior fossa, approximately half of which are intraventricular. The radiologi-

cal features consist of iso- to hypo-intensity on T1-weighted images and iso- to hyper-intensity on T2-weighted images with heterogeneous enhancement. Cystic components, calcification, or hemorrhage may be present. The lesions are less likely to be sub-ependymomas, which, even though many occur in the fourth ventricle, are much rarer, accounting for only 0.2–0.7% of intracranial neoplasms. Ependymomas also tend to be well-circumscribed and have minimal enhancement. Whereas 40% of choroid plexus neoplasms occur in the fourth ventricle, unlike Ependymomas, they tend to be highly vascular with intense contrast enhancement. Metastatic neoplasms occur rarely in the 4th ventricle and are more likely to manifest surrounding vasogenic edema. Meningiomas also occur rarely in the fourth ventricle, tend to be more globular in shape, and are iso- to hypo-intense on T1-weighted images.

Suggested Reading

- Smith AB, Smirniotopoulos JG, Horkanyne-Szakaly I. From the radiologic pathology archieves: intraventricular neoplasms: radiologic-pathologic correlation. Radiographics. 2013;33:21–43.

17. A 14-year-old female came to your office complaining of right periorbital headache with progressive visual loss. On examination, she has a slight right proptosis, visual acuity 20/70 in the right eye and 20/20 in the left eye, a right sided afferent pupillary defect. On her funduscopic examination, she has a few tiny pigmented nodules

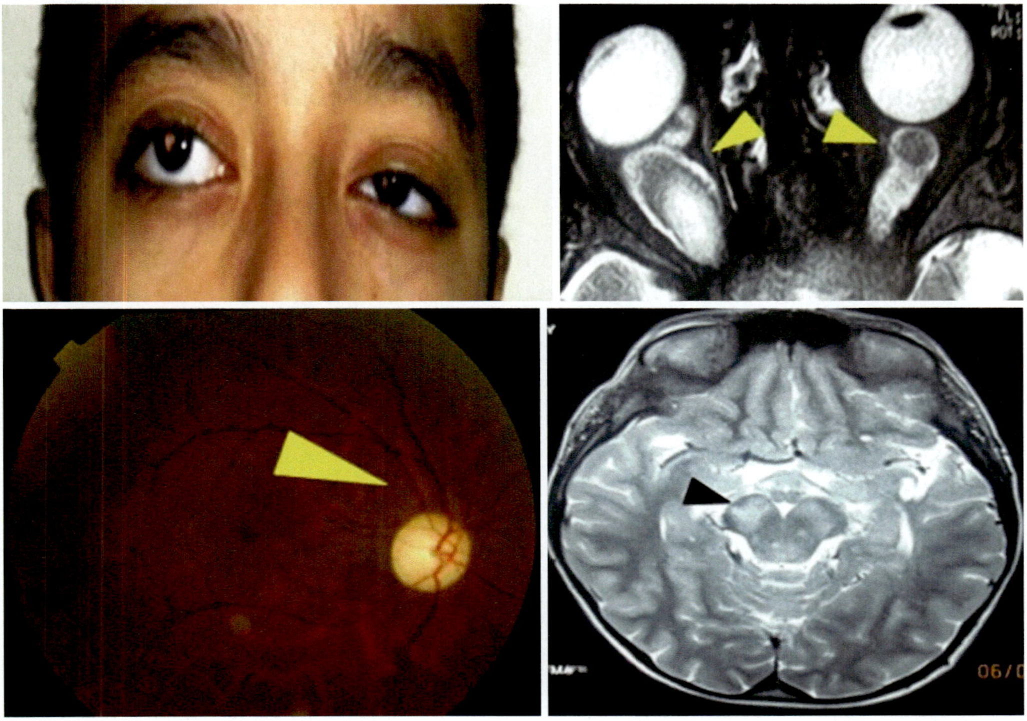

Figs. 19.10, 19.11, 19.12 and 19.13 Gliomas of both optic nerve in boy with NF type 1. ► https://openi.nlm.nih.gov/detailedresult.php?img=4189867_PAMJ-17-256-g001&query=optic+nerve+glioma&it=xg&lic=by&req=4&npos=28. (Handor H., Laghmari M., Hafidi Z., Daoudi R. W)

involving the iris. On her skin exam, she has multiple 2 cm, coffee-colored pigmented nevi are present on the trunk and lower extremities. Brain MRI is performed shown.

What is your most likely diagnosis?

A. Optic nerve glioma
B. Orbital Pseudo-tumor
C. Orbital rhabdomyosarcoma
D. Orbital sarcoidosis
E. Pseudo-tumor cerebri

Correct Answer is: A

The MRI shows optic nerve glioma. It is the most common CNS tumor associated with neurofibromatosis type 1 (NF1).

Diagnostic criteria for NF1, or von Recklinghausen disease, include having any two or more of:

(1) 6 or more café-au-lait spots, (2) two or more Lisch nodules (pigmented nodules on the iris), (3) optic glioma, (4) two or more neuro-fibromas or one plexiform neuro-fibroma, (5) a first degree relative with NF1, or (6) sphenoid dysplasia.

Majority of cases occurring in the first decade of life (peak incidence age 1–3), with over 90% of cases in the first two decades of life. 25% optic gliomas are associated with neurofibromatosis, and 15% of patients with NF1 will develop optic nerve and/or chiasmal tumors.

Manifestations of progressive visual loss in young children may be difficult to detect, and yearly routine ophthalmologic surveillance is recommended. Acquired strabismus or nystagmus in young children with NF1 should prompt immediate investigation for such a lesion.

Orbital sarcoidosis is one of the differential diagnosis of an optic nerve mass, but there is no skin and iris findings are found; patients may have chest x-ray abnormalities and elevated angiotensin converting enzyme.

19

Orbital Pseudo-tumor is an inflammatory disorder affecting the extraocular muscles, not the optic nerve.

Pseudo-tumor cerebri can cause pressure on the optic nerves and place vision at risk secondary to increased intracranial pressure; MRI findings may include optic nerve sheath edema; but skin and iris abnormalities are not seen.

Rhabdomyosarcoma is a rare soft tissue tumor that typically arises in the head and neck region or genitourinary tract, with 8% of tumors involving the orbit, but this tumor is not associated with the skin and iris findings as described, and most cases occur in children.

Suggested Reading

- Islam MP, Roach S. Neurocutaneous syndromes. In: RB Daroff, GM Fenichel, J Jankovic, JC Mazziotta, editors. Bradley's neurology in clinical practice. 6th ed. Elsevier; 2012. p. 1514–7.
- Elomrani F, Touri S, Ouziane I, et al. Orbital rhabdomyosarcoma with skin metastasis: a case report. BMC Res Notes. 2014;7:670.
- Van Stavern G. Metabolic, Hereditary, Traumatic, and Neoplastic Optic Neuropathies. Continuum (Minneap Minn). 2014;20(4):877–906.

18. A 17-year-old female is complaining of progressive hearing loss and gait instability for the last 2 years. On examination, she has significant bilateral sensorineural hearing loss, moderate bilateral lower motor neuron facial weakness, and a mildly wide-based gait with a positive Romberg testing with her eyes closed. She had an audiometry testing few years ago revealed significant bilateral hearing loss and hearing aids did not significantly help her. MRI is demonstrated (contrast and non-contrast).

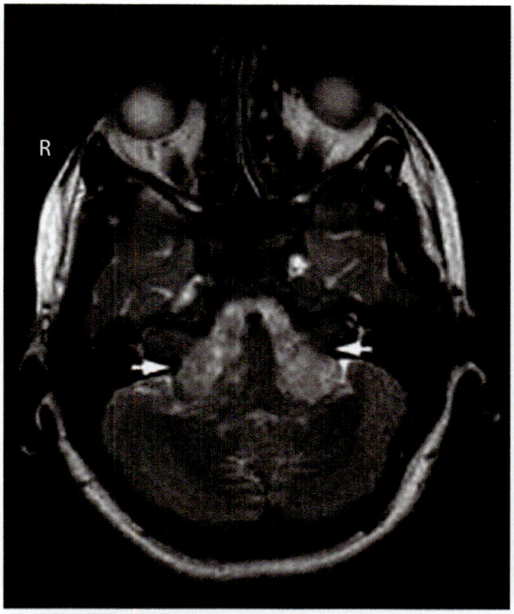

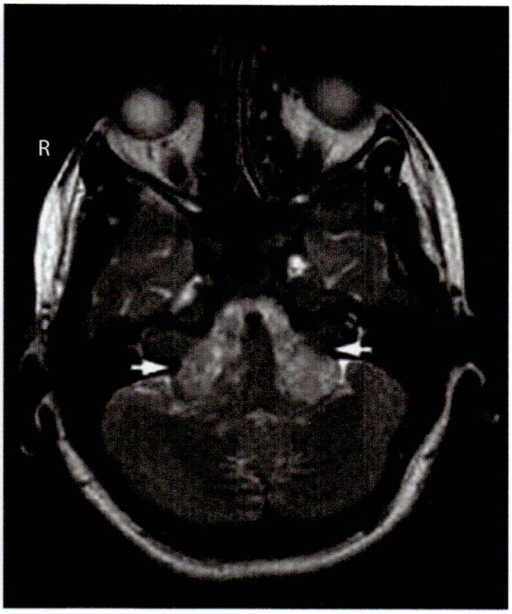

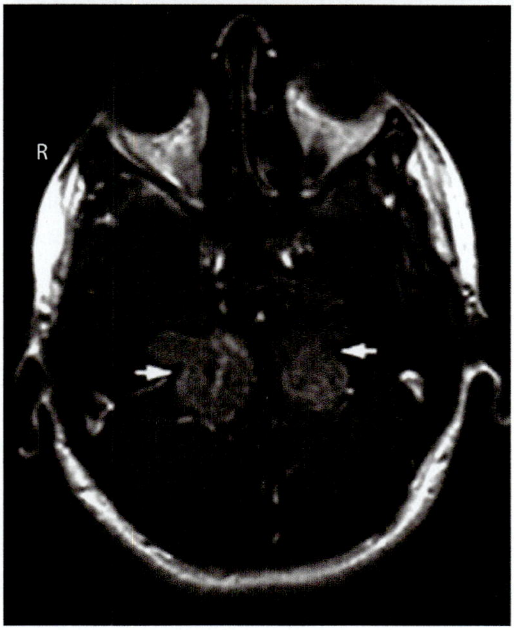

Figs. 19.14, 19.15 and 19.16 American Academy of Neurology Institute, produced by permission

What is your diagnosis?

A. Ataxia Telangiectasia
B. Neurofibromatosis type 2
C. Neurofibromatosis type I
D. Sturge-Weber syndrome
E. Tuberous Sclerosis Complex

Correct Answer is: B

NF2 is an autosomal dominant condition caused by mutation in the Merlin gene. Affected patients are at very high risk for acoustic neuromas (usually bilateral). Other features include juvenile cataracts

and increased risk for other tumors such as meningiomas and gliomas. On the other hand, NF2 cutaneous manifestations are not characteristic like NF1. The MRI shows large bilateral cerebellopontine angle lesions, which were consistent with acoustic neuromas. All of the other conditions listed are well-characterized neuro-cutaneous syndromes. Tuberous Sclerosis complex is associated with subependymal giant cell astrocytomas, but not acoustic neuromas.

Suggested Reading

- Mattox DE. Assessment and management of tinnitus and hearing loss. Continuum Lifelong Learning Neurol. 2006;12(4): 135–50.
- Nandhagopal R, et al. Teaching NeuroImages: vestibular schwannomas in neurofibromatosis type 2. Neurology. 2010;75.14.

19. You are seeing a 6-year-old boy in the ED with a history of progressive vomiting and headache for 3 days. He has no history of fever and has no previous history of headaches. Medical history is unremarkable. On examination, he is lethargic, he can speak but in a slow and staccato quality. He has gaze evoked nystagmus with attempts at horizontal gaze. Fundus exam is normal. Motor exam shows appropriate. He has normal tone and strength while in bed, but he is too unsteady to sit on his own. He has bilateral finger-nose-finger dysmetria. Brain MRI with a gadolinium-enhanced T1-weighted image is shown. **Which of the following tumors is most likely given the patient's age, neurologic findings and imaging results?**
    A. Dysembryoplastic Neuroepithelial tumor (DNET)
    B. Ganglioglioma
    C. Medulloblastoma
    D. Oligodendroglioma
    E. Pleomorphic Xanthoastrocytoma

19

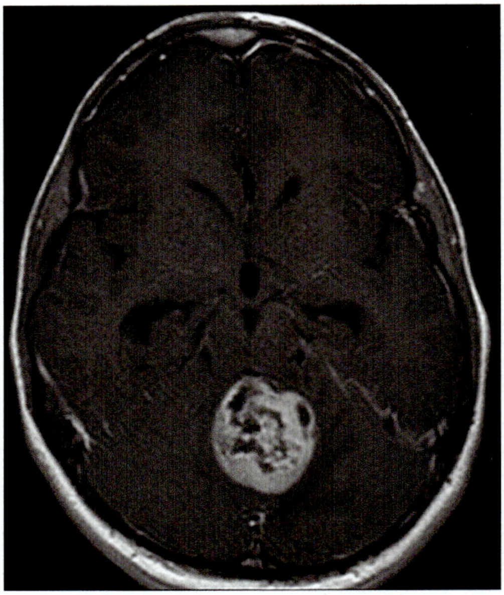

Fig. 19.17 American Academy of Neurology Institute, produced by permission

Correct Answer is: C

MRI shows signs of both midline and hemispheric cerebellar compromise and a diffusely enhancing mass in the region of the fourth ventricle. Medulloblastoma is the only tumor from the above list would occur in the posterior fossa. Posterior fossa is the most common area in almost 85% of primary brain tumors in children between the ages of 2 and 12. Medulloblastoma, juvenile pilocytic astrocytoma (JPA), and ependymoma and brainstem glioma are the four most common tumors in this region in childhood. The rest of tumors mentioned are supra-tentorial region tumors, mainly in the temporal lobes, and present with complex partial seizures or progressive focal motor deficits. Medulloblastoma is a primary neuroectodermal tumor (PNET) of the posterior fossa, usually in the region of the cerebellar vermis or 4th ventricle. 90% occur in children under the age of 10. These are rapidly growing tumors, usually with a short period of time between symptom onset

and diagnosis. The most presenting symptoms are headache, vomiting, unsteady gait and torticollis or stiff neck. Limb dysmetria is also noted. Papilledema occurs in 2/3 of patients due to hydrocephalus secondary to obstruction of outflow through the compressed 4th ventricle or cerebral aqueduct. In this setting, limb spasticity and/or brisk reflexes may also be present. The overall 5-year survival rate is approximately 40%, though this number is higher in children who undergo a gross total resection. Craniospinal irradiation and chemotherapy are commonly utilized after surgery. Dissemination through the neuro axis is possible, including drop metastases to the spinal cord and nerve roots.

Suggested Reading

- Fenichel GM. Clinical pediatric neurology. 6th ed. Philadelphia: Saunders Elsevier; 2009. p. 237–40.
- Dhall G. Medulloblastoma. J Child Neurol. 2009;24(11):1418–30.

20. You are evaluating a 7-year-old boy with 3-week history of headaches. He has generalized upon awaking in the morning headache. He complains of increased difficulty seeing the blackboard in school and while reading. His physical exam is remarkable for short stature. On neurological examination he has restricted peripheral vision, visual acuity in the right is 20/30 and left eye is 20/40 with signs of optic atrophy bilaterally.

What is your most likely diagnosis?

A. Hypothalamic hamartoma
B. Pituitary apoplexy
C. Craniopharyngioma
D. Optic neuritis

Correct Answer is: C

Craniopharyngioma is a supra-sellar tumor that compresses the medial aspect of the optic chiasm and hypothalamus. Peak age is 6–14 years, and the symptom onset is insidious and progression is slow. Progressive visual impairment (bi-temporal hemianopia in 50%), delayed sexual maturation, growth delay and diabetes insipidus are the most common symptoms. Headache and papilledema occur in 25% secondary to hydrocephalus.

Hypothalamic hamartoma is a non-progressive, benign tumor that results in a syndrome characterized by medically refractory seizures (including gelastic seizures), developmental delays and psychiatric symptoms.

Pituitary apoplexy is caused by a hemorrhage into the pituitary gland causing a sudden onset of headache, ophthalmoplegia, altered mental status and hormonal dysfunction. Eye pain and blurred vision that can progress to partial or total blindness in hours to days. In adults it is monocular, but in children up to 50% of the cases are binocular.

Suggested Reading

- Zada G, Lopes BS, Mukundan S Jr, Laws E Jr. Craniopharyngiomas. In Atlas of Sellar and Parasellar Lesions. Springer International Publishing; 2016. p. 197–210.

21. This is a histopathologic specimen from an 8-year-old boy with intractable epilepsy underwent temporal lobectomy.

Which statement below is incorrect regarding this tumor?

A. Most common location is the temporal lobe
B. This lesion often has a cortical or juxta-cortical location
C. Floating neurons are characteristic of this lesion
D. It is a WHO grade I tumor
E. on MRI, it has a heterogeneous contrast-enhancing pattern

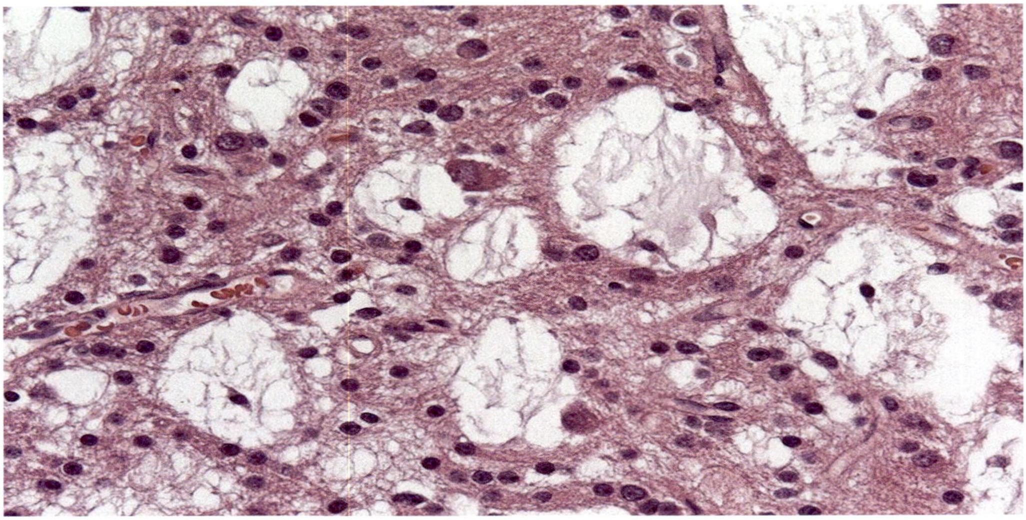

Fig. 19.18 Dyembryoplastic Neuroepithelial tumour (DNET). (Own work. Sbrandner. W)

Correct Answer is: E
This is typical pathologic features of dysembryoplastic neuroepithelial tumor (DNET), showing prominent clear spaces that seem to contain ganglion cells. In between these clear spaces, there are multiple cells and a glial component that resembles an oligodendroglioma. DNET is a benign superficial tumor that is an important cause of refractory seizures in children. These tumors are located in the cortical or juxta-cortical region, most commonly in the temporal lobe. The MRI shows a nodular or cystic lesion that is hyperintense on T2-weighted images and does not enhance with contrast. It grows very slowly, and macroscopically, it has a multinodular architecture, with mucinous cysts. Histologically, it is seen as multiple areas in which ganglion cells appear to float within mucin-filled spaces ("floating neurons"). In between these nodules, there is a component with more glial characteristics, sometimes resembling an oligodendroglioma. At the edges of these lesions, there may be cortical dysplasia. DNET is a WHO grade I tumor, and surgical resection is helpful for the cure or control of the seizures.

Suggested Reading

- Prayson RA, GoldblumJR. Neuropathology. 1st ed. Philadelphia: Elsevier; 2005.
- Ropper AH, Samuels MA. Adams and Victor's principles of neurology. 9th ed. New York: McGraw-Hill; 2009.
- Comprehensive Review in Clinical Neurology: A Multiple-Choice Question Book for the Wards and Boards © 2011 Wolters Kluwer Health Lippincott Williams & Wilkins. All rights reserve.

22. Which of the following pineal region tumors is most likely to have an excellent prognosis?
    A. Embryonal carcinoma
    B. Mixed germ cell tumor
    C. Yolk sac tumor
    D. Germinoma

Correct Answer is: D
Germinoma has the best prognosis of all the choices. Non-germinomatous germ cell

19

tumors include teratoma, embryonal carcinoma, yolk sac tumor, choriocarcinoma, and mixed germ cell tumor. Mature teratoma may also have an excellent prognosis, but this is not one of the answer choices. Choriocarcinoma and mixed germ cell tumors both have intermediate prognoses.

Embryonal carcinoma and Yolk sac tumor are a non-germinomatous germ cell tumor with a poor and worst prognosis.

Mixed germ cell tumor is a non-germinomatous germ cell tumor with an intermediate prognosis.

Suggested Reading

- Dhall G. Medulloblastoma. J Child Neurol. 2009;24(11):1418–30.
- Wells EM, Packer RJ. Pediatric brain tumors. Continuum: Lifelong Learning Neurol. 2015;21(2):373–96.
- Cohen KJ, Heideman RL, Zhou T, Holmes EJ, Lavey RS, Bouffet E, Pollack IF. Temozolomide in the treatment of children with newly diagnosed diffuse intrinsic pontine gliomas: a report from the Children's Oncology Group. Neuro-Oncology. 2011;13(4):410–6.
- Fujimaki T. Central nervous system germ cell tumors: classification, clinical features, and treatment with a historical overview. J Child Neurol. 2009;24(11):1439–45.
- Frappaz D, Center CF, Szathmari A, Valsijevic A, Mottolese C. The management of pineal tumors as a model for a multidisciplinary approach in neuro-oncology. Neurochirurgie. 2015;61(2):208–11.
- Faure-Conter C. Tumoral markers in tumors of the pineal region. Neurochirurgie 2015;61(2):143–5.
- Daras M, Kaley TJ. Benign brain tumors and tumors associated with phakomatoses. Continuum: Lifelong Learning Neurol. 2015;21(2):397–414.
- Pajtler KW, Witt H, Sill M, et al. Molecular classification of ependymal tumors across All CNS Compartments, Histopathological Grades, and Age Groups. Cancer Cell. 2015;27:728–43.
- Thompson YY, Ramaswamy V, Diamandis P, Daniels C, Taylor MD. Posterior fossa ependymoma: current insights. Childs Nerv Syst. 2015;31(10):1699–706.
- Korshunov A, Witt H,Hielscher T, Benner A, Remke M, Ryzhova M, Milde T, Bender S, Wittmann A, Schettler A, Kulozik AE, Witt 0, Deimling AV, Lichter P, Pfister S. Molecular staging of intracranial ependymoma in children and adults. J Clin Oncol. 2010;28(19):3182–90.
- Collins P, Jones DTW, Giannini C. Pilocytic astrocytoma: pathology, molecular mechanisms, and markers. Acta Neuropathol. 2015;129(6):775–88.

23. Corticosteroids are used for the treatment of intracranial hypertension associated with which of the following etiologies?
    - A. Traumatic brain injury
    - B. Intracerebral hemorrhage
    - C. Ischemic stroke
    - D. Acute obstructive hydrocephalus
    - E. Brain tumors

Correct Answer is: E

Corticosteroids are used for the treatment of intracranial hypertension associated with primary brain tumors and metastasis to the brain. Corticosteroids are beneficial in vasogenic cerebral edema as is seen with intracranial tumors, either primary or metastatic. However, the exact mechanism of action of steroids in vasogenic edema is not well understood. Available evidence suggests that corticosteroids are not useful in the management of other conditions commonly associated with cerebral edema such as traumatic brain injury, intracerebral hemorrhage, or ischemic stroke. This is explained in part by the difference in the type of edema seen in the latter conditions. Acute obstructive hydrocephalus requires a neurosurgical intervention.

Suggested Reading

- Suarez JI. Critical care neurology and neurosurgery. In: Totowa, NJ editor. 1st ed. Humana Press; 2004.
- Comprehensive Review in Clinical Neurology: A Multiple-Choice Question Book for the Wards and Boards ©2011 Wolters Kluwer Health Lippincott Williams & Wilkins. All rights reserved.

24. Which of the following tumors does not typically present with seizures?
    - A. Ganglioglioma
    - B. Dysembryoplastic neuroepithelial tumor
    - C. Oligodendroglioma
    - D. Ependymoma
    - E. Astrocytoma

Correct Answer is: D

Seizures are not common with Ependymoma. Ependymoma is the third most common CNS tumor in children, and 90% occur intracranially, most commonly in the infra-tentorial region, typically in the fourth ventricle. Hydrocephalus is the most common manifestations because those tumors obstruct the CSF flow because of their location and cause increased intracranial pressure. Ependymomas in the supra-tentorial region occur in the periventricular region, but they may uncommonly be more superficial.

Ependymomas can also occur in the spinal cord, more commonly in adults. Ganglioglioma, dysembryoplastic neuroepithelial tumors, oligodendrogliomas, and astrocytomas frequently present with seizures.

Suggested Reading

- Bradley WG, Daroff RB, Fenichel GM, et al. Neurology in clinical practice. 5th ed. Philadelphia: Elsevier; 2008.
- Prayson RA, Goldblum JR. Neuropathology. 1st ed. Philadelphia: Elsevier; 2005.
- Comprehensive Review in Clinical Neurology: A Multiple-Choice Question Book for the Wards and Boards ©2011 Wolters Kluwer Health Lippincott Williams & Wilkins. All rights reserved.

25. You are evaluating an 11-year-old boy with a history of headaches. On examination, he has restriction of voluntary up gaze and his pupils are more responsive to accommodation than to light. Hyper-intense enhancing mass in the pineal region is noted on T2 flair MRI.

    What is your next step in management?
    - A. Biopsy of the mass
    - B. Surgical resection followed by chemotherapy
    - C. Surgical resection followed by chemotherapy and radiation
    - D. Serum levels of beta human chorionic gonadotropin (beta-HCG) and alpha fetoprotein (AFP) levels in serum and cerebrospinal fluid
    - E. Recheck MRI in 1 month

Correct Answer is: D

Pineoblastoma, pineal parenchymal tumor, germ cell tumor, and astrocytoma are common pineal region tumors in the pediatric age group. Beta -HCG and AFP levels in the serum and CSF should be checked before performing a biopsy on some suspected germ cell tumors, because biopsy or surgery can be avoided.

Germinomas are often associated with slight elevation of beta-HCG, usually under 25 international units (IU) per liter.

Choriocarcinoma (nongerminomatous germ cell tumor) is typically associated with elevations in beta-HCG while yolk sac tumors are associated with AFP elevation.

Mixed germ cell tumors may have elevations in both AFP and beta-HCG while teratomas, particularly mature teratomas, are often non- secreting.

When a pineal region tumor is noted, and a germ cell tumor suspected, the first step in management is measurement of beta-HCG and AFP levels in CSF and serum. If beta-HCG are elevated to at least 50 IU/L, and/ or AFP is elevated, a biopsy is often not necessary and the diagnosis of non germinomatous germ cell tumor can be made.

Serum and CSF levels of AFP and beta HCG should be obtained. If these levels are normal biopsy might be necessary.

Surgical resection is important in the management of mature teratomas, but its role in prolonging survival in germinomas and other nongerminomatous germ cell tumors is unclear.

Again, serum and CSF levels of AFP and beta HCG should be obtained initially. Surgical resection is important in management of mature teratomas, while others are treated with chemotherapy and radiation alone.

Serum and CSF levels of AFP and beta HCG should be obtained; a follow up MRI is not the best option.

Suggested Reading

- Dhall G. Medulloblastoma. J Child Neurol. 2009;24(11):1418–30.
- Wells EM, Packer RJ. Pediatric brain tumors. Continuum: Lifelong Learning Neurol. 2015;21(2):373–96.
- Cohen KJ, Heideman RL, Zhou T, Holmes EJ, Lavey RS, Bouffet E, Pollack IF. Temozolomi de in the treatment of children with newly diagnosed diffuse intrinsic pontine gliomas: a report from the Children's Oncology Group. Neuro-Oncology. 2011;13(4):410–6.
- Fujimaki T. Central nervous system germ cell tumors: classification, clinical features, and treatment with a historical overview. J Child Neurol. 2009;24(11):1439–45.
- Frappaz D, Conter CF, Szathmari A. Valsijevic A. Mottolese C. Themanagement of pineal tumors as a model for a multidisciplinary approach in neuro-oncology. Neurochirurgie. 2015;61(2):208–11.
- Faure-Conter C. Tumoral Markers in Tumors of the Pineal Region Neurochirurgie. 2015;61(2):143–5.
- Daras M, Kaley TJ. Benign brain tumors and tumors associated With phakomatoses. Continuum: Lifelong Learning in Neurol. 2015;21(2):397–414.
- Pajtler KW, Witt H, Sill M, et al. Molecular classification of ependymal tumors across All CNS Compartments, Histopathologi cal Grades, and Age Groups. Cancer Cell. 2015;27:728–43.
- Thompson YY, Ramaswamy V, Diamandis P, Daniels C, Taylor MD. Posterior fossa ependymoma: current insights. Childs Nerv Syst. 2015;31(10):1699–706.
- Korshunov A. Witt H, Hielscher T, Benner Remke M, Ryzhova M, Milde T, Bender S, Wittmann A, Schettler A, Kulozik AE, Witt 0, Deimling AV, Lichter P, Pfister S. Molecular Staging of lntracranial Ependymoma in Children and Adults. J Clin Oncol. 2010;28(19):3182–90.
- Collins P, Jones DTW, Giannini C. Pilocytic astrocytoma: pathology, molecular mechanisms, and markers. Acta Neuropathol. 2015;129(6):775–88.
- Recht LO, van den Bent M, Shih H. Management of low grade glioma. Wen PY, Loeffler JS, Eichler AF, editors. Up-to-date 2015.
- Quaglietta L, Vitale V, Verrico A, Migliorati R, Ozek M, Cinalli G, Maixner W, Sainte-Rose C. Treatment of Medulloblastoma: Chemotherapy. In: Posterior Fossa Tumors in Children. Cham: Springer International Publishing; 2015. p. 349–61.
- Nolan CP, DeAngelis LM. Neurological complications of chemotherapy and radiation therapy. Wen PY, ed. Continuum: Lifelong Learning in Neurol 2015;21(2).
- Legault G, Allen JC. Germ cell tumors and other pineal region tumors. In: Packer RJ, Schiff D, editors. Neuro-Oncology. 1st ed.

Hoboken: Wiley-Blackwell; 2012. p. 95–102.
- Alexiou GA, Varela M, Prodromou N. Management of pineal region tumours in children. J Solid Tumors. 2012;2(2).
- Packer, RJ. Embryonal Tumors. In: Packer RJ, Schiff D, editors. Neuro-Oncology. 1st ed. Hoboken: Wiley-Blackwell; 2012. p. 157–66.

26. A newborn girl with megaencephaly has a prenatal ultrasound showed mass growing in both lateral ventricles.
What is the most likely diagnosis?
A. Ependymoma
B. Craniopharygioma
C. Teratoma
D. Meningioma

Correct Answer is: C
Intracranial teratomas account for 50% of all congenital brain tumors. Teratomas are benign tumors and consist of all 3 germinal layers. Brain teratomas are also commonly located in the pineal, supra-cellar and cerebellar regions. Other less common congenital tumors include astrocytomas, choroid plexus papilloma, primitive neuroectodermal tumors, rhabdoid tumors, and medulloblastomas.

Congenital ependymomas are very rare but do occur in the ventricles.

Congenital craniopharygiomas are rare and located in near the pituitary stalk.

Congenital meningiomas are extremely rare and do not develop in the ventricles.

Suggested Reading

- Severino M. Congenital tumors of the central nervous system. Neuroradiology. 2010. 52(6):531–48.

19

27. You are seeing a 9-year-old boy for his headache. You examined him and you noted that, he has limited voluntary up gaze and when he attempted to follow your finger upwards, his eyes were noted to retract. His MRI shows a heterogeneously enhancing pineal region tumor. You ordered alpha fetoprotein (AFP) and beta human chorionic gonadotropin (beta HCG) in serum and cerebrospinal fluid. AFP is markedly elevated while beta HCG is within normal limits. You started him on carboplatin and etoposide, alternating with ifosfamide and etoposide. Although AFP levels normalize, tumor growth is noted on imaging.
What is the most likely cause?
A. Regrowth of the patient's existing germinom
B. Regrowth of the patient's existing nongerminomatous germ cell tumor
C. Growing teratoma syndrome
D. Growing germinoma syndrome

Correct Answer is: C
This is a presentation of nongerminomatous germ cell tumor based on the boys' initial labs, and imaging findings. Typically, germinomas are associated with mild elevations in beta HCG. Yolk sac tumors and choriocarcinomas are both nongerminomatous germ cell tumors. Yolk sac tumors are associated with high levels of AFP while choriocarcinomas are associated with high levels of beta hCG. The boy is most likely having a yolk sac tumor because his elevated AFP and normal beta HCG. These are often treated with a combination of radiation and chemotherapy. Growing teratoma syndrome occurs in about 21% of intracranial nongerminomatous germ cell tumors, usually during treatment. Often, growth on MRI, accompanied by normalization of serum and CSF markers is noted. This is typically managed with maximal surgical resection and radiotherapy.

Germinomas are typically associated with mild elevations in beta HCG, not marked elevations of AFP.

Normalization of serum and CSF AFP levels with growth on imaging is consistent with growing teratoma syndrome; regrowth of the original tumor would be associated with continued increases in AFP.

The patient's most probable initial diagnosis is nongerminomatous germ cell tumor. Growing germinoma syndrome does not exist.

Suggested Reading

- Jozwiak S, Migone N, Ruggieri M. The tuberous sclerosis complexs. In: Ruggieri M, Pascual Castroviejo I, Di Rocco C, editors. Neurocutaneous disorders Phakomatoses and Hamartoneoplastic syndromes. Morlenbach: Springer-Verlag/Wien; 2008. p. 181–227.
- Tabori U, Laberge A-M, Ellezam B, Carret A-S. Cancer predisposition in children with braintumors. In: Scheinemann K, Bouffet E, editors. Pediatric Neuro-Oncology. New York: Springer; 2015. p. 69–89.
- Gorlin, RJ. Nevoid basal cell carcinoma. In: Ruggieri M, Pascual-Castroviejo I, Di Rocco C, editors. Neurocutaneous disorders Phakomatoses and Hamartoneoplastic syndromes. Morlenbach: Springer/Wien; 2008. p. 669–94.
- Chan TSY, Wang X, Spence T, Taylor MD, Huang A. Embryonal brain cell tumors. In: Scheinemann K, Bouffet E, editors. Pediatric Neuro-Oncology. New York: Springer; 2015. p. 127–38.
- Lee J, Johnston DL. Chemotherapy. In: Scheinemann K, Bouffet E, editors. Pediatric Neuro-Oncology. New York: Springer; 2015. p. 69–89.

28. You are seeing an 18-year-old female with a history of gradually progressive unsteadiness and hearing loss in the left ear. An MRI is obtained and is shown below.

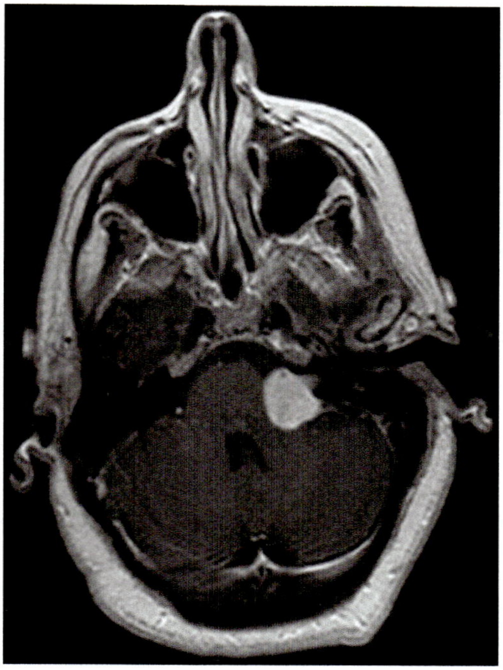

Fig. 19.19 Vestibular schwannoma. ► RadsWiki. (RadsWiki. Wikipedia)

What is your most likely diagnosis?

A. Vestibular schwannoma
B. Oligodendroglioma
C. Cerebellar hemangioblastoma
D. Ependymoma
E. Metastatic lesion

Correct Answer is: A

The MRI shows a vestibular schwannoma. Schwannoma occur commonly in the fourth and fifth decades, and they are on the vestibular portion of cranial nerve VIII. They grow in the cerebellopontine angle, and may compress the brain stem and erode into the internal auditory meatus. They grow slowly and they are either asymptomatic, or present with hearing loss, tinnitus, and in some cases cerebellar findings given that the cerebellar peduncles are compressed. On imaging, they are circumscribed isointense tumors with contrast

enhancement. The location and radiologic appearance of the tumor as shown in the figure, distinguish it from the other choices. It is extra-axial (not within the brain parenchyma) and is not within the ventricular system. This is not a location typical for metastatic lesions. Given the clinical and radiologic findings, this patient does not have an oligodendroglioma, cerebellar hemangioblastoma, ependymoma, or metastatic tumor.

Suggested Reading

- Bradley WG, Daroff RB, Fenichel GM, et al. Neurology in clinical practice. 5th ed. Philadelphia: Elsevier; 2008.
- Prayson RA, Goldblum JR. Neuropathology. 1st ed. Philadelphia: Elsevier; 2005.
- Comprehensive Review in Clinical Neurology: A Multiple Choice Question Book for the Wards and Boards © 2011 Wolters Kluwer Health Lippincott Williams & Wilkins. All rights reserved.

29. Primary CNS lymphoma occurs more frequently in patients with AIDS but may also be diagnosed in immunocompetent patients. What is the difference between the CNS lymphoma in the patient populations?
    - A. Association with Epstein Barr virus
    - B. Findings on cytology
    - C. Response to steroids
    - D. B-cell origin
    - E. M RI findings

Correct Answer is: A
Primary CNS lymphoma (PCNSL) is more frequently diagnosed in immunocompromised patients, especially in patients with AIDS. Almost all of these cases are associated with Epstein-Barr virus (EBV), and CSF EBV PCR is helpful in the diagnosis. In contrast, PCNSL in immunocompetent patients is not commonly associated with EBV. In general, PCNSL in immunocompromised patients occurs at earlier ages than in those who are immunocompetent. It is not possible to differentiate PCNSL in immunocompromised patients versus immunocompetent patients only on the basis of imaging, CSF findings, or cytology. There is no clear evidence of differences in response to steroids in either group.

Suggested Reading

- Comprehensive Review in Clinical Neurology: A Multiple-Choice Question Book for the Wards and Boards ©2011 Wolters Kluwer Health Lippincott Williams & Wilkins. All rights reserved.

30. The medulloblastomas are responsible for great percentage of tumors during childhood.
    What is the INCORRECT option about these tumors?
    - A. Typically, they originate at the cerebellar vermis
    - B. They are pathologically different from the PNETs (primitive neuroectodermal tumors)
    - C. Use of ventriculo-peritonea l derivation can lead to peritoneal metastasis
    - D. There is no difference in survival rate between partial or total resection, but only if a surgical procedure is followed by radiotherapy0 Radiation of the entire neuro-axis is normally recommended.

Correct Answer is: D
Studies show that groups of patients treated by radical or gross total resection showed much higher postoperative survival, so it's incorrect to affirm only radiotherapy affects the survival rate. All the other options are correctly describe medulloblastomas.

Suggested Reading

- Raimondi AJ, Tomita T. Medulloblastoma in childhood: comparative results of partial and total resection. Childs Brain. 1979;5(3):310–28.

31. Regarding the prognosis of oligodendrogliomas, which of the following is correct?
    - A. Chromosome 1p and 19q deletions confer a worse prognosis
    - B. Younger patients have better survival
    - C. p16 gene deletion is associated with better outcomes
    - D. p53 mutations occur in more than 50% of the cases
    - E. The prognosis in oligodendrogliom. as is worse than in astrocytomas

Correct Answer: B

The prognosis in oligodendrogliomas is better than in astrocytomas. Other factors that influence prognosis include age of the patient (better survival with younger patients), pre-surgical performance status (worse prognosis with poorer baseline functional and neurologic status), bulk of resection (the greater the extent of resection the better), and genetic alterations.

Important genetic alterations are chromosome 1p and 19q co-deletions, which occur in 50–80% of the cases, and are associated with a better prognosis, enhanced survival, and better response to chemotherapy, radiation therapy, or both. Mutation of p53 is not typically seen in oligodendrogliomas, and its presence suggests the possibility of an astrocytic neoplasm. Deletion of the chromosomal region p16 is more commonly seen in anaplastic astrocytomas and glioblastomas, and is associated with progression. Treatment of oligodendrogliomas involves surgical resection, chemotherapy, and radiation therapy. The chemotherapy used includes temozolomide, which has replaced PCV (procarbazine, lomustine, and vincristine).

Suggested Reading

- Bradley WG, Daroff RB, Fenichel GM, et al. Neurology in clinical practice. 5th ed. Philadelphia: Elsevier; 2008.
- Prayson RA, Goldblum JR. Neuropathology. 1st ed. Philadelphia: Elsevier; 2005.
- Comprehensive Review in Clinical Neurology: A Multiple-Choice Question Book for the Wards and Boards ©2011 Wolters Kluwer Health Lippincott Williams & Wilkins. All rights reserved.

32. Which of the following is incorrect regarding brain metastases?
    - A. They are more common than primary brain tumors
    - B. Hemorrhagic metastasis can be seen with melanomas, non-small cell carcinomas, and renal cell carcinomas
    - C. The majority are infra-tentorial
    - D. Multiple metastatic lesions can be seen with small cell carcinomas and melanomas
    - E. Steroids are used to treat surrounding edema in brain metastasis

Correct Answer is: C

Metastatic lesions are more common than primary brain tumors. 80% of brain metastases are supra-tentorial and 20% infra-tentorial. Infra-cranial metastatic lesion can affect the skull and dura and brain parenchyma or produce a meningeal carcinomatosis. The most common Lung is the most common source of metastasis to the brain, followed by breast and then melanoma. Gastrointestinal tumors (especially colon and rectum), kidney cancer and tumors originating from the gallbladder, liver, thyroid, testicle, uterus, ovary, and pancreas may produce brain metastasis.

Prostate, esophagus, oropharynx, and skin (other than melanoma) tumors are rare tumors to have parenchymal brain metastases. Colon and pelvic cancers have a tendency to spread to the posterior fossa. Metastatic lesions can be multiple or single. Small cell carcinomas and melanomas can have multiple metastases. Those that are frequently found as single metastasis originate from the kidney, breast, thyroid, or adenocarcinoma of the lung. Hemorrhagic metastases are seen with melanoma, choriocarcinomas, non-small cell carcinomas, thyroid carcinomas, and renal cell carcinomas. Metastasis in the brain can cause seizure, focal neurologic findings, headaches, and sometimes with increased intracranial pressure. Symptom onset is typically relatively rapid and abrupt rather than gradual. The treatment of brain metastasis includes brain irradiation, surgical intervention for solitary metastasis in some cases, and chemotherapy. Steroids play a significant role in the treatment of surrounding edema.

Suggested Reading

- Prayson RA, Goldblum JR. Neuropathology. 1st ed. Philadelphia: Elsevier; 2005.
- Comprehensive Review in Clinical Neurology: A Multiple-Choice Question Book for the Wards and Boards ©2011 Wolters Kluwer Health Lippincott Williams & Wilkins. All rights reserved.

33. Which of the following is recommended for a patient with choroid plexus carcinoma?
    A. Screening for somatic and germline mutations in the gene coding for the protein neurofibromin
    B. Screening for somatic and germline mutations in the gene cording for the protein hamartin
    C. Screening for somatic and germline mutations in the gene coding for the protein p53
    D. Screening for somatic and germline mutations in the gene coding for the protein tuberin

19

Correct Answer is: C
Choroid plexus carcinoma occurs in patients with Li Fraumeni syndrome. There are two sets of diagnostic criteria for this disorder.

In the Classic Li Fraumeni Syndrome Diagnostic criteria, a patient must have all of the following:(1) presence of a sarcoma diagnosed prior to age 45 years (2) presence of a 1st degree relative with any cancer before the age of 45. (3) A 1st or 2nd degree relative with any cancer before age 45 years OR with a sarcoma at any time.

The Compete diagnostic criteria for Li Fraumeni are slightly different. In this case, a diagnosis of Li Fraumeni can be made in 1 of 4 circumstances: (1) the patient has at least 1 tumor typical of LFS diagnosed prior to age 46 (brain tumor, adrenocortical carcinoma, leukemia, bronco alveolar cancer, soft tissue sarcoma, osteosarcoma, or premenopausal breast cancer) WITH > 1 1st or 2nd degree relative with a tumor typical for LFS before age 56, or the presence of multiple tumors. (2) The patient has many tumors,>2 within the disease spectrum, and > 1 occurring prior to age 46. (3) The patient has adrenocortical carcinoma or a tumor of the choroid plexus.

It is suggested that screening for mutations in TP53 should be performed in (1) individuals meeting criteria for the syndrome (2) women with breast cancer before age 30 with no BRCA1 or BRCA 2 mutations (3) people with adrenocortical carcinoma (4) people with choroid plexus carcinoma or (5) people with childhood sarcoma.

Ewings sarcoma is an exception to the latter. Thus, a patient with a choroid plexus carcinoma should be screened for germline mutations in the TP53 gene.

Mutations in the NF1 gene lead to neurofibromatosis type 1. This gene encodes neurofibromin. This syndrome is associated with gliomas including those affecting the optic pathway and brainstem.

Mutations in the tuberous sclerosis complex 1 (TSC1) gene encode for the protein hamartin. This is associated with tuberous sclerosis complex a syndrome associated with sub-ependymal giant cell astrocytoma (SEGA) and sub-ependymal nodules.

Mutations in the tuberous sclerosis complex 2 (TSC2) gene encode for the protein tuberin. This is also associated with tuberous sclerosis complex. Mutations the NF2 gene lead to dysfunction of the protein merlin, associated with neurofibromatosis type 2. Bilateral vestibular schwannomas are characteristic of this disorder and a diagnosis of neurofibromatosis type 2 can be made in the presence of this alone. Ependymomas are also characteristic of this syndrome.

Suggested Reading

- Jozwiak S, Migone N, Ruggieri M. The tuberous sclerosis complexes. In: Ruggieri M, Pascual Castroviejo I, Di Rocco C, editors. Neurocutaneous disorders Phakomatoses and Hamartoneoplastic syndromes. Morlenbach: Springer-Verlag/Wien; 2008. p. 181–227.
- Tabori U, Laberge A-M, Ellezam B, Carret A-S.Cancer predisposition in children with brain tumors. In: Scheinemann K, Bouffet E, editors. Pediatric Neuro-Oncology. New York: Springer; 2015. p. 69–89.
- Gorlin, RJ. Nevoid basal cell carcinoma. In: Ruggieri M, Pascual-Castroviejo I, Di Rocco C, editors. Neurocutaneous disorders Phakomatoses and Hamartoneoplastic syndromes. Morlenbach: Springer-Verlag/Wien; 2008. p. 669–94.
- Chan TSY, Wang X, Spence T, Taylor MD, Huang A. Embryonal brain cell tumors. In: Scheinemann K, Bouffet E, editors. Pediatric Neuro-Oncology. New York: Springer; 2015. p. 127–38.
- Lee J, Johnston DL. Chemotherapy. In: Scheinemann K, Bouffet E, eds. Pediatric Neuro-Oncology. New York: Springer; 2015. p. 69–89.
- Glass TD, Cochrane D, Rassekh SR, Goddard K, Hukin J. Growing teratoma syndrome in intracranial non germinomatous germ cell tumors (iNGGCTs): a risk for secondary malignant transformation- a report of two cases. Child Nerv Syst. 2014;30(5). p. 953–7.
- Bartels U, Singhal A. Central nervous system germ cell tumors. In: Scheinemann K, Bouffet E, editors. Pediatric Neuro-Oncology. New York: Springer; 2015. p. 149–62.
- Mach SC, Ramaswamy V, Wang X, Remke M, Sin-Chan P, Chan WSY, Bertrand KC, Merino D, Zayne K, Huang A, Taylor MD. Basic science of pediatric brain tumors. In: Scheinemann K, Bouffet E, editors. Pediatric Neuro-Oncology. New York: Springer; 2015. p. 59–67.
- Jones DTW, Korshunov A. Pfister SM, Tayllor MD, Northcott PA. Medulloblastoma and CNS primitive neuroectodermal tumors. In: Cagle PT, Matthias KA, Zagzag D, editors. Molecular pathology of nervous system tumors. New York: Springer; 2015. p. 121–42.
- Vanan Ml, Mehta V, Eisenstat DD. Diffuse intrinsic pontine glioma. In: Scheinemann K, Bouffet E, editors. Pediatric Neuro-Oncology. New York: Springer; 2015. p. 117–26.
- Rutkowski S, Bode U, Deinlein F, Ottensmeier H, Warmuth-Metz M, Soeroenson N,Grade N, Emser A. Pietsch T, Wolff JE, Kortmann RD, Kuehl J. Treatment of early childhood medulloblastoma by post-operative chemotherapy alone. N Eng J Med. 2005;352(10):978.
- Geyer JR, Sposto R, Jennings M, Boyett JM, Axtell RA, Brieger D, Broxso E, Donahue B, Finlay JL, Goldwein JW, Heier LA, Johnson DM, Mazewski C, Miller DC, Packer R, Puccetti D, RadcliffeJ, Tao ML, Shiminski-Maher T. Multiagent chemo-

therapy and deferred radiotherapy in infants with malignant brain tumors: a report from the Children's Cancer Group. J Clin Oncol. 2005;23(30):7621.
- Wells EM, Packer RJ. Pediatric Brain Tumors. Continuum: Lifelong Learning Neurol. 2015;21(2):373–96.
- Fleming AJ. Rare tumors of the central nervous system in children. In: Scheinemann K, Bouffet E, editors. Pediatric Neuro-Oncology. New York: Springer; 2015. p. 185–94.
- Evans DW. Li-Fraumeni syndrome. In: Up-to-date, Wen PY, Ross ME (Ed), Up-to-date, Waltham, MA (Accessed on November 22 2015).
- Ichimura K, Nishikawa R, Matsutani M. Molecular markers in pediatric neuro-oncology. Neuro Oncology. 2012;14(Suppl 4):iv90–9. doi:▶ https://doi.org/10.1093/neuonc/nos204.
- Vora NL. Melanoma and BRAF. eMedicine. ▶ http://emedicine.medscape.com/article/2045059-overview (▶ http://emedicine.medscape.com/article/2045059-overview). Updated January 14 2014. Accessed November 23 2015.
- Daras M, Kaley TJ. Benign brain tumors and tumors associated with phakomatoses. Continuum: Lifelong Learning in Neurol. 2015;21(2):373–96.

34. You are evaluating a 6-year-old girl for her unsteady gait. On exam, she is noted to have eyelid retraction and voluntary up-gaze restriction. An MRI is performed and an enhancing pineal region mass is noted. Serum and CSF alpha fetoprotein (AFP) levels are normal. Serum beta HCG is slightly elevated at a concentration of 20 international units per liter.
What is the most likely diagnosis?
A. Yolk sac tumor
B. Mature teratoma
C. Germinoma
D. Choriocarcinoma
E. Embryonal carcinoma

Correct Answer is: C
Slight elevation of beta HCG accompanied by normal AFP levels are consistent with germinoma.

Yolk sac tumor is a non-germinomatous germ cell tumor typically associated with elevated levels of AFP, although beta HCG may also be mildly elevated.

Mature teratomas tend not to secrete beta HCG or AFP, while choriocarcinomas tend to secrete high levels of beta HCG alone. Embryonal carcinoma may secrete both beta HCG and AFP.

Yolk sac tumors are typically associated with elevated levels of AFP although beta HCG can be mildly elevated.

Mature teratomas are usually not associated with elevations in AFP or beta HCG, although this can occur.

Choriocarcinoma is typically associated with more marked elevations of beta HCG; milder elevations occur in patients with germinoma.

Embryonal carcinoma is a non germinomatous germ cell tumor subtype which is associated with elevations in both AFP and beta HCG.

35. This is a histopathologic specimen form an intraventricular mass biopsied form a 5-year-old.
Which of the following is incorrect regarding this lesion?
Most common location is in the lateral ventricles
A. CSF production may be increase
B. It may present with hydrocephalus and features of increased intracranial pressure
C. It is a WHO grade II tumor
D. It is more common in children

Correct Answer is: C
The slide shows a proliferation of epithelial cells in a papillary pattern lining fibro-vascular cores, consistent with choroid plexus papilloma, which is a WHO grade I tumor. Choroid plexus pap-

19

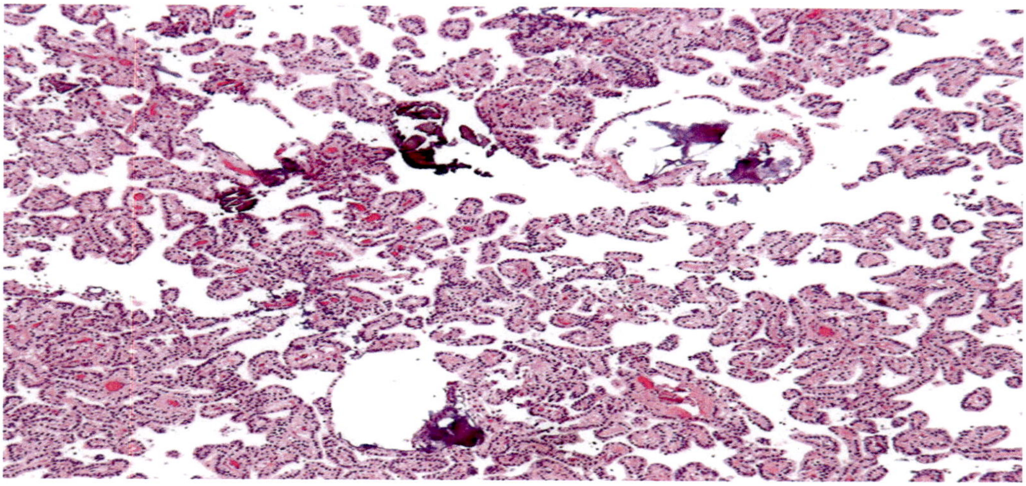

Fig. 19.20 Micrograph of a choroid plexus papilloma. H&E stain. (Own work. Nephron. Wikipedia)

illoma is a childhood tumor, the most common location is the lateral ventricles, followed by the fourth ventricle and then the third ventricle. They are either asymptomatic, or present with hydrocephalus and manifestations of increased intracranial pressure, sometimes due to a combination of obstructed flow and increased CSF production. Choroid plexus papilloma is circumscribed mass composed of epithelium lining fibro-vascular cores, resembling normal choroid plexus. In contrast to papilloma, choroid plexus carcinomas are invasive, with nuclear pleomorphism, demonstrating atypia, mitosis, and necrosis. Choroid plexus papilloma can be surgically resected and considered low grade or WHO grade I. Choroid plexus carcinomas are higher grade (WHO grade III), and after surgical resection, radiotherapy and chemotherapy may be needed.

Suggested Reading

- Prayson RA. Goldblum JR. Neuropathology. 1st ed. Philadelphia: Elsevier; 2005.
- Ropper AH, Samuels MA. Adams and Victor's principles of neurology. 9th ed. New York: McGraw-Hill; 2009.
- Comprehensive Review in Clinical Neurology: A Multiple-Choice Question Book for the Wards and Boards © 2011 Wolters Kluwer Health Lippincott Williams & Wilkins. All rights reserved.

Neuro-Ophthalmology

Y. M. Awaad, *Absolute Pediatric Neurology*, https://doi.org/10.1007/978-3-319-78801-2_20

1. A 16-year-old boy is complaining of increasingly blurry vision for the past 8 weeks. His right eye was affected first, but was soon bilateral. He has no past medical history of eye or vision difficulty before. Family history is positive for a grandfather with macular degeneration, both paternal grandparents with cataracts, and an uncle who has had "poor vision" for most of his life. He occasionally smokes cigarettes, but does not drink alcohol or take recreational drugs. He is a high school student and is currently taking AP English and AP math. On examination, his vision is 20/400 OD and 20/200 OS, normal reactive pupils, extraocular motility, and intraocular pressure. Funduscopic examination is shown below:
You ordered visual field testing. His visual field testing is below:

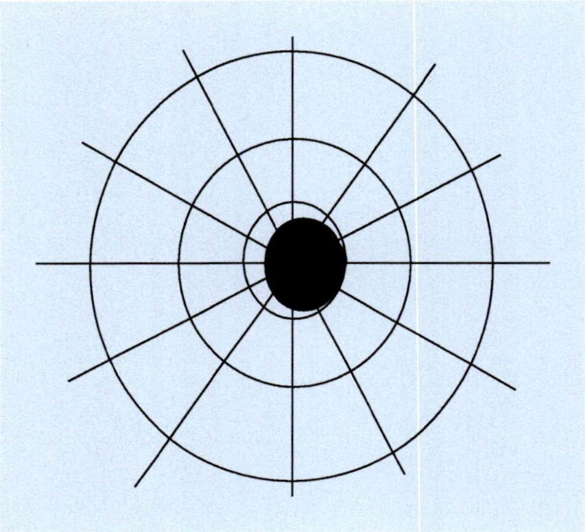

Fig. 20.1 Goldmann visual field record showing a ceentrocaecal scotoma, i.e. a central scotoma involving the blind spot. (Own work. RobertB3009)

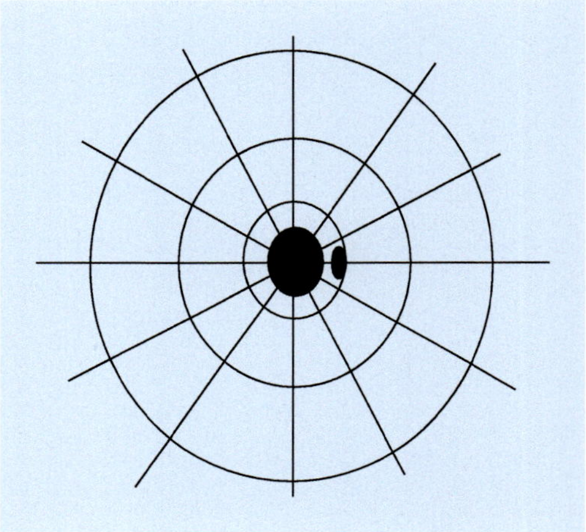

Fig. 20.2 Goldmann visual field record showing a macular or central scotoma. (Own work. RobertB3009)

You have never seen a central scotoma quite as large as his.
His likely diagnosis is:
A. Leber's hereditary optic neuropathy
B. Methanol toxicity
C. Pseudo tumor cerebri
D. Nicotine-induced visual loss
E. Neuromyelitis optica

Correct Answer is: A
Leber hereditary optic neuropathy (LHON) is an inherited form of vision loss. Usually it begins in the teens or twenties, but it can appear in early childhood or later in adulthood in rare cases. Males are more affected than females.

The first symptoms of LHON are usually blurring and clouding of vision. These vision problems can start unilateral or simultaneously in both eyes; if vision loss is unilateral, the other eye is usually affected within several weeks or months. Over time, vision in both eyes worsens with a severe loss of acuity and color vision. It affects mainly central vision and this is reflected in the very large central scotomata seen on the visual field testing. Vision loss results from the death of cells in the optic nerve, showing as an irregularly shrunken and pale optic nerve head on the funduscopic exam.

20

Suggested Reading

- Finsterer J. Inherited mitochondrial neuropathies. J Neurol Sci. 2011; 304(1–2):9–16.
- Yen MY, Wang AG, Wei YH. Leber's hereditary optic neuropathy: a multifactorial disease. Prog Retin Eye Res. 2006;25(4):381–96.

2. Concerning ophthalmoplegic migraine:
   A. The paresis of the oculomotor nerve may develop up to 4 days after the headache begins
   B. The headache can last up to a week
   C. Has been reclassified by the International Classification of Headache Disorders II as a cranial neuralgia and not a subset of migraine
   D. All of the above

Correct Answer is: D
The new reclassification of the ophthalmologic migraine is a cranial neuralgia and not a complicated migraine. The third nerve palsy is present and the headache typically lasts at least a week. Typically the ophthalmoplegia develops 3–5 days after development of the headache. Brain MRI can show gadolinium enhancement of the third nerve.

Suggested Reading

- Roy et al. Childhood steroid responsive ophthalmoplegic migraine. J Pediatr Neurosci. 2011;6(1):69–71.

3. Which statement below is incorrect regarding the differences between Optic Pathway Gliomas (OPGs) accompanied with neurofibromatosis type 1 (NF1) as compared to sporadic?
   A. Test of visual acuity is not useful in OPG screening in NF 1
   B. OPG associated with NF1 are less aggressive
   C. NF-1 associated OPGs rarely invade the optic radiations
   D. Bilateral OPG are seen more frequently in the setting of NF1

Correct Answer is: A
Optic Pathway Gliomas (OPGs) are low-grade pilocytic astrocytoma. One third of children having an OPG have been affected by NF1, with an OPG prevalence of up to one quarter in the NF population. In NF1 tumors are less aggressive and rarely invade the optic radiations. Bilateral OPGs are common with NF1 than with sporadic occurrence. Visual acuity assessment is a useful way to identify patients with OPGs in either setting.

Suggested Reading

- Ophthalmological assessment of children with neurofibromatosis type 1. Catherine Cassiman & Eric Legius & Werner Spileers & Ingele Casteels. Eur J Pediatr. 2013;172:1327–33. doi ► https://doi.org/10.1007/s00431-013-2035-2.
- National Institutes of Health Consensus Development Conference Statement: neurofibromatosis. Bethesda, July 13–15, 1987. Neurofibromatosis. 1988;1(3):172–8.

4. You are evaluating a 5-week-old baby boy who was admitted for jaundice and phototherapy. The nurse noticed dysconjugate gaze. His physical exam is normal except he is jaundiced. He has no trouble feeding, but appears sluggish. The child displays abnormal ocular alignment with transitory shifts of alignment from convergence to divergence. His neurological exam is unremarkable. What do you tell his family?
   A. Consult a pediatric ophthalmologist to rule out retinoblastoma

B. Non- paralytic strabismus secondary to kernicterus
C. The child will require corrective surgery before 6 months of age
D. This is normal

Correct answer is: D
Poor ocular coordination is common in newborns and infants. By 3–4 weeks of age, Ocular alignment occurs and consistent alignment by 3 months. However, is not uncommon for it to take as long as 5 months. Severe brain injury can cause signs of poor feeding, weak or high-pitched cry, lethargy, hypotonia and opisthotonic posturing.

At 5 weeks of age it is not possible to determine treatment or even if treatment will be required in the future.

Suggested Reading

- Wan MJ, Vanderveen DK. Eye disorders in newborn infants (excluding retinopathy of prematurity). Archives of Disease in Childhood-Fetal and Neonatal Edition, fetal neonatal-2014. 2014.

5. A 9-week old infant has a persistent left head tilt and misalignment of the eyes.
Where is the location of his neurological deficit?
A. Retina
B. Left oculomotor nerve
C. Medial to the red nucleus in the midbrain
D. Right trochlear nerve

Correct answer is: D
Local fourth cranial nerve trauma at birth can cause congenital superior oblique palsy, but many cases are idiopathic. The infant tilts the head away from the affected side in attempt to maintain the eyes in alignment. The significant ocular manifestation is hypertropia of the affected eye in the field of the impaired superior oblique muscle.

The fibers of the oculomotor nucleus pass medially to the red nucleus before exiting the midbrain as the third cranial nerve. Lesion in the region of the red nucleus may present with signs of third nerve palsy, not fourth nerve (trochlear) palsy.

Third nerve palsy presents with exotropia because of medial rectus impairment. The third nerve also innervates the superior rectus, inferior rectus and inferior oblique.

Retinal disease does not typically present with ocular misalignment.

Suggested Reading

- Yang HK, Kim H, Hwang JM. Congenital superior oblique palsy and trochlear nerve absence: a clinical and radiological study. Ophthalmology. 2012;119(1):170–77.

6. A 7-year-old girl with moderate to severe developmental delays was referred to you for a new onset of "problems moving her eye". On examination, vision was reduced in the left eye with limited mobility in all directions. The left pupil is sluggish with a white component. No abnormalities were noted in the right eye.
What is your next step in management?
A. Contact pediatric oncologist for immediate referral
B. Contact ophthalmologist for immediate referral
C. MRI with contrast of the anterior visual pathways
D. Send her back to her primary care physician

Correct answer is: B
Retinoblastoma is the only malignant intraocular tumor of childhood. Immediate referral to an ophthalmologist is crucial because surgical removal is the first treatment step. A neurological consultation is required when visual tumor symptomatology is accompanied with neurological syndromes, such as Sturge-Weber, neurofibromatosis and 13q deletion syndrome. Leukocoria is the most recognized initial feature in retinoblastoma. The pupil appears white in sunlight or flash photography.

Funduscopic examination will establish the diagnosis. High-resolution MRI is important for pre-surgical assessment. CT is no longer recommended. Surgery followed by chemotherapy and radiation therapy is the treatment of choice.

Suggested Reading

- Abramson DH, Frank CM, Susman M, Whalen MP, Dunkel IJ, Boyd NW. Presenting signs of retinoblastoma. J Pediat. 1998;132(3):505–8.

7. A 10-month-old boy was referred by his pediatrician because he recently stopped visual tracking and a nystagmus was noted. On examination, he has sluggish pupillary response and the rest of his neurological exam is within normal limits.
   What is your diagnosis?
   A. Retinoblastoma
   B. Craniopharyngioma
   C. Kearns-Sayre syndrome
   D. Leber Congenital amaurosis

Correct answer is: D
Leber congenital amaurosis is a retinal dystrophy and is the most common genetic cause of congenital visual impairment. The impairment starts in the first 3–4 months of life followed by nystagmus and sluggish pupillary responses. Visual acuity will rarely be better than 20/400 when they get older. Mid-facial hypoplasia and mental retardation can be associated in some children.

Retinoblastoma manifestation are unilateral progressive visual loss in a young child and strabismus. The first most common sign is leucocoria, in which the white tumor reflects light and blocks view of the red colored retina.

Craniopharygioma is the most common non-glial tumor in children and usually occurs between the ages of 6–14. There is a 1–2-year history of progressive visual loss, delayed sexual maturation growth failure and bitemporal hemianopia.

Kearns-Sayre syndrome is a mitochondrial disorder, it is a triad of symptoms including: progressive external ophthalmoplegia, onset before age 20 and one of the following; short stature, pigmentary retinopathy, cerebellar ataxia, heart block, cerebellar ataxia, and elevated cerebrospinal protein.

Suggested Reading

- Weleber RG, Francis PJ, Trzupek KM, Beattie C.Leber congenital amaurosis. 2013.

8. 16-year-old female came to your office with history of right upper and lower facial weakness for 1 month. Taste aberration and right hyperacusis are also reported. A blink reflex is performed with the following results: stimulating the right side: absent right R1 and R2 potentials, and normal left R2; stimulating the left side: normal left R1 and R2 potentials, and absent right R2.
   Where is the site of the lesion?
   A. left facial
   B. left trigeminal
   C. right facial
   D. right medullary
   E. right trigeminal

Correct Answer is: C
This is a right facial nerve lesion. Stimulating the affected side results in absence of ipsilateral R1 and R2 potentials, but a normal contralateral R2 potential; whereas stimulating the unaffected side results in a normal ipsilateral R1 and R2, but absent contralateral R2 suggesting a unilateral facial lesion.

Suggested Reading

- Misulis KE, Head TC. Essentials of clinical neurophysiology. 3rd ed. Philadelphia: Butterworth-Heinemann; 2003.
- Preston DC, Shapiro BE. Electromyography and neuromuscular disorders. 1st ed. Philadelphia: Butterworth-Heinemann; 1998.

Neurophysiology/ Localization

Y. M. Awaad, *Absolute Pediatric Neurology*, https://doi.org/10.1007/978-3-319-78801-2_21

21

1. What test can be used in your office to determine if a patient has conductive verses a sensorineural hearing loss?
   - A. Rinne test
   - B. Weber test
   - C. Ask her to repeat words that test high, medium and low frequency sounds
   - D. Tympanometry

Correct Answer is: A

The Rinne test: activating a tuning fork and holding the base against the mastoid process to determine if bone conduction is perceived, then when the patient reports the sound has faded the tuning fork is held 1 inch for the ipsilateral ear. Since air conduction is more sensitive than the bone conduction, the vibratory sound should still be heard twice as long as the bone conduction. Impaired air conduction response with normal bone conduction indicates a conductive hearing loss.

The Weber test: compares bone conduction in the two ears. The tuning fork is activated and placed at the center of the forehead and the patient is asked if one side is louder than the other.

Informal testing of hearing frequencies is helpful to determine if there is a Sensorineural hearing deficit. Tympanometry with pneumatic testing determines if there is abnormalities of the external ear and normal movement of the tympanic memory, and will only determine if immobile tympanic membrane is contributing to hearing loss.

Suggested Reading

- Nunez DA, Qi L. Tests for hearing. Logan Turner's Diseases of the Nose, Throat and Ear: Head and Neck Surgery. 2015;375.

2. A 9-year-old boy is complaining for the last 5 weeks of vertigo symptoms, including the sensation of the floor suddenly moving that causes him to suddenly lurch to one side.
   Which symptom is indicative of a central etiology?
   - A. Hearing loss
   - B. Tinnitus
   - C. Ataxia with eye closes
   - D. Hoarseness

Correct Answer is: D

When other cranial nerve affection is associated with vertigo, this indicates central pathology. Hoarseness is caused by the ten-cranial nerve injury. Etiologies of central vertigo include migraine, multiple sclerosis, seizure, stroke/TIA and tumor.

Hearing loss is a peripheral eighth cranial nerve affection and not central. Causes of peripheral vertigo include; benign positional vertigo, vestibular neuronitis, labyrinthitis, Meiere's disease and vestibular nerve tumor (schwannoma or meningioma).

Tinnitus is a peripheral eighth cranial nerve impairment and not central.

Maintaining balance without visual input, but normal with eyes open, is characteristic of a disorder of peripheral sensory input. Ataxic gait is a sign of central pathology.

Suggested Reading

- Thompson T, Amedee R. Vertigo: a review of common peripheral and central vestibular disorders. Ochsner J. 2009;9(1):20–6.

3. Which of the following tests would be most helpful What test will be helpful in diagnosing a 6-year-old male presenting with frequent starring episode that can be provoked in the office by having him hyperventilate?
   - A. MRI of brain
   - B. EEG
   - C. Evoked Potential
   - D. Positron Emission Tomography

Correct Answer is: B

The diagnostic EEG pattern for childhood absence epilepsy is a 3 per-second spike and-wave.

No abnormal brain structure on neuroimaging has been recognized in children with generalized epilepsies, including absence. Generalized epilepsy is considered ion channelopathy.

Evoked potential studies measure the response time (and strength) of a stimulation of a sensory nerve pathway to reach the brain. This test detects the slowing of electrical conduction most commonly caused by demyelination along sensory pathways.

PET scans measure local cerebral glucose metabolism and provides a representative image. This test can be helpful in identifying an epileptic focus in an individual with focal onset seizures. Cerebral tissue that has epileptic potential is often metabolically dysfunctional, and when inactive, is hypometabolic.

Suggested Reading

- Camfield P, Camfield C. Epileptic syndromes in childhood: clinical features, outcomes, and treatment. Epilepsia. 2002;43(Suppl 3):27–32.

4. A 12-year-old female is complaining of bilateral rhythmic contractions of her palate.

   Where do you locate the lesion?

   A. Central tegmental tract
   B. Basal ganglia
   C. Cerebellum
   D. Frontal lobe

Correct Answer is: A

Palatal myoclonus is a segmental myoclonus. The pathology is almost exclusively located in brainstem lesions of the central tegmental tract or the dentate-olivary pathways. Brainstem tumor and stroke are the most common etiologies.

Basal ganglia pathology leads to failure in suppressing the unwanted movements (Huntington's disease) or delay in initiating movements (Parkinson's disease).

Cerebellum pathology leads in impairment in coordination of motor movements and manifest as ataxia or dysarthria.

Frontal lobe lesion has different manifestations based on the affected location. Lesions in the motor planning and supplementary motor areas of the frontal cortex may lead to a deficit in executing motor actions and control over voluntary actions.

Suggested Reading

- Hirano M, Hatzoglou V, Karimi S, Young RJ. Hypertrophic olivary degeneration resulting from posterior fossa masses and their treatments. Clin Imaging. 2015;39(5):787–90.

5. What is the EEG finding in a 10-year-old boy that presented with acute onset of fever, headache, lethargy with subsequent development of hemiparesis and has focal seizures, and has multiple cold sores on his skin?

   A. General Epileptiform discharges
   B. Normal EEG
   C. per second spike and wave formations
   D. Periodic lateralizing epileptiform discharges

Correct Answer is: D

Herpes simplex virus (HSV) is the single most common cause of non-epidemic cases of encephalitis. A presumptive diagnosis of HSV encephalitis can be based on the presence of periodic lateralizing epileptiform discharges. MRI Classically, there is focal abnormalities in the temporal and inferior frontal lobes on the MRI. Only about 20% have a history of labial infections.

About 80% manifest focal neurological symptoms that include hemiparesis, cranial nerve deficits, visual field loss, aphasia and focal seizures.

Primary generalized epilepsies have generalized EEG patterns and not in encephalitis.

Essentially all persons with encephalitis will have focal EEG findings.

High voltage 3 per second spike and wave complexes are diagnostic for absence epilepsy.

Suggested Reading

- Cappellari AM, Tardini G, Bona AR, Belli M, Triulzi F, Fossali EF. Teaching NeuroImages: infantile herpes simplex encephalitis. Neurology. 2014;83(7):e85–6.

6. A 2-week-old infant is seen by his pediatrician because of distended abdomen. By mother's report, he has had a few bowel movements, but not having the normal bowel movements that his siblings has at his age. On examination, he has a distended abdomen with hypoactive bowel sounds. X-ray of the abdomen shows dilated loops of bowel with excessive fecal material. A diagnosis of Hirschsprung's disease is suspected after additional testing.
All of the following is correct expect?
   - A. It consists of the myenteric plexus, located between the outer and inner smooth muscle layers of the gastrointestinal tract, and the sub mucous plexus, located between the circular muscle layer and the mucosa
   - B. The myenteric plexus is predominantly involved in gut motility
   - C. The sub-mucous plexus is predominantly involved in secretory functions of the gastrointestinal tract
   - D. Hirschsprung's disease is due to congenital absence of the submucous plexus
   - E. Hirschsprung's disease is often focal, though rare cases involve the entire colon

Correct Answer is: D
Hirschsprung's disease is due to congenital absence of the myenteric plexus. The enteric nervous system consists of the myenteric (or Auerbach's) plexus that is located between the outer and inner smooth muscle layers of the gastrointestinal tract and the sub-mucous (or Meissner's) plexus, which is located between the circular muscle layer and the mucosa. The myenteric plexus is predominantly involved in gut motility, whereas the sub-mucous plexus is involved in secretory functions. Together, the myenteric and sub-mucous plexus control the function of the gastrointestinal tract. Hirschsprung's disease is due to maldevelopment of the myenteric plexus. Most commonly, focal congenital absence of the myenteric plexus in the internal anal sphincter or recto sigmoid junction occurs, though in rare cases, the myenteric plexus may be absent throughout the gastrointestinal system. Segments of the colon that lack myenteric plexus cannot relax, leading to fecal retention and distention of proximal colonic segments. Some cases of Hirschsprung's disease are due to mutations in the RET protooncogene.

Suggested Reading

- Comprehensive Review in Clinical Neurology: A Multiple-Choice Question Book for the Wards and Boards © 2011 Wolters Kluwer Health Lippincott Williams & Wilkins. All rights reserved.

7. Which one of the following is derived from the neural crest cells?
   - A. Cerebellum
   - B. Meninges
   - C. Autonomic ganglia
   - D. Olfactory bulb
   - E. Optic nerve

Correct Answer is: C
The peripheral nervous system including autonomic ganglia, chromaffin cells in adrenal medulla and melanocytes are derived from neural crest cells, which are derived from neural tube after fusion.

Suggested Reading

- Mowzoon N, Flemming KD. Neurology board review: an illustrated study guide. Rochester: Mayo Clinic Scientific; 2007. Print.

8. Which stage of sleep is characterized by sleep spindles and K complexes?
   A. Wakefulness
   B. Stage 1
   C. Stage 2
   D. Stage3

Correct Answer is: C
Wakefulness/Drowsiness produces primarily alpha waves. Stage 1 is characterized by low amplitude waves with sharp waves over the vertex. There are slow eye movements.

Stage 2 is noted by the presence of K complexes and sleep spindles.

Stage 3 is characterized by slow waves with large amplitudes (delta waves). REM sleep is noted by low EMG tone, rapid eye movements, and saw tooth waves.

Suggested Reading

- Rundell 0H, Jones, RK. Polysomnography methods and interpretations. Otolaryngol Clin North Am. 1990;23(4):583–92.
- De Gennaro L, Ferrara M. Sleep spindles: an overview. Sleep Med Rev. 2003;7(5):423–40.

9. All of the following are an activation procedure used during EEG recording except?
   A. Hyperventilation
   B. Sleep deprivation prior to the EEG
   C. Noxious stimulation
   D. Photic stimulation
   E. Recording during sleep

Correct Answer is: C
EEG represents the recording along the scalp of electrical l activity that is produced by the firing of pyramidal neurons within the cerebral cortex. EEG recording is based on differential amplification, in which the difference in voltage between two sites is compared with each recording channel. This recording helps in the evaluation and diagnosis of abnormalities in brain electrical activity, but is also useful in the evaluation of other neurologic conditions. Patients undergoing an evaluation for "spells" will often have an EEG to determine the presence or absence of epileptogenic activity. During a routine recording, various procedures are utilized to enhance potentially abnormal electrical activity. These so-called activation procedures include hyperventilation, photic stimulation, sleep deprivation prior to the EEG, and recording during sleep. Noxious stimulation is not part of the EEG activation procedures. Hyperventilation may produce generalized slowing or no effect in normal subjects; however, in certain epilepsies, such as absence epilepsy, hyperventilation may activate epileptiform discharges and even seizures.

Photic stimulation is performed with various frequencies, and may be helpful to induce epileptiform activity and seizures, most commonly myoclonic seizures, in individuals with photosensitive epilepsies. Sleep deprivation may also enhance epileptogenic activity. Furthermore, seizures may occur predominantly (or exclusively) during sleep in certain epilepsy syndromes, and EEG abnormalities may not be seen in the awake patient. Therefore, an EEG may be incomplete without a sleep recording.

21

Suggested Reading

- Tatum WO, Husain AM, Benbadis SR, et al. Handbook of EEG Interpretation, Demos Medical Publishing, LLC; 2008.
- Comprehensive Review in Clinical Neurology: A Multiple-Choice Question Book for the Wards and Boards ©20 11 Wolters Kluwer Health Lippincott Williams & Wilkins. All rights reserved.

10. A healthy 3-year-old female has been evaluated because her "strange behavior". The mother reports that her daughter sometimes rocks back and forth and makes strange faces for periods of time ranging from a few seconds to minutes. During those spells, she completely ignores everyone. You reviewed a video of an event, which shows while she is sitting on the couch rocking forward and back she is making repetitive smiling motions with her mouth for approximately 40 s. There are no particular events that precede the rocking and face behaviors, she seems to do them somewhat randomly at various times of day. Her general and neurological examinations are normal. Her labs including, serum electrolytes, calcium, and an EEG are normal.

    What is your next test to order?

    A. Sleep-deprived EEG
    B. Reassure the mother this is normal stimulating/soothing behavior
    C. Obtain lumbar puncture
    D. CT scan head
    E. Brain MRI

Correct Answer is: A

The clinical presentation could be difficulty to differentiate between repetitive soothing/stimulating behaviors and complex partial seizures. Rocking, head pounding, nail biting, thumb sucking, masturbating, hair pulling, and facial tics can represent neurologically benign behavior in some children who use these behaviors to relieve tension for self-soothing. These behaviors can also be seen in other disorders such as autism and OCD. In this case, since these behaviors seem to happen more randomly, and the child is non-responsive during the events, your suspicion would be raised to rule out a seizure disorder. Unfortunately, in many cases of complex partial seizures, the exam, blood work, and even EEG are normal. A sleep-deprived EEG is more sensitive and might be a good next step before referring the child to a neurologist or referring her for video EEG.

11. Which of the following definitions of neural tube defects is incorrect?

    A. Meningocele-isolated meningeal protrusion
    B. Myelomeningocele-protrusion of spinal cord and meninges
    C. Diastematomyelia-splitting of the spinal cord into two portions by a midline septum
    D. Diplomyelia-duplication of the spinal cord
    E. Sacral agenesis-isolated absence of the sacral spinal cord

Correct Answer is: E

Sacral agenesis is absence of the sacrum, rather than absence of the sacral spinal cord, and is frequently associated with other malformations. The neural tube defects (NTDs) include meningocele, myelomeningocele, diastematomyelia, diplomyelia, and sacral agenesis. Caudal NTDs result from failure of fusion of the posterior neuropore at day 26 of gestation. Meningocele is isolated protrusion of the meninges into a bony defect within the vertebral column. This protrusion is typically covered by skin. It is not usually associated

with neurologic deficits, and if neurologic deficit is found, myelomeningocele should be suspected.

Myelomeningocele (also known as spinal dysraphism or rachischisis) is protrusion of potentially all layers of intraspinal contents through a bony defect: spinal cord, nerve roots, and meninges. Either the spinal cord may be exposed or a thin membrane may cover the protrusion. They most often occur in the lumbosacral region but can occur at any level. This is a clinically severe NTD associated with hydrocephalus, motor and sensory abnormalities of the legs, and bowel/bladder dysfunction. Myelomeningocele occurs in association with Chiari II malformations. Diastematomyelia is splitting of the spinal cord into two portions by a midline septum. Diplomyelia is duplication of the spinal cord and is distinguished from diastematomyelia by the presence of two central canals each surrounded by gray and white matter as in a normal spinal cord. Sacral agenesis, or absence of the whole (or in some cases parts of) the sacrum, classically occurs in association with a variety of other urogenital, gastrointestinal, and spinal cord abnormalities. It has been associated with maternal insulin-dependent diabetes. Autosomal dominant forms associated with homeobox gene mutations have been identified. Clinical manifestations range from mild motor deficits to severe sensory and motor deficits and bowel and bladder dysfunction. Management of NTDs involves surgical approaches and management of complications including hydrocephalus and bowel and bladder dysfunction.

Suggested Reading

- Comprehensive Review in Clinical Neurology: A Multiple-Choice Question Book for the Wards and Boards © 2011 Wolters Kluwer Health Lippincott Williams & Wilkins. All rights reserved.

12. Which of the following EEG patterns is associated with epilepsy?
    A. Temporal rhythmic delta activity
    B. Stimulus-induced, rhythmic, periodic ictal discharges (SIRPIDs)
    C. Wicket spikes
    D. Burst suppression
    E. Triphasic waves

Correct Answer is: A

Temporal rhythmic delta activity (TIRDA) is usually associated with temporal lobe epilepsy.

Wicket spikes are usually a normal finding and not associated with epilepsy. SIRPIDs are usually seen in critically ill patients, even those without neurological problems.

Triphasic waves are commonly seen with hepatic or renal dysfunction or encephalopathy.

13. Which one of the following neurological abnormalities is caused by failure of closure of posterior neuropore?
    A. Anencephaly
    B. Spina bifida
    C. Lissencephaly
    D. Dandy-Walker syndrome
    E. Holoprosencephaly

Correct Answer is: B

Neural tube closure occurs around 4th week of gestation, anterior neuropore closes at day 25; failure leads to encephalocele and anencephaly. Posterior neuropore closes at day 27; failure leads to spina bifida or myelomeningocele.

Suggested Reading

- Mowzoon N, Flemming KD. Neurology board review: an illustrated study guide. Rochester: Mayo Clinic Scientific; 2007. Print.

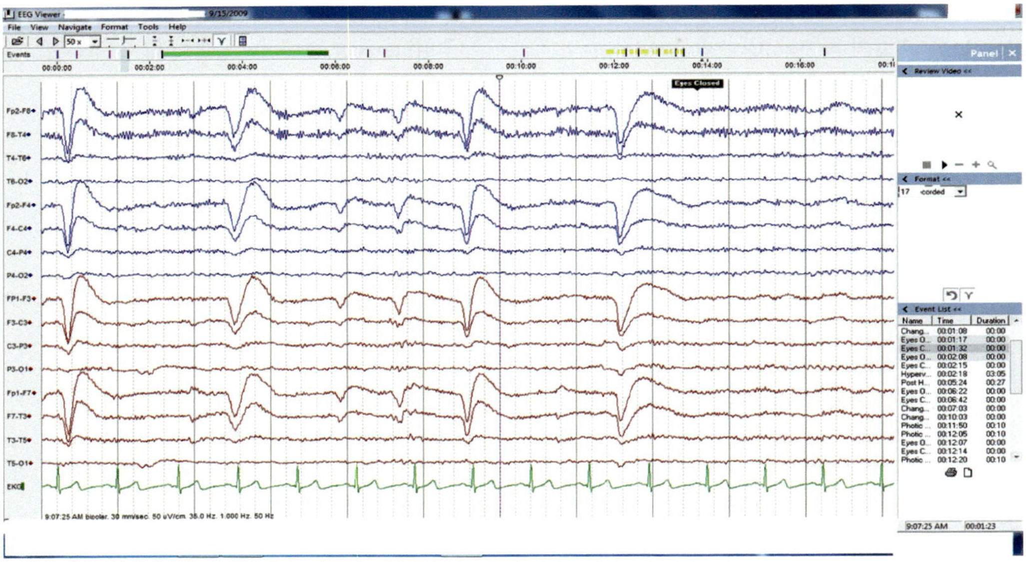

Fig. 21.1 EEG of brain and heart action on closing the eyes. (Own work. Otoomuch. Wikipedia)

14. Which of the following is correct regarding the EEG in the figure below?
    - A. There is poor reactivity of the posterior background.
    - B. The patient has an occipital seizure.
    - C. The posterior background shows Li-frequencies.
    - D. The patient is sleeping
    - E. An eye closure is recorded during this EEG page

Correct Answer is: E
There is a normal reactivity of the posterior background after an eye closure. Alpha rhythm (8 and 13 Hz), is a normal finding seen in the posterior head regions in normal people when they are awake, more prominent with eye closure, and attenuating with eye opening. Failure of attenuation with eye opening and reactivity with eye closure may be a sign of abnormality.

By 3 years of age, alpha rhythm of 8 Hz is seen in normal children, and it increases with age. A voltage asymmetry of >50% between sides is abnormal.

The posterior background is the first feature usually analyzed when reading an EEG. There are no spikes or other epileptiform discharges seen in the figure and therefore no evidence of an occipital seizure. The posterior background has Alpha-frequencies (in this case around 9 Hz) and not Li-frequencies. This patient has good reactivity of the background rhythm, suggesting an awake patient. There are no sleep structures visualized.

Suggested Reading

– Tatum WO, Husain AM, Benbadis SR, et al. Handbook of EEG Interpretation.

15. A 12-year-old boy came to the office after he had a generalized seizure preceded by left side eye and head deviation.
    Where do you locate the seizure focus?
    - A. Hypothalamus
    - B. Right frontal lobe
    - C. Left frontal lobe
    - D. Right temporal lobe
    - E. Left temporal lobe

Correct Answer is: B

Lateralization signs and symptoms during epileptic seizures are helpful to locate the seizure focus side, and this will help to classify the epilepsy correctly and also help in the pre-surgical evaluation of drug resistant patients. Auras are a focal discharge, which activate the area responsible for generation of the patient's aura at the beginning of the clinical (but not necessarily the electrographic) seizure. Thus, auras are good clue for the seizure origin. Some seizures do not start with an aura, but other semiological signs may point toward the origin of these seizures. Eyes and head version, characterized strictly by a forced and involuntary movement leading to an unnatural position of the head toward one side, are associated with a seizure focus in the contralateral hemisphere, and more specifically in the frontal region in the frontal eye fields and motor areas anterior to the precentral gyrus. The association of version with the contralateral hemisphere is more robust if the version occurs immediately prior to the secondarily generalized tonic-clonic phase. In this case, it is clear that the seizure is coming from the right frontal region.

Suggested Reading

- Harvey AS, Freeman J L. Epilepsy in hypothalamic hamartoma: clinical and EEG features. Semin Pediatr Neural. 2007;14(2):60–4.
- Loddenkemper T, Kotagal P. Lateralizing signs during seizures in focal epilepsy. Epilepsy Behav. 2005;7:1–17.
- Comprehensive Review in Clinical Neurology: a Multiple-Choice Question Book for the Wards and Boards ©2011 Wolters Kluwer Health Lippincott Williams & Wilkins. All rights reserved.

16. The father of a 16-year-old male descript his son seizure that begin with asymmetric tonic posturing with right arm extension at the elbow with the fist clenched and left arm flexion at the elbow. Then he had a generalized tonic-clonic (GTC) seizures.
Where is the seizure focus location?
    A. Right temporal lobe
    B. Left temporal lobe
    C. Right supplementary motor area
    D. Left supplementary motor area
    E. Right occipital lobe

Correct Answer is: D

There is asymmetric tonic posturing during a seizure, which is characteristic of seizures arising from the supplementary motor area (SMA). This specific case describes the "figure of 4 sign," in which the extended arm is contralateral to the seizure focus. Therefore, this patient's seizures originate in the left SMA.

Addendum: "the figure of 4" sign is an arm flexed at the elbow and a contralateral arm that is extended - the ictal focus is ipsilateral to the flexed arm and contralateral to the extended / dystonic arm.

Suggested Reading

- Harvey AS, Freeman JL. Epilepsy in hypothalamic hamartoma: clinical and EEG features. Semin. Pediatr Neurol. 2007;14(2):60–4.
- Loddenkemper T, Kotagal P. Lateralizing signs during seizures in focal epilepsy. Epilepsy Behav. 2005;7:1–17.
- Comprehensive Review in Clinical Neurology: A Multiple-Choice Question Book for the Wards and Boards ©2011 Wolters Kluwer Health Lippincott Williams & Wilkins. All rights reserved.

17. Which one of the following is true regarding myelination of the central nervous system?
    A. Myelination of axons is done by Schwann cells
    B. Myelination starts at 6 weeks of gestation

C. Extensor plantar response in infants is an abnormal finding
D. Bulk of myelination is done in the 3rd trimester
E. All cranial nerves myelinate prenatally

Correct Answer is: D
Myelination in central nervous system is done by oligodendrocytes and occurs as early as 14 weeks of gestation and continues to adulthood. Bulk of active myelination begins at third trimester and continues to about 2 years postnatally. Corticospinal tract myelinates throughout first 2 years of life: extensor plantar response is present at birth and disappears sometime during this development. Poor myelination of cortical pathways is responsible for lack of cortical control over motor function at birth and is responsible for primitive reflexes present at birth, such as grasp reflex. Optic nerve myelinates postnatally; most other cranial nerves myelinate prenatally. Certain subcortical association fibers (especially of frontal cortex) do not complete myelination until early adulthood.

Suggested Reading

- Mowzoon N, Flemming KD. Neurology board review: an illustrated study guide. Rochester: Mayo Clinic Scientific; 2007. Print.

18. Which is most likely to be the last reflex to disappear in an infant with normal development?
    A. Galant reflex
    B. Tonic neck reflex
    C. Landau reflex
    D. Crossed adduction
    E. Moro reflex

Correct Answer is: C
Galant reflex (Lateral incurvature of the trunk) appears at birth and disappears by 4–6 months of age. When the spine is stroked or tapped with the infant lying in a prone position, the hips move toward the touch.

The tonic neck reflex, or "fencing posture," is present at birth, and disappears by 5–6 months of age. When the baby's head is turned to the side, the ipsilateral arm and leg extend and the contra lateral arm and leg flex.

The Landau reflex does not typically appear until 5–10 months of age, and may persist until 24 months. It is a postural reflex elicited by holding the baby in a prone position. When moving the baby's head downward (flexion), the legs will follow, moving downward by flexion at the hip.

Crossed adduction appears at birth, and resolves by approximately 7 months of age. When testing a patellar reflex, there is adduction of the contralateral leg.

The Moro reflex appears at birth, and disappears at 5–6 months of age. With a sudden stimulus, both arms will extend.

19. Regarding the pharmacokinetics of phenytoin.which of the following is correct?
    A. It is predominantly renally metabolized
    B. It is exclusively metabolized by the liver
    C. It has zero-order (nonlinear) kinetics
    D. It is a hepatic enzyme inhibitor
    E. It has first-order (linear) kinetics

Correct Answer is: C
Phenytoin is used for the treatment of partial and/or generalized tonic clonic (GTC) seizures (primary or secondary). Its primary mechanism of action is inhibition of voltage-dependent neuronal sodium channels. It undergoes predominantly liver metabolism, although there

is also minimal renal metabolism. Patients who are in low-protein disease states (such as liver failure, etc.) need to be followed with free phenytoin levels because of less available protein for binding, making the total levels unreliable. It is important to understand that phenytoin exhibits nonlinear (zero-order) kinetics, as the metabolic pathways responsible for its metabolism become saturated. This means that when the dose of phenytoin is increased beyond a certain point, its plasma concentration at steady state will no longer increase in a proportionate manner, rather small dose changes may result in a large/toxic increment in plasma concentrations. In general, phenytoin approaches zero-order kinetics at total levels >10–15 Mg/ml and small dose increments can potentially cause large increases in the serum level.

Idiosyncratic reactions caused by phenytoin include aplastic anemia, Stevens-Johnson syndrome, and hepatic failure. Other side effects include thrombocytopenia, lymphadenopathy, gingival hyperplasia, acne, coarse facial features (also called "phenytoin facies," from hypertrophy of subcutaneous facial tissue), hirsutism, purple glove syndrome (with intravenous administration), nystagmus, ataxia, dysarthria, diplopia, nausea, dizziness, and drowsiness. Phenytoin can also cause folate deficiency and increased vitamin D metabolism, resulting in premature osteoporosis.

Chronically, its use has been associated with a usually mild peripheral neuropathy and with cerebellar, but not cortical atrophy. Acutely, the IV form can cause phlebitis, pain, burning, hypotension, and cardiac conduction abnormalities. Phenytoin is a liver enzyme inducer, so it can increase metabolism of many other drugs. There are variations of calculating loading and correcting doses of phenytoin. A general simple formula for calculating a supplementing (or loading) IV bolus of phenytoin is as follows: (target total phenytoin level - current total phenytoin level) x (kilogram body weight x volume of distribution). The therapeutic range for phenytoin is 10–20 Mg/ml. The range for volume of distribution for phenytoin is 0.5–1 L/kg, with an average of 0.8 L/kg often used. If we insert the numbers from the case into the formula, the calculation will be as follows: $(15-10) \times (75 \times 0.8) = 300$ mg. An accurate reassessment of new levels can be obtained by checking free and total levels approximately 2 h after the IV load.

Suggested Reading

- Ahn JE, Cloyd JC, Brundage RC, et al. Phenytoin half-life and clearance during maintenance therapy in adults and elderly patients with epilepsy. Neurology. 2008;71(1):38–43.
- Ropper AH, Samuels MA. Adams and Victor's Principles of Neurology, 9th ed. New York: McGraw-Hill; 2009.
- Schachter SC. Review of the mechanisms of action of antiepileptic drugs. CNS Drugs. 1995;4:469–77.
- Comprehensive Review in Clinical Neurology: A Multiple-Choice Question.
- Book for the Wards and Boards ©2011 Wolters Kluwer Health Lippincott Williams & Wilkins. All rights reserved.

20. Deficiency of which of the following neurotransmitters has been implicated in the pathogenesis of Narcolepsy?
    A. Noradrenaline
    B. Acetylcholine
    C. Serotonin
    D. Histamine
    E. Hypocretin

Correct Answer is: E

Hypocretin, also known as orexin, is deficient in the cerebrospinal fluid of most narcoleptics with cataplexy.

21

Suggested Reading

- Blumenfeld H. Neuroanatomy through clinical cases. 1st ed. Sunderland: Sinauer Associates; 2002.

21. Which of the following is most likely to be true of benign focal epilepsy with central mid temporal spikes?
    A. Lifelong treatment with anti-epileptic medications is often necessary
    B. Seizures usually occur during the daytime while the child is awake
    C. Children with this disorder may complain of facial numbness or may be observed drooling
    D. EEG findings are used to determine whether to continue, discontinue, or start anti-epileptic medications

Correct Answer is: C
Benign rolandic epilepsy (Benign focal epilepsy with centrotemporal spikes), accounts for 15% of childhood epilepsy. It begins between 7 and 9 years of age. Its name is referring to the typical EEG findings. Diphasic or triphasic sharp waves tend to occur in the mid temporal and central areas. The clinical presentation includes, speech arrest, hypersalivation, unilateral facial twitching, and paresthesias inside the mouth.

Treatment with anti-epileptic medications is often not necessarily. Seizures tend to occur at night and most patients have under 10 seizures total. Typically, remission occurs within 2–4 years of onset of seizures. Most are in remission by age 16. Treatment may be necessary in patients who have more frequent seizures, or in those with generalized seizures.

75% of seizures occur either during the night, or when the patient wakes. On EEG studies, epileptiform activity is more prominent during N-REM sleep.

EEG activity typical of benign focal epilepsy with centrotemporal spikes may occur in individuals who do not have known seizures. Also, in patients who do have clinical and EEG findings characteristic of this form of epilepsy, the EEG abnormalities may persist even after the seizures have stopped. Thus, decisions on whether to start or stop anti-epileptic drugs are not based on EEG findings.

22. Regarding embryonal nervous system development, which of the following statements is correct?
    A. Vertebral bodies arise from ectodermal cells of the neural plate
    B. Neural crest cells give rise to the peripheral nervous system
    C. Failure of fusion of the posterior neuropore leads to disorders such as anencephaly
    D. Failure of fusion of the anterior neuropore leads to disorders such as spina bifida
    E. The notochord gives rise to chromaffin cells of the adrenal medulla

Correct Answer is: B
The main embryonal layer giving rise to the nervous system is the ectoderm. In early stages of nervous system development, a structure known as the neural plate forms. The notochord, a layer of mesodermal cells in contact with the ectoderm, induces formation of the neural plate from the ectoderm and later signals differentiation of various cell types mediated by inductive signals. The notochord later gives rise to the vertebral column. The neural plate forms a structure known as the neural tube through a process called neurulation. Neurulation involves proliferation and migration of ectodermal cells and invagination, folding, and fusion of the neural plate in a specific pattern. An important step in neurulation includes the formation of a midline groove along which the lateral margins of the neural plate fold.

These lateral margins start to fuse in the center, so that for a period of time, there are openings at each end, the anterior and posterior neuropore.

Fusion then reaches the neuropores, the anterior one first, then the posterior one, and the neural tube is thus formed. The ventral and dorsal aspects of the neural tube each give rise to specific cell populations and ultimately specific parts of the nervous system. As mentioned, mesodermal cells of the notochord provide signals for differentiation to cells in the ventral aspect of the neural tube. These signals include sonic hedgehog protein and bone morphogenetic proteins, of which several types have been identified. Neurulation occurs at 3–6 weeks' gestation, and failure of crucial processes at any stage leads to a variety of abnormalities, collectively known as neural tube defects. As mentioned earlier, the neural plate undergoes fusion to form the neural tube in different areas at different times, and failure to fuse at each site results in specific defects. Abnormal rostral fusion at the anterior neuropore leads to abnormalities such as encephalocele or anencephaly, whereas abnormal caudal fusion (at the posterior neuropore) leads to disorders such as spina bifida. Following neurulation, the neural tube undergoes segmentation into three vesicles, in a process called specification, whereby different segments begin to acquire cell types and characteristics specific to the CNSstructure that will eventually arise from them. The three segments include the prosencephalon, mesencephalon, and rhombencephalon. The prosencephalon subsequently forms the telencephalon, which gives rise to the cerebral hemispheres, as well as the diencephalon, which forms the hypothalamus and thalamus. The rhombencephalon gives rise to the brain stem. Abnormalities during specification, which occurs at 5–6 weeks of gestation, lead to disorders such as septo-optic dysplasia. As the nervous system becomes more organized and specific areas more specialized, neuronal migration begins along specific routes, and abnormalities of neuronal proliferation and migration in turn lead to specific developmental abnormalities. The peripheral nervous system (including the autonomic ganglia) forms from neural crest cells that are derived from the neural tube after it fuses. In addition to peripheral nervous system structures, neural crest cells give rise to the chromaffin tissue of the adrenal medulla and melanocytes.

23. Which of the following anticonvulsants binds to synaptic vesicle protein SV2A?
    A. Levetiracetam
    B. Topiramate
    C. Lamotrigine
    D. Ethosuximide
    E. Perampanel

Correct Answer is: A

Levetiracetam binds to synaptic vesicle protein SV2A, which decreases calcium influx into the presynaptic terminal. The drug also blocks high voltage activated calcium channels and affects gamma aminobutyric acid (GABA) function. It is unclear, however, how these actions relate to its anticonvulsant effect.

Topiramate has multiple mechanisms of action, blocking sodium channels, calcium channels, kainate receptors, and a-amino-3-hydroxyl-5-methyl-4-i soxazole-proprionate (AMPA) glutamate receptors, while enhancing GABA activity.

Lamotrigine also has multiple mechanisms of action, blocking sodium channels and high voltage activated calcium channels.

Ethosuximide blocks thalamic T-type calcium channels, and likely inhibits sodium currents.

21

Perampanel is a new anticonvulsant with a novel mechanism of action, acting as a non-competitive AMPA glutamate receptor antagonist.

Suggested Reading

- Stafstrom CE. Mechanisms of action of antiepileptic drugs: the search for synergy. Curr Opin Neurol. 23:157–63.

24. Which of the cell types forms the blood-brain barrier and help in neuronal migration during development?
    A. Astrocytes
    B. Oligodendrocytes
    C. Microglia
    D. Neurons

Correct Answer is: A
Three cellular elements of the brain microvasculature compose the BBB: endothelial cells, astrocyte end-feet, and pericytes.

Astrocytes are one type of glia cells, responsible for the development and framework of the neurons. They outnumber neurons 5:1 and contiguously tile the entire CNS. They also form part of the blood-brain barrier.

Suggested Reading

- Ballabh P, Braun A, Nedergaard M. The blood-brain barrier: an overview: structure, regulation, and clinical implications. Neurobiol Dis. 2004 Jun;16(1):1–13.

25. Regarding embryonal nervous system development, which of the following statements is correct?
    A. The rhombencephalon gives rise to the cerebral hemispheres
    B. The mesencephalon gives rise to the hypothalamus and thalamus
    C. The prosencephalon gives rise to the telencephalon, which ultimately forms the cerebral hemispheres
    D. The diencephalon gives rise to the midbrain
    E. The prosencephalon gives rise to the telencephalon, which ultimately forms the brain stem

Correct Answer is: C
The main embryonal layer giving rise to the nervous system is the ectoderm. In early stages of nervous system development, a structure known as the neural plate forms. The notochord, a layer of mesodermal cells in contact with the ectoderm, induces formation of the neural plate from the ectoderm and later signals differentiation of various cell types mediated by inductive signals. The notochord later gives rise to the vertebral column. The neural plate forms a structure known as the neural tube through a process called neurulation. Neurulation involves proliferation and migration of ectodermal cells and invagination, folding, and fusion of the neural plate in a specific pattern. An important step in neurulation includes the formation of a midline groove along which the lateral margins of the neural plate fold. These lateral margins start to fuse in the center, so that for a period of time, there are openings at each end, the anterior and posterior neuropore. Fusion then reaches the neuropores, the anterior one first, then the posterior one, and the neural tube is thus formed. The ventral and dorsal aspects of the neural tube each give rise to specific cell populations and ultimately specific parts of the nervous system. As mentioned, mesodermal cells of the notochord provide signals for differentiation to cells in the ventral aspect of the neural tube. These signals include sonic hedgehog protein and bone morphogenetic proteins, of which several types have been identified. Neurulation occurs at 3–6 weeks' gesta-

tion, and failure of crucial processes at any stage leads to a variety of abnormalities, collectively known as neural tube defects. As mentioned earlier, the neural plate undergoes fusion to form the neural tube in different areas at different times, and failure to fuse at each site results in specific defects. Abnormal rostral fusion at the anterior neuropore leads to abnormalities such as encephalocele or anencephaly, whereas abnormal caudal fusion (at the posterior neuropore) leads to disorders such as spina bifida. Following neurulation, the neural tube undergoes segmentation into three vesicles, in a process called specification, whereby different segments begin to acquire cell types and characteristics specific to the CNS structure that will eventually arise from them. The three segments include the prosencephalon, mesencephalon, and rhombencephalon. The prosencephalon subsequently forms the telencephalon, which gives rise to the cerebral hemispheres, as well as the diencephalon, which forms the hypothalamus and thalamus. The rhombencephalon gives rise to the brain stem. Abnormalities during specification, which occurs at 5–6 weeks of gestation, lead to disorders such as septa-optic dysplasia. As the nervous system becomes more organized and specific areas more specialized, neuronal migration begins along specific routes, and abnormalities of neuronal proliferation and migration in turn lead to specific developmental abnormalities. The peripheral nervous system (including the autonomic ganglia) forms from neural crest cells that are derived from the neural tube after it fuses. In addition to peripheral nervous system structures, neural crest cells give rise to the chromaffin tissue of the adrenal medulla and melanocytes.

26. In the setting of a fetus with a neural tube defect (NTD), which of the following statements regarding prenatal diagnosis is incorrect?
    A. Fetoprotein level is elevated in maternal serum
    B. A-Fetoprotein level is elevated in amniotic fluid
    C. Acetylcholinesterase is elevated in amniotic fluid and increases sensitivity and specificity of NTD screening
    D. There is little utility in prenatal ultrasonography in the detection of NTDs
    E. When a NTD is detected prenatally, karyotyping to assess for trisomies and other genetic defects may be indicated

Correct Answer is: D
Neural tube defects (NTDs) can be detected by prenatal ultrasonography. Prenatally, in the setting of most NTDs, serum maternal A-fetoprotein level is elevated. A-Fetoprotein is a normal component of fetal CSF, and leakage into the amniotic fluid from an open neural tube leads to elevated amniotic A-fetoprotein level. The extent of elevation correlates with the severity of the NTD. Elevations in amniotic fluid acetylcholinesterase levels also occur, and combined with an elevated fetoprotein level, increase sensitivity and specificity in prenatal screening. Ultrasonography also can be used to detect NTDs and characterize them.

Prenatal MRI is also used in some cases to assess the extent of the abnormality, aiding in prognostication of neurologic function in life. When an NTD is detected with screening, and/or other abnormalities are detected on ultrasonography, fetal karyotyping to assess for trisomy 13, 18, and others may be done to assist in management of the pregnancy.

27. Regarding neural tube defects resulting from failure of fusion of the anterior neuropore, which of the following statements is correct?
    - A. Failure of fusion of the anterior neuropore leads to spina bifida
    - B. Failure of fusion of the anterior neuropore leads to anencephaly and encephalocele
    - C. Anterior neuropore defects typically occur from insults in the last trimester of gestation
    - D. Anencephaly may be occult and diagnosed in early childhood or even adolescence
    - E. Encephalocele is incompatible with life

Correct Answer is: B

The neural plate fuses to form the neural tube at different locations and at different times, and failure of fusion at these various locations leads to various neural tube defects. Failure of anterior neuropore fusion rostrally, leads to anencephaly and encephalocele. By day 26 of gestation, the anterior neuropore fuses and abnormalities in neurulation leading to these disorders therefore likely occur at or prior to this time (weeks 1–4 gestation).

Anencephaly is the complete absence of both cerebral hemispheres. Because the underlying mesoderm also fails to properly differentiate, a large cranial vault defect (in skull, meninges, and skin) also occurs. This is most often not compatible with life, and most such infants are still born; in rare cases in which the infant is born alive, death occurs soon after birth.

Encephalocele is defined by herniation of neural tissues (hamartomatous brain tissue, without recognizable architecture) into a midline defect in the skull. Encephaloceles are most often located in the occipital area and less often in frontal areas. Clinically, they appear as round, protuberant, fluctuant masses covered by an opaque membrane or normal skin. They are compatible with life although they cause multiple complications. Associated clinical features include microcephaly, developmental delay (which is more severe in occipital as compared with frontal encephaloceles), and invariably hydrocephalus. Chromosomal aberrations commonly seen in patients with encephaloceles include trisomy 13 and trisomy 18.

Occipital encephaloceles should be distinguished from cranial meningocele in which only leptomeninges and CSF are herniated through a skull defect.

28. Which of the following is not a risk factor for the occurrence of neural tube defects?
    - A. Male gender
    - B. Folate deficiency
    - C. Exposure to retinoic acid
    - D. Exposure to valproic acid
    - E. Maternal diabetes

Correct Answer is: A

Several risk factors for neural tube defects (NTDs) have been identified. NTDs are more common in females. Folate is involved in various pathways of nucleic acid synthesis and DNA methylation reactions, and maternal folate deficiency is a well-established risk factor for NTD. Therefore, prenatal and perinatal maternal supplementation with 0.4 mg folic acid is recommended. Teratogens associated with NTDs include retinoic acid (vitamin A or the acidic form, tretinoin, found in acne medications). Other teratogens associated with NTDs include anti-epileptics, particularly valproic acid and carbamazepine, which may lead to NTDs by affecting folate metabolism. Other risk factors for NTDs include maternal diabetes and history of a prior pregnancy resulting in an infant with an NTD.

29. At 9 months, an infant is typically able to:
    A. Take three steps unaided
    B. Scribble with a crayon
    C. Remove clothing
    D. Have a pincer grasp
    E. Stack two cubes

Correct Answer is: D
While the timing of developmental stages may vary greatly between children, a general timeline of important milestones follows:

- **3 Months:**
  - Puts hands together.
  - Has a social smile, recognizes parents.
  - Laughs.
- **4 Months:**
  - Rolls from tummy to back.
- **6 Months:**
  - Sits unsupported.
  - Rolls in both directions.
  - Begins to crawl.
  - Reaches and passes objects from one hand to another.
  - Babbles with strings of vowel and consonant sounds.
- **9 Months:**
  - May develop stranger anxiety.
  - Stands unassisted.
  - Has pincer grasp.
- **12 Months:**
  - Walks.
  - Scribbles.
  - Says "mama" and "dada".
- **15 Months:**
  - Stacks two cubes.
  - Runs.
  - Removes clothing.
  - Has a 6-word vocabulary

30. Regarding normal cerebral cortex architecture, which of the following statements is incorrect?
    A. Normal cerebra l cortex has six layers
    B. Pyramidal cells are the most common type of cortical neurons
    C. Granular cells are found in higher numbers in sensory cortex
    D. Different cortical and subcortical areas project to and receive projections from specific cortical layers
    E. Betz cells function predominantly as interneurons and are found in secondary association cortices

Correct Answer is: E
Betz cells are the upper motor neurons of the nervous system; these are large cells found in the primary motor cortex. The majority of the cerebral cortex (>90%) consists of neocortex (also known as isocortex), a six-layered cortex (as opposed to more primitive cortex with less numbers of layers, as occurs in the paleocortex (found in olfactory and limbic cortices) and archicortex, seen in the hippocampus). The six layers of the neocortex are molecular layer (layer I), external granular cell layer (layer II), external pyramidal cell layer (layer III), internal granular cell layer (layer IV), internal pyramidal cell layer (layer V), and multiform layer (layer VI). Cortico-cortical efferents (projections from one area of cortex to another) arise mainly in layer III and project predominantly to layers II and III. Layers I, IV, and VI receive the majority of thalamic efferents. Layer V gives rise to corticostriate projections (from cortex to striatum), and layer VI gives rise to corticothalamic projections (from cortex to thalamus). Pyramidal cells constitute the largest number of cortical neurons and are found in high-

21

est numbers in cortical areas that give rise to efferents; granular (or stellate) cells function predominantly as cortical interneurons and predominate in regions involved in sensory function or integration (secondary association cortices, etc.). Betz cells are the upper motor neurons of the nervous system; these are large cells found in layer V of the primary motor cortex. Formation of gyri and sulci normally occurs between weeks 20 and 36 of gestation. Abnormalities in this process can lead to a variety of malformations of cortical development.

31. What is the most useful treatment for an 8-year-old boy who has continues paroxysmal EEG discharges throughout sleep and presents with hyperactivity, learning disabilities and occasional severe behavioral out bursts?
    - A. Risperidone
    - B. Carbamazepin
    - C. Valproic acid
    - D. Phenytoin
    - E. ACTH

Correct Answer is: E
Electrical status epilepticus during slow wave sleep (ESES) is characterized by sleep induced paroxysmal EEG activity and is associated with neuropsychological dysfunction and behavioral disorders. Most children with isolated epileptiform EEG activity restricted to sleep do not have daytime clinical seizures. Seizure types during wakeful include atypical absence, myoclonic and akinetic. High dose steroids and ACTH are the most useful treatment. Standard anticonvulsants are rarely effective and anti-psychotic medications are not indicated.

Suggested Reading

- Smith S. EEG in the diagnosis, classification, and management of patients with epilepsy. J Neural Neurosurg Psychiatry. 2005;76:ii2–7.

32. A 15-year-old boy has a large right hemispheric tumor resection recently. He is admitted to inpatient rehabilitation, and his progress is being hindered by his lack of awareness of the left side of his body. He barely acknowledges the presence of weakness on the left side of his body; in fact, he largely does not recognize the left side of his body as being his own. **This is consistent with:**
    - A. A lesion in the dominant hemisphere parietal region involving the primary somatosensory cortex
    - B. A lesion in the nondominant hemisphere primary visual cortex
    - C. A lesion in the nondominant frontal lobe
    - D. A lesion in the nondominant hemisphere parietal region involving the primary somatosensory cortex
    - E. A lesion in the dominant hemisphere angular gyrus

Correct Answer is: D
This boy exhibits anosognosia, or a lack of awareness of an acquired neurologic deficit, and hemispatial neglect syndrome, consistent with a lesion in the nondominant hemisphere involving the primary somatosensory cortex (area SI). A lesion in the thalamus can also lead to a neglect syndrome.

33. A 17-year-old football player is brought by the EMS after he had a traumatic brain injury, sustained when he was tackled to the ground by an opposite player. He develops a fever of 102.2 °F (39 °C), which is unrelated to an infection or inflammation. **The fever is most likely due to a lesion of which of the following?**
    - A. Pre-optic Nucleus
    - B. Arcuate nucleus
    - C. Lateral hypothalamus
    - D. Paraventricular nucleus
    - E. Posterior nucleus

Correct Answer is: A
The pre-optic nucleus controls heat loss, and lesions in this area would produce a fever. The hypothalamus regulates body temperature. Core body temperature, the temperature of the deep tissues of the body, is detected by thermoreceptors located within the anterior hypothalamus. The anterior hypothalamus also contains neurons responsible for initiating reflexes, such as vasodilation and sweating, which are designed to reduce body temperature. Heat-producing reflexes, such as shivering, and heat-maintenance reflexes, such as vasoconstriction, are initiated by neurons located within the posterior hypothalamus. The posterior hypothalamus regulates catecholamine secretion. The paraventricular nucleus regulates TSH secretion. The lateral hypothalamus regulates thirst, and the arcuate nucleus exerts neuroendocrine control of prolactin secretion.

Suggested Reading

- Mowzoon N, Flemming KD. Neurology board review: an illustrated study guide. Rochester: Mayo Clinic Scientific; 2007. Print.

34. Which of the following statements is incorrect regarding cortical development?
    A. The cerebral hemispheres form from a single layer of columnar epithelium located in the sub-ependymal region known as the primary germinal zone
    B. Cells of the marginal zone proliferate and migrate along a scaffold formed by the processes of radial glia
    C. The most superficial cortical layers form from cells that migrate first (the cortex forms outside-in)
    D. Neuron types include pyramidal neurons, cortical granular or stellate neurons, and Betz cells
    E. Glial cell types include astrocytes, oligodendrocytes, ependyma, and microglia

Correct Answer is: C
The cortex forms inside-out: cells that migrate out first form deeper layers, whereas cells that migrate later form more superficial structures. The cerebral hemispheres form from an initially single layer of columnar epithelium located in the sub-ependymal region known as the ventricular zone (or primary germinal zone). Cells in this layer are pluripotential and frequently divide. Another layer, the sub-ventricular zone, consists of cells known as radial glia, which send out processes that extend all the way to the pial membrane at the cortical surface. Yet another, more superficial layer, the marginal zone, forms by the fifth week of gestation. Cells leave the marginal zone and migrate along the radial glial processes in two waves, one at approximately 6 weeks' gestation and the other at 11 weeks' gestation, peaking at weeks 12–14. Cells destined to form layers 2–6 of the cortex originate in this second wave. The cortex develops inside-out, such that cells in the earliest portion of migration form deeper layers, whereas cells that migrate later form more superficial structures. Several factors influence neurogenesis (formation of neurons, including pyramidal neurons, cortical granular or stellate neurons, Betz cells, and others) and gliogenesis (formation of glia, including astrocytes, oligodendrocytes, ependyma, and microglia), as well as cell migration. These include regulatory proteins, transcription factors, and neurotransmitters, each varying with the stage of development. Cajal-Retzius cells are a group of stellate neurons found in the cortex prior to arrival of the first wave of cells. These cells secrete GABA and acetylcholine and express several products including US1 and Reelin, genes necessary for neuronal migration along radial glia. All six layers of the cortex are identifiable by 27 weeks' gestation.

Short Q/A

Y. M. Awaad, *Absolute Pediatric Neurology*, https://doi.org/10.1007/978-3-319-78801-2_22

1. All the following are components of or functionally related to the basal ganglia EXCEPT
   A. caudate nucleus
   B. red nucleus
   C. Sub-thalamic nucleus
   D. putamen
   E. substantia nigra

Correct Answer is: B

2. All the following statements concerning spina bifida are correct EXCEPT
   A. spina bifida occurs after failure of closure of the posterior arch of one or more vertebrae
   B. in spina bifida, the defect occurs most frequently at sacral and lumbar levels of the spinal cord
   C. in spina bifida occulta, the meningeal herniation extends far above the defect in the verbal arch
   D. failure of closure of the caudal neuropore typically results in myelomeningocele
   E. myelomeningocele is frequently accompanied by obstruction to the flow of cerebrospinal fluid

Correct Answer is: C

3. All the following events occur during the process of retrograde degeneration EXCEPT
   A. a displacement of the nucleus toward the periphery of the cell
   B. an initial swelling of the cell body
   C. a proliferation of Nissl granules
   D. degeneration of process along the axon distal to the lesion
   E. an initial accumulation of mitochondria in the axoplasm at the nodes of Ranvier

Correct Answer is: C

4. Which of the following statements concerning ligand-gating of neuronal membrane channels is true?
   A. The normal triggering mechanism for gating involves non-specific binding by large classes of molecules.
   B. Channels are opened when a given molecule selectively binds with the gating molecule
   C. Ligand- gating is triggered by changes in the electrical potential across the membrane
   D. The channels are constructed of a mixture of proteins and lipids
   E. The gating molecule shows no conformational change during the gating process

Correct Answer is: B

5. After the occurrence of an action potential, there is a repolarization of the membrane.
   The principal explanation for this event is that
   A. potassium channels have been opened
   B. sodium channels have been opened
   C. potassium channels have been inactivated
   D. the membrane becomes impermeable to all ions
   E. there has been a sudden influx of calcium

Correct Answer is: A

6. Which of the following statements concerning sodium channels is true?
   A. They are opened when the membrane is hyperpolarized
   B. They display a high conductance in the resting membrane

C. They open rapidly following depolarization of the membrane
D. They are rapidly activated by tetrodotoxin

Correct Answer is: C

7. Epileptiform activity is believed to include the activation of
A. AMPA receptors alone
B. Glutamate receptors alone
C. metabotropic receptors alone
D. both AMPA and glutamate receptors
E. both AMPA and metabotropic receptors

Correct Answer is: D

8. All the following are usually classified as excitatory transmitters EXCEPT
A. glumate
B. acetylcholine
C. substance P
D. leucine
E. Aspartate

Correct Answer is: D

9. All of the following are drugs that affect central cholinergic synapses EXCEPT
A. atropine
B. scopolamine
C. haloperidol
D. Physostigmine
E. Hemicholinium

Correct Answer is: C

10. All of the following are common effects of a lesion of the pyramidal system EXCEPT
A. loss of volitional movement of the limb(s) contralateral to the lesion
B. spasticity
C. hypotonia of the limb(s) ipsilateral to the lesion
D. a positive Babinski sign
E. a reduction in the size of the internal capsule on the side ipsilateral to the lesion

Correct Answer is: C

11. Unilateral deafness may result from a lesion of
A. The auditory cortex of one side
B. The lateral lemniscus of one side
C. Cranial nerve VIII on one side
D. The medial geniculate
E. The medial lemniscus

Correct Answer is: C

12. A man is unable to move his eyes downward. The lesion is most likely situated in the
A. medulla
B. basilar aspect of the pons
C. pontine tegmentum
D. midbrain
E. cerebellum

Correct Answer is: D

13. Spasticity may result from a lesion of
A. ventral horn cells
B. corpus callosum
C. postcentral gyrus
D. internal capsule
E. substantia nigra

Correct Answer is: D

14. The Klüver-Bucy syndrome is typically associated with lesions of the
A. septal area
B. amygdale
C. cingulated gyrus
D. medial hypothalamus
E. lateral hypothalamus

Correct Answer is: B

15. All the following events are likely to occur during a seizure or as a consequence of seizure activity EXCEPT
    A. synchronization of synaptic activity
    B. a decrease in GABA receptors
    C. an increase in NMDA receptors
    D. an increase in extracellular concentration of calcium ions
    E. a change in noradrenergic innervations of the epileptogenic region

Correct Answer is: D

16. Head CT of a 5-years-old child. What procedure has this patient most likely undergone?

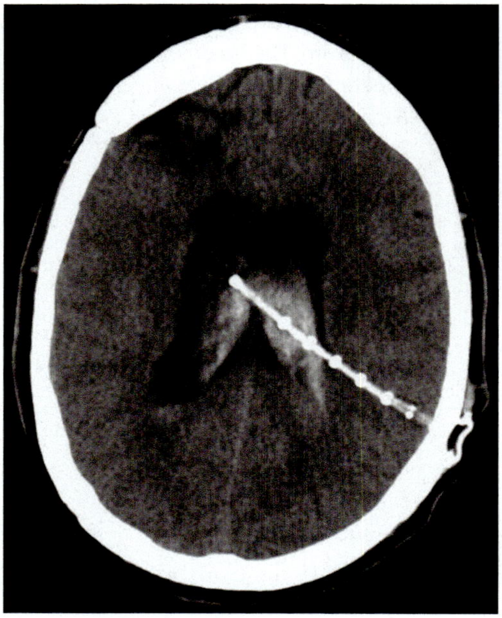

Fig. 22.1 A ventriculoperitoneal shunt as seen on CT imaging. (Own work. James Heilman, MD. Wikipedia)

    A. Recanalization of superior sagittal sinus
    B. Removal of left parietal tumor
    C. Removal of right parietal tumor
    D. Removal of subdural hematoma
    E. Ventriculo-peritoneal shunting

Correct Answer is: E

17. The cerebellar abnormality shown is most consistent with which of the following?
    A. arachnoid cyst
    B. Chiari type II malformation
    C. cystic hemangioblastoma with mural nodule
    D. Dandy-Walker malformation
    E. post-surgical changes

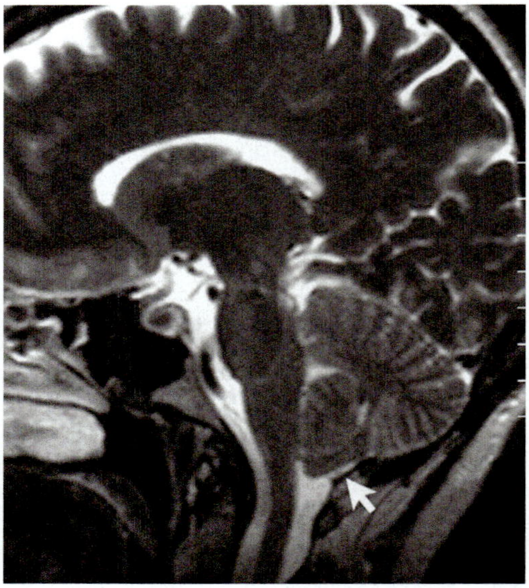

Fig. 22.2 A T2-weighted sagittal MRI scan, from a patient with Chiari-like symptomatology, demonstrating tonsillar herniation less than 3 mm. Dimensions of the posterior fossa in patients symptomatic for Chiari I malformation but without cerebellar tonsillar descent. (*Cerebrospinal Fluid Research* 2005, 2:11. doi: ▶ https://doi.org/10.1186/1743-8454-2-11. Raymond F Sekula Jr., Peter J Jannetta, Kenneth F Casey, Edward M Marchan, L Kathleen Sekula and Christine S McCrady. Wikipedia)

Correct Answer is: B

18. The proton density MRI shown was obtained on a five-year-old with quadriparesis. What is the most likely diagnosis?
    A. Binswanger's disease
    B. ceroid lipofuscinosis
    C. herpetic encephalitis
    D. Leigh's disease
    E. metachromatic leukodystrophy

Correct Answer is: E

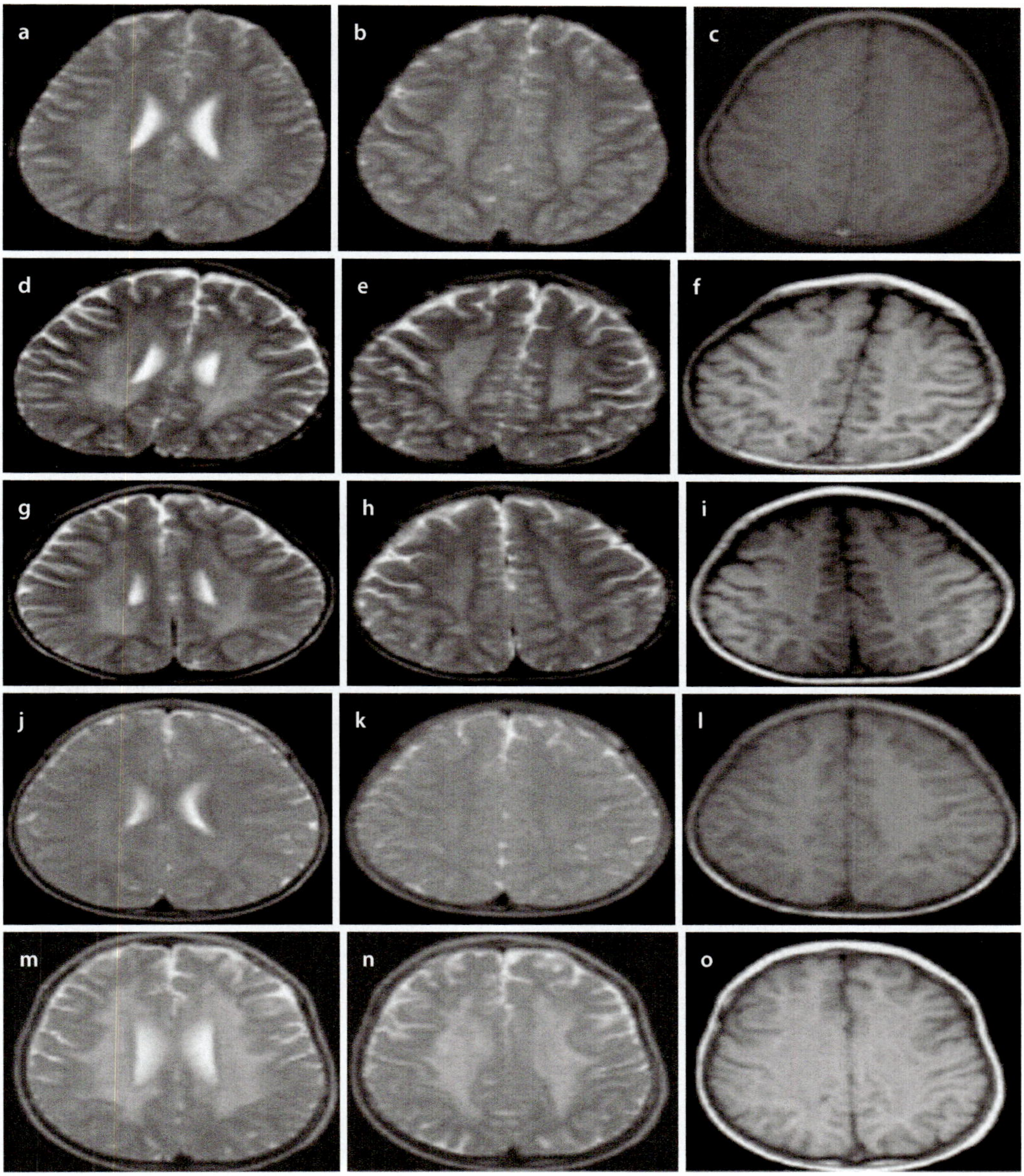

Fig. 22.3 Cranial MRIs of our patients. **a**-**c** represents patient 1, **d**-**f** patient 2, **g**-**i** patient 3, **j**-**l** patient 4, and **m**-**o** patient 5. **a**, **d**, **g**, **j**, **m** Hypointense radially oriented stripes and dots seen within the hyperintense cerebral white matter (resembling tiger skin) on T2-weighted axial imaging. **b**, **e**, **h**, **k**, **n** Hypointense dots resembling leopard skin seen on T2-weighted axial imaging at the level of centrum ovale. **c**, **f**, **i**, **l**, **o** Iso to hyperintense dots seen in the cerebral white matter on T1-weighted imaging. This pattern of dysmyelination resembles the skin of tiger (radial stripes) and leopard (dots), the so-called tigroid and leopard pattern of dysmyelination in metachromatic leukodystrophy. (Liaw, Hsiang-Ru, et al. "Late infantile metachromatic leukodystrophy: Clinical manifestations of five Taiwanese patients and Genetic features in Asia." *Orphanet Journal of Rare Diseases* 10.1 (2015): 1. HR Liaw, HF Lee, CS Chi. Wikipedia)

19. The MRI showed that of a young man. What is the most likely diagnosis of this patient?
    A. Chiari type I malformation
    B. Machado-Joseph disease
    C. Olivopontocerebellar atrophy
    D. Spinocerebellar ataxia type 6
    E. Supracerebellar arachnoid cyst

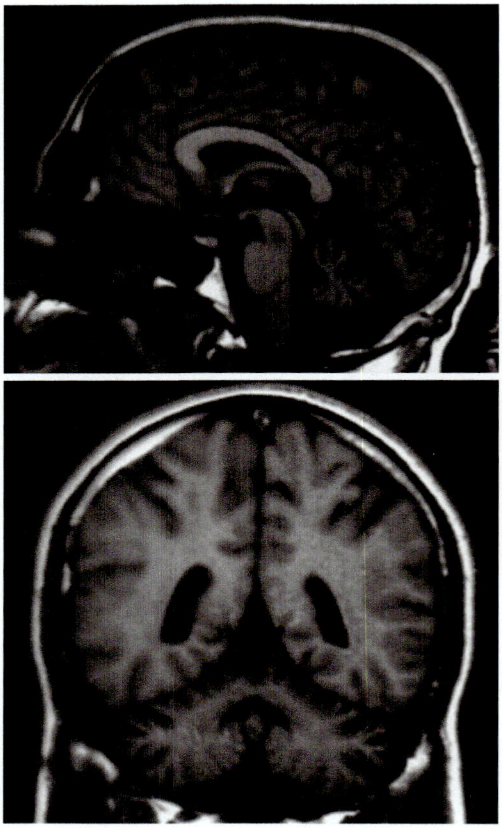

Figs. 22.4 and 22.5 Brain MRI images of the younger patient (II-14) at age 25 years old, showing cerebellar atrophy. (Nicolaou et al. *BMC Medical Genetics* 2008 9:28 doi: ▶ https://doi.org/10.1186/1471-2350-9-28. Nicolaou et al. Wikipedia)

Correct Answer is: D

20. An18-year-old girl presents with headache, nausea, and vomiting. Physical examination reveals marked papilledema. A subsequent MRI scan shows a four-cm diameter mass in the right parietal lobe. Biopsy is performed. Based on the morphologic features shown in the figure, what is the most likely diagnosis?
    A. Astroblastoma
    B. Ependymoma
    C. Fibrillary astrocytoma
    D. Gemistocytic astrocytoma
    E. Oligodendoglioma

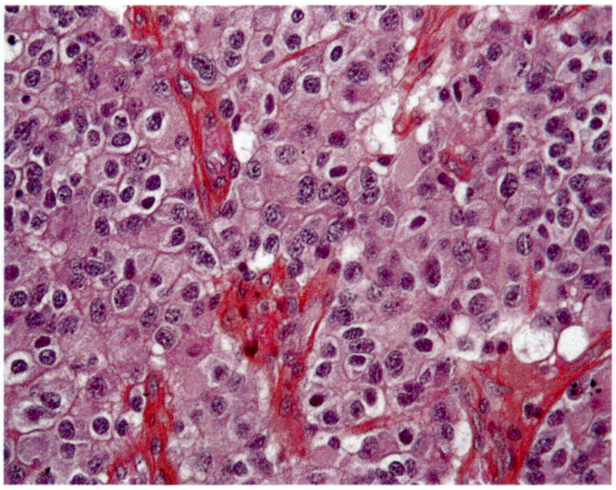

Fig. 22.6 High magnification micrograph of an **oligodendroglioma**. (H&E stain. Own work. Nephron. Wikipedia)

Correct Answer is: E

21. MRI image of a 16-year-old girl who is having seizures postpartum are shown. What is the most likely diagnosis?
    A. Adrenoleukodystrophy
    B. Bilateral hemorrhages
    C. Primary CNS angiitis
    D. Reversible posterior leukoencephalopathy syndrome
    E. Terminal area of non-myelination

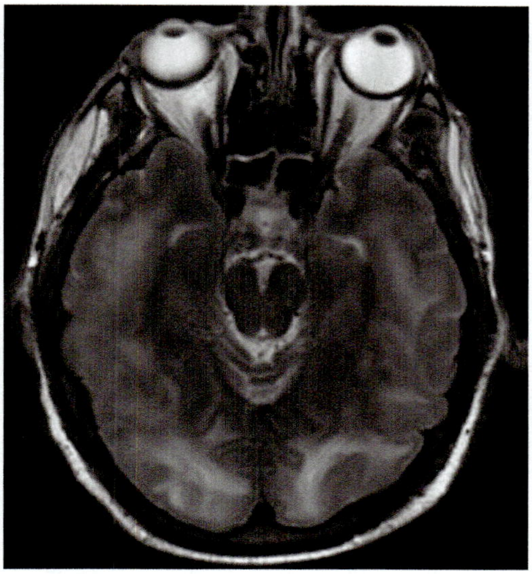

Fig. 22.7 Magnetic resonance image showing multiple cortico-subcortical areas of hyperintense signal involving the occipital and parietal lobes bilaterally and pons in a patient with posterior reversible encephalopathy syndrome. Near fatal posterior reversible encephalopathy syndrome complicating chronic liver failure and treated by induced hypothermia and dialysis: a case report. (*J Medical Case Reports* 2009, 3:6623. doi: ► https://doi.org/10.1186/1752-1947-3-6623. Rashmi Chawla, Daniel Smith and Paul E Marik. Wikipedia)

Correct Answer is: D

22. A 2-year-old boy presents with seizures. Head CT is shown. The findings are consistent with which of the following?
    A. Communicating hydrocephalus
    B. Hydrocephalus "ex vacuo"
    C. Lobar atrophy
    D. Microvascular disease
    E. Multiple sclerosis

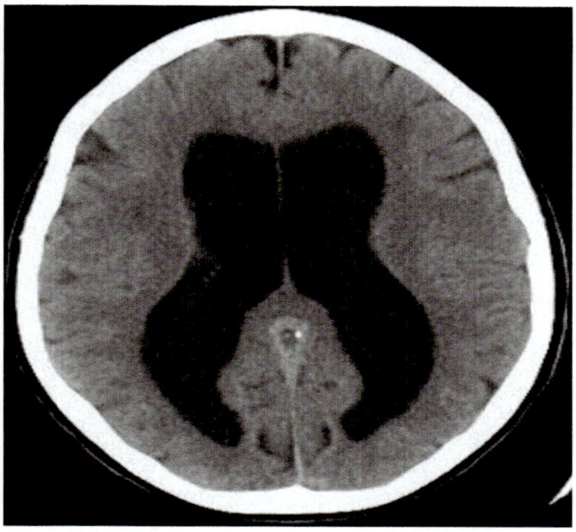

Fig. 22.8 Hydrocephalus as seen on a CT scan of the brain. The black areas in the middle of the brain are abnormally large and filled with fluid. (Lucien Monfils. Wikipedia)

Correct Answer is: A

23. The histopathology of a pineal tumor removed from a 16-year-old man is shown. What is the most appropriate diagnosis?
    A. Astrocytoma
    B. Germinoma
    C. Pinealoma
    D. Pineoblastoma
    E. Pineocytoma

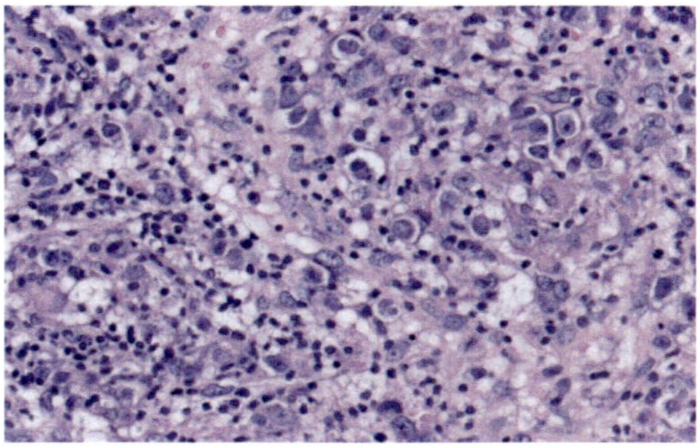

Fig. 22.9 Histology of a Germinoma (HE stain, ×200 magnification). (Own work. Jensflorian. Wikipedia)

Correct Answer is: B

24. A 13-year-old girl has a seven-year history of complex partial seizures. MRI scan reveals a hypo intense lesion in the left mesial temporal lobe. Based on the image shown, what is the most appropriate diagnosis?
    A. Dysembryoplastic neuroepithelial tumor
    B. Fibrillary astrocytoma
    C. Glioblastoma
    D. Pilocytic astrocytoma
    E. Pleomorphic xanthoastrocytoma

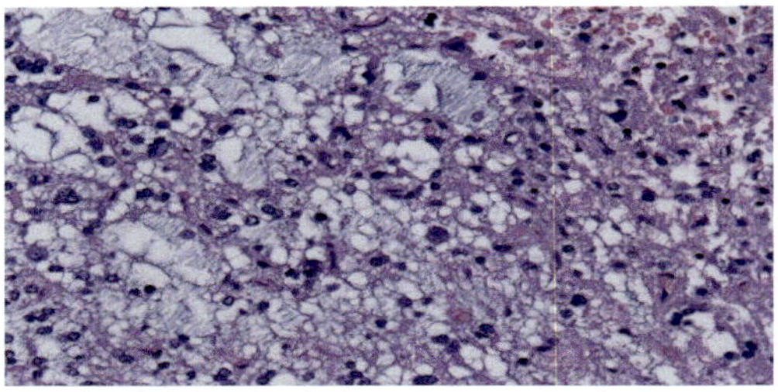

Fig. 22.10 Dysembryoplastic neuroepithelial tumor (HE stain, histology). (Own work. Jensflorian. Wikipedia)

Correct Answer is: A

25. What is the most likely diagnosis for the findings shown of an adolescent boy with leg numbness and blurry vision?
    A. Diffuse axonal injury
    B. Metastatic melanoma
    C. Multiple sclerosis
    D. vasculitis
    E. vertebral artery dissection

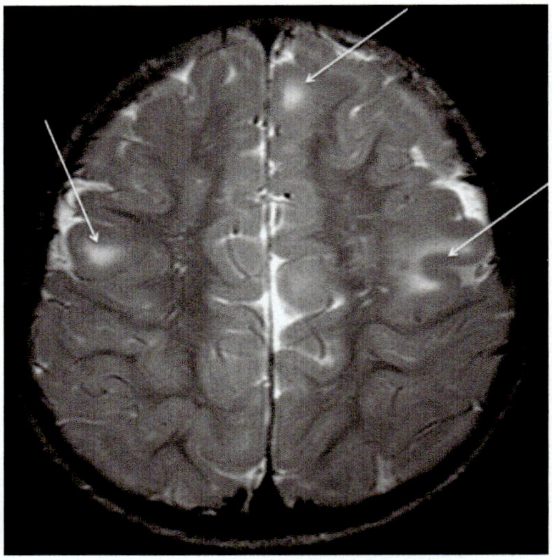

Fig. 22.11 TUBEROUS SCLEROSIS. ILAE.org. EpilepsyDiagnosis.org, Diagnostic Manual

Correct Answer is: C

26. An image of the choroid plexus of the lateral ventricle trigone (glomus choroideum) is shown. The cells identified by the arrow represent the cell of origin for which of the following neoplasms?
    A. Choroid plexus papilloma
    B. Germinoma
    C. Glomus tumor
    D. Meningiomz
    E. Teratoma

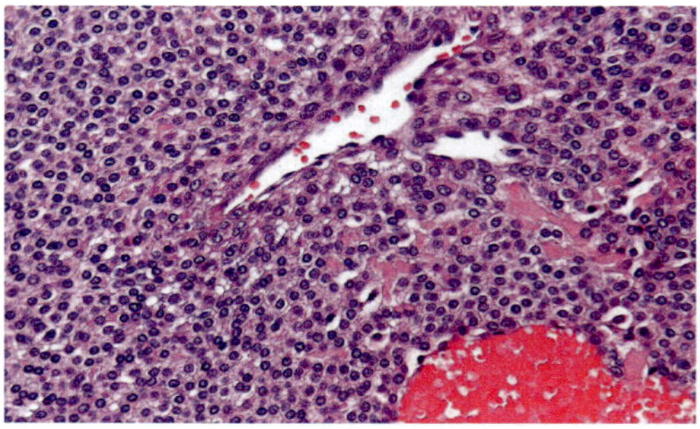

Fig. 22.12 Very high magnification micrograph of a **glomus tumour**, also written **glomus tumor**. H&E stain. (Own work.Nephron. Wikipedia)

Correct Answer is: C

27. The catheter arteriogram shown is that of a 3-month-old infant who has congestive heart failure and increased intracranial pressure. What is the most likely diagnosis?
   A. Anterior communicating artery aneurysm
   B. Hemangioblastoma
   C. Mycotic aneurysm
   D. Posterior communicating aneurysm
   E. Vein of Galen aneurysm

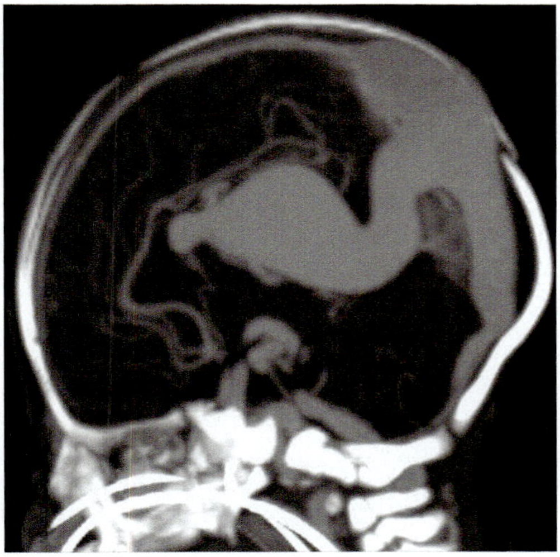

Fig. 22.13 Maximum-intensity projection from a CT cerebral angiogram showing an aneurysmal deep venous structure which drains to the vein of Galen, and then to an abnormal falcine sinus. (Radiopaedia. Dr. Laughlin Dawes. Wikipedia)

Correct Answer is: E

28. A 16-year-old woman presents with seizure disorder. Her brain MRI is shown. What is the most likely diagnosis?
   A. Bilateral strokes
   B. Epidermoid
   C. Mesial temporal sclerosis
   D. Middle fossa arachnoid cyst
   E. Previous viral encephalitis

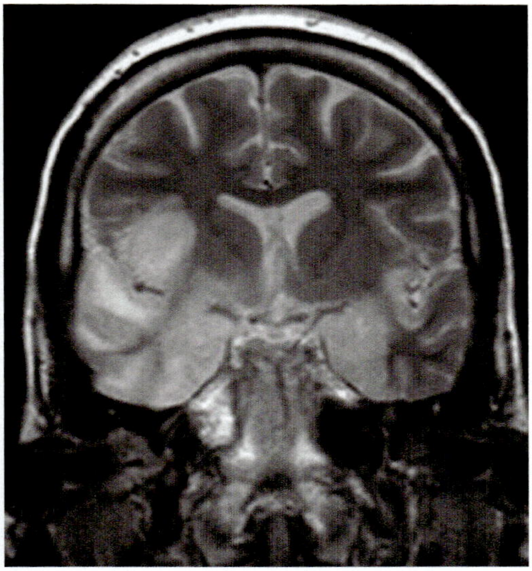

Fig. 22.14 HSV encephalitis. This coronal T2-weighted MR image shows high signal in the temporal lobes including hippocampal formations and parahippogampal gyrae, insulae, and right inferior frontal gyrus. The right gyrus rectus and the columns of the fornices were also involved (not shown). There was no associated hemorrhage or enhancement. There was moderate mass-effect. (▶ http://www.radpod.org/2007/03/24/herpes-simplex-encephalitis. dr Laughlin Dawes. Wikipedia)

Correct Answer is: E

22

29. Axial and sagittal T1-weighted images of a 5-week-old child are shown. What is the most likely diagnosis?
   - A. arachnoid cyst
   - B. Chiari type II malformation
   - C. Dandy-Walker malformation
   - D. epidermoid tumor
   - E. mega cistern magna

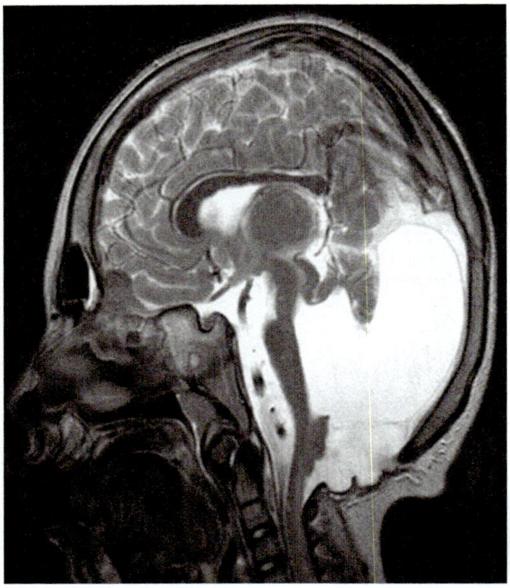

Fig. 22.15 Variant DWS with dysplasia of the pons and cerebellum in an 8-year old. T2 weighted sagittal MRI. (Hellerhoff. Wikipedia)

Correct Answer is: C

30. A 24-year-old woman presents with intractable headache and a fourth ventricular tumor. Based on the accompanying micrographs shown, what is the most likely diagnosis?
   - A. Ependymoma
   - B. Medulloblastoma
   - C. Meningioma
   - D. Oligodendroglioma
   - E. Primitive neuroectodermal tumor

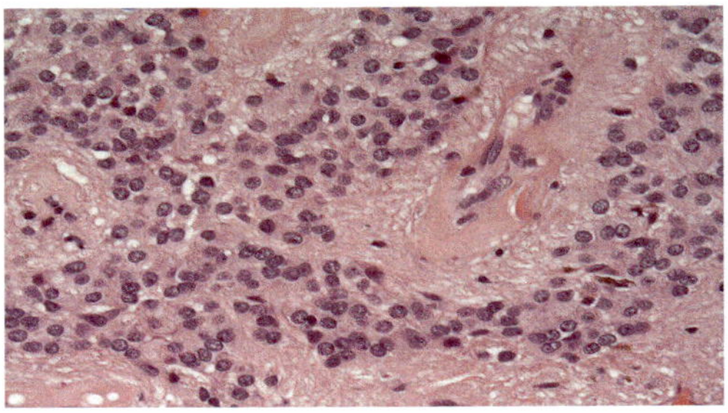

Fig. 22.16 Haematoxylin&Eosin stained paraffin section of an ependymoma (WHO Grade II). (Own work. Sbrandner. Wikipedia)

Correct Answer is: A

31. Based on the MR image shown of a 17-year-old boy with seizures, what is the most likely diagnosis?
   - A. Abscess
   - B. Cerebral cavernous angioma
   - C. Intracranial hemorrhage
   - D. Pleomorphic xanthoastrocytoma
   - E. Porencephalic cyst

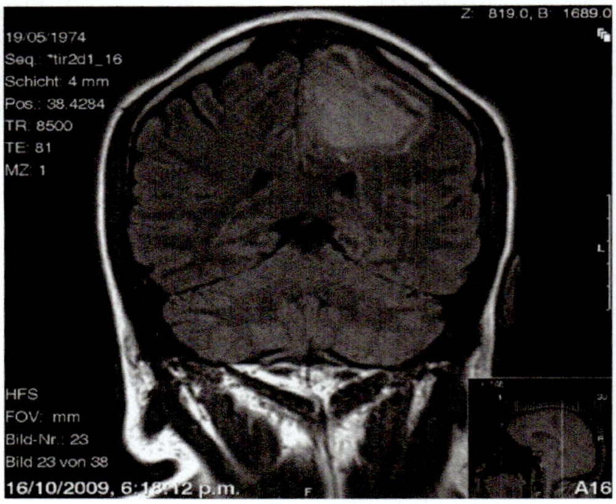

Fig. 22.17 Brain coronal section with an Intracranial hemorrhage (left hemisphere), from a MRI. (Own work. Jlguenego. Wikipedia)

Correct Answer is: C

32. The sagittal T1-weighted MR image shown, for an 18-year-old woman with weakness of both upper and lower extremities, indicates a need for which of the following?
    A. CT scan with intravenous contrast
    B. Omnipaque®
    C. Radiation therapy
    D. Spinal angiography
    E. Surgical exploration

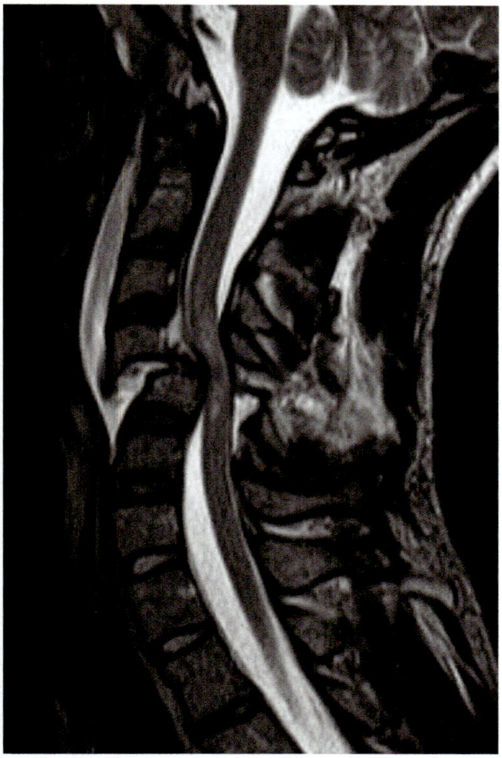

Fig. 22.18 Cervical Spine MRI of patient with SCI: C4 fracture and dislocation, spinal cord compression. (Own work. Андрей Королев 86. Wikipedia)

Correct Answer is: E

33. The S1 dorsal root ganglia are most frequently located at which of the following locations?
    A. distal to the intervertebral foramen
    B. proximal to the intervertebral foramen
    C. within the intervertebral foramen
    D. within the spinal cord dorsal horn
    E. within the spinal cord ventral horn

Correct Answer is: B
According to the anatomy and radiographic studies, the S1 dorsal root ganglia are intra-spinal and proximal to the intervertebral foramen in 71% of individuals. This is in contrast to cervical and thoracic dorsal root ganglia, which are typically located within the intervertebral foramen and lumbar dorsal root ganglia, which are intra-spinal 3% of the time at L3 and L4, and 11% to 38% of the time at L5.

Suggested Reading

- Levin K. Diseases of the nerve roots. Continuum Lifelong Learn Neurol 2008;14(3):134–55.

Sleep Disorders

Y. M. Awaad, *Absolute Pediatric Neurology*, https://doi.org/10.1007/978-3-319-78801-2_23

23

1. A 12-year-old boy complaining of difficulty falling asleep at night for last few months, and he is irritable and inattentive at school. He reports that his legs tingle when he lies down to sleep and he has to keep moving them around to get the feeling to go away. The mother has noticed that he kicks his legs frequently when he sleeps. Otherwise he has no other medical problems and takes no medications. His general and neurological examinations are normal.
What laboratory studies should you order to further evaluate his condition?
A. NCV
B. SSEP
C. Liver function tests
D. Ferritin
E. Fasting glucose

Correct Answer is: D
The presentation is typical of restless legs syndrome, which is estimated to occur in 2% of children 8–17 years of age. It is characterized by an urge to move the legs, unpleasant sensations, relieved by movement, and symptoms are worse at night. Primary RLS is idiopathic, while secondary RLS is caused by several conditions, including iron deficiency, pregnancy, renal disease, neuropathy, medications (including neuroleptics and serotonin re-uptake inhibitors). Genetic factors have an important role. The condition interferes with falling asleep, thereby causing insomnia. Most patients have periodic limb movements (stereotyped limb movements lasting 0.5–5 s recurring in 20–40 s intervals. In children with RLS, secondary causes should be sought, the most common of which is iron deficiency. Ferritin level below 50 warrants a trial of iron replacement. Dopamine agonists (ropinirole, pramipexole) are an effective treatment, as relative CNS dopamine deficiency seems to be the underlying etiology in primary RLS.

Suggested Reading

- Lipton J, Becker RE, Kothare SV. Insomnia of childhood. Curr Opin Pediatr. 2008;20(6):641–9.

2. A 7-year-old boy wakes up at night screaming for the past 3 months, which happens several times nightly. An hour after falling asleep he sits up in bed, with open eyes and begins screaming, is tremulous, sweaty and appears frightened. The episode stops after a few minutes and he goes back to sleep. Last night he got out of bed and ran around the house while screaming. His family cannot console him during the fits and he cannot remember what happened the following morning. His family reports that snores loudly at night and sometimes gasps for air. Past medical history is remarkable for episodes of recurrent otitis media as a child, for which he had myringotomy tubes placed. His early development was normal, but he is hyperactive and inattentive in second grade. On examination, he is a mouth breather and has enlarged tonsils.
What is his best treatment option?
A. Parental reassurance
B. Adenotonsillectomy
C. Benzodiazepine
D. Oxygen
E. SSRI

Correct Answer is: B
The clinical presentation is typical of sleep terrors (aka night terrors, pavor nocturnus), which are a form of non-REM parasomnias occurring during slow wave sleep. They affect about 3% of children, with peak incidence at 5–7 years of age, usually resolving by adolescence. The manifestations are characterized by

marked autonomic nervous system activation: tachycardia, tachypnea, tremulousness, mydriasis, and sweating. Facial expression of intense fear is associated with uncontrollable shouting, screaming, gasping, moaning, and agitation. Most children remain in bed during the events, but sometimes will walk or run during them. Their duration typically last one to several minutes, sometimes up to half an hour. The child cannot be consoled and attempts to awaken the child make them more intense. Differential diagnosis includes nightmares (briefer, second half of the night, consolable, dream recollection), seizures (1–2-min stereotyped hyper-motor activity), panic attacks, and cluster headaches. They can be exacerbated by acute stress, sleep deprivation, and some medications (stimulants, sedative-hypnotics, neuroleptics, antihistamines). Studies have shown that sleep disordered breathing and restless legs syndrome-periodic limb movement disorder can increase sleep terrors; treatment of these conditions can significantly improve the terrors. Signs and symptoms of obstructive sleep apnea are present in this boy and should be addressed.

Suggested Reading

- Mason T, Pack A. Sleep terrors in childhood. J Pediatr. 2005;147(3):388–92.

3. A 15-year-old female came to your office complaining of six episodes of hypersomnia in the last six months. She is an excellent academic student, well adjusted, and enjoys many extracurricular activities between the episodes. During the episodes, she is fatigued over several days, and then sleeps almost continuously for over a week but awakens to eat compulsively. On three occasions she sent sexually suggestive text messages to classmates which greatly disturbed her because this was not of her character. Her physical and neurological examination is normal. You order routine labs and a brain MRI which are all normal.
An EEG during the episode may show:
   A. Generalized slowing of background activity
   B. Slow spike and wave
   C. Electrographic status of slow wave sleep
   D. Central-temporal spike and wave discharges
   E. Frontal spikes

Correct Answer is: A
Klein-Levin syndrome is a rare disorder featuring recurrent episodes of excessive sleepiness and prolonged total sleep time. Usually, the onset is in late adolescence, but younger and older children cases have been reported. The excessive sleepiness and true hypersomnia can develop suddenly, but symptoms typically have a gradual onset of 1–7 days. During spells of hypersomnia, patients rarely leave their beds and sleep continuously. In addition to excessively long sleep episodes, abnormal behaviors, including but not limited to compulsive and excessive overeating and sexually acting out behavior can occur. Compulsive overeating and hyper sexuality are not present with each episode. Usually, physical examination is normal. Also, brain MRI is typically normal. Routine EEG obtained during attacks may show generalized slowing of the background or may be unremarkable.

Suggested Reading

- Sheldon et al. Principles of practice of pediatric sleep medicine. 2005.

4. A 10-year-old boy with a history of ADHD came for an evaluation. His family reports that he is constantly moving, always on the go and cannot

sit still at bedtime. He told his family that he has to move otherwise his legs would feel funny. He told you that he feels like there are bugs crawling on his legs and this sensation keeps him up at night, and if he walks or runs his legs feel better.

One of the criteria for Restless leg syndrome is that he has to relate a description in his own words that is consistent with leg discomfort.

All the criteria below for definite childhood restless leg syndrome are true except:

A. An urge to move the legs, usually accompanied or caused by uncomfortable and unpleasant sensations in the legs.
B. The urge to move or unpleasant sensations begin or worsen during periods of rest or inactivity such as lying down or sitting.
C. The urge to move or unpleasant sensations are partially or totally relieved by movement, such as walking or stretching, at least as long as the activity continues.
D. The urge to move or unpleasant sensations are worse in the evening or night than during the day, or only occur during the evening or night.
E. Ferritin levels must be lower than the 5th percentile.

Correct Answer is: E

The Criteria for Restless Leg syndrome is below.

Essential diagnostic criteria (adults)

1. An urge to move the legs, usually accompanied or caused by uncomfortable and unpleasant sensations in the legs
2. The urge to move or unpleasant sensations begin or worsen during periods of rest or inactivity such as lying down or sitting
3. The urge to move or unpleasant sensations are partially or totally relieved by movement, such as walking or stretching, at least as long as the activity continues
4. The urge to move or unpleasant sensations are worse in the evening or night than during the day, or only occur during the evening or night

Definite childhood restless legs syndrome (RLS)

1. The child meets all four essential adult criteria, *and*
2. The child relates a description in his or her own words that is consistent with leg discomfort

OR

1. The child meets all four essential adult criteria and has two of three following
   A. sleep disturbance for age
   B. biological parent or sibling with definite RLS
   C. polysomnographically documented periodic limb movement index of five or more per hour of sleep

Probable childhood RLS

1. The child meets all four essential adult criteria for RLS except criterion 4 (the urge to move or sensations are worse in the evening or at night than during the day), *And*
2. The child has a biological parent or sibling with definite RLS

OR

1. The child is observed to have behavioral manifestations of lower extremity discomfort when sitting or

   Lying, accompanied by motor movement of the affected limbs; the discomfort has characteristics of adult criteria 2, 3, and 4, *And*
2. The child has a biological parent or sibling with definite RLS

Adapted from: Allen RP, Pichhietti D, Hening WA, et al. Restless legs syndrome: diagnostic criteria, special considerations, and epidemiology.

A report from the restless legs syndrome diagnosis and

epidemiology workshop at the National Institutes of Health. Sleep Medicine 2003; 4:101–119.

Suggested Reading

- Kotagal S, et al. Childhood-onset restless legs syndrome. Ann Neurol. 2004;56:803–7.

5. A 17-year-old boy is complaining of excessive daytime sleepiness for the past 2 years. He goes to bed at 8:30 p.m. and falls asleep quickly but still feels tired upon awakening. He is not a restless sleeper and does not snore. He school grades are dropping, and his teachers complained of him falling asleep in class on several occasions. He takes short naps during his lunch period and on the bus ride home from school, after which he feels rested for a couple of hours. Another neurologist has evaluated her 2 months ago after having a seizure like event versus syncope. While he was joking around with his friends, suddenly he dropped his head to his chest and he was not able to respond for about 15 s. A polysomonogram (PSG) followed by multiple sleep latency test (MSLT) is ordered. The PSG shows an increased proportion of stage 1 sleep. The MSLT shows a mean sleep latency of 4 min and presence of REM sleep in 3 of the 5 naps.
What is the most appropriate recommendation to address this boy's daytime sleepiness?
   A. Start melatonin 1 h before bedtime
   B. Otolaryngologist referral for a tonsillectomy
   C. Start atomoxetine 80 mg daily
   D. Start fluoxetine 20 mg daily
   E. Start modafinil 100 mg daily in the morning

Correct Answer is: E
This boy clinical scenario and even the sleep studies are indicative of Narclepsy. The best treatment option is a stimulant to help him out the overcome his sleep disorder.

6. A 5-year-old boy has been evaluated for nocturnal spells, in which he wakes up and repeatedly screams, "No! Ow!" His family reports that on awakening he will have dilated pupils and his heart races, but no stereotyped movements have been noted. Try to comfort him, makes him more agitated. Those spells started 5 months ago and they are infrequent, occurring once every 2–3 weeks, usually within 2 h of his going to bed. They are about 10 min in duration, and then he goes back to sleep. He does not seem to remember the events in the morning. His family reports that he snores most nights, but a polysomnogram did not demonstrate sleep apnea.
What is the most appropriate treatment?
   A. Clonazepam
   B. Reassurance
   C. Clonidine
   D. Carbamazepine
   E. Referral to psychiatry

Correct Answer is: B
Parasomnias are "undesirable physical events or experiences that occur during entry into sleep, within sleep, or during arousals from sleep", according to the International Classification of Sleep Disorders (ISCD-2). They are classified as: (1) disorders of arousal from non-rapid eye movements (NREM) sleep; (2) parasomnias usually associated with REM sleep; and (3) other parasomnias. While the nightmares are the exception, they are associated with REM sleep, most of the pediatric parasomnias are disorders of arousal from NREM sleep, including sleepwalking, confusional arousals, and sleep terrors. Sleepwalking peaks at 11–12 years old, males and females are equally affected. Most children who sleepwalk appear calm; however, they are at risk for injury. Children, generally infants and toddlers, with confusional arousals are more agitated. They may

have their eyes open or closed and may cry or call out and thrash around for 5–15 min before returning to restful sleep, often becoming more agitated with attempts to console them. Sleep terrors are more dramatic still, with affected children appearing intensely fearful, showing evidence of autonomic activation (mydriasis, diaphoresis, tachycardia, and hyperventilation). Sleep terrors affect approximately 3% of children between the ages of 4–12 years, with peak prevalence between 5 and 7 years. Since sleepwalking, confusional arousals, and sleep terrors all arise out of NREM sleep, they tend to occur in the first third of the night when NREM sleep is most prevalent. Several studies showed that arousal parasomnias have a genetic predisposition. Sleep deprivation, a stimulating sleep environment, intrinsic sleep disorders (e.g. obstructive sleep apnea, periodic limb movements in sleep), and certain medications are known triggers.

The differential diagnosis includes epilepsy, particularly nocturnal frontal lobe epilepsy. Parasomnias can often be diagnosed on clinical grounds, but in some cases, sleep-deprived EEG, ambulatory continuous EEG, and/or inpatient video EEG monitoring may be necessary to clarify the diagnosis. Overnight polysomnography is indicated if there is concern for an intrinsic sleep disorder.

Treatment consists of reassurance, caffeine-free beverages, and minimizing sleep deprivation. Parents should be instructed not trying to wake the child during an episode and, when appropriate, about instituting safety measures. Scheduled anticipatory awakenings and/or low-dose clonazepam given at bedtime can be helpful in children with frequent parasomnias.

Suggested Reading

- Mason TBA, Pack AI. Pediatric parasomnias. In Sleep 2007;30(2):141–51.

7. Parents of a 6-year-old boy awakens several times a week on their son's piercing scream. He sits up in bed, looking afraid, flushed, sweating and breathing heavily. He is confused and disoriented. He goes back to sleep several minutes later and does not remember the event the next day. His physical and neurological examination is normal.

   What is your most likely diagnosis?

   A. Temporal lobe epilepsy
   B. Central sleep apnea
   C. Electrical status epilepticus of sleep
   D. Sleep terrors
   E. Benign epilepsy with centrotemporal spikes

Correct Answer is: D

Sleep terrors (night terrors, pavor nocturnus) occur during slow wave sleep, typically in the first third of the night and last seconds to minutes. Fearful behavior and sympathetic hyperactivity are typical. Sleep deprivation can be a trigger.

8. A 5-year-old girl has been evaluated of possible seizures. She has several episodes every month where she awakens screaming, flails her limbs and cannot be consoled. She has "pounding heart" and she sweats profusely during the episodes. She has been having those episodes for the past 4 months, though more often over the past month or so. They occur almost about 2 h after she falls asleep, last up to 20 min, and then she is back asleep. Sometimes she has more than 1 spell per night. No color change or incontinence is associated. She cannot recall anything about the episodes the following morning. Her general and neurologic examination are normal.

What is your explanation for these episodes?

A. nightmares
B. nocturnal frontal lobe epilepsy
C. psychogenic non-epileptic events
D. REM behavior disorder
E. sleep terrors

Correct Answer is: E

Paroxysmal events are very common referrals to pediatric and adult neurologists, mainly to rule out seizure. There are many paroxysmal non-epileptic events, some of which are unique to the pediatric age group. A detailed history of the episodes might be the single most important aspect of the evaluation and can often allow a specific diagnosis without the need for further testing. In fact, without an appropriately acquired history, ancillary testing often leads to an incorrect diagnosis as it is recognized that up to 3% of the population will have interictal epileptiform features on an EEG without having epileptic seizures. Video-recording of the event by the family can be very helpful. Events that occur during sleep can be quite distressful to the child and the entire family. Parasomnias are sleep related disorders occurring during REM and non-REM sleep leading to complete or partial arousals. Examples include nightmares, night terrors, sleepwalking and confusional arousals. Night terrors in particular are very common in young children, occurring in up to 5% of children ages 3–5 years. They occur in non-REM slow wave sleep (stage 3) and as such occur usually 60–120 min after sleep onset (and occasionally during subsequent entries into these stages of sleep later at night.) They do not occur at sleep-wake transitions, Seizures on the other hand usually occur just after entering sleep or immediately prior to awakening. Sleep terrors have a sudden onset, and the child appears terrified, with screaming, thrashing, sweating, and tachycardia. Usually the child appears awake with eyes open, but he is still asleep and cannot communicate effectively and cannot respond consistently to the family. Family often confuse the events with nightmares, but unlike nightmares (which occur in REM sleep), child cannot be aroused and do not report having had a dream. The night terror episode is usually several minutes in length, often up to 15–20 min, after which the child returns back to sleep and wakes up the next morning usually well rested (unlike the parents) without remembering the event. Although there have been many theories about the reasons for night terrors (including emotional stressors and occasionally in adults prescription drugs or alcohol use), most often there is no immediate cause identified and a family history of similar or other parasomnias is common. Treatment is often not indicated unless the events are occurring multiple times per week and impairing the quality of the sleep of the rest of the household. Searching for co-morbid sleep disorders including obstructive sleep apnea is important. Medications used with varying degrees of success have included iron supplementation (even if not frankly iron deficient), melatonin, clonidine and benzodiazepines. Often, reassurance is all that is needed. Nocturnal frontal lobe epilepsy, sometimes involving chiefly the supplementary motor cortex. Adding to the diagnostic confusion is the potential that there may never be any associated events during wakefulness. These are typically short (less than 1–2 min) abrupt arousals sometime accompanied by vocalizations, but not the same degree of persistent screaming. Hyperkinetic motor manifestations dominate the episodes, but can also be more subtle.

Multiple episodes throughout the night are commonly reported. In most

23

cases, an accurate history and/or video recording of the events will allow clear differentiation between these events and parasomnias. Psychogenic non-epileptic seizures can be challenging to distinguish from epileptic seizures as they can occur at apparent sleep wake transitions (though the patient may not have actually fallen asleep prior to the event onset). These events are not very common in children of this age, typically not until near the end of the first decade of life. REM behavior disorder involves the lack of REM atonia and leads to acting out of dreams. This is not common in children and in adults can be the first presentation of an impending neurodegenerative disorder like Parkinson disease. The patient can be typically woken from the spell and will recall the detail of the dream on most occasions.

Suggested Reading

- Drazkowski JF, Chung SS. Differential diagnosis of epilepsy. Continuum Lifelong Learning Neurol. 2010;16(3):36–56.

9. A 9-year-old boy with a six months history of increasing daytime sleepiness and falling asleep in unusual places. His family reported that he has weekly episodes of staring and unresponsiveness at times with facial twitching. His brain MRI is normal. He has a normal awake and sleep EEG. He has been taking ethosuximide for 2 weeks and has been having more episodes. The family also reported that he has become irritable and is having behavioral problems at school.

   What is the likely diagnosis?

   A. Substance abuse
   B. Benign Rolandic epilepsy
   C. Conversion disorder
   D. Narcolepsy
   E. Absence epilepsy

Correct Answer is: D

Recording REM on a routine EEG is abnormal. This indicates either extreme sleep deprivation or a potential diagnosis of narcolepsy. Excessive daytime sleepiness is the most common presenting feature of narcolepsy in children (though narcolepsy is certainly not the most common reason for excessive daytime sleepiness in children). The diagnosis is not confirmed until the additional core features of the disorder such as cataplexy, sleep paralysis and hypnagogic hallucinations develop in the teenage or early adult years. Disturbed nighttime sleep, automatic behavior and short-term memory problems are subtle features of the disorder in children.

The EEG in absence or benign Rolandic epilepsy should show representative interictal discharges and not epochs of REM sleep, but excessively sleepiness is not typically a feature of either conditions.

Conversion disorder and substance abuse should always be considered in atypical cases of altered responsiveness or excessive sleepiness, though onset at the age of nine would be highly unusual for either.

Suggested Reading

- Macleod S, Ferrie C, Zuberi SM. Symptoms of narcolepsy in children misinterpreted as epilepsy. Epileptic Disord. 2005;7(1):13–7.

10. A 17-year-old senior high school student comes to your clinic with complaints of daytime sleepiness which are causing him to fall asleep in the classroom for the last year, despite having adequate night sleep. He reported that he would likely doze *off* pretty quickly if he is sitting in a chair in a quiet room. He adds that at times he will find himself nodding *off* in front of the computer, and that

just before nodding *off* he will write nonsensical sentences which he will discover only once he awakens from nodding *off*. He mentioned, brief naps help. He denies ever falling down or having weakness in the knees from laughing or other strong emotion. He often gets tired while driving at night, he pulls over and exercise, or roll down the window to stay awake. He has no hallucinations right as he is going to sleep or as he is waking up, but reports that at times he does wake up, unable to move for a few seconds, which is very scary. No snoring has been reported, but he wakes up feeling tired. He sleeps at least 7 h at night, with more on weekends. **What medicine can be used to treat this disorder?**

A. Stimulants-modafinil, armodafinil, dextroamphetamine, methamphetamine and methylphenidate
B. Sodium oxybate
C. Tricyclic anti-depressants
D. SSRIs and SNRIs

Correct Answer is: All of the above

11. A 16-year-old boy is complaining of having a hard time waking up in the morning at 7 a.m. to go to school, and that he finds it difficult to fall asleep before 2 a.m. in the morning. He sometimes falls asleep in class, and does not yet drive. After he comes home back form school he feels tired, and occasionally naps, but says that cross country practice has him revved up until about 5 or 6 pm. He does not have trouble sleeping on the weekends, and you ask him to keep a sleep log over the next 4 weeks. His sleep log showing 6 h of sleep on weekdays, and 10–11 h of sleep on the weekends. He does not drink caffeinated beverages, and gets daily exercise with cross country practice. He does not have a TV in his bedroom, and doesn't work on the computer or do homework after 10 pm. He is not snoring. Physical exam including blood pressure shows a fit young adolescent with no apparent deficits. He is not feeling depressed, and says in general, he likes school.
What is your diagnosis?

A. Circadian rhythm disorder, delayed phase type
B. obstructive sleep apnea
C. shift work disorder
D. typical adolescent behavior, without pathology
E. occult alcohol abuse

Correct Answer is: A
Delayed sleep phase syndrome can be manifested in teenagers and young adults. This presentation is classic. Obstructive sleep apnea, is not ruled out, but in a young, physically fit individual who does not snore, it is much less likely. Shift work disorder is an excess of sleepiness experienced whenever a person is working when they would ordinarily be sleeping, which does not fit the above clinical presentation. As it is not typical adolescent behavior without pathology, and a sleepy teenage driver is a potent mix (looking forward a year or two if this behavior is not diagnosed and treated). Occult alcohol abuse is much lower on the differential, and while possible, hardly the most likely diagnosis, and should manifest with other symptoms (headache, frequent urination, decreased school performance, etc.).

12. Which of the following statements regarding sleep phenomena is not correct?

A. Sleep paralysis is a feature of narcolepsy
B. Hypnagogic hallucinations occur on falling asleep

C. Hypnopompic hallucinations occur on waking up from sleep
D. Patients have recollection of nightmares
E. REM sleep behavior disorder (RBD) is associated with excessive atonia during REM sleep

23

Correct Answer is: E
REM sleep behavior disorder (RBD) is characterized by REM without atonia and by the appearance of complex motor activity during which the patient acts out dreams. Dream content is usually violent with associated movements (e.g. Punching, kicking, and running). Sleep paralysis is a feature of narcolepsy and is characterized by a transient paralysis during sleep onset or on awakening; the patient is fully conscious during these events. Hypnagogic hallucinations occur at sleep onset and are seen in patients with narcolepsy, and hypnopompic hallucinations occur on awakening from sleep. A nightmare is a complicated dream that becomes frightening toward the end. Patients with nightmares usually remember their dream in detail, and occurs in the last third of the night, and there is much less autonomic activity as compared to sleep terrors. When patients are awakened from nightmares, they tend to have good intellectual l function and are not confused.

Suggested Reading

- American Academy of Sleep Medicine. International classification of sleep disorders, 2nd ed. Diagnostic and coding manual, Westchester, IL: American Academy of Sleep Medicine; 2005.
- Bradley WG, Daroff RB, Fenichel GM, et al. Neurology in clinical practice, 5th ed. Philadelphia, PA: Elsevier; 2008. Comprehensive review in clinical neurology: a multiple choice question book for the wards and boards ©2011 Wolters Kluwer Health Lippincott Williams & Wilkins. All rights reserved.

13. A mother of a 9 years old boy complaining that her son sleepwalks "frequently", at least 3–4 times per month. She has difficulty to arouse him during these times, and he has had odd behaviors while sleepwalking, urinating in corners of the house. He does not recall the episodes. He has good sleep hygiene, getting 10 h of sleep at night, with regular bedtimes. He has no snoring. Family is history is positive of his father also was a sleepwalker as a child.
What is the most important consideration in this case?
A. having the child wear diapers when sleeping
B. ensuring the child is not drinking before bedtime
C. avoiding afternoon naps
D. making sure the house *is* safe for the child during his sleepwalking episodes
E. locking him in the room where he is sleeping

Correct Answer is: D
Making sure the house is safe for the child during his sleepwalking episodes, protecting the child from any harm while sleepwalking is of at most importance. Benzodiazepines are occasionally used with severe (i.e. nightly) sleepwalking for a few months, with subsequent tapers. The other measures are either unnecessary, counterproductive, or not as important of considerations.

Suggested Reading

- Bhargava S. Diagnosis and management of common sleep problems in children. Pediatr Rev. 32(3);91–9, 201.
- Duysse DJ, Strollo PJ, Black JE, et al. "Chapter 22: sleep disorders" in the

American Psychiatric Publishing Textbook of Psychiatry, 5th Ed.
- Hales RE, Yudofsky SC, Gabbard GO, editors. American Psychiatric Publishing, 2011.

14. Which of the following is TRUE regarding sleep?
    A. newborns spent 90% of their sleep in REM
    B. duration of sleep decreases during adolescence
    C. stage 3 and 4 sleep peaks during adolescence
    D. number of night-time awakenings decreases as adulthood progresses
    E. stage 2 Non-REM and REM sleep increases as adulthood progresses

Correct Answer is: C
Adolescence marks the peak of "deep" sleep, adolescents and they do not tend to sleep more as newborns, and newborns spend approximately 50% of their sleep in REM-like sleep. Duration of sleep actually increases during adolescence. Number of awakenings, as well as the amount of "light" stage 1 sleep, increases as you progress in later adulthood.

15. A 5-year-old girl has frequent episodes of inconsolable crying shortly after falling asleep. Her family have noted that her pupils appear large and her heart races. She appears very scared and confused and will not react to her family's attempts to comfort her.
    This girl most likely has:
    A. Nocturnal seizures
    B. Nocturnal panic attacks
    C. Sleep terrors
    D. REM sleep behavior disorder
    E. Sleep-onset association disorder

Correct Answer is: C
This is a typical presentation of childhood sleep terrors.

16. Which of the following statements is true regarding the differentiation of frontal lobe seizures from sleep disorders?
    A. Seizures tend to occur fewer times per night than episodes due to sleep disorders
    B. Events occurring within the first 30 min of sleep are more likely to be seizures
    C. Episodes of dystonic posturing are less likely to be seizure
    D. Seizures tend to be of longer duration than episodes due to sleep disorders
    E. None of the above

Correct Answer is: B
Seizures occur during the first 30 min of sleep rather than sleep-related disorders.
Other different manifestations are: Frontal lobe seizures are more likely in younger patients, while sleep disorders are often evident at older adults. Seizures are brief, less than 2 min duration. Episodes related to sleep disorders are more likely to be prolonged, lasting more than 10 min. Episodes that cluster, with 3 events occurring per night more likely to be seizures. Events related to sleep disorders commonly occur 1–2 times per night. Auras are more common with seizure activity. Wandering outside of the bedroom is uncommon with seizure activity. Directed behaviors (e.g. dressing, preparing food) are uncommon with seizure activity. Stereotyped movements, dystonic posturing, tonic limb extension, and cramping are more common with seizure activity. Recall of events may occur with Seizure activity, and is uncommon with sleep disorders.

Suggested Reading

- Derry et al. Distinguishing sleep disorders from seizures: diagnosing bumps in the night. Arch Neurol. 2006;63(5):705–9. Erratum in: Arch Neurol. 2006;63(7):1037.

	Sleep disorder	Frontal lobe seizure
Age of onset	More likely in older patients, 55 years of age	More likely in younger J,-patients
Duration	More likely if prolonged, >10 min	More likely if brief: <2 min
Clusters	Commonly 1–2 events per night	More likely to have multiple events (2:3 per night)
Timing	May occur at any time during the night	Likely within 30 min of sleep Onset
Aura	Uncommon	Common
Wandering outside of the bedroom	Common	Uncommon
Directed behavior (i.e. dressing)	Common	Uncommon
Dystonic posturing, tonic limb extension, or cramping	Uncommon	Common
Stereotyped behavior	Uncommon	Common
Recall of events	Uncommon	May occur
Speech during event	More likely to have no speech, sounds: only, or single words, if coherent speech is present, there is often no recall	If coherent speech present, it is more likely to be recalled
Epileptiform EEG abnormalities	Absent	Present, although may be difficult to detect on scalp recordings

17. A 17-year-old student complains of difficulty staying awake in classroom. He reports having always been sleepy during the daytime since his early teenage years. He gets about 7 h of sleep nightly. He feels more alert after taking a short nap. Recently, he has developed spells of sudden falling down when laughing or being angry. He denies loss of consciousness during those episodes.

The patient most likely has:

A. Psychogenic unresponsiveness
B. Syncopal events
C. Narcolepsy
D. Complex partial seizures
E. Idiopathic hypersomnia

Correct Answer is: C

Excessive daytime sleepiness and cataplexy are classical features of narcolepsy. Narcolepsy is a classic tetrad: (1) excessive daytime sleepiness, (2) cataplexy, (3) hypnagogic or hypnopompic hallucinations, (4) sleep paralysis. Excessive daytime sleepiness – often the first symptom in adolescence or early adulthood. Cataplexy – sudden, transient loss of muscle tone with associated hyporeflexia or areflexia, provoked by an emotional stimulus such as laughter, surprise, anger. Partial or complete muscle atonia (sparing of respiratory and extraocular muscles). Sleep paralysis – occur mostly upon awakening but

also at sleep onset and resolves spontaneously or with sensory stimuli (touching patient, calling person's name). Hypnogogic and hypnopompic hallucinations – mostly visual hallucinations at transition between sleep and wakefulness; auditory, tactile, vestibular hallucinations also possible.

Suggested Reading

- Mowzoon N, Flemming KD. Neurology board review: an illustrated study guide. Rochester, MN: Mayo Clinic Scientific, 2007. Print.

18. Which chromosome is associated with Narcolepsy?
    - A. chromosome 2
    - B. chromosome 4
    - C. chromosome 6
    - D. chromosome 13
    - E. chromosome 18

Correct Answer is: C
A mutation in chromosome 6 is strongly associated with narcolepsy-cataplexy. Although this mutation is seen in 90% to 100% of patients with narcolepsy, it also occurs in as many as 50% of people without narcolepsy.

Suggested Reading

- Chromosomes and their associated diseases: Kaufman DM. (2007). Clinical neurology for psychiatrists, 6th ed. Philadelphia: W.B. Saunders.

19. At what time during the night does REM sleep occur?
    - A. right when a person falls asleep
    - B. in the middle of the cycle
    - C. in the second half of the night, in the morning hours
    - D. in the first half of the night, in the evening hours
    - E. none of the above

Correct Answer is: C
REM sleep is characterized by a mixed voltage EEG, which looks similar to Stage 1 sleep, with rapid phasic eye movements. Muscle tone should be absent, except for intermittent phasic muscle twitches.

Suggested Reading

- Duysse DJ, Strollo PJ, Black JE, et al. "Chapter 22: sleep disorders" in The American Psychiatric Publishing Textbook of Psychiatry, 5th ed. Hales RE, Yudofsky SC, Gabbard GO, editors. American Psychiatric Publishing, 2011.

20. A 15-year-old boy is having episodes of walking around his house in the middle of the night. Once, during such an episode, he took the garbage out of his house and placed it in front of his neighbor's door. His neighbor tried to talk to him, but he did not respond. When the neighbor shook him, the boy suddenly changed his behavior, started to scream, and became violent and confused. You diagnosed him with a sleep disorder. **Which of the following is correct?**
    - A. He has a REM parasomnia
    - B. He has confusional arousals
    - C. He has narcolepsy
    - D. During these episodes, the EEG shows slow-wave sleep
    - E. He has sleep terrors

Correct Answer is: D
The boy has sleepwalking which is a non-REM parasomnia. Parasomnias have been classified into REM parasomnias, arousal disorders, sleep-wake transition disorders, and other parasomnias. Arousal disorders include confusional arousals, sleepwalking, and sleep terrors. The latter three are non-REM parasomnias arising from slow-wave sleep or

stage III sleep (previously known as stage III and stage IV sleep; now they are combined into stage III sleep).

Sleepwalking consists of a group of complex behaviors resulting in walking during sleep. It is more commonly in children, but can present in adolescents and adults, and a positive family history has been reported in many cases. Sleepwalking occurs more commonly in the first third of the sleep, and patients have complex motor behaviors, with amnesia of the episode. These patients are difficult to arouse, and may become confused and exhibit violent behavior when this is attempted. Confusional arousals are a non-REM parasomnia occurring in children, in which the patient is confused following an arousal from slow-wave sleep. The clinical scenario of this boy is not consistent with narcolepsy, nor with sleep terrors.

Suggested Reading

- American Academy of Sleep Medicine. International classification of sleep disorders, 2nd ed. Diagnostic and coding manual. Westchester, IL: American Academy of Sleep Medicine; 2005.
- Bradley WG, Daroff RB, Fenichel GM, et al. Neurology in clinical practice, 5th ed. Philadelphia, PA: Elsevier; 2008.

21. A 17-year-old female has been evaluated for possible pseudo-seizures. During the episodes she falls suddenly to the floor and loses her muscle tone completely, and she cannot move for 30–40 s. These events usually come after emotional triggers, frequently laughter. She is completely conscious during these events. She complains of being very sleepy during daytime, having multiple episodes of falling asleep during the day, after which she feels refreshed.
    What is your the most likely diagnosis?
    A. Gelastic seizures
    B. Narcolepsy with cataplexy
    C. Pseudo-seizures
    D. Kleine-Levin syndrome
    E. Idiopathic hypersomnia

Correct Answer is: B
This is the clinical presentation of narcolepsy with cataplexy. Narcolepsy is characterized by excessive sleepiness, cataplexy, sleep paralysis, and hypnagogic and hypnopompic hallucinations. Narcolepsy patients complain of sleep attacks, in which they have an irresistible desire to fall asleep during inappropriate circumstances. The sleep attacks last 15–30 min, and the patient feels refreshed afterward. Even though cataplexy is associated with narcolepsy, not all patients with narcolepsy have cataplexy. Cataplexy is an episode of sudden loss of tone of voluntary muscles, except respiratory and ocular muscles.

During these attacks, the patients may fall and be cannot move, and deep tendon reflexes are decreased or absent. Patients are fully conscious. Cataplectic attacks are triggered by emotional events, such as laughter or anger. This patient does not have pseudo-seizures, nor gelastic seizures. This patient does not have Kleine-Levin syndrome, which is a recurrent hypersomnia, characterized by recurrent episodes of hypersomnia occur weeks or months apart. The episodes can last several days and sometimes weeks, occurring several times per year, and these patients sleep for prolonged periods of time, 18–20 h, waking only to eat and void. During these episodes, patients may have

disrupted behaviors, such as irritability, aggressiveness, confusion, hyper sexuality, and a voracious appetite. In between episodes, patients have normal behavior and sleep pattern. This patient does not have idiopathic hypersomnia, which is characterized by long-term inability to obtain adequate sleep, in which the patients have excessive sleepiness and the etiology is thought to be abnormal neurologic control of the sleep-wake system. Insomnia patients, they sleep for long periods of time, but they do not feel refresh afterward. The diagnosis is made only when no other medical or psychiatric condition can explain the hypersomnia.

Suggested Reading

- American Academy of Sleep Medicine. International classification of sleep disorders, 2nd ed. Diagnostic and coding manual, Westchester, IL: American Academy of Sleep Medicine; 2005.
- Bradley WG, Daroff RB, Fenichel GM, et al. Neurology in clinical practice, 5th ed. Philadelphia, PA: Elsevier; 2008.
- Comprehensive review in clinical neurology: a multiple-choice question book for the Wards and Boards ©201 1 Wolters Kluwer Health Lippincott Williams & Wilkins. All rights Reserved.

22. Regarding narcolepsy with cataplexy, which of the following is incorrect?
    - A. CSF hypocretin levels are increased
    - B. During cataplexy, muscle tone is lost and patients are hyporeflexic or areflexic
    - C. Sleep paralysis is frequent
    - D. Mean sleep latency test (MSLT) needs to be performed to help make the diagnosis
    - E. B-hydroxybutyrate is approved for the treatment of narcolepsy with cataplexy

Correct Answer is: A
Loss of hypocretin neurons in the lateral hypothalamus might be associated with narcolepsy with cataplexy, and hypocretin CSF levels are low in these patients. Patient's loss their muscle tone during the attack and they have hypo- or areflexia. Usually, they have sleep paralysis accompany the attack. You can diagnose narcolepsy with on clinical grounds; however, polysomnogram and mean sleep latency test (MSLT) can provide information to support the diagnosis by detecting a mean sleep latency of less than 8 min and two or more sleep-onset REM periods (SOREMPs). R-hydroxybutyrate has been approved for the treatment of sleepiness and cataplexy that is associated with narcolepsy. However, tricyclic antidepressants or serotonin reuptake inhibitors can be used for treatment.

Suggested Reading

- American academy of sleep medicine. International classification of sleep disorders, 2nd ed. Diagnostic and coding manual, Westchester, IL: American Academy of Sleep Medicine; 2005.
- Bradley WG, Daroff RB, Fenichel GM, et al. Neurology in clinical practice, 5th ed. Philadelphia, PA: Elsevier; 2008.

23. A 14-year-old boy wakes up in the middle of the night with frightening dreams of a big monster eating his little sister. On awaking, he recalls the dream well and does not look confused.
    What is your diagnosis?
    - A. Nightmares
    - B. REM sleep behavior disorder
    - C. Sleep terrors
    - D. Confusional arousals
    - E. Non-REM parasomnia

23

Correct Answer is: A
This presentation of a nightmare, in which is a complicated dream that becomes frightening toward the end. Nightmares should be differentiated from sleep terrors. Nightmares can be recalled by the patients in detail, it occurs in the last third of the night, and patients have much less autonomic activity as compared to sleep terrors. When patients are awakened from nightmares, they are not confused and tend to have good intellectual function. Sleep terrors occur more commonly in children, and patients wake up screaming or crying, with prominent accompanied autonomic and behavioral manifestations of intense fear, as well as confusion on awakening. Sleep terrors occur in the first third of the night. Confusional arousals are a non-REM parasomnia occurring in children, in which the patient is confused following an arousal from slow-wave sleep. The boy's clinical presentation is not consistent with REM sleep behavior disorder or a non-REM parasomnia.

Suggested Reading

- American Academy of Sleep Medicine. International classification of sleep disorders, 3rd ed. Diagnostic and coding manual, Westchester, IL: American Academy of Sleep Medicine; 2014.
- Bradley WG, Daroff RB, Fenichel GM, et al. Neurology in clinical practice, 5th ed. Philadelphia, PA: Elsevier; 2008. Comprehensive review in clinical neurology: a multiple choice question book for the Wards and Boards ©2011 Wolters Kluwer Health Lippincott Williams & Wilkins. All rights reserved.

24. In adolescents the entire sleep period tends to phase delay; the sleep period in later adulthood tends to:
    A. phase delay as well
    B. maintain sleep habits as in middle adulthood
    C. phase advance
    D. consist of sleep similar to a newborn's in stages and amount
    E. none of the above

Correct Answer is: C
There is a gradual change between middle and late adulthood. Newborn's sleep is profoundly different from an adult in later adulthood. Newborns spend approximately 50% of their sleep time in a stage of sleep resembling REM sleep, which rapidly decreases in the first year of life. Delta waves are most prominent in the sleep of newborns, whereas most adults late in life have very little delta wave "deep" sleep.

Suggested Reading

- Duysse DJ, Strollo PJ, Black JE, et al. "Chapter 22: sleep disorders" in the American Psychiatric Publishing Textbook of Psychiatry, 5th Ed.
- Hales RE, Yudofsky SC, Gabbard GO, editors. American Psychiatric Publishing, 2011.

25. An 18-year-old male complains of fatigue, increased daytime somnolence, and periodic sudden loss of muscle tone. Polysomnography confirms the diagnosis of narcolepsy. **Narcolepsy is associated with which of the following?**
    A. Decreased adenosine levels in the reticular formation
    B. Increased discharge of noradrenergic neurons in the locus ceruleus
    C. Hypothalamic dysfunction with decreased CSF levels of orexins
    D. Increased discharge of serotonergic neurons in the midbrain Raphe

Correct Answer is: C
Narcolepsy is associated with low CSF levels of the orexins and a defect in one of the receptors for orexins (hypocretins) in the hypothalamus. Adenosine

induces sleep, and serotonin agonists suppress sleep. Fatal familial insomnia is a progressive prion disease, characterized by worsening insomnia, impaired autonomic and motor functions, dementia, and death.

Suggested Reading

- Mowzoon N, Flemming KD. Neurology board review: an illustrated study guide. Rochester, MN: Mayo Clinic Scientific, 2007. Print.

26. Which type of seizure is activated in REM sleep?
    A. Partial seizures
    B. Tonic-clonic
    C. Tonic
    D. Myoclonic
    E. None of the above

Correct Answer is: E
Partial seizures show a complex relationship with sleep, and the relationship may be dictated by the location of the focus. Data indicate a protective effect of REM sleep. Generalized tonic-clonic seizures are associated with NREM sleep, or as in JME, soon after awakening. Tonic seizures are activated by NREM sleep. Myoclonic seizures are activated soon after awakening. REM sleep appears to be protective against the occurrence of seizures. Seizures are most common in Stage 2 sleep.

Suggested Reading

- Ng M, Pavlova M. Why are seizures rare in rapid eye movement sleep? Review of the frequency of seizures in different sleep stages.
- Epilepsy Res Treat. 2013; E pub 2013 Jun 18. Derry CP and Duncan S. Sleep and epilepsy. Epilepsy Behav. 2013;26(3):394–404.

27. You are seeing a 7-year-old boy with a history of increasing daytime sleepiness and falling asleep in unusual places for the last 3 months. He has occasional episodes of staring and unresponsiveness at times with facial twitching. Brain MRI is normal. Routine EEG is normal with waking and REM sleep recorded. He has been taking ethosuximide for last 4 weeks and but has been having more episodes. He has become irritable and is having behavioral problems at school.
    What is your likely diagnosis?
    A. Absence epilepsy
    B. Benign rolandic epilepsy
    C. Conversion disorder
    D. **Narcolepsy**
    E. Substance abuse

Correct Answer is: D
It is unusual and abnormal to record REM on a routine EEG. This suggests either extreme sleep deprivation or a potential diagnosis of narcolepsy. Excessive daytime sleepiness if by far the most common presenting feature of narcolepsy in children (though narcolepsy is certainly not the most common reason for excessive daytime sleepiness in children). The diagnosis is not finalized until the additional core manifestations of the disorder such as cataplexy, sleep paralysis and hypnagogic hallucinations develop in the teenage or early adult years. Other subtle features of the disorder in children may include disturbed nighttime sleep, automatic behavior and short-term memory problems.

Excessively sleepiness is not typically a feature of either absence or benign Rolandic epilepsy, and the EEG in these epilepsy syndromes should show representative inter-ictal discharges and not epochs of REM sleep.

Conversion disorder and substance abuse should always be considered in atypical cases of altered responsiveness or excessive sleepiness, though the onset at age 7 would be highly unusual for either.

Suggested Reading

- Macleod S, Ferrie C, Zuberi SM. Symptoms of narcolepsy in children misinterpreted as epilepsy. Epileptic Disord. 2005;7(1):13–7.

23

28. You are evaluating a 16-year-old female for day time sleepiness. She goes to sleep at 11 PM and waking at 7 AM and feels refreshed when she awakes. She does not drink caffeine. She has difficulty remaining awake during her classes which has her concerned she may fail some classes. She has a normal physical neurologically exams and she has a BMI of 24.3. She had a previously normal polysomnogram.

What is the next best step in evaluation and management?

A. Overnight oximetry
B. Uvulopalatopharyngoplasty
C. Mandibular advancement
D. **Overnight polysomnography with multiple sleep latency test**
E. Continuous positive air pressure

Correct Answer is: B

Daytime sleepiness is the most common symptom of narcolepsy. Given her previous normal polysomnogram as well as lack of risk factors for obstructive sleep apnea, she should have narcolepsy excluded.

Suggested Reading

- Scammell TE. Narcolepsy. N Engl J Med. 2015;373(27):2654–62.

29. An 18-year-old male is brought to the emergency room by his roommate. He was asleep on the coach, when he suddenly screamed and thrashed violently about shaking his head. The spell was 5 s long. His past medical history is remarkable of epilepsy in the past 10 years of age. His seizures have all occurred while he is sleeping and are similar to the recent event. He takes Ox carbamazepine, but missed his doses for the past few days. His family history is remarkable of similar seizures in his father, paternal uncle and his brother.

What is the best way to make a specific diagnosis?

A. Clinical presentation
B. CSF lactate level
C. Inter-ictal epileptiform pattern on EEG
D. MRI of the brain
E. Skin biopsy

Correct Answer is: A

Autosomal dominant nocturnal frontal lobe epilepsy is a focal epilepsy characterized by frequent, violent, brief seizures at night, usually beginning in childhood. A gene for ADNFLE is on chromosome 20 and associated with the nicotinic acethycholine receptor. The diagnosis is based on clinical grounds as well as genetic testing for the more common variants.

Inter-ictal frontal lobe EEG's discharges are not findings specific to this syndrome. CSF studies and skin biopsy are considerations in progressive epilepsies or those associated with prominent developmental delay or cognitive decline, or acute/subacute onset, and would not be expected to be helpful in defining an idiopathic epilepsy syndrome.

Suggested Reading

- Kurahashi H, Hirose S. Autosomal dominant nocturnal frontal lobe epilepsy. 2002 May 16 [Updated 2015 Feb 19]. In: Pagon RA, Adam MP, Ardinger HH, et al. editors. GeneReviews® [Internet]. Seattle (WA): University of Washington, Seattle; 1993–2015. Available from: ► http://www.ncbi.nlm.nih.gov/books/NBK1169/.
- Rudzinski LA, Shih JJ. "The classification of seizures and epilepsy syndromes." Continuum. 2010;16(3):15–35.

30. You are seeing an 18-year-old female with the diagnosis of narcolepsy for her recent sudden spells of bilateral skeletal muscle weakness triggered by intense, usually "positive", emotions such as laughter and excitement. She has one of her spells in the office and she became arefexic. Respiratory muscles are spared and she did not loss her consciousness.
Which of the following statements is FALSE?
   A. 85% to 95% of patients with narcolepsy with cataplexy are positive for HLA-DQB1*0602
   B. cataplexy usually develops within a few months or years of the onset of sleepiness
   C. children with very frequent cataplexy attacks should be tested for Niemann-Pick disease type C
   D. loss of consciousness is common in cataplexy
   E. low or absence of cerebrospinal fluid hypocretin levels have been found in more than 90% of patients with narcolepsy with cataplexy

Correct Answer is: D
Loss of consciousness does not happen in cataplexy. The other statements are correct.

Suggested Reading

- Silber MH, editor. Sleep medicine in clinical practice. London: Taylor & Francis; 2004. p. 92–3.

Spinal Cord

Y. M. Awaad, *Absolute Pediatric Neurology*, https://doi.org/10.1007/978-3-319-78801-2_24

1. A 3-day-old baby has weakness of the right arm since birth. He was delivered vaginally but it was complicated by shoulder dystocia. Birthweight was 4500 gm. The mother had gestational diabetes. Immediately after birth his right arm was weak and areflexic, but over time he has improved. Now, he has normal grasp and finger extension, but is unable to flex at the elbow or abduct at the shoulder and the biceps reflex is absent.
In addition to range of motion exercises, what is your recommendation at this time?
   A. Observation only
   B. MRI of the cervical spine
   C. Splint to the elbow to maintain flexion
   D. Nerve conduction velocity study
   E. Surgical exploration for nerve grafting

Correct Answer is: A
Brachial plexus palsy is a flaccid paresis of an upper extremity due to traumatic stretching of the brachial plexus during birth. The incidence is 0.38–3 per 1000 live births. The most significant risk factor is high birth weight, and it is 3 times more frequently specially with birth weight > 4500 gm. Breech delivery is another risk factor. Maternal factors include diabetes mellitus, obesity, excessive weight gain, age > 35 years, maternal pelvic anatomy, and primiparity are also risk factors. Shoulder dystocia is a strong predictor for brachial plexus injury. Clavicle and humerous fractures, facial nerve injury, cephalhematoma, and torticollis are usually associated injuries. Injuries include neurapraxia, neuroma, rupture, and avulsion. Erb's palsy (Upper plexus injury (C5 and C6) is the most common type. In these patients, the adducted and internally rotated at the shoulder, extended at the elbow, flexed at the wrist, and extended at the fingers (the waiter's tip poistion). Total plexus injury is second most common type and it results in long term disability. The majority (70–95%) of patients make complete spontaneous recovery. Evaluation using electromyography, nerve conduction studies, somatosensory evoked potentials, and MRI of the cervical spine can be utilized if recovery at 3 months is not complete, although the best timing of these studies is controversial. The primary goal of management is to maintain passive range of motion, maintain joints, and muscle strength. Indications for surgical exploration and reconstruction of the brachial plexus include failure of recovery of elbow flexion and shoulder abduction from the 3rd to the 6th month of life. It might take up to 2 years for complete recovery.

Suggested Reading

- Zafeiriou DI, Psychogiou K. Obstetrical brachial plexus palsy. Pediatr Neurol. 2008;38:235–42.

2. A 10-year-old girl came with a 3 days' history of weakness in the lower extremities and bladder control difficulty. She had an episode of loss of vision in her right eye one year ago which resolved in several weeks. She has a mild afferent pupillary defect and 20/80 vision in her right eye. Tendon reflexes in her lower extremities were increased and she had extensor plantar responses. Sensory level was not appreciated.
Which of the following antigens is useful in the diagnosis of this patient?
   A. Acetylcholine receptor (AChR)
   B. Aquaporin 4 channel (AQP4)
   C. Voltage gated calcium channel (VGCC)
   D. Alpha-4-beta integrin (ά4β1)
   E. Anti-Muscle specific kinase antibody (MuSK)

Correct Answer is: B

The integrin protein is important in cell signaling in glial neuronal interactions. The AChR is the primary ion channel in the neuromuscular junction and is important in impulse transmission as is the calcium channel. The MuSK antibody is associated with a form of Myasthenia. Although the role of the aquaporin channel is incompletely understood, it is associated with neuromyelitis optica and distinct from multiple sclerosis.

Suggested Reading

- Roemer SF, et al. Pattern-specific loss of aquaporin-4 immunoreactivity distinguishes neuromyelitis optica from multiple sclerosis. Brain 2007;130: 1194–205.
- Kira J. Neuromyelitis optica and Asian phenotype of multiple sclerosis. Ann N Y Acad Sci 2008;1142; 58–71.

3. A 10-year-old boy is referred to neurologist for constant tingling over his right shoulder and the lateral aspect of his proximal arm. He has mildly diminished pain and temperature sense in the same distribution as the tingling. Spinal MRI is shown below:

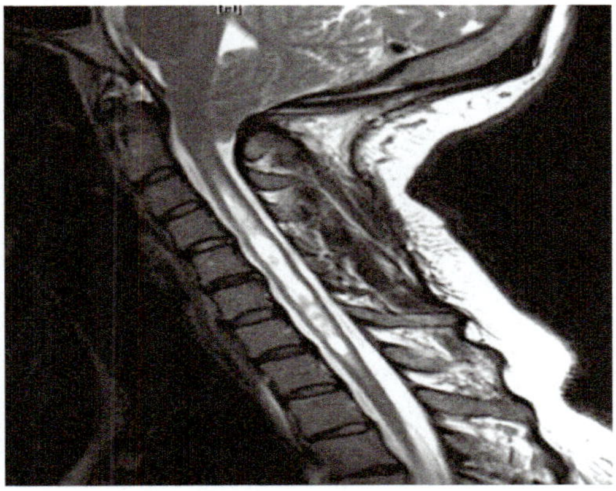

Fig. 24.1 Siringomielia. Own work. Luciobgomes. Wikipedia

Most likely he has:

A. Anterior spinal artery infarction
B. Ependymoma
C. Epidural abscess
D. Syringomyelia
E. Multiple sclerosis

Correct Answer is: D

Syringomyelia is a spinal cord condition which is secondary to of other congenital abnormalities (e.g., tethered cord or hydrocephalus) or trauma. It is a longitudinal "hole" in the spinal cord. The shape and size of the "hole" generally determines the symptoms and signs that result. A "suspended sensory loss", particularly one that is unilateral, like the "cape" sensory changes described in this case, is characteristic of a syrinx. The MRI scan shown demonstrates the 2–3 vertebral level extent of this intrinsic cord lesion.

Suggested Reading

- Vandertop WP. Syringomyelia. Neuropediatrics. 2014;45(1):3–9.

4. An 8-year-old boy presents with gradually progressive difficulty running for the past 2 years. He referred the problem to intermittent low back pain, which is worsened by activity but does not radiate. He has also had intermittent urinary incontinence for the last 4 months. On examination, he has normal bulk but mildly increased tone in his distal lower extremities and mild weakness in ankle dorsiflexion bilaterally. He has normal sensory examination. Deep tendon reflexes are 2+ in the upper extremities and 3+ in the lower extremities. Plantar responses are flexor bilaterally. Rectal tone is normal. He has lumbar levoscoliosis and a sacral hemangioma. He elevates his left shoulder and hip while walking but maintains a narrow base. Spinal MRI shows a

low-lying conus medullaris at L3 and an L4 hemi-vertebra with associated levoscoliosis. **Surgical treatment is most likely to lead to improvement in the following symptoms except?**

A. Scoliosis
B. Weakness
C. Bladder function
D. Pain
E. Spasticity

24

Correct Answer is: A

Tethered cord syndrome (TCS) is a constellation of motor and sensory findings that are attributable to excessive tension on the spinal cord. The majority of cases are associated with spinal dysraphism; however, TCS can also occur when an intradural process (e.g. abnormal thickened, shortened filum terminale, lipoma of the filum, fibrous adhesions) interferes with normal ascension of the conus with respect to the vertebral column. It can present at any age. Infants usually have cutaneous stigmata of spina bifida occulta, such as nevi, lipomas, tufts of hair, hemangiomas, and dermal sinuses. Other alarming signs include urinary dribbling, anorectal malformations, orthopedic deformities of the lower extremities, and scoliosis. Children and adolescents may be asymptomatic or may present with slowly progressive motor and sensory deficits. The clinical picture may also include varying degrees of weakness; patchy sensory deficits; scoliosis; non-dermatomal pain in the low back, perineum, and/or legs; bladder or less frequently bowel incontinence; orthopedic deformities of the lower extremities; and gait disturbances. MRI is the study of choice, as it can detect both the level of the conus and the cause of the tethering. Surgical untethering should be done in symptomatic patients, which results in pain relief in almost all cases and stabilization of neurologic decline in up to 90% of patients. Scoliosis progression after surgical tethering was noted in one cohort in long term follow up. However, there was improvement in muscle strength, gait, and spasticity. The role of surgery in asymptomatic patients remains less clear.

Suggested Reading

- Bowman RM, Mohan A, et al. Tethered cord release: a long term study in 114 patients. J Neurosurg Pediatr. 2009;3(3):181–7.

5. A 6-year-old girl came to ER after she was struck by a car while she was crossing the street. Paramedics found her to be awake, but distraught and complaining of neck pain. They immobilized her head and neck in neutral position before transferring her too ER. On examination, she has normal breathing l, normal vital signs, and moving all four extremities equally. Radiographs of the cervical spine show abnormal widening of the interspace at C1-C2.
Which of the following is the ideal next step in management?

A. Emergency tracheostomy
B. Continued immobilization of the head and neck, careful observation, and neurosurgical consultation.
C. fluoroscopy Lumbar puncture to exclude subarachnoid hemorrhage
D. Ophthalmology consultation for dilated fundus examination
E. Flexion and extension views of the neck under

Correct Answer is: B

Cervical spine (C-spine) injuries in prepubertal children are relatively uncommon in comparison to older age groups. In young children, C-spine injuries are usually occurring at the cranio-cervical junction or upper vertebral segments

C1-C4. Severe disruption of ligaments or other soft supporting tissues without obvious abnormalities of the vertebrae on radiographs may occur in children. However, selected MR sequences are sensitive to such soft tissue injuries, if indicated. Children who are unresponsive, intoxicated, have abnormal findings on neurological examination, or neck pain should remain immobilized until C-spine stability has been determined by the appropriate studies. The use of corticosteroid as neuroprotection following spinal injury remains contentious.

Suggested Reading

- Platzer P, Jaindl M, Thalhammer G, et al. Cervical spine injuries in pediatric patients. J Trauma. 2007;62:389–96.
- Hall ED, Springer JE. Neuroprotection and acute spinal cord injury: a reappraisal. NeuroRx. 2004;1:80–100.

6. A 14-year-old boy came to the emergency department with progressive weakness for 10-h while he was seated in his classroom. He described it as a stinging sensation in his arms that progressed to numbness and weakness to the level of his upper chest. He has not urinated for several hours and he wakes only with assistance. He has moderate hypertonia in his upper extremities and his lower extremities are flaccid. Formal strength testing reveals (R/L): biceps 4/4, triceps 3/3, and wrist extension 4/4, with all other muscle groups tested being grade 0. He has a sensory level at T2, and deep tendon reflexes are absent throughout. MRI of the spine shows an ill-defined intramedullary hyperintensity extending from C5 to T2 without significant cord expansion or enhancement. MRI of the head is normal. CSF studies are normal, and no oligoclonal bands are detected.

What is the most appropriate treatment at this time?

A. IVIG 0.5 g/kg I.V. daily × 4 days
B. Methylprednisolone 500 mg I.V.B.I.D × 5 days
C. Prednisone 40 mg P.O. daily with a slow taper
D. Cyclophosphamide 800 mg/m2 I.V. every 4 weeks
E. Interferon-β – 1a 30 μg I.M. every week

Correct Answer is: B

Transverse myelitis (TM) is a heterogeneous disorder. It occurs as an idiopathic or secondary to a wide array of inflammatory (post-infectious, demyelinating), metabolic, and vascular processes. Inflammatory demyelinating lesions, as seen in clinically isolated syndrome, multiple sclerosis, and neuromyelitis optica, are the most common cause of TM. Acute treatment for those demyelinating conditions is a high-dose, intravenous corticosteroids for 3–5 days. A subsequent oral steroid taper over 4–6 weeks is recommended for patients with acute disseminated encephalomyelitis. Long-term therapy with immunosuppressants may decrease the relapse rate for patients with NMO. Non-demyelinating forms of transverse myelitis must be treated according to the underlying etiology, e.g. parenteral cyanocobalamin (vitamin B12) supplementation for subacute combined degeneration.

Suggested Reading

- Brinar VV, Habek M, et al. Current concepts in the diagnosis of transverse myelopathies. Clin Neurol Neurosurg. 2008;110:919–27.
- Pohl D. Epidemiology, immunopathogenesis and management of pediatric central nervous system inflammatory demyelinating conditions. Curr Opin Neurol. 2008;21:366–72.

7. A 16 yr. old girl presents with hands tingling after a "deep belly laugh" for the last 6 months. Her imaging is shown below:

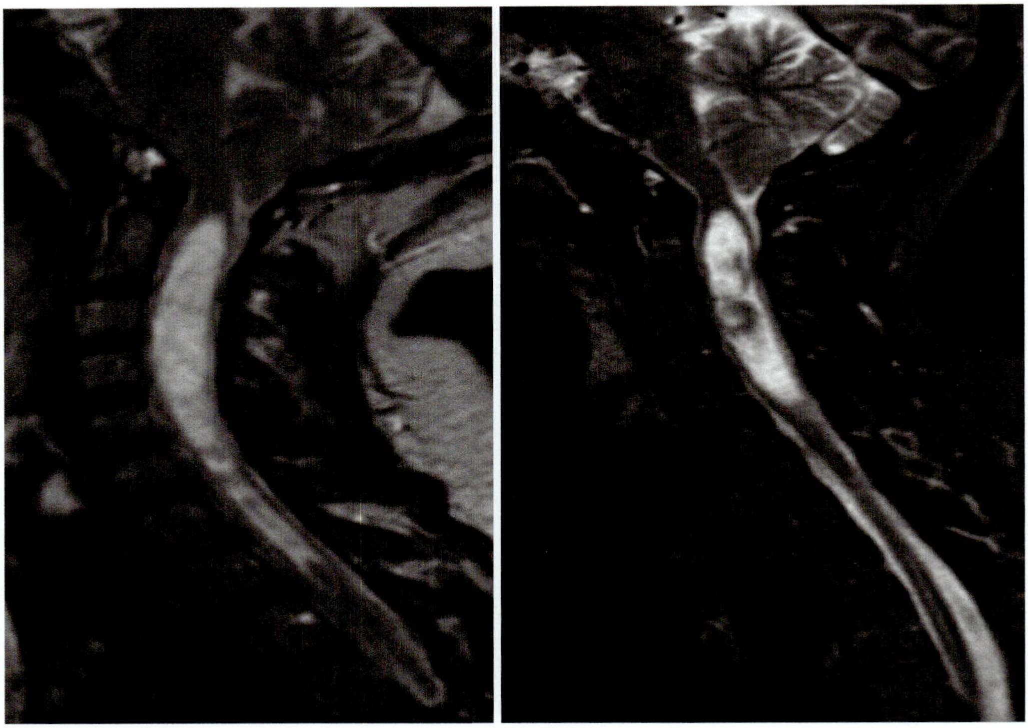

2006 2014

Figs. 24.2 and 24.3 Imágenes cortesía de la Chiari & Scoliosis & Syringomyelia Foundation. Las imágenes obtenidas por MR se tomaron antés y después de la Sección del Filum Terminale. Own work. Chiari & Scoliosis & Syringomyelia Foundation

What is the most likely diagnosis?

A. Klippel-Feil syndrome
B. Transverse myelitis
C. Platybasia
D. Chiari 1 malformation with syringomyelia
E. Intramedullary cervical spinal cord tumor

Correct Answer is: D

The "deep belly laugh" is a Valsalva maneuver which caused paresthesias secondary to the dilated space within the cervical cord or syrinx. The MRI image on the top shows the presence of septations in the syrinx indicating a congenital etiology. Chiari 1 malformations is a deviation of the cerebellar tonsil down through the formen magnum. When associated with a syringomyelia, the Chiari is felt to be symptomatic and surgical intervention is indicated. Other common symptoms could include occipital headaches, early morning headache, and headaches brought on by coughing or sneezing. Patients may experience difficulty swallowing due to decreased gag and parasthesias of the shoulders and hands.

Klippel-Feil syndrome is a triad of short neck, low posterior hair line and limited

neck movement. It involves fusion of cervical vertebrae. Platybasia involves flattening of the base of the skull, frequently seen in patients with bony dysplasias. Transverse myelitis was not shown on imaging which would appear patchy increased T2 signal in the cord. This image shows the syringomyelia which is similar in signal to CSF and not consistent with transverse myelitis.

Suggested Reading

- Fernandez A, et al. Malformations of the craniocervical junction (chiari type I and syringomyelia: classification, diagnosis and treatment). BMC Musculoskelet Disord. 2009;10(Suppl 1).

8. A 12-year-old boy complains of low back pain for the past 6 months and developed recently problems with urinary incontinence, often times occurring when he is walking upstairs. He was seen by a urologist, and urodynamic studies showed detrusor hyperreflexia. Past medical history is otherwise unremarkable. Review of systems is pertinent for constipation. His vital signs are normal. General examination shows mild thoracolumbar scoliosis and a small capillary hemangioma overlying the lumbar spine. Mental status, cranial nerves, strength and sensation are within normal limits. Deep tendon reflexes are 2+ in the upper extremities and 3+ in the lower extremities. Plantar responses are extensor bilaterally. He has a normal gait but he has trouble with tandem gait.

   Which of the following is most likely to be found on spine MRI?

   A. Cauda equina compression
   B. Diastematomyelia
   C. Syringomyelia
   D. Chiari malformation
   E. Tethered spinal cord

Correct Answer is: E

Tethered cord syndrome (TCS) is a spectrum of congenital anomalies secondary to an abnormally low position of the conus medullaris that may lead to neurological, musculoskeletal, urological, or gastrointestinal abnormalities. Most commonly TCS is associated with spinal dysraphism. The signs and symptoms correlate with the radiological findings showing the conus medullaris is anatomically lower than the L2 vertebra or below the L 1–2 disc space. However, some patients with signs and symptoms of TCS with a normal conus medullaris position. The clinical presentation is broad and different with age at presentation as well as underlying cause. Toddlers and young children have clumsy gait, regression in motor function or bladder control, or arrest in achievement of developmental milestones. Foot deformities, scoliosis, non-segmental sensory loss and pain in the back and lower extremities are also common features.
In the late childhood and teenage years, pain in the lumbosacral region, perineum, and legs is the predominant symptom. Progression of scoliosis, constipation and urinary incontinence are common. Urodynamic studies usually demonstrate detrusor hyperreflexia. MRI demonstrates a thickened filum terminale (>2 mm) and a conus positioned below the L2 level. Supine and prone MRI demonstrate lack of motion of the spinal cord. Surgical detethering of the cord is an effective treatment, particularly if performed early.

Suggested Reading

- Hertzler DA, DePowell JJ, Stevenson CB, Mangano FT. Tethered cord syndrome: a review of the literature from embryology to adult presentation. Neurosurg Focus. 2010;29:1–9.

9. A 12-year-old girl complained of pain between her shoulder blades during school. Later that day she had sudden

loss of strength in both arms and both legs, she could not stand and she was carried out of the shower. In the emergency department, a lumbar puncture was performed and cerebrospinal fluid was normal except for 24 lymphocytes/mm^3. Her condition remains unchanged and a week later her examination shows the following; decreased pin and temperature appreciation below C-4 spinal level with intact vibratory, position, and touch sensation. She has no reflexes in the flaccid upper extremities and increased reflexes in the lower extremities with bilateral Babinski. She has a neurogenic bladder and bowel. Her spine MRI of the spine are shown.

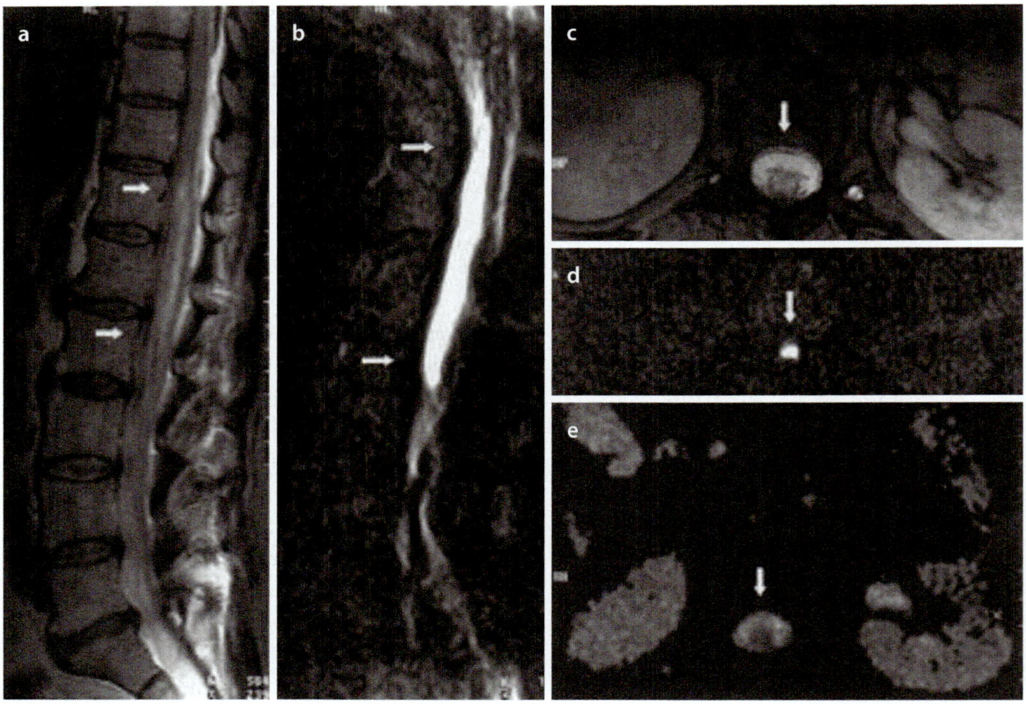

Fig. 24.4 T2-weighted sagittal **a** and transverse **c** MRI 30 h after symptom onset show a hyperintense lesion with edematous expansion in the central portion of the lumbar cord and the conus medullaris. Diffusion-weighted MRI demonstrates strong hyperintensity on sagittal **b** and transverse **d** images ($b = 1000$ s/mm^2) and a reduced apparent diffusion coefficient (ADC) 0.49×10^{-5} cm^2/s on calculated maps of the ADC **e**, confirming the ischemic pathology. (Neuroimages. Neurology **June 13, 2000** vol. 54 no. 11 **2195.** Figures Only ***Free***)

What is the most likely diagnosis?

A. Neuromyelitis optica
B. Acute transverse myelitis
C. Spinal cord infarction
D. Multiple sclerosis
E. Viral infection of the spinal cord

Correct Answer is: C

The classical presentation of anterior spinal artery infarction is:

- **Sudden onset of transient back or neck pain.**
- **Rapidly progressive flaccid and arreflexic paraplegia or tetraplegia in acute period.**

- Spasticity below the lesion with extensor plantar responses will follow.
- Loss of pain and temperature below level.
- Preservation of proprioception, light touch and vibration sensation.
- Autonomic dysfunction and bladder dysfunction.
- Painful dysesthesias below the level of the lesion.

The sensory changes are what separate this from demyelinating disease such as Devic's neuromyelitis optica, multiple sclerosis and acute transverse myelitis. Viral infections of the spine (poliomyelitis) usually spare the sensory system but frequently is associated with pain in the affected extremities.

Suggested Reading

- Love BB. Spinal cord vascular syndromes, In: Noseworthy JH, editor. Neurological therapeutics principles and practice. 2nd ed. Informa healthcare; 2006.

10. A 13-year-old female has been seen for headaches which began one a year ago. They occur 3–4 days per week, are located in the occipital area, and last for several hours unless she takes Tylenol. Occasionally they are triggered by coughing or sneezing. She has no associated nausea, vomiting, sensitivity to light or sound, and dizziness but says sometimes objects look like they are jiggling when she has the pain. Past medical history is otherwise normal and family history is noncontributory. Examination is normal except for hyperreflexia in the lower extremities.
What is the most common secondary complications could have happened?

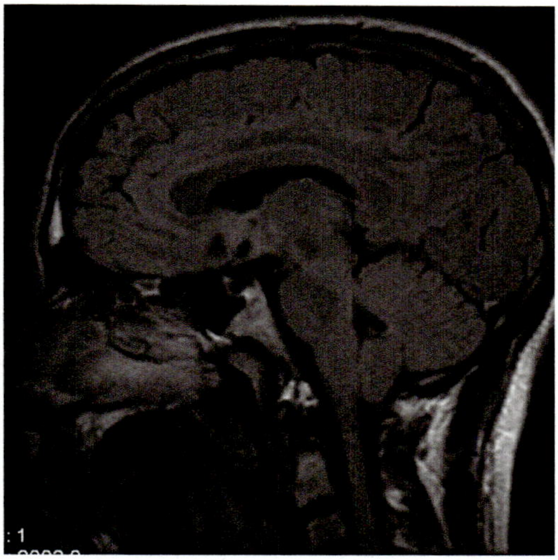

Fig. 24.5 Image of a Type 1 Arnold-Chiari Malformation. The cerebellum has descended 7 mm and there are herniated cerebellar tonsils into the foramen magnum. Basket of Puppies

A. Hemicord syndrome
B. Spinal stenosis
C. Syringomyelia
D. Spinal cord infarction
E. Transverse myelitis

Correct Answer is: C
The patient has a Chiari I malformation. Chiari malformation was first described by Hans Chiari in 1891. It is defined as cerebellar tonsil extension below the foramen magnum. Severity ranges from a morphological asymptomatic finding to a clinical Chiari. There appears to be evolution of the condition over time, the number of symptomatic patients increasing with age. Patients with this malformation have the risk of developing a dilation of the central canal (syrinx or hydromyelia). Abnormal CSF flow at the level of the foramen magnum is due to underdevelopment of the mesodermal occipital somite, resulting in a smaller posterior fossa. How this results in dilation of the central canal is not well

understood? Neurosurgical decompression of the posterior fossa via a suboccipital craniectomy, often combined with laminectomy to the level of the tonsillar herniation, with duraplasty or dural scoring is the optimal treatment of the condition. Surgical complication rate is much higher if the subarachnoid membrane is invaded.

24

Suggested Reading

- Navarro R, Olavarria G, et al. Surgical results of posterior fossa decompression for patients with Chiari I malformation. Childs Nerv Syst. 2004;20:349–56.
- Eule JM, Erickson MA, O'Brien MF, Handler M. Chiari I malformation associated with syringomyelia and scoliosis. A 20-year review of surgical and nonsurgical treatment in a pediatric population. Spine 2002;27:1451–5.

11. One week-old baby boy born at full term has weakness of the left arm since birth. No movements has been noted at the shoulder and does not flex at the elbow, but he has active elbow extension. Wiggle his fingers and has a grasp reflex in the hand. No respiratory difficulty was reported. His pupils are symmetric and there is no ptosis. He has normal tone and movements in the other limbs.
What is your next step in management at this time?
   - A. Immobilize the right arm in a splint
   - B. MRI of the cervical cord and left shoulder
   - C. Nerve conduction and EMG studies of the left arm
   - D. Micro neurosurgical intervention
   - E. Physiotherapy for gentle range of motion exercises

Correct Answer is: E
Brachial plexus birth palsy (BPBP) occurs in 0.4–4 per 1000 live births. Perinatal risk factors include macrosomia, multiparous pregnancies, and previous deliveries resulting in BPBP, prolonged labor, breech delivery, and assisted and difficult deliveries. 50% of patients have 1 or more of these risk factors, which demonstrate that the etiology of BPBP is not yet fully known. In children, the extent of brachial plexus injury differs greatly, and therefore the prognosis does as well. Between 66% and 92% have a mild injury and recover completely, usually within the first 2 months. Those with only C5-C6 involvement have classic Erb's palsy (46%) and have the most favorable prognosis. The most severely affected babies have a flail extremity, Horner's syndrome, and hemi-diaphragmatic paralysis. Early evaluation and intervention is warranted for babies with a more severe form of BPBP, since spontaneous recovery is unlikely. In this case, patient has a mild form, so the best management is observation with gentle range of motion exercises to prevent contractures.

Suggested Reading

- Hale HB, Bae DS, Waters PM. Current concepts in the management of brachial plexus birth palsy. J Hand Surg 2010;35A:322–31.

12. An 8-year-old boy came to your office with a history of difficulty running that has been gradually progressive over the past 2 years. He attributes this problem to intermittent low back pain, which is worsened by activity but does not radiate. Also, in the past 6 months he had intermittent urinary incontinence. He has normal bulk but mildly increased tone in his distal lower

extremities and mild weakness in ankle dorsiflexion bilaterally. Sensory examination is normal. Deep tendon reflexes are 2+ in the upper extremities and 3+ in the lower extremities. He has bilateral flexor plantar responses. Rectal tone is normal. He has lumbar levoscoliosis and a sacral hemangioma. He elevates his right shoulder and hip while walking but maintains a narrow base. MRI spine shows a low-lying conus medullaris at L3 and an L4 hemivertebra with associated levoscoliosis. **Surgical treatment is most likely to lead to improvement in which of this patient's symptoms?**

A. Pain
B. Spasticity
C. Scoliosis
D. Bladder function
E. Weakness

Correct Answer is: A
Tethered cord syndrome (TCS) is a constellation of motor and sensory findings that are attributable to excessive tension on the spinal cord. The majority of cases are associated with spinal dysraphism; however, TCS can also occur when an intradural process (e.g. abnormal thickened, shortened filum terminale, lipoma of the filum, fibrous adhesions) interferes with normal ascension of the conus with respect to the vertebral column. It can present at any age. Infants usually have cutaneous stigmata of spina bifida occulta, such as nevi, lipomas, tufts of hair, hemangiomas, and dermal sinuses. Other alarming signs include urinary dribbling, anorectal malformations, orthopedic deformities of the lower extremities, and scoliosis. Children and adolescents may be asymptomatic or may present with slowly progressive motor and sensory deficits. The clinical picture may also include varying degrees of weakness; patchy sensory deficits; scoliosis; non-dermatomal pain in the low back, perineum, and/or legs; bladder or less frequently bowel incontinence; orthopedic deformities of the lower extremities; and gait disturbances. MRI is the study of choice, as it can detect both the level of the conus and the cause of the tethering. Surgical untethering should be done in symptomatic patients, which results in pain relief in almost all cases and stabilization of neurologic decline in up to 90% of patients. Scoliosis progression after surgical tethering was noted in one cohort in long term follow up. However, there was improvement in muscle strength, gait, and spasticity. The role of surgery in asymptomatic patients remains less clear.

Suggested Reading

- Bowman RM, Mohan A, et al. Tethered cord release: a long term study in 114 patients. J Neurosurg Pediatr. 2009;3(3):181–7.
- Lew SM, Kothbauer KF. Tethered cord syndrome: an updated review. Pediatr Neurosurg. 2007;43:236–248.

13. A 12-year-old boy presents with walking difficulty, which has been progressive over the last few months. He has been dragging his feet on the ground and has tripped and fallen several times. Recently, he complained of urinary urgency and has had occasional incontinence. Workup by his pediatrician was negative including routine blood work and UA. He has increased tone and brisk deep tendon reflexes in both lower extremities with spastic gait. Spine MRI shown below.

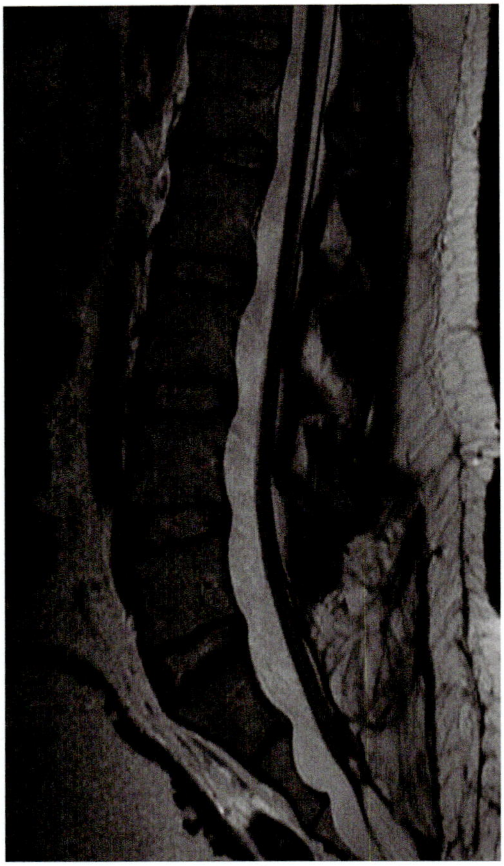

Fig. 24.6 Tethered Cord. American Academy of Neurology Institute, produced by permission

What is the most likely diagnosis?

A. Spinal Meningioma
B. Subacute Combined Degeneration of the Cord
C. Tethered Cord
D. Spinal AVM
E. Transverse Myelitis

Correct Answer: C

The MRI shows tethered cord with low lying conus ending much lower than normal S2-S3 level and also rules out the other options listed above. The cauda Equine includes the terminal spinal cord, spinal roots from T12 to S5 and the filum terminale, which is a fibrous band that anchors the lower tip of the spinal cord to the sacrum. In adults, the spinal cord ends around the level of L1. Tethered cord syndrome occurs in association with the spectrum of spinal dysraphisms which include spina bifida occulta, meningocele, myelomeningocle, diastematomyelia, intraspinal lipoma, sacral agenesis and fibrosis of the filum terminale, leading to abnormal fixation of the lower end of the spinal cord. The different rate of growth of the vertebral column and the spinal cord leads to the stretching of the spinal cord. In milder cases, symptoms might appear in childhood with progressive stretching of the cord. However if severe it can be symptomatic at birth. Symptoms can include myelopathy with upper motor neuron type weakness with increased tone and brisk reflexes as well as bladder dysfunction. Neurosurgical de-tethering procedures can improve the symptoms.

Suggested Reading

- Swaiman KF, Ashwal S, Ferriero DM. Pediatric neurology principles and practice, 4th ed. Philadelphia: Mosby Elsevier; 2006.
- Gruener G, Biller J. Spinal cord anatomy, localization and overview of spinal cord syndromes. Continuum Lifelong Learning Neurol. 2008;14(3):11–35.

14. A 4-year-old girl has been admitted to the hospital for evaluation of weakness 3 days. Initially weakness involved her left arm but one day later it worsened to involve the right arm and both legs. She complains of pain in the left shoulder. Past medical history is remarkable for fever and cough 2 week ago while shopping with her grandmother; symptoms resolved within 2 days. No medication was taken. Her examination is remarkable for 3/5 power in all limbs. It is difficult to elicit dep tendon reflexes in the upper extremities and are brisk

in the lower extremities. She has plantar flexor response and sensation is intact. MRI of the cervical spine is obtained and a sagittal T2-weighted sample is shown.

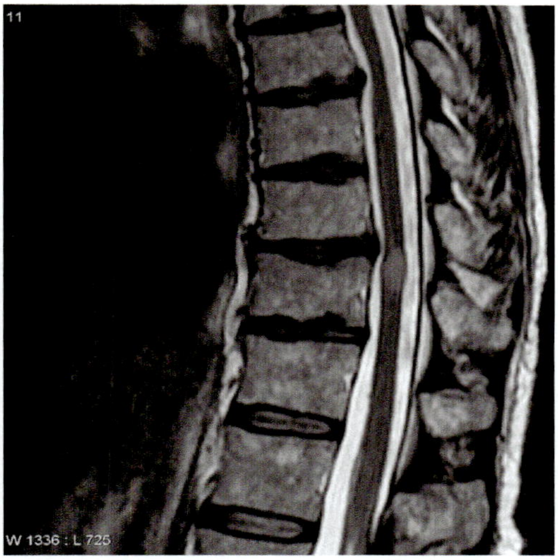

Fig. 24.7 Transverse myelitis, this 53 year old woman rapidly developed neurological symptoms, which resolved over the course of weeks. Followup MRI three months later demonstrated significant reduction is the size of the lesion. It is felt to be consistent with transverse myelitis. (► http://radiopaedia.org/cases/transversemyelitis and ► http://radiopaedia.org/uploads/radio/0001/3690/TM_01.jpg. Frank Gaillard. Wikipedia)

Would will be your initial treatment?

A. acyclovir
B. high-dose methylprednisolone
C. plasmapheresis
D. intravenous immunoglobulin infusions
E. surgical drainage of syrinx

Correct Answer: B

The presentation and MRI findings are consistent with acute transverse myelitis (ATM). ATM, a subgroup of different conditions that cause transverse spinal cord syndromes, is an inflammatory and usually idiopathic spinal cord condition. Diagnosis of idiopathic ATM is established according to criteria which include a clinical picture of bilateral symptoms and signs attributable to spinal cord disease, existence of focal cord inflammation by MRI and cerebrospinal fluid studies, and exclusion of other diseases, especially cord compression and disease-associated ATM, (e.g, Sjögren disease). Idiopathic ATM patients have motor, sensory and autonomic dysfunctions with acute or subacute onset, progressing to nadir in 4 h to 21 days, with full or partial recovery in most cases. Acute treatment to stop inflammation with corticosteroids is required as well as early appropriate symptomatic therapies. Recent discovery of novel biomarkers has set apart specific inflammatory and autoimmune myelopathies, namely paraneoplastic myelitis and neuromyelitis optica spectrum diseases, the diagnosis of which is important to establish therapeutic strategies.

Suggested Reading

- Sá MJ. Acute transverse myelitis: a practical reappraisal. Autoimmun Rev. 2009;9(2):128–31.

15. Physical complications of spina bifida include which of the following?
   A. Allergy to latex
   B. Leg weakness and paralysis
   C. Club foot
   D. (B) and (C)
   E. (A) (B) and (C)

Correct answer: E

68% of children with spina bifida have latex allergy, ranging from mild to life-threatening. The common use of latex in medical facilities makes this a particularly serious concern. Leg paralysis or weakness and orthopedic abnormalities such as club foot, hip dislocation or scoliosis, and urinary and bowel control problems are frequently present.

24

16. A 14-year-old girl presents with progressive lower extremity numbness and weakness bilaterally, walking difficulty for 2 months. She reports worsening over the past 3 days, when she woke up this morning she was unable to move her legs and felt numb from her upper chest down. Examination shows mild weakness and areflexia in both upper extremities, and significant weakness with spasticity and hyperreflexia in the lower extremities. She has a sensory level at T2. Sagittal MRI is shown below.

Which of the following is the most likely diagnosis?

A. Spinal cord infarct
B. Acute transverse myelitis
C. Epidural hematoma
D. Cord compression from a metastatic tumor
E. Meningioma with spinal cord compression

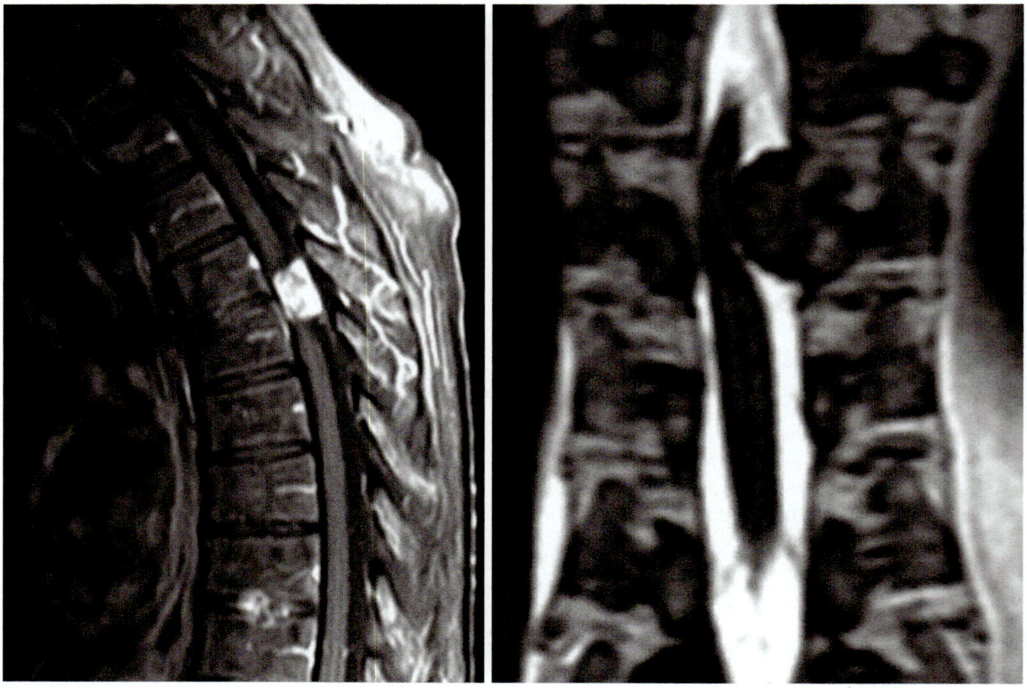

Figs. 24.8 and 24.9 Meningeom im Spinalkanal MRT. Links T1 sagittal mit Kontrastmittel, rechts T2 coronar. Own work. Hellerhoff. Wikipedia

Correct answer: E
MRI shows an intradural extramedullary tumor compressing the spinal cord. The tumor is located at the C7 to T1 vertebral level and is dural based. Meningiomas are one of the most common intradural extramedullary tumors. They are non-glial neoplasms that are usually benign and can cause neurologic problems due to compression. Neurologic symptoms progress very gradually and may compensate for the degree of compression because they grow slowly. Sometimes large tumors causing significant compression without prominent manifestations on clinical examination. The presentation is not acute to subacute so the patient does not have transverse myelitis nor a spinal cord infarct, with MRI findings showing a parenchymal cord lesion and not an extramedullary mass.

A spinal cord infarct may be sudden in onset and usually affects the anterior cord (anterior spinal artery), causing primarily bilateral weakness and pain and temperature loss rather than vibration and position loss (dorsal columns are relatively spared). Acute transverse myelitis progresses over hours or a few days rather than months. A metastatic tumor has a subacute presentation with prominent back pain. Because metastatic tumors develop more rapidly, the patient would have more symptoms and neurologic deficits than this patient has for the degree of compression seen on this MRI. An epidural hematoma also presents rapidly with an acute compressive myelopathy syndrome manifesting as spinal shock, usually with no evidence of spasticity or hyperreflexia on presentation.

Suggested Reading

- Comprehensive review in clinical neurology: a multiple choice question book for the wards and boards

17. A 5-month-old baby is brought to his PCP for a well-child visit. PCP found on examination that the child has a small, midline tuft of hair over the lower lumbar region. The rest of his physical examination is otherwise entirely normal. On annual follow-up at 3 years of age, the child continues to have normal development and a normal neurologic examination. **What statement regarding this child is correct?**
    A. On the basis of the finding of this tuft of hair, it can be concluded that he will eventually have significant cognitive delay, even if he has developed normally up until the age of 3 years
    B. On the basis of the finding of this tuft of hair, it can be concluded that he will eventually have significant motor and cognitive delay even if he has developed normally up until the age of 3 years
    C. This tuft of hair signifies a possible underlying defect in the posterior bony component of the vertebral column
    D. This tuft of hair signifies the presence of a myelomeningocele
    E. On the basis of the finding of this tuft of hair, it can be concluded that abnormalities in the spinal cord will definitely be seen on imaging

Correct answer is: D
The patient's history and examination are consistent with spina bifida occulta. This is a defect in the bony components along the posterior aspect of the vertebral column. It can be asymptomatic, but an abnormal conus medullaris and filum terminale are possible. The presence of a hair tuft, implying underlying spina bifida occulta, but not necessarily imply impending cognitive or motor delay. In fact, when early neurologic development is normal, it will typically continue to be so. However, associated neurologic deficits may portend future neurologic impairment. When there is associated neurologic deficits in a child with a tuft of hair over the lumbar region but with no other evidence of neural tube defect, the disorder is named occult spinal dysraphism. In this case, a variety of developmental abnormalities may be seen involving the spinal cord or roots and posterior fossa, and associated findings may include dermoid or epidermoid cysts, intraspinal or cutaneous lipomas, and tethered cord. Diastematomyelia, or dividing of the spinal cord, may also be seen. Rarely, a sinus tract connects the dura with the surface of the skin. In occult spinal dysraphism, neurologic manifestations vary widely and may range from mild motor deficits and ankle hyporeflexia to bowel and bladder

dysfunction, sensory loss, and paraparesis or paraplegia. Although patients may be initially asymptomatic, these neurological deficits can develop suddenly and be irreversible.

24

18. You are evaluating a previously healthy 17-year-old girl presents to the ED with difficulty walking for 2 days. She reports having difficulty moving or feeling her legs. Also she has difficulty urinating. On neurological exam, she has 3/5 weakness in both legs, ¾ reflexes in the bilateral patella reflexes, and 5 beats of clonus in the right Achilles reflex. There is a pinprick sensation loss at the level of the umbilicus.
What is the next best step in management?
A. Electromyography examination
B. MRI brain with and without gadolinium
C. MRI thoracic spine with and without gadolinium
D. MRI cervical spine with and without gadolinium
E. Lumbar puncture

Correct answer is: C
The clinical history and exam is suggestive of transverse myelitis. Given the sensory level at T10, a thoracic localization should be deduced. MRI of the brain and cervical spine would be useful in evaluating for possible underlying multiple sclerosis, but would not be used for the treatment of this acute presentation. Lumbar puncture should follow imaging. Electromyography does not have a role in the diagnosis of transverse myelitis.

Suggested Reading

- Wingerchuk DM, Weinshenker BG. Acute disseminated encephalomyelitis, transverse myelitis, and neuromyelitis optica. Continuum (Minneap Minn). 2013;19(4 Multiple Sclerosis):944–67

19. The most severe form of spina bifida is which of the following:
A. Spina bifida occulta
B. Myeloschisis
C. Meningocele
D. Myelomeningocele
E. Arnold-Chiari II malformation

Correct answer: B
In myeloschisis, the affected area is a flattened, plate-like mass of nervous tissue with no overlying membrane.

The exposure of these nerves and tissues makes the infant more prone to life-threatening infections such as meningitis. Spina bifida occulta is the least severe form and may be asymptomatic. Many individuals with spina bifida have an associated abnormality of the cerebellum, called the Arnold Chiari II malformation in which, the back portion of the brain is displaced from the back of the skull down into the upper neck.

Static Encephalopathy/ Cerebral Palsy/ Rehabilitation

Y. M. Awaad, *Absolute Pediatric Neurology*, https://doi.org/10.1007/978-3-319-78801-2_25

1. A 2-year-old premature boy, he was 26 weeks of gestation and his birth weight was 750 grams. He had retrolental fibroplasia but did not require laser surgery. At 2 years, he has sever global developmental delay and he is unable to walk or talk. On examination, he has remarkable hypotonia, athetois and dysmetria. Brain MRI is shown.

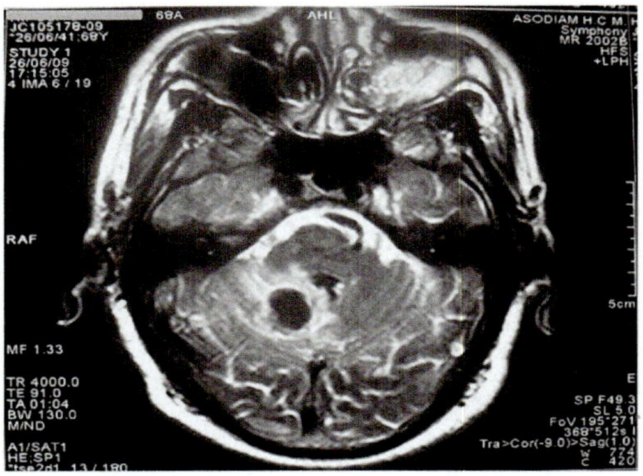

Fig. 25.1 Head MRI showing deep intracerebral hemorrhage due to bleeding within the cerebellum, approximately 30 h old: same patient as TAC craneo ECV.jpg, Head MRI stroke.JPG and Head CT stroke.jpg. (Own work. Bobjgalindo. Wikipedia)

What is the most likely cause of his condition?

A. Intraventricular hemorrhage
B. Neonatal streptococcal meningitis
C. Ischemia
D. Congenital toxoplasmosis
E. Neonatal herpes simplex infection

Correct Answer is: C
Cerebellum abnormalities on the MRI became more recognizable by the clinician evaluating children with cerebral palsy or developmental delay. This boy's birth weight was under 1000 grams and gestational age of less than 28 weeks makes the child extremely vulnerable to cerebellar injury. Cerebellar abnormalities can be presented in about 60% in such children with cerebral palsy. Those abnormalities do not see in the more mature premature. The reason for this abnormality is not clear, however the common marked loss of white matter volume would strongly suggest ischemia occurred and most likely contributed. Others suggest parenchymal hemorrhage as a main factor but the variety of injury observed suggest other possibilities, mainly ischemia.

Suggested Reading

- Bodensteiner JB, Johnsen SD. MRI findings in children surviving extremely premature delivery and extremely low birth weight with cerebral palsy. J Child Neurology. 2006;21(9):743–7.

2. A 15-month-old girl with decreased usage of her right hand in the last 4 months of age which was noted by her family. Her pediatrician diagnosed her as a right hemiparesis at 1 year of age. The mother had no complication during pregnancy and there was no history of prenatal or perinatal problems. Her birth weight was 6 pounds 5 ounces. She was discharged 1 day form the hospital. Her development was normal. She says a few words and understands many. On examination, her height, weight and head circumference just below the 2nd percentile. She is bright, alert and attentive. Cranial nerves exam was normal. Visual fields are intact to distraction. She has decreased usage of her right arm and leg. Right thumb is abducted and grasping with the right hand is crude. Tone is increased and tendon reflexes are exaggerated in the right limbs and her right plantar response is extensor.
What is your explanation for her neurological condition?

A. Congenital CMV infection
B. Lissencephaly
C. Postnatal cerebral infarction
D. Hemiparesis cerebral palsy
E. Fetal alcohol syndrome

Correct Answer is: D

She has cerebral palsy (hemi paretic type), which statistically is most likely prenatal in origin. Brain MRI is essential to determine if further evaluation is indicated. Limited further evaluation may be indicated if the child has a schizencephaly. On the other hand, a full hematologic evaluation of the mother and the child in the presence of a pre-natal infarction. The chances of CMV causing hemiparesis is less likely but would be suggested by malformation and calcification. Hearing and urine screening for CMV is of great help. Because the child has a benign neonatal course, the post-natal injury is not likely.

Suggested Reading

- Oskoui M, Shevell MI. Profile of pediatric hemiparesis. J Child Neurol. 2005;20(6):471.

3. A 2-day old baby boy who is one of an identical twin born at 27-week gestation. Birth weight was 800 grams. A routine head ultrasound testing was done and showed a small intraventricular hemorrhage but no evidence of ventricular enlargement or parenchymal damage. His identical twin sibling has a normal ultrasound. His family is asking about his prognosis.

   What statement is the most accurate one?

   A. He is no more likely than his sibling to have cerebral palsy or mental delay
   B. He is no more likely than his sibling to have mental delay but more likely to have cerebral palsy.
   C. He is more likely than his sibling to have cerebral palsy or mental delay
   D. He is more like than his sibling to have mental delay but not cerebral palsy
   E. The results at this gestational age are indeterminate

Correct Answer is: C

The studies referenced below indicate that intraventricular hemorrhage may be a radiological marker indicating wider spread insult. Thus, in a very low weight premature it may indicate a less favorable outcome.

Suggested Reading

- Inder TE. Neurodevelopmental impact of low-grade intraventricular hemorrhage in very preterm infants. J Pediatr. 2006;149(2):152–4.
- Patra K, Wilson-Costello D, Taylor G, Mercuri-Minich N, Hack M. Grades I-II Intraventricula hemorrhage in extremely low birth weight infants: Effects on neurodevelopment. J Pediatr. 2006;149(2):169–73.

4. A 30-week premature infant has a severe intraventricular hemorrhage and hydrocephalus at 3 weeks of age. He has been stable and recently came off the respirator. On examination, his anterior fontanelle is full but not firm. Sutures are not spread. Head growth has been normal.

   What is your advice to the family at this time?

   A. The patient needs an immediate ventriculo-peritoneal shunt and her prognosis is good.
   B. The patient needs an immediate ventriculo-peritoneal shunt but despite intervention her prognosis is very bad.
   C. The patient will only need medical management with acetazolamide and/or furosemide but despite treatment her prognosis is bad.
   D. The patient should be monitored with ultrasound and may need a drainage procedure; prognosis is indeterminant.
   E. The patient will only need medical management with acetazolamide and/or furosemide and with this treatment her prognosis is good

Correct Answer is: D
Prematurity has detrimental effects the brain. The complication of hemorrhage and consequent hydrocephalus is certainly undesirable. The practical issue is the relative risk of drainage and possible infection versus watching carefully and allowing additional damage to the brain.

Suggested Reading

- Casey AT, Kimmings EJ, Kleinlugtebeld AD, Taylor WA, Harkness WF, Hayward RD. The long-term outlook for hydrocephalus in childhood. A ten-year cohort study of 155 patients. Pediatr Neurosurg. 1007;27(2):63–70.
- Brouwer A, Groenendaal F, van Haastert IL, Rademaker K, Hanlo P, de Vries L. Neurodevelopmental outcome of preterm infants with severe intraventricular hemorrhage and therapy for post-hemorrhagic ventricular dilatation. J Pediatr. 2008;152(5):648–54.
- Peretta P, Ragazzi P, Carlino CF, Gaglini P, Cinalli G. The role of Ommaya reservoir and endoscopic third ventriculostomy in the management of post-hemorrhagic hydrocephalus of prematurity. Childs Nerv Sys. 2007;23(7):765–71.

5. A 5-year-old boy with a history of delayed development, mainly motor milestones. He stared walking independently at 2 years of age and continues to walk and run on his toes. He is getting faster with time and there has been no worsening of his gait pattern. He was 32 weeks gestation, his mother had preterm labor and gestational diabetes. He went home after 2 weeks of life and had some mild difficulties with feeding and weight gain initially.

   His mother reports that he has no seizures and he has normal social and cognitively abilities. On your examination, he is an alert and interactive young boy, who states his name, age, and birth date, knows his colors, and can count to 20. Cranial nerve exam is normal. Upper extremities show normal strength and tone, with some fine motor clumsiness for his given age. Lower extremities show increased tone at the ankles, with some limitation of dorsiflexion, more subtle increases in tone are noted bilaterally in the hip adductors and hamstrings. Reflexes are 2+ in the upper extremities and 3+ in the lower extremities. He has mildly crouched gait at both knees and on his toes (less so in his orthotics). Brain MRI is shown.

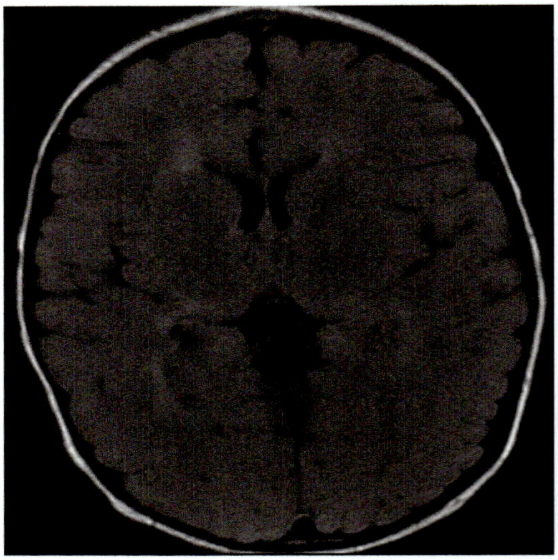

Fig. 25.2 Cation, PVL. American Academy of Neurology Institute, produced by permission

What is the most likely diagnosis?
A. arginase deficiency
B. bilateral closed lip schizencephaly
C. cerebral palsy
D. dopa responsive dystonia
E. idiopathic toe walking

Correct Answer is: C
This boy has a delayed motor development, but no regression or daytime fluctuation, and evidence of mild lower extremity spasticity and brisk reflexes. He

has a history of mild prematurity, and MRI findings of mild hyperintense signal on T2 FLAIR images of the periventricular white matter, all those findings are most consistent with a diagnosis of cerebral palsy.

Cerebral palsy is one of the neurodevelopmental disability disorders of childhood. It is not a specific etiologic diagnosis, rather a descriptive term for a disorder of motor control (affecting movement, tone or posture) causing activity limitation that is non-progressive in nature, resulting from an injury to or malformation of the brain at its early formative stages. Rarely, loss of motor function with time, which is typically secondary to complications of under treated spasticity (such as joint contractures or scoliosis) or rapid changes in weight or height during puberty rather than inherent progression of neurologic disease. CP refers only to the motor dysfunction seen; it does not confer (though is often associated with) cognitive impairment, hearing loss, strabismus or epilepsy. It happens in 1–3 out of 1000 live births, prematurity is the most common risk factor, which raises incidence to 4–10% if born with very low birth weight and up to 20% risk if born at 24–26 weeks gestational age.

Nonetheless, full term infants represent more the half of all cases of cerebral palsy. The potential etiologies includes brain malformations or genetic disorders, post-natal brain injury at a young age (CNS infection, accidental or non-accidental trauma, kernicterus), prenatal factors (maternal chorioamnionitis, intrauterine growth retardation, toxin exposure, congenital infections, maternal trauma), perinatal brain injury (hypoxic-ischemic encephalopathy, neonatal stroke, traumatic brain injury, intracranial hemorrhage) and brain injury related to prematurity (periventricular leukomalacia and intraventricular hemorrhage). CP has been classified based on the location and type of motor control difficulty. Spastic forms are the most common, and can involve the legs primarily (most common type affecting premature infants) called diplegic CP, involve one-half of the body (usually from unilateral hemorrhagic or ischemic stroke or unilateral brain malformation) called hemiplegic CP or involve all four extremities (often from HIE in a term infant or severe diffuse traumatic injury) called quadriparetic CP. Various degrees of dyskinesia (dystonic and choreoathetoid movements) often accompany the spasticity, especially in cases where there is prominent basal ganglia injury. Ataxic and hypotonic subtype are diagnoses of exclusion after a thorough evaluation for other primary cerebellar or lower motor neuron disorders are excluded. Neuroimaging is useful in the evaluation of the child with cerebral palsy if the etiology has not been established from the history. MRI is superior than CT scan because it provides more detail of the white matter and often shows abnormal white matter signal or volume, or in the case of hemiparetic CP evidence of old focal infarction or malformation of cortex. If the history and neuroimaging do not determine a specific structural abnormality, or not consistent with a static process, metabolic and genetic testing can be considered.

In this case, there is no sign of cortical malformation present, which argues against polymicrogyria as the etiology. Arginase deficiency presents much differently than the other urea cycles disorders, with onset of progressive spastic paraplegia, intellectual deterioration, and hyperactivity. Episodes of acute encephalopathy and seizures are unusual. Dopa-responsive dystonia is most commonly caused by mutations in GTP cyclohydrolase and presents with dystonic spasms, commonly isolated to the legs initially and leading to a gait pattern that may mimic that seen in cerebral palsy. Two-thirds of cases manifest a classic diurnal variation, with progressive worsening over the course

of the day, which would not be typical with cerebral palsy. It is important to remember to ask this question in the history, especially if there is a hint that motor symptoms are worsening. Idiopathic toe-walking manifests early in childhood (usually in the first 1–2 years of life) and shows a preference to be on the toes (in standing or with slow walking), that tends to lessen with attempts to run. No other upper motor neuron findings should be present on exam and neuroimaging studies are normal.

Suggested Reading

- Oskoui M, Shevell MI. Cerebral palsy and the transition from pediatric to adult care. Continuum Lifelong Learning Neurol. 2009;15(6):64–77. Ashwal S, Russman BS, Blasco PA, et al. Practice parameter: diagnostic assessment of the child with cerebral palsy. Report of the Quality Standards Subcommittee of the American Academy of Neurology and the Practice Committee of the Child Neurology Society. Neurology. 2004;62(6):851–63.

6. The Surveillance of Cerebral Palsy in Europe (SCPE) reported the following incidence of co-morbidities in children with CP:
   A. Active seizures 20%
   B. Mental disadvantage (IQ < 50) 70%
   C. Active seizures 50%
   D. Mental disadvantage (IQ < 50) 30%
   E. Both (A) and (D)

Correct Answer is: E
The SCPE reported an incidence of 20% active seizures and 30% mental disadvantage (IQ < 50) in their cerebral palsy population.

7. Which of the following statements regarding cerebral palsy is true?
   A. Hemiplegic cerebral palsy is often due to placental embolisms
   B. Hemiplegic cerebral palsy involves the right hemisphere in >80% of cases
   C. Symptoms are identifiable at birth
   D. It is commonly related to obstetrical procedures
   E. None of the above

Correct Answer is: A
Cerebral palsy is caused by intrauterine injury (i.e. infarcts), unrelated to complications of delivery. Symptoms are usually identified after 6 months of age, or later in patients with the choreoathetotic subtype. An initial, but often overlooked, feature is the demonstration of hand dominance within the first year. Cognition is most often normal, with intellectual disability in 20–25% of patients. Cerebral palsy may be characterized by the following subtypes:

- **Paraplegic (44%), caused by injury in the centrum semiovale, typically superior and lateral to the caudate. Lesions affect the lower extremity corticospinal tract fibers more so than upper extremity fibers.**
- **Hemiplegic (33%), often caused by placental emboli, periventricular hemorrhagic infarcts, and malformations. In approximately 70% of cases, the left hemisphere is affected due to flow through the patent ductus arteriosus entering the left carotid artery. Approximately 50% of children will have seizures.**
- **Quadriplegic (6%), caused by malformations and hypoxic-ischemic injury.**
- **Choreoathetotic (12%), previously caused by Rh incompatibility leading to kernicterus. Presently, most cases are due to idiopathic injuries of the basal ganglia.**
- **Ataxic (4%), most often caused by genetic disorders.**

Suggested Reading

- Fenichel GM. Clinical Pediatric Neurology.5th edition. Philadelphia: Elsevier Saunders; 2005. p. 239–40, 269–70.
- Nass R. Developmental disabilities. In: Bradley WG, Daroff RB, Fenichel GM, Jankovic J, editors. Neurology in Clinical Practice. 4th ed. Elsevier, Inc.; 2004. p. 1791–810.

8. An infant with epileptic encephalopathy came to your office for evaluation. On examination, he is micro cephalic and has prominent developmental delay. His CSF analysis showed, glucose level was 30 mg/dl, whereas the level of serum glucose was 112 mg/dl. The rest of his CSF tests are normal. **Which statement is correct regarding his condition?**
   A. It is caused by deficiency in the glucose transporter type 1
   B. Brain MRI usually suggests the diagnosis
   C. Ketogenic diet has been shown to be ineffective for seizure control
   D. Phenobarbital is the treatment of choice
   E. It is inherited in an X-linked fashion

Correct Answer is: A
This is the clinical presentation of a glucose transporter type 1 (GLUT-1) deficiency. The brain utilizes glucose as its primary source of energy. In fasting conditions, glycogen is exhausted within minutes, and since amino acids and fat cannot be used for the production of energy in the brain, ketones become the alternative fuel. Glucose crosses the blood brain barrier facilitated by GLUT-1, which is a membrane-bound protein encoded by the SLC2A 1 gene on chromosome 1p35–31.3. It is inherited in an autosomal dominant syndrome and causes a defect in glucose transport across the blood-brain barrier and into brain cells, manifesting as an epileptic encephalopathy with infantile-onset seizures, developmental delay, microcephaly, and complex movement disorders. CSF glucose level is low with a normal serum glucose level, and other CSF studies are normal, excluding other causes of hypoglycorrhachia (such as CNS infection). EEG may show 2.5–4 Hz spikes and waves and the interictal EEG findings may improve with glucose. Neuroimaging does not show specific abnormalities. Later-onset forms with episodic movement disorders and ataxia have been described. A ketogenic diet should be started as soon as the diagnosis is suspected, since this treatment option improves seizure control and the abnormal movements; however, it is less effective for the psychomotor impairment.

Suggested Reading

9. The diagnosis of cerebral palsy (CP) is divided into four major classifications which include which of the following:
   A. Hemiparetic, spastic diplegia, ataxic, and athetoid
   B. Hemiplegic, spastic diplegia, ataxic, and athetoid
   C. Hemiplegic, quadriplegic, dyskinetic, and athetoid
   D. Hemiplegic, diplegic, ataxic, and mixed
   E. Spastic, ataxic, athetoid/ dyskinetic and mixed

Correct Answer is: E
Quadriplegia, which is secondary to spinal cord injury or traumatic brain injury, should not be confused with spastic quadriplegia. Also, tardive dyskinesia not to be confused with dyskinetic cerebral palsy, or the condition of (paralytic) "diplegia" with spastic diplegia.

10. Which of the following statements about CP are true?
   A. The intellectual level among people with CP varies from genius to intellectually impaired, as it does in the general population.
   B. Therapies used to treat tight muscles due to spasticity may include surgical lengthening procedures, Botox, and orthotics.
   C. Individuals with CP have a shortened life expectancy
   D. CP is a progressive disorder because symptoms can become more severe due to subdural damage.

Correct Answer is: (A) and (B)
In spite of a great number of CP individuals have mental disadvantage, their intellectual level varies from genius to intellectually impaired just it does in the general population. Spasticity may be treated surgically, pharmacologically or with the use of appropriate orthotics. Individuals with CP usually have normal life expectancies. CP is a static neurologic disorder.

11. A 2-hour-old baby is admitted to NICU after being delivered by emergency C-section at full term to a 35-year-old female. Pregnancy was uncomplicated until the day of delivery when the mother had vaginal bleeding secondary of placental abruption. At delivery, Apgar scores were 2 at 1 min and 3 at 5 min. Resuscitated was done and the baby was placed on mechanical ventilation. On examination, he has decreased tone, minimal response to stimulation, sluggish pupillary, oculo-cephalic, and corneal reflexes. **What is the best treatment you can use to minimize the likelihood of the future development of cerebral palsy?**
    A. Indomethacin
    B. Dextromethorphan
    C. Moderate hypothermia
    D. Magnesium sulfate
    E. Phenytoin

Correct Answer is: C
Damaging the developing brain for any reason can cause death or permanent disability such as cerebral palsy. Term infants could suffer hypoxic-ischemic encephalopathy (HIE) about 3 per 1000 live-born infants in developed countries, higher in the developing world. Perinatal asphyxia can cause a million deaths worldwide. In the past physicians traditionally provided supportive care with little expectation that their interventions would salvage brain tissue or have an effect on the final outcome. However, in the last 5 years this situation has changed because of the publication of positive results from several controlled trials of therapeutic moderate hypothermia for term infants with neonatal HIE. This led wider clinical application of therapeutic hypothermia for neonatal encephalopathy. These advances in treatment are based on knowledge gained from clinical observation of babies with asphyxia and extensive laboratory research with experimental models. Data from these experiments led to a heuristic model in which hypoxia-ischemia triggers a delayed series of events that lead to cell death in the brain. This period of delay, or latent interval, suggested that post-insult interventions could be protective if started in time. Studies show that improves Survival without cerebral palsy or other disability is about 40% if moderate hypothermia within 6 h of asphyxia has been applied, also death or neurological disability will be reduced by nearly 30%.

Suggested Reading

- Johnston MV, Fatemi A, Wilson MA, Northington F. Treatment advances in neonatal neuroprotection and neurointensive care. In Lancet Neurol 2011;10:372–82.

12. A 5-year-old boy has been evaluated for toe walking. The mother went into labor at 32 weeks gestation. He was admitted to the neonatal intensive care unit for observation, he did not require intubation and was discharged home at 3 weeks of age. His early milestones were on target except he walked at 18 months of age. He has been toeing walking ever since. His toe walking has improved over time, but he still is not consistently able to pedal a bicycle with training wheels. He has no other medical complications. He speaks in

full sentences, can write his name and enjoys playing video games. Head circumference is at the 5th percentile. On examination, speech is mildly dysarthric. He has increased tone in both legs, with slightly limited passive leg extension and foot dorsiflexion. Arm strength, bulk and tone are normal. He has increased deep tendon reflexes in both lower extremities. He is a slow walker, unsteady with a mildly crouched appearance and he walks on the balls of his feet. Brain MRI axial T2 sample is shown.

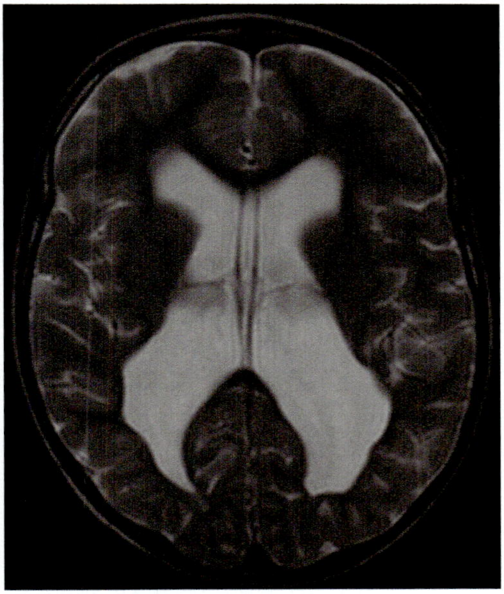

Fig. 25.3 American Academy of Neurology Institute, produced by permission

What is most likely diagnosis?

A. cerebral palsy
B. Charcot-Marie-Tooth disease type X
C. limb-girdle muscular dystrophy
D. pervasive developmental disorder
E. Sanfilippo disease

Correct Answer is: A

The boy has spasticity in his both lower extremities which is a long standing and non-progressive by history. This indicates a static upper motor neuron disorder. Limb-girdle muscular dystrophy and Charcot-Marie-Tooth disease type X (CMT-X) are disorders of the lower motor neuron and would not be expected to lead to spasticity. Although CMT-X can rarely have associated white matter changes and extensor plantar responses, distal weakness and sensory loss expected with this disorder are absent. No evidence of gray matter damage (cognition, language or social skills) making pervasive developmental disorder (PDD) and San Filippo disease inappropriate choices. Cerebral palsy is one of the neurodevelopmental disability disorders of childhood. It is not a specific etiologic diagnosis, rather a descriptive term for a disorder of motor control (affecting movement, tone or posture) causing activity limitation that is non-progressive in nature, resulting from an injury to or malformation of the brain at its early formative stages. Rarely, loss of motor function with time, which is typically secondary to complications of under treated spasticity (such as joint contractures or scoliosis) or rapid changes in weight or height during puberty rather than inherent progression of neurologic disease. CP refers only to the motor dysfunction seen; it does not confer (though is often associated with) cognitive impairment, hearing loss, strabismus or epilepsy. It happens in 1–3 out of 1000 live births, prematurity is the most common risk factor, which raises incidence to 4–10% if born with very low birth weight and up to 20% risk if born at 24–26 weeks gestational age.

Nonetheless, full term infants represent more the half of all cases of cerebral palsy. The potential etiologies includes brain malformations or genetic disorders, post-natal brain injury at a young age (CNS infection, accidental or non-accidental trauma, kernicterus), prenatal factors (maternal chorioamnionitis, intrauterine growth retardation, toxin exposure, congenital infections, maternal trauma),

perinatal brain injury (hypoxic-ischemic encephalopathy, neonatal stroke, traumatic brain injury, intracranial hemorrhage) and brain injury related to prematurity (periventricular leukomalacia and intraventricular hemorrhage). CP has been classified based on the location and type of motor control difficulty. Spastic forms are the most common, and can involve the legs primarily (most common type affecting premature infants) called diplegic CP, involve one-half of the body (usually from unilateral hemorrhagic or ischemic stroke or unilateral brain malformation) called hemiplegic CP or involve all four extremities (often from HIE in a term infant or severe diffuse traumatic injury) called quadriparetic CP. Various degrees of dyskinesia (dystonic and choreoathetoid movements) often accompany the spasticity, especially in cases where there is prominent basal ganglia injury. Ataxic and hypotonic subtype are diagnoses of exclusion after a thorough evaluation for other primary cerebellar or lower motor neuron disorders are excluded.
Neuroimaging is useful in the evaluation of the child with cerebral palsy if the etiology has not been established from the history. MRI is superior than CT scan because it provides more detail of the white matter and often shows abnormal white matter signal or volume, or in the case of hemiparetic CP evidence of old focal infarction or malformation of cortex. If the history and neuroimaging do not determine a specific structural abnormality, or not consistent with a static process, metabolic and genetic testing can be considered.

25

Suggested Reading

- Oskoui M, Shevall MI. Cerebral palsy and the transition from pediatric to adult care. Continuum. 2009;15(6):64–77.
- Ashwal S, Russman BS, Balsco PA. Practice parameter: diagnostic assessment of the child with cerebral palsy: Report of the Quality Standards Subcommittee of the American Academy of Neurology and the Practice Committee of the Child Neurology Society. Neurology. 2004;62(6):851–63.

13. A 16-month-old girl is being evaluated for delayed motor development. She stared sitting (10 months) and began army-crawling at 15 months. She cannot pull to stand, cruise, or walk. When you held her upright, she beards weight, but stand on her tip-toes. She was born premature at 27 weeks gestation, she was on a ventilator for 6 weeks in the NICU. She had bilateral subependymal hemorrhages which resolved on follow up ultrasound testing. On examination, she has severe spasticity in both lower extremities, 3+ reflexes at the knees and non-sustained clonus at both ankles. She has a crossed adductor response and scissors her legs when held upright.

What might you see on her MRI?

A. Bilateral subdural effusions
B. Communicating hydrocephalus
C. Diffuse cystic encephalomalacia
D. Noncommunicating hydrocephalus
E. Periventricular white matter injury

Correct Answer is: E
Cerebral palsy (CP) can occur secondary to a varieties of central nervous system abnormalities, which can occur pre-, peri-, or postnatally. By definition, CP excludes progressive or degenerative disorders. Brain MRI is currently the most commonly radiological used method of

investigating for cause of CP. A number of abnormalities can be identified, including periventricular white matter injury (leukomalacia), diffuse encephalopathy (including cystic encephalomalacia), focal ischemic lesions, and malformations. This is true in 80–90% of patients. Periventricular leukomalacia is the most common abnormality seen in patients with spastic diplegic type of CP, which is the predominant type of CP seen in babies born prematurely.

Suggested Reading

- Robinson MN, Peake LJ, et al. Magnetic resonance imaging findings in a population-based cohort of children with cerebral palsy. Dev Med Child Neurol. 2009;51(1):39–45.

14. An 8-year-old girl came to the ER with her mother for evaluation of headaches. She has right hemiplegia and developed headaches a month ago, which have worsened over time then became constant. She vomits with the severe headache. She never had headaches before, but does have history of complex partial epilepsy and she is on carbamazepine. Her mother has a history of migraine headaches. On examination, she is obtunded, appears ill, and has spasticity of her right limbs with a hemiparetic gait. Fundus exam was difficult to perform. Carbamazepine level is within normal therapeutic limits. She has normal CBC, electrolytes with sodium level 129 mEq/L. Head CT scan is shown. No previous images are available for comparison.
Which of the following is the most likely cause of her headaches and obtundation?

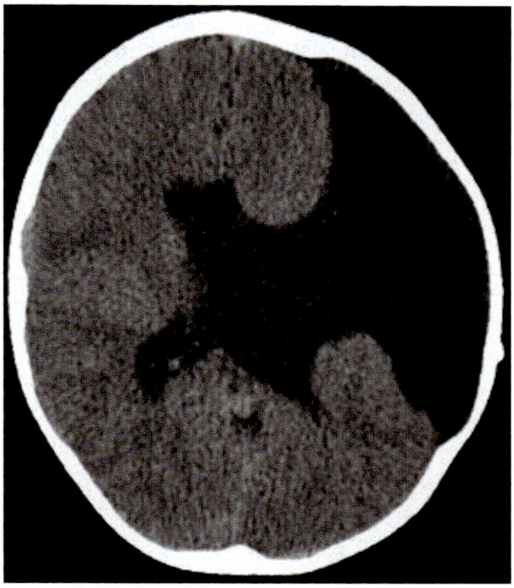

Fig. 25.4 Axial CT scan showing schizencephaly in a 6-year old child. (Hellerhoff. Wikipedia)

A. Carbamazepine toxicity
B. Hydrocephalus
C. Hyponatremia
D. Migraine headaches
E. Subclinical seizures

Correct Answer is: B
This child has schizencephaly (open-lipped type) as the cause of her cerebral palsy. This condition can be complicated by hydrocephalus. The fluid accumulation is causing mass effect, with a midline shift to the right side. It is helpful to compare the head scan with prior scans if possible, as significant changes in CSF flow dynamics related to the underlying malformation can be subtle, yet cause significant clinical problems.

Carbamazepine toxicity can be associated with headaches but also with diplopia and ataxia, which are not present. The mild hyponatremia may be due to carbamazepine therapy but is not likely

low enough to be causing problems. Migraine headaches are a diagnosis of exclusion. Subclinical seizures are not a common cause of headaches.

Hydrocephalus can complicate schizencephaly, particularly in the "open-lipped" form. Some patients also have septo-optic dysplasia, with agenesis of the septum pellucidum and optic nerve hypoplasia.

25

Suggested Reading

Maeda T, Akaishi M, Shimizu M, et al. The subclassification of schizencephaly and its clinical characterization. Brain Dev. 2009;31:694–701.

15. A 5-year-old boy has cerebral palsy came for his regular follow up visit. He was premature at 32 weeks gestation and had both hypoxic ischemic injury and grade 3 intraventricular hemorrhage requiring VP shunt. His treatment includes PT 4 days/week and 10 mg baclofen four times a day. He is doing his PT and taking his medicine religiously, but still he has increased tone and often appears uncomfortable because of muscle contractions which cause twisting of his limbs and lateral torsion of his trunk. On examination, he has increased deep tendon reflexes and increased tone in all limbs, but minimal spasticity.
What is your next step in his management?
A. Obtain EEG
B. Prescribe dantrolene
C. Assess for shunt malfunction
D. Prescribe diazepam
E. Prescribe trihexyphenidy

Correct Answer is: E
Cerebral palsy is the most common motor disability in childhood. Patients with CP usually have mixed muscle tone, some muscle groups have low tone and others have increased tone. Definition of hypertonia is abnormally increased resistance to externally imposed movement at a joint. Spasticity, dystonia, and rigidity, alone or in combination can cause hypertonia. It is important to differentiate between these syndromes because each may require different treatments. Spasticity is the most common etiology of hypertonia in children with cerebral palsy. It is a velocity-dependent resistance of a muscle to stretch and is defined as having one or both of the following: (1) resistance to externally imposed movement increases with increasing speed of stretch and varies with the direction of joint movement, and/or (2) resistance to externally imposed movement rises rapidly above a threshold speed or joint angle. On examination, upper motor signs (hyperreflexia, clonus, Babinski response) are present. Children who continue to have problems with hypertonia despite adequate spasticity treatment may have dystonia or rigidity. This boy has the typical features of dystonia, in which co-contraction of agonist and antagonist muscle groups result in twisting and abnormal postures. In the child whose etiology is undetermined, a trial of carbidopa-levodopa is given, as some have "dopa-responsive dystonia". Otherwise, trihexyphenidyl is used, starting at 2.5 mg/day and titrating up slowly to 60–80 mg/day.

Suggested Reading

Deon LL, Gaebler-Spira D. Assessment and treatment of movement disorders in children with cerebral palsy. Orthop Clin N Am. 2010;41:507–17.

16. A 10-year-old boy with a spastic diplega on daily physiotherapy, he has trouble ambulating without support in addition to painful muscle spasms. His family asked you for any other treatment options. He is taking oral baclofen 20 mg QID, which has provided modest benefit. On

examination, he has significant spasticity with marked increase in adductor tone.

What is your response to the family?

A. Oral Dantrolene
B. Oral Diazepam
C. Botulinum toxin type A
D. Selective dorsal rhizotomy
E. Intrathecal baclofen pump

Correct Answer is: C

Cerebral palsy (CP) is the most common cause of motor disability in children, with a prevalence of 3.6 per 1000 in 8-year-old children. The majority of children with CP are affected by spasticity, but it is only 1 component of the multifaceted motor disability of CP and may not be the main factor interfering with function. The decision to use anti-spasticity medications requires careful assessment of the patient's other impairments (e.g. weakness, movement disorders). Reasons to treat spasticity include reducing pain and muscle spasms, facilitating brace use, improving posture, minimizing contractures and deformity, facilitating mobility and dexterity, and improving patient ease of care. A multidisciplinary panel systematically reviewed relevant literature from 1966 to 2008 and generated practice parameter regarding pharmacologic treatment of spasticity in children and adolescents with cerebral palsy. For localized or egmental spasticity, botulinum toxin type A is established as an effective treatment to reduce spasticity in the upper or lower extremities. For generalized spasticity, baclofen and diazepam are probably effective, tizanidine is possibly effective, and there was insufficient data on the use of dantrolene. Intrathecal baclofen therapy use in generalized spasticity became very popular. In this patient with segmental spasticity, botulinum toxin is the preferred treatment option.

Suggested Reading

- Delgado MR, Hirtz D, et al. Practice parameter: pharmacologic treatment of spasticity in children and adolescents with cerebral palsy (an evidence-based review). Neurology. 2010;74:336–43.

Toxic Encephalopathy

Y. M. Awaad, *Absolute Pediatric Neurology*, https://doi.org/10.1007/978-3-319-78801-2_26

26

1. A 16 year old girl came to the ER by EMS in a coma. Her mother reported that her daughter became overly weight and health conscious for the past year and she is using her job money to buy vitamins and other supplements. The mother is concerned that her daughter eats these supplements instead of food. The girl was adequately oxygenated and had a normal heart rate, so the attending physician ordered a stat MRI scan. There is an increased signal in the striatum, thalamus, and internal capsule bilaterally on the T1-weighted images. The T2-weighted images showed white matter abnormalities and MR spectroscopy demonstrated elevated glutamine and glutamate in the white matter. Blood work shows highly elevated liver function tests and a serum ammonia of 360 mcg/dl. **The supplements she has taken most likely include:**
   A. Kava kava
   B. Ginko biloba
   C. Vitamin B12
   D. Selenium
   E. Chinese red rice

Correct Answer is: A
The clinical presentation indicates hepatic encephalopathy because of the high ammonia level, MRI and MRS scans findings. Kava kava is an herbal derived from roots of the plant Piper methysticum, a member of the pepper family found in the Western and South Pacific. It has been proposed to be anxiolytic and used in patients with anxiety disorders and as treatment for insomnia, premenstrual syndrome and stress. Recently, the safety of kava products became in question because reports of liver injury. Other groups have argued that hepatotoxicity is related to the use of concomitant drugs or herbals. Furthermore, the literature on liver injury from kava kava has included several incomplete or overlapping reports, and causality was rarely well shown. Nevertheless, there are a small number of cases of severe hepatic injury arising during therapy that are convincing.

Suggested Reading

- Teschke R, Schulze J, Schwarzenboeck A, Eickhoff A, Frenzel C. Herbal hepatotoxicity: suspected cases assessed for alternative causes. Eur J Gastroenterol Hepatol. 2013;25(9):1093–8.
- Binesh N, Huda A, Thomas MA, Wyckoff N, Bugbee M, Han S, Rasgon N, Davanzo P, Sayre J, Guze B, Martin P, Fawzy F. Hepatic encephalopathy: a neurochemical, neuroanatomical, and neuropsychological study. J Appl Clin Med Phys. 2006;7(1):86–96.

2. A foster parents brought their 5-year-old boy for an evaluation of developmental delay. The boy came to their home 2 months ago and they are not able to provide any medical history. He tends to eat toys, paper, wood and clay.
   What tests should you be ordered?
   A. EEG
   B. Lead level
   C. Liver function tests
   D. Brain MRI
   E. Thyroid function tests

Correct Answer is: B
Lead is one of the most common environmental toxin. There is a clear correlation between highly elevated serum lead levels, clinical symptoms, and cognitive deficits. In the past decades blood levels have dramatically fallen (from 15 ug/dl to 2.7 in 1991 to 1994), still there is big number of children who may have blood levels equal or greater than 10ug/dl. The current guidelines recommend screening of all children with identifiable risk factors including children

living in housing before 1950, children of ethnic or racial minority groups who may be exposed to lead containing food remedies, children who have emigrated (or adopted) from countries where lead poisoning is prevalent, children with iron deficiency, children exposed to contaminated dust or soil, children with developmental delay whose oral behavior places them at risk for lead exposure, children whose parents are expose to lead (vocationally, avocationally, and during home renovation), children of low income families and victims of abuse and neglect.

Suggested Reading

- Practice parameter: Evaluation of the child with global developmental delay: report of the Quality Standards subcommittee of the American Academy of Neurology and the practice committee of the Child Neurology Society, Shevell M, Ashwal S Neurology 2003;60:367–80.
- Davioli CT, Chisolm JJ. Childhood Lead Poisoning. In: Capute AJ, Accardo PJ, editors. Developmental disabilities in infancy and childhood. Vol. 1. 2nd ed. Baltimore: Brooke's publishing.1996. 232–3.

3. A 13-year-old boy was admitted to the emergency department with abnormal movements for the last 3 h. He stayed home with his family and he was acting normally, without any signs of sickness. After having his dinner with the family, he started "acting strange", and had twitching movements of his extremities. He has a history of mild depression and migraine headaches, and he takes 50 mg of amitriptyline at bedtime. One day ago, his neurologist added sertraline, 50 mg once daily. He took his first dose tonight with dinner. In the emergency department, he has a temperature of 102 F, pulse of 125, and oxygen saturations of 98% on room air. Currently he is lethargic with mildly dilated but reactive pupils, normal tone, but prominent shivering movements. DTRs are brisk in all limbs with clonus at both knees and ankles. A urine toxicology screen is normal. Serum comprehensive metabolic profile is normal. LP is performed and shows 5 WBC/hpf, 0 RBC/ hpf with normal protein and glucose.
What is most appropriate treatment for this patient?
A. IV acyclovir
B. Oral bromocriptine
C. Oral cyproheptadine
D. IV dantrolene
E. IV fosphenytoin

Correct Answer is: C
The patient has serotonin syndrome which can be diagnosed by having at least three of the following clinical findings: agitation, mental status changes, myoclonus, hyperreflexia, diaphoresis, shivering, tremor, diarrhea, incoordination and fever. The syndrome can occur soon after the addition of, or increase in dose of a serotonergic agent. You have to exclude other etiologic causes (such as substance abuse or withdrawal, metabolic derangement or infectious cause) and mandates that an antipsychotic drug (with dopaminergic blocking properties) has not recently been started or dose increased. Antidepressant medications (both serotonin specific reuptake inhibitors such as sertraline and tricyclic antidepressants such as amitriptyline), stimulants (especially amphetamine-based), triptans and ergotamine based compound for acute abortive migraine treatment, lithium, and the monamine oxidase inhibitors such as selegiline (typically used as an antiparkonsonian medication in adults) can lead to serotonin excess in pediatric neurology patients. Recreational drugs such as "Ecstasy" and cocaine also place a

patient at risk. Typically, a combination of two agents with serotonergic properties is required to produce the syndrome, though recent cases occurring with SSRI's in isolation have been reported.

In this case, there was no neuroleptic use, treatments for neuroleptic malignant syndrome, such as dantrolene or bromocriptine would not be appropriate. The patient does not have herpes encephalitis because the acute onset of symptoms without a viral prodrome and a normal CSF profile. The patient's clinical presentation is not suggestive of a seizure, making fosphenytoin an incorrect choice.

Physicians have to inform patients who are taking any serotonergic medications to watch for the symptoms and signs noted above, especially if two agents are being used together. The only combination that is clearly contraindicated are SSRI's and MAO inhibitors. The risk of prescribing triptans with either antidepressants or stimulant medication is controversial, and it has to be on case to case bases.

Most cases of serotonin syndrome occur in the first 24–48 h. For milder cases, stopping of the offending agent(s) is adequate treatment. More involved cases can be treated with benzodiazipines or cyproheptadine (a 5HT-2 antagonist) administered orally or via nasogastric tube. The syndrome itself usually resolves within 24 h of discontinuation of the offending medication.

26

Suggested Reading

- Seminars in Pediatric Neurology.10(1); 2003.

4. A 2-year-old girl was admitted to the hospital because of her vomiting and lethargy for 4 days. Her past medical history is negative. 3 months ago she began to have irritability, which was attributed to her constipation and recent move to a different house. The family moved into an older home 3 months ago, which they have been renovating. She have no fever. Her white blood cell count is normal but she has microcytic anemia. Her optic disc margins are obscure.

What is your the most likely diagnosis?

A. Glioblastoma
B. Lead poisoning
C. Pseudo tumor cerebri
D. Bacterial meningitis
E. Migraine headaches

Correct Answer is: B

This is a clinical presentation of an encephalopathy which is insidious in onset. Lead encephalopathy may present with increased intracranial pressure. There may also be nuchal rigidity secondary to tonsillar herniation. The initial picture maybe confused with meningitis or a case of increased intracranial pressure like space occupying lesions. Rarely, there may be cerebellar ataxia and 6th and 7th cranial nerve palsies. Peripheral neuritis from axonal degeneration may be present in older children or adults. Classically the presentation maybe insidious. The child may be pale, irritable, and listless with decreased appetite. Vomiting and epigastic pain are common. Radiographic findings are characteristic. There may be dense, radiopaque band at the metaphyses of numerous long bones. The patient does not have bacterial meningitis because she is afebrile with a normal white blood cell count.

Suggested Reading

- Menke J. Toxic and Nutritional disorders. In: Menke J, Sarnat H, Maria BL, editors. Child Neurology. 7th ed. Philadelphia: Lippincott Williams and Wilkins. 2006; pp. 703–5.

5. A 3-year-old girl was admitted to the Emergency Department for altered consciousness. She was found her in bed room, pale, disoriented, and unable to walk. She has become progressively more lethargic, and is barely arousable at the time of her arrival at the ED. No recent illnesses or injuries have been reported by her family and has had normal development. When you examined her, she was normotensive and afebrile, but mildly tachycardic. She grimaced and withdrew her hands to deep pain, but she did not open her eyes. All four extremities appear to move equally. She has pinpoint pupils. Further history with the family indicates that the child's grandmother (also living in the same home) is on oxycodone hydrochloride for chronic pain. According to the child's family, her grandmother has a bad habit of leaving her medication around the house. **Which of the following medications should be administered?**
   A. Clonidine
   B. Naloxone
   C. Flumazenil
   D. Apomorphine
   E. Propranolol

Correct Answer is: B
Opiate overdoses are characterized by depressed consciousness, decreased respiratory drive, and miosis, and can lead to hypothermia, bradycardia, and hypotension if sufficient amounts are ingested. Respiratory support may be required. Naloxone reverses the pharmacological effects of opiates by binding to opioid receptors (specifically with preferential binding to the μ-opioid receptor) as a competitive antagonist. When injected intravenously, it acts quickly (1 min), but has a relatively short duration of action (less than 1 h), and so additional doses may be required to counter-act the opiate effect.

Suggested Reading

Glatstein M, Finkelstein Y, Scolnick D. Accidental methadone ingestion in an infant: report and review of the literature. Pediatr Emerg Care. 2009;25:109–11.

6. A 10-year-old boy has the history of developmental delayed, attention deficit hyperactivity disorder and obsessive compulsive disorder brought by his family to the emergency department with gradual onset of abnormal movements of the neck, shoulders and back described by the family as "stiffening" and "rolling" movements. He has the movements during awaking and disappeared during sleep. His psychiatrist started him on quetiapine 50 mg/day as a "mood stabilizer", 3 days later the family noticed those abnormal movements. He had been taking escitlopram for the past 6 months without any side-effects. He has no intercurrent illnesses, fever/rash, muscle soreness/weakness/fatigue, urinary difficulties or mental status changes. He is healthy and interactive but distractible, with moderately severe spasmodic torticollis and generalized dystonia of the trunk. **What is your best treatment option?**
   A. Propranolol
   B. Phenytoin
   C. Metoclopramide
   D. Diphenhydramine
   E. Bromocriptine

Correct Answer is: D
This is a clinical presentation of drug-induced acute dystonia, induced by quetiapine fumarate (Seroquel®), a psychotropic agent belonging to a chemical class, the dibenzothiazepine derivatives, indicated for bipolar disorder (including maintenance treatment), mania, depression, and schizophrenia. Extrapyramidal side-effects are common with use of this medication, including dystonia and

choreo-athetosis. Serotonin syndrome and neuroleptic malignant syndrome can occur with the combination therapy with selective serotonin re-uptake inhibitors (SSRIs). Different medications can be used on an empiric basis to find one or a combination that is effective for a specific patient. It should be noted that not all patients will respond similarly to the same medications.

Suggested Reading

- Dressler D, Benecke R.Diagnosis and management of acute movement disorders. J Neurol. 2005;252(11):1299–306.
- Pierre JM. Extrapyramidal symptoms with atypical antipsychotics: incidence, prevention and management. Drug Saf. 2005;28(3):191–208.
- Rodnitzky RL. Drug-induced movement disorders in children and adolescents. Expert Opin Drug Saf. 2005;4(1):91–102.

7. When the nervous system is potentially vulnerable to toxic, infectious, and immune disorders, the blood-nerve barrier is most likely not intact at which of the following locations?
   - A. cauda equina
   - B. dorsal root ganglion
   - C. median nerve
   - D. spinal motor nerve root
   - E. spinal sensory nerve root

Correct Answer is: B
The dorsal root ganglion is where the blood-nerve barrier (analogous to the blood-brain barrier) is least intact, which may be important in the development of, for example, herpes zoster infections involving the nervous system or their reactivation, as well as immune-mediated ganglionopathies.

Suggested Reading

- Levin K. Diseases of the nerve roots. Continuum Lifelong Learn Neurol. 2008;14(3):134–55
- Weerasuriya A, Mizisin AP. The blood-nerve barrier: structure and functional significance. Methods. Mol Biol. 2011;686:149–73.
- Kanda T. Biology of the blood-nerve barrier and its alteration in immune-mediated neuropathies. J Neurol Neurosurg Psychiatry. 2013;84:208–12.

8. A 14-year-old boy complained to his family that he cannot "feel with his hands". The child has been moved recently to the states from an African country and lives with his aunt who is his legal guardian. His medical and family history is not available. He is underweight but muscular young boy. In spite of he has persistent cough he is not taking any medications since he moved to his aunt's house. The child recalls taking medication for several months because of his cough. On examination, he has reduced sensation in a glove and-stocking distribution. He has mild weakness in wrist and ankle flexors and extensors. DTR's are within normal limits with the exception of absent ankle reflexes.
   What is the most likely diagnosis?
   - A. Hereditary sensory and autonomic neuropathy type I
   - B. Isoniazid toxicity
   - C. Hereditary tyrosinemia
   - D. Congenital hypomyelinating neuropathy

Correct Answer is: B
Glove-and-stocking neuropathy can be caused by different medications including isoniazid, nitrofuratin, vincristine and zidovudine. The child came from Africa. Africa has the highest rate of tuberculosis in the world (1382 cases per 100,000) and has a persistent cough. His sensory lose is highly suggestive of a drug induced pyridoxine deficiency. Pyridoxine taken along with isoniazid can prevent neuropathy but has mini-

mal effect on rate of recovery after the neuropathy is present.

Hereditary sensory and autonomic neuropathy type I begin in the second decade of life and presents with lancinating pains in the legs and ulcerations of the feet.

The major clinical features of hereditary tyrosinemia are liver failure and Fanconi syndrome associated with peripheral dysesthesias or paralysis.

The clinical features in congenital hypomyelinating neuropathy are similar to acute infantile spinal muscular atrophy and presents in the newborn period.

Suggested Reading

- Mafukidze AT, Calnan M, Furin J. Peripheral neuropathy in persons tuberculosis and other comorbid disease. J Clin Tuberc Other Mycobact Dis. 2015.

9. A 6-year-old boy was brought to the emergency department because he was found to be agitated with delirium. He was recovering from chickenpox under the care of his grandmother because his parents were away on a vacation. His grandmother was giving him analgesics for discomfort and a low-grade fever. Three days later he began vomiting, became lethargic and confused. The ED attending admitted him to the pediatric ICU where he developed decorticate posturing and he was obtunded. He has hyperammonemia and elevated liver enzymes.
   What was the cause of this clinical course?
   A. Varicella encephalitis
   B. Cerebral hemorrhage
   C. Cerebral vasculitis
   D. Salicylate administration

Correct Answer is: D
This is a clinical presentation of Reye syndrome. It occurs with salicylate (aspirin) use for symptomatic relief during viral illness. There is an even higher rate when administered in children with chickenpox. The incidence of Reye syndrome decreased after the reduction aspirin use in children. The progression from symptom onset to hepatic failure, cerebral edema and death can occur rapidly, and has been reported to occur in less than 24 h.

Encephalitis has a less progressive course and with focal neurological symptoms. Liver involvement is not common.

Cerebral hemorrhage is not associated with varicella infections and most commonly would presents with focal neurological symptoms. Liver involvement is not common.

Vasculitis is not commonly seen in varicella infections and would present in a more gradual onset with focal neurological symptoms. Severe liver involvement is not commonly associated with vasculitis.

Suggested Reading

- Glasgow JFT, Middleton B. Reye syndrome- insights on causation and prognosis. Arch Dis Child. 2001;85(5):351–53.

10. All the following are known side effect of carbamazepine except?
    A. A Dizziness
    B. Nystagmus
    C. Drowsiness
    D. Hypernatremia
    E. Nausea

Correct Answer is: D
Carbamazepine is used for partial or secondarily generalized tonic-clonic (GTC) seizures, although it is important to remember that it can rarely worsen some generalized epilepsies (including myoclonic and absence epilepsies), similar to phenytoin. Its primary mode of action is via blockade of sodium chan-

nels, which leads to a decrease/prevention of repetitive firing in depolarized neurons. Side effects include dizziness, vertigo, fatigue, drowsiness, diplopia, nystagmus, headache, nausea, vomiting, elevated liver function tests, hyponatremia, and ataxia. Serious idiosyncratic reactions include Stevens-Johnson syndrome, leukopenia, and aplastic anemia.

26

Carbamazepine undergoes liver metabolism with renal excretion of metabolites, so caution is advised with kidney or liver failure.

Carbamazepine is also a hepatic enzyme inducer, and undergoes auto-induction. The dose must be titrated up gradually to allow tolerance to develop to its CNS side effects, but also to avoid early toxicity as carbamazepine "auto- induces" the hepatic enzymes responsible for its own metabolism. If carbamazepine is started at too high of a dose, or titrated too fast, the result would be elevated carbamazepine levels with accompanying toxicity early on, as the hepatic enzymes responsible for carbamazepine's metabolism have not been fully activated (auto-induced) yet. It is therefore important to remember that carbamazepine's half-life decreases from 30 h to 10 to 20 h after the first few days to weeks of use.

Auto-induction is completed after 3–5 weeks of a fixed dosing regimen. Plasma concentrations decrease in the first 1 to 2 months, and during this time, the dose of carbamazepine should be gradually increased. Therefore, carbamazepine would not be a good option if quick control of new-onset, frequent seizures was desired. Of note, oxcarbazepine does not undergo auto- induction and can be titrated faster. Oxcarbazepine is a structural derivative of carbamazepine, and is reduced to 10- monohydroxy carbamazepine and unlike carbamazepine does not undergo oxidation to epoxide. Carbamazepine on the other hand is oxidized to 10, 11- carbamazepine epoxide, which is the principal metabolite of carbamazepine. It is important to remember that the 10, 11-carbamazepine epoxide is pharmacologically active and responsible for many of the side effects seen with carbamazepine use. Because of these differences, oxcarbazepine has less side effects, overall, as compared to carbamazepine. Oxcarbazepine has less liver enzyme induction, no auto-induction (and can thus be titrated more rapidly), and is used for the same seizure types as carbamazepine, having the same mechanism of action, metabolic pathways, and side-effect profile. Approximately 30% of patients who have a history of a rash with carbamazepine will also develop a rash when exposed to oxcarbazepine. Valproic acid inhibits the metabolism of the pharmacologically active 10, 11-carbamazepine epoxide (the principal metabolite of carbamazepine). Thus, although the carbamazepine level may be normal, the patient may experience toxicity because of elevated 10, 11-carbamazepine epoxide levels. The 10, 11-carbamazepine epoxide is not routinely measured, but can be ordered specifically if there are concerns about toxicity.

Suggested Reading

- Koch MW, Polman SK. Oxcarbazepine versus carbamazepine monotherapy for partial onset seizures. Cochrane Database Syst Rev.2009; CD006453.
- Porter RJ. How to initiate and maintain carbamazepine therapy in children and adults. Epilepsia. 1987;28(Suppl 3):S59-S63.
- Purcell TB, Mc Pheeters RA, Feil M, et al. Rapid oral loading of carbamazepine in the emergency department. An Emerg Med. 2007;50(2):121–26.

- Tudur SM, Marson AG, Clough HE, et al. Carbamazepine versus phenytoin monotherapy for epilepsy. Cochrane Database Syst Rev. 2002;(2):CD001911.
- Comprehensive Review in Clinical Neurology: a multiple choice question Book for the Wards and Boards © 2011 Wolters Kluwer Health Lippincott Williams & Wilkins. All rights reserved.

11. Chronic lead exposure in children most commonly leads to:
   A. Neuropsychological symptoms
   B. Sensory neuropathy
   C. Motor neuropathy
   D. Optic neuropathy
   E. Ataxia

Correct Answer is: A Neuropsychological symptoms
Lead poisoning has differing clinical features based on age presentation. Children are more affected because they absorb lead more effectively compared to adults. CNS manifestations are more common in children, but peripheral symptoms are more common in adults. Neuropsychological effects, including irritability, fatigue, and impaired memory, attention, and intelligence are common in children with chronic exposure to lead. On the other hand, neuropathy is rare.

Motor or sensorimotor neuropathies with subacute and chronic exposures are more common in adults. Lead poisoning is caused by ingestion of paint chips, as lead-containing residential paints were used in homes built prior to 1978. Lead may also leach into drinking water from old lead-containing plumbing, and can be found in soil contaminated by vehicle exhaust or industrial emissions. Certain ceramics, cosmetics, jewelry, crystal, herbal medications, and other products may also contain lead. Blood levels are useful for detection of lead poisoning, and indicate exposure within the previous month. Paint chips can be demonstrate on X-rays within the GI tract or "lead lines" on skeletal films (indicative of bone growth arrest). Skeletal lead concentrations can be measured by X-ray fluorescence techniques. Treatment involves chelation therapy with dimercaptosucccinic acid (DMSA), calcium disodium ethylenediaminetetraacetic acid (CaNa2ETDA), and/or British anti-lewisite (BAL), depending upon the levels. BAL should be given prior to EDTA, however, as EDTA may increase the distribution of lead into the brain.

Suggested Reading

- Kathuria P. Lead toxicity.Medscape. ▶ http://emedicine.medscape.com/article/1174752-oveNiew. Updated 1/29/14. Accessed 4/11/14.
- Kumar N. Industrial and environmental toxins. Continuum. 2008;14(5):102–37.

12. Which of the following agents is most likely to cause hearing loss and ototoxicity.
   A. Vincristine
   B. Cyclophospham ide
   C. Methotrexat
   D. Cisplatin
   E. Lomustine

Correct Answer is: D
Cisplatin is known to cause ototoxicity and hearing loss. Cisplatin is usually used in treatment of medulloblastomas. Tinnitus, ototoxicity with hearing loss, kidney damage, and myelosuppression are common side effects. Peripheral neuropathy, seizures, and visual impairment are rare side effects.

Vincristine is a vinca alkaloid which used to treat both low and high grade gliomas and medulloblastomas. The most common side effects are constipation, diarrhea, and peripheral neuropathy; but, syndrome of inappropriate

antidiuretic hormone (SIADH), paralytic ileus, jaw pain, and seizures occur are less side effects.

Cyclophosphamide is a nitrogen mustard, it inhibits DNA replication. Sometimes it has been used to treat medulloblastoma. The most side effects are hemorrhagic cystitis, myelosuppression, nausea, vomiting, mucositis, or nasal congestion. Hepatotoxicity, SIADH, and sterility may occur as a rare side effects.

Methotrexate works on dihydrofolate reductase causing DNA and RNA synthesis inhibition. It has been used in the management of high grade gliomas and diffuse intrinsic pontine gliomas in addition to medulloblastoma. Methotrexate can cause myelosuppression, mucositis, and, in high doses, or when given intrathecally, it may cause neurotoxicity. Skin reactions are rare side effects.

Lomustine is a nitrosurea which ca be used for medulloblastoma. This has also been used for low grade gliomas and, in adults, has been used with procarbazine and vincristine in the treatment of grade III gliomas. This does not tend to cause hearing loss or ototoxicity.

Suggested Reading

- Jozwiak S, Migone N, Ruggieri M. The tuberous sclerosis complex. In: Ruggieri M, Pascual Castroviejo I, Di Rocco C, editors. Neurocutaneous disorders Phakomatoses and Hamartoneoplastic syndromes. Morlenbach: Springer-Verlag/Wien;2008. p. 181–227.
- Tabori U, Laberge A-M, Ellezam B, Carret A-S. Cancer predisposition in children with braintumors. In: Scheinemann K, Bouffet E, editors. Pediatric Neuro-Oncology. New York: Springer; 2015. p. 69–89.
- Gorlin, RJ. Nevoid basal cell carcinoma. In: Ruggieri M, Pascual-Castroviejo I, Di Rocco C, editors. Neurocutaneous disorders Phakomatoses and hamartoneoplastic syndromes. Morlenbach: Springer-Verlag/Wien; 2008. p. 669–694.
- Chan TSY, Wang X, Spence T, Taylor MD, Huang A. Embryonal brain cell tumors. In: Scheinemann K, Bouffet E, editors. Pediatric neuro-oncology. New York: Springer; 2015. p. 127–138.
- Lee J, Johnston DL. Chemotherapy. In: Scheinemann K, Bouffet E, editors. Pediatric neuro-oncology. New York:Springer; 2015. p. 69–89.
- Glass TD, Cochrane D, Rassekh SR, Goddard K, Hukin J. Growing teratoma syndrome in intracranial non germinomatous germ cell tumors (iNGGCTs): a risk for secondary malignant transformation- a report of two cases. Child Nerv Syst. 2014;30(5):953–7.
- Bartels U, Singhal A. Central nervous system germ cell tumors. In: Scheinemann K, Bouffet E, editors. Pediatric neuro-oncology. New York: Springer; 2015:149–62.
- Mach SC, Ramaswamy V, Wang X, Remke M, Sin-Chan P, Chan WSY, Bertrand KC, Merino D, Zayne K. Huang A. Taylor MD. Basic science of pediatric brain tumors. In: Scheinemann K, Bouffet E, editors. Pediatric neuro-oncology. New York: Springer; 2015. p. 59–67.
- Jones DTW, Korshunov A, Pfister SM, Tayllor MD, Northcott PA. Medulloblastoma and CNS primitive neuroectodermal tumors. In: Cagle PT, Matthias KA, Zagzag D, editors. Molecular pathology of nervous system tumors. New York: Springer; 2015:121–42.
- Vanan Ml, Mehta V, Eisenstat DD. Diffuse intrinsic pontine glioma. In: Scheinemann K, Bouffet E, editors. Pediatric neuro-oncology. New York: Springer; 2015. p. 117–26.
- Rutkowski S, Bode U, Deinlein F, Ottensmeier H, Warmuth-Metz M, Soeroenson N, Grade N, Emser A, Pietsch T, Wolff JE, Kortmann RD, Kuehl J. Treatment of early childhood medulloblastoma by post-operative chemotherapy alone. N Eng J Med. 2005;352(10):978.

- Geyer JR, Sposto R, Jennings M, Boyett JM, Axtell RA. Brieger D, Broxso E, Donahue B, Finlay JL, Goldwein JW, Heier LA, Johnson DM, Mazewski C, Miller DC, Packer R, Puccetti D, Radcliffe J, Tao ML, Shiminski-Maher T. Multiagent chemotherapy and deferred radiotherapy in infants with malignant brain tumors: a report from the Children's Cancer Group. J Clin Oneel. 2005;23(30):7621.
- Wells EM, Packer RJ. Pediatric Brain Tumors. Continuum: Lifelong Learning in Neurology 2015; 21(2):373–96.
- Fleming AJ. Rare tumors of the central nervous system in children. In: Scheinemann K, Bouffet E, editors. Pediatric Neuro-Oncology. New York: Springer; 2015. p. 185–94.
- Evans DW. Li-Fraumeni syndrome. In: Up-to-date, Wen PY, Ross ME, editors. Up-to-date, Waltham. Accessed on 22 Nov 2015.
- lchimura K, Nishikawa R, Matsutani M. Molecular markers in pediatric neuro-oncology. Neuro Oncology. 2012;14(Suppl 4):iv90–iv99. ▶ https://doi.org/10.1093/neuonc/nos204.
- 17. Vora NL. Melanoma and BRAF. eMedicine. ▶ http://emedicine.medscape.com/article/2045059-overview). Updated January 14 2014. Accessed 23 Nov 2015.
- Daras M, Kaley TJ. Benign brain tumors and tumors associated with phakomatoses. Continuum Lifelong Learn Neurology 2015;21(2):373–96.

13. Oxcarbazepine is a structural derivative of carbamazepine. Which of the following is true about oxcarbazepine in comparison to carbamazepine?
    - A. Is not metabolized to an epoxide
    - B. Is not a hepatic enzyme inducer
    - C. Indicated in both partial and generalized epilepsy
    - D. No risk of hyponatremia
    - E. No risk of rash as seen with carbamazepine

Correct Answer is: A
Oxcarbazepine is a structural derivative of carbamazepine, and is reduced to 10-monohydroxy-carbamazepine and unlike carbamazepine does not undergo oxidation to epoxide. Carbamazepine on the other hand is oxidized to 10, 11-carbamazepi ne epoxide, which is the principal metabolite of carbamazepine. 10, 11-carbamazepine epoxide is pharmacologically active and responsible for many of the side effects seen with carbamazepine use.

Oxcarbazepine has less side effects, overall, as compared to carbamazepine. It has less liver enzyme induction, no auto induction (and can thus be titrated more rapidly), and is used for the same seizure types as carbamazepine, having the same mechanism of action, metabolic pathways, and side-effect profile. There is a cross reaction between the two drugs in 30% of patients who have a history of a rash with carbamazepine when they have been exposed to oxcarbazepine. Valproic acid inhibits the metabolism of the pharmacologically active 10, 11-carbamazepine epoxide. Thus, although the carbamazepine level may be normal, the patient may experience toxicity because of elevated 10, 11- carbamazepine epoxide levels. The 10, 11-carbamazepine epoxide is not routinely measured, but can be ordered specifically if there are concerns about toxicity.

Suggested Reading

- Koch MW, Polman SK. Oxcarbazepine versus carbamazepine monotherapy for partial onset seizures. Cochrane Database Syst Rev. 2009;CD006453.
- Porter RJ. How to initiate and maintain carbamazepine therapy in children and adults. Epilepsia. 1987;28(Suppl 3):559–63.
- Purcell TB, Mc Pheeters RA, Feil M, et al. Rapid oral loading of carbamazepine in the emergency department. Ann Emerg Med. 2007;50(2):121–26.

- Tudur SM, Marson AG, Clough HE, et al. Carbamazepine versus phenytoin monotherapy for epilepsy. Cochrane Database Syst Rev.2002;(2):CD001911.
- Comprehensive Review in Clinical Neurology: a multiple choice question Book for the Wards and Boards ©2011 Wolters Kluwer Health Lippincott Williams & Wilkins. All rights reserved.

14. Of the medications listed below, which of the following would not lower the seizure threshold?
    A. Amoxapine
    B. Venlafaxine
    C. Mirtazapine
    D. Buspirone
    E. Diazepam

Correct Answer is: E
Buspirone, bupropion, the tricyclics, amoxapine, and clomipramine should all be avoided. Amoxapine, which is a TCA inhibiting NE and SHT reuptake, does lower the seizure threshold. Venlafaxine is an SNRI, and has also been shown to lower the seizure threshold. Diazepam is a benzodiazepine and may be used to treat seizures acutely, and would therefore not lower the seizure threshold.

Suggested Reading

- Lee, HW, Khoshbin S. Seizure Disorders Chapter 76, page 1050, Mass General Comprehensive Clinical Psychiatry.

15. Which of the following is true regarding carbamazepine?
    A. It inhibits its own metabolism
    B. For new-onset, frequent seizures, carbamazepine is a good option as initial antiepileptic therapy
    C. It has no effect on its own metabolism
    D. It induces its own metabolism
    E. It has no hepatic metabolism

Correct Answer is: D
Carbamazepine is used for partial or secondarily generalized tonic-clonic (GTC) seizures, it worsen some generalized epilepsies (including myoclonic and absence epilepsies), like phenytoin. It blocks sodium channels, which leads to a decrease/prevention of repetitive firing in depolarized neurons. Side effects include dizziness, vertigo, fatigue, drowsiness, diplopia, nystagmus, headache, nausea, vomiting, elevated liver function tests, hyponatremia, and ataxia. Stevens-Johnson syndrome, leukopenia, and aplastic anemia are some serious idiosyncratic reactions.

Carbamazepine undergoes liver metabolism with renal excretion of metabolites, dose adjustment has to be done in kidney or liver failure.

Carbamazepine is also a hepatic enzyme inducer, and undergoes autoinduction. The dose must be titrated up gradually to allow tolerance to develop to its CNS side effects, but also to avoid early toxicity as carbamazepine "autoinducer" the hepatic enzymes responsible for its own metabolism. If carbamazepine is started at too high of a dose, or titrated too fast, the result would be elevated carbamazepine levels with accompanying toxicity early on, as the hepatic enzymes responsible for carbamazepine's metabolism have not been fully activated (autoinducer) yet. It is therefore important to remember that carbamazepine's half-life decreases from 30 h to 10 to 20 h after the first few days to weeks of use.

Autoinduction is completed after 3–5 weeks of a fixed dosing regimen. Plasma concentrations decrease in the first 1 to 2 months, and during this time, the dose of carbamazepine should be gradually increased. Therefore, carbamazepine would not be a good option if quick control of new-onset,

frequent seizures was desired. Of note, oxcarbazepine does not undergo auto-induction and can be titrated faster. Oxcarbazepine is a structural derivative of carbamazepine, and is reduced to 10-monohydroxy-carbamazepine and unlike carbamazepine does not undergo oxidation to epoxide. Carbamazepine on the other hand is oxidized to 10, 11-carbamazepi ne epoxide, which is the principal metabolite of carbamazepine. 10, 11-carbamazepine epoxide is pharmacologically active and responsible for many of the side effects seen with carbamazepine use.

Oxcarbazepine has less side effects, overall, as compared to carbamazepine. It has less liver enzyme induction, no auto induction (and can thus be titrated more rapidly), and is used for the same seizure types as carbamazepine, having the same mechanism of action, metabolic pathways, and side-effect profile. There is a cross reaction between the two drugs in 30% of patients who have a history of a rash with carbamazepine when they have been exposed to oxcarbazepine. Valproic acid inhibits the metabolism of the pharmacologically active 10, 11-carbamazepine epoxide. Thus, although the carbamazepine level may be normal, the patient may experience toxicity because of elevated 10, 11- carbamazepine epoxide levels. The 10, 11-carbamazepine epoxide is not routinely measured, but can be ordered specifically if there are concerns about toxicity.

Suggested Reading

- Koch MW, Polman SK. Oxcarbazepine versus carbamazepine monotherapy for partial onset seizures. Cochrane Database Syst Rev. 2009;CD006453.
- Porter RJ. How to initiate and maintain carbamazepine therapy in children and adults. Epilepsia. 1987;28(Suppl 3):S59-S63.
- Purcell TB, Mc Pheeters RA, Feil M, et al. Rapid oral loading of carbamazepine in the emergency department. An Emerg Med. 2007;50(2):121–6.
- Tudur SM, Marson AG, Clough HE, et al. Carbamazepine versus phenytoin monotherapy for epilepsy. Cochrane Database Syst Rev. 2002;(2):CD001911.

16. An 18-year-old male was brought to the ED by his college peers because of his bizarre behavior, specifically being seen wandering around campus. On examination, blood pressure is 180/90 mm Hg and pulse is 110 beats/min. He is diaphoretic, agitated, but responding to internal visual stimuli. His pupils are dilated, both arms tremor, and there is diffuse myoclonus. **What is the most likely cause of his symptoms?**
    A. Cocaine intoxication
    B. Ethanol withdrawal
    C. N-hexane inhalation
    D. MDMA (ecstasy) intoxication
    E. Opiate withdrawal

Correct Answer is: D
The boy is presenting with a hyperactive encephalopathy and systemic signs of both hyper-adrenergic activity (tachycardia, hypertension) and excessive serotonin activity (hallucinations, tremor). Of the options listed above, MDMA intoxication is most likely to cause this constellation of symptoms (increased catecholamine and serotonin activity).

Suggested Reading

- Brust JC. Abused agents: acute effects, withdrawal, and treatment. Continuum. 2004;10:14–47.

17. You are evaluating a 17-year-old male with a history of progressive sensory loss and paresthesia affecting his

hands and feet and gait unsteadiness for 3 months. You examined him and you demonstrated that, he has loss of pinprick and temperature sensation up to the knee bilaterally; decreased vibratory sense at the great toe bilaterally; trace reflexes throughout; and a positive Romberg test.

Abuse of which of the following agents is the reason for his symptoms?

A. N-hexane
B. Ethanol
C. Heroin
D. MDMA (ecstasy)
E. Nitrous oxide

26

Correct Answer is: A

Distal symmetric polyneuropathy primarily affecting small fibers, resulting in sensory loss that involves pain and temperature more so than vibration or joint position sense is commonly seen with inhaling n-hexane or related compounds (also known as "huffing"). Those syndrome could be rapid and progress over weeks, sometimes resembling Guillain-Barre syndrome. While ethanol abuse can be associated with neuropathy, this is more of a chronic process than the subacute pattern described here. Nitrous oxide abuse can also be associated with distal paresthesia and sensory loss though examination findings typically show more involvement of vibration and joint position sense (due to posterior column dysfunction) as opposed to the findings described here.

Suggested Reading

- Weimer LH. Spinal and neuromuscular complications of substance abuse. Continuum. 2004;10:115–43.

Traumatic Brain Injury

Y. M. Awaad, *Absolute Pediatric Neurology*, https://doi.org/10.1007/978-3-319-78801-2_27

27

1. A 1 month old baby has been colicky after he was discharged from the regular nursery. He has a normal eating pattern, is growing, fixes and follows his mother's face, startles in response to loud noise. He has attacks of crying vigorously during which he pulls his legs up and appears to be uncomfortable. His mother cannot console him during those attacks, but eventually, he falls asleep and wakes up fine. His primary care physician assured the mother that he will outgrow these attacks.

His parents decide to go out for dinner. They are grateful to the 17 year old girl who lives next door, as she has agreed to stay with the baby to give them a well-deserved respite. When they come home, they pay the girl and thank her. As soon as she left, they go into the baby's room and notice the baby looks very pale and is breathing irregularly. They turn on the light and try to arouse the baby, but he does not wake up. The mother screams as the father calls 9-1-1.

He is rushed by ambulance to the hospital. His exam reveals a comatose infant with stable vital signs and retinal hemorrhages. His skin, chest, abdomen, and limbs appear normal. A head CT scan shows left occipital, right temporal, and bifrontal intraparenchymal hemorrhages and a moderate amount of subarachnoid blood. **You ordered a:**

A. Lumbar puncture
B. Stat head MRI
C. Spine MRI
D. Serum S100b
E. Skeletal survey

Correct Answer is: E

The most likely diagnosis is Shaken baby syndrome. The clinical presentation of retinal hemorrhages, subarachnoid blood, and locations of intraparenchymal blood indicates a traumatic brain injury, and the social story is suspicious for but never diagnostic of non-accidental trauma. You cannot assume that shaking, if it occurred, was the only traumatic event or that the circumstances that led to the baby's current state constituted an isolated incident. Skeletal survey is typically performed in children in whom non-accidental trauma is suspected.

Suggested Reading

- Preer G, Sorrentino D, Newton AW. Child abuse pediatrics: prevention, evaluation, and treatment. Curr Opin Pediatr. 2012;24(2):266–73.

2. A 4-month-old girl was seen by paramedics because she vomited and then stopped breathing at home. The mother's boyfriend had been babysitting for the evening while the mother worked. He left the house suddenly when the mother returned. The baby had no prior history for significant health problems. However, her mother reported that she currently has an upper respiratory infection and has not been sleeping well. In the Emergency Room, the child is breathing regularly, but is unresponsive. A head CT reveals a small amount of acute subdural bleeding in the interhemispheric fissure. **What is you're the most appropriate next step in evaluation?**

A. Funduscopic examination
B. Wrist X-ray for bone age determination
C. Serum copper and ceruloplasmin levels
D. Cortisol serum level
E. DNA mutation analysis for osteogenesis imperfecta

Correct Answer is: A

Shaken baby syndrome and non-accidental trauma, are common, and accounts for a large proportion of traumatic brain injury (TBI) cases in children younger than 2 years of age. Usually, the history at presentation does not match the pattern of physical injury. Symptoms are non-specific, including vomiting, apnea, seizures, and depressed consciousness. Subdural hemorrhage, mainly in the interhemispheric fissure, is the single most common feature with brain imaging, but cerebral contusions, stroke, and hypoxic-ischemic injury may also occur. Other problems may include retinal hemorrhage, injury to the cervical spine or abdomen, and fractures.

Suggested Reading

- Chiesa A, Duhaime AC. Abusive head trauma. Pediatr Clin N Am. 2009;56:317–31.

3. A 12-year-old boy experiences head to head trauma with another boy while playing basketball. The boy lay motionless on the ground, while the second boy walked away without difficulty. Referees and coaches found him able to open his eyes to shout, but unable to verbally respond for at least 2 min. He vomited on the field, but then was able to stand and walk to the sidelines with his coaches' assistance.

   Which one of the following is correct?

   A. Basketball is the sport most likely to result in concussion (mild traumatic brain injury) in the US, as defined as an incidence rate for all children participating in the sport.
   B. Neuropsychological tests 1 week after the incident may show a decline compared to pre-injury baseline values.
   C. This boy should be evaluated by his coach, and sent home with his older brother.
   D. Concussion occurs as a result of penetrating forces applied to the brain.
   E. After the first concussion, the risks associated with a second concussion are lower.

Correct Answer is: B

Concussion (or mild traumatic brain injury) associated with official sports is common in children and teenagers. Ice hockey and American football appear to have the highest incidence rates. It has been established that athletes (both pediatric and adult) under-report the occurrence of symptoms resulting from concussion. More time to recover to baseline is needed for younger athletes, and more conservative return-to-play decisions are appropriate for the pediatric age group. Children with one concussion are at higher risk for a second concussion. Neuropsychological testing may reveal deficits even in the absence of reported symptoms.

Suggested Reading

- Meehan WP III, Bachur RG. Sport-related concussion. Pediatrics. 2009;123:114–23.

4. A 13 year old football player came to the office 14 days after sustaining a concussion while playing football. No loss of consciousness was reported but he was stunned after getting hit head to head. He has not played for 10 days and would like to return to play. His physical examination was unremarkable on examination. However he has difficulty with serial 7's and recalling 3/3 words. He has delay in processing information. At baseline he is an above average student. His family would like to know the risk factors for concussion.

What is your response?

A. Female sex is a risk factor for concussion
B. Prior concussions are a risk factor for concussion
C. The rate of concussion is higher in practice than in games
D. The football helmet decreases the rate of concussions
E. Mouth guards decrease the risk of concussion

Correct Answer is: B

Concussions counts for 8.9% of high school athletic injuries and 5.8% of collegiate athletic injuries, with an incidence of 0.23 per 1000 and 0.43 per 1000 athlete exposures, respectively. Female sex confers an increased risk of concussion. While overall rates of concussion at the high school and collegiate levels are higher in male athletes, when sports are examined where the men's and women's games are similar (including soccer and basketball), female athletes have a higher risk of concussion. Multiple prospective studies have identified a history of prior concussion as a risk factor for subsequent concussion. In high school athletes, a greater-than-twofold increase in concussion rate was seen with history of concussion, even when adjusting for sport contact level, grade, and body mass index. Helmets reduce the acceleration of the head from collisions and decrease severe head injuries, but the rate and severity of concussion are not affected by different helmets. Mouth guards in multiple sports and face shields in ice hockey decrease dental and orofacial injuries but have no effect on concussion risk.

Suggested Reading

- Scopaz KA. Risk modifiers for concussion and prolonged recovery. Sports Health. 2013;5(6):537–41.

27

5. A 9 year old was climbing a tree when she missed a branch and fell 18 feet onto the grass below onto her back. She had a brief loss of consciousness. She was transferred to the emergency room wherein route she had a GCS of 12. In the Emergency Department she vomited several times. She has headache. Vital signs were normal. She was agitated. She did not have neck point tenderness. On neurological examination she had a normal funduscopic examination and pupillary response. However she did not fix and follow and did not blink to threat. Opticokinetic nystagmus was absent. The rest of the neurological examination was nonfocal. Head CT was negative for bleed or fracture. She was evaluated by ophthalmology and his examination did not reveal any abnormalities. Three hours later she was able to track a pen light. **The most likely reason for the visual disturbance is:**

A. Ocular migraine
B. Post-traumatic Transient Cortical Blindness
C. Conversion reaction
D. Retinal detachment
E. Posterior reversible encephalopathy syndrome

Correct Answer is: B

Post-traumatic transient cortical blindness following a head injury is a distinct phenomenon first described by Bodian. It usually occurs in children after a mild head injury with occipital trauma being the most common cause. Visual loss can be complete (blindness) or partial (able to see light). The examination can be normal. The majority of cases resolve within hours.

Suggested Reading

- Gleeson et al. Post traumatic transient cortical blindness in children: a report of four cases and a review of the literature. J Accid Emerg Med. 1994;11:250–52.

6. A three-week-old boy came to the Emergency Department with decreased oral intake. He was born full term. The mother has gestational diabetes so he was large for gestational age. The delivery was complicated requiring vacuum extraction and forceps delivery. He was admitted to the newborn nursery for 2 days and then discharged home. Over the past several days he has not been breast feeding as vigorously and has had a decreased amount of diapers. He was lethargic but was arousable. Ophthalmological examination revealed retinal hemorrhages. The rest of the examination was unremarkable. **Which of the following statements is true?**
   A. Retinal hemorrhages can be seen in full-term newborn infants after vaginal delivery
   B. Subdural hematomas cannot be an indication to a difficult delivery
   C. Extracranial injuries such as caput succedaneum and cephal-hematomas are uncommon as birth related cranial injury
   D. Complicated skull fractures are not associated with serious intracranial pathology
   E. Epidural hematomas are not seen in traumatic births

Correct Answer is: A
Many different injuries can happened during the birth process. Extracranial injuries are common including caput succedaneum, cephal-hematomas and sub-galeal hematomas. In general skull fractures are either linear or depressed and complicated fractures indicate serious intracranial pathology. Epidural and subdural hematomas, subarachnoid hemorrhage, and intracerebral hemorrhage have all been reported. Subdural hematomas are common with a difficulty delivery or a large for gestational age. Retinal hemorrhages are seen in 11–40% of full-term newborn infants after vaginal delivery and are seen more commonly after complicated or traumatic births such as a vacuum extraction.

Suggested Reading

- Swaiman. Pediatric Neurology Principles and Practice. 1996.

7. A 3-month-old boy was seen in the emergency department 30 min after he stopped breathing and had a seizure at her daycare. His stepfather says that he rolled off of the couch onto the ground, cried briefly, then stopped breathing, became cyanotic and stiff. This lasted 3 min and then he became limp and unarousable. In the emergency department, his vital signs are stable. There is no external evidence of trauma. He does not arouse with vigorous physical stimulation. Anterior fontanelle is bulging and tight. Pupils are 4 mm and sluggish, oculocephalic reflexes are intact. Fundus examination shows bilateral retinal hemorrhages. Muscle tone and tendon reflexes are decreased. Head CT is obtained, showing extra axial effusions and a subdural hemorrhage in the left frontotemporal area. Shaken infant syndrome (Non-accidental trauma) is suspected. **Which of the following metabolic conditions must be excluded as an alternative explanation?**
   A. Glutaric acidemia
   B. Menkes disease
   C. Leigh's disease
   D. Maple syrup urine disease
   E. Neonatal adrenoleukodystrophy

Correct Answer is: A
The clinical presentation supported by the history, exam, and CT findings suggestive of shaken baby syndrome (SBS),

a cause of non-accidental head injury (NAHI). It is estimated that 25% to 50% of all children under 2 years of age admitted to the hospital with a history of head trauma are abuse victims. It is difficult to categorize head trauma as non-accidental without a perpetrator's confession, NAHI is often a diagnosis of exclusion. Shaken baby syndrome is one of the most difficult causes of NAHI to diagnose. External bruising is not seen in a significant minority (21%) of fatal NAHI cases and a history of previous maltreatment can be absent in up to 40% of all cases. SBS refers to a constellation of inflicted injuries mostly seen in young children (mean age about 4 months), caused by violent shaking, and is typically characterized by subdural hematomas and retinal hemorrhages. On the other hand, retinal hemorrhages can be seen in other conditions, including osteogenesis imperfect, homozygous protein C deficiency, Terson syndrome (intraocular bleeding associated with acute intracranial hemorrhage), Hermansky-Pudlak syndrome (an autosomal recessive condition characterized by albinism and platelet abnormalities), hemorrhagic disease of the newborn, and Glutaric Acidemia type 1.

Suggested Reading

- Togioka BM, Arnold MA, et al. Retinal hemorrhages and shaken baby syndrome: an evidence based review. J Emerg Med. 2009;37:98–106.

8. A 15-year-old boy was seen at the hospital with severe headache leading to unconsciousness. CT scan of the head in the Emergency Department showed subarachnoid hemorrhage, with a significant amount of blood in the cisterns at the base of the brain. There was no evidence for intra-parenchymal hemorrhage or ischemic stroke. The boy was participating in skateboarding competitions. He always attempting risky jumps that are avoided by other skateboarders. He has had multiple falls in the past, but has never been lost consciousness. He is otherwise healthy. Toxicology screen was negative and no history for substance abuse, an angiogram shows an aneurysm of the supraclinoid portion of the left internal carotid artery, perhaps secondary to earlier traumatic injury.
In order to prevent secondary complications from vasospasm in this patient, which of the following medications should be administered?
   - A. Heparin
   - B. Nimodipine
   - C. Clonidine
   - D. Phenytoin
   - E. Propranolol

Correct Answer is: B
Ruptured intracranial aneurysms are relatively rare in the patients less than 18 years of age. In contrast to adult patients, in whom sporadic saccular aneurysms predominate, aneurysms in children are more diverse, including giant, fusiform, dissecting or infectious aneurysms. Posterior cerebral circulation is usually more involved. Familial predisposition is 10%. The prognosis in children may be more favorable relative to that seen in adults even with severe subarachnoid hemorrhage (SAH). Many complications following SAH are possible, including hydrocephalus, seizures, syndrome of inappropriate anti-diuretic hormone (SIADH) or vasospasm leading to ischemic infarction. Nimodipine is approved by FDA for prevention of vasospasm in this condition.

Suggested Reading

- Lasjaunias P, Wuppalapati S, Alvarez H, Rodesch G, Ozanne A. Intracranial aneurysms in children aged under 15 years: review of 59 consecutive children with 75 aneurysms. Childs Nerv Syst. 2005;21:437–50.

9. A 16-year-old boy was drinking alcohol with his cousin, at a picnic in a public park. A fight between the patient and his cousin ensued, and the patient was struck in the head with a baseball bat, with immediate loss of consciousness. He was taken to the Emergency Department, and on examination he had an enlarged and non-reactive right pupil, and no motor response on the left side of the body. An emergency head CT scan is shown.

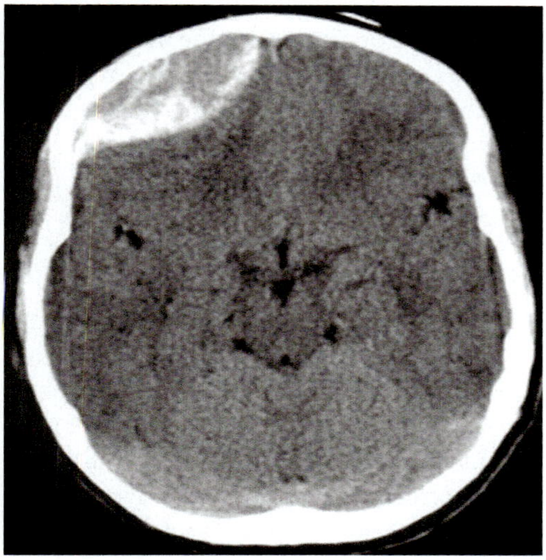

Fig. 27.1 Non-contrast CT scan of an acute epidual hematoma, right fronto-temporal area, due to trauma. (Own work. Jpogi. Wikipedia)

Which of the following is the best management approach?

A. ICU admission, careful observation, and serial head CT scans.
B. ICU admission with osmotic therapy for increased intracranial pressure.
C. Surgical evacuation of the hematoma as soon as possible.
D. A loading dose of Fosphenytoin I.V.
E. ICU admission, with hyperventilation to pCO2 25

Correct Answer is: C
The peak incidence of epidural hematoma (EDH) is in the second decade. EDH are relatively not ommon in the elderly. Non-operative management with careful ICU observation and serial brain imaging is an option for those patients who are awake and responsive, without focal deficits, and with a maximal EDH thickness of less than 10–15 mm. Others should be considered for surgical treatment as soon as possible.

Suggested Reading

- Bullock MR, Chesnut R, Ghajar J, et al. Surgical management of acute epidural hematomas. Neurosurgery. 2006;58(Suppl):S2–7.

10. An 8-year-old girl was transferred to the Emergency Department after she was struck by a car while running across the street. At the scene, EMS found her to be awake, but distraught and complaining of neck pain. She was transported with her head and neck immobilized in neutral position. Upon examination, she is breathing well, has stable vital signs, and appears to be moving all four extremities equally. Cervical spine radiology shows abnormal widening of the interspace at C1-C2. **What is your next step in management?**

A. Lumbar puncture to exclude subarachnoid hemorrhage
B. Urgent tracheostomy
C. Continued immobilization of the head and neck, careful observation, and neurosurgical consultation.
D. Flexion and extension views of the neck under fluoroscopy
E. Ophthalmology consultation for dilated fundus examination

Correct Answer is: C
Cervical spine (C-spine) injuries in prepubertal children are relatively not common in comparison to older age groups. In young children, C-spine injuries are most likely to occur at the cranio-cervical junction or upper vertebral segments C1-C4. Children may have severe Disruption of ligaments or other soft supporting tissues may occur in children without obvious abnormalities of the vertebrae on radiographs. Such soft tissue injuries can be detected by selected MR sequences, if indicated. C-spine stability has to be determined by the appropriate studies if the children are unresponsive, intoxicated, have abnormal findings on neurological examination, or if they have a neck pain, and they should remain immobilized. The role of corticosteroid administration for neuroprotection following spinal injury remains contentious.

27

Suggested Reading

- Platzer P, Jaindl M, Thalhammer G, et al. Cervical spine injuries in pediatric patients. J Trauma. 2007;62:389–96.
- Hall ED, Springer JE. Neuroprotection and acute spinal cord injury: a reappraisal. NeuroRx. 2004;1:80–100.

11. A 16-year-old boy who is a goalie on a field hockey team is knocked to the ground and strikes his head. He lost consciousness and doesn't respond immediately. He became conscious after a few seconds. His coach helped him to get up and walked him to the sideline. Upon evaluation he was confused and he did not recall the injury. He felt dizzy and has a headache. Half an hour later, a repeat examination is performed. He still does not recall the event, but is no longer dizzy or unsteady on his feet but still having headache. Family took him to the ER where a head CT scan is performed and is normal. Past medical history is remarkable for migraine headaches. **What is your diagnoses?**
    - A. moderate traumatic brain injury
    - B. confusional migraine
    - C. grade 1 concussion
    - D. grade 2 concussion
    - E. grade 3 concussion

Correct Answer is: E
The most likely diagnosis in this case is grade 3 concussion. According to AAN Practice Parameters, concussion is a trauma induced alteration in mental status that may or may not involve loss of consciousness. The practice parameter using a scale to help differentiate the severity of the concussion. Scales were reviewed and a grading scale adopted that was dependent on the duration of the symptoms and the absence or presence of loss of consciousness. Grade 1 concussion has transient symptoms without loss of consciousness and symptoms lasting less than 15 min. A grade 2 concussion has symptoms lasting more than 15 min without loss of consciousness. A grade 3 concussion is loss of consciousness of any duration. While he has a history of migraines, the fact that he experienced loss of consciousness would make this diagnosis incorrect. Moderate TBI occurs when a patient has a Glasgow Coma Scale of 9–12 with prolonged loss of consciousness and/or neurologic deficit.

Suggested Reading

- Practice Parameter: the management of concussion in sport. Neurology. 1997;48(3):581–85.
- Geocadin RG. Traumatic brain injury. In: Bhardwaj A, Mirski MA, Ulatowski JA, editors. Handbook of neurocritical care.

12. A 5-month old baby was seen by a pediatric neurologist for evaluation. His mother noticed that he is not

grasping with his left hand as much as he is with his right hand. Neurological exam showed a healthy child without dysmorphic features. He has normal truncal tone and he makes eye contact with objects presented to him. He has a strong grasp on the right but cannot grasp objects on the left. He can lift his arm but does not use his hand muscles. He has normal symmetric tone proximally in the arms, and decreased distally in the left arm. Biceps reflexes are present bilaterally. The left pupil is also smaller than the right, and does not dilate well upon turning the light off.

Which of the following features from the birth history would be most anticipated?

A. Traction on the infant's neck as a complications from shoulder dystocia.
B. Right middle cerebral artery infarction in the infant.
C. Perinatal asphyxia to the infant.
D. Left arm presentation during a difficult vaginal birth.
E. Traumatic right subdural hematoma during vaginal delivery

Correct Answer is: D

The baby has asymmetric left arm weakness. Localization to an upper or lower motor neuron cause has to be determined. Cortical injury, including trauma, arterial stroke or diffuse hypoxic-ischemic insult can easily be excluded because there are no features of upper motor neuron disease on exam. The remaining choices represent mechanisms for the two most common obstetrically related brachial plexopathies, affecting up to 2 per 1000 live births, Erb's palsy, the most common of these, arises from injury to the upper plexus (C5/6) due to traction of the head away from the shoulder, stretching the upper trunk of the brachial plexus. Children with Erb's palsy present with weakness of shoulder abduction, elbow flexion and arm supination and babies hold their arms in an adducted and internally rotated position ("waiter's tip position"). On the other hand, a Klumpke palsy can result from hyper-abduction of the affected arm, often in association with a challenging arm presentation during delivery. Infants present with intact proximal arm strength but weakness of the hand if C8/T1 roots got affected. A congenital Horner syndrome may also result from the second order neurons for sympathetic supply to the pupil dilator muscle arising at the C8/T1 level of the spinal cord.

Suggested Reading

Ferrante MA. Brachial Plexopathies. CONTINUUM: Lifelong Learning in Neurol. 2014;20(5):1323–42.

13. A 15-year-old male lost unconsciousness for about 20 s after being hit in the head by another player during a hockey game. He was dazed for another 15 min after regaining consciousness.

What is the correct statement regarding neuropsychological testing for concussion per AAN's guidelines?

A. Standardized Assessment of Concussion (SAC) has the highest sensitivity in detecting subtle cognitive deficits.
B. Commonly used cognitive evaluation tools include the "stick drop" test and the King-Devick Test of visual tracking.
C. Cognitive restructuring is the standard method of neuropsychological assessment immediately after a concussive head injury.
D. The most appropriate use of pre-injury clinical tools is as a source of data to be included as part of a comprehensive neurologic evaluation.

E. Standard neuropsychological tests can be administered and interpreted by a trained non-neuropsychologist.

Correct Answer is: D

Stick drop test "the clinical reaction time" and the King-Devick Test of visual tracking along with balance tests such as the Balance Error Scoring System (BESS) are used for physical evaluation and not cognitive evaluation. Common preinjury cognitive tests include computerized tools such as the Axon Sports Computerized Cognitive Assessment Tool (CCAT) and the Immediate Post-Concussion Assessment and Cognitive Testing (ImPACT) assessment tool, and paper-and-pencil tools such as the Standardized Assessment of Concussion (SAC). In general, none of the preinjury evaluation tool has been shown to be superior over another. Preinjury cognitive assessment is useful both in assessing the severity of effects of concussion and recovery of symptoms as compared to baseline. However it is not specific and should be used as part of a comprehensive neurologic evaluation.

Although neuropsychological testing may be administered by a trained non-neuropsychologist, only a neuropsychologist should interpret them.

Cognitive restructuring is not a test for evaluation but a form of brief psychological counseling that consists of education, reassurance, and reattribution of symptoms. Although are no specific studies using cognitive restructuring specifically in sports concussions, it has been shown to be effective in decreasing the development of chronic post-concussion syndrome in patients with mild traumatic brain injury.

Suggested Reading

- Giza C, et al. Summary of evidence-based guideline update: evaluation and management of concussion in Sports. Report of the Guideline Development Subcommittee of the American Academy of Neurology. Neurol. 2013;80:2250.
- Scorza K, Raleigh M, O'Connor F. Current Concepts in Concussion: evaluation and Management. Am Fam. Physician. 2012;85(2):123.
- Kutcher J, Giza C. Sports Concussion Diagnosis and Management. Continuum Lifelong Learning Neurol. 2014;20(6):1552.

14. A 14 year old boy had a sudden sharp, throbbing pain in his left upper arm 1 week ago and the pain did not disappeared. He was not able to play on the basketball team since that time. Pain does not disappear by rest, and activity aggravates his discomfort. He has some improvement in his pain in the past 3 days. On examination there is weakness in shoulder muscles, triceps and his wrist extensors. He has good strength in wrist flexion.
What is his diagnosis and where is the lesion?
  A. Upper brachia! Plexus – Brachial Plexitis
  B. Upper and lower brachia! Plexus
  C. Spinal cord compression – C4-C6
  D. Spinal cord compression C8-T1

Correct Answer is: A

Sudden onset of acute pain without trauma at the time, is an indication of a brachial neuritis. The clinical presentation indicate that the axillary and radian nerves (via roots C4-C6; upper plexus) are affected based on the muscle impairment distribution. Even though the boy plays basketball, there was no impact near the time of the pain onset.

Median and ulnar nerves that innervate the wrist flexors contribute to the Lower brachial Plexus roots.

Although C4-C6 nerves are involved, the clinical course of spinal cord

compression in most cases would be more gradual.

C8-T1 contribute to the lower brachia! Plexus branches only and therefore would not be consistent with the symptoms in this case.

Suggested Reading

- Tharin BD, Jonathan AK, York GE, Ritter JL. Brachia! Plexopathy: a Review of Traumatic and Non-traumatic Causes. Am J Neonatology. 2014;202(1):W67–75.

15. A child that develops right-sided ipsilateral ptosis, miosis, and facial anhidrosis after a fall from a ladder.
Most likely has injury to which area?
A. Right maxillary bone
B. Right temporal cortex
C. Left foramen ovale
D. Right brachial plexus

Correct Answer is: D
Falling from a high places with an outstretched arm to attempt to break the fall, can cause neuropraxis (stretching) of the brachial plexus. Horner syndrome results from the sympathetic denervation associated with the trauma to the brachial plexus and nerve roots. At birth, brachial plexus injury is secondary to neuroblastoma tumor invasion can also cause Horner syndrome.

Right maxillary bone fracture may damage the maxillary branch of the fifth cranial nerve causing sensory deficits in the area.

Right temporal bone impact or fracture can be result in concussion or intracranial hemorrhage. The patient has no altered mental status or contralateral sensory motor symptoms.

The mandibular branch of the fifth cranial nerve passed through the foramen ovale and compression would result in sensory disturbances in that region.

Suggested Reading

- Jeffery AR, Ellis FJ, Repka MX, Buncic JR. Pediatric Horner syndrome. J AAPOS. 1998;2(3):159–67.

16. A 9 year-old boy was evaluated by you after he received multiple organ trauma in an automobile accident. Brain CAT scan shows sign of cerebral edema. Caloric testing was performed by instilling 5 cc's of cool water into the right external auditory canal. 10 s later both eyes deviated to the right side, but was followed by a fast component back to the left.
What is your interpretation of this test result?
A. This is an indication of cerebral trauma
B. There is involvement of the brainstem injury
C. There is a pending brain herniation
D. This is a normal finding

Correct Answer is: D
Irrigation of the external auditory canal with cold-water produces a slow component movement toward the ipsilateral side of the stimulated ear, and then a fast nystagmus (corrective movement) in the opposite direction. This requires an intact vestibular nerve, brainstem vestibular nuclei, medial longitudinal fasciculus abducens nuclei, trochlear nerve and oculomotor nuclei. Severe cerebral trauma without significantly increased intracranial pressure typically does not result in brainstem nuclei dysfunction. Brainstem injury in the medulla and/or pontine regions will result in abnormal ocular response. The test results are normal in this clinical presentation. Brain herniation causing pressure on the brainstem and lead to dysfunction of the nuclei and/or exiting cranial nerves resulting in reduction or absent function of vestibular, abducens,

trochlear and/or oculomotor nuclei. If we have no response to caloric testing, this would suggest severe brainstem damage/injury and may contribute to a diagnosis of brain death.

Suggested Reading

- Buttner-Ennever J. A review of otolith pathways to brainstem and cerebellum. Ann NY Acad Sci. 1999;871:51–64.

27

17. A 4-year-old girl has been evaluated for super sensitive hearing. The child covers her ears or runs to another room when the vacuum is started or the television is turned loud. When a sudden loud noise occurs, she appears to be in physical pain for few seconds. She has a normal development.
Which of the following conditions may have predisposed him to this problem?
A. Pervasive Developmental disorder
B. Bell's Palsy
C. Ototoxicity form medication
D. Frequent middle ear infections

Correct Answer is: B
Chorda tympani branch of the seventh cranial nerve can be affected in Bell's palsy. It innervates the stapedius muscle and can limit the movement of the bony ossicles when loud noises are present. Inability of the chorda tympani to innervate the muscle results in greater movement of the ossicles and a greater amplitude is transmitted to the inner ear causing hyperacusis.

Children with pervasive developmental disorders can have hearing or sound sensitivities, but it is not a primary behavioral disturbance. The child in this case has normal language development.

Sensorineural hearing deficits, not hyperacusis can be the result of Ototoxicity form medications. Frequent middle ear infections can result in ossification of the cartilaginous connections between the bones, limits the ossicles movement and results in hearing loss.

Suggested Reading

- Nemholt SS, Schmidt JH, Wedderkopp N, Baguley DM. Prevalence of tinnitus and/or hyperacusis in children and adolescents: study protocol for a systematic review. BMJ open. 2015;5(1):e006649.

18. A large infant (10.5 pounds) was delivered to a mother with a history of gestational diabetes. The delivery was prolonged and difficult.
The baby sustained an Erb-Duchenne paralysis, resulting from traumatic evulsion of:
A. C4-CS
B. CS-C6
C. C6-C7
D. C7-C8
E. C8-T1

Correct Answer is: B
Erb-Duchenne paralysis is due to traumatic avulsion of C5-C6 nerve roots, typically occurred at birth due to traction on the head during delivery of the shoulder. The injury results in loss of shoulder abduction and elbow flexion, and loss of the biceps and brachioradialis reflexes. The arm is held in an internally rotated, extended position, with pronation of the forearm – often referred to as the "waiter's tip" position.

19. A 14-year-old boy falls while skateboarding and hits the side of his head against the side curb. He did not have his helmet on. He had a minor scalp laceration that stops bleeding within 5 min. Initially, he is alert, but he suddenly he lost his consciousness 20 min later. A bystander sees him collapse and calls 911. Head CT scan is shown below.

What blood vessel most likely has been damaged?

A. Great vein of Galen
B. Middle meningeal artery
C. Inferior cerebellar artery
D. Bridging veins

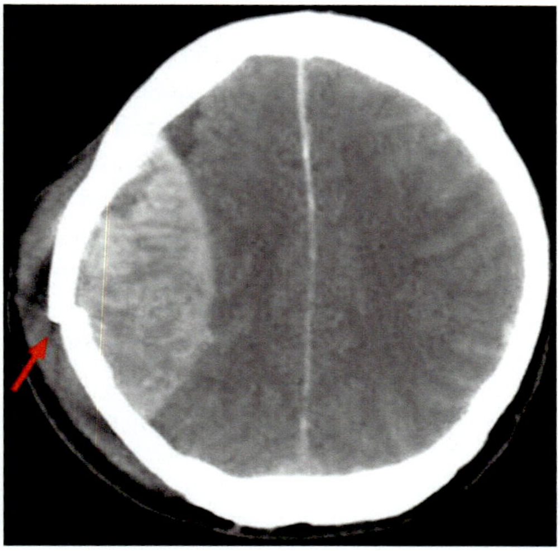

Fig. 27.2 Epidurales Hämatom bei Fraktur (Pfeil) der Schädelkalotte. (Own work. Hellerhoff. Wikipedia)

Correct Answer is: B

This is the classic presentation of an epidural hematoma presenting with the "lucid period" and lens-shaped area on the CT scan. Hematoma can compress intracranial structures and impinge on CN III, lead to a fixed and dilated pupil on the side of the injury; the eye will also be directed down and out because of unopposed CN IV and CN VI innervation. The most serious complication is uncal herniation, leading to respiratory arrest as the medullary structures are compressed in the foramen magnum. The patient sustained damage to his left temple area, which is where the middle meningeal artery runs along the temporal bone.

Trauma in general does affect the great vein of Galen, however it may be damaged in cases of thrombosis.

Trauma also does not damage the Inferior cerebellar artery which may cause a subarachnoid hemorrhage.

Subdural hemorrhages can be the result of the damage to bridging veins, where bleeding occurs beneath the dura.

Bleeding from the veins of the cavernous sinus would be slow and lead to progression of symptoms over a longer period of time.

20. A 15-year-boy was involved in a motor vehicle accident 6 months ago and suffered sustained head trauma, multiple craniofacial surgeries were done. His past medical history is remarkable for chronic sinusitis. He now presents with fever and change in mental status. B rain MRI is shown. **Which of the following is correct regarding this condition?**

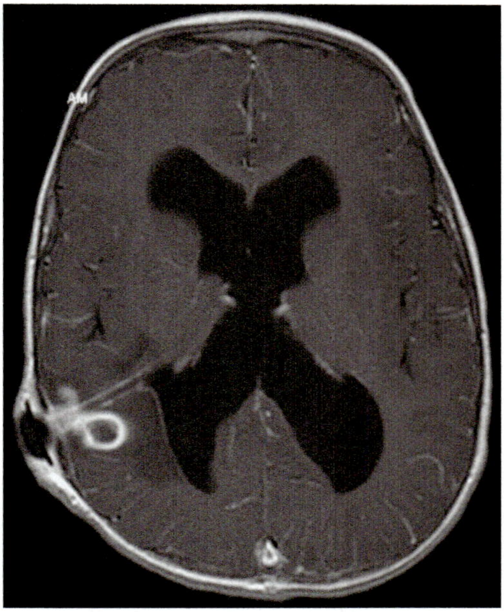

Fig. 27.3 MRI (T1 + contrast): showing a small ring-enhancing lesion with mild surrounding edema adjacent to the ventricular catheter and ventricular dilatation. (Jamjoom et al. *Cases Journal* 2009 2:110. ► https://doi.org/10.1186/1757-1626-2-110. Brain abscess formation as a CSF shunt complication: a case report. Aimun AB Jamjoom, Abrar R Waliuddin and Abdulhakim B Jamjoom. Wikipedia)

A. It can be polymicrobial
B. Highly active antiretroviral therapy is the treatment of choice
C. CSF shows atypical lymphocytes with monoclonal B cells
D. He should be treated with pyrimethamine and sulfadiazine
E. It is caused by mycobacteria

Correct Answer is: A
There is a small ring-enhancing lesion with mild surrounding edema adjacent to the ventricular catheter and ventricular dilatation on his MRI. The history and the clinical findings are consistent with brain abscesses. This lesion originate from invasion of brain parenchyma by bacterial organisms, commonly polymicrobial, with a combination of streptococci, staphylococci, enterobacteria, and anaerobes. The bacterial agents spread via hematogenous routes or from a contiguous infected site, such as the sinuses, ears, or teeth. They also can be encountered after open trauma or neurosurgical interventions. Patients may present with fever, headaches, neck stiffness, focal neurologic findings, and altered mental status. The diagnosis is made on the basis of clinical suspicion and the presence of risk factors, along with clinical and radiologic findings, with the MRI showing ring enhancing lesions with surrounding edema. Lumbar puncture may be contraindicated in the presence of mass effect; however, if a CSF sample is obtained, there may be increased WBC and protein levels, with normal to decreased glucose level. Atypical lymphocytes and monoclonal B cells are seen in lymphoproliferative disorders and not in brain abscesses.

27

Suggested Reading

- Comprehensive Review in Clinical Neurology: a Multiple Choice Question Book for the Wards and Boards © 2011 Wolters Kluwer Health Lippincott Williams & Wilkins. All rights reserved.

21. A 10-year-old boy falls off and fractures the proximal humerus. After the removal of the cast, he is noted to have weakness of the arm, and he was referred for neurologic consultation. On examination, he is able to abduct the arm up to around 30°, but not beyond that. Sensory examination reveals a small area of hypoesthesia on the lateral aspect of the upper arm, but is otherwise normal. Arm adduction, forearm pronation, and forearm, wrist, and finger extension, are of normal strength.
What is the most likely diagnosis in this patient?
A. Axillary neuropathy
B. Radial neuropathy
C. Posterior cord lesion
D. C8 radiculopathy
E. Middle trunk lesion

Correct Answer is: A
This is the classic presentation of axillary neuropathy based on the patient's history and examination. Axillary neuropathies occur secondary to a fractures at the surgical neck of the humerus and with anterior shoulder dislocations. The axillary nerve is a continuation of the posterior cord, and carries predominantly CS and C6 fibers. The axillary nerve innervates the deltoid muscle, which is the main arm abductor, particularly between 30° and 90° (supraspinatus significantly contributes to arm abduction in the first 30° of abduction and the trapezius contributes to greater than 90°). The deltoid has three heads: (1) the anterior head, which is involved arm flexion (in front of the body), assisted by serratus anterior, (2) the lateral head, which along with the anterior head is mainly involved in arm abduction to the side and slightly anteriorly,

and (3) the posterior head, which is involved in posterior movement of the abducted arm. The axillary nerve also innervates teres minor, which externally rotates the arm along with infraspinatus. The axillary nerve provides sensory innervation to the upper lateral arm through the upper lateral brachial cutaneous nerve. Intact arm abduction in the first 30° suggests the supraspinatus is of normal strength. In addition, there is intact sensation over the posterolateral arm, territory innervated by the C8 nerve root through the lateral and posterior cutaneous nerves to the arm (radial nerve branches). These findings make a C8 radiculopathy unlikely. Intact strength of radial nerve-innervated muscles excludes a posterior cord lesion and a radial neuropathy intact strength of predominantly C7-innervated muscles excludes a middle trunk lesion.

Suggested Reading

- Russell SM. Examination of Peripheral Nerve Injuries. New York: Thieme; 2006.
- Comprehensive Review in Clinical Neurology: A Multiple Choice Question Book for the Wards and Boards ©2011 Wolters Kluwer Health Lippincott Williams & Wilkins. All rights reserved.

22. A 9-year-old boy presents with impaired abduction of the left eye. The rest of his neurologic examination was normal.
The most likely cause is:
   A. Trauma
   B. Malignancy
   C. Foville syndrome
   D. Milard-Gubler syndrome
   E. Gradenigo's syndrome

Correct Answer is: A
Trauma is the most frequent cause of childhood-onset abducens palsies, occurring in 40% of cases. Malignancy is the second most cause of abducens nerve palsies in children, it occurs in 13% of cases. Primary brainstem gliomas are a common etiology. Isolated abducens weakness may be the initial sign of illness. Foville syndrome is an abducens and facial nerve palsies with contralateral hemiplegia, also most commonly caused by basilar artery infarcts. The lesion is in the caudal tegmental pons, potentially affecting the abducens nucleus or para-pontine reticular formation (PPRF), facial cranial nerve or nucleus, and corticospinal tract. A normal motor examination in this patient makes this syndrome unlikely. Millard-Gubler syndrome consists of a facial nerve palsy with contralateral hemiparesis, classically caused by basilar artery infarcts of the caudal ventral pons involving the cranial nerve nucleus or fascicle and corticospinal tract. Later descriptions of the syndrome included abducens nerve palsies, as well. The isolated abducens weakness in this patient makes this syndrome unlikely. Gradenigo's syndrome is the paralysis of the abducens nerve due to osteitis of the petrous pyramid, secondary to middle ear infections or mastoiditis. The classic triad of symptoms includes diplopia, periorbital unilateral pain due to trigeminal nerve involvement, and persistent otorrhea. This syndrome is rare in the current age of antibiotic use.

Suggested Reading

- Pedroso JL, et al. Gradenigo's syndrome: beyond the classical trial of diplopia, facial pain and otorrhea. Case Rep Neurol. 2011;3(1):45–47.
- Sweeney PJ, Hanson MR. Cranial neuropathies. In: Bradley WG, Daroff RB, Fenichel GM, Ankovic J, editors. Neurology in Clinical Practice. 4rth ed. Elsevier, Inc.; 2004. p. 2107–23.

23. Late complications from head injury include all of the following except:
    A. Hormone disturbances
    B. Seizures
    C. Postconcussion syndrome
    D. Posttraumatic hydrocephalus
    E. Cluster headaches

Correct Answer is: E
Cluster headaches are not typically a complication of head injury.

27

24. A 17-year-old girl is involved in a motorcycle accident while riding with her boyfriend. She did not have her helmet on. Her boyfriend was wearing a helmet. However, he suffered lung contusions, left sided pneumothorax, multiple fractures, and splenic laceration. The boyfriend remained comatose, and his examination a few days after admission demonstrated multiple petechial hemorrhages all over his skin, particularly in the axillary region. The patient died a few days later. On autopsy, the brain showed multiple diffuse petechial hemorrhages.
    How do you explain the neuropathologic findings?
    A. Fat embolization
    B. Diffuse axonal injury
    C. Meningococcal meningitis
    D. Coup and countercoup injury
    E. SAH

Correct Answer is: A
Fat embolism, is most frequently occurred after fractures of long bones such as the femur which results from fat droplets entering the circulation usually in the setting of surgery or trauma. Fat micro-particles from the bone marrow travel in the venous system to the lungs and spread systemically. The typical clinical presentation is agitation, delirium, coma, respiratory distress, anemia, thrombocytopenia, and generalized petechial rash, often concentrated in the axilla, sub-conjunctival area, and palate. Multiple petechial hemorrhages can be seen in the gray and white matter of the brain on autopsy. This clinical presentation of petechial hemorrhages after multiple fractures is not consistent with the other options.

Suggested Reading

- Posner JB, Saper CB, Schiff ND, Plum F. Plum and Postern's Diagnosis of Stupor and Coma, 4rth ed. New York, NY: Oxford University Press; 2007.
- Comprehensive Review in Clinical Neurology: A Multiple-Choice Question Book for the Wards and Boards ©2011 Wolters Kluwer Health Lippincott Williams & Wilkins. All rights reserved.

25. A 16-year-old girl is complaining of chronic headaches, problems falling asleep, scary dreams, and poor school performance for the last few months. She lost interest in school activities, in socializing with friends, and has been increasingly irritable, moody and angry. She told you that her father had been killed in a car accident 6 months ago, also she broke up with her boyfriend after numerous fights 3 months ago. She has been afraid to drive in a car and has had recurring nightmares about her father's death. Her headaches are not migraine in nature, and the rest of her neurological examination is normal.
    What is her diagnosis?
    A. Depression
    B. Post-traumatic stress disorder
    C. Bipolar disorder
    D. Insomnia
    E. Learning disability

Correct Answer is: B
Stressful events that lead to both emotional and physical consequences can be experienced by all children and adolescents. Usually the reactions to

stressful events are generally brief and associated with full recovery, the exposure to catastrophic or repeated traumatic events can lead to unconscious mental dissociation, an emotional numbing to deaden or block the pain and trauma. It is important to realize that since younger children have limited verbal skills and non-specific ways of reacting to stress, they may not always fully meet the DSM-IV-TR criteria (designed for adults) for post-traumatic stress disorder. Behavioral lability is more common in children than adults, and fewer criteria may be necessary to establish a diagnosis.

Suggested Reading

- American Academy of Child and Adolescent Psychiatry Work Group on Quality Issues. Practice parameters for the assessment and treatment of children and adolescents with posttraumatic stress disorder. J Am Acad Child Adolesc Psychiatry. 1998;37(10 Suppl):4S–26S.
- American Psychiatric Association. Diagnostic and statistical manual of mental disorders DSM-IV-TR. 4rth ed. Washington, D.C.: American Psychiatric Association; 2000.

26. A 16-year-old boy presents with a closed traumatic head injury.
    Which of the following is the strongest predictor of poor outcome?
    A. Presence of convexity subarachnoid hemorrhage on head CT
    B. Bilateral dilated unreactive pupils
    C. Glasgow coma scale of 10 after full resuscitation
    D. Midline shift on head CT
    E. Unilateral compression of ambient cistern on head CT

Correct Answer is: B
The major predictors of outcome after severe traumatic brain injury are GCS score after full resuscitation, age, pupillary reactivity, CT findings, and presence of major extracranial injury. Bilateral dilated unreactive pupils predict poor outcome and, when present, is the strongest predictor.

Suggested Reading

- Mangat HS. Severe traumatic brain injury. Continuum (Minneap Minn), 2012;18:532–46.

27. You are seeing a football player who has an episode of convulsion with loss of consciousness for 60 s after colliding with another player. Imaging is negative. He was admitted for observation. The following morning, he is back to his baseline, but complaining of mild headache, but with an entirely intact mental status.
    What is the appropriate statement regarding management of his convulsion?
    A. He should be started on an antiepileptic drug and continued on it for 30 days.
    B. He does not need medication for seizure prophylaxis but should be monitored under concussion protocol.
    C. He would benefit from antiepileptic drug prophylaxis for 7 days even though his imaging is normal.
    D. He should undergo continuous EEG monitoring to detect any underlying epileptiform discharges
    E. Seizure prophylaxis for 7 days post-injury will substantially reduce the risk of him developing late-onset posttraumatic epilepsy

Correct Answer is: B
Patient should be in the concussion protocol as recommended by the American Academy of Neurology guidelines for evaluation and management of concussion in sports because he suffered concussive convulsion. The risk of early

posttraumatic seizures ranges between 10% and 20%. Patient's imaging does not suggest any penetrative injury or intracranial contusions, which would otherwise place him at high risk for recurrent early post-traumatic seizures and therefore benefit from short-term seizure prophylaxis for 7 days. Continuous EEG would not be necessary either given no obvious injuries that put him at risk for seizures. There is no evidence to suggest that early institution of anti-epileptic medication helps prevent the occurrence of late-onset post-traumatic epilepsy (usually defined as seizures more than 1 week removed from the traumatic insult.)

Suggested Reading

- Mangat HS. Continuum (Minneap Minn). 2012;18(3):542–6.
- Giza CC, Kutcher JS, Ashwal S MH, et al. Summary of evidence-based guideline update: evaluation and management of concussion in sports: report of the Guideline Development Subcommittee of the American Academy of Neurology. Neurol. 2013;80(24):2250–57.

Vascular

Y. M. Awaad, *Absolute Pediatric Neurology*, https://doi.org/10.1007/978-3-319-78801-2_28

1. You are evaluating a 3-year-old boy in the ED for his lethargy. His family reported that he has been irritable, sleepy most of the day and he cannot get up and walk one day before his admission to the ER. His past medical history is unremarkable and his development is on target. On examination, he is lethargic, and difficult to arouse. He has drooling, intact gag, some inward deviation of his right eye, and no papilledema. He moves all four extremities equally, but overall has a paucity of movement. DTRs are decreased, but toes are up-going bilaterally. An urgent CT head is ordered, followed by a CT Venogram.

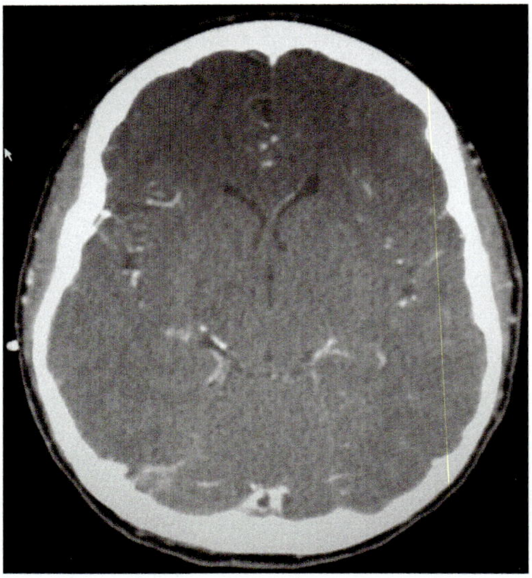

Fig. 28.1 CT Venogram of the brain showing a filling defect in the Sagital Sinus. Most likely a Thrombus. self-made. (Heather. Wikipedia)

What is the most likely diagnosis?

A. CNS vasculitis
B. Carbon monoxide poisoning
C. Mitochondrial disorder
D. Inferior sagittal sinus thrombosis
E. None of the above

Correct Answer is: D

There is an absence of signal in the inferior sagittal sinus on the CT Venogram. The incidence of cerebral venous sinus thrombosis (CVST) is approximately 67 per 100,000 children per year. The differential diagnosis of cerebral venous sinus thrombosis includes malignancy, nephrotic syndrome, congenital heart disease, rheumatologic disorders such as Lupus, infection, hypercoagulable disorders, medications and genetic disorders, head injury, and recent surgery. Clinical manifestations include lethargy, irritability, seizures, and symptoms of increased intracranial pressure, mutism, vomiting, headache, coma and death.

In CNS vasculitis, MRI findings typically include multifocal cortical and subcortical white and grey matter lesions.

The Globus pallidus is preferentially involved in carbon monoxide poisoning, not the bilateral thalami. Mitochondrial disorders typically involve the basal ganglia on MRI as well.

Suggested Reading

- Rodríguez-Fanjul J, et al. Deep vein thrombosis: rare cases of diagnoses in a pediatric emergency department. Pediatr Emerg Care. 2011;27(5):417–9.
- Kanakkande A, et al. Deep vein thrombosis in children. Pediatr Rep. 2013;5(2):48–9.
- Sé bire B, et al. Cerebral venous sinus thrombosis in children: risk factors, presentation, diagnosis and outcome. Brain. 2005;128:477–89.
- deVeber G, et al. Canadian pediatric ischemic stroke study group. Cerebral sinovenous thrombosis in children. N Engl J Med. 2001;345(6):417–23.

2. You were asked to see a 7-month-old baby for her developmental delay and seizure-like spells. She is a full- term baby, and was born without complications.

She never has been able to roll over or sit, does not consistently visually regard or track objects, and does not reach for objects with her hands, but does put her hands in her mouth. Head circumference is at 5th percentile, but there are no dysmorphic features. Her pupils are reactive to light but she does not track. She has symmetric facial movements upon crying. She has decreased muscle tone in her neck and shoulder girdle, but increased in the hands and ankles. Tendon reflexes are brisk, with bilateral ankle clonus. Her side picture is shown below.

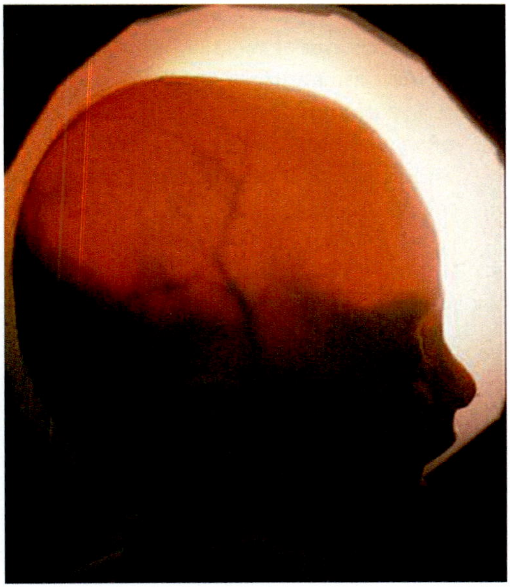

Fig. 28.2 Head illumination showing Hydranecephaly. ► http://neuropathology-web.org/chapter3/images3/3-8l.jpg. Dimitri Agamanolis, M.D. Department of Pathology, Akron Children's Hospital, One Perkins Square, Akron, Ohio, 44,308, USA. Wikipedia.

What is the most likely mechanism to account for her condition?

A. Congenital infection
B. Inborn error of metabolism
C. Migrational brain anomaly
D. Perinatal hemorrhage
E. Prenatal ischemia

Correct Answer is: E

Hydranencephaly is characterized by severe dysgenesis of the cerebral hemispheres, with relative preservation of the thalamus, cerebellum and brainstem. The affected areas are usually localized within the territories of the middle cerebral arteries. Vasculopathy with carotid artery occlusion has been suggested as the reason of hydranencephaly. This has been supported by the distribution of the marked hemispheric destruction observed in those patients. Experiments entailing ligation of both the common carotid arteries and the jugular veins in monkeys during early gestation resulted in subsequent cerebral dysgenesis and focal destruction, with the regions supplied by the anterior and middle cerebral arteries being reduced to thin transparent membranes. The tissues supplied by the posterior cerebral arteries, which receive collateral blood flow from the vertebrobasilar system through the posterior communicating arteries, were usually mainly preserved. These findings support the proposed pathologic process in hydranencephaly.

Suggested Reading

- Tsai JD, Kuo HT, Chou IC. Hydranencephaly in Neonates. Pediatr Neonatol. 2008;49(4):154–7.

3. You are seeing an 8-year-old female in the ED who has complex partial status epilepticus, fluctuating confusion and intermittent clonic movements of her right arm and leg. She has normal birth history and early development. At age 5 years, she started having generalized tonic-clonic seizures, easy fatigability, generalized muscle weakness, and intermittent headaches. She has mild, bilateral sensorineural hearing loss, and she failed a school hearing

screen. Her family history is remarkable of her mother has migraine headaches and hypertrophic cardiomyopathy of unknown etiology. On examination, her height and weight are both <3rd percentile. She has a left homonymous hemi-anopsia, proximal muscle weakness, and hypoactive reflexes. Her EEG shows intermittent theta slowing in the right posterior head region. Brain MR shows lacunar infarcts of both putamen, as well as an infarction of the right occipital cortex. Her serum creatinine kinase is 540 IU/L (elevated), and her serum lactate is 4.2 (elevated).

What other complications are expected in this patient?

A. Arthritis
B. Asthma
C. Diabetes mellitus
D. Heliotropic rash
E. Precocious puberty

Correct Answer is: C
This is a clinical presentation of MELAS, which is a mitochondrial disorder characterized by the triad of encephalopathy (seizures, dementia, or both), lactic acidosis, and stroke-like episodes. Short stature, cognitive impairment, sensorineural hearing loss, migraines, depression, cardiomyopathy, cardiac conduction defects, and diabetes mellitus are secondary manifestations. Age of onset ranges from 2 to 60 years, but almost 70% of patients present between the ages of 2–20 years. The disorder is typically caused by an A-to-G transition (m.3243 A > G) in the gene that encodes mitochondrial tRNA $^{(Leu)}$; hence, it is inherited via the mothers. Brain MRI usually demonstrates asymmetric lesions of the occipital and parietal lobes that mimic ischemia, except that they are usually restricted to the cortex without respect for particular vascular territories. Those patients have normal MR angiography, but MR spectroscopy may show a decrease in the N-acetyl aspartate signal and a high lactate peak. Muscle biopsy reveals scattered, vacuolated muscle fibers with a clear surrounding rim on hematoxylin-eosin staining; basophilic inclusions on Gomori trichrome staining; and scattered ragged-red fibers on succinate dehydrogenase staining. Molecular testing can be performed on blood leukocytes, skin fibroblasts, urine sediment cells, and buccal mucosa, with the latter 2 sources carrying the highest mutation loads. Treatment consists of symptomatic management and supplementation with a "mitochondrial cocktail," consisting of some combination of creatine, coenzyme Q10, alpha-lipoic acid, riboflavin, thiamine, vitamin C, vitamin E, and biotin. There are no curative treatments for MELAS.

Suggested Reading

- Sproule DM, Kaufmann P. Mitochondrial encephalopathy, lactic acidosis, and stroke-like episodes: basic concepts, clinical phenotype, and therapeutic management of MELAS syndrome. Ann NY Acad Sci. 2008;1142:133–58.

4. You are seeing a 10-year-old boy in the PICU who has sudden headache, followed by rapid depressed level of consciousness and right-side body weakness. He has no recent history of fever, trauma, or systemic illness. He is not taking any medications. On examination, you were able to arouse him with deep pain, but he had a gaze preference to his right and lack of motor response to the right arm or leg. Urgent brain CT showed a large intraparenchymal bleeding within the left parieto-occipital region with evidence of herniation of brain tissue from left to right under the falx. A neurosurgeon

was called and an emergency craniotomy was performed to evacuate the hemorrhage, followed by an angiography showed an arteriovenous malformation (AVM) in the left parietal midline region fed predominately by the left posterior cerebral artery.
What symptom would be present in this child before the AVM rupture?

A. Episodes of left sided weakness
B. Learning disability
C. Migraine with aura
D. No symptoms prior to the hemorrhage
E. Simple partial sensory seizures

Correct Answer is: D
AVM is the most common cause of non-traumatic intra-parenchymal brain hemorrhage in children after the newborn period. There are no symptoms prior to the hemorrhage itself in 75–80% of children and adolescents. There is a higher likelihood of hemorrhage into the posterior fossa or deep cerebral structures, and the bleeding itself is often more massive from AVM bleeding in adults. The morbidity and mortality with hemorrhage from AVMs in children is high, and a proactive approach to treatment is usually recommended when they are discovered. Surgical treatment should be individualized to the circumstances of each case, but can include craniotomy with surgical excision, endovascular embolization, or stereotactic radiosurgery (or some combination of these).

Suggested Reading

Niazi TN, Klimo P Jr., Anderson RC, Raffel C. Diagnosis and management of arteriovenous malformations in children. Neurosurg Clin N Am. 2010;21:443–56.

5. You are evaluating a 1-month-old boy for his remarkable developmental delay and rapidly enlarging head size. He has unremarkable prenatal and perinatal histories. He has a full and enlarged fontanelle. Head circumference is 45 cm. He does not fixate or follow. He has increased tone, hyperactive reflexes and no purposeful motor activity. Head MRI scan is shown.

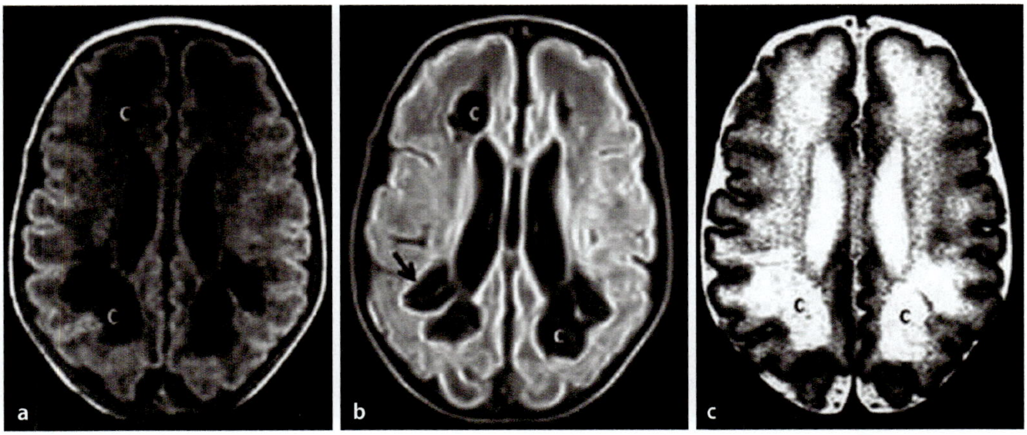

Fig. 28.3 (**a–c**) A 31-day-old infant born preterm (31 weeks) shows mild-to-moderate hypoxic ischemic injury. The infant also had refractory hypoglycemia. **a** Axial T1WI at the level of lateral ventricles shows frontal and posterior periventricular white matter cysts. **b** Axial fluid-attenuated inversion recovery (FLAIR) and T2WI at the level of lateral ventricles show frontal and posterior periventricular white matter cysts **c** with gliosis (*arrows*). (Indian Journal of Radiology and Imaging. Year: 2016;26(3):316–27)

What is your most likely explanation for his condition?

A. Migration brain disturbance
B. X-linked aqueduct stenosis
C. Prenatal vascular brain injury
D. Brain injury from herpes encephalitis
E. Congenital virus infection

Correct Answer is: C
Patients with this clinical picture are always a challenge to the child neurologist. Therapeutic futility rules. Recognizing the underlying vascular insult leading to the severe cortical insult may not obviate a shunt for a rapidly expanding head but it puts the objectives and limitation of any intervention in proper perspective.

28

Suggested Reading

- Jung JH, Graham JM Jr., Schultz N, Smith DW. Congenital hydranencephaly/porencephaly due to vascular disruption in monozygotic twins. Pediatrics. 1984;73(4):467–9.

6. A 29- week gestation infant has been doing well since birth. She is on CPAP with no need for inotropic medications or antibiotics, but it was very. A routine ultrasound performed on her second day of life is shown.

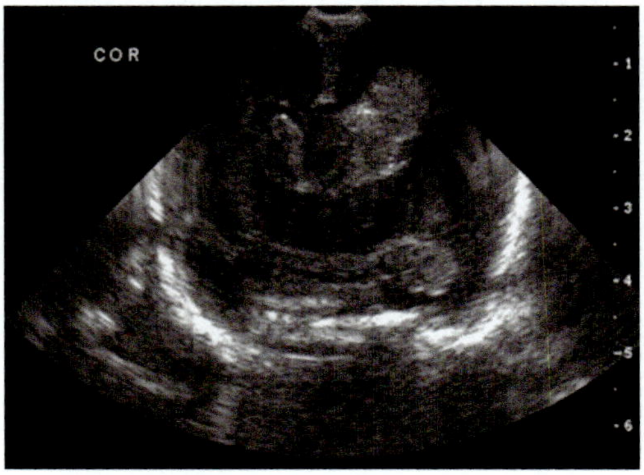

Fig. 28.4 Ultra Sound showing grade 3 IVH. With permission from med-ed.virginia.edu. Free for residents and students

This condition puts this baby at highest risk for which of the following neurological conditions?

A. Deafness
B. Cerebral palsy
C. Cortical visual impairment
D. Epilepsy
E. Autism

Correct Answer is: B
The ultra sound shows grade 3 IVH (germinal matrix hemorrhage with IVH filling and distending lateral ventricles). This hemorrhage is secondary to immaturity of the germinal matrix vessels which are thought to rupture due to high central venous pressures transmitted to the region during or following birth during vaginal delivery, need for high pressure ventilation or other interventions. Both grade 3 and 4 IVH have approximately 50% chance of producing post-hemorrhagic hydrocephalus that requires treatment in the neonatal period. In addition, grade 3 IVH is associated with 50% chance of cerebral palsy and developmental delay.

Suggested Reading

- Allan WC, Vohr BR, Makuch RW, Katz KH, and Ment LR. Antecedents of cerebral palsy in a multicenter trial of indomethacin for intraventricular hemorrhage. Arch Pediatr Adolesc Med. 1997;151:580–5.

7. You are seeing a 14-year-old boy in the ER for his sudden onset of headache and left face and extremities weakness. When he woke up in the morning, he noticed the symptoms which improved after 1 h, but worsened again 4 h later. He has unremarkable past medical history and takes no medications. He is afebrile, pulse 85/min, BP 95/65, respirations 18/min. He has mild weakness of the lower left face, and more dense paralysis of his left upper and lower extremities. He lost sensation in his left

face and limbs. DTRs are brisk on the left side, with extensor plantar response. A bolus of IV fluids was given and his BP rises to 130/80. A brain MRI is shown.

An MRA demonstrates narrowing and beading of the right middle and anterior cerebral arteries. He is started on low-dose aspirin.

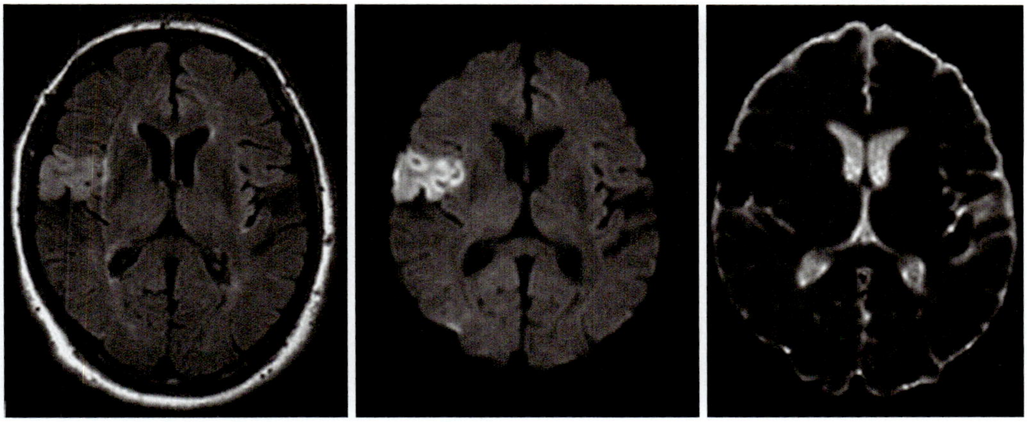

Fig. 28.5 MRI with FLAIR, DWI, and ADC showing an established infarction in the right frontal lobe matching the CTP-delineated ischemic core. (Permission by Hindawi. Free access)

What is your next step in management?

A. Hypothermia
B. Prednisone
C. Warfarin
D. Verapamil
E. Phenylephrine

Correct Answer is: B

This is a case of acute ischemic stroke in the right anterior and middle cerebral arteries territory. The findings of stenosis and beading are typical of inflammatory vasculitis. The vasculitis can be a primary CNS disease or secondary to a variety of inflammatory (lupus, Behcet's, Sjogren, dermatomyositis, scleroderma, polyarteritis nodosa, Kawasaki disease, HSP, Wegener's, Churg-Strauss, and inflammatory bowel disease) or infectious (bacterial, viral, fungal, spiorochete) conditions. Primary CNS vasculitis is divided into large-medium vessel and small vessel types. The boy has the large-medium vessel variety. Headache and acute focal motor or sensory deficits are typical presentations. Brain and leptomeningeal biopsy are not typically needed if the classic findings of inflammatory vasculitis have been demonstrated by the angiogram. Patients with neurocognitive dysfunction at presentation, multifocal T2 hyper-intense lesions on MRI, and evidence of distal stenosis on angiography are at higher risk of progressive disease and should be treated aggressively (induction with monthly IV cyclophosphamide and high-dose steroids for 6 months followed by oral mycophenalate mofetil or oral azathioprine for 18 months. Patients who do not have the high-risk profile are often treated with an antiplatelet agent combined with high-dose steroids for 3 months.

Suggested Reading

- Elbers J, Benseler SM. Central nervous system vasculitis in children. Curr Opin Rheumatol. 2008;20(1); 47–54.

8. You are seeing a 12-year-old trisomy 21 girl in the ED for her transient weakness episode of her right hand and face along with difficulty speaking, all of which resolved spontaneously after an hour. The event occurred when she was upset and crying after being struck in the head by a baseball at school. She had a history of infantile spasms when she was 1 year old, which resolved after treatment. She has had migraine headaches for several years. She has the typical features of trisomy 21, but no focal deficits. Her brain MRI and MRA are shown.

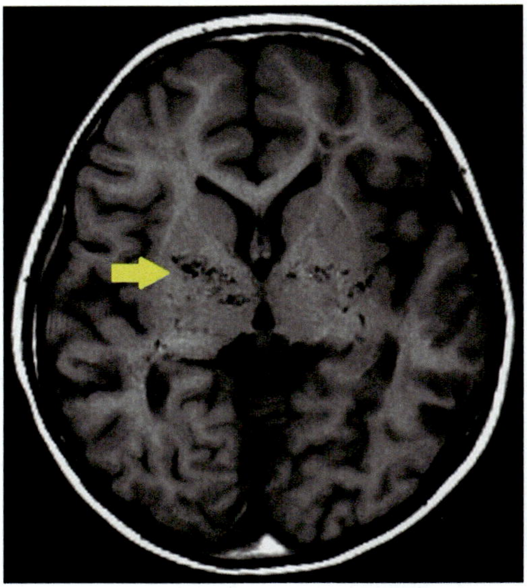

Fig. 28.6 T1-weighted MR image of moyamoya disease. Flow void in the basal ganglia is indicated by the arrow. Own work. (Takuma-sa. Wikipedia)

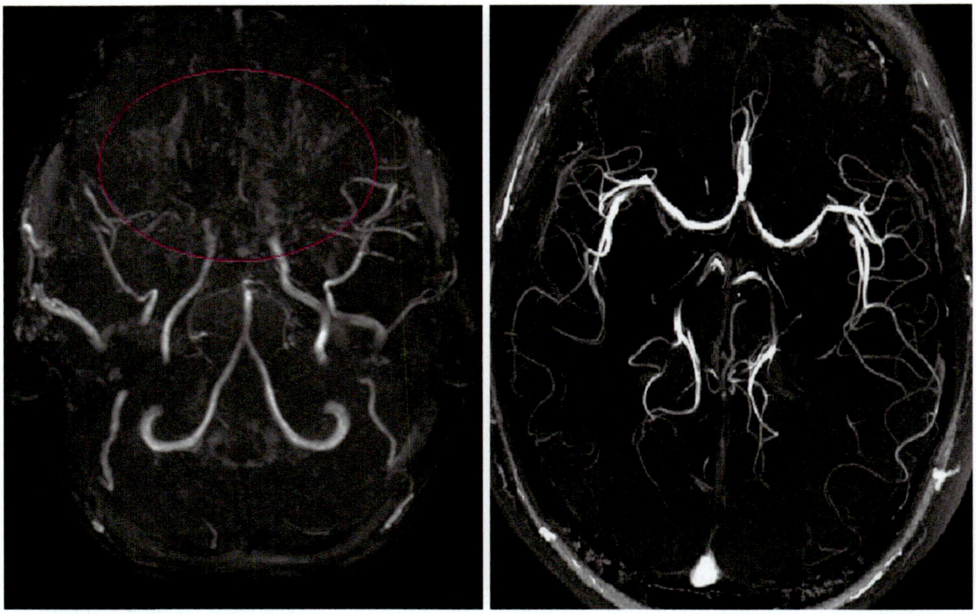

Fig. 28.7 (Left) MIP reconstructed MR angiography of a 11 year old girl with en:Moya moya disease. (Right) healthy patient, for comparison. (*Left image*) own work by commons:User:MBq, (*Right image*) ► https://commons.wikimedia.org/wiki/File:Mra-mip.jpg. commons:User:MBq, commons:User:SBarnes. Wikipedia

What is the most likely diagnosis?

A. Atlantoaxial dislocation
B. Partial seizure
C. Moya Moya syndrome
D. Breath-holding spell
E. Traumatic arterial dissection

Correct Answer is: C

Moya Moya syndrome is a cerebrovascular condition which lead to stroke in affected patients secondary to progressive stenosis of the intracranial internal carotid arteries and their proximal vessels. Development of compensatory collateral small blood vessels near the apex of the carotid arteries occur secondary to the stenosis. Patients at increased risk include, people with history of radiotherapy to the head or neck, trisomy 21, neurofibromatosis type 1, and sickle cell disease. The most presenting manifestations are, migraine-like headaches, ischemic symptoms such as hemiparesis, aphasia, and cognitive impairment. Less frequent presenting symptoms include visual deficits, syncope, seizures, and cerebral hemorrhage. Ischemic symptoms are often precipitated by hyperventilation from crying, dehydration and exertion. Choreiform movements can develop secondary to the dilated collateral vessels in the basal ganglia. The vascular stenosis is due to a combination of hyperplasia of smooth muscle cells and luminal thrombosis. If no treatment has been provided, most patients will progress over time and are therefore at high risk of stroke. Medical treatment options such as antiplatelet agents, anticoagulation, and calcium channel blockers seem to be less effective than surgical revascularization procedures, either direct or indirect (e.g. encephalo-duroarterio-synangiosis).

Suggested Reading

- Scott RM, Smith ER. Moya Moya disease and Moya Moya syndrome. NEJM. 2009;360(12);1226–37.

9. You are seeing a 7-year-old black boy, with sickle cell disease in the ED after developing right-sided weakness and numbness. MRI shows a small stroke in the left fronto-parietal region. MR angiogram shows narrowing of the left middle cerebral artery, and peak systolic velocities of the left middle cerebral artery on transcranial Doppler are 230 cm/s.

What is the most appropriate step for secondary stroke prevention?

A. anticoagulation with warfarin, goal international normalized ratio (INR) of 2–3
B. dual antiplatelet therapy with aspirin and clopidogrel
C. intracranial angioplasty and stenting
D. permissive hypertension with goal systolic BP greater than 160 mmHg
E. transfusion with goal HbS fraction of less than 30%

Correct Answer is: E

Sickle cell disease patients are at high risk for stroke due to narrowing of the distal internal carotid artery and major intracranial vessels. This is a non-atherosclerotic vasculopathy, possibly related to trauma from sickled red blood cells.

The treatment of choice for stroke prevention in sickle cell disease patients is transfusion to maintain an HbS fraction below 30%. Transfusions are typically begun when MCA velocities on transcranial Doppler exceed 200 cm/s.

The use of antiplatelet, or anticoagulant therapy, in sickle cell disease is complex, since patients often develop a Moya Moya like pattern, where ischemic strokes are more common in younger patients and hemorrhagic stroke risk increases with age and disease severity.

The roles of intracranial angioplasty and stenting, as well as blood pressure goals, are unclear in this setting.

Suggested Reading

- Roach ES, Golomb MR, Adams R, et al. Management of stroke in infants and children. Stroke. 2008;39(9):2644–91.
- Adams RJ. Big strokes in small persons. Arch Neurol. 2007;64:1567–74.

10. An 18-year-old African-American boy is seen in the ED for acute onset of right-sided weakness and numbness. There is mild expressive aphasia and right hemiparesis on his examination. MR Angiogram is shown.

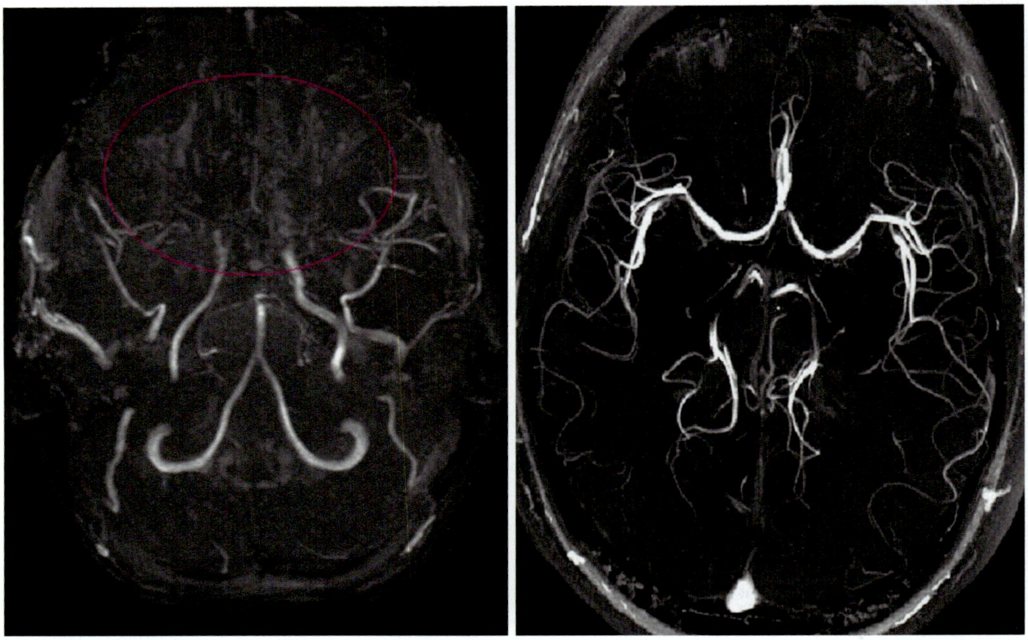

Fig. 28.8 (Left) MIP reconstructed MR angiography of a 11 year old girl with en:Moya moya disease. (Right) healthy patient, for comparison. (*Left image*) own work by commons:User:MBq, (*Right image*) ► https://commons.wikimedia.org/wiki/File:Mra-mip.jpg. commons:User:MBq, commons:User:SBarnes. Wikipedia

What is most likely diagnoses?

A. bilateral carotid artery dissection
B. fibromuscular dysplasia
C. moya Moya syndrome
D. paradoxical embolism to the left middle cerebral artery
E. reversible cerebral vasoconstriction syndrome

Correct Answer is: C

The abrupt abnormality in the distal internal carotid arteries is highly suggestive of Moya Moya syndrome, a progressive non-atherosclerotic vasculopathy. Although idiopathic Moya Moya disease is seen almost exclusively in Asian populations, secondary forms can be seen in several systemic conditions, including African-Americans with sickle cell disease. The visualized portions of the carotid arteries appear normal, so fibromuscular dysplasia or bilateral carotid artery dissections would be less likely. Both distal carotid arteries are abnormal, so an embolic process to the left middle cerebral artery would not explain the imaging findings. Reversible cerebral vasoconstriction syndrome is an idiopathic condition affecting more distal cerebral arteries.

Suggested Reading

- Roach ES, Golomb MR, Adams R, et al. Management of stroke in infants and children. Stroke. 2008;39(9):2644–91.
- Scott RM, Smith ER. Moyamoya disease and moyamoya syndrome. N Engl J Med. 2009;360:1226–37.

28

11. What is the estimated annual risk of hemorrhage in a 13-year-old boy who is admitted to the hospital for evaluation of a seizure which involved twitching and tingling of his right hand, followed by 12 h of weakness and sensory loss in the hand? His MRI and MRA are shown.

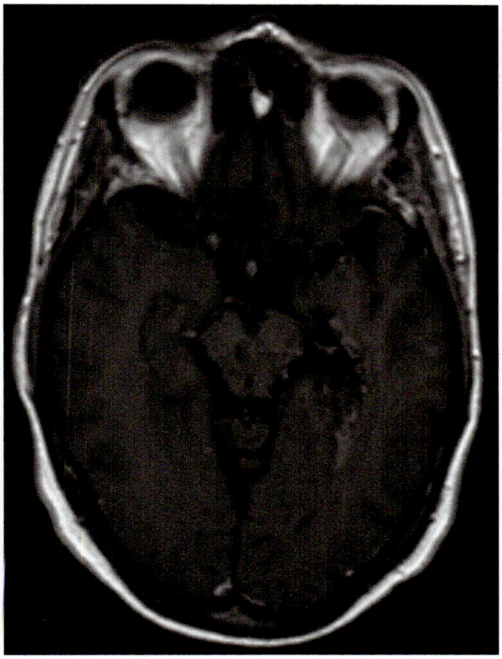

Fig. 28.9 Arteriovenöse Malformation des Gehirns in der MRT T1 KM axial. Own work. (Hellerhoff. Wikipedia)

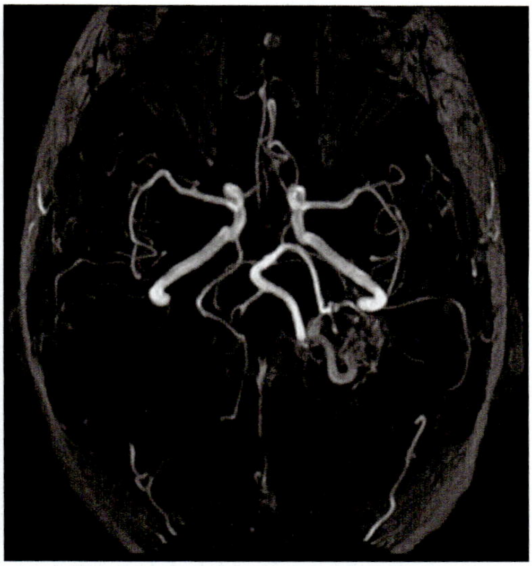

Fig. 28.10 Arteriovenöse Malformation im Gehirn: MRT TOF gedrehte MIP-Projektion. Own work. (Hellerhoff. Wikipedia)

A. 2–4%
B. 5–10%
C. 15–20%
D. 30%
E. 50%

Correct Answer is: A
There is a lack of high quality data however, a systematic review of the epidemiology and natural history of AVM's showed an annual risk of first hemorrhage of about 2%.

Suggested Reading

- Wilkins RH. Natural history of intracranial vascular malformations: a review. Neurosurgery. 1985;16(3):421–30.
- Al-Shahi R, Warlow C. A systematic review of the frequency and prognosis of arteriovenous malformations of the brain in adults. Brain. 2001;124:1900–26.

12. An 18-year-old female has an acute onset of weakness of the right arm and expressive aphasia. Her MRI shows acute ischemia in a segment of the left MCA. **Of the following infectious agents, which is most likely to be responsible for her condition?**
A. cytomegalovirus
B. echovirus
C. mycoplasma
D. parvovirus
E. varicella-zoster virus

Correct Answer is: E

Varicella-zoster virus (VZV) has been associated with stroke at almost any age and not all patients have a preceding rash. In one study of 30 patients, rash occurred in 19 (63%); CSF pleocytosis in 20 (67%); and imaging abnormalities in 29 (97%). Angiography in 23 patients revealed abnormalities in 16 (70%). Large and small arteries were involved in 15 (50%), small arteries in 11 (37%), and large arteries in only 4 (13%) of 30 patients. Average time from rash to neurologic symptoms and signs was 4.1 months and from neurologic symptoms and signs to CSF virology analysis was 4.2 months.

CSF of 9 (30%) patients contained VZV DNA while 28 (93%) had anti-VZV IgG antibody in CSF; in each of these patients reduced serum/CSF ratio of VZV IgG confirmed intrathecal synthesis. VZV vasculopathy is caused by a productive viral infection in arteries, as evidenced by the presence of multinucleated giant cells, Cowdry A inclusion bodies and herpes virus particles. Postmortem virology analysis reveals VZV antigen in cerebral vessels.

28

Suggested Reading

- Nagel MA, Cohrs RJ, Mahalingam R, et al. The varicella zoster virus vasculopathies: clinical, CSF, imaging, and virologic features. Neurology. 2008;70(11):853–60.

13. You are seeing a 14-month-old boy in the ED who has a left-sided focal motor seizure 2 h ago. He has been sleepy and has not moved his left limbs since then. He fell 1 foot off of a couch onto a carpeted floor an hour prior to the seizure, but he did not lost his consciousness. On examination, he has a port-wine birthmark involving the right upper eyelid and forehead. **What are you going to see on his MRI scan?**
    - A. arteriovenous malformation in the left frontal region
    - B. cerebral contusion in the left frontal region
    - C. leptomeningeal vascular malformation in the left posterior region
    - D. multiple cerebral cavernous malformations
    - E. subdural hematoma in the left frontotemporal region

Correct Answer is: C

The boy has Sturge-Weber syndrome (SWS), which is a congenital capillary-venous vascular malformation involving the brain (leptomeningeal angioma), skin (capillary malformation) and eye. Seizure in infancy is a very common presentation in patients with brain involvement. Neurologic deficits can be acquired slowly over time, or as the result of stroke-like episodes associated with seizures and/or migraines.

Toddlers and young children are particularly prone to stroke-like episodes triggered by falls with minor head injury. SWS brain involvement should be suspected in any newborn with a port-wine birthmark in the V1 distribution (forehead to 1 side and/or upper eyelid). A PWB of any size in that location has approximately a 10% to 20% risk of SWS brain involvement. However, the risk increases with the size, extent, and bilaterally of the birthmark. Approximately 10% of those with typical SWS brain involvement will have no birthmark or eye involvement.

SWS brain involvement is diagnosed by visualization of the typical leptomeningeal vascular malformation on contrast enhanced T1-weighted MRI imaging. Associated dilation and enhancement of the choroid plexus (glomus) on the involved side is also often present in older children and adults; dilated deep draining venous vessels underlying the effected cortical region may also be seen. Cortical and subcortical calcification which develop over time are best seen on head CT.

Suggested Reading

- Comi AM. Presentation, diagnosis, pathophysiology, and treatment of the neurological features of Sturge-Weber syndrome. Neurologist. 2011;17(4): 179–84.

14. You are seeing a 7-day postpartum 18-Year-old girl, after having a full-term baby. She complains of severe headache and blurred vision. On arrival, her BP is 160/95; heart rate 90; temperature 37.5 °C. She has a generalized tonic-clonic seizure while she in the ER. Brain MRI is shown.

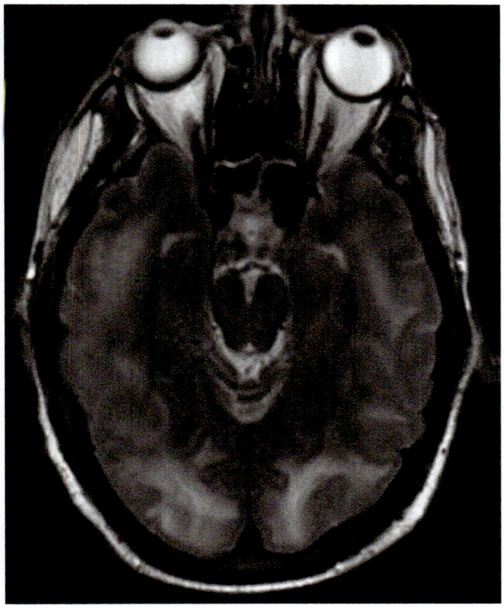

Fig. 28.11 Magnetic resonance image showing multiple cortico-subcortical areas of hyperintense signal involving the occipital and parietal lobes bilaterally and pons in a patient with posterior reversible encephalopathy syndrome. Near fatal posterior reversible encephalopathy syndrome complicating chronic liver failure and treated by induced hypothermia and dialysis: a case report. (J Medical Case Reports 2009, 3:6623. 10.1186/1752-1947-3-6623. Rashmi Chawla, Daniel Smith and Paul E Marik. Wikipedia)

What is the most likely etiology of the imaging findings shown?

A. arteriovenous malformation
B. basilar artery thrombosis
C. posterior reversible encephalopathy syndrome
D. reversible cerebral vasoconstriction syndrome
E. venous sinus thrombosis

Correct Answer is: C
Posterior reversible encephalopathy syndrome (PRES) is very common in a young women with pre-eclampsia or eclampsia. This is secondary to impaired cerebral autoregulation and increased cerebral blood flow volume in the pregnant state. The symmetric hyper-intensities seen in FLAIR in the posterior regions of the cerebrum are the most common and characteristic imaging finding in this syndrome.

Suggested Reading

- Oehm E, Hetzel A, Els T, et al. Cerebral hemodynamics and autoregulation in reversible posterior leukoencephalopathy syndrome caused by pre-/eclampsia. Cerebrovasc Dis. 2006;22(2–3):204–8.

15. Which of the following clinical manifestations is more prevalent in children with moyamoya disease?

A. dystonia
B. intracerebral hemorrhage
C. ischemic cerebrovascular events
D. optic disk abnormalities
E. subarachnoid hemorrhage

Correct Answer is: C
Seventy to eighty percent of Moya Moya disease children can present with ischemic episodes in the form of transient ischemic attacks or strokes that are frequently recurrent, involving the

anterior brain circulation because of a predilection of the involvement of the terminal portions of the internal carotid arteries. Posterior circulation events can occur through the involvement of the vertebra-basilar system, but these events are much less common. Signs are often provoked by periods of hyperventilation, e.g., after crying, coughing, straining, or playing on a wind instrument.

(The reduced partial pressure of carbon dioxide [Paco2] results in reduced cerebral blood flow because of vasoconstriction. The fall in cerebral blood flow compromises the already reduced cerebral perfusion to the point of causing clinical manifestations, which can include dysarthria, aphasia, hemiparesis, or seizures.) Atypical presenting signs include syncope, para-paresis, visual disturbance, and involuntary movements. Children with frontal lobe involvement may also develop long-term intellectual impairment.

Suggested Reading

- Currie S, Raghavan A, Batty R, et al. Childhood moyamoya disease and moyamoya syndrome: a pictorial review. Pediatr Neurol. 2011;44(6): 401–13.

16. You are evaluating an 18-year-old female for her sudden onset of headaches. You ordered a non-contrast CT scan, which is shown. Her NIH Stroke Scale is reported to be 2.
On neurologic examination, which of the following findings is most likely?
    A. complete right homonymous hemianopia
    B. forced gaze deviation to the left
    C. left hemiparesis with some effort against gravity
    D. severe aphasia
    E. severe sensory loss involving the right face, arm, and leg

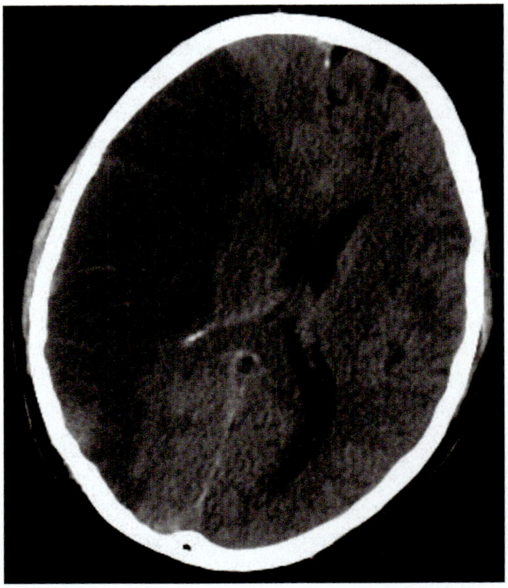

Fig. 28.12 CT-scan of the brain with a RIGHT MCA infarct. Own work. (Lucien Monfils. Wikipedia)

Correct Answer is: C
The CT scan shows a right -side infarct in the distribution of the MCA; therefore, the preferred response is left homonymous hemianopia.

Suggested Reading

- NIH Stroke Scale. ► www.ninds.nih.gov.

17. Which of the following is true regarding septic cavernous sinus thrombophlebitis?
    A. CSF usually shows a lymphocytic pleocytosis
    B. CSF usually shows a polymorphonucleocyte pleocytosis
    C. engorgement of ophthalmic veins leads to proptosis and chemosis
    D. infection is usually from extension from the mastoid air cells
    E. vision loss due to optic neuropathy is uncommon

Correct Answer is: C
Vision loss is common and rarely recovers completely. CSF is typically normal

unless there is an associated meningitis or subdural empyema. Venous congestion of ophthalmic and retinal veins leads to proptosis, chemosis, orbital edema, and retinal hemorrhage. Involvement of mastoid air cells is more common with septic lateral sinus thrombosis.

Suggested Reading

Ropper AH, Samuels MA. Infections of the nervous system (bacterial, fungal, spirochetal, parasitic) and sarcoidosis. In: Ropper AH, Samuels MA, editors. Adams and Victor's principles of neurology. 9th ed. New York: McGraw-Hill; 2009.

18. You are evaluating a 3-day-old infant who has a congestive heart failure which has been refractory to medical management. He has impaired renal function, with hydrops fetalis. You ordered a head ultrasound, showed an abnormal vascular structure. Brain CTA is obtained and shown here.

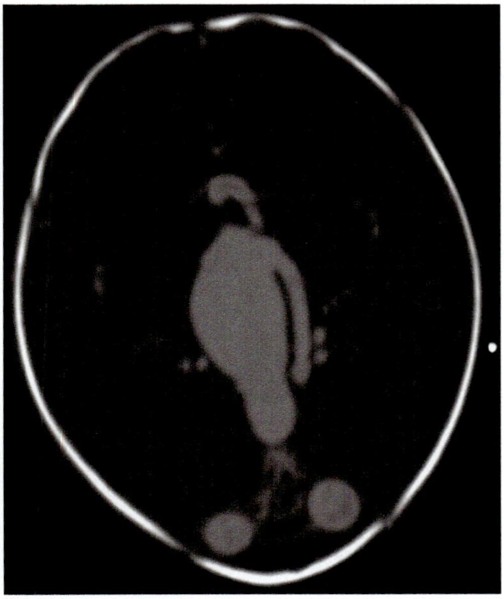

Fig. 28.13 Axial image from CTA showing arteriovenous communication in vein of Galen malformation. Radiopaedia. (Dr. Laughlin Dawes. Wikipedia)

What is the best treatment option?

A. anticoagulation using enoxaparin
B. continued medical management with surgical intervention planned for 5 to 6 months of age
C. endovascular embolization performed urgently
D. placement of a ventriculo-peritoneal shunt
E. surgical removal of the abnormality

Correct Answer is: C

This is a presentation of a vein of Galen malformation (VGM). High-output cardiac failure and neurologic symptoms secondary to cerebral venous congestion and abnormal CSF flow are the most pathophysiological consequences of VGM. The severity of the symptoms is variable and dependent on the underlying angioarchitecture of the VGM as well as the age of the child. Neonates typically present with congestive heart failure; but infants present with hydrocephalus; and the older children or adults present with headache and, frequently, with signs and symptoms of subarachnoid hemorrhage. The development of endovascular therapy, together with a comprehensive multidisciplinary approach in the intensive care units, has significantly improved the poor prognosis of patients with VGM.

Despite advances in micro-neurosurgery, complete removal of the lesion in newborns is rarely achieved or advised because of the hemodynamic instability and location of the lesion, poor myelination of the brain parenchyma and cerebral venous hypertension. Thus, surgical treatment is now reserved for the evacuation of intracranial hematomas and the treatment of hydrocephalus, or in cases of embolization failure.

Medical treatment with diuretics, inotropes, and other cardiovascular agents is used only to relieve symptoms of cardiovascular instability and

renal insufficiency until the patient can undergo embolization.

Most of the newborns with VGM need immediate treatment. The main goal in the newborn with high-output cardiac failure is to decrease the flow in the VGM and therefore reduce the cardiac output failure, improve the coronary perfusion, and increase the blood flow to the renal arteries.

Suggested Reading

Hoang S, Choudhri O, Edwards M, Guzman R. Vein of Galen malformation. Neurosurg Focus. 2009;27(5): E8.

28

19. Which of the following CSF findings is most reliable for differentiating SAH from a traumatic lumbar puncture?
    - A. A relative CSF leukocytosis will be present in cases of SAH.
    - B. The presence of xanthochromia indicates SAH.
    - C. A twofold or greater decrease in the number of RBCs from tube 1 to tube 4 is always due to a traumatic tap.
    - D. A positive CSF clotting assay is consistent with a traumatic tap.
    - E. All of the above is equally useful.

Correct Answer is: B

Xanthochromia is the presence of a yellowish coloration to the supernatant of centrifuged CSF samples. It secondary to the breakdown of hemoglobin first to oxyhemoglobin and then to bilirubin. Methemoglobin may also be produced, but like bilirubin, it occurs after oxyhemoglobin is generated. These latter molecules have a yellowish tint and characteristic spectrophotometric absorption curves. Typically, oxyhemoglobin will appear within 2 h of SAH and reach a peak concentration between 24 and 46 h. Bilirubin does not appear until approximately 10 h after SAH. Although the presence of xanthochromia remains the most reliable method for differentiating between a traumatic lumbar puncture and an SAH, its presence is not pathognomonic for SAH. Recent studies have demonstrated that xanthochromia begins to develop immediately after mixing of blood and CSF as seen in traumatic lumbar puncture. The degree of xanthochromia correlates with the amount of bleeding induced by trauma. Clinically, recent studies have established that in the presence of a traumatic lumbar puncture and an RSC concentration of 10,000 RSC per L, xanthochromia cannot be reliably used to confirm SAH. Conversely, xanthochromia in the setting of RSC concentrations 5000 RSC per L is a reliable indicator of SAH. The method of comparing RSC counts in the first and fourth tubes has been shown to be an unreliable means of differentiating these two entities. None of the other methods listed has been shown to be reliable.

Suggested Reading

1200 Questions to Help You Pass the Emergency Medicine Boards © 2012 Wolters Kluwer Health Lippincott Williams & Wilkins. All rights reseNed.

20. You are evaluating a 7- year-old female because sub-acutely she is not able to move her left eye. While you are examining her, her right eye follows your hand movements, but left eye moves only minimally. The pupillary response is absent in the left eye but it is normal in the right eye. The rest of cranial nerves are normal. She has non-focal neurological exam. Her left eye is swollen and erythematous. She had fever 2 days ago, and seemed excessively tired today and complained of a headache.
    What is your most likely diagnosis?
    - A. Encephalitis
    - B. Cavernous sinus thrombosis
    - C. Retinal vein occlusion
    - D. Eye trauma

Correct Answer is: B

The typical history is, development of fever, malaise, and frontal headache following dental procedures. However, infection can also originate from the face, nose or paranasal sinuses as well. Proptosis, orbital congestion, ptosis, external ophthalmoplegia, pupillary paralysis, and blindness may follow the initial symptoms. The infection begins in one cavernous sinus and may spread to the other. If untreated, it may extend to the meninges. Even with vigorous antibiotic treatment, the mortality rate is 15%.

Encephalitis presents with altered mental status and seizures. Retinal vein occlusion is rare in children and young adults. The presenting symptoms are rapid onset blurred vision or loss of vision. There was no evidence described of trauma to head or eye. Trauma would not be associated with fever and would not typically present with intra-ocular muscle paralysis.

Suggested Reading

- Press CA, Lindsay A, Stence NV, Fenton LZ, Bernard TJ, Mirsky DM. Cavernous sinus thrombosis in children imaging characteristics and clinical outcomes. Stroke. 2015;46(9):2657–60.

21. You are evaluating a 3-year-old girl in the hospital with an acute onset hemiparesis. She has a remarkable past medical history of four transient ischemic attacks. Her previous workups for hematological etiologies were normal and there were no signs of inflammatory conditions. The diagnosis of Moya Moya is suspected.
    What study could make a definitive diagnosis in her condition?
    A. MRI of the base of the brain
    B. Positron Emission Tomography
    C. Magnetic resonance angiography
    D. Angiography

Correct Answer is: D

The characteristic "puff of smoke" can be imaged by MRA or CT angiogram but a definitive diagnosis requires arteriographic demonstration of bilateral stenosis in the distal internal carotid arteries with collateral development in the basal ganglia and meninges. It is important to rule out an underlying vasculopathy and coagulopathy.

MRI in this condition would identify cerebral regions affected by ischemia but does not image arteries.

PET scan are not typically utilized to evaluate cause of stroke or vascular disorders.

MRA is an adequate non-invasive arterial imaging mode, but the detection and resolution quality is not sufficient for a definitive diagnosis.

Suggested Reading

- Hackenberg A, Plecko B, Khan N. OP26-2867: Recurrent stroke in toddlers and hemiplegic or atypical migraine in school aged children: Think of Moya Moya. Europ J Pediatr Neurol. 2015;19:59.

22. A 6 -year-old boy is brought to the ED after a recent right ischemic middle cerebral artery stroke. He has no history of fever or any sickness. He has normal cognitive and motor development. Family history is remarkable for deep vein thrombosis in his father.
    What laboratory test is most likely to aid in identifying the etiology of this child's stroke?
    A. Serum triglyceride
    B. Serum cholesterol
    C. Plasma Protein C and S
    D. Muscle biopsy

Correct Answer is: C

A history of deep vein thrombosis or a positive family history for deep vein thrombosis are the risk factors for a prothrombotic state in a child. Protein C

or Protein S deficiency, antithrombin III deficiency, factor V Leiden mutation and antiphospholipid antibody syndrome are the most common hypercoagulable states in children.

Serious atherosclerosis formation causing stroke in children as a consequence of hypertriglyceridemia is rare.

Certain mitochondrial disorders are associated with stroke in children, but are accompanied with preexisting cognitive and motor deficits. Mitochondrial conditions include mitochondrial encephalopathy, Lactic acidosis and stroke (MELAS).

Suggested Reading

- Doan D, Barreto A, Gildersleeve K, Sarraj A, Butler I. Comparison of Hypercoagulable Evaluation in Perinatal and Pediatric Ischemic Stroke (P2. 261). Neurology. 2015;84(14 Suppl):P2–261.

23. An 8 -year-old boy suffered a minor ischemic stroke, during an episode of vasculitis, involving the right lateral lemniscus.
What sensory disturbance will she likely experience once she recovers?
A. Left visual field deficient
B. Right visual field deficit
C. Leaf ear hearing loss
D. Right ear hearing loss
E. No auditory of visual deficit

Correct Answer is: E
The auditory portion of the eighth cranial nerve transmits information to the ipsilateral cochlear nuclei in the medulla. Each cochlear nucleus sends information to both superior olivary nuclei and therefore bilateral representation of hearing occurs through the remainder of the ascending pathways. Both lateral lemniscus carries information from both superior olivary nuclei to the inferior colliculi. Even complete destruction of one lateral lemniscus would still allow the other side to carry bilateral auditory information to higher processing centers.

Visual information travels through the optic nerve to the lateral geniculate body and then to the occipital lobe.

Auditory information is transmitted with bilateral representation before the lateral lemniscus pathways.

Suggested Reading

- Celesia GG. Hearing disorders in brainstem lesions. Handbook Clin Neurol. 2014;129:509–36.

24. What do you expect as a diagnosis in a 5 -year-old female with a history of frequent ear infections and tonsillitis that presented with fever, right neck tenderness and subsequent rapid onset of a right-sided hemiplegia?
A. Moya Moya disease
B. Protein C deficiency
C. Cervical arteritis
D. Sickle cell anemia

Correct Answer is: C
Children with chronic tonsillitis and otitis media with cervical lymphadenopathy can have an occlusion of cervical portions of the internal carotid arteries. Reduction in lumen diameter and turbulence in flow, which increases the risk of thromboembolism generation can occur secondary to cervical arteritis which is a local inflammatory vasculitis.

Moya Moya is a slowly progressive non-inflammatory vasculopathy that most commonly results in the occlusion of the internal carotid arteries. Rapid onset of a hemiplegia can occur but not associated with fever and neck tenderness.

Protein C deficiency is a hereditary condition that causes hyper-coagulability and increases risk of stroke. Activated protein C inactivates coagulation

factors Va and VIIIa and normal levels aids in the coagulation hemodynamic balance. A deficit in protein C production results in a high risk of vascular thromboembolism formation.

Jaundice, pallor, weakness and fatigability from chronic anemia are the most common presentations of sickle cell anemia. Forty percent of patients can have strokes at some time in their lives affected individuals. Dehydration is the most commonly known cause of a sickle cell crisis that can cause cerebral hypo perfusion or stroke.

Suggested Reading

- Weiss PF. Pediatric vasculitis. Pediatr Clin North Am. 2012;59(2):407–23.

25. Which of the following has not been associated with increased risk of venous thrombosis that may involve the CNS?
    - A. Anti-phospholipid antibody syndrome
    - B. Acquired factor VIII deficiency
    - C. G20210 A prothrombin polymorphism
    - D. Antithrombin III deficiency
    - E. Factor V Leiden

Correct Answer is: B

Acquired hemophilia (Acquired factor VIII deficiency) leads to increased risk of hemorrhage rather than thrombosis. Anti-phospholipid antibody syndrome (APLS) and most of the so-called hereditary thrombophilias, including G20210 A prothrombin polymorphism, mutation in the methylene tetrahydrofolate reductase gene (leading to hyper-homocysteinemia), and factor V Leiden, as well as others including anti-thrombin III, protein C, and protein S deficiency, lead to venous thrombosis. Therefore, venous sinus thrombosis is the most common neurologic manifestation of these disorders. However, arterial ischemia in the form of venous infarction is seen, as are paradoxical emboli to the cerebral vasculature from the venous system through an intracardiac right to-left shunt. Other causes of both venous and arterial thrombosis include malignancy, heparin-induced thrombocytopenia, systemic vasculitis and myeloproliferative diseases (such as essential thrombocythemia, polycythemia rubra vera, and others). APLS is a disorder of thrombosis resulting from the presence of circulating antibodies against phospholipid bound proteins such as anti-cardiolipin antibodies and lupus anticoagulant antibodies. In addition to venous and less commonly arterial thrombosis, other neurologic manifestations seen in APLS include chorea, headaches, and seizures.

Suggested Reading

- Comprehensive review in clinical neurology: a multiple-choice question book for the wards and boards © 2011 Wolters Kluwer Health Lippincott Williams & Wilkins. All rights reserved.

26. A patient has a large intracranial hemorrhage. On examination, he has a left fixed dilated pupil and he has hemiparesis on the right side.
    Which type of herniation does this patient have?
    - A. Uncal herniation
    - B. Subfalcine herniation
    - C. Tonsillar herniation
    - D. Central transtentorial herniation
    - E. Transcalvarial herniation

Correct Answer is: A

Uncal herniation produces mass effect and pressure over the ipsilateral midbrain, affecting the ipsilateral cranial nerve III nucleus, and the corticospinal fibers. The mass effect compresses parasympathetic fibers that mediate

miosis, resulting in mydriasis. Since the corticospinal tract has not decussated at the level of the midbrain, patients have a contralateral hemiparesis. Occasionally, the uncal herniation will lead to displacement of the midbrain against the contralateral Kernohan's notch, resulting in a contralateral compression of the corticospinal tract, and therefore an ipsilateral hemiparesis. The other types of herniation syndromes do not include an ipsilateral dilated pupil with contralateral hemiparesis.

Suggested Reading

- Posner JB, Saper CB, Schiff ND, Plum F. Plum and Postern's diagnosis of stupor and coma, 4th ed. New York: Oxford University Press; 2007.
- Comprehensive review in clinical neurology: a multiple-choice question book for the wards and boards ©2011 Wolters Kluwer Health Lippincott Williams & Wilkins. All rights reserved.

28

27. An 18-year-old man hit his head on a rock while he was rafting with his father. He had no helmet on. His father noticed that the boy was slightly confused immediately after the head trauma, but he came back to normal after few minutes. Few hours later he became lethargic and his right side was not moving properly. He was taken to the emergency room of a local hospital. The CT scan showed an epidural hematoma. **What is the vessel ruptured and through which foramen does it enter the skull?**
    A. Jugular vein, through the jugular foramen
    B. Middle meningeal artery, through the foramen lacerum
    C. Jugular vein, through the foramen spinosum
    D. Carotid artery, through the carotid canal
    E. Middle meningeal artery, through the foramen spinosum

Correct Answer is: E
Epidural hematoma is most commonly caused by head trauma, leading to rupture of the middle meningeal artery, which passes through the foramen spinosum. Rupture of this artery results in accumulation of blood in the epidural space. The appearance on CT is lenticular shaped or biconvex. Clinically, patients may present with a brief loss of consciousness followed by a lucid interval and subsequent deterioration over hours.

The jugular vein passes through the jugular foramen; however, injury to it is not the cause of epidural hematomas.

The carotid artery passes through the carotid canal and runs in the foramen lacerum; however, injury to this structure is not the cause of epidural hematomas.

Suggested Reading

- Blumenfeld H. Neuroanatomy through Clinical Cases, 1st ed. Sunderland: Sinauer; 2002. Suarez JI.
- Critical care neurology and neurosurgery, 1st ed. Totowa: Humana Press; 2004.
- Comprehensive review in clinical neurology: a multiple-choice question book for the wards and boards ©2011 Wolters Kluwer Health Lippincott Williams & Wilkins. All rights reserved.

28. Which of the following is correct regarding thrombosis of the venous sinuses?
    A. Diplopia with a sixth cranial nerve palsy is specific for cavernous sinus thrombosis
    B. Headache is present in less than 50% of cases

C. Increased intracranial pressure is uncommon
D. Superior sagittal sinus thrombosis may produce bilateral thalamic venous infarcts
E. Seizures are more common in venous infarcts as compared to arterial infarcts

Correct Answer is: E
Venous sinus thrombosis is associated with seizures in 40% of patients, it is a higher percentage than that in patients with arterial strokes. In patients with venous sinus thrombosis, Headache is the most common symptom in adults (about 90%). Given the occlusion of venous drainage along with hemorrhagic infarct and edema, patients may develop increased intracranial pressure. Diplopia caused by a sixth cranial nerve palsy has non-localizing value and may be a manifestation of increased intracranial pressure. In patients with venous infarcts, focal neurologic findings will be present depending on the area affected along the thrombosed venous sinus. Thrombosis of the deep venous system may lead to deep venous infarcts, including bilateral thalamic infarcts. This is not seen with superior sagittal sinus thrombosis, which instead can lead to infarcts in the para-sagittal cortex bilaterally along the sinus.

Suggested Reading

- Ropper AH, Samuels MA. Adams and Victor's principles of neurology, 9th ed. New York: McGraw Hill; 2009.
- Stam J. Thrombosis of the cerebral veins and sinuses. N Engl J Med. 2005;352: 1791–8.
- Comprehensive review in clinical neurology: a multiple-choice question book for the wards and boards ©2011 Wolters Kluwer Health Lippincott Williams & Wilkins. All rights reserved.

29. You are seeing a newborn baby in the NICU, who has a high-output cardiac failure at birth. His head circumference has been increased in size and a cranial ultrasound is pending.
What is your treatment of choice in this condition?
A. Ventroperitoneal shunt placement
B. Aggressive treatment of cardiac disease
C. Embolization of cerebral vein
D. Close observation and monitoring

Correct Answer is: C
Vein of Galen malformation is actually a median prosencephalic arteriovenous fistula (ANF) that dilates, it is associated with hydrocephalus secondary to venous hypertension or compression of the aqueduct of Sylivis. This is the most common antenatal diagnosed intracranial malformation. The median prosencephalic vein is a precursor to the development of the vein of Galen and typically regresses before 40 weeks gestation. On auscultation of the skull, a cranial bruit can be heard. Cardiac symptoms are present due to the large left-to-right shunting through the cerebral arteriovenous fistula.

Embolization of the AV fistula resolves the cardiac failure and will gradually allow cerebrospinal fluid to flows more normally as the venous pressure subsides.

A ventro-peritoneal shunt does not address the etiology of the increased ventricular pressure. In fact, reducing ventricular pressure may allow more rapid expansion of the arteriovenous fistula.

Since the high-out cardiac cycle is compensatory and survival depends on it, aggressive treatment to resolve it would be harmful.

This condition does not typically resolve spontaneously. The infant would have a cardiac failure without intervention.

Suggested Reading

- Sheth RD, Tiznado-Garcia E. 2011. Vein of Galen malformation.

30. You are evaluating a 16 -year-old male for his progressive double vision and left eye pain for 2 days. He has incomplete left eye ptosis and ophthalmoplegia, but his visual acuity is preserved. Sensation in the face on the left is diminished in the V1 and V2 distribution. The rest of the neurological examination is normal.
Where is lesion causing this clinical presentation?
A. Cerebral peduncle
B. Superior orbital fissure
C. Cavernous sinus
D. Orbital apex
E. Central pons

Correct Answer is: C
This is a clinical picture of a cavernous sinus thrombosis. Infection is the main cause of the cavernous sinus thrombosis, and causes ipsilateral ptosis and ophthalmoplgia by involving CN III, IV, and VI. Ipsilateral loss of sensation is due to involvement of V1 and V2 of the trigeminal nerve which traverse through the cavernous sinus as well. Visual acuity is usually preserved, but can be affected late in the course with progressing infection. Antibiotics based on the underlying infection is the treatment of choice.

Superior orbital fissure syndrome is similar to cavernous sinus syndrome, however, the V2 portion of the trigeminal nerve exits the skull via the foramen rotundum after traversing through the cavernous sinus, and thus does not cross the superior orbital fissure.

Orbital apex syndrome is also similar to cavernous sinus syndrome, but has early involvement of the optic nerve, thus resulting in loss of visual acuity.

Lesions of the cerebral peduncle of the midbrain and the central pons would affect motor tracts and result in weakness.

Suggested Reading

- Brazis PW, et al. Localization in clinical neurology. 6th ed. Chapter 8: the localization of lesions affecting the ocular motor system. 2011. p. 184–206.

31. A healthy 10- year- old female had been crying after skinning her knee on the playground. She devolved sudden onset of left face, arm, hand, and leg weakness and numbness, which resolved completely in 30 min. She has a normal MRI, and angiography was ordered.

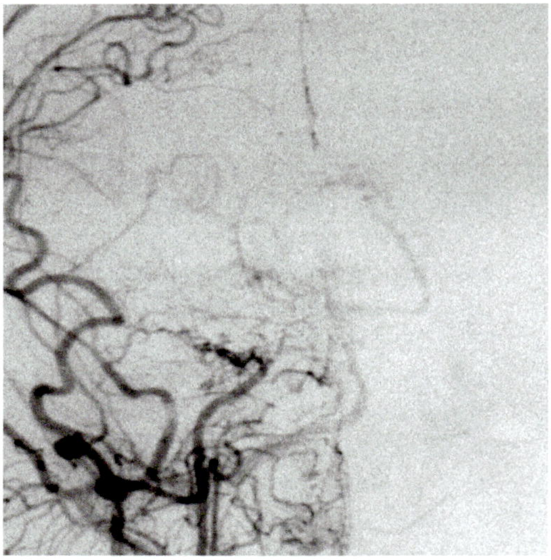

Fig. 28.14 Right ICA DSA in patient with moya moya disease. (Dr. Frank Gaillard. Wikipedia)

The most likely diagnosis is:
A. Carotid dissection
B. Moyamoya disease
C. Vasculitis
D. Fibromuscular dysplasia
E. Non-vascular cause of symptoms

Correct Answer is: B
There is a stenosis of the supra-clinoid Right **ICA with the development of collateral circulation on the angiogram, consistent with Moya Moya disease. Moya Moya disease consists of progressive non-atherosclerotic bilateral stenosis of the distal internal carotid arteries and**

trunks of the anterior and middle cerebral arteries. Collaterals develop at the base of the brain, with a characteristic "puff of smoke" appearance on angiography. Data suggest, however, that the classic "puff of smoke" may only be evident in approximately 30% of cases. Intra-cranial aneurysms may also be present. The disease is most common in Japanese girls, and may be of autosomal recessive inheritance. The same angiographic pattern can also be seen with a number of conditions, however, including sickle cell anemia, basilar meningitis, tuberous sclerosis, and many others. Hence, Moya Moya may be considered as a descriptive term for the vascular process rather than a specific disease. Symptoms in children tend to be ischemic, while manifestations in adults tend to be hemorrhagic. Moya Moya can cause TIA, infarcts, headaches, seizures, movement disorders, cognitive decline, and hemorrhages. TIAs may be precipitated by crying or hyperventilation.

Suggested Reading

- Biller J, Love BB. Vascular diseases of the nervous system. In: Bradley WG, Daroff RB, Fenichel GM, Jankovic J, editors. Neurology in clinical practice. 4th ed. Elsevier, Inc.; 2004. p. 1197–250.
- Simon RP, et al. Clinical neurology. 4th ed. Stamford: Appleton & Lange. p. 282–3.
- Images from: Shoukat S, et al. Moyamoya disease: a clinical spectrum, literature review and case series from a tertiary care hospital in Pakistan. BMC Neurol. 2009;9:15.

32. Which of the following is standard of care for primary stroke prevention in children with sickle cell.
    A. Chronic transfusion therapy
    B. Aspirin
    C. Warfarin
    D. Hydroxyurea
    E. None of the above; no preventative treatment has been shown to be effective

Correct Answer is: A
Substitution of amino acid at position number 6 of the b-polypeptide chain of hemoglobin, with valine in place of glutamic acid is the etiology for sickle cell anemia. It is an autosomal recessive disorder, and it is more common African or African American patients. Hemoglobin S, is an abnormal hemoglobin which is less soluble, more viscous, and forms polymers when deoxygenated, which leads to a characteristic sickle shape of the red cell and membrane rigidity. The abnormal cells adhere to vessel walls causing vaso-occlusive crises with severe pain, often in the back, chest, and extremities. Strokes usually occur in early childhood. In children, typically it is an ischemic stroke, while initial strokes in adults are most often hemorrhagic. Proximal arterial stenosis with a Moya Moya pattern may be evident. The risk of ischemic stroke is increased with a prior TIA, elevated systolic blood pressure, low hemoglobin levels, and frequent or recent acute chest syndromes. Risk factors for hemorrhagic stroke include low hemoglobin levels and elevated white blood cell counts. Only chronic transfusion therapy has been shown to dramatically reduce the risk of initial strokes in high-risk children.

33. A 4-year-old girl came with acute onset of flaccid weakness of the left side of her body, and inability to talk. She is lethargic, on stimulation she awakens and shows visual regard. Her past medical history is significant for complex congenital heart disease, including transposition of the great vessels, and underwent an arterial switch procedure at 15 months of age, with no complications. She has no history of recent illnesses or injuries. Head CT shows a hypodense region in the distribution of the right middle cerebral artery (MCA), and CT angiography shows a sharp cutoff of blood flow distal to the right MCA origin.

What test is most likely to identify the etiology of this stroke?

A. Echocardiogram
B. Factor V Leiden mutation analysis
C. Erythrocyte sedimentation rate
D. Holter monitor
E. Protein C level

Correct Answer is: A
Acute ischemic stroke in children has many causes, but congenital heart disease is the most common. Many different cardiac conditions may be responsible, for example right-to-left intra-cardiac shunting of blood flow, increases the risk of emboli entering the cerebral circulation. Other causes include hemoglobinopathies (such as sickle cell disease), acquired vasculopathies (such as Moya-Moya syndrome), systemic illness (such as varicella), and multiple hypercoagulable states.

28

Suggested Reading

- Roach ES. Etiology of stroke in children. Semin Pediatr Neurol. 2000;7:244–60.

34. Which of the following is not considered as a predictive variable of outcome in patients with intra-parenchymal hemorrhage?

A. Serum glucose level
B. Age
C. Volume of the hematoma
D. Location of the hematoma
E. Glasgow Coma Scale (GCS)

Correct Answer is: A
The intracerebral hemorrhage (ICH) score is a well-validated scoring system for predicting the outcome of patients with intra-parenchymal hemorrhage in 30 days after the event. The score ranges from 0 (least severe with low expected mortality) to 6 (the worst possible score with death likely). The total ICH Score is the sum of the points of the 5 various variables which are considered as predictors of outcome in ICH. These variables are Glasgow Coma Scale (GCS), age, location of hematoma, volume of hematoma and presence or absence of intraventricular hemorrhage. Serum glucose level was not shown to be a predictive of 30-day outcome.

GCS
3–4 = 2 pts
5–12 = 1 pt.
13–15 = 0 pts

ICH Volume
$>30\ cm^3 = 1$ pt.
$<30\ cm^3 = 0$ pts

IVH
Yes = 1 pt.
No = 0 pts

Location
Infratentorial = 1 pt.
Supratentorial = 0 pts

Age
>80 yrs = 1 pt.
<80 yrs = 0 pts

Suggested Reading

- Hemphill JC 3rd, Bonovich DC, Besmertis L, et al. The ICH score: a simple, reliable grading scale for intracerebral hemorrhage. Stroke. 2001;32:891–7.

Correction to: Absolute Pediatric Neurology

Yasser M. Awaad

Correction to:

Y. M. Awaad, *Absolute Pediatric Neurology*, https://doi.org/10.1007/978-3-319-78801-2

The author, Dr. Awaad's affiliation has been corrected as below:
Bloomfield Hills, MI
USA

The updated online version of the book can be found at https://doi.org/10.1007/978-3-319-78801-2

Y. M. Awaad, *Absolute Pediatric Neurology*, https://doi.org/10.1007/978-3-319-78801-2_29

Supplementary Information

Y. M. Awaad, *Absolute Pediatric Neurology*, https://doi.org/10.1007/978-3-319-78801-2

Index

D

E

F

G

M

N

O

P

Q

R

S

X

Y

Z

Printed by Printforce, the Netherlands